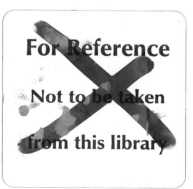

The GALE
ENCYCLOPEDIA of
MEDICINE

THIRD EDITION

The GALE
ENCYCLOPEDIA of
MEDICINE

THIRD EDITION

VOLUME

4

N-S

JACQUELINE L. LONGE, PROJECT EDITOR

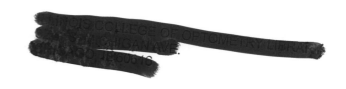

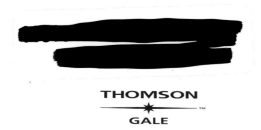

THOMSON

★

GALE

Detroit • New York • San Francisco • San Diego • New Haven, Conn. • Waterville, Maine • London • Munich

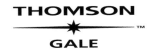

THE GALE ENCYCLOPEDIA OF MEDICINE, THIRD EDITION

Project Editor
Jacqueline L. Longe

Editorial
Shirelle Phelps, Laurie Fundukian, Jeffrey Lehman, Brigham Narins

Editorial Support Services
Luann Brennan, Grant Eldridge, Andrea Lopeman

Rights Acquisition Management
Shalice Caldwell-Shah

Imaging
Randy Bassett, Lezlie Light, Dan Newell, Christine O'Bryan, Robyn V. Young

Product Design
Tracey Rowens

Composition and Electronic Prepress
Evi Seoud, Mary Beth Trimper

Manufacturing
Wendy Blurton, Dorothy Maki

Indexing
Factiva

LIBRARY OF CONGRESS CATALOGING-IN-PUBLICATION DATA

The Gale encyclopedia of medicine / Jacqueline L. Longe, editor.– 3rd ed.
   p. ; cm.
   Includes bibliographical references and index.
   ISBN 1-4144-0368-2 (set hardcover : alk. paper) – ISBN 1-4144-0369-0 (v. 1 : hardcover : alk. paper) – ISBN 1-4144-0370-4 (v. 2 : hardcover : alk. paper) – ISBN 1-4144-0371-2 v. 3 : hardcover : alk. paper) – ISBN 1-4144-0372-0 (v. 4 : hardcover : alk. paper) – ISBN 1-4144-0373-9 (v. 5 : hardcover : alk. paper)
   1. Internal medicine–Encyclopedias.
   [DNLM: 1. Internal Medicine–Encyclopedias–English. 2. Complementary Therapies–Encyclopedias–English. WB 13 G151 2005] I. Title: Encyclopedia of medicine. II. Longe, Jacqueline L. III. Gale Group.
   RC41.G35 2006
   616'.003–dc22
                                                        2005011418

This title is also available as an e-book
ISBN 1-4144-0485-9 (set)
Contact your Gale sales representative for ordering information.
ISBN 1-4144-0368-2 (set)
1-4144-0369-0 (Vol. 1)
1-4144-0370-4 (Vol. 2)
1-4144-0371-2 (Vol. 3)
1-4144-0372-0 (Vol. 4)
1-4144-0373-9 (Vol. 5)

Printed in China
10 9 8 7 6 5 4 3 2 1

CONTENTS

List of Entries vii

Introduction.. xxi

Advisory Board... xxiii

Contributors xxv

Entries

Volume 1: A-B... 1

Volume 2: C-F..693

Volume 3: G-M...1533

Volume 4: N-S...2569

Volume 5: T-Z...3621

Organizations.. 4037

General Index 4061

LIST OF ENTRIES

A

Abdominal ultrasound
Abdominal wall defects
Abortion, partial birth
Abortion, selective
Abortion, therapeutic
Abscess incision & drainage
Abscess
Abuse
Acetaminophen
Achalasia
Achondroplasia
Acid phosphatase test
Acne
Acoustic neuroma
Acrocyanosis
Acromegaly and gigantism
Actinomycosis
Acupressure
Acupuncture
Acute kidney failure
Acute lymphangitis
Acute poststreptococcal
  glomerulonephritis
Acute stress disorder
Addiction
Addison's disease
Adenoid hyperplasia
Adenovirus infections
Adhesions
Adjustment disorders
Adrenal gland cancer
Adrenal gland scan
Adrenal virilism
Adrenalectomy
Adrenocorticotropic hormone test
Adrenoleukodystrophy
Adult respiratory distress syndrome
Aging

Agoraphobia
AIDS tests
AIDS
Alanine aminotransferase test
Albinism
Alcoholism
Alcohol-related neurologic disease
Aldolase test
Aldosterone assay
Alemtuzumab
Alexander technique
Alkaline phosphatase test
Allergic bronchopulmonary
  aspergillosis
Allergic purpura
Allergic rhinitis
Allergies
Allergy tests
Alopecia
Alpha$_1$-adrenergic blockers
Alpha-fetoprotein test
Alport syndrome
Altitude sickness
Alzheimer's disease
Amblyopia
Amebiasis
Amenorrhea
Amino acid disorders screening
Aminoglycosides
Amnesia
Amniocentesis
Amputation
Amylase tests
Amyloidosis
Amyotrophic lateral sclerosis
Anabolic steroid use
Anaerobic infections
Anal atresia
Anal cancer
Anal warts
Analgesics, opioid

Analgesics
Anaphylaxis
Anemias
Anesthesia, general
Anesthesia, local
Aneurysmectomy
Angina
Angiography
Angioplasty
Angiotensin-converting enzyme
  inhibitors
Angiotensin-converting enzyme
  test
Animal bite infections
Ankylosing spondylitis
Anorectal disorders
Anorexia nervosa
Anoscopy
Anosmia
Anoxia
Antacids
Antenatal testing
Antepartum testing
Anthrax
Antiacne drugs
Antiandrogen drugs
Antianemia drugs
Antiangina drugs
Antiangiogenic therapy
Antianxiety drugs
Antiarrhythmic drugs
Antiasthmatic drugs
Antibiotic-associated colitis
Antibiotics, ophthalmic
Antibiotics, topical
Antibiotics
Anticancer drugs
Anticoagulant and antiplatelet
  drugs
Anticonvulsant drugs
Antidepressant drugs, SSRI

Antidepressant drugs
Antidepressants, tricyclic
Antidiabetic drugs
Antidiarrheal drugs
Antidiuretic hormone (ADH) test
Antifungal drugs, systemic
Antifungal drugs, topical
Antigas agents
Antigastroesophageal reflux
    drugs
Antihelminthic drugs
Antihemorrhoid drugs
Antihistamines H-2 blockers
Antihistamines
Antihypertensive drugs
Anti-hyperuricemic drugs
Anti-insomnia drugs
Anti-itch drugs
Antimalarial drugs
Antimigraine drugs
Antimyocardial antibody test
Antinausea drugs
Antinuclear antibody test
Antiparkinson drugs
Antiprotozoal drugs
Antipsychotic drugs, atypical
Antipsychotic drugs
Anti-rejection drugs
Antiretroviral drugs
Antirheumatic drugs
Antiseptics
Antispasmodic drugs
Antituberculosis drugs
Antiulcer drugs
Antiviral drugs
Anxiety disorders
Anxiety
Aortic aneurysm
Aortic dissection
Aortic valve insufficiency
Aortic valve stenosis
Apgar testing
Aphasia
Aplastic anemia
Appendectomy
Appendicitis
Appetite-enhancing drugs
Apraxia
Arbovirus encephalitis
Aromatherapy
Arrhythmias
Art therapy
Arterial embolism
Arteriovenous fistula

Arteriovenous malformations
Arthrography
Arthroplasty
Arthroscopic surgery
Arthroscopy
Asbestosis
Ascites
Aspartate aminotransferase test
Aspergillosis
Aspirin
Asthma
Astigmatism
Aston-Patterning
Ataxia-telangiectasia
Atelectasis
Atherectomy
Atherosclerosis
Athlete's foot
Athletic heart syndrome
Atkins diet
Atopic dermatitis
Atrial ectopic beats
Atrial fibrillation and flutter
Atrial septal defect
Attention-deficit/Hyperactivity disor-
    der (ADHD)
Audiometry
Auditory integration training
Autism
Autoimmune disorders
Autopsy
Aviation medicine
Ayurvedic medicine

B

Babesiosis
Bacillary angiomatosis
Bacteremia
Bacterial vaginosis
Bad breath
Balance and coordination tests
Balanitis
Balantidiasis
Balloon valvuloplasty
Barbiturate-induced coma
Barbiturates
Bariatric surgery
Barium enema
Bartholin's gland cyst
Bartonellosis
Battered child syndrome
Bedsores

Bed-wetting
Behcet's syndrome
Bejel
Bence Jones protein test
Bender-Gestalt test
Benzodiazepines
Bereavement
Beriberi
Berylliosis
Beta blockers
Beta$_2$-microglobulin test
Bile duct cancer
Biliary atresia
Binge-eating disorder
Biofeedback
Bipolar disorder
Bird flu
Birth defects
Birthmarks
Bites and stings
Black lung disease
Bladder cancer
Bladder stones
Bladder training
Blastomycosis
Bleeding time
Bleeding varices
Blepharoplasty
Blood clots
Blood count
Blood culture
Blood donation and registry
Blood gas analysis
Blood sugar tests
Blood typing and crossmatching
Blood urea nitrogen test
Blood-viscosity reducing drugs
Body dysmorphic disorder
Boils
Bone biopsy
Bone density test
Bone disorder drugs
Bone grafting
Bone growth stimulation
Bone marrow aspiration and
    biopsy
Bone marrow transplantation
Bone nuclear medicine scan
Bone x rays
Botulinum toxin injections
Botulism
Bowel preparation
Bowel resection
Bowel training

Brain abscess
Brain biopsy
Brain tumor
Breast biopsy
Breast cancer
Breast implants
Breast reconstruction
Breast reduction
Breast self-examination
Breast ultrasound
Breech birth
Bronchiectasis
Bronchiolitis
Bronchitis
Bronchodilators
Bronchoscopy
Brucellosis
Bruises
Bruxism
Budd-Chiari syndrome
Buerger's disease
Bulimia nervosa
Bundle branch block
Bunion
Burns
Bursitis
Byssinosis

C

Caffeine
Calcium channel blockers
Campylobacteriosis
Cancer therapy, definitive
Cancer therapy, palliative
Cancer therapy, supportive
Cancer
Candidiasis
Canker sores
Carbohydrate intolerance
Carbon monoxide poisoning
Carcinoembryonic antigen test
Cardiac blood pool scan
Cardiac catheterization
Cardiac rehabilitation
Cardiac tamponade
Cardiomyopathy
Cardiopulmonary resuscitation
  (CPR)
Cardioversion
Carotid sinus massage
Carpal tunnel syndrome
Cataract surgery

Cataracts
Catatonia
Catecholamines tests
Catheter ablation
Cat-scratch disease
Celiac disease
Cell therapy
Cellulitis
Central nervous system depressants
Central nervous system infections
Central nervous system stimulants
Cephalosporins
Cerebral amyloid angiopathy
Cerebral aneurysm
Cerebral palsy
Cerebrospinal fluid (CSF) analysis
Cerumen impaction
Cervical cancer
Cervical conization
Cervical disk disease
Cervical spondylosis
Cervicitis
Cesarean section
Chagas' disease
Chancroid
Charcoal, activated
Charcot Marie Tooth disease
Charcot's joints
Chelation therapy
Chemonucleolysis
Chemotherapy
Chest drainage therapy
Chest physical therapy
Chest x ray
Chickenpox
Child abuse
Childbirth
Children's health
Chiropractic
Chlamydial pneumonia
Choking
Cholangitis
Cholecystectomy
Cholecystitis
Cholera
Cholestasis
Cholesterol test
Cholesterol, high
Cholesterol-reducing drugs
Cholinergic drugs
Chondromalacia patellae
Choriocarcinoma
Chorionic villus sampling
Chronic fatigue syndrome

Chronic granulomatous disease
Chronic kidney failure
Chronic obstructive lung disease
Circumcision
Cirrhosis
Cleft lip and palate
Clenched fist injury
Club drugs
Clubfoot
Cluster headache
Coagulation disorders
Coarctation of the aorta
Cocaine
Coccidioidomycosis
Coccyx injuries
Cochlear implants
Cognitive-behavioral therapy
Cold agglutinins test
Cold sore
Colic
Colon cancer
Colonic irrigation
Colonoscopy
Color blindness
Colostomy
Colposcopy
Coma
Common cold
Common variable immunodeficiency
Complement deficiencies
Computed tomography scans
Concussion
Condom
Conduct disorder
Congenital adrenal hyperplasia
Congenital amputation
Congenital bladder anomalies
Congenital brain defects
Congenital heart disease
Congenital hip dysplasia
Congenital lobar emphysema
Congenital ureter anomalies
Congestive cardiomyopathy
Conjunctivitis
Constipation
Contact dermatitis
Contraception
Contractures
Cooling treatments
Coombs' tests
Cor pulmonale
Corneal abrasion
Corneal transplantation
Corneal ulcers

List of Entries

Corns and calluses
Coronary artery bypass graft surgery
Coronary artery disease
Coronary stenting
Corticosteroids systemic
Corticosteroids, dermatologic
Corticosteroids, inhaled
Corticosteroids
Cortisol tests
Cosmetic dentistry
Costochondritis
Cough suppressants
Cough
Couvade syndrome
Cox-2 inhibitors
Craniosacral therapy
Craniotomy
C-reactive protein
Creatine kinase test
Creatinine test
Creutzfeldt-Jakob disease
Cri du chat syndrome
Crohn's disease
Croup
Cryoglobulin test
Cryotherapy
Cryptococcosis
Cryptosporidiosis
CT-guided biopsy
Culture-fair test
Cushing's syndrome
Cutaneous larva migrans
Cutaneous T-cell lymphoma
Cutis laxa
Cyanosis
Cyclic vomiting syndrome
Cyclosporiasis
Cystectomy
Cystic fibrosis
Cystinuria
Cystitis
Cystometry
Cystoscopy
Cytomegalovirus antibody screening
  test
Cytomegalovirus infection

D

Dacryocystitis
Death
Debridement
Decompression sickness

Decongestants
Deep vein thrombosis
Defibrillation
Dehydration
Delayed hypersensitivity skin test
Delirium
Delusions
Dementia
Dengue fever
Dental trauma
Depo-Provera/Norplant
Depressive disorders
Dermatitis
Dermatomyositis
DES exposure
Detoxification
Deviated septum
Diabetes insipidus
Diabetes mellitus
Diabetic foot infections
Diabetic ketoacidosis
Diabetic neuropathy
Dialysis, kidney
Diaper rash
Diaphragm (birth control)
Diarrhea
Diets
Diffuse esophageal spasm
DiGeorge syndrome
Digitalis drugs
Dilatation and curettage
Diphtheria
Discoid lupus erythematosus
Disk removal
Dislocations and subluxations
Dissociative disorders
Diuretics
Diverticulosis and diverticulitis
Dizziness
Doppler ultrasonography
Down syndrome
Drug metabolism/interactions
Drug overdose
Drug therapy monitoring
Drugs used in labor
Dry mouth
Duodenal obstruction
Dysentery
Dysfunctional uterine bleeding
Dyslexia
Dysmenorrhea
Dyspepsia
Dysphasia

E

Ear exam with an otoscope
Ear surgery
Echinacea
Echinococcosis
Echocardiography
Ectopic pregnancy
Edema
Edwards' syndrome
Ehlers-Danlos syndrome
Ehrlichiosis
Elder Abuse
Electric shock injuries
Electrical nerve stimulation
Electrical stimulation of the brain
Electrocardiography
Electroconvulsive therapy
Electroencephalography
Electrolyte disorders
Electrolyte supplements
Electrolyte tests
Electromyography
Electronic fetal monitoring
Electrophysiology study of the heart
Elephantiasis
Embolism
Emergency contraception
Emphysema
Empyema
Encephalitis
Encopresis
Endarterectomy
Endocarditis
Endometrial biopsy
Endometrial cancer
Endometriosis
Endorectal ultrasound
Endoscopic retrograde
  cholangiopancreatography
Endoscopic sphincterotomy
Enemas
Enlarged prostate
Enterobacterial infections
Enterobiasis
Enterostomy
Enterovirus infections
Enzyme therapy
Eosinophilic pneumonia
Epidermolysis bullosa
Epididymitis
Epiglottitis
Episiotomy

Epstein-Barr virus test
Erectile dysfunction treatment
Erectile dysfunction
Erysipelas
Erythema multiforme
Erythema nodosum
Erythroblastosis fetalis
Erythrocyte sedimentation rate
Erythromycins
Erythropoietin test
Escherichia coli
Esophageal atresia
Esophageal cancer
Esophageal disorders
Esophageal function tests
Esophageal pouches
Esophagogastroduodenoscopy
Evoked potential studies
Exercise
Exophthalmos
Expectorants
External sphincter electromyography
Extracorporeal membrane
  oxygenation
Eye and orbit ultrasounds
Eye cancer
Eye examination
Eye glasses and contact lenses
Eye muscle surgery
Eyelid disorders

F

Face lift
Factitious disorders
Failure to thrive
Fainting
Familial Mediterranean fever
Familial polyposis
Family therapy
Fanconi's syndrome
Fasciotomy
Fasting
Fatigue
Fatty liver
Fecal incontinence
Fecal occult blood test
Feldenkrais method
Female genital mutilation
Female sexual arousal disorder
Fetal alcohol syndrome
Fetal hemoglobin test
Fever evaluation tests

Fever of unknown origin
Fever
Fibrin split products
Fibrinogen test
Fibroadenoma
Fibrocystic condition of the breast
Fibromyalgia
Fifth disease
Filariasis
Finasteride
Fingertip injuries
Fish and shellfish poisoning
Fistula
Flesh-eating disease
Flower remedies
Fluke infections
Fluoroquinolones
Folic acid deficiency anemia
Folic acid
Follicle-stimulating hormone test
Folliculitis
Food allergies
Food poisoning
Foot care
Foreign objects
Fracture repair
Fractures
Fragile X syndrome
Friedreich's ataxia
Frostbite and frostnip
Fugu poisoning

G

Galactorrhea
Galactosemia
Gallbladder cancer
Gallbladder nuclear medicine scan
Gallbladder x rays
Gallium scan of the body
Gallstone removal
Gallstones
Gammaglobulin
Ganglion
Gangrene
Gas embolism
Gastrectomy
Gastric acid determination
Gastric emptying scan
Gastrinoma
Gastritis
Gastroenteritis
Gastrostomy

Gaucher disease
Gay and lesbian health
Gender identity disorder
Gender reassignment surgery
Gene therapy
General adaptation syndrome
General surgery
Generalized anxiety disorder
Genetic counseling
Genetic testing
Genital herpes
Genital warts
Gestalt therapy
Gestational diabetes
GI bleeding studies
Giardiasis
Ginkgo biloba
Ginseng, Korean
Glaucoma
Glomerulonephritis
Glucose-6-phosphate dehydrogenase
  deficiency
Glycogen storage diseases
Glycosylated hemoglobin test
Goiter
Gonorrhea
Goodpasture's syndrome
Gout drugs
Gout
Graft-vs.-host disease
Granuloma inguinale
Group therapy
Growth hormone tests
Guided imagery
Guillain-Barré syndrome
Guinea worm infection
Gulf War syndrome
Gynecomastia

H

Hair transplantation
Hairy cell leukemia
Hallucinations
Hammertoe
Hand-foot-and-mouth disease
Hantavirus infections
Haptoglobin test
Hartnup disease
Hatha yoga
Head and neck cancer
Head injury
Headache

Hearing aids
Hearing loss
Hearing tests with a tuning fork
Heart attack
Heart block
Heart failure
Heart murmurs
Heart surgery for congenital defects
Heart transplantation
Heart valve repair
Heart valve replacement
Heartburn
Heat disorders
Heat treatments
Heavy metal poisoning
Heel spurs
Heimlich maneuver
Heliobacteriosis
Hellerwork
Hematocrit
Hemochromatosis
Hemoglobin electrophoresis
Hemoglobin test
Hemoglobinopathies
Hemolytic anemia
Hemolytic-uremic syndrome
Hemophilia
Hemophilus infections
Hemoptysis
Hemorrhagic fevers
Hemorrhoids
Hepatitis A
Hepatitis B
Hepatitis C
Hepatitis D
Hepatitis E
Hepatitis G
Hepatitis virus tests
Hepatitis, alcoholic
Hepatitis, autoimmune
Hepatitis, drug-induced
Herbalism, traditional Chinese
Herbalism, Western
Hereditary fructose intolerance
Hereditary hemorrhagic
  telangiectasia
Hernia repair
Hernia
Herniated disk
Hiccups
High-risk pregnancy
Hirschsprung's disease
Hirsutism
Histiocytosis X

Histoplasmosis
Hives
Hodgkin's disease
Holistic medicine
Holter monitoring
Holtzman ink blot test
Homeopathic medicine, acute
  prescribing
Homeopathic medicine, constitu-
  tional prescribing
Homeopathic medicine
Homocysteine
Hookworm disease
Hormone replacement therapy
Hospital-acquired infections
Human bite infections
Human chorionic gonadotropin
  pregnancy test
Human leukocyte antigen test
Human-potential movement
Huntington disease
Hydatidiform mole
Hydrocelectomy
Hydrocephalus
Hydronephrosis
Hydrotherapy
Hyperaldosteronism
Hyperbaric Chamber
Hypercalcemia
Hypercholesterolemia
Hypercoagulation disorders
Hyperemesis gravidarum
Hyperhidrosis
Hyperkalemia
Hyperlipoproteinemia
Hypernatremia
Hyperopia
Hyperparathyroidism
Hyperpigmentation
Hypersensitivity pneumonitis
Hypersplenism
Hypertension
Hyperthyroidism
Hypertrophic cardiomyopathy
Hyphema
Hypnotherapy
Hypocalcemia
Hypochondriasis
Hypoglycemia
Hypogonadism
Hypokalemia
Hypolipoproteinemia
Hyponatremia
Hypoparathyroidism

Hypophysectomy
Hypopituitarism
Hypospadias and epispadias
Hypotension
Hypothermia
Hypothyroidism
Hypotonic duodenography
Hysterectomy
Hysteria
Hysterosalpingography
Hysteroscopy
Hysterosonography

I

Ichthyosis
Idiopathic infiltrative lung diseases
Idiopathic primary renal hematuric/
  proteinuric syndrome
Idiopathic thrombocytopenic
  purpura
Ileus
Immobilization
Immune complex test
Immunodeficiency
Immunoelectrophoresis
Immunoglobulin deficiency
  syndromes
Immunologic therapies
Immunosuppressant drugs
Impacted tooth
Impedance phlebography
Impetigo
Implantable cardioverter-defibrillator
Impotence
Impulse control disorders
In vitro fertilization
Inclusion conjunctivitis
Incompetent cervix
Indigestion
Indium scan of the body
Induction of labor
Infant massage
Infection control
Infectious arthritis
Infectious mononucleosis
Infertility drugs
Infertility therapies
Infertility
Influenza
Inhalation therapies
Insecticide poisoning
Insomnia

Insulin resistance
Intermittent claudication
Intermittent explosive disorder
Intersex states
Interstitial microwave thermal
 therapy
Intestinal obstructions
Intestinal polyps
Intrauterine growth retardation
Intravenous rehydration
Intravenous urography
Intussusception
Ipecac
Iron deficiency anemia
Iron tests
Irritable bowel syndrome
Ischemia
Isolation
Itching
IUD

J

Japanese encephalitis
Jaundice
Jaw wiring
Jet lag
Jock itch
Joint biopsy
Joint fluid analysis
Joint replacement
Juvenile arthritis

K

Kaposi's sarcoma
Kawasaki syndrome
Keloids
Keratitis
Keratosis pilaris
Kidney biopsy
Kidney cancer
Kidney disease
Kidney function tests
Kidney nuclear medicine scan
Kidney stones
Kidney transplantation
Kidney, ureter, and bladder x-ray
 study
Kinesiology, applied
Klinefelter syndrome
Knee injuries

Kneecap removal
KOH test
Korsakoff's syndrome
Kyphosis

L

Labyrinthitis
Laceration repair
Lacrimal duct obstruction
Lactate dehydrogenase isoenzymes
 test
Lactate dehydrogenase test
Lactation
Lactic acid test
Lactose intolerance
Laparoscopy
Laryngeal cancer
Laryngectomy
Laryngitis
Laryngoscopy
Laser surgery
Laxatives
Lead poisoning
Learning disorders
Leeches
Legionnaires' disease
Leishmaniasis
Leprosy
Leptospirosis
Lesch-Nyhan syndrome
Leukemia stains
Leukemias, acute
Leukemias, chronic
Leukocytosis
Leukotriene inhibitors
Lice infestation
Lichen planus
Lichen simplex chronicus
Life support
Lipase test
Lipidoses
Lipoproteins test
Liposuction
Listeriosis
Lithotripsy
Liver biopsy
Liver cancer
Liver disease
Liver encephalopathy
Liver function tests
Liver nuclear medicine scan
Liver transplantation

Low back pain
Lower esophageal ring
Lumpectomy
Lung abscess
Lung biopsy
Lung cancer, non-small cell
Lung cancer, small cell
Lung diseases due to gas or chemical
 exposure
Lung perfusion and ventilation scan
Lung surgery
Lung transplantation
Luteinizing hormone test
Lyme disease
Lymph node biopsy
Lymphadenitis
Lymphangiography
lymphedema
Lymphocyte typing
Lymphocytic choriomeningitis
Lymphocytopenia
Lymphogranuloma venereum
Lysergic acid diethylamide (LSD)

M

Macular degeneration
Magnesium imbalance
Magnetic field therapy
Magnetic resonance imaging
Malabsorption syndrome
Malaria
Malignant lymphomas
Malignant melanoma
Malingering
Mallet finger
Mallory-Weiss syndrome
Malnutrition
Malocclusion
MALT lymphoma
Mammography
Mania
Marfan syndrome
Marijuana
Marriage counseling
Marshall-Marchetti-Krantz
 procedure
Massage therapy
Mastectomy
Mastitis
Mastocytosis
Mastoidectomy
Mastoiditis

Maternal to fetal infections
Maxillofacial trauma
Measles
Meckel's diverticulum
Mediastinoscopy
Meditation
Medullary sponge kidney
Melioidosis
Ménière's disease
Meningitis
Meningococcemia
Menopause
Men's health
Menstrual disorders
Mental retardation
Mental status examination
Mesothelioma
Metabolic acidosis
Metabolic alkalosis
Methadone
Methemoglobinemia
Microphthalmia and anophthalmia
Mifepristone
Migraine headache
Mineral deficiency
Mineral toxicity
Minerals
Minnesota multiphasic personality
    inventory (MMPI-2)
Minority health
Minoxidil
Miscarriage
Mitral valve insufficiency
Mitral valve prolapse
Mitral valve stenosis
Moles
Monkeypox
Monoamine oxidase inhibitors
Mood disorders
Motion sickness
Movement disorders
Movement therapy
Mucopolysaccharidoses
Mucormycosis
Multiple chemical sensitivity
Multiple endocrine neoplasia
    syndromes
Multiple myeloma
Multiple personality disorder
Multiple pregnancy
Multiple sclerosis
Multiple-gated acquisition (MUGA)
    scan
Mumps

Munchausen syndrome
Muscle relaxants
Muscle spasms and cramps
Muscular dystrophy
Mushroom poisoning
Music therapy
Mutism
Myasthenia gravis
Mycetoma
Mycobacterial infections, atypical
Mycoplasma infections
Myelodysplastic syndrome
Myelofibrosis
Myelography
Myers-Briggs type indicator
Myocardial biopsy
Myocardial resection
Myocarditis
Myoglobin test
Myomectomy
Myopathies
Myopia
Myositis
Myotonic dystrophy
Myringotomy and ear tubes
Myxoma

N

Nail removal
Nail-patella syndrome
Narcolepsy
Narcotics
Nasal irrigation
Nasal packing
Nasal papillomas
Nasal polyps
Nasal trauma
Nasogastric suction
Nasopharyngeal culture
Naturopathic medicine
Nausea and vomiting
Near-drowning
Necrotizing enterocolitis
Neonatal jaundice
Nephrectomy
Nephritis
Nephrotic syndrome
Nephrotoxic injury
Neuralgia
Neuroblastoma
Neuroendocrine
    tumorsNeurofibromatosis

Neurogenic bladder
Neurolinguistic programming
Neurologic exam
Neutropenia
Night terrors
Nitrogen narcosis
Nocardiosis
Nongonococcal urethritis
Non-nucleoside reverse transcriptase
    inhibitors
Nonsteroidal anti-inflammatory
    drugs
Noroviruses
Nosebleed
Numbness and tingling
Nutrition through an intravenous line
Nutrition
Nutritional supplements
Nystagmus

O

Obesity surgery
Obesity
Obsessive-compulsive disorder
Obstetrical emergencies
Occupational asthma
Oligomenorrhea
Omega-3 Fatty Acids
Onychomycosis
Oophorectomy
Ophthalmoplegia
Oppositional defiant disorder
Optic atrophy
Optic neuritis
Oral contraceptives
Oral hygiene
Orbital and periorbital cellulitis
Orchitis
Orthopedic surgery
Orthostatic hypotension
Osteoarthritis
Osteochondroses
Osteogenesis imperfecta
Osteomyelitis
Osteopathy
Osteopetroses
Osteoporosis
Ostomy
Otitis externa
Otitis media
Otosclerosis
Ototoxicity

Ovarian cancer
Ovarian cysts
Ovarian torsion
Overactive bladder
Overhydration
Oxygen/ozone therapy

P

Pacemakers
Paget's disease of bone
Paget's disease of the breast
Pain management
Pain
Palpitations
Pancreas transplantation
Pancreatectomy
Pancreatic cancer, endocrine
Pancreatic cancer, exocrine
Pancreatitis
Panic disorder
Pap test
Papilledema
Paracentesis
Paralysis
Paranoia
Parathyroid hormone test
Parathyroid scan
Parathyroidectomy
Paratyphoid fever
Parkinson disease
Parotidectomy
Paroxysmal atrial tachycardia
Parrot fever
Partial thromboplastin time
Paruresis
Patau syndrome
Patent ductus arteriosus
Pellagra
Pelvic exam
Pelvic fracture
Pelvic inflammatory disease
Pelvic relaxation
Pelvic ultrasound
Penicillins
Penile cancer
Penile prostheses
Percutaneous transhepatic
  cholangiography
Perforated eardrum
Perforated septum
PericardiocentesisPericarditis
Perinatal infection

Periodic paralysis
Periodontal disease
Peripheral neuropathy
Peripheral vascular disease
Peritonitis
Pernicious anemia
Peroxisomal disorders
Personality disorders
Pervasive developmental disorders
Pet therapy
Peyronie's disease
Pharmacogenetics
Phenylketonuria
Pheochromocytoma
Phimosis
Phlebotomy
Phobias
Phosphorus imbalance
Photorefractive keratectomy and
  laser-assisted in-situ keratomileusis
Photosensitivity
Phototherapy
Physical allergy
Physical examination
Pica
Pickwickian syndrome
Piercing and tattoos
Pilates
Pinguecula and pterygium
Pinta
Pituitary dwarfism
Pituitary tumors
Pityriasis rosea
Placenta previa
Placental abruption
Plague
Plasma renin activity
Plasmapheresis
Plastic, cosmetic, and reconstructive
  surgery
Platelet aggregation test
Platelet count
Platelet function disorders
Pleural biopsy
Pleural effusion
Pleurisy
Pneumococcal pneumonia
Pneumocystis pneumonia
Pneumonia
Pneumothorax
Poison ivy and poison oak
Poisoning
Polarity therapy
Polio

Polycystic kidney disease
Polycystic ovary syndrome
Polycythemia vera
Polydactyly and syndactyly
Polyglandular deficiency syndromes
Polyhydramnios and
  oligohydramnios
Polymyalgia rheumatica
Polymyositis
Polysomnography
Porphyrias
Portal vein bypass
Positron emission tomography
  (PET)
Post-concussion syndrome
Postmenopausal bleeding
Postpartum depression
Postpolio syndrome
Post-traumatic stress disorder
Prader-Willi syndrome
Precocious puberty
Preeclampsia and eclampsia
Pregnancy
Premature ejaculation
Premature labor
Premature menopause
Premature rupture of membranes
Prematurity
Premenstrual dysphoric disorder
Premenstrual syndrome
Prenatal surgery
Prepregnancy counseling
Presbyopia
Priapism
Prickly heat
Primary biliary cirrhosis
Proctitis
Progressive multifocal
  leukoencephalopathy
Progressive supranuclear palsy
Prolactin test
Prolonged QT syndrome
Prophylaxis
Prostate biopsy
Prostate cancer
Prostate ultrasound
Prostatectomy
Prostate-specific antigen test
Prostatitis
Protease inhibitors
Protein components test
Protein electrophoresis
Protein-energy malnutrition
Prothrombin time

List of Entries

Proton Pump Inhibitors
Pseudogout
Pseudomonas infections
Pseudoxanthoma elasticum
Psoriasis
Psoriatic arthritis
Psychiatric confinement
Psychoanalysis
Psychological tests
Psychosis
Psychosocial disorders
Psychosurgery
Ptosis
Puberty
Puerperal infection
Pulmonary alveolar proteinosis
Pulmonary artery catheterization
Pulmonary edema
Pulmonary embolism
Pulmonary fibrosis
Pulmonary function test
Pulmonary hypertension
Pulmonary valve insufficiency
Pulmonary valve stenosis
Pyelonephritis
Pyloric stenosis
Pyloroplasty
Pyruvate kinase deficiency

 Q

Q fever
Qigong

 R

Rabies
Radial keratotomy
Radiation injuries
Radiation therapy
Radical neck dissection
Radioactive implants
Rape and sexual assault
Rashes
Rat-bite fever
Raynaud's disease
Recompression treatment
Rectal cancer
Rectal examination
Rectal polyps
Rectal prolapse

Recurrent miscarriage
Red blood cell indices
Reflex sympathetic dystrophy
Reflex tests
Reflexology
Rehabilitation
Reiki
Reiter's syndrome
Relapsing fever
Relapsing polychondritis
Renal artery occlusion
Renal artery stenosis
Renal tubular acidosis
Renal vein thrombosis
Renovascular hypertension
Respiratory acidosis
Respiratory alkalosis
Respiratory distress syndrome
Respiratory failure
Respiratory syncytial virus
   infection
Restless legs syndrome
Restrictive cardiomyopathy
Reticulocyte count
Retinal artery occlusion
Retinal detachment
Retinal hemorrhage
Retinal vein occlusion
Retinitis pigmentosa
Retinoblastoma
Retinopathies
Retrograde cystography
Retrograde ureteropyelography
Retrograde urethrography
Reye's syndrome
Rheumatic fever
Rheumatoid arthritis
Rhinitis
Rhinoplasty
Riboflavin deficiency
Rickets
Rickettsialpox
Ringworm
Rocky Mountain spotted fever
Rolfing
Root canal treatment
Rosacea
Roseola
Ross River Virus
Rotator cuff injury
Rotavirus infections
Roundworm infections
Rubella test
Rubella

S

Sacroiliac disease
Salivary gland scan
Salivary gland tumors
Salmonella food poisoning
Salpingectomy
Salpingo-oophorectomy
Sarcoidosis
Sarcomas
Saw palmetto
Scabies
Scarlet fever
Scars
Schistosomiasis
Schizoaffective disorder
Schizophrenia
Sciatica
Scleroderma
Sclerotherapy for esophageal varices
Scoliosis
Scrotal nuclear medicine scan
Scrotal ultrasound
Scrub typhus
Scurvy
Seasonal affective disorder
Seborrheic dermatitis
Secondary polycythemia
Sedation
Seizure disorder
Selective serotonin reuptake
   inhibitors
Self-mutilation
Semen analysis
Seniors' health
Sensory integration disorder
Sepsis
Septic shock
Septoplasty
Serum sickness
Severe acute respiratory syndrome
   (SARS)
Severe combined immunodeficiency
Sex hormones tests
Sex therapy
Sexual dysfunction
Sexual perversions
Sexually transmitted diseases
Sexually transmitted diseases cultures
Shaken baby syndrome
Shiatsu
Shigellosis
Shin splints

Shingles
Shock
Shortness of breath
Shy-Drager syndrome
Shyness
Sick sinus syndrome
Sickle cell disease
Sideroblastic anemia
Sigmoidoscopy
Sildenafil citrate
Silicosis
Sinus endoscopy
Sinusitis
Situs inversus
Sitz bath
Sjögren's syndrome
Skin biopsy
Skin cancer, non-melanoma
Skin culture
Skin grafting
Skin lesion removal
Skin lesions
Skin pigmentation disorders
Skin resurfacing
Skull x rays
Sleep apnea
Sleep disorders
Sleeping sickness
Small intestine biopsy
Smallpox
Smelling disorders
Smoke inhalation
Smoking
Smoking-cessation drugs
Snoring
Somatoform disorders
Sore throat
South American blastomycosis
Speech disorders
Spina bifida
Spinal cord injury
Spinal cord tumors
Spinal instrumentation
Spinal stenosis
Splenectomy
Splenic trauma
Sporotrichosis
Sports injuries
Sprains and strains
Sputum culture
St. John's wort
Stanford-Binet intelligence scales
Stapedectomy
Staphylococcal infections

Staphylococcal scalded skin
    syndrome
Starvation
Stem cell transplantation
Stillbirth
Stockholm syndrome
Stomach cancer
Stomach flushing
Stomatitis
Stool culture
Stool fat test
Stool O & P test
Strabismus
Strep throat
Streptococcal antibody tests
Streptococcal infections
Stress reduction
Stress test
Stress
Stridor
Stroke
Stuttering
Subacute sclerosing panencephalitis
Subarachnoid hemorrhage
Subdural hematoma
Substance abuse and dependence
Sudden cardiac death
Sudden infant death syndrome
Suicide
Sulfonamides
Sunburn
Sunscreens
Superior vena cava syndrome
Surfactant
Swallowing disorders
Sydenham's chorea
Sympathectomy
Syphilis
Systemic lupus erythematosus

T

Tai chi
Tapeworm diseases
Tardive dyskinesia
Tarsorrhaphy
Tay-Sachs disease
Technetium heart scan
Teeth whitening
Temporal arteritis
Temporomandibular joint disorders
Tendinitis
Tennis elbow

Tensilon test
Tension headache
Testicular cancer
Testicular self-examination
Testicular surgery
Testicular torsion
Tetanus
Tetracyclines
Tetralogy of Fallot
Thalassemia
Thallium heart scan
Thematic apperception test
Therapeutic baths
Therapeutic touch
Thoracentesis
Thoracic outlet syndrome
Thoracic surgery
Thoracoscopy
Threadworm infection
Throat culture
Thrombocytopenia
Thrombocytosis
Thrombolytic therapy
Thrombophlebitis
Thymoma
Thyroid biopsy
Thyroid cancer
Thyroid function tests
Thyroid hormones
Thyroid nuclear medicine scan
Thyroid ultrasound
Thyroidectomy
Thyroiditis
Tilt table test
Tinnitus
Tissue typing
Tonsillectomy and adenoidectomy
Tonsillitis
Tooth decay
Tooth extraction
Tooth replacements and restorations
Toothache
Topical Anesthesia
TORCH test
Torticollis
Total parenteral nutrition
Tourette syndrome
Toxic epidermal necrolysis
Toxic shock syndrome
Toxoplasmosis
Trabeculectomy
Tracheoesophageal fistula
Tracheotomy
Trachoma

Traction
Traditional Chinese medicine
Trager psychophysical integration
Transcranial Doppler
  ultrasonography
Transesophageal echocardiography
Transfusion
Transhepatic biliary catheterization
Transient ischemic attack
Transposition of the great arteries
Transurethral bladder resection
Transvaginal ultrasound
Transverse myelitis
Traumatic amputations
Traveler's diarrhea
Tremors
Trench fever
Trichinosis
Trichomoniasis
Tricuspid valve insufficiency
Tricuspid valve stenosis
Trigeminal neuralgia
Trigger finger
Triglycerides test
Triple screen
Tropical spastic paraparesis
Troponins test
Tubal ligation
Tube compression of the esophagus
  and stomach
Tube feedings
Tuberculin skin test
Tuberculosis
Tularemia
Tumor markers
Tumor removal
Turner syndrome
2,3-diphosphoglycerate test
Typhoid fever
Typhus
Tzanck preparation

 U

Ulcer surgery
Ulcerative colitis
Ulcers (digestive)
Ultraviolet light treatment
Umbilical cord blood banking
Undescended testes
Upper GI exam
Ureteral stenting

Urethritis
Uric acid tests
Urinalysis
Urinary anti-infectives
Urinary catheterization
Urinary diversion surgery
Urinary incontinence
Urine culture
Urine flow test
Uterine fibroid embolization
Uterine fibroids
Uveitis

 V

Vaccination
Vaginal pain
Vagotomy
Valsalva maneuver
Valvular heart disease
Varicose veins
Vasculitis
Vasectomy
Vasodilators
Vegetarianism
Vegetative state
Velopharyngeal insufficiency
Vena cava filter
Venography
Venous access
Venous insufficiency
Ventricular aneurysm
Ventricular assist device
Ventricular ectopic beats
Ventricular fibrillation
Ventricular septal defect
Ventricular shunt
Ventricular tachycardia
Vesicoureteral reflux
Vibriosis
Vision training
Visual impairment
Vitamin A deficiency
Vitamin B$_6$ deficiency
Vitamin D deficiency
Vitamin E deficiency
Vitamin K deficiency
Vitamin tests
Vitamin toxicity
Vitamins
Vitiligo

Vitrectomy
Vocal cord nodules and polyps
Vocal cord paralysis
von Willebrand disease
Vulvar cancer
Vulvodynia
Vulvovaginitis

 W

Waldenstrom's macroglobulinemia
Warts
Wechsler intelligence test
Wegener's granulomatosis
Weight loss drugs
West Nile Virus
Wheezing
Whiplash
White blood cell count and
  differential
Whooping cough
Wilderness medicine
Wilms' tumor
Wilson disease
Wiskott-Aldrich syndrome
Withdrawal syndromes
Wolff-Parkinson-White
  syndrome
Women's health
Wound culture
Wound flushing
Wounds

X

X-linked agammaglobulinemia
X rays of the orbit

 Y

Yaws
Yellow fever
Yersinosis
Yoga

Z

Zoonosis

PLEASE READ—IMPORTANT INFORMATION

The *Gale Encyclopedia of Medicine* is a medical reference product designed to inform and educate readers about a wide variety of disorders, conditions, treatments, and diagnostic tests. Thomson Gale believes the product to be comprehensive, but not necessarily definitive. It is intended to supplement, not replace, consultation with a physician or other healthcare practitioner. While Thomson Gale has made substantial efforts to provide information that is accurate, comprehensive, and up-to-date, Thomson Gale makes no representations or warranties of any kind, including without limitation, warranties of merchantability or fitness for a particular purpose, nor does it guarantee the accuracy, comprehensiveness, or timeliness of the information contained in this product. Readers should be aware that the universe of medical knowledge is constantly growing and changing, and that differences of medical opinion exist among authorities. Readers are also advised to seek professional diagnosis and treatment for any medical condition, and to discuss information obtained from this book with their healthcare provider.

INTRODUCTION

The third edition of the *Gale Encyclopedia of Medicine (GEM3)* is a one-stop source for medical information on over 1,750 common medical disorders, conditions, tests, and treatments, including high-profile diseases such as AIDS, Alzheimer's disease, cancer, and heart attack. This encyclopedia avoids medical jargon and uses language that laypersons can understand, while still providing thorough coverage of each topic. The *Gale Encyclopedia of Medicine 3* fills a gap between basic consumer health resources, such as single-volume family medical guides, and highly technical professional materials.

SCOPE

More than 1,750 full-length articles are included in the *Gale Encyclopedia of Medicine 3*, including disorders/conditions, tests/procedures, and treatments/therapies. Many common drugs are also covered, with generic drug names appearing first and brand names following in parentheses, eg. acetaminophen (Tylenol). Throughout the *Gale Encyclopedia of Medicine 3*, many prominent individuals are highlighted as sidebar biographies that accompany the main topical essays. Articles follow a standardized format that provides information at a glance. Rubrics include:

Disorders/Conditions	Tests/Treatments
Definition	Definition
Description	Purpose
Causes and symptoms	Precautions
Diagnosis	Description
Treatment	Preparation
Alternative treatment	Aftercare
Prognosis	Risks
Prevention	Normal/Abnormal results
Resources	Resources
Key terms	Key terms

In recent years there has been a resurgence of interest in holistic medicine that emphasizes the connection between mind and body. Aimed at achieving and maintaining good health rather than just eliminating disease, this approach has come to be known as alternative medicine. The *Gale Encyclopedia of Medicine 3* includes a number of essays on alternative therapies, ranging from traditional Chinese medicine to homeopathy and from meditation to aromatherapy. In addition to full essays on alternative therapies, the encyclopedia features specific **Alternative treatment** sections for diseases and conditions that may be helped by complementary therapies.

INCLUSION CRITERIA

A preliminary list of diseases, disorders, tests and treatments was compiled from a wide variety of sources, including professional medical guides and textbooks as well as consumer guides and encyclopedias. The general advisory board, made up of public librarians, medical librarians and consumer health experts, evaluated the topics and made suggestions for inclusion. The list was sorted by category and sent to *GEM3* medical advisers, for review. Final selection of topics to include was made by the medical advisors in conjunction with the Thomson Gale editor.

ABOUT THE CONTRIBUTORS

The essays were compiled by experienced medical writers, including physicians, pharmacists, nurses, and other health care professionals. *GEM3* medical advisors reviewed the completed essays to insure that they are appropriate, up-to-date, and medically accurate.

HOW TO USE THIS BOOK

The *Gale Encyclopedia of Medicine 3* has been designed with ready reference in mind.

- Straight **alphabetical arrangement** allows users to locate information quickly.

- Bold faced terms function as **print hyperlinks** that point the reader to related entries in the encyclopedia.

- **Cross-references** placed throughout the encyclopedia direct readers to where information on subjects without entries can be found. Synonyms are also cross-referenced.

- A list of **key terms** are provided where appropriate to define unfamiliar terms or concepts.

- Valuable **contact information** for organizations andsupport groups is included with each entry.

The appendix contains an extensive list of organizations arranged in alphabetical order.

- **Resources section** directs users to additional sources of medical information on a topic.

- A comprehensive **general index** allows users to easily target detailed aspects of any topic, including Latin names.

GRAPHICS

The *Gale Encyclopedia of Medicine 3* is enhanced with over 675 illustrations, including photos, charts, tables, and customized line drawings.

ADVISORS

A number of experts in the library and medical communities provided invaluable assistance in the formulation of this encyclopedia. Our advisory board performed a myriad of duties, from defining the scope of coverage to reviewing individual entries for accuracy and accessibility. The editor would like to express her appreciation to them.

MEDICAL ADVISORS

Rosalyn Carson-DeWitt, M.D.
Durham, NC

Larry I. Lutwick M.D., F.A.C.P.
Director, Infectious Diseases
VA Medical Center
Brooklyn, NY

Samuel Uretsky, Pharm.D.
Pharmacist
Wantagh, NY

CONTRIBUTORS

Margaret Alic, Ph.D.
Science Writer
Eastsound, WA

Janet Byron Anderson
Linguist/Language Consultant
Rocky River, OH

Lisa Andres, M.S., C.G.C.
Certified Genetic Counselor and Medical Writer
San Jose, CA

Greg Annussek
Medical Writer/Editor
New York, NY

Bill Asenjo, Ph.D.
Science Writer
Iowa City, IA

Sharon A. Aufox, M.S., C.G.C.
Genetic Counselor
Rockford Memorial Hospital
Rockford, IL

Sandra Bain Cushman
Massage Therapist, Alexander Technique Practitioner
Charlottesville, VA

Howard Baker
Medical Writer
North York, Ontario

Laurie Barclay, M.D.
Neurological Consulting Services
Tampa, FL

Jeanine Barone
Nutritionist, Exercise Physiologist
New York, NY

Julia R. Barrett
Science Writer
Madison, WI

Donald G. Barstow, R.N.
Clincal Nurse Specialist
Oklahoma City, OK

Carin Lea Beltz, M.S.
Genetic Counselor and Program Director
The Center for Genetic Counseling
Indianapolis, IN

Linda K. Bennington, C.N.S.
Science Writer
Virginia Beach, VA

Issac R. Berniker
Medical Writer
Vallejo, CA

Kathleen Berrisford, M.S.V.
Science Writer

Bethanne Black
Medical Writer
Atlanta, GA

Jennifer Bowjanowski, M.S., C.G.C.
Genetic Counselor
Children's Hospital Oakland
Oakland, CA

Michelle Q. Bosworth, M.S., C.G.C.
Genetic Counselor
Eugene, OR

Barbara Boughton
Health and Medical Writer
El Cerrito, CA

Cheryl Branche, M.D.
Retired General Practitioner
Jackson, MS

Michelle Lee Brandt
Medical Writer
San Francisco, CA

Maury M. Breecher, Ph.D.
Health Communicator/Journalist
Northport, AL

Ruthan Brodsky
Medical Writer
Bloomfield Hills, MI

Tom Brody, Ph.D.
Science Writer
Berkeley, CA

Leonard C. Bruno, Ph.D.
Medical Writer
Chevy Chase, MD

Diane Calbrese
Medical Sciences and Technology Writer
Silver Spring, Maryland

Richard H. Camer
Editor
International Medical News Group
Silver Spring, MD

Rosalyn Carson-DeWitt, M.D.
Medical Writer
Durham, NC

Lata Cherath, Ph.D.
Science Writing Intern
Cancer Research Institute
New York, NY

Linda Chrisman
Massage Therapist and Educator
Oakland, CA

Lisa Christenson, Ph.D.
Science Writer
Hamden, CT

Geoffrey N. Clark, D.V.M.
Editor
Canine Sports Medicine
    Update
Newmarket, NH

Rhonda Cloos, R.N.
Medical Writer
Austin, TX

Gloria Cooksey, C.N.E
Medical Writer
Sacramento, CA

Amy Cooper, M.A., M.S.I.
Medical Writer
Vermillion, SD

David A. Cramer, M.D.
Medical Writer
Chicago, IL

Esther Csapo Rastega, R.N.,
    B.S.N.
Medical Writer
Holbrook, MA

Arnold Cua, M.D.
Physician
Brooklyn, NY

Tish Davidson, A.M.
Medical Writer
Fremont, California

Dominic De Bellis, Ph.D.
Medical Writer/Editor
Mahopac, NY

Lori De Milto
Medical Writer
Sicklerville, NJ

Robert S. Dinsmoor
Medical Writer
South Hamilton, MA

Stephanie Dionne, B.S.
Medical Writer
Ann Arbor, MI

Martin W. Dodge, Ph.D.
Technical Writer/Editor
Centinela Hospital and Medical
    Center
Inglewood, CA

David Doermann
Medical Writer
Salt Lake City, UT

Stefanie B. N. Dugan, M.S.
Genetic Counselor
Milwaukee, WI

Doug Dupler, M.A.
Science Writer
Boulder, CO

Thomas Scott Eagan
Student Researcher
University of Arizona
Tucson, AZ

Altha Roberts Edgren
Medical Writer
Medical Ink
St. Paul, MN

Karen Ericson, R.N.
Medical Writer
Estes Park, CO

L. Fleming Fallon Jr., M.D.,
    Dr.PH
*Associate Professor of Public
    Health*
Bowling Green State University
Bowling Green, OH

Faye Fishman, D.O.
Physician
Randolph, NJ

Janis Flores
Medical Writer
Lexikon Communications
Sebastopol, CA

Risa Flynn
Medical Writer
Culver City, CA

Paula Ford-Martin
Medical Writer
Chaplin, MN

Janie F. Franz
Writer
Grand Forks, ND

Sallie Freeman, Ph.D., B.S.N.
Medical Writer
Atlanta, GA

Rebecca J. Frey, Ph.D.
*Research and Administrative
    Associate*
East Rock Institute
New Haven, CT

Cynthia L. Frozena, R.N.
Nurse, Medical Writer
Manitowoc, WI

Jason Fryer
Medical Writer
San Antonio, TX

Ron Gasbarro, Pharm.D.
Medical Writer
New Milford, PA

Julie A. Gelderloos
Biomedical Writer
Playa del Rey, CA

Gary Gilles, M.A.
Medical Writer
Wauconda, IL

Harry W. Golden
Medical Writer
Shoreline Medical Writers
Old Lyme, CT

Debra Gordon
Medical Writer
Nazareth, PA

Megan Gourley
Writer
Germantown, MD

Jill Granger, M.S.
Senior Research Associate
University of Michigan
Ann Arbor, MI

Alison Grant
Medical Writer
Averill Park, NY

Elliot Greene, M.A.
*former president, American
    Massage Therapy Association*
Massage Therapist
Silver Spring, MD

Peter Gregutt
Writer
Asheville, NC

Laith F. Gulli, M.D.
M.Sc., M.Sc.(MedSci), M.S.A.,
    Msc.Psych, MRSNZ
FRSH, FRIPHH, FAIC, FZS
DAPA, DABFC, DABCI
*Consultant Psychotherapist in
    Private Practice*
Lathrup Village, MI

Kapil Gupta, M.D.
Medical Writer
Winston-Salem, NC

Maureen Haggerty
Medical Writer
Ambler, PA

Clare Hanrahan
Medical Writer
Asheville, NC

Ann M. Haren
Science Writer
Madison, CT

Judy C. Hawkins, M.S.
Genetic Counselor
The University of Texas Medical
   Branch
Galveston, TX

Caroline Helwick
Medical Writer
New Orleans, LA

David Helwig
Medical Writer
London, Ontario

Lisette Hilton
Medical Writer
Boca Raton, FL

Katherine S. Hunt, M.S.
Genetic Counselor
University of New Mexico Health
   Sciences Center
Albuquerque, NM

Kevin Hwang, M.D.
Medical Writer
Morristown, NJ

Holly Ann Ishmael, M.S.,
   C.G.C.
Genetic Counselor
The Children's Mercy Hospital
Kansas City, MO

Dawn A. Jacob, M.S.
Genetic Counselor
Obstetrix Medical Group of
   Texas
Fort Worth, TX

Sally J. Jacobs, Ed.D.
Medical Writer
Los Angeles, CA

Michelle L. Johnson, M.S., J.D.
*Patent Attorney and Medical
   Writer*
Portland, OR

Paul A. Johnson, Ed.M.
Medical Writer
San Diego, CA

Cindy L. A. Jones, Ph.D.
Biomedical Writer
Sagescript Communications
Lakewood, CO

David Kaminstein, M.D.
Medical Writer
West Chester, PA

Beth A. Kapes
Medical Writer
Bay Village, OH

Janet M. Kearney
Freelance writer
Orlando, FL

Christine Kuehn Kelly
Medical Writer
Havertown, PA

Bob Kirsch
Medical Writer
Ossining, NY

Joseph Knight, P.A.
Medical Writer
Winton, CA

Melissa Knopper
Medical Writer
Chicago, IL

Karen Krajewski, M.S., C.G.C.
Genetic Counselor
Assistant Professor of Neurology
Wayne State University
Detroit, MI

Jeanne Krob, M.D., F.A.C.S.
Physician, writer
Pittsburgh, PA

Jennifer Lamb
Medical Writer
Spokane, WA

Richard H. Lampert
Senior Medical Editor
W.B. Saunders Co.
Philadelphia, PA

Jeffrey P. Larson, R.P.T.
Physical Therapist
Sabin, MN

Jill Lasker
Medical Writer
Midlothian, VA

Kristy Layman
Music Therapist
East Lansing, MI

Victor Leipzig, Ph.D.
Biological Consultant
Huntington Beach, CA

Lorraine Lica, Ph.D.
Medical Writer
San Diego, CA

John T. Lohr, Ph.D.
*Assistant Director, Biotechnology
   Center*
Utah State University
Logan, UT

Larry Lutwick, M.D., F.A.C.P.
Director, Infectious Diseases
VA Medical Center
Brooklyn, NY

Suzanne M. Lutwick
Medical Writer
Brooklyn, NY

Nicole Mallory, M.S.
Medical Student
Wayne State University
Detroit, MI

Warren Maltzman, Ph.D.
*Consultant, Molecular
   Pathology*
Demarest, NJ

Adrienne Massel, R.N.
Medical Writer
Beloit, WI

Ruth E. Mawyer, R.N.
Medical Writer
Charlottesville, VA

Richard A. McCartney M.D.
*Fellow, American College of
   Surgeons*
*Diplomat American Board of
   Surgery*
Richland, WA

Bonny McClain, Ph.D.
Medical Writer
Greensboro, NC

Sally C. McFarlane-Parrott
Medical Writer
Ann Arbor, MI

Mercedes McLaughlin
Medical Writer
Phoenixville, CA

Alison McTavish, M.Sc.
Medical Writer and Editor
Montreal, Quebec

Liz Meszaros
Medical Writer
Lakewood, OH

Betty Mishkin
Medical Writer
Skokie, IL

Barbara J. Mitchell
Medical Writer
Hallstead, PA

Mark A. Mitchell, M.D.
Medical Writer
Seattle, WA

Susan J. Montgomery
Medical Writer
Milwaukee, WI

Louann W. Murray, PhD
Medical Writer
Huntington Beach, CA

Bilal Nasser, M.Sc.
Senior Medical Student
Universidad Iberoamericana
Santo Domingo, Domincan
  Republic

Laura Ninger
Medical Writer
Weehawken, NJ

Nancy J. Nordenson
Medical Writer
Minneapolis, MN

Teresa Odle
Medical Writer
Albaquerque, NM

Lisa Papp, R.N.
Medical Writer
Cherry Hill, NJ

Lee Ann Paradise
Medical Writer
San Antonio, TX

Patience Paradox
Medical Writer
Bainbridge Island, WA

Barbara J. Pettersen
Genetic Counselor
Genetic Counseling of Central
  Oregon
Bend, OR

Genevieve Pham-Kanter, M.S.
Medical Writer
Chicago, IL

Collette Placek
Medical Writer
Wheaton, IL

J. Ricker Polsdorfer, M.D.
Medical Writer
Phoenix, AZ

Scott Polzin, M.S., C.G.C.
Medical Writer
Buffalo Grove, IL

Elizabeth J. Pulcini, M.S.
Medical Writer
Phoenix, Arizona

Nada Quercia, M.S., C.C.G.C.
Genetic Counselor
Division of Clinical and
  Metabolic Genetics
The Hospital for Sick Children
Toronto, ON, Canada

Ann Quigley
Medical Writer
New York, NY

Robert Ramirez, B.S.
Medical Student
University of Medicine &
  Dentistry of New Jersey
Stratford, NJ

Kulbir Rangi, D.O.
Medical Doctor and Writer
New York, NY

Esther Csapo Rastegari, Ed.M.,
  R.N./B.S.N.
Registered Nurse, Medical Writer
Holbrook, MA

Toni Rizzo
Medical Writer
Salt Lake City, UT

Martha Robbins
Medical Writer
Evanston, IL

Richard Robinson
Medical Writer
Tucson, AZ

Nancy Ross-Flanigan
Science Writer
Belleville, MI

Anna Rovid Spickler, D.V.M., Ph.D.
Medical Writer
Moorehead, KY

Belinda Rowland, Ph.D.
Medical Writer
Voorheesville, NY

Andrea Ruskin, M.D.
Whittingham Cancer Center
Norwalk, CT

Laura Ruth, Ph.D.
*Medical, Science, & Technology
  Writer*
Los Angeles, CA

Karen Sandrick
Medical Writer
Chicago, IL

Kausalya Santhanam, Ph.D.
Technical Writer
Branford, CT

Jason S. Schliesser, D.C.
Chiropractor
Holland Chiropractic, Inc.
Holland, OH

Joan Schonbeck
Medical Writer
Nursing
Massachusetts Department of
  Mental Health
Marlborough, MA

Laurie Heron Seaver, M.D.
Clinical Geneticist
Greenwood Genetic Center
Greenwood, SC

Catherine Seeley
Medical Writer

Kristen Mahoney Shannon, M.S., C.G.C.
Genetic Counselor
Center for Cancer Risk Analysis
Massachusetts General Hospital
Boston, MA

Kim A. Sharp, M.Ln.
Writer
Richmond, TX

Judith Sims, M.S.
Medical Writer
Logan, UT

Joyce S. Siok, R.N.
Medical Writer
South Windsor, CT

Jennifer Sisk
Medical Writer
Havertown, PA

Patricia Skinner
Medical Writer
Amman, Jordan

Genevieve Slomski, Ph.D.
Medical Writer
New Britain, CT

Stephanie Slon
Medical Writer
Portland, OR

Linda Wasmer Smith
Medical Writer
Albuquerque, NM

Java O. Solis, M.S.
Medical Writer
Decatur, GA

Elaine Souder, PhD
Medical Writer
Little Rock, AR

Jane E. Spehar
Medical Writer
Canton, OH

Lorraine Steefel, R.N.
Medical Writer
Morganville, NJ

Kurt Sternlof
Science Writer
New Rochelle, NY

Roger E. Stevenson, M.D.
Director
Greenwood Genetic Center
Greenwood, SC

Dorothy Stonely
Medical Writer
Los Gatos, CA

Liz Swain
Medical Writer
San Diego, CA

Deanna M. Swartout-Corbeil, R.N.
Medical Writer
Thompsons Station, TN

Keith Tatarelli, J.D.
Medical Writer

Mary Jane Tenerelli, M.S.
Medical Writer
East Northport, NY

Catherine L. Tesla, M.S., C.G.C.
Senior Associate, Faculty
Dept. of Pediatrics, Division of Medical Genetics
Emory University School of Medicine
Atlanta, GA

Bethany Thivierge
Biotechnical Writer/Editor
Technicality Resources
Rockland, ME

Mai Tran, Pharm.D.
Medical Writer
Troy, MI

Carol Turkington
Medical Writer
Lancaster, PA

Judith Turner, B.S.
Medical Writer
Sandy, UT

Amy B. Tuteur, M.D.
Medical Advisor
Sharon, MA

Samuel Uretsky, Pharm.D.
Medical Writer
Wantagh, NY

Amy Vance, M.S., C.G.C.
Genetic Counselor
GeneSage, Inc.
San Francisco, CA

Michael Sherwin Walston
Student Researcher
University of Arizona
Tucson, AZ

Ronald Watson, Ph.D.
Science Writer
Tucson, AZ

Ellen S. Weber, M.S.N.
Medical Writer
Fort Wayne, IN

Ken R. Wells
Freelance Writer
Laguna Hills, CA

Jennifer F. Wilson, M.S.
Science Writer
Haddonfield, NJ

Kathleen D. Wright, R.N.
Medical Writer
Delmar, DE

Jennifer Wurges
Medical Writer
Rochester Hills, MI

Mary Zoll, Ph.D.
Science Writer
Newton Center, MA

Jon Zonderman
Medical Writer
Orange, CA

Michael V. Zuck, Ph.D.
Medical Writer
Boulder, CO

Nail infections *see* **Onychomycosis**

Nail-patella syndrome

Definition

Nail-patella syndrome, is a genetic disease of the connective tissue that produces defects in the fingernails, knee caps, and kidneys.

Description

Nail-patella syndrome is also known as Fong Disease, Hereditary Onycho-Osteodysplasia (H.O.O.D.), Iliac Horn Disease, and Turner-Kieser syndrome. Patients who have nail-patella syndrome may show a variety of physical defects. The hallmark features of this syndrome are poorly developed fingernails, toenails, and patellae (kneecaps). Other common abnormalities include elbow deformities, abnormally shaped pelvis bone (hip bone), and kidney (renal) disease.

Less common medical findings include defects of the upper lip, the roof of the mouth, and unusual skeletal abnormalities. Skeletal abnormalities may include poorly developed scapulae (shoulder blades), sideways bent fingers (clinodactyly), clubfoot, scoliosis, and unusual neck bones. There are also other effects, such as thickening of the basement membrane in the skin and of the tiny clusters of capillaries (glomeruli) in the kidney. Scientists have recognized an association between nail-patella syndrome and **colon cancer**. Nail-patella syndrome is associated with open-angle **glaucoma**, which, if untreated, may lead to blindness. Patients may also have **cataracts**, drooping eyelids (**ptosis**), or corneal problems such as glaucoma.

People with nail-patella syndrome may display only a few or many of the recognized signs of this disease. Symptoms vary widely from person to person. Signs even vary within a single family with multiple affected members.

The incidence of nail-patella syndrome is approximately one in 50,000 births. This disorder affects males and females equally. It is found throughout the world and occurs in all ethnic groups. The strongest risk factor for nail-patella syndrome is a family history of the disease.

Causes and symptoms

Nail-patella syndrome has been recognized as an inherited disorder for over 100 years. It is caused by mutations in a gene known as LIM Homeobox Transcription Factor 1-Beta (LMX1B), located on the long arm of chromosome 9.

The LMX1B gene codes for a protein that is important in organizing embryonic limb development. Mutations in this gene have been detected in many unrelated people with nail-patella syndrome. Scientists have also been able to interrupt this gene in mice to produce defects similar to those seen in human nail-patella syndrome.

Nail-patella syndrome is inherited in an autosomal dominant manner. This means that possession of only one copy of the defective gene is enough to cause disease. When a parent has nail-patella syndrome each of their children has a 50% chance to inherit the disease-causing mutation.

A new mutation causing nail-patella syndrome can also occur, causing disease in a person with no family history. This is called a sporadic occurrence and accounts for approximately 20% of cases of nail-patella syndrome. The children of a person with sporadic nail-patella syndrome are also at a 50% risk of developing signs of the disorder.

Medical signs of nail-patella syndrome vary widely between patients. Some patients with this disorder do not display symptoms. These patients are discovered to have the nail-patella syndrome only when genetic studies trace their family history. Scientists are now working to learn what causes different people to display such different symptoms of nail-patella syndrome.

The most obvious sign associated with nail-patella syndrome is absent, poorly developed, or unusual fingernails. Fingernail abnormalities are found in over 80% of patients with this disorder. Abnormalities may be found in one or more fingernails. Only rarely are all fingernails affected. This disease most commonly affects the fingernails of the thumbs and index fingers. The pinky fingernail is least likely to be affected. Fingernails may be small and concave with pitting, ridges, splits, and/or discoloration. Toenails are less often affected. The lunulae, or light-colored crescent moons, at the base of the fingernail bed next to the cuticle are sometimes triangularly-shaped in people with nail-patella syndrome.

Kneecap abnormalities are the second most common sign associated with this disorder. Either or both kneecaps may be missing or poorly formed. If present, kneecaps are likely to be dislocated. The knees of people with nail-patella syndrome may have a square appearance. Besides the kneecap, other support structures including bones, ligaments, and tendons may also be malformed. These support structures stabilize the knee, therefore patients with some leg malformations may have difficulty in walking.

The hip bones of approximately 80% of patients with nail-patella syndrome have unusual bony projections called posterior iliac horns. These bony projections, or spurs, are internal and not obvious unless they are detected on x ray. This unusual pelvic anatomy is not associated with any other disease.

Kidney disease is present in at least 30% of people with nail-patella syndrome. Biopsy shows lesions that resemble those of inflammation of the clusters of capillaries in the kidneys (glomerulonephritis), but without any infection present. Kidney failure is the most dangerous consequence of nail-patella syndrome. It occurs in about 30% of patients who have kidney involvement. An early sign of kidney involvement is the presence of protein or blood in the urine (chronic, benign proteinuria and hematuria.) Kidney involvement is progressive, so early diagnosis and treatment of renal disease is important. Kidney disease has been reported in children with nail-patella syndrome, but renal involvement more commonly develops during adulthood.

Various skeletal symptoms may occur. Patients with nail-patella syndrome may not be able to fully straighten their arms at the elbow. This may create a webbed appearance at the elbow joint. Patients may have sideways bent fingers, poorly developed shoulder blades, **clubfoot**, hip dislocation, unusual neck bones, or **scoliosis**.

Eye problems may be present and vary from person to person. Nail-patella syndrome is associated with open angle glaucoma. Open angle glaucoma is caused by fluid blocked into the front chamber of the eye. This blocked fluid builds increasing pressure into the eye. If untreated, this increased pressure may lead to permanent damage of the optic nerve and irreversible blindness. Some patients with nail-patella syndrome have ptosis, or drooping eyelids. Nail-patella syndrome has also been associated with abnormalities of the cornea, cataracts, and **astigmatism**. Additionally, the irises of the eye may be multicolored, possibly displaying a clover-shaped pattern of color.

Diagnosis

As of early 2001, **genetic testing** for nail-patella syndrome is available only through research institutions that are working to further characterize this disorder. Genetic testing cannot predict which signs of the disease will develop. Nor can genetic testing predict the severity of disease symptoms. Improved genetic testing for nail-patella syndrome is anticipated in the future.

Diagnosis of this disease is most often made on visual medical clues such as the characteristic abnormalities of the fingernails and kneecaps. Diagnosis is confirmed by x-ray images of the affected bones and, when indicated, kidney biopsy. The bony pelvic spurs found in 80% of patients with nail-patella syndrome are not associated with any other disease.

Prenatal diagnosis for nail-patella syndrome by third-trimester ultrasound was documented in 1998. Prenatal diagnosis via genetic testing of cells obtained by chorionic villus sampling was reported the same year. As of 2001, prenatal genetic testing for nail-patella syndrome is not yet widely available. There is controversy surrounding the use of prenatal testing for such a variable disorder. Prenatal testing cannot predict the extent of an individual's disease.

Treatment

Treatment is usually not necessary. Treatment, when required, depends on each patient's specific symptoms. Severe kidney disease is treated with dialysis or a kidney transplant. Patients receiving kidney transplants do not develop nail-patella type renal complications in their new kidney.

A wheelchair may be required if walking becomes painful due to bone, tendon, ligament, or muscle defects. **Orthopedic surgery** may be necessary for congenital clubfoot deformity. Manipulation or surgery may be required to correct hip dislocation. Cataracts are also surgically treated. Medical treatment at early signs of glaucoma prevents progression of the disease to blindness.

Genetic counseling is offered to persons who have the disease. Parents with this disease have a 50% chance of passing it to each of their children. As of 2001, current genetic testing technology cannot predict the severity or scope of an individual's symptoms.

Because many possible manifestations of nail-patella syndrome exist, patients are advised to pursue extra medical care including regular **urinalysis** and special eye exams. Children with nail-patella syndrome should be screened for scoliosis.

Prognosis

Survival among patients with nail-patella syndrome is not decreased unless a they exhibit renal complications. It is estimated that 8% of individuals with nail-patella syndrome who come to medical attention eventually die of kidney disease.

Resources

BOOKS

Berkow, R., M. H. Beers, A. J. Fletcher, and R. M. Bogin. *The Merck Manual of Medical Information - Home Edition.* McGraw-Hill, 2004.

OTHER

Gene Clinics. < http://www.geneclinics.org >.
OMIM—Online Mendelian Inheritance in Man. < http://www3.ncbi.nlm.nih.gov/Omim >.

John T. Lohr, PhD
Judy C. Hawkins, MS

Nail removal

Definition

Nail removal is a form of treatment that is sometimes necessary following traumatic injuries or recurrent infections in the area of the nail. There are nonsurgical as well as surgical methods of nail removal.

Purpose

Nails are removed only when necessary to allow the skin beneath the nail (the nail bed) to heal or in some cases, to remove a nail that has been partially pulled out in an accident. In the case of toenails, it is occasionally necessary to remove the nail of the large toe due to a chronic condition caused by badly fitted shoes. In general, however, doctors prefer to try other forms of treatment before removing the nail. Depending on the cause, nail disorders are usually treated with oral medications; applying medicated gels or creams directly to the skin around the nail; avoiding substances that irritate the nail folds; surgical lancing of abscesses around the nail; or injecting **corticosteroids** under the nail fold.

The most common causes of nail disorders include:

• Trauma. The nails can be damaged by nail biting, using the fingernails as tools, and incorrect use of nail files and manicure scissors as well as by accidents and **sports injuries**.

• Infections. These include fungal infections under the nails, bacterial infections of cuts or breaks in the nail folds, or infections of the nails themselves caused by *Candida albicans*. Inflammation of the nail folds is called paronychia.

• Exposure to harsh detergents, industrial chemicals, hot water, and other irritants. People who work as dishwashers are especially vulnerable to separation of the nail itself from the nail bed (onycholysis).

• Systemic diseases and disorders. These include **psoriasis**, anemia, and certain congenital disorders.

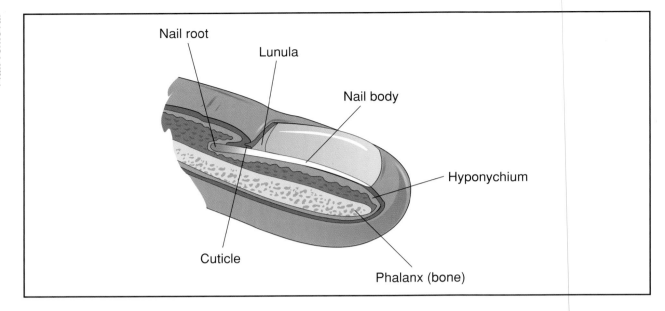

Nail root

Lunula

Nail body

Hyponychium

Cuticle

Phalanx (bone)

The physiology of the human fingernail. The most common causes of nail disorders include trauma, infections, exposure to harsh detergents, hot water and other irritants, systemic diseases and disorders, and allergic reactions to nail polish, nail polish remover, and nail glue. *(Illustration by Electronic Illustrators Group.)*

- Allergic reactions to nail polish, polish remover, or the glue used to attach false nails.

Precautions

In the case of infections, it is necessary to distinguish between fungal, bacterial, and candidal infections before removing the nail. Cultures can usually be obtained from pus or tissue fluid from the affected nail.

Description

Surgical nail removal

If necessary, the surgeon can remove the nail at its base with an instrument called a needlepoint scalpel. In a few cases, the nail may need to be pulled out (avulsed) from its matrix.

Nonsurgical nail removal

Nails can be removed by applying a mixture of 40% urea, 20% anhydrous lanolin, 5% white wax, 25% white petroleum jelly, and silica gel type H.

Preparation

For nonsurgical nail removal, the nail fold is treated with tincture of benzoin and covered with adhesive tape. The nail itself is thickly coated with

---

KEY TERMS

Avulse—To pull or tear away forcibly. In some cases, a surgeon must remove a nail by avulsing it from its matrix.

Matrix—The tissue at the base of the nail, from which the nail grows.

Nail bed—The layer of tissue underneath the nail.

Onycholysis—The separation of a nail from its underlying bed. Onycholysis is a common symptom of candidal infections of the nail or of exposure to harsh chemicals and detergents.

Paronychia—Inflammation of the folds of skin that surround a nail.

---

the urea mixture, followed by a layer of plastic film and adhesive tape. The mixture is left on the nail for five to 10 days, after which the nail itself can be removed.

Aftercare

Aftercare of surgical removal is similar to the care of any minor surgical procedure. Aftercare of the urea paste method includes applying medication for the specific infection that is being treated.

Risks

Risks from either procedure are minimal.

Normal results

Normal results include the successful removal of the infected or damaged nail.

Resources

BOOKS

Baden, Howard P. "Diseases of the Nails." In *Conn's Current Therapy, 1996*, edited by Robert E. Rakel. Philadelphia: W. B. Saunders Co., 1996.

Rebecca J. Frey, PhD

Nalidixic acid *see* **Urinary anti-infectives**

Narcissistic personality disorder *see* **Personality disorders**

Narcolepsy

Definition

Narcolepsy is a disorder marked by excessive daytime sleepiness, uncontrollable sleep attacks, and cataplexy (a sudden loss of muscle tone, usually lasting up to half an hour).

Description

Narcolepsy is the second-leading cause of excessive daytime sleepiness (after obstructive sleep apnea). Persistent sleepiness and sleep attacks are the hallmarks of this condition. The sleepiness has been compared to the feeling of trying to stay awake after not sleeping for two or three days.

People with narcolepsy fall asleep suddenly—anywhere, at any time, maybe even in the middle of a conversation. These sleep attacks can last from a few seconds to more than an hour. Depending on where they occur, they may be mildly inconvenient or even dangerous to the individual. Some people continue to function outwardly during the sleep episodes, such as talking or putting things away. But when they wake up, they have no memory of the event.

Narcolepsy is related to the deep, dreaming part of sleep known as rapid eye movement (REM) sleep. Normally when people fall asleep, they experience 90 minutes of non-REM sleep, which is then followed by REM sleep. People with narcolepsy, however, enter REM sleep immediately. In addition, REM sleep occurs inappropriately throughout the day.

There has been debate over the incidence of narcolepsy. It is thought to affect between one in every 1,000 to 2,000 Americans. The known prevalence in other countries varies, from one in 600 in Japan to one in 500,000 in Israel. Reasons for these differences are not clear.

Causes and symptoms

In 1999 researchers identified the gene that causes narcolepsy. The gene allows cells in the hypothalamus (the part of the brain that regulates sleep behavior) to receive messages from other cells. When this gene is abnormal, cells cannot communicate properly, and abnormal sleeping patterns develop.

The disorder sometimes runs in families, but most people with narcolepsy have no relatives with the disorder. Researchers believe that the inheritance of narcolepsy is similar to that of heart disease. In heart disease, several genes play a role in being susceptible to the disorder, but it usually does not develop without an environmental trigger of some sort.

While the symptoms of narcolepsy usually appear during the teens or 20s, the disease may not be diagnosed for many years. Most often, the first symptom is an overwhelming feeling of fatigue. After several months or years, cataplexy and other symptoms appear.

Cataplexy is the most dramatic symptom of narcolepsy. It affects 75% of people with the disorder. During attacks, the knees buckle and the neck muscles go slack. In extreme cases, the person may become paralyzed and fall to the floor. This loss of muscle tone is temporary, lasting from a few seconds to half an hour, but frightening. The attacks can occur at any time but are often triggered by strong emotions, such as anger, joy, or surprise.

Other symptoms of narcolepsy include:

- sleep attacks: short, uncontrollable sleep episodes throughout the day
- sleep **paralysis**: a frightening inability to move shortly after awakening or dozing off
- auditory or visual **hallucinations**: intense, sometimes terrifying experiences at the beginning or end of a sleep period

- disturbed nighttime sleep: tossing and turning, nightmares, and frequent awakenings during the night

Diagnosis

If a person experiences both excessive daytime sleepiness and cataplexy, a diagnosis may be made on the patient history alone. Laboratory tests, however, can confirm a diagnosis. These may include an overnight polysomnogram—a test in which sleep is monitored with electrocardiography, video, and respiratory parameters. A Multiple Sleep Latency Test, which measures sleep latency (onset) and how quickly REM sleep occurs, may be used. People who have narcolepsy usually fall asleep in less than five minutes.

If a diagnosis is in question, a genetic blood test can reveal the existence of certain substances in people who have a tendency to develop narcolepsy. Positive test results suggest, but do not prove, the existence of narcolepsy.

Narcolepsy is a complex disorder, and it is often misdiagnosed. It takes 14 years, on average, for an individual to be correctly diagnosed.

Treatment

There is no cure for narcolepsy. It is not progressive, and it is not fatal, but it is chronic. The symptoms can be managed with medication or lifestyle adjustment. Amphetamine-like stimulant drugs are often prescribed to control drowsiness and sleep attacks. A drug called sodium oxybate (Xyrem) was tested for use in 2004 and was shown to reduce daytime sleepiness as well as cataplexy attacks when used along with stimulants. Patients who do not like taking high doses of stimulants may choose to take smaller doses and "manage" their lifestyles, such as by napping every few hours to relieve daytime sleepiness. Antidepressants are often effective in treating symptoms of abnormal REM sleep.

With the recent discovery of the gene that causes narcolepsy, researchers are hopeful that therapies can be designed to relieve the symptoms of the disorder.

Prognosis

Narcolepsy is not a degenerative disease, and patients do not develop other neurologic symptoms. However, narcolepsy can interfere with a person's ability to work, play, drive, and perform other daily activities. In severe cases, the disorder prevents people from living a normal life, leading to depression and a loss of independence.

KEY TERMS

Cataplexy—A symptom of narcolepsy in which there is a sudden episode of muscle weakness triggered by emotions. The muscle weakness may cause the person's knees to buckle, or the head to drop. In severe cases, the patient may become paralyzed for a few seconds to minutes.

Hypnagogic hallucinations—Dream-like auditory or visual hallucinations that occur while falling asleep.

Hypothalamus—A part of the forebrain that controls heartbeat, body temperature, thirst, hunger, body temperature and pressure, blood sugar levels, and other functions.

Sleep paralysis—An abnormal episode of sleep in which the patient cannot move for a few minutes, usually occurring on falling asleep or waking up. Often found in patients with narcolepsy.

Resources

PERIODICALS

Siegel, Jeremy M. "Narcolepsy." *Scientific American* January 2000. < http://www.sciam.com/2000/0100issue/0100siegel.html >.

"Xyrem Study for EDS in Narcolepsy Shows Positive Data Across All Measures." *Pain & Central Nervous System Week* January 14, 2004: 69.

ORGANIZATIONS

American Sleep Disorders Association. 1610 14th St. NW, Suite 300, Rochester, MN 55901. (507) 287-6006.

Narcolepsy Network. PO Box 42460, Cincinnati, OH 45242. (973) 276- 0115.

National Center on Sleep Disorders Research. Two Rockledge Centre, 6701 Rockledge Dr., Bethesda, MD 20892. (301) 435-0199.

National Sleep Foundation. 1522 K St., NW, Suite 500, Washington, DC 20005. (202) 785-2300. < http://www.sleepfoundation.org >.

Stanford Center for Narcolepsy. 1201 Welch Rd-Rm P-112, Stanford, CA 94305. (415) 725-6517.

University of Illinois Center for Narcolepsy Research. 845 S. Damen Ave., Chicago, IL 60612. (312) 996-5176.

OTHER

"Stanford Researchers Nab Narcolepsy Gene For SleepDisorders." *Stanford University Medical Center.* [cited August 5, 1999]. < http://www.stanford.edu/%7Edement/ngene.html >.

Michelle Lee Brandt
Teresa G. Odle

Narcotics

Definition

Narcotics are natural opioid drugs derived from the Asian poppy *Palaver somniferous* or semi-synthetic or synthetic substitutes for these drugs.

Purpose

Narcotics are drugs that dull the sense of **pain** and cause drowsiness or sleep. They are the most effective tool a physician has to relieve severe pain. Narcotics are also given pre-operatively to relieve **anxiety** and induce anesthesia. Other common uses are to suppress **cough** and to control very severe **diarrhea**. In large doses, they can suppress the ability to breathe and cause **coma** and **death**. Narcotics are also taken illegally for recreational use.

Precautions

Narcotics should only be taken under the direction of a physician. These drugs depress the central nervous system and should not be taken with other drugs, such as alcohol, **barbiturates**, **antihistamines**, and **benzodiazepines** that also depress the central nervous system.

Opioids are broken down by the liver. Individuals with liver damage may not detoxify these substances as rapidly as healthy individuals, leading to potential accidental overdose. Street narcotics are of uncertain strength and may be contaminated with toxic chemicals or contain a mixture of drugs that can cause life-threatening reactions.

Description

Natural narcotics are derived directly from the sap of the unripe seed pods of the opium poppy. Morphine and codeine are the most familiar natural narcotics and are the narcotics most frequently used in medical settings. Often they are prescribed in combination with other non-narcotic drugs. Heroin is a semi-synthetic narcotic. It has no medical or legal uses. Other completely synthetic narcotics are made in the laboratory. These include drugs with medical uses such as fentanyl and oxycodone and illegal "designer drugs" synthesized for recreational use. Some man-made narcotics are hundreds of times more potent than natural narcotics.

Narcotics depress the central nervous system. They work by binding chemically with receptors in a way that blocks the transmission of nerve impulses. These drugs do not cure the source of the pain; they simply block the individual's perception of pain. When used to treat cough or diarrhea, they slow or block muscle contractions.

Morphine (Roxanol, Dura morphine, morphine sulfate, morphine hydrochloride) is the most commonly used medical narcotic for managing moderate to severe pain. It can be also be used to control extreme diarrhea caused by **cholera** or similar diseases. Morphine sulfate is a white powder that dissolves in water. It is usually given by injection into a muscle or intravenously by injection into a vein. When given intravenously, its effect occurs almost immediately. Individuals given morphine regularly have a high potential for developing dependence on the drug. Morphine can cause withdrawal symptoms if stopped abruptly. It is not a common street drug.

More codeine is prescribed medically than any other narcotic. Concentrations of codeine in the sap of the opium poppy are low, so most codeine is manufactured by chemical alteration of morphine. For pain control, codeine is combined with other non-narcotic painkillers such as **aspirin** (Empirin with Codeine,) **acetaminophen** (Tylenol with Codeine) or non-steroid anti-inflammatory drugs. These combination painkillers are manufactured as tablets (most common) or liquids and come in a variety of strengths based on the amount of codeine they contain. Codeine is also found in some cough syrups (Robitussin A-C, for example) and is used to control dry cough. Occasionally codeine is used to control severe diarrhea, although diphenoxylate (Lomotil) is used more often.

In Canada, certain low-dose codeine pain relievers are sold without prescription. In the United States pain medication with codeine requires a prescription. The likelihood of physical or psychological dependence on codeine is much lower than with morphine.

Hydromorphone (Dilaudid) is a narcotic synthetically produced from morphine. It is available in tablets or as an injectable solution and used for pain relief. It is one of the most common pain relievers prescribed for patients who are terminally ill, because it combines high effectiveness with low side effects.

Mederidine (Demerol) was originally developed to treat **muscle spasms** but is as of 2005 used mainly for pain relief. It is manufactured as tablets of varying strengths. Another synthetic pain relief narcotic whose use parallels mederidine is propoxyphene. When combined with aspirin this narcotic is known under the brand name Darvon.

Oxycodone (Oxycontin), a synthetic narcotic used for pain relief, is manufactured both alone and with aspirin (Percodan) or acetaminophen (Percoset) in tablets of various strengths. OxyContin is a controlled release formula of oxycodone that controls pain continuously for 12 hours at a time. Oxycodone has a high potential for prescription drug and street **abuse**. Hydrocodone with acetaminophen (Vicodin) is another synthetic narcotic whose use and potential abuse parallels oxycodone.

Fentanyl (Sublimaze, Actiq, Duragesic) is used as a surgical anesthetic. It is available as an injectable solution and as a skin patch.

Methadone is a synthetic narcotic used mainly as a substitute for heroin in heroin withdrawal treatment, although it does have pain-killing properties. Methadone, when taken by mouth (liquid, wafers, tablets) provides little of the euphoria of heroin, but it blocks heroin cravings and withdrawal symptoms.

The first international attempts to control narcotic drugs were made in 1909 with the formation of the Opium Commission Forum, which developed the first international drug control treaty in 1912. In the early 2000s narcotics are regulated internationally by the International Narcotics Control Board (INCB), established in 1961. The INCB regulates the cultivation of raw materials to make narcotics and natural and man-made drugs. **Cocaine** and **marijuana** also fall under the board's control, although they are not technically narcotics. Narcotic drugs are also regulated by federal and state governments. In law enforcement, the term narcotics is extended to include other, mainly illicit drugs such as cocaine that have little medical use.

Preparation

No special preparation is required before being treated with narcotics, although, as with all medications, individuals should tell their physician about all prescription and non-prescription drugs, supplements, and herbal remedies that they are taking, as certain medications may enhance the effects of narcotics.

Aftercare

When an individual is prescribed narcotics regularly for an extended period, tolerance may develop. With tolerance, the individual must take higher and higher doses to achieve the same level of pain control. In some cases, when narcotics are stopped abruptly, withdrawal symptoms may develop. These include:

KEY TERMS

Tapering—Gradually reducing the amount of a drug when stopping it abruptly would cause unpleasant withdrawal symptoms.

- anxiety
- irritability
- rapid breathing
- runny nose
- sweating
- vomiting and diarrhea
- confusion
- shaking
- lack of appetite

In order to prevent withdrawal symptoms, the dose of narcotics can be gradually diminished, a process known as tapering, until they can be discontinued completely without unpleasant effects. Individuals may also be treated with the drug cloindine (Catapres) to relieve some withdrawal symptoms.

Risks

All narcotics have the potential to become physically and psychologically addictive. When used regularly, tolerance can develop. Abuse and dependence on narcotic prescription drugs in an increasing problem among the elderly particularly and among members of the middle class generally.

Overdose and withdrawal symptoms and reactions caused by contamination with other drugs or toxic chemicals are common reasons for drug-related visits to the emergency room by individuals using street narcotics recreationally. Overdose is treated with the drug naloxone (ReVia). Naloxone blocks and reverses the effects of narcotics. When given intravenously it is effective within one to two minutes.

Normal results

When used as prescribed, narcotics are a generally safe and effective way to relieve pain and control cough and severe diarrhea. Individuals should not be afraid they will develop an **addiction** after a short-term course of narcotics following a dental or medical procedure, provided that they follow their physician's instructions for taking the drugs.

Resources

ORGANIZATION

National Institute on Drug Abuse/National Institutes of Health. 6001 Executive Boulevard, Room 5213, Bethesda, MD 20892-9561. (301) 443-1124. < http://www.nida.nih.gov >.

United States Drug Enforcement Administration. Dr Mailstop: AXS, 2401 Jefferson Davis Highway, Alexandria, VA 22301. (202) 307-1000. < http://www.dea.gov >.

OTHER

"Narcotics." United States Drug Enforcement Administration (undated) [cited March 25, 2005] < http://www.usdoj.gov/dea/concern/narcotics.html >.

National Institute on Drug Abuse. February 4, 2005 [cited March 25, 2005]. < http://www.nida.nih.giv/Research Report/Prescription/Prescription.html >

Stephens, Everett. *Toxicity, Narcotics* January 7, 2005 [cited March 25, 2005]. < http://www.emedicine.com/emerg/topic330.htm >.

Tish Davidson, A. M.

Nasal culture *see* **Nasopharyngeal culture**

Nasal irrigation

Definition

Nasal irrigation is the practice of flushing the nasal cavity with a sterile solution. The solution may contain **antibiotics** or steroid medications.

Purpose

Nasal irrigation is used to clear infected sinuses or may be performed after surgery to the nose region. It may be performed by adding antibiotics to the solution to treat **nasal polyps**, nasal septal deviation, allergic nasal inflammation, chronic sinus infection, and swollen mucous membranes. One benefit of nasal irrigation in treating these conditions is that it usually lowers the amount of medication that the patient must take by mouth.

Irrigation is also used to treat long-term users of inhalants, such as illicit drugs (**cocaine**), or such occupational toxins as paint fumes, sawdust, pesticides, and coal dust.

Nasal irrigation may also be used in occupational medicine to monitor workers for exposure to airborne glass fibers, asbestos, and similar materials.

Precautions

Nasal irrigation should not be performed on people who have frequent nosebleeds; have recently had nasal surgery; or whose gag reflex is impaired, as fluid may enter the windpipe.

Description

Nasal irrigation can be performed by the patient at home or by a medical professional. A forced-flow instrument, such as a syringe, is filled with a warm saline solution. The solution can be commercially prepared (Ayr, NaSal) or can be prepared by the patient, using one half teaspoon salt with each eight ounces of warm water. Occasionally, antibiotics or steroids are added to the solution to kill bacteria and aid healing of irritated membrane. The syringe is then directed into the nostril. The irrigation solution loosens encrusted material in the nasal passage, and drainage takes place through the nose. The patient leans over a catch basin during irrigation, into which the debris flows. Irrigation continues until all debris is cleared from the passage. Nasal irrigation can be performed up to twice daily, unless the irrigation irritates the mucous membrane.

Preparation

Before nasal irrigation, the patient is instructed not to open his or her mouth or swallow during the procedure. Opening the mouth or swallowing may cause infectious material to move from the nasal passage into the sinuses or the ear.

Risks

Complications of nasal irrigation include irritation of the nasal passages due to extreme temperature of the irrigation solution. Rarely, irrigation fluid may enter the windpipe in people with a poor gag reflex.

Resources

BOOKS

Beers, Mark H., MD, and Robert Berkow, MD., editors. "Hypersensitivity Reactions." Section 12, Chapter 148 In *The Merck Manual of Diagnosis and Therapy.* Whitehouse Station, NJ: Merck Research Laboratories, 2004.

PERIODICALS

Aukema, A. A., and W. J. Fokkens. "Chronic Rhinosinusitis: Management for Optimal Outcomes."

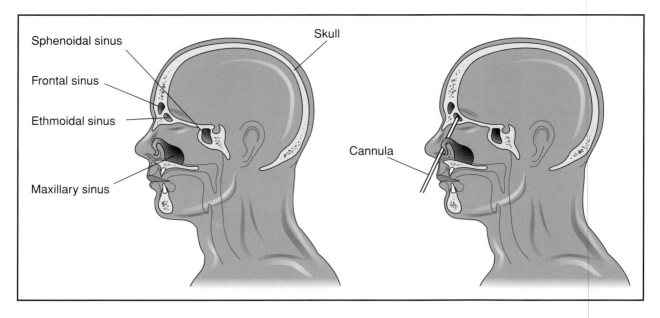

Labels: Sphenoidal sinus, Frontal sinus, Ethmoidal sinus, Maxillary sinus, Skull, Cannula

Because surgery in the nasal area has a high incidence rate for contamination with pathogenic bacteria, nasal irrigation is performed to remove loose tissue and prevent infection. The illustration (right) shows a cannula in place while the sinus passages are being flushed. *(Illustration by Electronic Illustrators Group.)*

KEY TERMS

Irrigation—In medicine, the practice of washing out or flushing a wound or body opening with a stream of water or another liquid.

Saline—A solution made from salt and water.

Treatments in Respiratory Medicine 3 (February 2004): 97–105.

Brown, C. L., and S. M. Graham. "Nasal Irrigations: Good or Bad?" *Current Opinion in Otolaryngology and Head and Neck Surgery* 12 (February 2004): 9–13.

Lavigne, F., M. K. Tulic, J. Gagnon, and Q. Hamid. "Selective Irrigation of the Sinuses in the Management of Chronic Rhinosinusitis Refractory to Medical Therapy: A Promising Start." *Journal of Otolaryngology* 33 (February 2004): 10–16.

Paananen, H., M. Holopainen, P. Kalliokoski, et al. "Evaluation of Exposure to Man-Made Vitreous Fibers by Nasal Lavage." *Journal of Occupational and Environmental Hygiene* 1 (February 2004): 82–87.

ORGANIZATIONS

American Academy of Family Physicians (AAFP). 11400 Tomahawk Creek Parkway, Leawood, KS 66211-2672. (800) 274-2237 or (913) 906-6000. < http:// www.aafp.org >.

American Academy of Otolaryngology, Head and Neck Surgery, Inc. One Prince St., Alexandria, VA 22314-3357. (703) 836-44 44. < http://www.entnet.org >.

Mary K. Fyke
Rebecca J. Frey, PhD

Nasal packing

Definition

Nasal packing is the application of gauze or cotton packs to the nasal chambers.

Purpose

The most common purpose of nasal packing is to control bleeding following surgery to the septum or nasal reconstruction and to treat chronic nosebleeds. Packing is also used to provide support to the septum after surgery.

Description

Packing is the placement of gauze or cotton into the nasal area. Packing comes in three forms: gauze, cotton balls, and preformed cotton wedges. Packing is usually coated with antibiotics and, sometimes, petrolatum. The end of the nose may be taped to keep the packings in place or to prevent the patient from pulling them out. In cases of surgery, packings are frequently removed within 24–48 hours following surgery. In the case of nosebleeds, packing is left in for extended periods of time to promote healing and to prevent the patient from removing scar tissue which might reopen the wound. If both sides of the nose are packed, the patient must breathe through his or her mouth while the packs are in place.

In patients who are chronic nose pickers, frequent bleeding is common and ulceration of nasal tissue is possible. To promote healing and to prevent nose picking, both sides of the nose are packed with cotton that contains **antibiotics**. The nose is taped shut with surgical tape to prevent the packing from being removed. The packing is left in the nose for seven to 10 days. If the wound is high up in the nasal cavity, gauze strips treated with petrolatum and antibiotics are used. The strips are placed into the nose one layer at a time, folding one layer on top of the other until the area is completely packed.

Local packing is a procedure used when only a small part of the nose must be packed. Typically, this occurs when one blood vessel is prone to bleeding, and there is no need to block breathing through the nose. Local packing is used when the pack can remain in place by itself. This situation can be found at the turbinates. Turbinates are folds of tissue on the insides of the nose. The folds are sufficiently firm to support packing. A small piece of gauze or cotton is wedged in between the turbinates where the blood vessel being treated is located. Local packing is left in place for up to 48 hours and then removed. The main advantage to this type of packing is that it enables the patient to breathe through his or her nose. Local packing is also more comfortable than complete packing, although the patient will still experience a sensation that something is in the nasal cavity. The patient must be instructed not to interfere with or probe the packing while it is in place.

A postnasal pack is used to treat bleeding in the postnasal area. This is a difficult area to pack. Packs used in this area are made from cotton balls or gauze that have been tied into a tubular shape with heavy gauge suture or umbilical tape. Long lengths of suture or tape are left free. The lengths of suture or tape are used to help position the pack during installation and to remove it. An alternative is to cut a vaginal tampon and reposition the strings. Balloons have been tried as a method to replace postnasal packing, but have not

KEY TERMS

Turbinate—Ridge-shaped cartilage or soft bony tissue inside the nose.

Ulcer—A sore on the skin or mucous tissue that produces pus and in which tissue is destroyed.

proved effective. After being tied, the pack is soaked with an antibiotic ointment. Generally, packs are formed larger than needed, so that they completely block the nasal passage. A catheter is passed through the nose and pulled out through the mouth. Strings from one end of the pack are tied to the catheter and the pack pulled into place by passing through the mouth and up the back of the nasal cavity. The pack is removed in a similar manner. Complications may occur if a pack compresses the Eustachian tube, causing ear problems. The ear should be examined to ensure that infection is not developing.

Packing of the anterior (front) part of the nose is also performed following surgery such as septoplasty and **rhinoplasty**. In these operations, the surgeon cuts through the skin flap covering cartilage and bone in the center, top, and bottom of the nose to correct the shape of the nose. At the conclusion of the surgery, the skin flap is sutured back into place. The purposes of packing are to absorb any drainage from the incision and mucus produced by nasal tissue, and to support the skin flap and cartilage. The packing used is either gauze or preformed adsorbent wedges of cotton. Both are usually treated with antibiotic to reduce the chance of infections at the incision site. Generally, there is little bleeding following septoplasty and rhinoplasty, and the incisions heal normally. These packs are left in place for 24 to 48 hours and then removed.

Aftercare

Ice chips or mouthwash can be used to moisten the mouth while packing is in place, as the mouth may be dry from breathing through it. Humidifiers may also help with breathing. After nasal packing, the nose should not be blown for two to three days.

Since one of the major reasons that packing is performed is to heal damage to nasal blood vessels from nose-picking, follow-up examination should be done to ensure that the patient is no longer practicing this habit. If the patient has restarted nose-picking, therapy to alter this behavior should be pursued. When the packing completely blocks the nasal cavity and prevents breathing through the nose, the patient should adjust to breathing through the mouth. In elderly patients, adjustment may be more difficult. This leads to a drop in the blood oxygen content and an increase in blood carbon dioxide levels (CO_2). This, in turn, can cause respiratory and cardiac complications, including a racing pulse.

Risks

Nasal packing could cause a lack of oxygen in those who have difficulty breathing through their mouths. Rarely, sinus infection or middle ear infection may occur.

Resources

BOOKS

Bluestone, C. D., S. E. Stool, and M. A. Kenna. *Pediatric Otolaryngology*. Philadelphia: W. B. Saunders Co., 1996.

John T. Lohr, PhD

Nasal papillomas

Definition

Nasal papillomas are **warts** located inside the nose.

Description

Two types of tumors can grow inside the nose: polyps and papillomas. By far the most common are polyps, which have smooth surfaces. On the contrary, papillomas have irregular surfaces and are, in fact, warts. Papillomas may be caused by the same viruses that cause warts elsewhere on the body. They are inside the nose, more often on the side near the cheek, and, because of their internal structure, they are much more likely to bleed than polyps.

There is a special type of nasal papilloma called an inverting papilloma because of its unique appearance. About 10 or 15% of these are or can become cancers.

Causes and symptoms

Like polyps, papillomas can plug up the nose and disable the sense of smell. Unlike polyps, papillomas often bleed.

Diagnosis

A **physical examination** with special instruments will detect these tumors.

Treatment

Because of the possibility of **cancer**, all nasal papillomas must be removed surgically and sent to the laboratory for analysis. If a cancer is present, further surgery may be necessary to guarantee that all of the cancer has been removed. The initial surgery can be done in an office setting by a specialist in head and neck surgery, also known as otorhinolaryngology and popularly abbreviated ENT (ear, nose, and throat). Cancer surgery is more extensive and often requires hospitalization.

Prognosis

For benign (non-cancerous) lesions, removal is curative, although they tend to recur, just like warts elsewhere. The cancerous papillomas may occasionally escape complete surgical removal and spread to adjacent or distant sites. The prognosis is then much more complex.

Resources

BOOKS

Ballenger, John Jacob. *Disorders of the Nose, Throat, Ear, Head, and Neck*. Philadelphia: Lea & Febiger, 1996.

J. Ricker Polsdorfer, MD

Nasal polyps

Definition

A polyp is the medical term for any overgrowth of tissue from the surface of a body organ. Polyps come in all shapes—round, droplet, and irregular being the most common. Nasal polyps are teardrop-shaped while growing and resemble peeled grapes when they have reached their full size. The condition of nasal polyps is sometimes called nasal polyposis.

Description

Nasal polyps tend to occur in people with respiratory **allergies**. Hay **fever** (**allergic rhinitis**) is an irritation of the membranes of the nose by airborne particles or chemicals. These membranes secrete mucus. When irritated, they can also grow polyps. The nose is not only a passageway for air to reach the lungs; it also provides the connection between the sinuses and the outside world. Sinuses are lined with mucous membranes, just like the nose. Polyps can easily obstruct the drainage of mucus from the sinuses. When any fluid in the body is trapped so it cannot flow freely, it becomes infected. The result, **sinusitis**, is a common complication of allergic **rhinitis**.

Nasal polyps may also develop in children with **cystic fibrosis**.

Causes and symptoms

Some people who are allergic to **aspirin** develop both asthma and nasal polyps.

Nasal polyps often plug the nose, usually one side at a time. People with allergic rhinitis are so used to having a stopped-up nose they may not notice the difference when a polyp develops. Other polyps may be closer to a sinus opening, so airflow is not obstructed, but mucus becomes trapped in the sinus. In this case, there is a feeling of fullness in the head, no sense of smell, and perhaps a **headache**. The trapped mucus will eventually get infected, adding **pain**, fever, and perhaps bloody discharge from the nose.

Diagnosis

A **physical examination** will identify most polyps. Small polyps located higher up or further back may be hidden from view, but they will be detected with more sophisticated medical instruments. The otorhinolaryngologist is equipped to diagnose nasal polyps. In order to perform the examination, the doctor must apply medicine to reduce congestion in the swollen membranes. Cotton balls soaked with one of these agents and left in the nostrils for a few minutes provide adequate shrinkage.

Treatment

Most polyps can be removed by the head and neck surgeon as an office procedure called a nasal

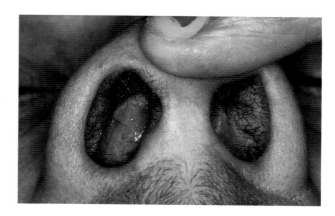

A nasal polyp inside patient's right nostril. *(Custom Medical Stock Photo. Reproduced by permission.)*

KEY TERMS

Allergen—Any substance that irritates only those who are sensitive (allergic) to it.

Asthma—Wheezing (labored breathing) due to allergies or irritation of the lungs.

Decongestant—Medicines that shrink blood vessels and consequently mucus membranes. Pseudoephedrine, phenylephrine, and phenylpropanolamine are the most common.

Polyposis—The medical term for the development of multiple polyps on a body part.

Sinus—Air-filled cavities surrounding the eyes and nose are lined with mucus-producing membranes. They cleanse the nose, add resonance to the voice, and partially determine the structure of the face.

---

polypectomy. Bleeding, the only complication, is usually easy to control. Nose and sinus infections can be treated with **antibiotics** and **decongestants**, but if airflow is restricted, the infection will recur.

Prognosis

Polyps may reappear as long as the allergic irritation continues. In addition, one study of patients who had undergone nasal polypectomy reported that 60% had a recurrence of nasal polyposis, and 47% were advised to have revision surgery. The risk of recurrence is higher among patients with **asthma**.

Prevention

If aspirin is the cause of the polyps, all aspirin containing medications must be avoided.

Since most nasal polyps are the result of allergic rhinitis, they can be prevented by treating this condition. New treatments have greatly improved control of hay fever. There are now several spray medicines that are quite effective. Spray cortisone-like drugs, usually beclomethasone (Beconase, Vancenase) or flunisolide (Nasalide), are the most popular. Over-the-counter nasal decongestants have an irritating effect similar to the allergy they are supposed to be treating. Continued use can bring more trouble than relief and result in an addiction to nose sprays. The resulting disease, rhinitis medicamentosa, is more difficult to treat than allergic rhinitis.

Allergists and ENT surgeons both treat allergic rhinitis with a procedure called desensitization. After identifying suspect allergens using one of several methods, they will give the patient increasing doses of those allergens in order to produce blocking antibodies that will impede the allergic reaction. This approach is effective in a number of patients, but the treatment may take a period of months to years.

Resources

BOOKS

Beers, Mark H., MD, and Robert Berkow, MD., editors. "Nose and Paranasal Sinuses: Polyps." Section 7, Chapter 86 In *The Merck Manual of Diagnosis and Therapy*. Whitehouse Station, NJ: Merck Research Laboratories, 2004.

PERIODICALS

Bikhazi, N. B. "Contemporary Management of Nasal Polyps." *Otolaryngologic Clinics of North America* 37 (April 2004): 327–337.

Drake-Lee, A. B. "Nasal Polyps." *Hospital Medicine* 65 (May 2004): 264–267.

Wynn, R., and G. Har-El. "Recurrence Rates after Endoscopic Sinus Surgery for Massive Sinus Polyposis." *Laryngoscope* 114 (May 2004): 811–813.

ORGANIZATIONS

American Academy of Allergy, Asthma and Immunology (AAAAI). 611 East Wells Street, Milwaukee, WI 53202. (800) 822-2762. < http://www.aaaai.org >.

American Academy of Otolaryngology–Head and Neck Surgery, Inc. One Prince Street, Alexandria, VA 22314-3357. (703) 836-4444. < http://entnet.org >.

J. Ricker Polsdorfer, MD
Rebecca J. Frey, PhD

Nasal trauma

Definition

Nasal trauma is defined as any injury to the nose or related structure that may result in bleeding, a physical deformity, a decreased ability to breathe normally because of obstruction, or an impaired sense of smell. The injury may be either internal or external.

Description

The human nose is composed of bone, soft tissue, and cartilage. It serves as a passageway for air to flow from the outside environment into the lower respiratory tract and lungs. At the same time, the nasal passages warm and humidify the air that enters the body.

Internal injuries to the nose typically occur when a foreign object (including the fingers) is placed in the nose or when a person takes in drugs of **abuse** (inhalants or **cocaine**) through the nose. External injuries to the nose are usually blunt force injuries related to sports participation, criminal violence, parental abuse, or automobile or bicycle accidents. This type of injury may result in a nasal fracture. The nasal bones are the most frequently fractured facial bones due to their position on the face, and are the third most common type of bone fracture in general after **fractures** of the wrist and collarbone. A force of only 30g is required to break the nasal bones, compared to 70g for the bones in the jaw and 200 g for the bony ridge above the eyes. The pattern of the fracture depends on the direction of the blow to the nose, whether coming from the front, the side, or above the nose. Although not life-threatening by itself, a fractured nose may lead to difficulties in breathing as well as facial disfigurement.

Fractures resulting from trauma to the nose may involve the bones of the septum (the partition of bone and cartilage dividing the two nostrils) as well as the bones surrounding the eyes. These bones include the nasal, maxilla, lacrimal, and frontal bones. Direct trauma to the bridge of the nose may also result in damage to a part of the base of the skull known as the cribriform plate. This injury in turn may allow cerebrospinal fluid to leak out of the skull and leave the body through the nose. Fractures may also damage the membranes that line the nasal passages, leading to possible formation of scar tissue, obstruction of the airway, and damage to the child's sense of smell.

In addition to fractures, external injuries of the nose include soft-tissue injuries resulting from bites (human and animal), insect stings, cuts, or scrapes. Penetrating injuries to the nasal area caused by air gun or BB pellets

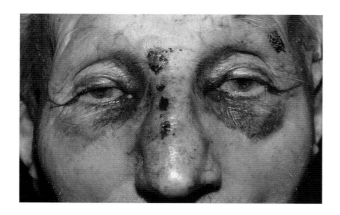

Fractured nose of an elderly patient. *(Photograph by Dr. P Marazzi. Photo Researchers. Reproduced by permission.)*

are also reported with increasing frequency in older children and adolescents. When fired at close range, these pellets can penetrate the skin and cheekbone and lodge in the nasal septum or the sinuses near the nose.

Lastly, nose **piercing** as a fashion trend is a type of intentional injury to the nose that has several possible complications, including infections of the cartilage and soft tissues in the nose; blockage of the airway due to a loosened stud or other nose ornament; and gastrointestinal emergencies caused by accidental swallowing of nose jewelry.

Causes and symptoms

Causes

External trauma to the nose may be accidental (transportation accidents, animal bites, air gun injuries, and **sports injuries**) or intentional (fights, criminal assault, domestic violence, nose piercing). Nasal injuries from athletic activities may result from contact with equipment (being hit in the face by a baseball, hockey ball, or other small ball hit at high speed, or by the bat or stick itself) or the bodies of other players (football, boxing, martial arts, rugby). Nasal injuries from piercing include bacterial infections of the skin and nasal cartilage, allergic reactions to the jewelry, tissue damage, and periodic bleeding.

In a few cases, external trauma to the nose may also be iatrogenic, or caused by medical care. Most of these injuries result from medical examination of the nose—particularly in emergency circumstances—or as complications of **plastic surgery**. In a few cases damage to the nose is caused by **radiation therapy** for **cancer**.

Internal injuries to the nose may be either mechanical (caused by **foreign objects** in the nose or by picking or scratching the tissues lining the nose) or chemical (caused by environmental irritants or **substance abuse**).

Chemical injuries to the nose are caused by accidental or purposeful breathing or sniffing of irritating substances. These may include tobacco smoke; household cleaners (ammonia and chlorine bleach) and furniture polish; ozone and other air pollutants; cocaine; and glue, paint thinners, solvents, and similar household products that produce toxic vapors. An increasingly common form of chemical injury to the nasal membranes in toddlers is alkali **burns** caused by leakage from small batteries placed in the nose. While chemical damage to the nose is usually accidental in younger children, it is more often the result of substance abuse in adolescents. Taking cocaine through the nose ("snorting") or inhalant abuse ("sniffing" or "huffing") are the most common causes of chemical damage to the nose in older children or teenagers.

Symptoms

The symptoms of physical trauma to the nose may include:

- Flattening or other deformation of the shape of the nose
- Infections of the cartilage or soft tissue
- Epistaxis or bleeding from the nose
- Crepitus. Crepitus is the crackling or crunching sound heard when the ends of a fractured bone are rubbed together
- Pain and tissue swelling
- Airway blockage from bleeding, fluid discharge, or tissue swelling
- **Rhinitis**. Rhinitis is an inflammation of the mucous membranes lining the nose. In the case of a fracture, rhinitis may lead to increased tear production in the eyes and a runny nose
- Septal hematoma. A septal hematoma is a mass of blood from torn tissue that may collect within the cartilage that divides the two nostrils. It may become infected and form an **abscess** that eventually destroys the cartilage
- Bruising or discoloration (ecchymosis) of the tissues around the eye
- Leakage of cerebrospinal fluid through the nostrils

Chemical trauma to the nose may result in:

- Runny nose and watering of the eyes
- Pain

- Loss of the sense of smell
- Nasal congestion and sneezing
- Reddening and swelling of the mucous membranes lining the nose
- Eventual destruction of the cartilage in the nasal septum and the tissues lining the nose

Some common irritants that may be encountered in the home and workplace include:

- cleaning solutions and powders
- ammonia
- environmental tobacco smoke
- bleach
- metalworking fluids
- ozone
- sulfur dioxide
- paint thinners
- arsenic
- chromic acid
- copper dust and mists

Sequelae following exposure to these chemicals are based not only on the concentration of the irritant but also on factors specific to the individual. Reactions vary among persons, even with similar exposures.

Diagnosis

Diagnosis of a fracture is normally based on a history of nasal trauma and clinical presentation. Epistaxis may or may not be present. An intranasal examination is performed in order to look for a septal hematoma that may result in serious consequences such as death of the septal cartilaginous tissue. The nose is also checked for tenderness, mobility, stability, and crepitance.

X rays are normally not indicated, however, in more severe fractures involving multiple bones, a computed tomography (CT) scan may be required. The physician should look for associated injuries such as periorbital (surrounding the eye) ecchymosis, watery eyes, or diplopia (double vision) that may indicate orbital injuries. In addition, dental fractures and a cerebrospinal fluid (CSF) leak should be looked for. CSF leaks indicate a more severe injury possibly involving an ethmoid bone fracture.

The physician may also ask for photographs taken prior to the injury in order to determine the extent of deformity. Photographs may also be taken to document the injury in regards to possible legal actions.

In order to diagnose trauma sustained by a chemical injury, a history of exposure to potentially toxic chemicals should be ascertained. In addition, the patient should also bring information related to the types of chemicals that he or she has been exposed to. If injury occurs in the workplace, Material Safety Data Sheets should be available in the employer's poison control center that list the chemical components of commercial materials. Measurements of air from the patient's work area may also be obtained. Symptomatic improvement on off-days followed by a subsequent return of symptoms when returning to work confirms that the illness is work related. The physician should perform an intranasal examination to determine the extent of the chemical injury. A **chest x ray** as well as a **pulmonary function test** may be ordered to determine if there is any subsequent lower respiratory tract involvement.

Treatment

Timing

Nasal injuries should be treated as promptly as possible to prevent complications. Batteries placed in the nose should be removed within 4 hours to prevent burns and other damage to the tissues from leaking chemicals. If a septal hematoma has developed, the doctor must remove it as quickly as possible to prevent infection or eventual death of the tissues in the nasal septum. Lastly, if the child has been bitten by an animal, the injury must be cleansed as soon as possible to lower the risk of **rabies**.

Treatment of nasal fractures is best performed during the first three hours after the injury. If this is impossible, management of a nasal fracture should be done within three to seven days. Timing is of utmost importance when treating nasal fractures because delays longer than seven to 10 days may allow the broken bones to set without proper alignment, or lead to such complications as scar tissue formation and airway obstruction. Poorly set nasal fractures usually require surgical correction.

Specific procedures

Foreign objects in the nose can be removed by nasal suction in most cases. Most nosebleeds are treated by 5–30 minutes of direct pressure on the nostrils, with the patient's head placed in an upright position. The doctor may also pack the nose with gauze coated with petroleum jelly. If the bleeding does not stop, or if it appears to originate in the upper nose, the doctor will consult a head and neck surgeon or an otolaryngologist for specialized evaluation of the bleeding.

Air gun or BB pellets that have penetrated the nose or nearby sinuses are generally removed with the help of an endoscope, which is a slender tubular instrument that allows the doctor to examine the inside of a body cavity.

Treatment of nasal fractures depends on the extent of the injury; the most difficult fractures to treat are those that involve the nasal septum. The doctor will usually reduce the fracture, which means that he or she will restore the damaged bones to their proper position and alignment. Although **local anesthesia** is usually sufficient for treating nasal fractures in adults and older teenagers, **general anesthesia** is usually given when treating these injuries in younger children.

Reductions of nasal fractures may be either open or closed. A closed reduction involves manipulation of the bones without cutting into the overlying skin. This type of reduction will be performed for fractures of the nasal bones that are limited in size and complexity. Open reductions are performed for more complex nasal fractures. In an open reduction, the nasal bones are moved back to their original location after the surgeon has made an incision in the overlying skin. This procedure is done for fractures involving dislocation of the septum as well as the nasal bones. In addition, an open reduction is necessary if the child has a septal hematoma or an open fracture in which the skin has been perforated. If a septal hematoma is present, the doctor will drain it and pack the nose to prevent subsequent accumulation of blood. The nasal bones are held in the proper position with external splints as well as the internal packing, and the splints are kept in place for 7–10 days. The patient will be given **antibiotics** to lower the risk of infection and may be referred to an otolaryngologist or plastic surgeon for further evaluation. Ice packs or cold compresses can be applied at home to lower swelling and ease discomfort.

In the case of animal bites, the patient may be given passive or active immunization against rabies if there is a chance that the dog or other animal is rabid. This precaution is particularly important for animal bites on the nose or other parts of the face, as the incubation period of the rabies virus is much shorter for bites on the head and neck than for bites elsewhere on the body.

Complications can arise following treatment and therefore follow-up is necessary. Problems that may occur resemble symptoms of nasal fractures. Others include infection, CSF leakage, scar tissue build-up, and a saddle nose deformity where the bridge of the nose is markedly depressed.

Treatment for trauma caused by irritant inhalation involves removing the patient from the contaminated area or decreasing exposure time. Other measures include using a saline nasal spray or topical steroids. For acute injuries oxygen or supportive treatment for any subsequent lower respiratory tract involvement may be administered.

If the injury is occupation-related, changes should be made in order to eliminate future incidents. These changes may include having the patient wear a respiratory protection device while working. In addition, the employer should be made aware of the situation and employ measures to prevent future incidents.

Prognosis

Most types of nasal trauma have a good prognosis. Nosebleeds or tissue damage caused by scratching or picking at the nose usually clear completely once these habits are stopped. Infections or allergic reactions caused by foreign objects in the nose or piercing usually clear up promptly after the object or piece of jewelry is removed. Nasal fractures that do not involve the nasal septum or other facial bones and receive prompt treatment generally heal without deformities of the nose, cartilage destruction, or other complications. More extensive facial fractures, however, may require a second operation to correct the positioning of the bones and restore the appearance of the nose.

The prognosis for soft-tissue injuries to the nose depends on the cause and extent of the injuries. Such tearing or crushing injuries as those caused by bites take longer to heal than simple cuts, and may require plastic surgery at a later date to restore the appearance of the nose.

Damage to the tissues lining the nose caused by exposure to tobacco smoke or other irritants in the environment is usually reversible once the patient is removed from contact with the irritating substance. Erosion or destruction of the nasal cartilage as a result of inhalant or cocaine abuse, however, usually requires surgical treatment.

Prevention

Although most cases of nasal trauma happen inadvertently, some measures can be employed in order to prevent injury. Patients should be aware of the symptoms of nasal fracture and should seek medical attention as soon as possible to prevent more invasive reductions. Protective equipment should also be worn when playing sports. Employees should also be aware of irritating chemicals in their workplace and appropriate measures should be taken to avoid exposure.

KEY TERMS

Crepitus—A crackling or crunching sound heard when the ends of a fractured piece of bone rub against each other.

Diplopia—The medical term for seeing double.

Ecchymosis (plural, ecchymoses)—The medical term for a bruise. Ecchymoses may develop around the eyes following a nasal fracture.

Epistaxis—The medical term for a nosebleed.

Hematoma—A localized collection of blood that accumulates in an organ, tissue, or body space as the result of leakage from a broken blood vessel. Hematomas sometimes develop within the nasal cartilage when the nose is fractured.

Iatrogenic—Referring to injuries caused by a doctor. Nasal trauma may occasionally result from a doctor's examination of the nose or complications from plastic surgery.

Otolaryngologist—A doctor who specializes in diagnosing and treating disorders of the ears, nose, and throat.

Reduce—To restore a part of the body to its normal position or place, as in treating a fracture or dislocation. The repositioning of the bone or body part is called a reduction.

Rhinitis—An inflammation of the mucous membranes that line the nasal passages.

Rhinoplasty—Plastic surgery of the nose to repair or change the shape of the nose.

Septal hematoma—A mass of extravasated blood that is confined within the nasal septum.

Septum—The partition of bone and cartilage in the nose that separates the two nostrils.

Resources

BOOKS

Beers, Mark H., MD, and Robert Berkow, MD., editors. "Fractures of the Nose." Section 7, Chapter 86 In *The Merck Manual of Diagnosis and Therapy*. Whitehouse Station, NJ: Merck Research Laboratories, 2004.

Jackler, Robert K., and Michael J. Kaplan. "Ear, Nose, and Throat." In *Current Medical Diagnosis and Treatment*, edited by Lawrence M. Tierney, Jr., et al. New York: Lange Medical Books/McGraw-Hill, 2001.

PERIODICALS

Alvi, A., T. Doherty, and G. Lewen. "Facial Fractures and Concomitant Injuries in Trauma Patients." *Laryngoscope* 113 (January 2003): 102–106.

Anderson, Carrie E., MD, and Glenn A. Loomis, MD. "Recognition and Prevention of Inhalant Abuse." *American Family Physician* 68 (September 1, 2003): 869–876.

Brinson, G. M., B. A. Senior, and W. G. Yarbrough. "Endoscopic Management of Retained Airgun Projectiles in the Paranasal Sinuses." *Otolaryngology and Head and Neck Surgery* 130 (January 2004): 25–30.

Kalavrezos, N. "Current Trends in the Management of Frontal Sinus Fractures." *Injury* 35 (April 2004): 340–346.

Mahajan, M., and N. Shah. "Accidental Lodgment of an Air Gun Pellet in the Maxillary Sinus of a 6-Year-Old Girl: A Case Report." *Dental Traumatology* 20 (June 2004): 178–180.

Ross, Adam T., MD, and Daniel G. Becker, MD. "Fractures, Nasal and Septal." *eMedicine* July 13, 2004. < http://www.emedicine.com/ent/topic159.htm >.

Rupp, Timothy J., MD, Marian Bednar, MD, and Stephen Karageanes, DO. "Facial Fractures." *eMedicine* August 29, 2004. < http://www.emedicine.com/sports/topic33.htm >.

Tu, A. H., J. A. Girotto, N. Singh, et al. "Facial Fractures from Dog Bite Injuries." *Plastic and Reconstructive Surgery* 109 (April 1, 2002): 1259–1265.

ORGANIZATIONS

American Academy of Family Physicians (AAFP). 11400 Tomahawk Creek Parkway, Leawood, KS 66211-2672. (800) 274-2237 or (913) 906-6000. < http://www.aafp.org >.

American Academy of Otolaryngology—Head and Neck Surgery. One Prince Street, Alexandria, VA 22314-3357. (703) 836-4444. < http://www.entnet.org >.

American College of Sports Medicine (ACSM). 401 West Michigan Street, Indianapolis, IN 46202-3233. (317) 637-9200. Fax: (317) 634-7817. < http://www.acsm.org >.

Laith Farid Gulli, M.D.
Robert Ramirez, B.S.
Rebecca J. Frey, PhD

Nasogastric suction

Definition

Nasogastric suction involves removing solids, liquids, or gasses from the stomach or small intestine by inserting a tube through the nose and suctioning the gastrointestinal material through the tube.

Purpose

Nasogastric suction may be done in the following situations:

- to decompress the stomach or small intestine when intestinal obstruction (**ileus**) is suspected
- prior to gastrointestinal operations
- to obtain a sample of the gastric contents for analysis
- to remove toxic substances
- to flush the stomach during gastrointestinal bleeding or poisonings

Nasogastric intubation, the insertion of a tube through the nose into the stomach or small intestine, is also done to temporarily feed certain patients. In this case, material is not suctioned out.

Precautions

Nasogastric tubes cannot be placed in patients who have blockages in their esophagus, enlarged esophageal veins or arteries that might bleed, or severe damage to the jaws and face. The tube cannot be inserted in a patient who is having convulsions, or who is losing or has lost consciousness unless a tube has been inserted into his or her airway (intubation).

Description

The patient sits upright while a lubricated tube is slipped through the nose and down the throat. The patient may be asked to sip water at a certain point in the procedure to facilitate the passage of the tube. If the tube is to be placed into the small intestine, the doctor may use an endoscope to help see where the tube is going. Once the tube is in place, material can be removed from the stomach or intestines with gentle suction.

There are several different types of nasogastric tubes, each with a different purpose. Tubes used for **stomach flushing** are called orogastric tubes and are the largest in diameter. Tubes that are threaded through the lower opening of the stomach (pylorus) and into the small intestine are stiffer and have a balloon tip. Other specialized tubes are used for long-term and short-term feeding.

Preparation

Little preparation is necessary for this procedure other than educating the patient as to what will happen. The patient should remove dental appliances before the nasogastric tube is inserted.

Aftercare

After the tube is removed, no special care is needed. The patient's throat may feel irritated from the presence of the tube.

Risks

The most serious risk is that the patient will inhale some of the stomach contents into the lungs (aspiration). This may lead to bronchial infections and aspiration **pneumonia**. There is also the chance that the tube will be misplaced in the windpipe (trachea), causing violent coughing. Irritation to the throat and esophagus can cause bleeding.

Normal results

Nasogastric suctioning is normally well tolerated by patients and is a temporary treatment, performed in conjunction with other therapies.

Resources

BOOKS

Berkow, Robert, editor. "Nasogastric or Intestinal Intubation." In *The Merck Manual of Diagnosis and Therapy*. Rahway, NJ: Merck Research Laboratories, 2004.

Tish Davidson, A.M.

Nasopharyngeal culture

Definition

A nasopharyngeal culture is used to identify pathogenic (disease-causing) organisms present in the nasal cavity that may cause upper respiratory tract symptoms.

Purpose

Some organisms that cause upper respiratory infections are carried primarily in the nasopharynx, or back of the nose. The person carrying these pathogenic bacteria may have no symptoms, but can still infect others with the pathogen and resulting illness. The most serious of these organisms is *Neisseriea meningitidis*, which causes **meningitis** or blood stream infection in infants. By culturing a sample from the nasopharynx, the physician can identify this organism, and others, in the asymptomatic carrier. The procedure can also be used as a substitute for a **throat culture** in infants, the elderly patient, the debilitated patient, or in cases where a throat culture is difficult to obtain.

Precautions

The technician taking the specimen should wear gloves to prevent spreading infectious organisms. The patient should not be taking **antibiotics**, as these drugs may influence the test results.

Description

The patient should **cough** before collection of the specimen. Then, as the patient tilts his or her head backwards, the caregiver will inspect the back of the throat using a penlight and tongue depressor. A swab on a flexible wire is inserted into the nostril, back to the nasal cavity and upper part of the throat. The swab is rotated quickly and then removed. Next, the swab is placed into a sterile tube with culture fluid in it for transport to the microbiology laboratory. To prevent contamination, the swab should not touch the patient's tongue or side of the nostrils.

When the sample reaches the laboratory, the swab will be spread onto an agar plate and the agar plate incubated for 24–48 hours, to allow organisms present to grow. These organisms will be identified and any pathogenic organisms may also be tested for susceptibility to specific antibiotics. This allows the treating physician to determine which antibiotics will be effective.

Alternative procedures

In most cases of upper respiratory tract infections, a throat culture is more appropriate than a nasopharyngeal culture. However, the nasopharyngeal culture should be used in cases where throat cultures are difficult to obtain or to detect the carrier states of *Harmophilus influenzae* and meningococcal disease.

Some researchers regard the immunoblot method as preferable to a standard culture to detect certain species of pneumococci and other organisms that cause **pneumonia**. The immunoblot method uses a membrane that changes color in response to a specific antigen-antibody reaction.

As of the early 2000s, polymerase chain reaction (PCR) analysis is considered more sensitive than standard culture in detecting *Bordetella pertussis*, the bacterium that causes **whooping cough**. PCR has the additional advantage of providing test results more rapidly than culture.

Preparation

The procedure of inserting the swab should be described to the patient, as there is a slight discomfort associated with taking the sample. Other than that, no special preparation is necessary.

Aftercare

None

Risks

There is little to no risk involved in a nasopharyngeal culture.

Normal results

Bacteria that normally grow in the nose cavity will be identified by a nasopharyngeal culture. These include nonhemolytic streptococci, alpha-hemolytic streptococci, some *Neisseria* species, and some types of staphylococci.

Abnormal results

Pathogenic organisms that might be identified by this culture include

- Group A beta-hemolytic streptococci
- *Bordetella pertussis*, the causative agent of whooping cough
- *Corynebacterium diptheriae*, the causative agent of diptheria
- *Staphylococcus aureus*, the causative agent of many staphylococcal infections.

Additional bacteria are abnormal if they are found in large amounts. These include

- *Haemophilus influenzae*, a causative agent for certain types of meningitis and chronic pulmonary disease.
- *Streptococcus pneumoniae*, a causative agent of pneumonia
- *Candida albicans*, the causative agent of thrush.

Resources

BOOKS

Byrne, J., D. F. Saxton, P. K. Pelikan, and P. M. Nugent. *Laboratory Tests, Implication for Nursing Care.* 2nd ed. Menlo Park, CA: Addison-Wesley Publishing Company.

PERIODICALS

Bronsdon, M. A., K. L. O'Brien, R. R. Facklam, et al. "Immunoblot Method to Detect *Streptococcus pneumoniae* and Identify Multiple Serotypes from Nasopharyngeal Secretions." *Journal of Clinical Microbiology* 42 (April 2004): 1596–1600.

Fry, N. K., O. Tzivra, Y. T. Li, et al. "Laboratory Diagnosis of Pertussis Infections: The Role of PCR and Serology." *Journal of Medical Microbiology* 53 (June 2004): 519–525.

ORGANIZATIONS

American Medical Association. 515 N. State St., Chicago, IL 60612. (312) 464-5000. <http://www.ama-assn.org>.

Centers for Disease Control and Prevention. 1600 Clifton Rd., NE, Atlanta, GA 30333. (800) 311-3435, (404) 639-3311. <http://www.cdc.gov>.

Cindy L. A. Jones, PhD
Rebecca J. Frey, PhD

Native American health *see* **Minority health**

Naturopathic medicine

Definition

Naturopathic medicine is a branch of medicine in which a variety of natural medicines and treatments are used to heal illness. It uses a system of medical diagnosis and therapeutics based on the patterns of chaos and organization in nature. It is founded on the premise that people are naturally healthy, and that healing can occur through removing obstacles to a cure and by stimulating the body's natural healing abilities. The foundations of health in natural medicine are diet, **nutrition**, homeopathy, physical manipulation, **stress** management, and **exercise**.

Naturopaths are general practitioners who treat a wide variety of illnesses. They believe in treating the "whole person"—the spirit as well as the physical body—and emphasize preventive care. They often recommend changes in diet and lifestyle to enhance the health of their patients.

Purpose

Naturopathic medicine is useful for treating chronic as well as acute diseases. It is sometimes used in conjunction with allopathic care to enhance wellness and relieve chronic symptoms, such as **fatigue** and **pain**. A naturopath treats a wide range of health problems, ranging from back pain to depression.

A naturopathic physician will spend extra time interviewing and examining the patient to find the underlying cause for a medical problem. Emotional and spiritual symptoms and patterns are included in the assessment. The naturopath often spends more time educating patients in preventive health, lifestyle, and nutrition than most M.D.s.

Description

Origins

People have always seen a connection to diet and disease, and many therapies are built around special **diets**. Naturopathy began in the eighteenth and nineteenth centuries, as the industrial revolution brought about unhealthy lifestyles, and the European custom of "taking the cure" at natural spas became popular. Benedict Lust, who believed deeply in natural medicine, organized naturopathy as a formal system of healthcare in the 1890s. By the early 1900s, it was flourishing.

The first naturopaths in the United States emphasized the healing properties of a nutritious diet, as did a number of their contemporaries. In the early twentieth century, for instance, John Kellogg, a physician and vegetarian, opened a sanitarium that used healing methods such as **hydrotherapy**, often prescribed by today's naturopaths. His brother Will produced health foods, such as corn flakes and shredded wheat. The Post brothers helped make naturopathic ideas popular and emphasized the value of whole grains over highly refined ones. Together with one of their employees, C.W. Post, they eventually went on to start the cereal companies that bear their names.

In the early 1900s, most states licensed naturopaths as physicians. There were 20 medical schools of naturopathic medicine. From early on, naturopathic physicians were considered "eclectic," since they drew on a variety of natural therapies and traditions for treating their patients.

In the 1930s, naturopathy dramatically declined for several reasons. Allopathic medicine finally stopped using therapies such as bloodletting and **heavy metal poisoning** as curatives. New therapies were more effective and less toxic. Allopathic medical schools became increasingly well-funded by foundations with links to the emerging drug industry. Also, allopathic physicians became much more organized and wielded political clout. Naturopathy has experienced a resurgence over the last 20 years, however. The lay public is aware of the connection between a healthy diet and lifestyle and avoiding chronic disease. In addition, conventional medicine is often unable to treat these chronic diseases. Patients are now health care consumers, and will seek their own resolution to health problems that cannot be resolved by conventional physicians. As a result, even medical groups which once considered naturopathy ineffective are now beginning to accept it.

Naturopathic medicine modalities include a variety of healing treatments, such as diet and clinical nutrition, homeopathy, botanical medicine, soft tissue and spinal manipulation, ultrasound, and therapeutic exercise. A naturopath provides complete diagnostic and treatment services in sciences such as obstetrics, pediatrics and obstetrics. Some are also licensed midwives.

Naturopaths consider health to be not just the absence of disease, but complete physical, mental and social well being. Naturopathic physicians often say that diseases must be healed not just by suppressing symptoms, but by rooting out the true cause. Symptoms are actually viewed as the body's natural efforts to heal itself and restore balance.

A typical office visit to a naturopath takes an hour. During the first visit, the doctor will ask detailed questions about the patient's symptoms, lifestyle, history of illness, and state of his or her emotions. The naturopath will take a complete medical history, and may order lab tests such as urine and blood tests. A naturopath may talk with the patient about the possible causes for an illness—poor diet, life stresses, occupational dangers, and mental, emotional, and spiritual problems. Naturopaths believe that even widely varying symptoms can sometimes be traced to one underlying cause. Often environmental or metabolic toxins or serious stress bring on an illness.

In some states, naturopaths prescribe pharmaceuticals. In these cases, naturopaths might prescribe natural medicines, such as natural hormones, glandular **thyroid hormones**, herbal extracts, **vitamins**, etc.

As with most doctors, treatment by a naturopath can range from one office visit to many. Some acute illnesses can be alleviated with one or two visits. Other chronic diseases need regular weekly or monthly attention. Clinical care provided by naturopathic physicians are covered by insurance in a number of states in the United States.

Preparations

There were about 1,500 naturopathic physicians in the United States practicing as of 2004; nearly 80% of these practitioners entered the profession following the revival of interest in naturopathy in the late 1970s. Consumers can find naturopaths by contacting the American Association of Naturopathic Physicians (AANP) or logging on to their web site. Naturopaths recommended by the AANP have met requirements for state licensure and have taken a national exam that qualifies them to practice. Qualified naturopaths can also be found through the local branch of the national or state association of naturopathic physicians. It is sometimes useful to request names from another health care provider who knows naturopathic practitioners in the community.

Some states license naturopathic physicians. As of late 2003, those states included Hawaii, Alaska, Washington, Oregon, Utah, Montana, Arizona, Connecticut, New Hampshire, Vermont, Maine, and Kansas, in addition to the territories of Puerto Rico and the Virgin Islands. Training via a correspondence school does not qualify a naturopath for licensure or to take the national qualifying examination.

Precautions

A good naturopath is always willing to work with the patient's other physicians or health care providers. To avoid **drug interactions** and to coordinate care, it is important for a patient to inform his or her allopathic doctor about supplements prescribed by a naturopath.

Many naturopaths give childhood vaccinations, but some do not. If a parent is concerned about this, it is best to go to an allopathic doctor for vaccinations.

Naturopaths are not licensed to perform major surgery, or prescribe **narcotics** and **antidepressant drugs**. They must involve an oncologist when treating a **cancer** patient.

Side effects

Although naturopathic remedies are from natural sources and pose much less risk than traditional drugs do, there are some side effects with the use of some. One problem they can pose is the interaction with prescription medicines. It is important for a patient to inform his or her allopathic physician about any natural remedies or herbs prescribed by a naturopath.

It is also important to note that the U.S. Food and Drug Administration considers medicinal herbs as dietary supplements, not drugs, and so are not subject to the same regulations as drugs are. Because they come from natural sources, the active ingredients may not always be in the same concentration from bottle to bottle, since plants naturally vary. To guard against using too little or too much of a natural remedy, use herbs and supplements recommended by a naturopath or those produced by well-respected companies.

Research and general acceptance

Medical research in naturopathy has increased dramatically in the United States within the last 10 years. Naturopathic research often employs case histories, summaries of practitioners' clinical observations, and medical records. Some U.S. studies have also met today's scientific gold standard; they were double-blind and placebo-controlled. Much naturopathic research has also been done in Germany, France, England, India, and China.

Some mainstream medical practitioners remain distrustful of naturopathy, however. Such problems as health-food store employees without naturopathic credentials giving health-related advice to customers, or occasional rare cases of infections caused by naturopathic injections, continue to damage the reputation of this form of alternative medicine.

Research in naturopathy tends to focus on single treatments used by naturopaths, rather than naturopathy as a whole. In 1998, an extensive review of such single treatment studies found that naturopathic healing methods were effective for 15 different medical conditions, including **osteoarthritis**, **asthma**, and middle ear infections. A study of 8,341 men with damaged heart muscles in 1996 revealed that supplementation with niacin, a B vitamin, was associated with an 11% reduced risk of mortality over 15 years. In 1996, a study showed **St. John's wort** was as effective as prescription antidepressants in relieving depression, and had fewer side effects.

Studies have also demonstrated benefits in the arena of **women's health** issues. In one classic 1993 study, women with cervical dysplasia or abnormal Pap smears were treated by naturopaths with topical applications of herbs and dietary supplements. These medications included Bromelian, an enzyme from the pineapple; bloodroot; marigold; and zinc chloride; and suppositories made from herbal and nutritional ingredients, such as **echinacea**, vitamin A, and vitamin E. Thirty eight of the 43 women in the study had normal Pap smears and normal tissue biopsies after treatment. The study concluded that these protocols might benefit the health of patients undergoing more traditional treatments for cervical dysplasia, such as **cryotherapy**.

Other more recent research has documented the benefits of such nutritional foods as soy in relieving hot flashes and vaginal dryness. **Nutritional supplements** prescribed by naturopaths to enhance women's health during **menopause** have also proven effective; in general, naturopathy appears to be as useful as conventional medicine for treating menopausal symptoms. Research shows vitamin E supplements are helpful for 50% of postmenopausal women with thinning vaginal tissue. Studies also reveal that bioflavonoids with vitamin C and gamma-oryzanol, a substance taken from rice bran oil, can relieve hot flashes.

Another area of women's health concerns that naturopathy has taken seriously is a growing preference for skin care and beauty products derived from natural sources rather than from chemical laboratories. Such products are often more beneficial to the skin and less likely to cause **rashes** or other allergic reactions.

Resources

BOOKS

Better Homes and Gardens. *Smart Choices in Alternative Medicine*. Meredith Books, 1999.

Pelletier, Dr. Kenneth R. *The Best Alternative Medicine*. Simon and Schuster, 2000.

PERIODICALS

Cramer, E. H., P. Jones, N. L. Keenan, and B. L. Thompson. "Is Naturopathy as Effective as Conventional Therapy for Treatment of Menopausal Symptoms?" *Journal of Alternatie and Complementary Medicine* 9 (August 2003): 529–538.

Engelhart, S., F. Saborowski, M. Krakau, et al. "Severe *Serratia liquefaciens* Sepsis Following Vitamin C Infusion Treatment by a Naturopathic Practitioner." *Journal of Clinical Microbiology* 41 (August 2003): 3986–3988.

Hudson, Tori. "Naturopathic Medicine, Integrative Medicine and Women's Health." *Townsend Letter for Doctors and Patients* November 2001: 136.

Hudson, Tori, N.D. "Six Paths to Menopausal Wellness." *Herbs for Health* January–February 2000: 47–50.

Lee, A. C., and K. J. Kemper. "Homeopathy and Naturopathy: Practice Characteristics and Pediatric Care." *Archives of Pediatric and Adolescent Medicine* 154, no. 1 (January 2000): 75–80.

Mills, E., R. Singh, M. Kawasaki, et al. "Emerging Issues Associated with HIV Patients Seeking Advice from Health Food Stores." *Canadian Journal of Public Health* 94 (September–October 2003): 363–366.

ORGANIZATIONS

The American Association of Naturopathic Physicians. 601 Valley Street, Suite 105, Seattle, WA 98109. (206) 298-0126. < http://www.naturopathic.org >.

Naturopathic Physicians Licensing Examination Board (NPLEX). P. O. Box 69657, Portland, OR 97201. (503) 250-9141. < http://www.nabne.org/html/index2.html >.

Barbara Boughton
Rebecca J. Frey, PhD

Naturopathy *see* **Naturopathic medicine**

Nausea and vomiting

Definition

Nausea is the sensation of being about to vomit. Vomiting, or emesis, is the expelling of undigested food through the mouth.

Description

Nausea is a reaction to a number of causes that include overeating, infection, or irritation of the throat or stomach lining. Persistent or recurrent nausea and vomiting should be checked by a doctor.

A doctor should be called if nausea and vomiting occur:

- after eating rich or spoiled food or taking a new medication
- repeatedly or for 48 hours or longer
- following intense **dizziness**

It is important to see a doctor if nausea and vomiting are accompanied by:

- yellowing of the skin and whites of the eyes
- **pain** in the chest or lower abdomen
- trouble with swallowing or urination
- **dehydration** or extreme thirst
- drowsiness or confusion
- constant, severe abdominal pain
- a fruity breath odor

A doctor should be notified if vomiting is heavy and/or bloody, if the vomitus looks like feces, or if the patient has been unable to keep food down for 24 hours.

An ambulance or emergency response number should be called immediately if:

- Diabetic **shock** is suspected
- Nausea and vomiting continue after other symptoms of viral infection have subsided
- The patient has a severe **headache**
- The patient is sweating and having chest pain and trouble breathing
- The patient is known or suspected to have swallowed a **drug overdose** or poisonous substance
- The patient has a high body temperature, **muscle cramps**, and other signs of heat exhaustion or heat stroke

- Nausea, vomiting, and breathing problems occur after exposure to a known allergen

Causes and symptoms

Persistent, unexplained, or recurring nausea and vomiting can be symptoms of a variety of serious illnesses. It can be caused by simply overeating or drinking too much alcohol. It can be due to **stress**, certain medications, or illness. For example, people who are given morphine or other opioid medications for pain relief after surgery sometimes feel nauseated by the drug. Such poisonous substances as arsenic and other heavy metals cause nausea and vomiting. Morning sickness is a consequence of pregnancy-related hormone changes. **Motion sickness** can be induced by traveling in a vehicle, plane, or on a boat. Many patients experience nausea after eating spoiled food or foods to which they are allergic. Patients who suffer migraine headache often experience nausea. **Cancer** patients on **chemotherapy** are nauseated. **Gallstones**, **gastroenteritis** and stomach ulcer may cause nausea and vomiting. These symptoms should be evaluated by a physician.

Nausea and vomiting may also be psychological in origin. Some people vomit under such conditions of emotional stress as family arguments, academic tests, airplane travel, losing a job, and similar high-stress situations. In addition, some eating disorders are characterized by self-induced vomiting.

Diagnosis

Diagnosis is based on the severity, frequency, and duration of symptoms, and other factors that could indicate the presence of a serious illness.

Diagnosis is based on the taking of a careful patient history. In some cases, the doctor may order laboratory tests or imaging studies to determine the presence of drugs or poisonous substances in the patient's blood or urine, or evidence of head injuries or abnormalities in the digestive tract. If the nausea and vomiting appear to be related to **anxiety**, stress, or an eating disorder, the doctor may refer the patient to a psychiatrist for further evaluation.

Treatment

Getting a breath of fresh air or getting away from whatever is causing the nausea can solve the problem. Eating olives or crackers or sucking on a lemon can calm the stomach by absorbing acid and excess fluid. Coke syrup is another proven remedy.

Vomiting relieves nausea right away but can cause dehydration. Sipping clear juices, weak tea, and some sports drinks help replace lost fluid and minerals without irritating the stomach. Food should be reintroduced gradually, beginning with small amounts of dry, bland food like crackers and toast.

Medications that are given to relieve nausea and vomiting are called antiemetics. Meclizine (Bonine), a medication for motion sickness, also diminishes the feeling of queasiness in the stomach. Dimenhydrinate (Dramamine), another motion-sickness drug, is not effective on other types of nausea and may cause drowsiness.

Newer drugs that have been developed to treat postoperative or postchemotherapy nausea and vomiting include ondansetron (Zofran) and granisetron (Kytril). Another treatment that has been found to lower the risk of nausea after surgery is intravenous administration of supplemental fluid before the operation.

Alternative treatment

Advocates of alternative treatments suggest biofeedback, acupressure and the use of herbs to calm the stomach. Biofeedback uses **exercise** and deep relaxation to control nausea. Acupressure (applying pressure to specific areas of the body) can be applied by wearing a special wristband or by applying firm pressure to:

- the back of the jawbone
- the webbing between the thumb and index finger
- the top of the foot
- the inside of the wrist
- the base of the rib cage

Acupuncture is another alternative treatment found to be effective in relieving nausea. A few people, however, experience nausea as a side effect of acupuncture.

Chamomile (*Matricaria recutita*) or lemon balm (*Melissa officinalis*) tea may relieve symptoms. Ginger (*Zingiber officinale*), another natural remedy, can be drunk as tea or taken as candy or powered capsules.

Prevention

Massage, **meditation**, yoga, and other relaxation techniques can help prevent stress-induced nausea. Anti-nausea medication taken before traveling can prevent motion sickness. Sitting in the front seat,

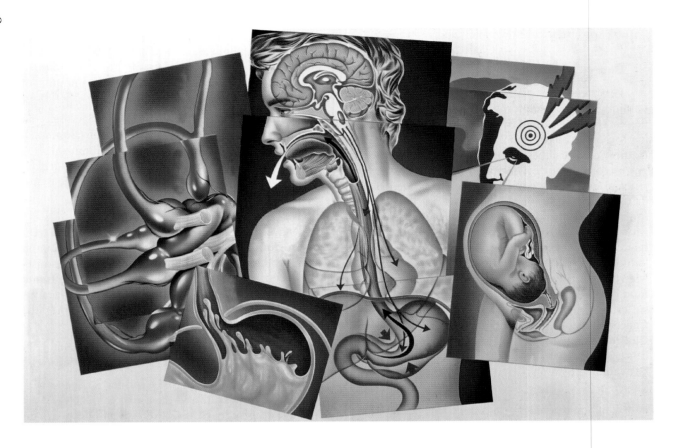

These illustrations depict the mechanism and causes of vomiting in the human body. An impulse from the brain stimulates the vomiting center (top center) in the brain stem. Nerve impulses sent to the stomach, diaphragm, and abdominal wall (bottom center) result in stomach's contents being expelled. Other causes of vomiting include raised pressure in the skull due to injury or tumor (upper right), and hormonal changes during pregnancy. *(Illustration by John Bavosi, Custom Medical Stock Photo. Reproduced by permission.)*

KEY TERMS

Acupuncture—A treatment technique associated with traditional Chinese medicine, in which thin needles are inserted into specific points located along energy channels in the human body known as meridians.

Antiemetic—A preparation or medication that relieves nausea and vomiting. Coke syrup, ginger, and motion sickness medications are examples of antiemetics.

Dehydration—Loss of fluid and minerals following vomiting, prolonged diarrhea, or excessive sweating.

Diabetic coma—Reduced level of consciousness that requires immediate medical attention.

Emesis—The medical term for vomiting.

focusing on the horizon, and traveling after dark can also minimize symptoms.

Food should be fresh, properly prepared, and eaten slowly. Overeating, tight-fitting clothes, and strenuous activity immediately after a meal should be avoided.

Vomiting related to emotional upsets may be avoided by forms of psychotherapy that teach patients to manage stress in healthier ways.

Resources

BOOKS

American Psychiatric Association. *Diagnostic and Statistical Manual of Mental Disorders*. 4th ed., revised. Washington, DC: American Psychiatric Association, 2000.

Beers, Mark H., MD, and Robert Berkow, MD., editors. "Functional Vomiting." Section 3, Chapter 21

In *The Merck Manual of Diagnosis and Therapy.* Whitehouse Station, NJ: Merck Research Laboratories, 2002.

Pelletier, Dr. Kenneth R. *The Best Alternative Medicine, Part I: Western Herbal Medicine.* New York: Simon and Schuster, 2002.

PERIODICALS

Ali, S. Z., A. Taguchi, B. Holtmann, and A. Kurz. "Effect of Supplemental Pre-Operative Fluid on Postoperative Nausea and Vomiting." *Anaesthesia* 58 (August 2003): 780–784.

Cepeda, M. S., J. T. Farrar, M. Baumgarten, et al. "Side Effects of Opioids During Short-Term Administration: Effect of Age, Gender, and Race." *Clinical Pharmacology and Therapeutics* 74 (August 2003): 102–112.

Chung, A., L. Bui, and E. Mills. "Adverse Effects of Acupuncture. Which Are Clinically Significant?" *Canadian Family Physician* 49 (August 2003): 985–989.

O'Brien, C. M., G. Titley, and P. Whitehurst. "A Comparison of Cyclizine, Ondansetron and Placebo as Prophylaxis Against Postoperative Nausea and Vomiting in Children." *Anaesthesia* 58 (July 2003): 707–711.

Quinla, J. D., and D. A. Hill. "Nausea and Vomiting of Pregnancy." *American Family Physician* 68 (July 1, 2003): 121–128.

Ratnaike, R. N. "Acute and Chronic Arsenic Toxicity." *Postgraduate Medical Journal* 79 (July 2003): 391–396.

Tan, M. "Granisetron: New Insights Into Its Use for the Treatment of Chemotherapy-Induced Nausea and Vomiting." *Expert Opinion in Pharmacotherapy* 4 (September 2003): 1563–1571.

Tiwari, A., S. Chan, A. Wong, et al. "Severe Acute Respiratory Syndrome (SARS) in Hong Kong: Patients' Experiences." *Nursing Outlook* 51 (September-October 2003): 212–219.

Walling, Anne D. "Ginger Relieves Nausea and Vomiting During Pregnancy." *American Family Physician* 64 (November 15, 2001): 1745.

ORGANIZATIONS

American Gastroenterological Association (AGA). 7910 Woodmont Ave., 7th Floor, Bethesda, MD 20814. (310) 654-2055. < http://www.gastro.org/index.html >. aga001@aol.com.

Maureen Haggerty
Rebecca J. Frey, PhD

Nberg disease *see* **Osteopetroses**

NCV *see* **Electromyography**

Near-drowning

Definition

Near-drowning is the term for survival after suffocation caused by submersion in water or another fluid. Some experts exclude from this definition cases of temporary survival that end in death within 24 hours, which they prefer to classify as drownings.

Description

An estimated 15,000–70,000 near-drownings occur in the United States each year (insufficient reporting prevents a better estimate). The typical victim is young and male. Nearly half of all drownings and near-drownings involve children less than four years old. Home swimming pools pose the greatest risk for children, being the site of 60–90% of drownings in the 0–4 age group. Teenage boys also face a heightened risk of drowning and near-drowning, largely because of their tendency to behave recklessly and use drugs and alcohol (drugs and alcohol are implicated in 40–50% of teenage drownings). Males, however, predominate even in the earliest age-groups, possibly because young boys are often granted more freedom from supervision than young girls enjoy, making it more likely that they will stumble into danger and less likely that they will attract an adult's attention in time for a quick rescue. Roughly four out of five drowning victims are males.

Causes and symptoms

The circumstances leading to near-drownings (and drownings also) cannot be reduced to a single scenario involving nonswimmers accidentally entering deep water. On many occasions, near-drownings are secondary to an event such as a **heart attack** that causes unconsciousness or a head or spinal injury that prevents a diver from resurfacing. Near-drownings, moreover, can occur in shallow as well as deep water. Small children have drowned or almost drowned in bathtubs, toilets, industrial-size cleaning buckets, and washing machines. Bathtubs are especially dangerous for infants six months to one year old, who can sit up straight in a bathtub but may lack the ability to pull themselves out of the water if they slip under the surface.

A reduced concentration of oxygen in the blood (hypoxemia) is common to all near-drownings. Human life, of course, depends on a constant supply of oxygen-laden air reaching the blood by way of the lungs. When drowning begins, the larynx (an air passage) closes involuntarily, preventing both air and water from entering the lungs. In 10–15% of cases, hypoxemia results because the larynx stays closed. This is called "dry drowning." Hypoxemia also occurs in "wet drowning," the 85–90% of cases where the larynx relaxes and water enters the lungs. The physiological mechanisms that produce hypoxemia in wet drowning are different for freshwater and saltwater, but only a small amount of either kind of water is needed to damage the lungs and interfere with the body's oxygen intake. All of this happens very quickly: within three minutes of submersion most people are unconscious, and within five minutes the brain begins to suffer from lack of oxygen. Abnormal heart rhythms (cardiac dysrhythmias) often occur in near-drowning cases, and the heart may stop pumping (cardiac arrest). An increase in blood acidity (acidosis) is another consequence of near-drowning, and under some circumstances near-drowning can cause a substantial increase or decrease in the volume of circulating blood. Many victims experience a severe drop in body temperature (**hypothermia**).

The signs and symptoms of near-drowning can differ widely from person to person. Some victims are alert but agitated, while others are comatose. Breathing may have stopped, or the victim may be gasping for breath. Bluish skin (**cyanosis**), coughing, and frothy pink sputum (material expelled from the respiratory tract by coughing) are often observed. Rapid breathing (tachypnea), a rapid heart rate (tachycardia), and a low-grade fever are common during the first few hours after rescue. Conscious victims may appear confused, lethargic, or irritable.

Diagnosis

Diagnosis relies on a **physical examination** of the victim and on a wide range of tests and other procedures. Blood is taken to measure oxygen levels and for many other purposes. Pulse oximetry, another way of assessing oxygen levels, involves attaching a device called a pulse oximeter to the patient's finger. An electrocardiograph is used to monitor heart activity. X rays can detect head and neck injuries and excess tissue fluid (**edema**) in the lungs.

Treatment

Treatment begins with removing the victim from the water and performing **cardiopulmonary resuscitation (CPR)**. One purpose of CPR—which, of course, should be attempted only by people trained in its use—is to bring oxygen to the lungs, heart, brain, and other organs by breathing into the victim's mouth. When the victim's heart has stopped, **CPR** also attempts to get the heart pumping again by pressing down on the victim's chest. After CPR has been performed and emergency medical help has arrived on the scene, oxygen is administered to the victim. If the victim's breathing has stopped or is otherwise impaired, a tube is inserted into the windpipe (trachea) to maintain the airway (this is called endotracheal intubation). The victim is also checked for head, neck, and other injuries, and fluids are given intravenously. Hypothermia cases require careful handling to protect the heart.

In the emergency department, victims continue receiving oxygen until blood tests show a return to normal. About one-third are intubated and initially need mechanical support to breathe. Rewarming is undertaken when hypothermia is present. Victims may arrive needing treatment for cardiac arrest or cardiac dysrhythmias. Comatose patients present a special problem: although various treatment approaches have been tried, none have proved beneficial. Patients can be discharged from the emergency department after four to six hours if their blood oxygen level is normal and no signs or symptoms of near-drowning are present. But because lung problems can arise 12 or more hours after submersion, the medical staff must first be satisfied that the patients are willing and able to seek further medical help if necessary. Admission to a hospital for at least 24 hours for further observation and treatment is a must for patients who do not appear to recover fully in the emergency department.

Prognosis

Neurological damage is the major long-term concern in the treatment of near-drowning victims. Patients who arrive at an emergency department awake and alert usually survive with brain function intact, as do about 90% of those who arrive mentally impaired (lethargic, confused, and so forth) but not comatose. **Death** or permanent neurological damage is very likely when patients arrive comatose. Early rescue of near-drowning victims (within five minutes of submersion) and prompt CPR (within less than 10 minutes of submersion) seem to be the best guarantees of a complete recovery. An analysis of 715 patients admitted to emergency departments in 1971–81 revealed that 69% recovered completely, 25% died, and 6% survived but suffered permanent neurological damage.

Prevention

Prevention depends on educating parents, other adults, and teenagers about water safety. Parents must realize that young children who are left in or near water without adult supervision even for a short time can easily get into trouble, not just at the beach or next to a swimming pool, but in bathtubs and around toilets, buckets, washing machines, and other household articles where water can collect. Research on swimming pool drownings involving young children shows that the victims have usually been left unattended less than five minutes before the accident. Experts consider putting up a fence around a home swimming pool an essential precaution, and estimate that 50–90% of child drownings and near-drownings could be prevented if fences were widely adopted. The fence should be at least five feet high and unclimbable, have a self-closing and self-locking gate, and completely surround the pool.

Pool owners—and, indeed, all other adults—should consider learning CPR. Everyone, of course, should follow the rules for safe swimming and boating. Those who have a medical condition that can cause a seizure or otherwise threaten safety in the water are advised always to swim with a partner. And of course, people need to be aware that alcohol and drug use substantially increase the chances of an accident.

The danger of alcohol and drug use around water is a point that requires special emphasis where teenagers are concerned. Teenagers can also benefit from CPR training and safe swimming and boating classes.

Resources

BOOKS

Modell, Jerome H. "Drowning and Near-Drowning." In *Harrison's Principles of Internal Medicine*, edited by Anthony S. Fauci, et al. New York:McGraw-Hill, 1997.

Howard Baker

Nearsightedness *see* **Myopia**

Necrotizing enterocolitis

Definition

Necrotizing enterocolitis is a serious bacterial infection in the intestine, primarily of sick or premature newborn infants. It can cause the death (necrosis) of intestinal tissue and progress to blood poisoning (septicemia).

Description

Necrotizing enterocolitis develops in approximately 10% of newborns weighing less than 800 g (under 2 lbs). It is a serious infection that can produce complications in the intestine itself—such as ulcers, perforations (holes) in the intestinal wall, and tissue necrosis—as well as progress to life-threatening septicemia. Necrotizing enterocolitis most commonly affects the lower portion of the small intestine (ileum). It is less common in the colon and upper small bowel.

Causes and symptoms

The cause of necrotizing enterocolitis is not clear. It is believed that the infection usually develops after the bowel wall has already been weakened or damaged by a lack of oxygen, predisposing it to bacterial invasion. Bacteria proliferate in the bowel and cause a deep infection that can kill bowel tissue and spread to the bloodstream.

Necrotizing enterocolitis almost always occurs in the first month of life. Infants who require **tube feedings** may have an increased risk for the disorder. A number of other conditions also make newborns susceptible, including **respiratory distress syndrome**, congenital heart problems, and episodes of apnea (cessation of breathing). The primary risk factor, however, is **prematurity**. Not only is the immature digestive tract less able to protect itself, but premature infants are subjected to many stresses on the body in their attempt to survive.

Early symptoms of necrotizing enterocolitis include an intolerance to formula, distended and tender abdomen, **vomiting**, and blood (visible or not) in the stool. One of the earliest signs may also be the need for mechanical support of the infant's breathing. If the infection spreads to the bloodstream, infants may develop lethargy, fluctuations in body temperature, and periodically stop breathing.

Diagnosis

The key to reducing the complications of this disease is early suspicion by the physician. A series of x rays of the bowel often reveals the progressive condition, and blood tests confirm infection.

Treatment

Over two-thirds of infants can be treated without surgery. Aggressive medical therapy is begun as soon as the condition is diagnosed or even suspected. Tube feedings into the gastrointestinal tract (enteral **nutrition**) are discontinued, and tube feedings into the veins (parenteral nutrition) are used instead until the condition has resolved. Intravenous fluids are given for several weeks while the bowel heals.

Some infants are placed on a ventilator to help them breathe, and some receive transfusions of platelets, which help the blood clot when there is internal bleeding. **Antibiotics** are usually given intravenously for at least 10 days. These infants require frequent evaluations by the physician, who may order multiple abdominal x rays and blood tests to monitor their condition during the illness.

Sometimes, necrotizing enterocolitis must be treated with surgery. This is often the case when an infant's condition does not improve with medical therapy or there are signs of worsening infection.

The surgical treatment depends on the individual patient's condition. Patients with infection that has caused serious damage to the bowel may have portions of the bowel removed. It is sometimes necessary to create a substitute bowel by making an opening (**ostomy**) into the abdomen through the skin, from which waste products are discharged temporarily. But many physicians are avoiding this and operating to remove diseased bowel and repair the defect at the same time.

Postoperative complications are common, including wound infections and lack of healing, persistent **sepsis** and bowel necrosis, and a serious internal bleeding disorder known as disseminated intravascular coagulation.

Prognosis

Necrotizing enterocolitis is the most common cause of death in newborns undergoing surgery. The average mortality is 30–40%, even higher in severe cases.

Early identification and treatment are critical to improving the outcome for these infants. Aggressive nonsurgical support and careful timing of surgical intervention have improved overall survival; however, this condition can be fatal in about one-third of cases. With the resolution of the infection, the bowel may begin functioning within weeks or months. But infants need to be carefully monitored by a physician for years because of possible future complications.

About 10–35% of all survivors will eventually develop a stricture, or narrowing, of the intestine that occurs with healing. This can create an intestinal obstruction that will require surgery. Infants may also be more susceptible to future bacterial infections in the

---

---

gastrointestinal tract and to a delay in growth. Infants with severe cases may also suffer neurological impairment.

The most serious long-term gastrointestinal complication associated with necrotizing enterocolitis is short-bowel, or short-gut, syndrome. This refers to a condition that can develop when a large amount of bowel must be removed, making the intestines less able to absorb certain nutrients and enzymes. These infants gradually evolve from tube feedings to oral feedings, and medications are used to control the malabsorption, **diarrhea**, and other consequences of this condition.

Prevention

In very small or sick premature infants, the risk for necrotizing enterocolitis may be diminished by beginning parenteral nutrition and delaying enteral feedings for several days to weeks.

Some have suggested that breast milk provides substances that may be protective, but there is no evidence that this reduces the risk of infection. A large multicenter trial showed that steroid drugs given to women in preterm labor may protect their offspring from necrotizing enterocolitis.

Sometimes necrotizing enterocolitis occurs in clusters, or outbreaks, in hospital newborn (neonatal) units. Because there is an infectious element to the disorder, infants with necrotizing enterocolitis may be isolated to avoid infecting other infants. Persons caring for these infants must also employ strict measures to prevent spreading the infection.

Resources

OTHER

Neonatology on the Web. < http://www.neonatology.org >.

Caroline A. Helwick

Necrotizing fasciitis *see* **Flesh-eating disease**

Neisseria gonorrheae infection *see*
  Gonorrhea

Neisseria meningitidis bacteremia *see*
  Meningococcemia

Nelfinavir *see* **Protease inhibitors**

Neonatal jaundice

Definition

Neonatal **jaundice** (or hyperbilirubinemia) is a higher-than-normal level of bilirubin in the blood. Bilirubin is a by-product of the breakdown of red blood cells. This condition can cause a yellow discoloration of the skin and the whites of the eyes called jaundice.

Description

Bilirubin, a by-product of the breakdown of hemoglobin (the oxygen-carrying substance in red blood cells), is produced when the body breaks down old red blood cells. Normally, the liver processes the bilirubin and excretes it in the stool. Hyperbilirubinemia means there is a high level of bilirubin in the blood. This condition is particularly common in newborn infants. Before birth, an infant gets rid of bilirubin through the mother's blood and liver systems. After birth, the baby's liver has to take over processing bilirubin on its own. Almost all newborns have higher than normal levels of bilirubin. In most cases, the baby's systems continue to develop and can soon process bilirubin. However, some infants may need medical treatment to prevent serious complications which can occur due to the accumulation of bilirubin.

Causes and symptoms

In newborn infants, the liver and intestinal systems are immature and cannot excrete bilirubin as fast as the body produces it. This type of hyperbilirubinemia can cause jaundice to develop within a few days after birth. About one-half of all newborns develop

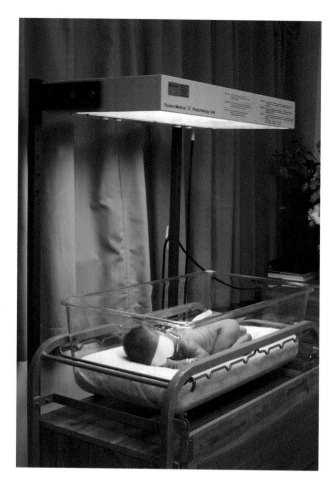

A newborn baby undergoes phototherapy with visible blue light to treat his jaundice. *(Photograph by Ron Sutherland, Photo Researchers, Inc. Reproduced by permission.)*

jaundice, while premature infants are much more likely to develop it. Hyperbilirubinemia is also more common in some populations, such as Native American and Asian. All infants with jaundice should be evaluated by a health care provider to rule out more serious problems.

Hyperbilirubinemia and jaundice can also be the result of other diseases or conditions. Hepatitis, **cirrhosis** of the liver, and mononucleosis are diseases that can affect the liver. **Gallstones**, a blocked bile duct, or the use of drugs or alcohol can also cause jaundice.

Extremely high levels of bilirubin in infants may cause kernicterus, a form of brain damage. Signs of severe hyperbilirubinemia include listlessness, high-pitched crying, apnea (periods of not breathing), arching of the back, and seizures. If severe hyperbilirubinemia is not treated, it can cause **mental retardation**, hearing loss, behavior disorders, **cerebral palsy**, or **death**.

Diagnosis

The initial diagnosis of hyperbilirubinemia is based on the appearance of jaundice at physical examination. The child is often placed by an open window so he/she may be checked in natural light. Blood samples may be taken to determine the bilirubin level in the blood.

Treatment

Most cases of newborn jaundice resolve without medical treatment within two to three weeks, but should be checked by the health care provider. It is important that the infant is feeding regularly and having normal bowel movements. If bilirubin levels are extremely high, the infant may be treated with phototherapy—exposure of the baby's skin to fluorescent light. The bilirubin in the baby's skin absorbs the light and is changed to a substance that can be excreted in the urine. This treatment can be done in the hospital and is often done at home with special lights which parents can rent for the treatment. Treatment may be needed for several days before bilirubin levels in the blood return to normal. The baby's eyes are shielded to prevent the optic nerves from absorbing too much light. Another type of treatment uses a special fiberoptic blanket. There is no need to shield the baby's eyes with this treatment, and it can be done at home. In rare cases, where bilirubin levels are extremely high, the baby may need to receive a blood **transfusion**.

Prognosis

Most infants with hyperbilirubinemia and associated jaundice recover without medical treatment. **Photopherapy** is very effective in reducing bilirubin levels in the majority of infants who need it. There are usually no long-term effects on the child from the hyperbilirubinemia or the phototherapy. It is very rare that a baby may need a blood transfusion for treatment of this condition.

Prevention

There is no way to predict which infants will be affected by hyperbilirubinemia. Newborns should be breastfed or given formula frequently, and feedings should begin as soon as possible after delivery to increase activity of the baby's digestive system.

Resources

OTHER

D'Alessandro, Hellen Anne. *Biliary Atresia. The Virtual Hospital Page*. University of Iowa. < http://www.vh.org/Providers/Textbooks/ElectricGiNucs/Text/BiliaryAtresia.html >.

"Jaundice/Hyperbilirubinemia." < http://www2.medsch.wisc.edu/childrenshosp/Parents_of_Preemies/jaundice.html >

"Jaundice in Newborn (Hyperbilirubinemia)." < http://www.ivillage.com >.

"Neonatal Jaundice." < http://www.gi.vghtc.gov.tw/Teaching/Biliary/Jaundice/s13.htm >.

"Neonatology on the Web." < http://www.neonatology.org >.

Altha Roberts Edgren

Nephrectomy

Definition

Nephrectomy is the surgical procedure of removing a kidney or section of a kidney.

Purpose

Nephrectomy, or kidney removal, is performed on patients with **cancer** of the kidney (renal cell carcinoma); a disease in which cysts (sac-like structures) displace healthy kidney tissue (**polycystic kidney disease**); and serious kidney infections. It is also used to remove a healthy kidney from a donor for the purposes of **kidney transplantation**.

Precautions

Because the kidney is responsible for filtering wastes and fluid from the bloodstream, kidney function is critical to life. Nephrectomy candidates suffering from serious kidney disease, cancer, or infection usually have few treatment choices but to undergo the procedure. However, if kidney function is lost in the remaining kidney, the patient will require chronic dialysis treatments or transplantation of a healthy kidney to sustain life.

Description

Nephrectomy may involve removing a small portion of the kidney or the entire organ and surrounding tissues. In partial nephrectomy, only the diseased or infected portion of the kidney is removed. Radical nephrectomy involves removing the entire kidney, a section of the tube leading to the bladder (ureter), the gland that sits atop the kidney (adrenal gland), and the fatty tissue surrounding the kidney. A simple nephrectomy performed for transplant purposes requires removal of the kidney and a section of the attached ureter. A similar procedure is used to harvest cadaver kidneys, although both kidneys are typically removed at once (bilateral nephrectomy) and blood and cell samples for **tissue typing** are also taken.

The nephrectomy patient is administered **general anesthesia** and the surgeon makes an incision on the side or front of the abdomen. Muscle, fat, and tissue are cut away to reveal the kidney. The blood vessels connecting the kidney to the circulation are cut and clamped. Depending on the type of nephrectomy procedure being performed, the ureter, adrenal gland, and/or surrounding tissue may also be cut. The vessels and the ureter in the patient are then tied off and the incision is sewn up (sutured). The surgical procedure can take up to three hours, depending on the type of nephrectomy being performed.

Laparoscopic nephrectomy is a form of minimally-invasive surgery that utilizes instruments on long, narrow rods to view, cut, and remove the kidney. The surgeon views the kidney and surrounding tissue with a flexible videoscope. The videoscope and surgical instruments are maneuvered through four small incisions in the abdomen. Once the kidney is freed, it is secured in a bag and pulled through a fifth incision, approximately 3 in (7.6 cm) wide, in the front of the abdominal wall below the navel. Although this surgical technique takes slightly longer than a traditional nephrectomy, preliminary studies have shown that it promotes a faster recovery time, shorter hospital stays, and less post-operative **pain** for kidney donors.

Preparation

Prior to surgery, blood samples will be taken from the patient to type and crossmatch in case **transfusion**

is required during surgery. A catheter will also be inserted into the patient's bladder. The surgical procedure will be described to the patient, along with the possible risks.

Aftercare

Nephrectomy patients may experience considerable discomfort in the area of the incision. Patients may also experience **numbness**, caused by severed nerves, near or on the incision. Pain relievers are administered following the surgical procedure and during the recovery period on an as-needed basis. Although deep breathing and coughing may be painful due to the proximity of the incision to the diaphragm, breathing exercises are encouraged to prevent **pneumonia**. Patients should not drive an automobile for a minimum of two weeks.

Risks

Possible complications of a nephrectomy procedure include infection, bleeding (hemorrhage), and post-operative pneumonia. There is also the risk of kidney failure in a patient with impaired function or disease in the remaining kidney.

Normal results

Normal results of a nephrectomy are dependent on the purpose of the procedure and the type of nephrectomy performed. Immediately following the procedure, it is normal for patients to experience pain near the incision site, particularly when coughing or breathing deeply. Renal function of the patient is monitored carefully after nephrectomy surgery. If the remaining kidney is healthy, it will increase its functioning over time to compensate for the loss of the removed kidney.

Length of hospitalization depends on the type of nephrectomy procedure. Patients undergoing a laparoscopic radical nephrectomy may be released within two to four days after surgery. Traditional open nephrectomy patients are typically hospitalized for about a week. Recovery time will also vary, on average from three to six weeks.

Resources

ORGANIZATIONS

National Kidney Foundation. 30 East 33rd St., New York, NY 10016. (800) 622-9010. < http://www.kidney.org >.

Paula Anne Ford-Martin

Nephritic syndrome *see* **Glomerulonephritis**

Nephritis

Definition

Nephritis is inflammation of the kidney.

Description

The most prevalent form of acute nephritis is **glomerulonephritis**. This condition affects children and teenagers far more often than it affects adults. It is inflammation of the glomeruli, or small round filters located in the kidney. **Pyelonephritis** affects adults more than children, and is recognized as inflammation of the kidney and upper urinary tract. A third type of nephritis is hereditary nephritis, a rare inherited condition.

Causes and symptoms

Acute glomerulonephritis usually develops a few weeks after a strep infection of the throat or skin. Symptoms of glomerulonephritis include **fatigue**, high blood pressure, and swelling. Swelling is most notable in the hands, feet, ankles and face.

Pyelonephritis usually occurs suddenly, and the acute form of this disease is more common in adult women. The most common cause of this form of bacterial nephritis is the backward flow of infected urine from the bladder into the upper urinary tract. Its symptoms include **fever** and chills, fatigue, burning or frequent urination, cloudy or bloody urine, and aching **pain** on one or both sides of the lower back or abdomen.

Hereditary nephritis can be present at birth. The rare disease presents in many different forms and can

be responsible for up to 5% of end-stage renal disease in men.

Diagnosis

Diagnosis of nephritis is based on:

- the patient's symptoms and medical history
- physical examination
- laboratory tests
- kidney function tests
- imaging studies such as ultrasound or x rays to determine blockage and inflammation

Urinalysis can reveal the presence of:

- albumin and other proteins
- red and white blood cells
- pus, blood, or bacteria in the urine

Treatment

Treatment of glomerulonephritis normally includes drugs such as cortisone or cytotoxic drugs (those that are destructive to certain cells or antigens). **Diuretics** may be prescribed to increase urination. If high blood pressure is present, drugs may be prescribed to decrease the **hypertension**. Iron and vitamin supplements may be recommended if the patient becomes anemic.

Acute pyelonephritis may require hospitalization for severe illness. **Antibiotics** will be prescribed, with the length of treatment based on the severity of the infection. In the case of chronic pyelonephritis, a six-month course of antibiotics may be necessary to rid the infection. Surgery is sometimes necessary.

Treatment of hereditary nephritis depends of the variety of the disease and severity at the time of treatment.

Alternative treatment

Alternative treatment of nephritis should be used as a complement to medical care and under the supervision of a licensed practitioner. Some herbs thought to relieve symptoms of nephritis include cleavers (*Galium* spp.) and wild hydrangea.

Prognosis

Prognosis for most cases of glomerulonephritis is generally good. Ninety percent of children recover without complications. With proper medical treatment, symptoms usually subside within a few weeks, or at the most, a few months.

Pyelonephritis in the acute form offers a good prognosis if diagnosed and treated early. Follow-up urinalysis studies will determine if the patient remains bacteria-free. If the infection is not cured or continues to recur, it can lead to serious complications such as **bacteremia** (bacterial invasion of the bloodstream), hypertension, chronic pyelonephritis and even permanent kidney damage.

If hereditary nephritis is not detected or treated, it can lead to complications such as eye problems, deafness or kidney failure.

Prevention

Streptococcal infections that may lead to glomerulonephritis can be prevented by avoiding exposure to strep infection and obtaining prompt medical treatment for **scarlet fever** or other infection.

Pyelonephritis can best be avoided if those with a history of urinary tract infections take care to drink plenty of fluids, urinate frequently, and practice good hygiene following urination.

Hereditary nephritis can not be prevented, but research to combat the disease continues.

Resources

ORGANIZATIONS

American Kidney Fund AKF). Suite 1010,6110 Executive Boulevard, Rockville, MD 20852. (800) 638-8299. < http://216.248.130.102/Default.htm >.

National Kidney Foundation. 30 East 33rd St., New York, NY 10016. (800) 622-9010. < http://www.kidney.org >.

OTHER

"Glomerulonephritis." *National Institute of Diabetes and Digestive and Kidney Disease.* < http://www.niddk.nih.gov >.

Maureen Haggerty

Nephroblastoma *see* **Wilms' tumor**

Nephrocarcinoma *see* **Kidney cancer**

Nephrotic syndrome

Definition

Nephrotic syndrome is a collection of symptoms which occur because the tiny blood vessels (the glomeruli) in the kidney become leaky. This allows protein (normally never passed out in the urine) to leave the body in large amounts.

Description

The glomeruli (a single one is called a glomerulus) are tiny tufts of capillaries (the smallest type of blood vessels). Glomeruli are located in the kidneys, where they allow a certain amount of water and waste products to leave the blood, ultimately to be passed out of the body in the form of urine. Normally, proteins are unable to pass through the glomerular filter. Nephrotic syndrome, however, occurs when this filter becomes defective, allowing large quantities of protein to leave the blood circulation, and pass out or the body in the urine.

Patients with nephrotic syndrome are from all age groups, although in children there is an increased risk of the disorder between the ages of 18 months and four years. In children, boys are more frequently affected; in adults, the ratio of men to women is closer to equal.

Causes and symptoms

Nephrotic syndrome can be caused by a number of different diseases. The common mechanism which seems to cause damage involves the immune system. For some reason, the immune system seems to become directed against the person's own kidney. The glomeruli become increasingly leaky as various substances from the immune system are deposited within the kidney.

A number of different kidney disorders are associated with nephrotic syndrome, including:

- minimal change disease or MCD (responsible for about 80% of nephrotic syndrome in children, and about 20% in adults) MCD is a disorder of the glomeruli

- focal glomerulosclerosis

- membranous glomerulopathy

- membranoproliferative glomerulonephropathy

Other types of diseases can also result in nephrotic syndrome. These include diabetes, sickle-cell anemia, **amyloidosis**, systemic lupus erythematosus, **sarcoidosis**, leukemia, lymphoma, cancer of the breast, colon, and stomach, reactions to drugs (including **nonsteroidal anti-inflammatory drugs**, lithium, and street heroine), allergic reactions (to insect stings, snake venom, and poison ivy), infections (**malaria**, various bacteria, **hepatitis B**, herpes zoster, and the virus which causes **AIDS**), and severe high blood pressure.

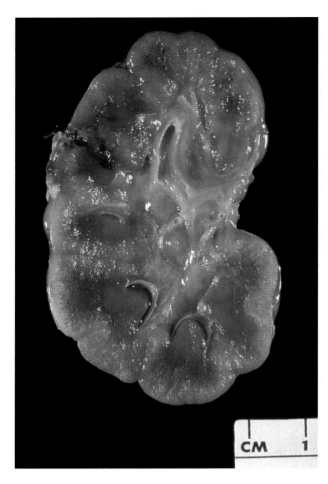

A specimen of a nephrotic human kidney. *(Custom Medical Stock Photo. Reproduced by permission.)*

Diagnosis

Diagnosis is based first on the laboratory examination of the urine and the blood. While the urine will reveal significant quantities of protein, the blood will reveal abnormally low amounts of circulating proteins. Blood tests will also reveal a high level of cholesterol. In order to diagnose one of the kidney disorders which cause nephrotic syndrome, a small sample of the kidney (biopsy) will need to be removed for examination. This biopsy can be done with a long, very thin needle which is inserted through the skin under the ribs.

Treatment

Treatment depends on the underlying disorder which has caused nephrotic syndrome. Medications which dampen down the immune system are a mainstay of treatment. The first choice is usually a steroid drug (such as prednisone). Some conditions may require even more potent medications, such as cyclophosphamide or cyclosporine. Treating the underlying conditions (lymphoma, cancers, heroine use, infections) which have led to nephrotic syndrome will often improve the symptoms of nephrotic syndrome as well. Some patients will require the use of specific medications to control high blood pressure. Occasionally, the quantity of fluid a patient is allowed to drink is restricted. Some patients benefit from the use of **diuretics** (which allow the kidney to produce more urine) to decrease swelling.

Prognosis

Prognosis depends on the underlying disorder. Minimal change disease has the best prognosis of all

The first symptom of nephrotic syndrome is often foamy urine. As the syndrome progresses, swelling (**edema**) is noticed in the eyelids, hands, feet, knees, scrotum, and abdomen. The patient feels increasingly weak and fatigued. Appetite is greatly decreased. Over time, the loss of protein causes the muscles to become weak and small (called muscle wasting). The patient may note abdominal **pain** and difficulty breathing. Because the kidneys are involved in blood pressure regulation, abnormally low or abnormally high blood pressure may develop.

Over time, the protein loss occurring in nephrotic syndrome will result in a generally malnourished state. Hair and nails become brittle, and growth is stunted. Bone becomes weak, and the body begins to lose other important nutrients (sugar, potassium, calcium). Infection is a serious and frequent complication, as are disorders of blood clotting. Acute kidney failure may develop.

the kidney disorders, with 90% of all patients responding to treatment. Other types of kidney diseases have less favorable outcomes, with high rates of progression to kidney failure. When nephrotic syndrome is caused by another, treatable disorder (infection, allergic or drug reaction), the prognosis is very good.

Resources

ORGANIZATIONS

American Kidney Fund (AKF). Suite 1010, 6110 Executive Boulevard, Rockville, MD 20852. (800) 638-8299. < http://216.248.130.102/Default.htm >.

National Kidney Foundation. 30 East 33rd St., New York, NY 10016. (800) 622-9010. < http://www.kidney.org >.

Rosalyn Carson-DeWitt, MD

Nephrotoxic injury

Definition

Nephrotoxic injury is damage to one or both of the kidneys that results from exposure to a toxic material, usually through ingestion.

Description

The kidneys are the primary organs of the urinary system, which purifies the blood by removing wastes from it and excreting them from the body in urine. Every day, the kidneys filter about 45 gal (180 l) of blood, about four times as much as the amount that passes through any other organ. Because of this high volume, the kidneys are more often exposed to toxic substances in the blood and are very vulnerable to injury from those sources.

Each kidney contains over one million structures called nephrons. Each nephron consists of two parts: the renal corpuscle and the renal tubule. The renal corpuscle is where the blood is filtered. It is made up of a network of capillaries (the glomerulus) and the structure that surrounds these capillaries (Bowman's capsule). Blood flows into the glomerulus, where the liquid part of the blood (plasma) passes through the walls of the capillaries and into Bowman's capsule (blood cells and some proteins are too big to pass through and therefore remain in the blood vessels). The plasma, now called filtrate, contains substances that the body needs, such as water, glucose, and other nutrients, as well as wastes, excess salts, and excess water. When the filtrate moves from Bowman's

capsule into the renal tubules, about 99% of it is taken back up as the action of the tubules allows beneficial substances to be reabsorbed into the blood stream. The remaining filtrate is then passed to the bladder as urine.

When the kidneys are exposed to a toxic agent, either accidentally or intentionally (as in a suicide attempt), damage can occur in a number of different ways, depending upon the agent. One toxin may directly affect the glomerulus or the renal tubules, causing the cells of these structures to die. Another toxin may create other substances or conditions that result in the same cell death. Nephrotoxic injury can lead to acute renal failure, in which the kidneys suddenly lose their ability to function, or chronic renal failure, in which kidney function slowly deteriorates. If unchecked, renal failure can result in death.

Causes and symptoms

Several different substances can be toxic to the kidneys. These include:

- **antibiotics**, primarily **aminoglycosides**, sulphonamides, amphotericin B, polymyxin, neomycin, bacitracin, rifampin, trimethoprim, cephaloridine, methicillin, aminosalicylic acid, oxy- and chlorotetracyclines

- **analgesics**, including **acetaminophen** (Tylenol), all nonsteroidal anti-inflammatory drugs (e.g. **aspirin**, ibuprofen), all prostaglandin synthetase inhibitors

- contrast agents used in some diagnostic tests, such as sodium iodide

- heavy metals, such as lead, mercury, arsenic, and uranium

- anti-cancer drugs, such as cyclosporin, cisplatin, and cyclophosphamide

- methemoglobin-producing agents

- solvents and fuels, such as carbon tetrachloride, methanol, amyl alcohol, and ethylene glycol

- herbicides and pesticides

- overproduction of uric acid

Nephrotoxic injury is most commonly caused by drugs, primarily antibiotics, analgesics, and contrast agents. In some cases, such as with aminoglycosides and amphotericin B, the drug itself will damage the kidneys. In others, such as with methicillin, sulphonamides, and some contrast agents, the drug provokes an allergic reaction that destroys the kidneys. Some chemicals found in certain drugs and industrial agents damage the kidneys by converting the hemoglobin of red blood cells into methemoglobin, thereby interfering with the blood's transport of oxygen. In hospitals, the most common form of nephrotoxic injury is antibiotic nephropathy, which usually occurs when antibiotics are given to patients with already weakened kidneys. Analgesic nephropathy is another common form of nephrotoxic injury and occurs as a result of long-term abuse of analgesics, usually NSAIDs (e.g., ibuprofen). Analgesic nephropathy is most prevalent in women over 30. Lead nephropathy, arising from lead poisoning, and nephropathy, from ingestion of the solvent carbon tetrachloride, are also more common forms of nephrotoxic injury. Uric acid nephropathy is one form of nephropathy that is not caused by exposure to an external toxin; instead, it arises from the body's overproduction of uric acid, usually in persons with diseases of the lymph nodes or bone marrow.

Risk factors for nephrotoxic injury include:

- Age. The elderly are more likely to overdose on antibiotics or analgesics.

- Underlying **kidney disease**. Kidneys already weakened by conditions such as diabetes can be particularly susceptible to nephrotoxic injury.

- Severe **dehydration**.

- Prolonged exposure to heavy metals or solvents on the job or in the home.

- Presence of diseases that cause the overproduction of uric acid.

Symptoms of nephrotoxic injury are wide ranging and, in some cases, depend upon the type of toxin involved. In general, symptoms are similar to those of renal failure and include excess urea in the blood (azotemia), anemia, increased hydrogen ion concentration in the blood (acidosis), excess fluids in the body (**overhydration**), and high blood pressure (**hypertension**). Blood or pus may be present in the urine, as may uric acid crystals. A decrease in urinary output may also occur. If the toxin's effect on the kidneys remains unchecked, more serious symptoms of kidney failure may occur, including seizures and **coma**.

Diagnosis

Damage to the kidneys is assessed through a combination of physical examination, blood tests, urine tests, and imaging procedures. Diagnosis of nephrotoxic injury as the underlying cause results from a thorough investigation of the patient's history. Information regarding preexisting conditions, current prescriptions, and environmental exposures to toxins

---

KEY TERMS

Bowman's capsule—The structure surrounding the glomerulus.

Chelate—A chemical that binds to heavy metals in the blood, thereby helping the body to excrete them in urine.

Contrast agent—Substance ingested so as to highlight anatomical structures in x-ray imaging tests.

Diuretic—A drug that promotes the excretion of urine.

Glomerulus—A network of capillaries located in the nephron where wastes are filtered from the blood.

Methemoglobin—A compound formed from hemoglobin by oxidation.

Nephron—Basic functional unit of the kidney.

Nephrotoxin—Substance that is poisonous to the kidneys.

Renal failure—Disorder characterized by the kidney's inability to filter wastes from the blood. It may be acute (occuring suddenly and usually reversable) or chronic (developing slowly over time as a result of permanent damage).

---

aid the physician in determining what toxin, if any, has caused the kidneys to malfunction.

Treatment

Treatment of nephrotoxic injury takes place in the hospital and focuses on removing the toxin from the patient's system, while maintaining kidney function. Removal methods are targeted to specific toxins and may include the use of **diuretics** or chelates to enhance excretion of the toxin in urine, or, in extreme cases, the direct removal of toxins from the blood via hemodialysis or passing the blood over an absorbent substance such as charcoal. Support of kidney function depends on the extent of damage to the organs and ranges from monitoring fluid levels to dialysis.

Prognosis

The outcome of nephrotoxic injury is determined by the cause and severity of the damage. In cases where damage has not progressed beyond acute renal failure, kidney function can be fully restored once the toxin is removed from the system and equilibrium restored.

However, if permanent damage has resulted in chronic renal failure, lifelong dialysis or a kidney transplant may be required.

Prevention

Exposure to nephrotoxins can be minimized several different ways. When taking antibiotics or analgesics, recommended dosages should be strictly followed. Also, elderly patients on these medications (for example, those taking aspirin for heart problems or NSAIDs for arthritis) should be closely monitored to prevent accidental overdose. Health care workers should be aware of any underlying conditions, such as diabetes or **allergies** to antibiotics, that may heighten the effect of a potential nephrotoxin. When using solvents or handling heavy metals, procedures regarding their safe use should be employed.

Resources

ORGANIZATIONS

American Kidney Fund (AKF). Suite 1010, 6110 Executive Boulevard, Rockville, MD 20852. (800) 638-8299. < http://216.248.130.102/Default.htm >.
National Kidney Foundation. 30 East 33rd St., New York, NY 10016. (800) 622-9010. < http://www.kidney.org >.

Bridget Travers

Nerve conduction velocity testing *see* **Electromyography**

Neural hearing loss *see* **Hearing loss**

Neuralgia

Definition

Neuralgia is defined as an intense burning or stabbing pain caused by irritation of or damage to a nerve. The **pain** is usually brief but may be severe. It often feels as if it is shooting along the course of the affected nerve.

Description

Different types of neuralgia occur depending on the reason the nerve has been irritated. Neuralgia can be triggered by a variety of causes, including tooth decay, eye strain, or **shingles** (an infection caused by the herpes zoster virus). Pain is usually felt in the part of the body that is supplied by the irritated nerve.

Causes and symptoms

Neuralgia is caused by irritation or nerve damage from systemic disease, inflammation, infection, and compression or physical irritation of a nerve. The location of the pain depends on the underlying condition that is irritating the nerve or the location of the particular nerve that is being irritated.

Neuralgia can result from **tooth decay**, poor diet, eye strain, nose infections, or exposure to damp and cold. Postherpetic neuralgia is an intense debilitating pain felt at the site of a previous attack of shingles. **Trigeminal neuralgia** (also called tic douloureux, the most common type of neuralgia), causes a brief, searing pain along the trigeminal nerve, which supplies sensation to the face. The facial pain of migraine neuralgia lasts between 30 minutes and an hour and occurs at the same time on successive days. The cause is not known.

Glossopharyngeal neuralgia is an intense pain felt at the back of the tongue, in the throat, and in the ear—all areas served by the glossopharyngeal nerve. The pain may occur spontaneously, or it can be triggered by talking, eating, or swallowing (especially cold foods such as ice cream). Its cause is not known.

Occipital neuralgia is caused by a pinched occipital nerve. There are two occipital nerves, each located at the back of the neck, each supplying feeling to the skin over half of the back of the head. These nerves can be pinched due to factors ranging from arthritis to injury, but the result is the same: **numbness**, pain, or **tingling** over half the base of the skull.

Diagnosis

Neuralgia is a symptom of an underlying disorder; its diagnosis depends on finding the cause of the condition creating the pain.

To diagnose occipital neuralgia, a doctor can inject a small amount of anesthetic into the region of the occipital nerve. If the pain temporarily disappears, and there are no other physical reasons for the pain, the doctor may recommend surgery to deal with the pinched nerve.

Treatment

Glossopharyngeal, trigeminal, and postherpetic neuralgias sometimes respond to **anticonvulsant drugs**, such as carbamazepine or phenytoin, or to painkillers, such as **acetaminophen**. Trigeminal neuralgia may also be relieved by surgery in which the nerve is cut or decompressed. In some cases, compression neuralgia (including occipital neuralgia) can be relieved by surgery.

People with shingles should see a doctor within three days of developing the rash, since aggressive treatment of the blisters that appear with the rash can ease the severity of the infection and minimize the risk of developing postherpetic neuralgia. However, it is not clear whether the treatment can prevent postherpetic neuralgia.

If postherpetic neuralgia develops, a variety of treatments can be tried, since their effectiveness varies from person-to-person.

- antidepressants such as amitriptyline (Elavil)
- anticonvulsants (phenytoin, valproate, or carbamazepine)
- capsaicin (Xostrix), the only medication approved by the FDA for treatment of postherpetic neuralgia
- topical painkillers
- desensitization
- TENS (transcutaneous **electrical nerve stimulation**)
- dorsal root zone (DREZ) surgery (a treatment of last resort)

Alternative treatment

B-complex **vitamins**, primarily given by intramuscular injection, can be an effective treatment. A whole foods diet with adequate protein, carbohydrates, and fats that also includes yeast, liver, wheat germ, and foods that are high in B vitamins may be helpful. **Acupuncture** is a very effective treatment, especially for postherpetic neuralgia. Homeopathic treatment can also be very effective when the correct remedy is used. Some botanical medicines may also be useful. For example, black cohosh (*Cimicifuga racemosa*) appears to have anti-inflammatory properties based on recent research.

Prognosis

The effectiveness of the treatment depends on the cause of the neuralgia, but many cases respond to pain relief.

Trigeminal neuralgia tends to come and go, but successive attacks may be disabling. Although neuralgia is not fatal, the patient's fear of being in pain can seriously interfere with daily life.

Some people with postherpetic neuralgia respond completely to treatment. Most people, however, experience some pain after treatment, and a few receive no

---

KEY TERMS

Desensitization—A technique of pain reduction in which the painful area is stimulated with whatever is causing the pain.

Dorsal root entry zone (DREZ)—A type of nerve surgery for postherpetic neuralgia that is occasionally used when the patient can get no other pain relief. The surgery destroys the area where damaged nerves join the central nervous system, thereby interfering with inappropriate pain messages from nerves to the brain.

Glossopharyngeal neuralgia—Sharp recurrent pain deep in the throat that extends to the area around the tonsils and possibly the ear. It is triggered by swallowing or chewing.

Migraine neuralgia—A variant of migraine pain, also called cluster headache, in which severe attacks of pain affect the eye and forehead on one side of the face.

Occipital neuralgia—Pain on one side of the back of the head caused by entrapment or pinching of an occipital nerve.

Postherpetic neuralgia—Persistent pain that occurs as a complication of a herpes zoster infection. Although the pain can be treated, the response is variable.

Shingles—A painful rash with blisters that appears along the course of a nerve. It is caused by infection with herpes zoster virus.

TENS—The abbreviation for transcutaneous electrical nerve stimulation, a technique used to control chronic pain. Electrodes placed over the painful area deliver a mild electrical impulse to nearby nerve pathways, thereby easing pain.

Trigeminal neuralgia—Brief episodes of severe shooting pain on one side of the face caused by inflammation of the root of the trigeminal nerve. Also referred to as tic douloureux.

---

relief at all. Some people live with this type of neuralgia for the rest of their lives, but for most, the condition gradually fades away within five years.

Resources

PERIODICALS

Fields, H. "Treatment of Trigeminal Neuralgia." *The New England Journal of Medicine* 334 (April 1996): 1125-1126.

ORGANIZATIONS

American Chronic Pain Association. P.O. Box 850, Rocklin, CA 95677-0850. (916) 632-0922. < http:// members.tripod.com/~widdy/ACPA.html >.

National Chronic Pain Outreach Association. P.O. Box 274, Millboro, VA 24460. (540) 997-5004.

Trigeminal Neuralgia/Tic Douloureux Association. P.O. Box 340, Barnegat Light, NJ 08006. (609) 361-1014.

Carol A. Turkington

Neuroblastoma

Definition

Neuroblastoma is a type of **cancer** that usually originates either in the tissues of the adrenal gland or in the ganglia of the abdomen or in the ganglia of the nervous system. (Ganglia are masses of nerve tissue or groups of nerve cells.) Tumors develop in the nerve tissue in the neck, chest, abdomen, or pelvis.

Description

Neuroblastoma is one of the few cancer types known to secrete hormones. It occurs most often in children, and it is the third most common cancer that occurs in children. Approximately 7.5% of the childhood cancers diagnosed in 2001 were neuroblastomas, affecting one in 80,000 to 100,000 children in the United States. Close to 50% of cases of neuroblastoma occur in children younger than two years old. The disease is sometimes present at birth, but is usually not noticed until later. By the time the disease is diagnosed, it has often spread to the lymph nodes, liver, lungs, bones, or bone marrow. Approximately one-third of neuroblastomas start in the adrenal glands.

Demographics

According to some reports, African-American children develop the disease at a slightly higher rate than Caucasian children (8.7 per million compared to 8.0 per million cases diagnosed).

Causes and symptoms

The causes of neuroblastoma are not precisely known. Current research holds that neuroblastomas develop when cells produced by the fetus (neuroblast cells) fail to mature into normal nerve or adrenal cells and keep growing and proliferating. The first symptom of a neuroblastoma is usually an unusual growth or lump, found in most cases in the abdomen of the child, causing discomfort or a sensation of fullness and **pain**. Other symptoms such as **numbness** and **fatigue**, arise because of pressure caused by the tumor. Bone pain also occurs if the cancer has spread to the bone. If it has spread to the area behind the eye, the cancer may cause protruding eyes and dark circles around the eyes; in a few cases, blindness may be the presenting symptom. Or **paralysis** may result from compression of the spinal cord. **Fever** is also reported in one case out of four. High blood pressure, persistent **diarrhea**, rapid heartbeat, reddening of the skin and sweating occur occasionally. Some children may also have uncoordinated or jerky muscle movements, or uncontrollable eye movements, but these symptoms are rare. If the disease spreads to the skin, blue or purple patches are observed.

Diagnosis

A diagnosis of neuroblastoma usually requires blood and urine tests to investigate the nature and quantity of chemicals (neurotransmitters) released by the nerve cells. These are broken down by the body and released in urine. Additionally, scanning techniques are used to confirm the diagnosis of neuroblastoma. These techniques produce images or pictures of the inside of the body and they include computed tomography scan (CT scan) and **magnetic resonance imaging** (MRI). To confirm the diagnosis, the physician will surgically remove some of the tissue from the tumor or bone marrow (biopsy), and examine the cells under the microscope.

Treatment

The treatment team usually consists of an oncologist specialized in the treatment of neuroblastoma, a surgeon to perform biopsies and possibly attempt surgical removal of the tumor, a **radiation therapy** team and, if indicated, a **bone marrow transplantation** team.

Staging

Once neuroblastoma has been diagnosed, the physician will perform more tests to determine if the cancer has spread to other tissues in the body. This process, called staging, is important for the physician to determine how to treat the cancer and check liver and kidney function. The staging system for neuroblastoma is based on how far the disease has spread from its original site to other tissues in the body.

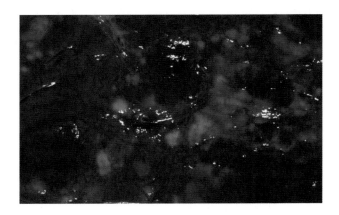

A neuroblastoma appearing at the surface of the liver. *(Custom Medical Stock Photo. Reproduced by permission.)*

Localized resectable (able to be cut out) neuroblastoma is confined to the site of origin, with no evidence that it has spread to other tissues, and the cancer can be surgically removed. Localized unresectable neuroblastoma is confined to the site of origin, but the cancer cannot be completely removed surgically. Regional neuroblastoma has extended beyond its original site, to regional lymph nodes, and/or surrounding organs or tissues, but has not spread to distant sites in the body. Disseminated neuroblastoma has spread to distant lymph nodes, bone, liver, skin, bone marrow, and/or other organs. Stage 4S (or IVS, or "special") neuroblastoma has spread only to liver, skin, and/or, to a very limited extent, bone marrow. Recurrent neuroblastoma means that the cancer has come back, or continued to spread after it has been treated. It may come back in the original site or in another part of the body.

Treatments are available for children with all stages of neuroblastoma. More than one of these treatments may be used, depending on the stage of the disease. The four types of treatment used are:

- surgery (removing the tumor in an operation)
- radiation therapy (using high-energy x-rays to kill cancer cells)
- **chemotherapy** (using drugs to kill cancer cells)
- bone marrow transplantation (replacing the patient's bone marrow cells with those from a healthy person)

Surgery is used whenever possible, to remove as much of the cancer as possible, and can generally cure the disease if the cancer has not spread to other areas of the body. Before surgery, chemotherapy may be used to shrink the tumor so that it can be more easily removed during surgery; this is called neoadjuvant chemotherapy. Radiation therapy is often used after surgery; high-energy rays (radiation) are used to kill as many of the remaining cancer cells as possible. Chemotherapy (called adjuvant chemotherapy) may also be used after surgery to kill remaining cells. Bone marrow transplantation is used to replace bone marrow cells killed by radiation or chemotherapy. In some cases the patient's own bone marrow is removed prior to treatment and saved for transplantation later. Other times the bone marrow comes from a "matched" donor, such as a sibling.

One novel approach to treatment of neuroblastomas is therapy with desferoxamine (DFO), which is ordinarily used to treat iron **poisoning**. DFO has been shown to have antitumor activity in neuroblastomas and other cancers of the central nervous system. It is thought that the drug works by lowering the increased iron levels in the body associated with cancer.

As of 2004, there are significant differences in treatment protocols for neuroblastoma between the major North American study group (Children's Oncology Group) and its European counterpart, the Société Internationale d'Oncologie Pédiatrique (SIOP). These differences include biopsy techniques, the timing and extent of surgery, chemotherapy dosages, and the types of salvage therapy employed.

Alternative treatment

No alternative therapy has yet been reported to substitute for conventional neuroblastoma treatment. Complementary therapies—such as retinoic acid therapy—have been shown to be beneficial to patients when administered after a conventional course of chemotherapy or transplantation.

Prognosis

The chances of recovery from neuroblastoma depend on the stage of the cancer, the age of the child at diagnosis, the location of the tumor, and the state and nature of the tumor cells evaluated under the microscope. Infants have a higher rate of cure than do children over one year of age, even when the disease has spread. In general, the prognosis for a young child with neuroblastoma is good: the predicted five-year survival rate is approximately 85% for children who had the onset of the disease in infancy, and 35% for those whose disease developed later.

Prevention

Neuroblastoma may be a genetic disease passed down from the parents. In 2004, a group of German

KEY TERMS

Adjuvant chemotherapy—Treatment of the tumor with drugs after surgery to kill as many of the remaining cancer cells as possible.

Adrenal gland—Gland located above each kidney consisting of an outer wall (cortex) that produces steroid hormones and an inner section (medulla) that produces other important hormones, such as adrenaline and noradrenaline.

Alternative therapy—A therapy is generally called alternative when it is used instead of conventional cancer treatments.

Biopsy—A small sample of tissue removed from the site of the tumor to be examined under a microscope.

Conventional therapy—Treatments that are widely accepted and practiced by the mainstream medical community.

Complementary therapy—A therapy is called complementary when it is used in addition to conventional cancer treatments.

Disseminated—Spread to other tissues.

Hormone—A substance produced by specialized cells that affects the way the body carries out the biochemical and energy-producing processes required to maintain health (metabolism.

Localized—Confined to a small area.

Neoadjuvant chemotherapy—Treatment of the tumor with drugs before surgery to reduce the size of the tumor.

Neuroblast cells—Cells produced by the fetus which mature into nerve cells and adrenal medulla cells.

Monoclonal antibody—A protein substance which is produced in the laboratory by a single population of cells. They are being tested as a possible form of cancer treatment.

Resectable cancer—A tumor that can be surgically removed.

Salvage therapy—Treatment measures taken late in the course of a disease after other therapies have failed. It is also known as rescue therapy.

Staging system—A system based on how far the cancer has spread from its original site, developed to help the physician determine how best to treat the disease.

Unresectable cancer—A tumor that cannot be completely removed by surgery.

researchers reported that a series of neuroblastomas demonstrated a consistent pattern of deletions and overrepresentations on chromosomes 3, 10, 17q, and 20. There is currently no known method for its prevention.

Special concerns

After completion of a course of treatment for neuroblastoma, physicians sometimes recommend that the child undergo an investigative operation. This procedure allows the treatment team to evaluate how effective treatment has been, and may offer an opportunity to remove more of the tumor if it is still present.

Resources

BOOKS

Alexander, F. "Neuroblastoma." *Urol. Clin. North. Am.* 27, August 2000, pp. 383-92.

Beers, Mark H., MD, and Robert Berkow, MD., editors. "Neuroblastoma." Section 19, Chapter 266 In *The Merck Manual of Diagnosis and Therapy*. Whitehouse Station, NJ: Merck Research Laboratories, 2004.

PERIODICALS

Alexander, F. "Neuroblastoma." *Urol. Clin. North. Am.* 27 (August 2000): 383–392.

Berthold, F., and B. Hero. "Neuroblastoma: current drug therapy recommendations as part of the total treatment approach." *Drugs* 59 (June 2000): 1261–1277.

Bockmuhl, U., X. You, M. Pacyna-Gengelbach, et al. "CGH Pattern of Esthesioneuroblastoma and Their Metastases." *Brain Pathology* 14 (April 2004): 158–163.

Dayani, P. N., M. C. Bishop, K. Plack, and P. M. Zeltzer. "Desferoxamine (DFO)—Mediated Iron Chelation: Rationale for a Novel Approach to Therapy for Brain Cancer." *Journal of Neurooncology* 67 (May 2004): 367–377.

Grosfeld, J. L. "Risk-based management of solid tumors in children." *American Journal of Surgery* 180 (November 2000):322–327.

Lau, J. J., J. D. Trobe, R. E. Ruiz, et al. "Metastatic Neuroblastoma Presenting with Binocular Blindness from Intracranial Compression of the Optic Nerves." *Journal of Neuroophthalmology* 24 (June 2004): 119–124.

Morgenstern, B. Z., A. P. Krivoshik, V. Rodriguez, and P. M. Anderson. "Wilms' Tumor and Neuroblastoma." *Acta Paediatrica Supplementum* 93 (May 2004): 78–84.

Pinkerton, C., R. Blanc, M. P. Vincent, C. Bergeron, B. Fervers, and T. Philip. "Induction chemotherapy in metastatic neuroblastoma—does dose influence response? A critical review of published data standards, options and recommendations (SOR) project of the National Federation of French Cancer Centres

(FNCLCC)." *European Journal of Cancer* 36 (September 2000): 1808–1815.

ORGANIZATIONS

The American Cancer Society. "After Diagnosis: A Guide for Patients and Families." "Caring for the Patient with Cancer at Home." "Understanding Chemotherapy: A Guide for Patients and Families." "Understanding Radiation Therapy: A Guide for Patients and Families."

National Cancer Institute. Office of Cancer Communications, 31 Center Drive, MSC 2580, Bethesda, MD 20892-2580. 800-422-6237. < http://cancernet.nci.nih.gov/clinpdq/pif/Neuroblastoma_Patient.html >.

National Institutes of Health & National Cancer Institute. *Young People With Cancer: A Handbook for Parents.* < http://www.cancernet.nci.nih.gov/young_people/yngconts.html >.

Lisa Christenson, PhD
Monique Laberge, PhD
Rebecca J. Frey, PhD

Neuroendocrine tumors

Definition

Neuroendocrine tumor refers to the type of cell that a tumor grows from rather than where that tumor is located. Neuroendocrine cells produce hormones or regulatory proteins, and so tumors of these cells usually have symptoms that are related to the specific hormones that they produce.

Description

Neuroendocrine cells have roles both in the endocrine system and the nervous system. They produce and secrete a variety of regulatory hormones, or neuropeptides, which include neurotransmitters and growth factors. When these cells become cancerous, they grow and overproduce their specific neuropeptide. Neuroendocrine tumors are generally rare. One type of neuroendocrine tumor is a carcinoid tumor. This type of tumor can occur in the intestinal tract, appendix, rectum, bronchial tubes, or ovary. Most carcinoid tumors secrete serotonin. When the blood concentration of this hormone is high enough, it causes carcinoid syndrome. This syndrome refers to a variety of symptoms that are caused by the excessive amount of hormone secreted rather than the tumor itself.

The total incidence of neuroendocrine tumors is thought to be between five and nine million people in the United States. It is possible that these tumors are underreported because they grow slowly and do not always produce dramatic symptoms.

Causes and symptoms

Many of the symptoms of carcinoid tumor are due to the hormones that the tumor secretes. These hormones can affect the whole body and cause what is referred to as carcinoid syndrome. The most common symptom of carcinoid syndrome is flushing, a sudden appearance of redness and warmth in the face and neck that can last from minutes to hours. Other symptoms of carcinoid syndrome are **diarrhea**, asthma-like symptoms and heart problems. Since most carcinoid tumors are found in the appendix, the symptoms are often similar to **appendicitis**, primarily **pain** in the abdomen. When these tumors are found in the small intestine, they can cause abdominal pain that is often initially diagnosed as bowel obstruction. Many patients have no symptoms and the carcinoids are found during routine endoscopy of the intestines.

Diagnosis

The diagnosis of carcinoid syndrome is made by the measurement of 5–hydroxy indole acetic acid (5–HIAA) in the urine. 5–HIAA is a breakdown (waste) product of serotonin. If the syndrome is diagnosed, the presence of carcinoid tumor is a given. When the syndrome is not present, diagnosis may be delayed, due to the vague symptoms present. Diagnosis can sometimes take up to two years. It is made by performing a number of tests, and the specific test used depends on the tumor's suspected location. The tests that may be performed include gastrointestinal endoscopy, **chest x ray**, computed tomography scan (CT scan), **magnetic resonance imaging**, or ultrasound. A biopsy of the tumor is performed for diagnosis. A variety of hormones can be measured in the blood as well to indicate the presence of a carcinoid.

Treatment

The only effective treatment for carcinoid tumor as of the early 2000s is surgical removal of the tumor. Although **chemotherapy** is sometimes used when metastasis has occurred, it is rarely effective. The treatment for carcinoid syndrome is typically meant to decrease the severity of symptoms. Patients should avoid **stress** as well as foods that bring on the syndrome. Some medications can be given for

KEY TERMS

Appendicitis—Inflammation of the appendix.

Growth factor—A local hormone produced by some cells that initiates growth.

Metastasis—The spread of disease from one part of the body to another, as when cancer cells appear in parts of the body remote from the site of the primary tumor.

Neurotransmitter—A chemical messenger used to transmit information in the nervous system.

symptomatic relief; for example, tumors of the gastrointestinal tract may be treated with octreotide (Sandostatin) or lanreotide (Somatuline) to relieve such symptoms as diarrhea and flushing. These drugs are known as somatostatin analogs.

Liver transplantation is a treatment option for patients with neuroendocrine tumors that have metastasized only to the liver. As of 2004, this approach is reported to offer patients long disease-free periods and relief of symptoms.

Prognosis

The prognosis of carcinoid tumors is related to the specific growth patterns of that tumor, as well as its location. For example, a group of researchers at the University of Wisconsin reported in 2004 that patients with gastrointestinal tumors in the hindgut had longer periods of disease-free survival than those with foregut or midgut cancers. For localized disease the five-year survival rate can be 94%, whereas for patients where metastasis has occurred, the average five-year survival rate is 18%. It is not unusual for patients with carcinoid tumors to live ten or fifteen years after the initial diagnosis.

Prevention

Neuroendocrine tumors such as carcinoid tumors are rare, and no information consequently is yet available on cause or prevention.

Resources

BOOKS

Beers, Mark H., MD, and Robert Berkow, MD., editors. "Carcinoid Tumors." Section 2, Chapter 17 In *The Merck Manual of Diagnosis and Therapy*. Whitehouse Station, NJ: Merck Research Laboratories, 2004.

PERIODICALS

Ahlman, H., S. Friman, C. Cahli, et al. "Liver Transplantation for Treatment of Metastatic Neuroendocrine Tumors." *Annals of the New York Academy of Sciences* 1014 (April 2004): 265–269.

Oberg, K., L. Kvols, M. Caplin, et al. "Consensus Report on the Use of Somatostatin Analogs for the Management of Neuroendocrine Tumors of the Gastroenteropancreatic System." *Annals of Oncology* 15 (June 2004): 966–973.

Singhal, Hemant, MD, and Alan A. Saber, MD. "Carcinoid Tumor, Intestinal." *eMedicine* April 13, 2004. < http:// www.emedicine.com/med/topic271.htm >.

Van Gompel, J. J., R. S. Sippel, T. F. Warner, and H. Chen. "Gastrointestinal Carcinoid Tumors: Factors That Predict Outcome." *World Journal of Surgery* 28 (April 2004): 387–392.

ORGANIZATIONS

Carcinoid Cancer Foundation, Inc. 1751 York Ave., New York, NY 10128. (212) 722-3132. < http:// www.carcinoid.org >.

Cindy L. A. Jones, PhD
Rebecca J. Frey, PhD

Neurofibromatosis

Definition

Neurofibromatosis (NF), or von Recklinghausen disease, is a genetic disease in which patients develop multiple soft tumors (neurofibromas). These tumors occur under the skin and throughout the nervous system.

Description

Neural crest cells are primitive cells which exist during fetal development. These cells eventually turn into:

- cells which form nerves throughout the brain, spinal cord, and body
- cells which serve as coverings around the nerves that course through the body
- pigment cells, which provide color to structures
- the meninges, the thin, membranous coverings of the brain and spinal cord
- cells which ultimately develop into the bony structures of the head and neck

In neurofibromatosis, a genetic defect causes these neural crest cells to develop abnormally. This results in numerous tumors and malformations of the nerves, bones, and skin.

Neurofibromatosis occurs in about one of every 4,000 births. Two types of NF exist, NF-1 (90% of all cases), and NF-2 (10% of all cases).

Causes and symptoms

Both forms of neurofibromatosis are caused by a defective gene. NF-1 is due to a defect on chromosome 17; NF-2 results from a defect on chromosome 22. Both of these disorders are inherited in a dominant fashion. This means that anybody who receives just one defective gene will have the disease. However, a family pattern of NF is only evident for about half of all cases of NF. The other cases of NF occur due to a spontaneous mutation (a permanent change in the structure of a specific gene). Once such a spontaneous mutation has been established in an individual, however, it is then possible to be passed on to any offspring. The chance of a person with NF passing on the NF gene to a child is 50%.

NF-1 has a number of possible signs and can be diagnosed if any two of the following are present:

- The presence of café-au-lait (French for coffee-with-milk) spots. These are patches of tan or light brown skin, usually about 5-15 mm in diameter. Nearly all patients with NF-1 will display these spots.

- Multiple freckles in the armpit or groin area.

- Ninty percent of patients with NF-1 have tiny tumors called Lisch nodules in the iris (colored area) of the eye.

- Neurofibromas. These soft tumors are the hallmark of NF-1. They occur under the skin, often located along nerves or within the gastrointestinal tract. Neurofibromas are small and rubbery, and the skin overlying them may be somewhat purple in color.

- Skeletal deformities, such as a twisted spine (scoliosis), curved spine (humpback), or bowed legs.

- Tumors along the optic nerve, which cause vision disturbance in about 20% of patients.

- The presence of NF-1 in a patient's parent, child, or sibling.

There are very high rates of speech impairment, learning disabilities, and attention deficit disorder in children with NF-1. Other complications include the development of a **seizure disorder**, or the abnormal accumulation of fluid within the brain (hydrocephalus).

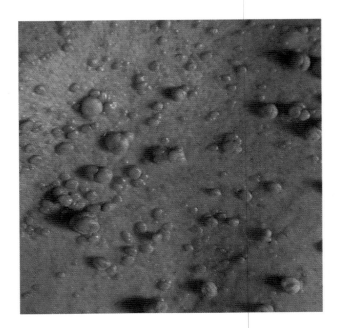

This person's skin has multiple soft tumors, or neurofibromas. Such tumors develop underneath the skin. *(Custom Medical Stock Photo. Reproduced by permission.)*

A number of cancers are more common in patients with NF-1. These include a variety of types of malignant brain tumors, as well as leukemia, and cancerous tumors of certain muscles (rhabdomyosarcoma), the adrenal glands (**pheochromocytoma**), or the kidneys (Wilms' tumor).

Patients with NF-2 do not necessarily have the same characteristic skin symptoms (café-au-lait spots, freckling, and neurofibromas of the skin) that appear in NF-1. The characteristic symptoms of NF-2 are due to tumors along the acoustic nerve. Interfering with the function of this nerve results in the loss of hearing; and the tumor may spread to neighboring nervous system structures, causing weakness of the muscles of the face, **headache**, **dizziness**, poor balance, and uncoordinated walking. Cloudy areas on the lens of the eye (called **cataracts**) frequently develop at an unusually early age. As in NF-1, the chance of brain tumors developing is unusually high.

Diagnosis

Diagnosis is based on the symptoms outlined above. Diagnosis of NF-1 requires that at least two of the listed signs are present. Diagnosis of NF-2 requires the presence of either a mass on the acoustic nerve or another distinctive nervous system tumor. An important diagnostic clue for either NF-1 or NF-2 is the presence of the disorder in a patient's parent, child, or sibling.

KEY TERMS

Chromosome—A structure within the nucleus of every cell, which contains genetic information governing the organism's development.

Mutation—A permanent change to the genetic code of an organism. Once established, a mutation can be passed on to offspring.

Neurofibroma—A soft tumor usually located on a nerve.

Tumor—An abnormally multiplying mass of cells.

Monitoring the progression of neurofibromatosis involves careful testing of vision and hearing. X-ray studies of the bones are frequently done to watch for the development of deformities. CT scans and MRI scans are performed to track the development/progression of tumors in the brain and along the nerves. Auditory evoked potentials (the electric response evoked in the cerebral cortex by stimulation of the acoustic nerve) may be helpful to determine involvement of the acoustic nerve, and EEG (electroencephalogram, a record of electrical currents in the brain) may be needed for patients with suspected seizures.

Treatment

There are no available treatments for the disorders which underlie either type of neurofibromatosis. To some extent, the symptoms of NF-1 and NF-2 can be treated individually. Skin tumors can be surgically removed. Some brain tumors, and tumors along the nerves, can be surgically removed, or treated with drugs (**chemotherapy**) or x-ray treatments (**radiation therapy**). Twisting or curving of the spine and bowed legs may require surgical treatment, or the wearing of a special brace.

Prognosis

Prognosis varies depending on the types of tumors which an individual develops. As tumors grow, they begin to destroy surrounding nerves and structures. Ultimately, this destruction can result in blindness, deafness, increasingly poor balance, and increasing difficulty with the coordination necessary for walking. Deformities of the bones and spine can also interfere with walking and movement. When cancers develop, prognosis worsens according to the specific type of **cancer**.

Prevention

There is no known way to prevent the approximately 50% of all NF cases which occur due to a spontaneous change in the genes (mutation). New cases of inherited NF can be prevented with careful **genetic counseling**. A person with NF can be made to understand that each of his or her offspring has a 50% chance of also having NF. When a parent has NF, and the specific genetic defect causing the parent's disease has been identified, tests can be performed on the fetus (developing baby) during pregnancy. Amniocentesis or chorionic villus sampling are two techniques which allow small amounts of the baby's cells to be removed for examination. The tissue can then be examined for the presence of the parent's genetic defect. Some families choose to use this information in order to prepare for the arrival of a child with a serious medical problem. Other families may choose not to continue the **pregnancy**.

Resources

ORGANIZATIONS

March of Dimes Birth Defects Foundation. 1275 Mamaroneck Ave., White Plains, NY 10605. (914) 428-7100. resourcecenter@modimes.org. < http://www.modimes.org >.

National Neurofibromatosis Foundation, Inc. 95 Pine St., 16th Floor, New York, NY 10005. (800) 323-7938. < http://nf.org >.

Neurofibromatosis, Inc. 8855 Annapolis Rd., #110, Lanham, MD 20706-2924. (800) 942-6825.

Rosalyn Carson-DeWitt, MD

Neurogenic arthropathy *see* **Charcot's joints**

Neurogenic bladder

Definition

Neurogenic bladder is a dysfunction that results from interference with the normal nerve pathways associated with urination.

Description

Normal bladder function is dependent on the nerves that sense the fullness of the bladder (sensory nerves) and on those that trigger the muscle movements that either empty it or retain urine (motor nerves). The reflex to urinate is triggered when the bladder fills to 300-500 ml. The bladder is then emptied when the contraction of the bladder wall muscles forces urine out through the urethra. The bladder, internal sphincters, and external sphincters may all be affected by nerve disorders that create abnormalities in bladder function.

There are two categories of neurogenic bladder dysfunction: overactive (spastic or hyper-reflexive) and underactive (flaccid or hypotonic). An overactive neurogenic bladder is characterized by uncontrolled, frequent expulsion of urine from the bladder. There is reduced bladder capacity and incomplete emptying of urine. An underactive neurogenic bladder has a capacity that is extremely large (up to 2000 ml). Due to a loss of the sensation of bladder filling, the bladder does not contract forcefully, and small amounts of urine dribble from the urethra as the bladder pressure reaches a breakthrough point.

Causes and symptoms

There are numerous causes for neurogenic bladder dysfunction and symptoms vary depending on the cause. An **overactive bladder** is caused by interruptions in the nerve pathways to the bladder occurring above the sacrum (five fused spinal vertebrae located just above the tailbone or coccyx). This nerve damage results in a loss of sensation and motor control and is often seen in **stroke**, Parkinson's disease, and most forms of spinal-cord injuries. An underactive bladder is the result of interrupted bladder stimulation at the level of the sacral nerves. This may result from certain types of surgery on the spinal cord, sacral spinal tumors, or congenital defects. It also may be a complication of various diseases, such as **syphilis**, **diabetes mellitus**, or **polio**.

Diagnosis

Neurogenic bladder is diagnosed by carefully recording fluid intake and urinary output and by measuring the quantity of urine remaining in the bladder after voiding (residual urine volume). This measurement is done by draining the bladder with a small rubber tube (catheter) after the person has urinated. Kidney function also is evaluated by regular laboratory testing of the blood and urine. **Cystometry** may be used to estimate the capacity of the bladder and the pressure changes within it. These measurements can help determine changes in bladder compliance in order to assess the effectiveness of treatment. Doctors may use a cystoscope to look inside the bladder and tubes that lead to it from the kidneys (ureters). **Cystoscopy** may be used to assess the loss of muscle fibers and elastic tissues and, in some cases, for removing small pieces of tissue for biopsy.

Treatment

Doctors begin treating neurogenic bladder by attempting to reduce bladder stretching (distension) through intermittent or continuous catheterization. In intermittent catheterization, a small rubber catheter is inserted at regular intervals (four to six times per day) to approximate normal bladder function. This avoids the complications that may occur when a catheter remains in the bladder's outside opening (urethra) continuously (an indwelling catheter). Intermittent catheterization should be performed using strict sterile technique (asepsis) by skilled personnel, and hourly fluid intake and output must be recorded. Patients who can use their arms may be taught to catheterize themselves.

Indwelling catheters avoid distension by emptying the bladder continuously into a bedside drainage collector. Individuals with indwelling catheters are encouraged to maintain a high fluid intake in order to prevent bacteria from accumulating and growing in the urine. Increased fluid intake also decreases the concentration of calcium in the urine, minimizing urine crystallization and the subsequent formation of stones. Moving around as much as possible and a low calcium diet also help to reduce stone formation.

Drugs may be used to control the symptoms produced by a neurogenic bladder. The unwanted contractions of an overactive bladder with only small volumes of urine may be suppressed by drugs that relax the bladder (anticholinergics) such as propantheline (Pro-Banthine) and oxybutynin (Ditropan). Contraction of an underactive bladder with normal bladder volumes may be stimulated with parasympathomimetics (drugs that mimic the action resulting from stimulation of the parasympathetic nerves) such as bethanechol (Urecholine).

Long-term management for the individual with an overactive bladder is aimed at establishing an effective spontaneous reflex voiding. The amount of fluid taken in is controlled in measured amounts during the waking hours, with sips only toward bedtime to avoid bladder distension. At regular intervals during the day (every four to six hours when fluid intake is two to three liters per 24 hours), the patient attempts to void using pressure over the bladder (Crede maneuver). The patient may also stimulate reflex voiding by abdominal tapping or stretching of the anal sphincter. The **Valsalva maneuver**, involving efforts similar to those used when straining to pass stool, produces an increase in intra-abdominal pressure that is sometimes adequate to completely empty the bladder. The amount of urine remaining in the bladder (residual volume) is estimated by a comparison of fluid intake and output. The patient also may be catheterized immediately following the voiding attempt to determine residual urine. Catheterization intervals are lengthened as the residual urine volume decreases and catheterization may be discontinued when urine residuals are at an acceptable level to prevent urinary tract infection.

For an underactive bladder, the patient may be placed on a similar bladder routine with fluid intake and output adjusted to prevent bladder distension. If an adequate voiding reflex cannot be induced, the patient may be maintained on clean intermittent catheterization.

Some individuals who are unable to control urine output (**urinary incontinence**) due to deficient sphincter tone may benefit from perineal exercises. Although this is a somewhat dated technique, male patients with extensive sphincter damage may be helped by the use of a Cunningham clamp. The clamp is applied in a horizontal fashion behind the glans of the penis and must be removed approximately every four hours for bladder emptying to prevent bacteria from growing in the urine and causing an infection. Alternation of the Cunningham clamp with use of a **condom** collection device will reduce the skin irritation sometimes caused by the clamp.

Surgery is another treatment option for incontinence. Urinary diversion away from the bladder may involve creation of a urostomy or a continent diversion. The surgical implantation of an inflatable sphincter is another option for certain patients. An indwelling urinary catheter is sometimes used when all other methods of incontinence management have failed. The long-term use of an indwelling catheter almost inevitably leads to some urinary tract infections, and contributes to the formation of urinary stones (calculi). Doctors may prescribe **antibiotics** preventively to reduce recurrent urinary tract infection.

Alternative treatment

The cause of the bladder problem must be determined and treated appropriately. If nerve damage is not permanent, homeopathy and **acupuncture** may help restore function.

Prognosis

Individuals with an overactive bladder caused by spinal cord lesions at or above the seventh thoracic vertebra, are at risk for sympathetic dysreflexia, a life-threatening condition which can occur when the

---

KEY TERMS

Anticholinergic—An agent that blocks certain nerve impulses.

Catheterization—Insertion of a slender, flexible tube into the bladder to drain urine.

Compliance—A term used to describe how well a patient's behavior follows medical advice.

Cystometry—A test of bladder function in which pressure and volume of fluid in the bladder are measured during filling, storage, and voiding.

Cystoscopy—A direct method of bladder study and visualization using a cystoscope (self-contained optical lens system). The cystoscope can be manipulated to view the entire bladder, with a guide system to pass it up into the ureters (tubes leading from the kidneys to the bladder).

Glans penis—The bulbous tip of the penis.

Motor nerves—Nerves that cause movement when stimulated.

Parasympathomimetic—An agent whose effects mimic those resulting from stimulation of the parasympathetic nerves.

Perineal—The diamond-shaped region of the body between the pubic arch and the anus.

Reflex—An involuntary response to a particular stimulus.

Sensory nerves—Nerves that convey impulses from sense organs to the higher parts of the nervous system, including the brain.

Sphincter—A band of muscles that surrounds a natural opening in the body; these muscles can open or close the opening by relaxing or contracting.

Ureter—A tube leading from one of the kidneys to the bladder.

Urethra—The tube that leads from the bladder to the outside of the body.

Urostomy—A diversion of the urinary flow away from the bladder, resulting in output through the abdominal wall. The most common method involves use of a portion of intestine to conduct the urine out through the abdomen and into an external pouch worn for urine collection.

---

bladder (and/or rectum) becomes overly full. Initial symptoms include sweating (particularly on the forehead) and **headache**, with progression to slow heart rate (bradycardia) and high blood pressure (**hypertension**). Patients should notify their physician promptly if symptoms do not subside after the bladder (or rectum) is emptied, or if the bladder (or rectum) is full and cannot be emptied.

Resources

ORGANIZATIONS

Bladder Health Council, American Foundation for Urologic Disease. 300 West Pratt St., Suite 401, Baltimore, MD 21201. (800) 242-2383 or (410) 727- 2908.

National Association for Continence. P.O. Box 8310, Spartanburg, SC 29305-8310. (800) 252-3337. <http://www.nafc.org>.

Simon Foundation for Continence. Box 835, Wilmette, IL 60091.

Kathleen D. Wright, RN

Neuroleptics *see* **Antipsychotic drugs**

▌Neurolinguistic programming

Definition

Neurolinguistic programming (NLP) is aimed at enhancing the healing process by changing the conscious and subconscious beliefs of patients about themselves, their illnesses, and the world. These limiting beliefs are "reprogrammed" using a variety of techniques drawn from other disciplines including **hypnotherapy** and psychotherapy.

Purpose

Neurolinguistic programming has been used to change the limiting beliefs of patients about their prospects of recovery from a wide variety of medical conditions including Parkinson's disease, **AIDS**, migraines, arthritis, and **cancer**. Practitioners claim to be able to cure most **phobias** in less than one hour, and to help in making lifestyle changes regarding **exercise**, diet, **smoking**, etc. NLP has also been used to treat **allergies**. In other fields, claimed benefits include improved relationships, communication, motivation, and business performance.

Description

Origins

NLP was originally developed during the early 1970s by linguistics professor John Grinder and psychology and mathematics student Richard Bandler, both of the University of California at Santa Cruz.

Studying the well-known psychotherapist Virginia Satir, the hypnotherapist Milton Erickson, the anthropologist Gregory Bateson, and others whom they considered "charismatic superstars" in their fields, Grinder and Bandler identified psychological, linguistic and behavioral characteristics that they said contributed to the greatness of these individuals. On the other hand, they found that persons experiencing emotional difficulties could be similarly identified by posture, breathing pattern, choice of words, voice tone, eye movements, body language, and other characteristics.

Grinder and Bandler then focused on using these indicators to analyze and alter patterns of thought and behavior. After publishing their findings in two books in 1975, Grinder and Bandler parted company with themselves, with a number of other collaborators, and with the University of California, continuing their work on NLP outside the formal world of academia. As a result, NLP split into a number of competing schools.

Popularized by television "infomercial" personality Anthony Robbins and others, NLP was quickly adopted in management and self-improvement circles. During the 1990s, there was growing interest in NLP's healing potential.

In a health-care context, practitioners of neurolinguistic programming first seek to identify the negative attitudes and beliefs with which a client has been "programmed" since birth. This is accomplished by asking questions and observing physical responses such as changes in skin color, muscle tension, etc. Then, a wide variety of techniques is employed to "reprogram" limiting beliefs. For example, clients with chronic illness such as AIDS or cancer might be asked to displace the despair and loss of identity caused by the disease by visualizing themselves in vigorous health. Treatment by NLP practitioners is often of shorter duration than that of other alternative practitioners, but NLP self-help seminars and courses can be quite expensive.

For those who wish to try self-treatment with NLP, a wide variety of books, audio tapes, and videos are available.

Precautions

NLP is particularly popular in the self-improvement and career-development fields, and some trainers and practitioners have little experience in its use for healing. Practitioners should be specifically asked about this.

Because NLP is intended to enhance the healing process, it should not be used independently of other healing methods. In all cases of serious illness, a physician should be consulted.

Side effects

NLP is believed to be generally free of harmful side effects.

Research and general acceptance

Although some physicians and mental health practitioners employ principles of neurolinguistic programming, the field is generally considered outside of mainstream medical practice and academic thinking.

Resources

ORGANIZATIONS

Association for NLP. PO Box 78, Stourbridge, UK DY8 2YP.

International NLP Trainers Association, Ltd. Coombe House, Mill Road, Fareham, Hampshire, UK PO16 0TN. (044) 01489 571171.

Society of Neuro-Linguistic Programming. PO Box 424, Hopatcong, NJ 07843. (201) 770-3600.

David Helwig

Neurologic bladder dysfunction *see*
Neurogenic bladder

Neurologic exam

Definition

A neurological examination is an essential component of a comprehensive **physical examination**. It is a systematic examination that surveys the functioning of nerves delivering sensory information to the brain and caring motor commands (Peripheral nervous system) and impulses back to the brain for processing and coordinating (Central nervous system).

Purpose

A careful neurological evaluation can help to determine the cause of impairment since a clinician can begin localizing the problem. Symptoms that

occur unexpectedly suggest a blood vessel or seizure problem. Those that are not so sudden suggest a possible tumor. Symptoms that have a waning course with recurrences and worsen over time suggest a disease that destroys nerve cells. Others that are chronic and progressive indicate a degenerative disorder. In cases of trauma, symptoms may be evident upon inspection and causes may be explained by third party witnesses. Some patients may require extensive neurological screening examination (NSE) and/or neurological examination (NE) to determine the cause. The NH will assist the clinician to diagnose illnesses such as seizure disorders, **narcolepsy**, migraine disorders, **dizziness**, and dementia.

Description

A neurological screening is an essential component of every comprehensive physical examination. In cases of neurological trauma, disease, or psychological disorders patients are usually given a very in-depth neurological examination. The examination is best performed in a systematic manner, which means that there is a recommended order for procedures.

Neurological screening examination

The NSE is basic procedure especially in patients who have a general neurological complaint or symptoms. The NSE consists of six areas of assessment:

- mental status: assessing normal orientation to time, place, space, and speech
- cranial nerves: checking the eyes with a special light source (ophthalmoscope), and also assessment of facial muscles strength and functioning
- motor: checking for tone, drift, heal, and toe and walking
- sensory: cold and vibration tests
- coordination: observing the patient walk and finger to nose testing
- reflexes: using a special instrument the clinician taps an area above a nerve to emit a reflex (usually movement of muscle groups)

Neurological examination

The NE should be performed on a patient suspected of having neurological trauma, neurological, or psychological diseases. The NE is performed in a systematic and comprehensive manner. The NE consists of several comprehensive and in-depth assessments of mental status, cranial nerves, motor examination, reflexes, sensory examination, and posture and walk-ing (gait) analysis.

MENTAL STATUS EXAMINATION (MSE). There are two types of MSE, informal and formal. The informal MSE is usually done when clinicians are obtaining historical information from a patient. The formal MSE is performed in a patient suspected of a neuro-logical problem. The patient is commonly asked his/her name, the location, the day, and date. Retentive memory capability and immediate recall can be assessed by determining the number of digits that can be repeated in sequence. Recent memory is typically examined by testing recall potential of a series of objects after defined times, usually within five and 15 minutes. Remote memory can be assessed by asking the patient to review in a coherent and chronological fashion, his or her illness or personal life events that the patient feels comfortable talking about. Patient recall of common historical or current events can be utilized to assess general knowledge. Higher function-ing (referring to brain processing capabilities) can be assessed by spontaneous speech, repetition, reading, naming, writing, and comprehension. The patient may be asked to perform further tasks such as identifica-tion of fingers, whistling, saluting, brushing teeth motions, combing hair, drawing, and tracing figures. These procedures will assess the intactness of what is called dominant (left-sided brain) functioning or higher cortical function referring to the portion of the brain that regulates these activities.

The MSE is particularly important in the specialty of psychotherapy. Psychotherapists recommend an in-depth MSE to all patients with possible organic (refer-ring to the body) or psychotic disorders. This exam-ination is also performed in a systematic and orderly manner. It is divided into several categories:

- Appearance: This assessment determines the patient's presentation, i.e., how the patient looks (clothes posture, grooming, and alertness).

- Behavior: This assesses the patient's motor (move-ments) activity such as walking, gestures, muscular twitching, and impulse control.

- Speech: the patient's speech can be examined con-cerning volume, rate of speech and coherence. Patients who exhibit latent or delayed speech can indicate depression, while a rapid or pressured speech may suggest possible **mania** or **anxiety**.

- Mood and affect: Normal mood is term euthymia. There is variation in mood presentations and patients may display a flat, labile, blunted, con-structed or inappropriate mood. The patient can

also be euphoric (elevated) or dysphoric (on the down side).

- Thought processes and content: This category is typically assessed by determining word usage (can indicate brain disease), thought stream (whether thoughts are slow, restricted, blocked, or overabun-dant), continuity of thought (referring to associa-tions among ideas), and content of thought (delusional thoughts).

- Perception: This assessment examines the patient's ability to hear, see, touch, taste, and smell. Certain psychological states may cause hearing and visual **hallucinations**. Impairments of smell and touch are usually caused by medical (organic) causes or as side effects from certain medications.

- Attention and concentration: This clinician assesses the patient's ability to focus on a specific task or activity. Abnormalities in attention and concentra-tion can indicate problems related to anxiety or hallucinations.

- Orientation: The patient is examined for orientation to time, place, and identification of self (asking the patient his/her name). Disturbances in orientation can be due to a medical condition (other than psy-chological), **substance abuse**, or as a side effect of certain medications such as those used to treat depression, anxiety or **psychosis** (since these medica-tions usually have a sedative affect).

- Memory: Patients are examined for remote, recent, and immediate memory capabilities. Remote and recent memory can be assessed by the patient's abil-ity to recall historical and current events. Immediate memory can be tested by naming three objects and asking the patient to repeat the named objects imme-diately, then after five and 15 minute intervals.

- Judgment: This category evaluates the patient's abil-ity to **exercise** appropriate judgment. It also deter-mines whether the patient has an understanding of consequences associated with their actions.

- Intelligence and information: The only precise mea-surement for this category can be obtained by admin-istering specialized intelligence tests, However a preliminary assessment of intelligence can be made based on the patient's fund of information, general knowledge, awareness of current events, and the ability for abstract thinking (thinking of unique concepts).

- Insight: Insight in the MSE pertains to the patient's awareness of their problem that prompted them to seek professional examination. Insight concerning the present illness can range from denial to fleeting admission of current illness.

CRANIAL NERVES (CN). Cranial nerves are specialized nerves that originate in the brain and connect to specialized structures such as the nose, eyes, muscles in the face, scalp, ear, and tongue.

- CNI: This nerve checks for visual capabilities. Patients are usually given the Snellen Chart (a chart with rows of large and small letters). Patients read letters with one eye at a time.

- CN III, IV, and VI: These nerves examine the pupillary (the circular center structure of the eye that light rays enter) reaction. The pupils get smaller, normally when exposed to the light. The eyelids are also examined for drooping or retraction. The eyeball is also checked for abnormalities in movement.

- CNV: The clinician can assess the muscles on both sides of the scalp muscles (the temporalis muscle). Additionally the jaw can be tested for motion resistance, opening, protrusion, and side-to-side mobility. The cornea located is a transparent tissue covering the eyeball and could be tested for intactness by lightly brushing a wisp of cotton directly on the outside of the eye.

- CNVII: Examination of CNVII assesses asymmetry of the face at rest and during spontaneous movements. The patient is asked to raise eyebrows, wrinkle forehead, close eyes, frown, smile, puff cheeks, purse lips, whistle, and contract chin muscles. Taste for the front and middle portions of the tongue can also be examined.

- CNVIII: Testing for this CN deals with hearing. The clinician usually uses a special instrument called a tuning fork and tests for air conduction and structural problems which can occur inside the ear.

- CN IX and X: These tests will evaluate certain structures in the mouth. The clinician will usually ask the patient to say "aah" and can detect abnormal positioning of certain structures such as the palatel-uvula. The examiner will also assess the sensation capabilities of the pharynx, by stimulating the area with a wooden tongue depressor, causing a gag reflex.

- CNXI: This nerve is usually examined by asking the patient to shrug shoulders (testing a muscle called the trapezius) and rotating the head to each side (testing a muscle called the sternocleidomastoid). These muscles are responsible for movement of the shoulders and neck. The test is usually done with resistance, meaning the examiner holds the area while the patient is asked to move. This is done to assess patient's strength in these areas.

- CNXII: This nerve tests the bulk and power of the tongue. The examiner looks for tongue protrusion and/or abnormal movements.

MOTOR EXAMINATION. The motor examination assesses the patient's muscle strength, tone, and shape. Muscles could be abnormally larger than expected (hypertrophy) or small due to tissues destruction (atrophy). It is important to assess if there is evidence of twitching or abnormal movements. Involuntary movements due to tics or myoclonus can be observed. Additionally, movements can be abnormal during maintained posture in neurological disorders such as Parkinson's disease. Muscle tone is usually tested by applying resistance to passive motion of a relaxed limb. Power is assessed for movements at each joint. Decreases or increases in muscle tone can help the examiner localize the affected area.

REFLEXES. The patient's reflexes are tested by using a special instrument that looks like a little hammer. The clinician will tap the rubber triangular shaped end in several different areas in the arms, knee, and Achilles heal area. The clinician will ask the patient to relax and gently tap the area. If there is a difference in response from the left to right knee, then there may be an underlying problem that merits further evaluation. A difference in reflexes between the arms and legs usually indicates of a lesion involving the spinal cord. Depressed reflexes in only one limb, while the other limb demonstrates a normal response usually indicates a peripheral nerve lesion.

SENSORY EXAMINATION. Although a very essential component of the NE, the sensory examination is the least informative and least exacting since it requires patient concentration and cooperation. Five primary sensory categories are assessed: vibration (using a tuning fork), joint position (examiner moves the limb side-to-side and in a downward position), light touch, pinprick, and temperature. Patients who have sensory abnormalities may have a lesion above the thalamus. Spinal cord lesions or disease can possibly be detected by pinprick and temperature assessment.

COORDINATION. The patient is asked to repetitively touch his nose using his index finger and then to touch the clinician's outstretched finger. Coordination can also be assessed by asking the patient to alternate tapping the palm then the back of one hand on the thigh. For coordination in the lower extremities on legs, the patient lies on his or her back and is asked to slide the heel of each foot from the knee down the shin of the opposite leg and to raise the leg and touch the examiners index finger with the great toe.

KEY TERMS

Corticospinal tract—A tract of nerve cells that carries motor commands from the brain to the spinal cord.

Gait—Referring to walking motions.

Reflex—A response, usually a movement, elicited by tapping on the nerve with a special hammer-like instrument.

Thalamus—A part of the brain that filters incoming sensory information.

WALKING (GAIT). Normal walking is a complex process and requires usage of multiple systems such as power, coordination and sensation working together in a coordinated fashion. The examination of gait can detect a variety of disease states. Decreased arm swinging on one side is indicative of corticospinal tract disease. A stooped down posture and short-stepped gait may suggest Parkinson's syndrome. A high stepped, slapping gait may be the result of a peripheral nerve disease.

Preparation

The MSE is the first step in a continuous assessment to determine the diagnosis a psychotherapist should take a detailed medical history in the process of ruling out a general medical condition. If a general medical disease is suspected, referral is indicated to rule out this category. Once a medical condition has been fully excluded the therapist can then localize the components of an abnormal MSE to determine the underlying psychological disorder. Once this is determined treatment may include, but is not limited to therapy sessions and/or medication. For neurological diseases the clinician will use information gained from the NE for ordering further tests. These tests may include a complete blood analysis, liver function tests, **kidney function tests**, hormone tests, and a lumbar puncture to determine abnormalities in cerebrospinal fluid. In cases of trauma (car accident, sports injury) the NE is a quick and essential component of emergency assessment. One a diagnosis is determined emergency measures may include further tests and/or surgery.

Aftercare

Care is usually specific once the final diagnosis has been determined. In psychological cases the treatment may include therapy and/or medication. In causes of an acute insult such as stroke or trauma, the patient is usually admitted to the hospital for appropriate treatment. Some neurological diseases are chronic and require conservative (medical) treatment and frequent follow-up visits for monitoring and stability or progression of the disease state. The MSE and NE are good diagnostic tools. Further testing using advanced technological procedures is usually required for definitive diagnosis and initiation of disease-specific treatment.

The outcome depends ultimately on the final diagnosis. Neurological diseases typically follow a chronic course. Situations that present as trauma may require surgical intervention and intensive care with an outcome usually proportional to extent of injuries. Psychological disorders may require long term (chronic) treatment and/or medication(s). Most neurological conditions require follow-up and periodic monitoring.

Resources

BOOKS

Behrman, Richard E., et al, editors. *Nelson Textbook of Pediatrics.* 16th ed. W. B. Saunders Company, 2000.

Goldman, Lee, et al. *Cecil's Textbook of Medicine.* 21st ed. W. B. Saunders Company, 2000.

Laith Farid Gulli, M.D.
Bilal Nasser, M.Sc.

Neuromuscular junction disease *see* **Myasthenia gravis**

Neuropathic bladder *see* **Neurogenic bladder**

Neutropenia

Definition

Neutropenia is an abnormally low level of neutrophils in the blood. Neutrophils are white blood cells (WBCs) produced in the bone marrow that ingest bacteria. Neutropenia is sometimes called agranulocytosis or granulocytopenia because neutrophils make up about 60% of WBCs and have granules inside their cell walls. Neutropenia is a serious disorder because it makes the body vulnerable to bacterial and fungal infections.

Description

The normal level of neutrophils in human blood varies slightly by age and race. Infants have lower counts than older children and adults, and African Americans have lower counts than Caucasians or Asians. The average adult level is 1500 cells/mm3 of blood. Neutrophil counts (in cells/mm3) are interpreted as follows:

- greater than 1000. Normal protection against infection
- 500–1000. Some increased risk of infection
- 200–500. Great risk of severe infection
- lower than 200. Risk of overwhelming infection; requires hospital treatment with antibiotics

Causes and symptoms

Causes

Neutropenia may result from three processes:

DECREASED WBC PRODUCTION. Lowered production of white blood cells is the most common cause of neutropenia. It can result from:

- medications that affect the bone marrow, including cancer drugs, chloramphenicol (Chloromycetin), anticonvulsant medications, and **antipsychotic drugs** (Thorazine, Prolixin, and other phenothiazines)
- hereditary and congenital disorders that affect the bone marrow, including familial neutropenia, cyclic neutropenia, and infantile agranulocytosis
- **cancer**, including certain types of leukemia
- radiation therapy
- exposure to pesticides
- vitamin B_{12} and folate (folic acid) deficiency

DESTRUCTION OF WBCS. WBCs are used up at a faster rate by:

- acute bacterial infections in adults
- infections in newborns
- certain **autoimmune disorders**, including **systemic lupus erythematosus** (SLE)
- penicillin, phenytoin (Dilantin), and sulfonamide medications (Benemid, Bactrim, Gantanol)

SEQUESTRATION AND MARGINATION OF WBCS. Sequestration and margination are processes in which neutrophils are removed from the general blood circulation and redistributed within the body. These processes can occur because of:

- hemodialysis

- felty's syndrome or **malaria**, the neutrophils accumulate in the spleen
- bacterial infections, the neutrophils remain in the infected tissues without returning to the bloodstream

Symptoms

Neutropenia has no specific symptoms except the severity of the patient's current infection. In severe neutropenia, the patient is likely to develop periodontal disease, oral and rectal ulcers, **fever**, and bacterial pneumonia. Fever recurring every 19–30 days suggests cyclical neutropenia.

Diagnosis

Diagnosis is made on the basis of a white blood cell count and differential. The cause of neutropenia is often difficult to establish and depends on a combination of the patient's history, genetic evaluation, **bone marrow biopsy**, and repeated measurements of the WBC.

Treatment

Treatment of neutropenia depends on the underlying cause.

Medications

Patients with fever and other signs of infection are treated for seven to 10 days with antibiotics. Nutritional deficiencies are corrected by green vegetables to supply **folic acid**, and by vitamin B supplements.

Medications known to cause neutropenia are stopped. Neutropenia related to pesticide exposure is treated by removing the patient from the contaminated environment.

Patients receiving **chemotherapy** for cancer may be given a blood growth factor called sargramostim (Leukine, Prokine) to stimulate WBC production.

Surgery

Patients with Felty's syndrome who have repeated infections may have their spleens removed.

Prognosis

The prognosis for mild or chronic neutropenia is excellent. Recovery from acute neutropenia depends on the severity of the patient's infection and the promptness of treatment.

KEY TERMS

Cyclical neutropenia—A rare genetic blood disorder in which the patient's neutrophil level drops below 500/mm3 for six to eight days every three weeks.

Differential—A blood cell count in which the percentages of cell types are calculated as well as the total number of cells.

Felty's syndrome—An autoimmune disorder in which neutropenia is associated with rheumatoid arthritis and an enlarged spleen.

Granulocyte—Any of several types of white blood cells that have granules in their cell substance. Neutrophils are the most common type of granulocyte.

Neutrophil—A granular white blood cell that ingests bacteria, dead tissue cells, and foreign matter.

Sargramostim—A medication made from yeast that stimulates WBC production. It is sold under the trade names Leukine and Prokine.

Sequestration and margination—The removal of neutrophils from circulating blood by cell changes that trap them in the lungs and spleen.

Resources

BOOKS

Linker, Charles A. "Blood." In *Current Medical Diagnosisand Treatment, 1998*, edited by Stephen McPhee, et al., 37th ed. Stamford: Appleton &Lange, 1997.

Rebecca J. Frey, PhD

Nevirapine *see* **Non-nucleoside reverse transcriptase inhibitors**

Nevus *see* **Moles**

Newborn life support *see* **Extracorporeal membrane oxygenation**

Niacin deficiency *see* **Pellagra**

Nicotine *see* **Smoking; Smoking-cessation drugs**

Nicotinic acid deficiency *see* **Pellagra**

Niemann-Pick disease *see* **Lipidoses**

Nifedipine *see* **Calcium channel blockers**

Night blindness *see* **Vitamin A deficiency**

Night terrors

Definition

Night terrors are a sleep disorder characterized by **anxiety** episodes with extreme panic, often accompanied by screaming, flailing, fast breathing, and sweating and that usually occur within a few hours after going to sleep.

Description

Night terrors occur most commonly in children between the ages of four and 12 but can also occur at all ages. Affected individuals usually suffer these episodes within a few hours after going to sleep. They appear to bolt up suddenly, and wake up screaming, sweating and panicked. The episode may last anywhere from five to 20 minutes. During this time, the individual is actually asleep, although the eyes may open. Quite often, nothing can be done to comfort the affected person. Very often, the person has no memory of the episode upon waking the next day.

Night terrors are differentiated from nightmares in that they have been shown to occur during Stage 4 of sleep, or in REM sleep, while nightmares can occur anytime throughout the sleep cycle.

Causes and symptoms

Suffering from night terrors seems to run in families. Extreme tension or **stress** can increase the incidence of the episodes. In adults, the use of alcohol also contributes to an increased incidence of night terrors. Episodes sometimes occur after an accident involving **head injury**. Other factors thought to contribute to episodic night terrors, but not actually cause them, include:

- medications
- excessive tiredness at bedtime
- eating a heavy meal prior to bedtime

drug abuse

Diagnosis

Night terrors are primarily diagnosed by observing the person suffering from an episode. The following symptoms are characteristic of a person suffering from a night terror:

- panic
- sweating
- gasping, moaning, crying or screaming during sleep
- little or no recollection of the episode upon awakening

Treatment

In most cases, the individual will still be asleep as the night terror episode happens and will prove difficult to awaken. The goal should be to help the affected person go back into a calm state of sleep. The lights should be turned on, and soothing comments should be directed at the person, avoiding brusque gestures such as shaking the person or shouting to startle them out of the episode. Any form of stress should be avoided.

Individuals affected by night terrors should be evaluated by a physician if they are really severe and occur frequently. A physician can recommend the best treatment for the particular circumstances of the night terrors. In some severe cases, the physician may prescribe a benzodiazepine tranquilizer, such as Diazepam, known to suppress Stage 4 of sleep. The physician may also refer the affected person for further evaluation by a sleep disorder specialist. It should be noted that episodic night terrors in children are normal and do not suggest the presence of psychological problems. In adults, night terrors are more likely to be related to a significant stress-related or emotional problem.

Prognosis

In children, night terror episodes in children usually end by the age of 12.

Prevention

If a child seems to have a regular pattern of night terror episodes, he should be gently awakened about 15 minutes before the episode usually happens. The child should be kept awake and out of the bed for a short period of time and then allowed to return to bed.

Since sleep deprivation is a strong trigger for night terror episodes, children should not be allowed to become overtired. Having children take a nap during the day may be useful.

Adults affected by night terror episodes should avoid stress, the consumption of alcohol and stimulants before going to sleep.

KEY TERMS

Benzodiazepines—A class of drugs that suppresses Stage 4 of sleep.

REM sleep—Rapid Eye Movement phase of sleep, a mentally active period during which dreaming occurs.

Sleep disorder—Any disorder that keep a person from falling asleep or staying asleep.

Resources

PERIODICALS

American Academy of Family Physicians. "Nightmares and Night Terrors in Children." October 2000.

Laberge, Luc, et al. "Development of Parasomnias from Childhood to Early Adolescence." *Pediatrics* July 2000: 67-74.

ORGANIZATIONS

American Sleep Disorders Association, 6301 Bandel Road Suite 101, Rochester, MN 55901. (507) 287-6008. < http://www.asda.org >.

National Foundation for Sleep and Related Disorders in Children. 4200 W. Peterson Suite 109, Chicago, IL 60646. (708) 971-1086.

Kim A. Sharp, M.Ln.

Nitrates *see* **Antiangina drugs**

Nitrofurantoin *see* **Urinary anti-infectives**

Nitrogen narcosis

Definition

Nitrogen narcosis is a condition that occurs in divers breathing compressed air. When divers go below depths of approximately 100 ft, increase in the partial pressure of nitrogen produces an altered mental state similar to alcohol intoxication.

Description

Nitrogen narcosis, commonly referred to as "rapture of the deep," typically becomes noticeable at 100 ft underwater and is incapacitating at 300 ft, causing stupor, blindness, unconsciousness, and even **death**. Nitrogen narcosis is also called "the martini effect" because divers experience an effect comparable to that from one martini on an empty stomach for every 50 ft of depth beyond the initial 100 ft.

Causes and symptoms

Nitrogen narcosis is caused by gases in the body acting in a manner described by Dalton's Law of partial pressures: the total pressure of a gas mixture is equal to the sum of the partial pressures of gases in the mixture. As the total gas pressure increases with increasing dive depth, the partial pressure of nitrogen increases and more nitrogen becomes dissolved in the blood. This high nitrogen concentration impairs the conduction of nerve impulses and mimics the effects of alcohol or **narcotics**.

Symptoms of nitrogen narcosis include: wooziness; giddiness; euphoria; disorientation; loss of balance; loss of manual dexterity; slowing of reaction time; fixation of ideas; and impairment of complex reasoning. These effects are exacerbated by cold, **stress**, and a rapid rate of compression.

Diagnosis

A diagnosis must be made on circumstantial evidence of atypical behavior, taking into consideration the depth of the dive and the rate of compression. Nitrogen narcosis may be differentiated from toxicity of oxygen, carbon monoxide, or carbon dioxide by the absence of such symptoms as **headache**, seizure, and bluish color of the lips and nail beds.

Treatment

The effects of nitrogen narcosis are totally reversed as the gas pressure decreases. They are typically gone by the time the diver returns to a water depth of 60 ft. Nitrogen narcosis has no hangover or lasting effects requiring further treatment. However, a doctor should be consulted whenever a diver has lost consciousness.

Prognosis

When a diver returns to a safe depth, the effects of nitrogen narcosis disappear completely. Some evidence exists that certain divers may become partially acclimated to the effects of nitrogen narcosis with frequency—the more often they dive, the less the increased nitrogen seems to affect them.

Prevention

Helium may be used as a substitute for nitrogen to dilute oxygen for deep water diving. It is colorless,

---

KEY TERMS

Compressed air—Air that is held under pressure in a tank to be breathed by underwater divers. A tank of compressed air is part of a diver's scuba (self-contained underwater breathing apparatus) gear.

Compression—An increase in pressure from the surrounding water that occurs with increasing diving depth.

Partial pressure—The pressure exerted by one of the gases in a mixture of gases. The partial pressure of the gas is proportional to its concentration in the mixture. The total pressure of the gas mixture is the sum of the partial pressures of the gases in it (Dalton's Law) and as the total pressure increases, each partial pressure increases proportionally.

---

odorless, tasteless, and chemically inert. However, it is more expensive than nitrogen and drains body heat from a diver. In diving with rapid compression, the helium-oxygen mixture may produce **nausea**, **dizziness**, and trembling, but these adverse reactions are less severe than nitrogen narcosis.

Nitrogen narcosis can be avoided by limiting the depth of dives. The risk of nitrogen narcosis may also be minimized by following safe diving practices, including proper equipment maintenance, low work effort, proper buoyancy, maintenance of visual cues, and focused thinking. In addition, no alcohol should be consumed within 24 hours of diving.

Resources

ORGANIZATIONS

American College of Hyperbaric Medicine. P.O. Box 25914-130, Houston, Texas 77265. (713) 528-0657. < http://www.hyperbaricmedicine.org >.

Divers Alert Network. The Peter B. Bennett Center, 6 West Colony Place, Durham, NC 27705. (800) 446-2671. < http://www.diversalertnetwork.org >.

Undersea and Hyperbaric Medical Society. 10531 Metropolitan Ave., Kensington, MD 20895. (301) 942-2980. < http://www.uhms.org >.

Bethany Thivierge

Nitroglycerin *see* **Antiangina drugs**

Nlein purpura *see* **Allergic purpura**

NMR *see* **Magnetic resonance imaging**

Nocardia asteroides infection *see*
Nocardiosis

Nocardiosis

Definition

Nocardiosis is a serious infection caused by a fungus-like bacterium that begins in the lungs and can spread to the brain.

Description

Nocardiosis is found throughout the world among people of all ages, although it is most common in older people and males. While people with poor immunity are vulnerable to this infection, it sometimes strikes individuals with no history of other diseases. Nocardiosis is rare in AIDS patients. It is not transmitted by person-to-person contact.

Causes and symptoms

Nocardiosis is caused by a bacterium of the *Nocardia* species—usually *N. asteroides*, an organism that is normally found in the soil. The incubation period is not known, but is probably several weeks.

The bacteria can enter the human body when a person inhales contaminated dust. Less often, people can pick up the bacteria in contaminated puncture wounds or cuts.

Symptoms

The infection causes a **cough** similar to **pneumonia** or **tuberculosis**, producing thick, sometimes bloody, sputum. Other symptoms include chills, night sweats, chest **pain**, weakness, loss of appetite and weight loss. Nocardiosis does not, however, respond to short-term **antibiotics**.

Complications

In about one-third of patients, the infection spreads from the blood into the brain, causing brain abscesses. This complication can trigger a range of symptoms including severe **headache**, confusion, disorientation, dizziness, nausea and seizures, and problems in walking. If a brain abscess ruptures, it can lead to **meningitis**.

About a third of patients with nocardiosis also have abscesses in the skin or directly underneath the

skin. They may also have lesions in other organs, such as the kidneys, liver, or bones.

Diagnosis

Nocardia is not easily identified from cultures of sputum or discharge. A doctor can diagnose the condition using special staining techniques and taking a thorough medical history. Lung biopsies or x rays also may be required. Up to 40% of the time, however, a diagnosis can't be made until an **autopsy** is done.

Treatment

Treatment of nocardiosis includes bed rest and high doses of medication for a period of 12 to 18 months, including sulfonamide drugs or a combination of trimethoprim-sulfamethoxazole (Bactrim, Septra). If the patient doesn't respond to these drugs, antibiotics such as ampicillin (Amcill, Principen) or erythromycin (E-Mycin, Eryc) may be tried.

The abscesses may need to be drained and dead tissue cut away. Other symptoms are treated as necessary.

Prognosis

Nocardiosis is a serious disease with a high mortality rate. If it has been diagnosed early and caught before spreading to the brain, the prognosis is better. Even with appropriate treatment, however, the **death** rate is still 50%. Once the infection reaches the brain, the death rate is above 80%. This outcome is most commonly seen in patients with a weakened immune system.

Resources

BOOKS

Orris, June, editor. *Handbook of Diseases.* Springhouse, PA: Springhouse Corp., 1996.

Carol A. Turkington

Nodule *see* **Skin lesions**

Non-Hodgkin's lymphomas *see* **Malignant lymphomas**

Non-melanoma skin cancer *see* **Skin cancer, non-melanoma**

Non-nucleoside reverse transcriptase inhibitors

Definition

This type of drug interferes with an enzyme that is key to the replication (reproduction) of the human **immunodeficiency** virus (HIV). The drug is designed to help suppress the growth of HIV, but does not eliminate it.

Purpose

This medication is used to treat patients with the HIV virus and **AIDS** in combination with one or more other AIDS drugs. Combining NRTIs with older drugs improves their ability to lower the levels of HIV in the bloodstream, and strengthens the immune system.

HIV becomes rapidly resistant to this class of drugs when they are used alone. However, in combination with older drugs, they can interfere with the virus's ability to become resistant because they attack the virus on several fronts. As the virus tries to evade one drug, another attacks. This combination can lower the level of HIV in the blood to undetectable levels.

Precautions

Patients should not discontinue this drug even if symptoms improve without consultation with a physician.

Description

Nucleoside analogues, the first class of HIV drugs to be developed, worked by incorporating themselves into the virus's DNA, making the DNA incomplete and therefore unable to create a new virus. Non-nucleoside inhibitors work at the same stage as nucleoside analogues, but act in a completely different way, preventing the conversion of RNA to DNA.

This class of drugs includes nevirapine (Viramune) and delavirdine (Rescriptor). It may take several weeks or months before the full benefits are apparent.

Depending on the drug prescribed, doses may start with a lower amount and be increased after a short period of time.

Risks

A mild skin rash is common; a severe skin rash can be a life threatening reaction. Other possible side effects include **fever**, blistering skin, mouth sores, aching joints, eye inflammation, **headache**, **nausea**, and tiredness.

Because the drug passes into breast milk, breast-feeding mothers should avoid the drug, or not nurse until the treatment is completed.

Resources

ORGANIZATIONS

National AIDS Treatment Advocacy Project. 580 Broadway, Ste. 403, New York, NY 10012. (888) 266-2827. < http://www.natap.org >.

Carol A. Turkington

Non-small cell lung cancer *see* **Lung cancer, non-small cell**

Non-A, non-B hepatitis *see* **Hepatitis C**

Non-tuberculous *see* **Mycobacterial infections, atypical**

Nonbacterial regional lymphaden *see* **Cat-scratch disease**

Noncholera vibrio infections *see* **Vibriosis**

Noneros *see* **Gastritis**

Nongonococcal urethritis

Definition

Any inflammation of the urethra not due to gonorrhea, almost always contracted through sexual intercourse and found far more often in men.

Description

Men between the ages of 15 and 30 who have multiple sex partners are most at risk for nongonococcal **urethritis** (NGU), which is believed to be the most common sexually transmitted disease in the United States.

Causes and symptoms

NGU is spread almost exclusively via sexual contact, and appears most often in men because a woman's urethra is less easily infected during sex. The infection is most often due to *Chlamydia trachomatis*, the organism that causes chlamydia. Those that aren't caused by *Chlamydia trachomatis* are usually due to another bacterium, *Ureaplasma urealyticum*. In 10% to 20% of NGU cases, the cause is unknown.

Symptoms appear within one to five weeks after infection, and include a slight clear discharge (the color of the discharge can vary from one patient to the next), and **itching** or burning during or after urination.

However, some men never develop symptoms, and women almost never show signs of infection. However, it's possible that symptoms of burning or itching in or around the vagina may be due to NGU.

The disease is communicable from the time of first infection until the patient is cured. Past infection doesn't make a person immune.

Diagnosis

Nongonococcal urethritis is diagnosed by excluding other causes, since inflammation that is not caused by **gonorrhea** is classified as NGU. A microscopic and/or culture test of the discharge or urine can reveal the infection.

Since many people are infected with both NGU and syphilis at the same time, infected patients also should have a test for **syphilis** before treatment for NGU begins, and three months after treatment ends.

Treatment

Antibiotics such as tetracycline or azithromycin will cure NGU; both sexual partners should be treated at the same time.

Patients taking tetracycline should avoid milk or milk products and take the medication at least one hour before or two hours after meals. On the last day of treatment, a male should have a urine test to make

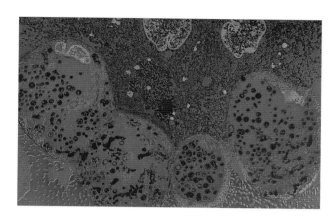

A microscopic image of non-specific urethritis. This sexually transmitted disease is usually caused by a bacterium of the genus Chlamydia. *(Custom Medical Stock Photo. Reproduced by permission.)*

KEY TERMS

Chlamydia—One of the most common sexually transmitted diseases in the United States. It causes discharge, inflammation and burning during urination. About half of the cases of nongonococcal urethritis are due to chlamydia.

Gonorrhea—A sexually transmitted disease that affects the genital mucous membranes of men and women.

Urethra—The tube that carries urine from the bladder through the outside of the body.

sure the infection has cleared. If it hasn't, he should take a second course of therapy. Men should use a **condom** during treatment and for several months after treatment is completed.

If urine tests indicate the infection is gone but symptoms persist, the doctor will check for signs of prostate inflammation.

Prognosis

NGU is completely curable with proper antibiotic treatment. Untreated, NGU can lead to sterility in both men and women, inflammation of the mouth of the uterus, and infections of the woman's internal sexual organs. An infection during **pregnancy** may lead to **pneumonia** or eye infections in the newborn child. Untreated men may develop swelling of the testicles and an infected prostate gland.

Prevention

People can prevent the spread of NGU by:

- using a condom
- limiting the number of sex partners
- washing the genital area after sex
- if infected, avoid sexual contact; take antibiotics, notify all partners

Resources

ORGANIZATIONS

American Social Health Association. P.O. Box 13827, Research Triangle Park, NC 27709. (800) 227-8922. < http://www.ashastd.org >.

OTHER

Sexually Transmitted Diseases Hotline. (800) 227-8922.

Carol A. Turkington

Nonsteroidal anti-inflammatory drugs

Definition

Nonsteroidal anti-inflammatory drugs are medicines that relieve **pain**, swelling, stiffness, and inflammation.

Purpose

Nonsteroidal anti-inflammatory drugs (NSAIDs) are prescribed for a variety of painful conditions, including arthritis, **bursitis**, **tendinitis**, **gout**, menstrual cramps, sprains, strains, and other injuries. They are also given to control the pain of **cancer** and the side effects of **radiation therapy**.

A group of researchers associated with the Women's Health Initiative reported in 2003 that regular use of **aspirin**, ibuprofen, and other NSAIDs may help to lower a woman's risk of developing **breast cancer**. Further clinical trials are needed, however, to confirm the group's findings.

Description

Nonsteroidal anti-inflammatory drugs relieve pain, stiffness, swelling, and inflammation, but they do not cure the diseases or injuries responsible for these problems. Two drugs in this category, ibuprofen and naproxen, also reduce **fever**. Some nonsteroidal anti-inflammatory drugs can be bought over the counter; others are available only with a prescription from a physician or dentist.

Among the drugs in this group are diclofenac (Voltaren), etodolac (Lodine), flurbiprofen (Ansaid), ibuprofen (Motrin, Advil, Rufen), ketorolac (Toradol), nabumetone (Relafen), naproxen (Naprosyn); naproxen sodium (Aleve, Anaprox, Naprelan); and oxaprozin (Daypro). They are sold as tablets, capsules, caplets, liquids, and rectal suppositories and some are available in chewable, extended-release, or delayed-release forms.

A newer group of NSAIDs known as **COX-2 inhibitors** are being used successfully to treat patients with allergic reactions to the older NSAIDs. Their name comes from the fact that they block an enzyme known as cyclooxygenase-2, or COX-2, which is involved in the inflammation pathway. The COX-2 inhibitors are also less likely to affect the patient's digestive tract. They include such drugs as celecoxib (Celebrex), rofecoxib (Vioxx), etoricoxib (Arcoxia), and valdecoxib (Bextra). With regard to cancer treatment, some studies indicate that the use of COX-2 inhibitors may postpone the need to prescribe narcotic medications for severe pain.

Recommended dosage

Recommended doses vary, depending on the patient, the type of nonsteroidal anti-inflammatory drug prescribed, the condition for which the drug is prescribed, and the form in which it is used. Always take nonsteroidal anti-inflammatory drugs exactly as directed. If using non-prescription (over-the-counter) types, follow the directions on the package label. For prescription types, check with the physician who prescribed the medicine or the pharmacist who filled the prescription. Never take larger or more frequent doses, and do not take the drug for longer than directed. Patients who take nonsteroidal anti-inflammatory drugs for severe arthritis must take them regularly over a long time. Several weeks may be needed to feel the results, so it is important to keep taking the medicine, even if it does not seem to be working at first.

When taking nonsteroidal anti-inflammatory drugs in tablet, capsule, or caplet form, always take them with a full, 8-ounce glass of water or milk. Taking these drugs with food or an antacid will help prevent stomach irritation.

Precautions

Nonsteroidal anti-inflammatory drugs can cause a number of side effects, some of which may be very serious (See Side effects). These side effects are more likely when the drugs are taken in large doses or for a long time or when two or more nonsteroidal anti-inflammatory drugs are taken together. Health care professionals can help patients weigh the risks of benefits of taking these medicines for long periods.

Do not take **acetaminophen**, aspirin, or other salicylates along with other nonsteroidal anti-inflammatory drugs for more than a few days unless directed to do so by a physician. Do not take ketorolac (Toradol) while taking other nonsteroidal anti-inflammatory drugs unless directed to do so by a physician.

Because older people are more sensitive than younger adults to nonsteroidal anti-inflammatory drugs, they may be more likely to have side effects. Some side effects, such as stomach problems, may also be more serious in older people.

Serious side effects are especially likely with one nonsteroidal anti-inflammatory drug, phenylbutazone. Patients age 40 and over are especially at risk of side effects from this drug, and the likelihood of serious side effects increases with age. Because of these potential problems, it is especially important to check with a physician before taking this medicine. Never take it for anything other than the condition for which it was prescribed, and never share it—or any other prescription drug—with another person.

Some nonsteroidal anti-inflammatory drugs can increase the chance of bleeding after surgery (including dental surgery), so anyone who is taking the drugs should alert the physician or dentist before surgery. Avoiding the medicine or switching to another type in the days prior to surgery may be necessary.

Some people feel drowsy, dizzy, confused, lightheaded, or less alert when using these drugs. Blurred vision or other vision problems also are possible side effects. For these reasons, anyone who takes these drugs should not drive, use machines or do anything else that might be dangerous until they have found out how the drugs affect them.

Nonsteroidal anti-inflammatory drugs make some people more sensitive to sunlight. Even brief exposure to sunlight can cause severe **sunburn**, **rashes**, redness, **itching**, blisters, or discoloration. Vision changes also may occur. To reduce the chance of these problems, avoid direct sunlight, especially from mid-morning to mid-afternoon; wear protective clothing, a hat, and sunglasses; and use a sunscreen with a skin protection factor (SPF) rating of at least 15. Do not use sunlamps, tanning booths or tanning beds while taking these drugs.

Special conditions

People with certain medical conditions and people who are taking some other medicines can have problems if they take nonsteroidal anti-inflammatory drugs. Before taking these drugs, be sure to let the physician know about any of these conditions:

ALLERGIES. Let the physician know about any **allergies** to foods, dyes, preservatives, or other substances. Anyone who has had reactions to nonsteroidal anti-inflammatory drugs in the past should also check with a physician before taking them again.

PREGNANCY. Women who are pregnant or who plan to become pregnant should check with their physicians before taking these medicines. Whether nonsteroidal anti-inflammatory drugs cause birth defects in people is unknown, but some do cause birth defects in laboratory animals. If taken late in **pregnancy**, these drugs may prolong pregnancy, lengthen labor time, cause problems during delivery, or affect the heart or blood flow of the fetus.

BREASTFEEDING. Some nonsteroidal anti-inflammatory drugs pass into breast milk. Women who are breastfeeding should check with their physicians before taking these drugs.

OTHER MEDICAL CONDITIONS. A number of medical conditions may influence the effects of nonsteroidal anti-inflammatory drugs. Anyone who has any of the conditions listed below should tell his or her physician about the condition before taking nonsteroidal anti-inflammatory drugs.

- stomach or intestinal problems, such as colitis or Crohn's disease
- liver disease
- current or past **kidney disease**; current or past kidney stones
- heart disease
- high blood pressure
- blood disorders, such as anemia, low **platelet count**, low white blood cell count
- bleeding problems
- diabetes mellitus
- hemorrhoids, rectal bleeding, or rectal irritation
- asthma
- Parkinson's disease
- epilepsy
- systemic lupus erythematosus

- diseases of the blood vessels, such as polymyalgia rheumatica and **temporal arteritis**
- fluid retention
- alcohol **abuse**
- mental illness.

People who have sores or white spots in the mouth should tell the physician about them before starting to take nonsteroidal anti-inflammatory drugs. Sores or white spots that appear while taking the drug can be a sign of serious side effects.

SPECIAL DIETS. Some nonsteroidal anti-inflammatory drugs contain sugar or sodium, so anyone on a low-sugar or low-sodium diet should be sure to tell his or her physician.

SMOKING. People who smoke cigarettes may be more likely to have unwanted side effects from this medicine.

USE OF CERTAIN MEDICINES. Taking nonsteroidal anti-inflammatory drugs with certain other drugs may affect the way the drugs work or increase the risk of unwanted side effects. (See Interactions.)

Side effects

The most common side effects are stomach pain or cramps, **nausea**, **vomiting**, **indigestion**, **diarrhea**, **heartburn**, **headache**, **dizziness** or lightheadedness, and drowsiness. As the patient's body adjusts to the medicine, these symptoms usually disappear. If they do not, check with the physician who prescribed the medicine.

Serious side effects are rare, but do sometimes occur. If any of the following side effects occur, stop taking the medicine and get emergency medical care immediately:

- swelling or puffiness of the face
- swelling of the hands, feet, or lower legs
- rapid weight gain
- fainting
- breathing problems
- fast or irregular heartbeat
- tightness in the chest

Other side effects do not require emergency medical care, but should have medical attention. If any of the following side effects occur, stop taking the medicine and call the physician who prescribed the medicine as soon as possible:

- severe pain, cramps, or burning in the stomach or abdomen
- convulsions
- fever
- severe nausea, heartburn, or indigestion
- white spots or sores in the mouth or on the lips
- rashes or red spots on the skin
- any unusual bleeding, including nosebleeds, spitting up or vomiting blood or dark material
- black, tarry stool
- chest pain
- unusual bruising
- severe headaches

A number of less common, temporary side effects are also possible. They usually do not need medical attention and will disappear once the body adjusts to the medicine. If they continue or interfere with normal activity, check with the physician. Among these side effects are:

- gas, bloating, or **constipation**
- bitter taste or other taste changes
- sweating
- restlessness, irritability, **anxiety**
- trembling or twitching

Some patients who have had problems with side effects from NSAIDs may benefit from **acupuncture** as an adjunctive treatment in **pain management**. A recent study done in New York found that older patients with lower back pain related to cancer reported that their pain was relieved by acupuncture with fewer side effects than those caused by NSAIDs.

Interactions

Nonsteroidal anti-inflammatory drugs may interact with a variety of other medicines. When this happens, the effects of the drugs may change, and the risk of side effects may be greater. Anyone who takes these drugs should let the physician know all other medicines he or she is taking. Among the drugs that may interact with nonsteroidal anti-inflammatory drugs are:

- blood thinning drugs, such as warfarin (Coumadin)
- other nonsteroidal anti-inflammatory drugs
- heparin
- tetracyclines
- cyclosprorine

KEY TERMS

Anemia—A lack of hemoglobin—the compound in blood that carries oxygen from the lungs throughout the body and brings waste carbon dioxide from the cells to the lungs, where it is released.

Bursitis—Inflammation of the tissue around a joint.

Colitis—Inflammation of the colon (large bowel.

COX-2 inhibitors—A class of newer NSAIDs that are less likely to cause side effects in the digestive tract. COX-2 inhibitors work by inhibiting the production of cyclooxygenase-2, an enzyme involved in inflammation.

Inflammation—Pain, redness, swelling, and heat that usually develop in response to injury or illness.

Salicylates—A group of drugs that includes aspirin and related compounds. Salicylates are used to relieve pain, reduce inflammation, and lower fever.

Tendinitis—Inflammation of a tendon, which is a tough band of tissue that connects muscle to bone.

- digitalis drugs
- lithium
- phenytoin (Dilantin)
- zidovudine (AZT, Retrovir).

NSAIDs may also interact with certain herbal preparations sold as dietary supplements. Among the herbs known to interact with NSAIDs are bearberry (*Arctostaphylos uva-ursi*), feverfew (*Tanacetum parthenium*), evening primrose (*Oenothera biennis*), and gossypol, a pigment obtained from cottonseed oil and used as a male contraceptive. In most cases, the herb increases the tendency of NSAIDs to irritate the digestive tract. It is just as important for patients to inform their doctor of herbal remedies that they take on a regular basis as it is to give the doctor a list of their other prescription medications.

Resources

BOOKS

Beers, Mark H., MD, and Robert Berkow, MD., editors. "Drug Therapy in the Elderly." Section 22, Chapter 304 In *The Merck Manual of Diagnosis and Therapy*. Whitehouse Station, NJ: Merck Research Laboratories, 2004.

Pelletier, Dr. Kenneth R. *The Best Alternative Medicine, Part I: Western Herbal Medicine*. New York: Simon and Schuster, 2002.

Wilson, Billie Ann, RN, PhD, Carolyn L. Stang, PharmD, and Margaret T. Shannon, RN, PhD. *Nurses Drug Guide 2000*. Stamford, CT: Appleton and Lange, 1999.

PERIODICALS

Birbara, C. A., A. D. Puopolo, D. R. Munoz, et al. "Treatment of Chronic Low Back Pain with Etoricoxib, A New Cyclo-Oxygenase-2 Selective Inhibitor: Improvement in Pain and Disability—A Randomized, Placebo-Controlled, 3-Month Trial." *Journal of Pain* 4 (August 2003): 307–315.

Gordon, D. B. "Nonopioid and Adjuvant Analgesics in Chronic Pain Management: Strategies for Effective Use." *Nursing Clinics of North America* 38 (September 2003): 447–464.

Graf, C., and K. Puntillo. "Pain in the Older Adult in the Intensive Care Unit." *Critical Care Clinics* 19 (October 2003): 749–770.

Harris, R. E., R. T. Chlebowski, R. D. Jackson, et al. "Breast cancer and Nonsteroidal Anti-Inflammatory Drugs: Prospective Results from the Women's Health Initiative." *Cancer Research* 63 (September 15, 2003): 6096–6101.

Hatsiopoulou, O., R. I. Cohen, and E. V. Lang. "Postprocedure Pain Management of Interventional Radiology Patients." *Journal of Vascular and Interventional Radiology* 14 (November 2003): 1373–1385.

Meng, C. F., D. Wang, J. Ngeow, et al. "Acupuncture for Chronic Low Back Pain in Older Patients: A Randomized, Controlled Trial." *Rheumatology (Oxford)* 42 (December 2003): 1508–1517.

Perrone, M. R., M. C. Artesani, M. Viola, et al. "Tolerability of Rofecoxib in Patients with Adverse Reactions to Nonsteroidal Anti-Inflammatory Drugs: A Study of 216 Patients and Literature Review." *International Archives of Allergy and Immunology* 132 (September 2003): 82–86.

Raffa, R. B., R. Clark-Vetri, R. J. Tallarida, and A. I. Wertheimer. "Combination Strategies for Pain Management." *Expert Opinion in Pharmacotherapy* 4 (October 2003): 1697–1708.

Small, R. C., and A. Schuna. "Optimizing Outcomes in Rheumatoid Arthritis." *Journal of the American Pharmaceutical Association* 43, no. 5, Supplement 1 (September-October 2003): S16–S17.

Stephens, J., B. Laskin, C. Pashos, et al. "The Burden of Acute Postoperative Pain and the Potential Role of the COX-2-Specific Inhibitors." *Rheumatology (Oxford)* 42, Supplement 3 (November 2003): iii40–iii52.

ORGANIZATIONS

U. S. Food and Drug Administration (FDA). 5600 Fishers Lane, Rockville, MD 20857. (888) 463-6332. < http://www.fda.gov >.

Nancy Ross-Flanigan
Rebecca J. Frey, PhD

Nontropical sprue *see* **Celiac disease**

Nonvenereal syphilis *see* **Bejel**

Norfloxac *see* **Fluoroquinolones**

Noroviruses

Definition

Noroviruses are a group of related, single-stranded RNA (ribonucleic acid) viruses that cause acute **gastroenteritis** in humans.

Description

Noroviral infection

Noroviruses are a major cause of viral gastroenteritis—an inflammation of the linings of the stomach and small and large intestines that causes **vomiting** and **diarrhea**. Viruses are responsible for 30–40% of all cases of infectious diarrhea and viral gastroenteritis is the second most common illness in the United States, exceeded only by the **common cold**.

Anyone can become infected with norovirus. During norovirus outbreaks there are high rates of infection among people of all ages. There are a large number of genetically-distinct strains of norovirus. Immunity appears to be specific for the norovirus strain and lasts for only a few months. Therefore norovirus infection can recur throughout a person s lifetime. Because of genetic (inherited) differences among humans, some people appear to be more susceptible to norovirus infection and may suffer more severe illness. People with type O blood are at the highest risk for severe infection.

Infected individuals are contagious from the first onset of symptoms until at least three days after full recovery. Some people may remain contagious for as long as two weeks after recovery.

Gastroenteritis

Gastroenteritis often is referred to as the stomach flu even though the flu is a respiratory illness caused by an **influenza** virus. Other common names for viral gastroenteritis include:

- food poisoning
- winter-vomiting disease
- non-bacterial gastroenteritis
- calicivirus infection.

The U.S. Centers for Disease Control and Prevention (CDC) estimate that noroviruses are responsible for some 23 million cases of acute gastroenteritis in the United States every year. Epidemiologists estimate that about 50,000 Americans are hospitalized annually and about 400 die as a result of norovirus infection. In developing countries noroviruses are a major cause of human illness.

Gastroenteritis caused by infection with a norovirus is rarely a serious illness. Typically an infected person suddenly feels very ill and may vomit many times in a single day. The symptoms, although quite unpleasant, usually last only 24–60 hours.

Transmission

Noroviruses are ubiquitous in the environment. They are highly contagious and are considered to be among the most infectious of viruses. The reasons for this include:

- Only a small number of viral particles—fewer than 100—are required for infection.
- Although noroviruses cannot reproduce outside of their human hosts, they can remain viable for weeks or even months on objects and surfaces.
- Human immunity to norovirus is short-lived and strain-specific.

Noroviruses are transmitted among people by a fecal-oral route, either by ingestion of food or water contaminated with feces or by contact with the vomit or feces of an infected person. Norovirus infection can occur by:

- consuming contaminated food or liquids
- hand contact with contaminated objects or surfaces, followed by hand contact with the mouth
- contact with an infected person, including caring for the sick person or sharing food or utensils
- aerosolized vomit that is swallowed or contaminates surfaces.

Environmental contamination or contact with infected clothing or linen also may be a source of transmission. Although there is no evidence that norovirus infection can occur via the respiratory system, the sudden and violent vomiting of noroviral gastroenteritis can lead to contamination of the surroundings and of public areas. Particles laden with virus can be suspended in the air and swallowed.

FOODBORNE TRANSMISSION. Noroviruses account for at least 50% of food-related outbreaks of gastroenteritis. A European study found that between 1995 and 2000 noroviruses were responsible for more than 85% of all foodborne non-bacterial gastroenteritis outbreaks. Restaurant or catered foods are common sources of norovirus transmission, with subsequent infection of household members. The majority of norovirus outbreaks occur via contamination by a food handler immediately before the food is consumed.

Foods that frequently are associated with norovirus outbreaks include:

- foods that are eaten without further cooking, including sandwiches, salads, and bakery products
- liquids such as salad dressing or cake icing in which the virus becomes evenly distributed
- food that is contaminated at its source, including oysters and clams from contaminated waters and raspberries irrigated with sewage-contaminated water
- food that becomes contaminated before distribution, including salads and frozen fruit.
- Shellfish, including oysters and clams, concentrate norovirus from contaminated water in their tissues. Steaming shellfish may not completely inactivate the virus.

WATERBORNE TRANSMISSION. There is widespread norovirus contamination of rivers and seas, often with more than one strain of the virus. Waterborne outbreaks of norovirus have been associated with:

- sewage-contaminated wells
- contaminated municipal water systems
- stream and lake water
- swimming pools and spas
- commercial ice.

Outbreaks

Norovirus infection can spread rapidly through daycare centers, schools, prisons, hospitals, nursing homes, camps, and other confined spaces. About 40% of group- or institutionally-related outbreaks of diarrhea are caused by norovirus. Outbreaks usually peak during the winter months.

Between July of 1997 and June of 2000, 232 norovirus outbreaks were reported to the CDC. It was determined that 57% of these outbreaks were due to foodborne transmission, 16% were spread by human contact, and 3% were due to waterborne transmission. The mode of transmission could not be determined in 23% of the outbreaks. Restaurants or catered food accounted for 36% of the outbreaks, 23% occurred

in nursing homes, 13% in schools, and 10% at resorts or on cruise ships. Outbreaks also have occurred at large family gatherings.

Cruise ships have become notorious for norovirus outbreaks among passengers and staff. Cruise ships and naval vessels are at increased risk for contamination when docking in regions that lack adequate sanitation and where contaminated food or water may be brought onboard. Outbreaks on cruise ships are exacerbated by close living quarters and the arrival of new, susceptible passengers every one to two weeks. Norovirus outbreaks have been reported to continue through more than 12 successive cruises on a single ship.

A study of 12 calicivirus outbreaks on cruise ships in 2002 found that 11 of the outbreaks were caused by noroviruses and seven of these were due to a previously unreported strain. In the same year, 10 out of 22 land-based outbreaks were attributed to this new strain.

Outbreaks of norovirus appear on the increase. In 2005 the CDC reported that norovirus outbreaks were increasing in hospitals, daycare centers, nursing homes, and schools across the country. The International Council of Cruise Lines reported that, although less than 1% of passengers become infected with norovirus each year, outbreaks on cruise ships also were on the increase. In the summer of 2004 an outbreak at Yellowstone National Park sickened 134 people. More than 1,100 people became ill in early 2004 after a norovirus outbreak at Las Vegas hotels. The following autumn more than 1,200 people became sick from a norovirus outbreak at a single Las Vegas hotel-casino.

Causes & symptoms

Norovirus strains

Noroviruses lack outer envelopes and their genetic material is carried as single-stranded RNA rather than DNA. Although noroviruses are not new, the extent of norovirus infection was not recognized until the 1990s. This has led to increased research on noroviruses and more monitoring of outbreaks.

Until 2004 noroviruses were commonly referred to as:

- Norwalk virus
- Norwalk-like viruses (NLVs)
- caliciviruses
- small, round-structured viruses (SRSVs).

Noroviruses are named after the original strain—the Norwalk virus—that caused an outbreak of gastroenteritis in a Norwalk, Ohio, school in 1968. The virus was identified in 1972. Since then many related viruses have been identified. In 2004 these viruses were grouped together in the genus *Norovirus* within the *Caliciviridae* family of viruses. Eight to ten distinct genogroups of norovirus have been found in various parts of the world. The most common genogroups are GI, GII, GIII, and GIV. Each of these groups can be further differentiated into at least 20 genetic clusters. Evidence suggests that noroviruses in different genetic clusters can recombine to form new, genetically-distinct noroviruses. GII strains, especially GII4, are the most prevalent. However the most common method of identifying noroviruses—the reverse transcription-polymerase chain reaction (RT-PCR)—may not always identify GII genetic clusters correctly.

The increased number of norovirus outbreaks in European countries in 2002—occurring in the spring and summer rather than in winter—were found to be associated with the emergence of a new variant of the GII4 strain. Increased international outbreaks in 2003 and 2004 also were caused by a GII4-related norovirus that was found to mutate rapidly. Mutations in the viral capsid—the virus s outer protective layer—were used to determine the predominant routes of norovirus transmission.

Symptoms

Symptoms of norovirus infection usually appear within 24–48 hours after exposure, with a median incubation period during outbreaks of 33–36 hours. However symptoms can occur as early as 12 hours or less after exposure.

Typical symptoms of norovirus infection are:

- **nausea**
- vomiting
- watery diarrhea without blood
- abdominal cramping.

Among children, vomiting is the predominant symptom, whereas diarrhea is more common in adults. Vomiting can be frequent and violent and may occur without warning.

Additional symptoms of norovirus infection may include:

- low-grade fever
- chills
- headache
- muscle aches
- fatigue.

Dehydration is the major risk from gastroenteritis caused by norovirus, particularly among infants, young children, the elderly, and those with underlying health conditions.Symptoms of dehydration include:

- dry mouth
- increased or excessive thirst
- low urine output
- nausea
- dizziness or faintness
- sunken eyes
- sunken fontanelle—the soft spot on an infant s head
- confusion.

As many as 30–50% of norovirus infections do not produce symptoms. It is not known whether individuals with asymptomatic infections can transmit the virus.

Diagnosis

Identifying noroviruses

Viral gastroenteritis usually is diagnosed on the basis of the symptoms. Many types of viruses cause gastroenteritis. Rotoviruses are a leading cause of gastroenteritis in children who then transmit the virus to adults. In addition to noroviruses, viral gastroenteritis in humans can be caused by another genus of viruses within the *Caliciviridae* family. Formerly known as the Sapporo-like virus, or classic or typical calicivirus, these now are grouped in the genus *Sapovirus*. Other genera in the *Caliciviridae* family are not pathogenic in humans. Some bacteria and parasites also cause illnesses that are similar to norovirus infection.

The cloning and sequencing of noroviruses in the early 1990s made it easier to identify norovirus outbreaks. RT-PCR is the most commonly used method for identifying norovirus. With this technique the virus s RNA is used as the template for transcribing the corresponding DNA using the enzyme reverse transcriptase. The DNA is amplified into many copies using the polymerase chain reaction. Many state public health laboratories use this method to detect norovirus in vomit and stools. The best identification usually comes from stool samples taken within 48–72 hours after the onset of symptoms; however norovirus can be detected in stool samples taken five days after the onset of symptoms and sometimes even in samples taken up to two weeks after recovery.

Norovirus from fecal samples can be visualized using electron microscopy. With immune electron microscopy (IEM), antibodies against norovirus are collected from blood serum and used to trap and visualize the virus from fecal samples. However these methods require high concentrations of norovirus in the stool, as well as a fourfold increase in norovirus-specific antibodies in blood samples taken during the acute or recovery phases of gastroenteritis.

Enzyme-linked immunosorbent assays may be used to detect noroviruses in fecal samples. In these assays noroviral-specific antibodies bound to the virus are detected by the reaction of an enzyme that is attached to the antibody. Nucleic acid probes that hybridize with noroviral RNA also can be used for virus detection in feces.

As of 2005 a Japanese chemical company was producing a reagent kit that can be used to detect norovirus in two hours rather than the 12–24 hours needed for conventional detection. Other simpler methods for rapidly identifying norovirus are under development.

Investigating outbreaks

Epidemiological studies often involve sequencing the norovirus RNA. This can help to determine whether outbreaks in different geographical locations are connected to each other and can help trace the source of the norovirus to contaminated food or water. CaliciNet is a database that stores the RNA sequences of all norovirus strains that cause gastroenteritis in the United States.

Criteria that are sometimes used to determine whether an outbreak of gastroenteritis is caused by a norovirus include:

• a mean incubation period of 24–48 hours

• a mean duration time for illness of 12–60 hours

• vomiting in more than 50% of patients

• failure to find a bacterial cause for the illness.

During investigations of norovirus outbreaks, food handlers may be asked to provide a stool sample and possibly a blood sample. Food rarely is tested for norovirus since each type of food requires a specific assay. However tests are used to detect the virus in shellfish. When large amounts—1–26 gal. (5–100 L)—of water are processed through specially designed filters, the norovirus can be concentrated and assayed by RT-PCR.

Treatment

Gastroenteritis caused by noroviruses usually resolves itself without treatment within a very few days. As of 2005 there are no medications or vaccines that are effective against the norovirus. Viruses are not affected by **antibiotics** and antidiarrheal medications may prolong the infection.

Norovirus infections should be treated by:

• drinking plenty of fluids, such as water and juice, to prevent dehydration caused by vomiting and diarrhea

• intravenous fluids if severe nausea prevents drinking, particularly in small children

• drinking oral rehydration fluids (ORFs) to prevent dehydration and to replace electrolytes (salt and **minerals**) and glucose

• avoiding alcohol and **caffeine** which can increase urination.

Commercially available ORFs include Naturalyte, Pedialyte, Infalyte, and Rehydralyte.

Juice, soda, and water do not replace lost electrolytes; nor do sports drinks replace nutrients and minerals lost through vomiting and diarrhea. Those taking **diuretics** should ask their healthcare provider whether to stop taking the medication during acute diarrhea.

Since the risk of dehydration is higher for infants and young children, the number of wet diapers per day should be closely monitored. Severely dehydrated children may receive rapid **intravenous rehydration** in a hospital or emergency-room setting.

A health care provider should be consulted if:

• symptoms of dehydration appear

• diarrhea persists for longer than a few days

• there is blood in the stool.

Alternative treatment

An infusion of meadowsweet (*Filipendula ulmaria*) may reduce nausea. Once the symptoms are reduced, slippery elm (*Ulmus fulva* may calm the digestive system. Castor oil packs placed on the abdomen can reduce inflammation and discomfort.

Homeopathic remedies for gastroenteritis include *Arsenicum album*, **ipecac**, and *Nux vomica*. Chinese patent herbal remedies include Po Chai and Pill Curing.

During recovery from viral gastroenteritis, live cultures of *Lactobacillus acidophilus*, found in live-culture yogurt or as powder or capsules, may be useful for restoring the native flora of the digestive tract.

Prognosis

Norovirus infection is followed by complete recovery and there are no known long-term health effects. Infected persons do not become long-term carriers of the virus. Dehydration is the most serious possible consequence of noroviral infection and can be fatal, particularly among older people with debilitating medical conditions or impaired immune systems.

Prevention

Noroviruses are difficult to destroy. They can survive freezing as well as temperatures as high as 140° F (60° C). Noroviruses can survive chlorine levels as high as 10 parts per million (ppm), far higher than the levels present in most public water systems. A 2004 study from the Netherlands found that inactivation of norovirus with 70% ethanol was inefficient and that sodium hypochlorite solutions were effective only at concentrations above 300 ppm.

The best prevention against noroviral infection is frequent, thorough hand washing with soap and water. All soaped hand surfaces should be rubbed vigorously for at least 10 seconds. The hands should be thoroughly rinsed under a stream of water. In particular hands always should be washed before handling food and after using the toilet or changing diapers.

Other important measures for preventing norovirus infection include:

- proper handling of cold foods
- careful washing of fruits and vegetables
- steaming oysters before eating, although even this may be insufficient for destroying norovirus
- taking particular care when handing the diapers of children with diarrhea
- properly disposing of sewage and diapers
- excluding sick infants and children from food preparation areas.

To prevent further transmission of norovirus:

- All surfaces exposed to vomit or otherwise contaminated should be immediately cleaned and disinfected with a solution of 10% bleach, followed by rinsing.
- Contaminated clothing and linens should be removed immediately and washed with hot water and detergent on the maximum machine cycle and with a minimum of handling, followed by machine drying.
- Vomit and feces should be discarded or flushed immediately and the toilet area should be kept clean.
- Exposed or contaminated food should be discarded.
- Masks may be worn while cleaning areas that have been badly contaminated with vomit or feces, such as in hospitals or nursing homes.

A 2004 study found that detergent-based cleaning with a cloth consistently failed to eliminate norovirus contamination. With fecal contamination, detergent-based cleaning, followed by cleaning with a combination hypochlorite/detergent formula containing 5000 ppm of available chlorine significantly reduced contamination. However norovirus still could be detected on as much as 28% of the surfaces. When this procedure failed to eliminate contamination, the virus was transmitted to the cleaner's hands. Contaminated fingers consistently transferred norovirus to up to seven different surfaces including doorknobs and telephones. However the contamination was diluted during secondary transmission and treatment with the combined bleach/detergent eliminated the virus without prior cleaning.

In situations where there is a periodic renewal of susceptible people, such as on cruise ships and at camps, the facility may have to be closed until cleaning is complete. Although many state and local health departments require that food handlers with gastroenteritis not return to work until 2–3 days following recovery, this may not be an adequate length of time to prevent noroviral transmission.

The prevention of norovirus outbreaks include reducing contamination of water supplies with human waste and using high-level chlorination—at least 10 ppm for more than 30 min. Surveillance of shorelines for potential sources of fecal contamination and for boats that are dumping human waste may help prevent shellfish-associated norovirus outbreaks.

In 2004 researchers at Washington University announced that they had succeeded in growing a mouse norovirus in the laboratory for the first time, with the goal of studying the virus and developing a vaccine against it. New surveillance systems also are being developed to detect norovirus outbreaks at an early stage.

Resources

BOOKS

Richman, Douglas D., et al., editors. *Clinical Virology*. 2nd ed. Washington, D.C.: ASM Press, 2002.

Antibody—A blood protein produced in response to foreign material such as a virus; the antibody attaches to the virus and destroys it.

Calicivirus—A member of the *Caliciviridae* family of viruses that includes noroviruses.

Capsid—The outer protein coat of a virus.

Gastroenteritis—An inflammation of the lining of the stomach and intestines, usually caused by a viral or bacterial infection.

Genetic cluster—A group of viral strains with very similar, yet distinct, nucleic acid sequences.

Genogroup—Related viruses within a genus; may be further subdivided into genetic clusters.

Reverse transcription-polymerase chain reaction; RT-PCR—A method of polymerase-chain-reaction amplification of nucleic acid sequences that uses RNA as the template for transcribing the corresponding DNA using reverse transcriptase.

DC 20013-1133. healthfinder@nhic.org. < http://www.healthfinder.gov/ >.
Office of Health Communication. National Center for Infectious Diseases. Centers for Disease Control and Prevention. Mailstop C-14, 1600 Clifton Road, Atlanta, GA 30333. 800-311-3435. < http://www.cdc.gov/ncidod/index.htm >.

OTHER

PM Medical Health News. *21st Century Complete Medical Guide to Gastroenteritis, Norwalk Virus, Norovirus, Authoritative Government Documents, Clinical References, and Practical Information for Patients and Physicians.* CD-ROM. Progressive Management, 2004.
Norovirus. Respiratory and Enteric Viruses Branch, National Center for Infectious Diseases. January 20, 2005 [cited February 21, 2005]. < http://www.cdc.gov/ncidod/dvrd/revb/gastro.norovirus.htm >.
"Norovirus Cultured for the First Time." *Public Library of Science Biology* 2.12 (2004). November 30, 2004 [cited February 26, 2005]. < http://www.plosbiology.org/plosonline/?request = get-document&doi = 10.1371%2Fjournal.pbio.0020445 >.

Margaret Alic, Ph.D.

Norplant *see* **Depo-Provera/Norplant**

Norwalk virus infection *see* **Gastroenteritis**

Nose injuries *see* **Nasal trauma**

Nose irrigation *see* **Nasal irrigation**

Nose job *see* **Rhinoplasty**

Nose packing *see* **Nasal packing**

Nose papillomas *see* **Nasal papillomas**

Nose polyps *see* **Nasal polyps**

PERIODICALS

Blevins, L. Zanardi, et al. "An Outbreak of Norovirus Gastroenteritis at a Swimming Club—Vermont, 2004." *MMWR. Morbidity and Mortality Weekly Report* 53, no. 34 (September 3, 2004): 793-5.
Centers for Disease Control and Prevention, National Center for Infectious Diseases. "Norwalk-Like Viruses: Public Health Consequences and Outbreak Management." *MMWR. Morbidity and Mortality Weekly Report* 50, no. RR-9 (June 1, 2001).
Kirkwood, Chris. "Viral Gastroenteritis in Europe: A New Norovirus Variant?" *The Lancet* 363, no. 9410 (February 28, 2004): 671-2.
Lopman, Ben, et al. "Increase in Viral Gastrocenteritis Outbreaks in Europe and Epidemic Spread of New Norovirus Variant." *The Lancet* 363, no. 9410 (February 28, 2004): 682-8.
"Norovirus; Cruise Ships Experience Increase in Norovirus Incidents." *Science Letter* February 22, 2005: 1140.
"Norovirus; Detergent Followed by Bleach/Detergent Reduces Norovirus Contamination." *Science Letter* December 14, 2004: 843.
"Norovirus Outbreak; Alterations to Norovirus Capsid Structure Explains 2002–2003 Outbreaks." *Science Letter* November 30, 2004: 1008.

ORGANIZATIONS

National Health Information Center. Office of Disease Prevention and Health Promotion. U.S. Department of Health & Human Services. P.O. Box 1133, Washington,

Nosebleed

Definition

A nosebleed is bleeding from the nose; the medical term for it is epistaxis.

Description

Unexpected bleeding from anywhere is cause for alarm. Persistent bleeding should always be investigated because it may be the earliest sign of **cancer**. Fortunately, nosebleeds are rarely a sign of cancer. A much more common cause of nosebleeds is injury from picking or blowing or fisticuffs. People with

Noosebleed

hay **fever** have swollen membranes that are fragile and more likely to bleed.

Most nosebleeds (about 90%) come from the front of the septum, that plane of cartilage that separates the nostrils. These are called anterior nosebleeds. The lower front part of the septum has a mass of blood vessels on either side called Kiesselbach's plexus that is easy to injure. Nosebleeds from the more remote reaches of the nose are called posterior nosebleeds. They are less common, are less likely to have a benign cause, and are much harder to manage.

Nosebleeds are most likely to occur in children between the ages of two and 10 years, in part because younger children frequently insert small objects in the nose or pick at the tissues lining the nose. Nosebleeds in adolescents may indicate **cocaineabuse**. Nosebleeds in older adults may result from arteriosclerosis or high blood pressure.

Causes and symptoms

Nosebleeds may result from a number of different causes:

- local infections (colds, sinus infections)
- systemic infections (**scarlet fever**, **typhoid fever**, malaria)
- drying of the membranes lining the nose, often during heating season in colder climates
- medications, most commonly, overuse of nasal decongestant sprays
- trauma (from **foreign objects** in the nose; scratching or picking with the fingers; or blunt trauma to the face)
- tumors in the nasopharynx or paranasal sinuses
- cocaine abuse
- bleeding disorders (leukemia, **liver disease**, **hemophilia** and other hereditary clotting disorders)

Treatment

The first treatment is to pinch the patient's nostrils together, have them sit forward, and ask them to stay that way for 5–10 minutes. This method usually stops nosebleeds originating in Kiesselbach's plexus. The patient should not tilt his or her head backward, as this position may cause blood to drip backward into the throat or windpipe. It is best to hold the head upright.

In the case of small children, the doctor may examine the inside of the nose to check for foreign bodies, evidence of scratching or picking, etc. Small foreign bodies (watch batteries, dried peas or beans, buttons, etc.) can be removed by suction if necessary. The doctor may also have to remove clotted blood by suction.

Bleeding that continues originates from the back of the nose in most cases and will flow down the throat. If that happens, emergency intervention is needed.

As an emergency procedure, the nose will be packed front and/or back with cotton gauze and a rubber balloon from a Foley catheter. This treatment is not comfortable. Having no place to flow, the blood should clot, giving the ear, nose and throat specialists (otorhinolaryngologists) a chance to find the source and permanently repair it. If the packing has to remain for any length of time, **antibiotics** and **pain** medication will be necessary—antibiotics because the sinuses will be plugged up and prone to infection. Nose packing may so interfere with breathing that the patient will need supplemental oxygen.

Newer options for controlling posterior nosebleeds include the use of Surgicel, Merocel, or other oxidized cellulose products that expand with moisture. These may control the bleeding without the need for bulky **nasal packing**.

Many bleeds are from small exposed blood vessels with no other disease. They can be destroyed by cautery, usually done by applying silver nitrate to the affected area. Larger vessels may not respond to cautery. The surgeon may have to tie them off, which is known as ligation. Another technique that is sometimes used with larger vessels is embolization, in which the doctor injects a chemical to block or close the blood vessel.

Alternative treatment

Estrogen cream, the same preparation used to revitalize vaginal tissue, can toughen fragile blood vessels in the anterior septum and forestall the need for cauterization. Botanical medicines known as styptics, which slow down and can stop bleeding, may be taken internally or applied topically. Some of the plants used are achillea (yarrow), trillium, geranium, and shepherd's purse (*capsella-bursa*). Homeopathic remedies can be one of the quickest and most effective treatments for epistaxis.

Prevention

Both before and after a nosebleed, the patient should blow the nose gently and avoid picking or

KEY TERMS

Cautery—The use of heat, electricity, or chemicals to destroy tissue.

Embolization—A technique for stopping bleeding by introducing a substance into larger blood vessels that blocks or closes them.

Epistaxis—The medical term for nosebleed.

Kiesselbach's plexus—An area on the anterior part of the nasal septum that has a rich supply of blood vessels and is a common site of nosebleeds. It is named for Wilhelm Kiesselbach, a nineteenth-century German otolaryngologist.

Septum—The partition that separates the two nostrils. It consists of membranes, cartilage, and bone.

Styptic—Any remedy with an astringent and hemostatic (stopping bleeding) quality.

American Academy of Otolaryngology—Head and Neck Surgery. One Prince Street, Alexandria, VA 22314-3357. (703) 836-4444. < http://www.entnet.org >.

J. Ricker Polsdorfer, MD
Rebecca J. Frey, PhD

Nosocomial infections *see* **Hospital-acquired infections**

NS *see* **Nephrotic syndrome**

NSAIDs *see* **Nonsteroidal anti-inflammatory drugs**

Nther's disease *see* **Porphyrias**

Nuclear magnetic resonance *see* **Magnetic resonance imaging**

Nucleoside analogs *see* **Antiretroviral drugs**

scratching the tissues that line it. Children with recurrent nosebleeds during heating season may benefit from the use of a cool-mist vaporizer to humidify the bedroom at night, or from the application of a small quantity of petroleum jelly to the inside of each nostril. Treatment of hay fever helps reduce the fragility of the tissues.

Resources

BOOKS

Beers, Mark H., MD, and Robert Berkow, MD., editors. "Epistaxis." Section 7, Chapter 86 In *The Merck Manual of Diagnosis and Therapy*. Whitehouse Station, NJ: Merck Research Laboratories, 2004.

PERIODICALS

Bhatnagar, R. K., and S. Berry. "Selective Surgicel Packing for the Treatment of Posterior Epistaxis." *Ear, Nose, and Throat Journal* 83 (September 2004): 633–634.

Gluckman, William, DO, and Robert Baricella, DO. "Epistaxis." *eMedicine* October 11, 2004. < http://emedicine.com/ped/topic1618.htm >.

Gurney, T. A., C. F. Dowd, and A. H. Murr. "Embolization for the Treatment of Idiopathic Posterior Epistaxis." *American Journal of Rhinology* 18 (September-October 2004): 335–339.

ORGANIZATIONS

American Academy of Family Physicians (AAFP). 11400 Tomahawk Creek Parkway, Leawood, KS 66211-2672. (800) 274-2237 or (913) 906-6000. < http://www.aafp.org >.

Numbness and tingling

Definition

Numbness and tingling are decreased or abnormal sensations caused by altered sensory nerve function.

Description

The feeling of having a foot "fall asleep" is a familiar one. This same combination of numbness and tingling can occur in any region of the body and may be caused by a wide variety of disorders. Sensations such as these, which occur without any associated stimulus, are called paresthesias. Other types of paresthesias include feelings of cold, warmth, burning, **itching**, and skin crawling.

Causes and symptoms

Causes

Sensation is carried to the brain by neurons (nerve cells) running from the outer parts of the body to the spinal cord in bundles called nerves. In the spinal cord, these neurons make connections with other neurons that run up to the brain. Paresthesias are caused by disturbances in the function of neurons in the sensory pathway. This disturbance can occur in the central nervous system (the brain and spinal cord), the nerve roots that are attached to the spinal cord, or the peripheral nervous system (nerves outside the brain and spinal cord).

Peripheral disturbances are the most common cause of paresthesias. "Falling asleep" occurs when the blood supply to a nerve is cut off—a condition called **ischemia**. Ischemia usually occurs when an artery is compressed as it passes through a tightly flexed joint. Sleeping with the arms above the head or sitting with the legs tightly crossed frequently cause numbness and tingling.

Direct compression of the nerve also causes paresthesias. Compression can be short-lived, as when a heavy backpack compresses the nerves passing across the shoulders. Compression may also be chronic. Chronic nerve compression occurs in entrapment syndromes. The most common example is **carpal tunnel syndrome**. Carpal tunnel syndrome occurs when the median nerve is compressed as it passes through a narrow channel in the wrist. Repetitive motion or prolonged vibration can cause the lining of the channel to swell and press on the nerve. Chronic nerve root compression, or radiculopathy, can occur in disk disease or spinal arthritis.

Other causes of paresthesias related to disorders of the peripheral nerves include:

- Metabolic or nutritional disturbances. These disturbances include diabetes, **hypothyroidism** (a condition caused by too little activity of the thyroid gland), alcoholism, **malnutrition**, and vitamin B_{12} deficiency.

- Trauma. Trauma includes injuries that crush, sever, or pull on nerves.

- Inflammation.

- Connective tissue disease. These diseases include arthritis, systemic lupus erythematosus (a chronic inflammatory disease that affects many systems of the body, including the nervous system), polyarteritis nodosa (a vascular disease that causes widespread inflammation and ischemia of small and medium-size arteries), and **Sjögren's syndrome** (a disorder marked by insufficient moisture in the tear ducts, salivary glands, and other glands).

- Toxins. Toxins include heavy metals (metallic elements such as arsenic, lead, and mercury which can, in large amounts, cause **poisoning**), certain **antibiotics** and **chemotherapy** agents, solvents, and overdose of pyridoxine (vitamin B_6).

- Malignancy.

- Infections. Infections include **Lyme disease**, human immunodeficiency virus (HIV), and leprosy.

- Hereditary disease. These diseases include Charcot-Marie-Tooth disease (a hereditary disorder that causes wasting of the leg muscles, resulting in malformation of the foot), porphyria (a group of inherited disorders in which there is abnormally increased production of substances called porphyrins), and Denny-Brown's syndrome (a hereditary disorder of the nerve root).

Paresthesias can also be caused by central nervous system disturbances, including stroke, TIA (transient ischemic attack), tumor, trauma, **multiple sclerosis**, or infection.

Symptoms

Sensory nerves supply or innervate particular regions of the body. Determining the distribution of symptoms is an important way to identify the nerves involved. For instance, the median nerve innervates the thumb, the first two fingers, half of the ring finger, and the part of the hand to which they connect. The ulnar nerve innervates the other half of the ring finger, the little finger, and the remainder of the hand. Distribution of symptoms may also aid diagnosis of the underlying disease. Diabetes usually causes a symmetrical "glove and stocking" distribution in the hands and feet. Multiple sclerosis may cause symptoms in several, widely separated areas.

Other symptoms may accompany paresthesias, depending on the type and severity of the nerve disturbance. For instance, weakness may accompany damage to nerves that carry both sensory and motor neurons. (Motor neurons are those that carry messages outward from the brain.)

Diagnosis

A careful history of the patient is needed for a diagnosis of paresthesias. The medical history should focus on the onset, duration, and location of symptoms. The history may also reveal current related medical problems and recent or past exposure to drugs, toxins, infection, or trauma. The family medical history may suggest a familial disorder. A work history may reveal repetitive motion, chronic vibration, or industrial chemical exposure.

The physical and neurological examination tests for distribution of symptoms and alterations in reflexes, sensation, or strength. The distribution of symptoms may be mapped by successive stimulation over the affected area of the body.

Lab tests for paresthesia may include blood tests and **urinalysis** to detect metabolic or nutritional abnormalities. Other tests are used to look for specific suspected causes. Nerve conduction velocity tests, **electromyography**, and imaging studies of the affected area may be employed. Nerve biopsy may be indicated in selected cases.

Treatment

Treatment of paresthesias depends on the underlying cause. For limbs that have "fallen asleep," restoring circulation by stretching, exercising, or massaging the affected limb can quickly dissipate the numbness and tingling. If the paresthesia is caused by a chronic disease such as diabetes or occurs as a complication of treatments such as chemotherapy, most treatments are aimed at relieving symptoms. Anti-inflammatory drugs such as **aspirin** or ibuprofen are recommended if symptoms are mild. In more difficult cases, **antidepressant drugs** such as amitriptyline (Elavil) are sometimes prescribed. These drugs are given at a much lower dosage for this purpose than for relief of depression. They are thought to help because they alter the body's perception of pain. In severe cases, opium derivatives such as codeine can be prescribed. Currently trials are being done to determine whether treatment with human nerve growth factor will be effective in regenerating the damaged nerves.

Alternative treatment

Several alternative treatments are available to help relieve symptoms of paresthesia. Nutritional therapy includes supplementation with B complex **vitamins**, especially vitamin B_{12} (intramuscular injection of vitamin B_{12} is most effective). Vitamin supplements should be used cautiously however. Overdose of Vitamin B_6 is one of the causes of paresthesias. People experiencing paresthesia should also avoid alcohol. **Acupuncture** and massage are said to relieve symptoms. Self-massage with aromatic oils is sometimes helpful. The application of topical ointments containing capsaicin, the substance that makes hot peppers hot, provides relief for some. It may also be helpful to wear loosely fitting shoes and clothing. None of these alternatives should be used in place of traditional therapy for the underlying condition.

Prognosis

Treating the underlying disorder may reduce the occurrence of paresthesias. Paresthesias resulting from damaged nerves may persist throughout or even beyond the recovery period. The overall prognosis depends on the cause.

KEY TERMS

Electromyography—A test that uses electrodes to record the electrical activity of muscle. The information gathered is used to diagnose neuromuscular disorders.

Motor nerve—Motor or efferent nerve cells carry impulses from the brain to muscle or organ tissue.

Nerve conduction velocity test—A test that measures the time it takes a nerve impulse to travel a specific distance over the nerve after electronic stimulation.

Nerve growth factor—A protein resembling insulin that affects growth and maintenance of nerve cells

Peripheral nervous system—The part of the nervous system that is outside the brain and spinal cord. Sensory, motor, and autonomic nerves are included.

Sensory nerves—Sensory or afferent nerves carry impulses of sensation from the periphery or outward parts of the body to the brain. Sensations include feelings, impressions, and awareness of the state of the body.

Prevention

Preventing the underlying disorder may reduce the incidence of paresthesias. For those with frequent paresthesias caused by ischemia, changes in posture may help.

Resources

PERIODICALS

McKnight, Jerry T., and Bobbi B. Adcock. "Paresthesias: A Practical Diagnostic Approach." *American Family Physician* 56 (December 1997): 2253-2260.

Richard Robinson

Nummular dermatitis *see* **Dermatitis**

Nutrition

Definition

Good nutrition can help prevent disease and promote health. There are six categories of nutrients that the body needs to acquire from food: protein, carbohydrates, fat, fibers, **vitamins** and **minerals**, and water.

Proteins

Protein supplies amino acids to build and maintain healthy body tissue. There are 20 amino acids considered essential because the body must have all of them in the right amounts to function properly. Twelve of these are manufactured in the body but the other eight amino acids must be provided by the diet. Foods from animal sources such as milk or eggs often contain all these essential amino acids while a variety of plant products must be taken together to provide all these necessary protein components.

Fat

Fat supplies energy and transports nutrients. There are two families of fatty acids considered essential for the body: the omega-3 and omega-6 fatty acids. Essential fatty acids are required by the body to function normally. They can be obtained from canola oil, flaxseed oil, cold-water fish, or fish oil, all of which contain **omega-3 fatty acids**, and primrose or black currant seed oil, which contains omega-6 fatty acids. The American diet often contains an excess of omega-6 fatty acids and insufficient amounts of omega-3 fats. Increased consumption of omega-3 oils is recommended to help reduce risk of cardiovascular diseases and **cancer** and alleviate symptoms of rheumatoid arthritis, **premenstrual syndrome**, **dermatitis**, and inflammatory bowel disease.

Carbohydrates

Carbohydrates are the body's main source of energy and should be the major part of total daily intake. There are two types of carbohydrates: simple carbohydrates (such as sugar or honey) or complex carbohydrates (such as grains, beans, peas, or potatoes). Complex carbohydrates are preferred because these foods are more nutritious yet have fewer calories per gram compared to fat and cause fewer problems with overeating than fat or sugar. Complex carbohydrates also are preferred over simple carbohydrates by diabetics because they allow better blood glucose control.

Fiber

Fiber is the material that gives plants texture and support. Although it is primarily made up of carbohydrates, it does not have a lot of calories and is usually not broken down by the body for energy. Dietary fiber is found in plant foods such as fruits, vegetables, legumes, nuts, and whole grains.

There are two types of fiber: soluble and insoluble. Insoluble fiber, as the name implies, does not dissolve in water because it contains high amount of cellulose. Insoluble fiber can be found in the bran of grains, the pulp of fruit and the skin of vegetables. Soluble fiber is the type of fiber that dissolves in water. It can be found in a variety of fruits and vegetables such as apples, oatmeal and oat bran, rye flour, and dried beans.

Although they share some common characteristics such as being partially digested in the stomach and intestines and have few calories, each type of fiber has its own specific health benefits. Insoluble fiber speeds up the transit of foods through the digestive system and adds bulk to the stools, therefore, it is the type of fiber that helps treat **constipation** or **diarrhea** and prevents colon cancer. On the other hand, only soluble fiber can lower blood cholesterol levels. This type of fiber works by attaching itself to the cholesterol so that it can be eliminated from the body. This prevents cholesterol from recirculating and being reabsorbed into the bloodstream. In 2003, the World Health Organization released a new report specifically outlining the link of a healthy diet rich in high-fiber plant foods to preventing cancer.

Vitamins and minerals

Vitamins are organic substances present in food and required by the body in a small amount for regulation of metabolism and maintenance of normal growth and functioning. The most commonly known vitamins are A, B_1 (thiamine), B_2 (riboflavin), B_3 (niacin), B_5 (pantothenic acid), B_6 (pyridoxine), B_7 (biotin), B_9 (folic acid), B_{12} (cobalamin), C (ascorbic acid), D, E, and K. The B and C vitamins are water-soluble, excess amounts of which are excreted in the urine. The A, D, E, and K vitamins are fat-soluble and will be stored in the body fat.

Minerals are vital to our existence because they are the building blocks that make up muscles, tissues, and bones. They also are important components of many life-supporting systems, such as hormones, oxygen transport, and enzyme systems.

There are two kinds of minerals: the major (or macro) minerals and the trace minerals. Major minerals are the minerals that the body needs in large amounts. The following minerals are classified as major: calcium, phosphorus, magnesium, sodium, potassium, sulfur, and chloride. They are needed to build muscles, blood, nerve cells, teeth, and bones. They also are essential electrolytes that the body requires to regulate blood volume and acid-base balance.

Unlike the major minerals, trace minerals are needed only in tiny amounts. Even though they can be found in the body in exceedingly small amounts, they are also very important to the human body. These minerals participate in most chemical reactions in the body. They also are needed to manufacture important hormones. The following are classified as trace minerals: iron, zinc, iodine, copper, manganese, fluoride, chromium, selenium, molybdenum, and boron.

Many vitamins (such as vitamins A, C, and E) and minerals (such as zinc, copper, selenium, or manganese) act as antioxidants. They protect the body against the damaging effects of free radicals. They scavenge or mop up these highly reactive radicals and change them into inactive, less harmful compounds. In so doing, these essential nutrients help prevent cancer and many other degenerative diseases, such as premature **aging**, heart disease, autoimmune diseases, arthritis, **cataracts**, **Alzheimer's disease**, and diabetes mellitus.

Water

Water helps to regulate body temperature, transports nutrients to cells, and rids the body of waste materials.

Origins

Unlike plants, human beings cannot manufacture most of the nutrients that they need to function. They must eat plants and/or other animals. Although nutritional therapy came to the forefront of the public's awareness in the late twentieth century, the notion that food affects health is not new. John Harvey Kellogg was an early health-food pioneer and an advocate of a high-fiber diet. An avowed vegetarian, he believed that meat products were particularly detrimental to the colon. In the 1870s, Kellogg founded the Battle Creek Sanitarium, where he developed a diet based on nut and vegetable products.

Purpose

Good nutrition helps individuals achieve general health and well-being. In addition, dietary modifications might be prescribed for a variety of complaints including **allergies**, anemia, arthritis, colds, depressions, **fatigue**, gastrointestinal disorders, high or low blood pressure, **insomnia**, headaches, **obesity**, **pregnancy**, premenstrual syndrome (PMS), respiratory conditions, and stress.

Nutritional therapy may also be involved as a complement to the allopathic treatments of cancer, diabetes, and Parkinson's disease. Other specific dietary measures include the elimination of food additives for attention deficit hyperactivity disorder (ADHD), gluten-free **diets** for schizophrenia, and dairy-free for chronic respiratory diseases.

A high-fiber diet helps prevent or treat the following health conditions:

- High cholesterol levels. Fiber effectively lowers blood cholesterol levels. It appears that soluble fiber binds to cholesterol and moves it down the digestive tract so that it can be excreted from the body. This prevents the cholesterol from being reabsorbed into the bloodstream.

- Constipation. A high-fiber diet is the preferred non-drug treatment for constipation. Fiber in the diet adds more bulk to the stools, making them softer and shortening the time foods stay in the digestive tract.

- Hemorrhoids. Fiber in the diet adds more bulk and softens the stool, thus, reducing painful hemorrhoidal symptoms.

- Diabetes. Soluble fiber in the diet slows down the rise of blood sugar levels following a meal and helps control diabetes.

- Obesity. Dietary fiber makes a person feel full faster.

- Cancer. Insoluble fiber in the diet speeds up the movement of the stools through the gastrointestinal tract. The faster food travels through the digestive tract, the less time there is for potential cancer-causing substances to work. Therefore, diets high in insoluble fiber help prevent the accumulation of toxic substances that cause cancer of the colon. Because fiber reduces fat absorption in the digestive tract, it also may prevent breast cancer.

A diet low in fat also promotes good health and prevents many diseases. Low-fat diets can help treat or control the following conditions:

- Obesity. High fat consumption often leads to excess caloric and fat intake, which increases body fat.

- Coronary artery disease. High consumption of saturated fats is associated with coronary artery disease.

- Diabetes. People who are overweight tend to develop or worsen existing diabetic conditions due to decreased insulin sensitivity.

- Breast cancer. A high dietary consumption of fat is associated with an increased risk of breast cancer.

Description

The four basic food groups, as outlined by the United States Department of Agriculture (USDA) are:

- dairy products (such as milk and cheese)
- meat and eggs (such as fish, poultry, pork, beef, and eggs)
- grains (such as bread cereals, rice, and pasta)
- fruits and vegetables

The USDA recommendation for adults is that consumption of meat, eggs, and dairy products should not exceed 20% of total daily caloric intake. The rest (80%) should be devoted to vegetables, fruits, and grains. For children age two or older, 55% of their caloric intake should be in the form of carbohydrates, 30% from fat, and 15% from proteins. In addition, saturated fat intake should not exceed 10% of total caloric intake. This low-fat, high-fiber diet is believed to promote health and help prevent many diseases, including heart disease, obesity, and cancer.

Allergenic and highly processed foods should be avoided. Highly processed foods do not contain significant amounts of essential trace minerals. Furthermore, they contain lots of fat and sugar as well as preservatives, artificial sweeteners and other additives. High consumption of these foods causes build up of unwanted chemicals in the body and should be avoided. Food allergies causes a variety of symptoms including food cravings, weight gain, bloating, and water retention. They also may worsen chronic inflammatory conditions such as arthritis.

Preparations

An enormous body of research exists in the field of nutrition. Mainstream Western medical practitioners point to studies that show that a balanced diet, based on the USDA Food Guide Pyramid, provides all of the necessary nutrients.

In 2004, the USDA was working on a revision of the Food Guide Pyramid to reflect changes in American lifestyle habits. The new eating guide was due for release in January 2005. The World Health Organization (WHO) also was weighing in on the obesity and nutrition issue, even struggling with objections from member nations that supply goods such as sugar, to endorse a global strategy in spring 2004 on diet, physical activity and health.

The Food Guide Pyramid recommends the following daily servings in six categories:

- grains: six or more servings
- vegetables: five servings
- fruits: two to four servings
- meat: two to three servings
- dairy: two to three servings
- fats and oils: use sparingly

Precautions

Individuals should not change their diets without the advice of nutritional experts or health care professionals. Certain individuals, especially children, pregnant and lactating women, and chronically ill patients, only should change their diets under professional supervision.

Side effects

It is best to obtain vitamins and minerals through food sources. Excessive intake of vitamins and mineral supplements can cause serious health problems. Likewise, eating too much of one type of food, as can happen with fad diets, can be harmful. The key to nutrition is moderation. If a person feels they are short on iron, for example, he or she should not go too far to the extreme in getting more iron through diet and supplements. A 2003 report said that too much stored iron in the body has possibly been linked with heart disease, cancer and diabetes.

The following is a list of possible side effects resulting from excessive doses of vitamins and minerals:

- vitamin A: **birth defects**, irreversible bone and liver damage
- vitamin B_1: deficiencies in B_2 and B_6
- vitamin B_6: damage to the nervous system
- vitamin C: affects the absorption of copper; diarrhea
- vitamin D: **hypercalcemia** (abnormally high concentration of calcium in the blood)
- phosphorus: affects the absorption of calcium
- zinc: affects absorption of copper and iron; suppresses the immune system

Research and general acceptance

Due to a large volume of scientific evidence demonstrating the benefits of the low-fat, high-fiber diet in disease prevention and treatment, these recommendations have been accepted and advocated by both complementary and allopathic practitioners.

Resources

BOOKS

U.S. Preventive Services Task Force Guidelines. "Counseling to Promote a Healthy Diet." *Guide to Clinical Preventive Services. 2nd ed.* < http://cpmcnet.columbia.edu/texts/gcps/gcps0066.html >.

PERIODICALS

Clapp, Stephen. "World Health Assembly Adopts Global Anti-obesity Strategy." *Food Chemical News* May 31, 2004: 26.

Halbert, Steven C. "Diet and Nutrtion in Primary Care: From Antioxidants to Zinc." *Primary Care: Clinics in Office Practice* December 1997: 825-843.

Mangels, Reed. "How Can You Avoid Having Too Much Iron?" *Vegetarian Journal* March-April 2003: 17.

Turner, Lisa. "Good 'n Plenty." *Vegetarian Times* February 1999: 48.

"U.N. Report Supports Key Role for Diet, Activity in Cancer Prevention." *Cancer Weekly* March 25, 2003: 154.

Vickers, Andrew, and Catherine Zollman. "Unconventional approaches to nutritional medicine." *British Medical Journal* November 27, 1999: 1419.

ORGANIZATIONS

American Association of Nutritional Consultants. 810 S. Buffalo Street, Warsaw, IN 46580. (888) 828-2262.

American Dietetic Association. 216 W. Jackson boulevard, Suite 800, Chicago, IL 60606-6995. (800) 366-1655. < http://www.eatright.org >.

Mai Tran
Teresa G. Odle

Nutrition through an intravenous line

Definition

Sterile solutions containing some or all of the nutrients necessary to support life, are injected into the body through a tube attached to a needle, which is inserted into a vein, either temporarily or for long-term treatment.

Purpose

Patients who cannot consume enough nutrients or who cannot eat at all due to an illness, surgery, or accident, can be fed through an intravenous (IV) line or tube. An IV can be used for as little as a few hours, to provide fluids to a patient during a short surgical procedure, or to rehydrate a patient after a viral illness.

Patients with more serious and long term illnesses and conditions may require months or even years of intravenous therapy to meet their nutritional needs. These patients may require a central **venous access** port. A specialized catheter (Silastic Broviac or Hickman) is inserted beneath the skin and positioned below the collarbone. Fluids can then be injected directly into the bloodstream for long periods of time. X rays are taken to ensure that the permanent catheter is properly positioned.

Precautions

Patients receiving IV therapy need to be monitored to ensure that the IV solutions are providing the correct amounts of fluids, **minerals**, and other nutrients needed.

Description

There are two types of IV, or parenteral, **nutrition**. Parenteral nutrition is that which is delivered through a system other than the digestive system. In this case, the nutrition is delivered through a vein. Partial parenteral nutrition (PPN) is given for short periods of time, to replace some of the nutrients required daily and only supplements a normal diet. **Total parenteral nutrition** (TPN) is given to someone who cannot eat anything and must receive all nutrients required daily through an intravenous line. Both of these types of nutrition can be performed in a medical facility or at the patient's home. Home parenteral nutrition (HPN) usually requires a central venous catheter, which must first be inserted in a fully equiped medical facility. After it is inserted, therapy can continue at home.

Basic IV solutions are sterile water with small amounts of sodium (salt) or dextrose (sugar) supplied in bottles or thick plastic bags that can hang on a stand mounted next to the patient's bed. Additional minerals, like potassium and calcium, **vitamins**, or drugs can be added to the IV solution by injecting them into the bottle or bag with a needle. These simple sugar and salt solutions can provide fluids, calories, and electrolytes necessary for short periods of time. If a patient requires intravenous feeding for more than a few days, additional nutrients like proteins and fats will be included. The amounts of each of the nutrients to be added will depend on the patient's age, medical condition, and particular nutritional requirements.

Preparation

A doctor orders the IV solution and any additional nutrients or drugs to be added to it. The doctor

KEY TERMS

Home parenteral nutrition (HPN)—Long-term parenteral nutrition, given through a central venous catheter and administered in the patient's home.

Intravenous—Into a vein; a needle is inserted into a vein in the back of the hand, inside the elbow, or some other location on the body. Fluids, nutrients, and drugs can be injected.

Parenteral—Not in or through the digestive system. Parenteral nutrition is given through the veins of the circulatory system, rather than through the digestive system.

Partial parenteral nutrition (PPN)—A solution, containing some essentail nutrients, is injected into a vein to supplement other means of nutrition, usually a partially normal diet of food.

Total parenteral nutrition (TPN)—A solution containing all the required nutrients including protein, fat, calories, vitamins, and minerals, is injected over the course of several hours, into a vein. TPN provides a complete and balanced source of nutrients for patients who cannot consume a normal diet.

also specifies the rate at which the IV will be infused. The IV solutions are prepared under the supervision of a doctor, pharmacist, or nurse, using sanitary techniques that prevent bacterial contamination. Just like a prescription, the IV is clearly labeled to show its contents and the amounts of any additives. The skin around the area where the needle is inserted is cleaned and sanitized. Once the needle is in place, it will be taped to the skin to prevent it from dislodging.

In the case of HPN, the IV solution is delivered to the patient's home on a regular basis and should be kept refrigerated. Each bag will have an expiration date, by which time the bag should be used. The solution should be allowed to be warmed to room temperature before intravenous nutrition begins.

Aftercare

Patients who have been on IV therapy for more than a few days may need to have foods reintroduced gradually to give the digestive tract time to start working again. After the IV needle is removed, the site should be inspected for any signs of bleeding or infection.

When using HPN, the catheter should be kept clean at all times. The dressings around the site should be changed at least once a week and the catheter site should be monitored closely for signs of redness, swelling, and drainage. The patient's extremities should be watched for swelling, which is a sign of nutritional imbalance.

Risks

There is a risk of infection at the injection site, and for patients on long term IV therapy, the risk of an infection spreading to the entire body is fairly high. It is possible that the IV solution may not provide all of the nutrients needed, leading to a deficiency or an imbalance. If the needle becomes dislodged, it is possible that the solution may flow into tissues around the injection site rather than into the vein. The patient should be monitored regularly, particulary if receiving HPN, as intravenous nutrition can potentially cause infection at the site of the catheter, high blood sugar, and low blood potassium, which can all be life-threatening.

Resources

OTHER

"Clinical Management: Parenteral Nutrition" In *Revised Intravenous Nursing Standards of Practice.* <http://www.ins1.org>.

Altha Roberts Edgren

Nutritional supplements

Definition

Nutritional supplements include **vitamins**, **minerals**, herbs, meal supplements, sports **nutrition** products, natural food supplements, and other related products used to boost the nutritional content of the diet.

Purpose

Nutritional supplements are used for many purposes. They can be added to the diet to boost overall health and energy; to provide immune system support and reduce the risks of illness and age-related conditions; to improve performance in athletic and mental activities; and to support the healing process during illness and disease. However, most of these products are treated as food and not regulated as drugs are.

Description

The Natural Nutritional Foods Association estimated that in 2003 nutritional supplements amounted to a $19.8 billion market in the United States. By category, vitamins provided $6.6 billion in sales, herbs $4.2 billion, meal supplements $2.5 billion, sports nutrition products $2.0 billion, minerals $1.8 billion, and specialty and other products totaling $2.7 billion. The nutritional supplement industry provides a huge array of products for consumer needs.

Vitamins

Vitamins are micronutrients, or substances that the body uses in small amounts, as compared to macronutrients, which are the proteins, fats, and carbohydrates that make up all food. Vitamins are present in food, but adequate quantities of vitamins may be reduced when food is overcooked, processed, or improperly stored. For instance, processing whole wheat grain into white flour reduces the contents of vitamins B and E, fiber, and minerals, including zinc and iron. The body requires vitamins to support its basic biochemical functions, and deficiencies over time can lead to illness and disease.

Vitamins are either water-soluble or fat-soluble. Water-soluble vitamins dissolve in water and pass through the body quickly, meaning that the body needs them on a regular basis. Water-soluble vitamins include the B-complex vitamins and vitamin C. Fat-soluble vitamins are stored in the body's fatty tissue, meaning that they remain in the body longer. Fat-soluble vitamins include vitamins A, D, E, and K.

The amount of vitamins needed by the body has been the subject of much research. The U.S. government has published recommended dietary allowances (RDAs) for each vitamin for the general population. These figures can be used as guidelines, but individuals may have different needs depending on gender, age, and health conditions.

Vitamins can be natural or synthetic. Natural vitamins are extracted from food sources, while synthetic vitamins are formulated in laboratory processes. The only vitamin for which there is a noted difference between the natural and synthetic forms is vitamin E. The natural form is labeled d-alpha-tocopherol while the synthetic form is named dl-alpha-tocopherol, with the extra "l" signifying laboratory production. Natural vitamin E has been shown to be slightly more absorbable by the body than the synthetic version, although for other vitamins no significant differences in absorption have been noted.

Minerals

Minerals are micronutrients and are essential for the proper functioning of the body. Cells in the body require minerals as part of their basic make-up and chemical balance, and minerals are present in all foods. Minerals can either be bulk minerals, used by the body in larger quantities, or trace minerals, used by the body in minute or trace amounts. Bulk minerals include sodium, potassium, calcium, magnesium, and phosphorus. Trace minerals include iron, zinc, selenium, iodine, chromium, copper, manganese, and others. Some studies have shown that the amount of minerals, particularly trace minerals, may be decreasing in foods due to mineral depletion of the soil caused by unsustainable farming practices and soil erosion. Supplemental minerals are available in chelated form, in which they are bonded to proteins in order to improve their absorption by the body.

Herbs

Herbal supplements are added to the diet for both nutritional and medicinal purposes. Herbs have been used for centuries in many traditional medicine systems, and as sources of phytochemicals, or substances found in plants that have notable effects in the body. Chinese medicine and **Ayurvedic medicine** from India, two of the world's oldest healing systems, use hundreds of herbal medications. Naturopathy and homeopathy, two other systems of natural healing, also rely on herbal preparations as their main sources of medication. The medicinal effects of herbs are getting scientific validation; about one-fourth of all pharmaceuticals have been derived directly from plant sources, including **aspirin** (found in willow bark), codeine (from poppy seeds), paclitaxel (Taxol), a patented drug for ovarian and **breast cancer** (from the Pacific Yew tree), and many others.

Herbs can supplement the diet to aid in overall health or to stimulate healing for specific conditions. For instance, ginseng is used as a general tonic to increase overall health and vitality, while **echinacea** is a popular herb used to stimulate the body's resistance to colds and infections. Herbs come in many forms. They can be purchased as capsules and tablets, as well as in tinctures, teas, syrups, and ointments.

Meal supplements

Meal supplements are used to replace or fortify meals. They may be designed for people with special needs, or for people with illnesses that may affect digestion capabilities and nutritional requirements. Meal supplements may contain specific blends of macronutrients, or proteins, carbohydrates, fats, and fiber. Some meal supplements consist of raw, unprocessed foods, or vegetarian or vegan options, or high protein and low fat composition. Meal supplements are available to support some popular diet programs. Meal supplements are often fortified with vitamins, minerals, herbs, and nutrient-dense foods.

Sports nutrition

Nutritional supplements may be designed to provide specialized support for athletes. Some of these consist of high-protein products, such as amino acid supplements, while other products contain nutrients that support metabolism, energy, and athletic performance and recovery. People engaging in intense athletic activity may have increased needs for water-soluble vitamins, antioxidants, and certain minerals, including chromium. Sports drinks contain blends of electrolytes (salts) that the body loses during exertion and sweating, as well as vitamins, minerals, and performance-supporting herbs.

Other nutritional supplements

Other nutritional supplements include nutrient-dense food products. Examples of these are brewer's yeast, spirulina (sea algea), bee pollen and royal jelly, fish oil and essential fatty acid supplements, colostrum (a specialty dairy product), psyllium seed husks (a source of fiber), wheat germ, wheatgrass, and medicinal mushrooms such as the shiitake and reishi varieties.

Specialty products may offer particular health benefits or are targeted for specific conditions. These products may consist of whole foods or may be isolated compounds from natural or synthetic sources. Examples include antioxidants, probiotics (supplements containing friendly bacteria for the digestive tract), digestive enzymes, shark cartilage, or other animal products, or chemical extracts such as the hormone DHEA (dehydroepiandrosterone) and coenzyme Q10, an antioxidant.

General guidelines

Considering average dietary needs and the prevalence of certain health conditions, some basic guidelines may provide the foundation for the effective use of nutritional supplements. First, a high quality, broad-spectrum multivitamin and mineral supplement, taken once per day, is recommended to provide a range of nutrients. This should contain the B-complex vitamins B6, B12, and **folic acid**, which may help prevent heart disease, and the minerals zinc and copper, which aid immunity. In addition to a multivitamin, antioxidants can be added to a supplementation routine. These include vitamin A (or beta-carotene), vitamin C, and vitamin E, and the mineral selenium. Antioxidants may have several positive effects on the body, such as slowing the **aging** process, reducing the risks of **cancer** and heart disease, and reducing the risks of illness and infection by supporting the immune system. Coenzyme Q10 is another antioxidant in wide usage, as studies have shown it may improve the health of the heart and reduce the effects of heart disease. Essential fatty acids, particularly omega-3, are also recommended as they are involved in many important processes in the body, including brain function. Calcium supplementation is recommended for the elderly and for women, to strengthen bones and prevent bone loss. Calcium supplements that are balanced with magnesium have a less constipating effect and are better absorbed.

After basic nutritional requirements are supported, supplements may be used to target specific needs and health conditions. For instance, athletes, men, women, children, the elderly, and vegetarians have differing needs for nutrients, and an informed use of supplements would take these differences into account. People suffering from health conditions and diseases may use specific supplements to target their condition and to support the body's healing capacity by providing optimal amounts of nutrients.

Recommended dosage

Dosages of nutritional supplements vary widely, depending on the product and individual needs. For vitamins and minerals, U.S. RDA's are essential guidelines. For other products, manufacturers' guidelines, consumer information sources such as nutritional books and magazines, and practitioners including nutritionists and naturopathic physicians may be consulted.

Precautions

Overall diet is an important first consideration for those considering nutritional supplementation. Healthy dietary habits can help optimize nutrition and the absorption of supplements, and nutritional supplements cannot substitute for a diet that is not nutritionally balanced in the first place. Supplements are best used moderately to supply any extra nutritional requirements. Sound **diets** contain a variety of wholesome foods. At least five servings per day of fruits and vegetables are recommended, as well as the inclusion of whole grains in the diet. Variety in the diet is important to provide a full range of vitamins and minerals. Overeating inhibits digestion and absorption of nutrients, while regular **exercise** contributes to sound nutrition, by improving metabolism and digestion. Drinking plenty of clean water prevents **dehydration**, improves digestion, and helps the body flush out impurities.

Generally, nutrients from food sources are more efficiently utilized by the body than isolated substances. For instance, fresh fruit and vegetable juice could be used to provide concentrated amounts of particular nutrients, such as vitamins A and C, to the diet. As another example, eating plenty of leafy green vegetables is a healthy option for those wishing to add calcium to the diet.

Vitamins and minerals are most easily digested with food. Fat-soluble vitamins should be taken with food that contains fat. Vitamins tend to work synergistically, meaning that they work together in order to be effective. For instance, vitamin E requires some of the B-complex vitamins and the minerals selenium and zinc for most effective absorption. Some minerals may not be absorbed or may inhibit each other when taken in improper ratios. Generally, a high quality, broad-spectrum vitamin and mineral supplement will be formulated to prevent unfavorable interactions.

Vitamin A can become toxic when taken in large amounts (over 100,000 International Units) on a daily basis over time, as can vitamin D. Substituting beta-carotene for vitamin A can alleviate this risk. Very large doses of minerals taken over long periods may have toxic effects in the body. Dosages far exceeding RDA's of vitamins are not recommended, nor are large doses of other supplements.

Consumers can make wise choices for nutritional supplementation by consulting professional nutritionists and naturopathic physicians. Nutritional supplements are best added into the diet slowly, starting with small dosages and working up to the manufacturers' recommended amounts over time. Also, some supplements, such as herbal medications that may stimulate processes in the body, are best taken intermittently, allowing the body occasional rest periods without the supplement. To avoid unfavorable interactions, nutritional supplements are best used moderately and individually, rather than taking handfuls of capsules and tablets for various needs and conditions at the same time. Finally, consumers should be wary of excessive or grandiose health claims made by manufacturers of nutritional supplements and rely on scientific information to validate these claims.

KEY TERMS

Antioxidants—A class of biochemicals that have been found to protect cells from free-radical damage.

Enzymes—Chemical catalysts that help initiate biochemical processes.

Essential fatty acids—Sources of fat in the diet, including omega-3 and omega-6 fatty acids.

Naturopathic physicians—Physicians specializing in the treatment of disease using a variety of natural methods and plant-based medicines.

Side effects

Some nutritional supplements can cause upset stomach and allergic reactions, including **rashes**, flushing, **nausea**, sweating, and headaches.

Interactions

Herbal preparations and nutritional supplements may interact unfavorably with pharmaceutical drugs. For instance, some nutritional supplements recommended for nervous system function may not be recommended for those taking pharmaceutical antidepressants, such as taking 5-HTP, a nutritional supplement for the brain, or the herb **St. John's Wort**, with prescription antidepressants. Vitamin C should not be taken with aspirin, as it can irritate the stomach and limit absorption. Minerals should be taken in proper proportions to prevent unfavorable interactions; large amounts of zinc may deplete the body of the mineral copper, while too much calcium adversely affects the magnesium levels in the body. Balanced mineral supplements are recommended to alleviate these interactions.

Resources

BOOKS

Balch, Phyllis A. *Prescription for Nutritional Healing*. East Rutherford, NJ: Penguin Group Inc., 2005.

Firshein, Richard. *The Nutraceutical Revolution: 20 Cutting-Edge Nutrients to Help You Design Your Own Perfect Whole-Life Program*. East Rutherford, NJ: Penguin Group Inc., 1999.

Hudson, Tori. *Women's Encyclopedia of Natural Medicine*. New York: McGraw-Hill, 1999.

Weil, Andrew. *Eating Well for Optimum Health: The Essential Guide to Bringing Health and Pleasure Back to Eating*. New York: Harper Trade, 2001.

PERIODICALS

Natural Health http://www.naturalhealthmag.com.

ORGANIZATIONS

Center for Science in the Public Interest. 1875 Connecticut Avenue NW, Suite 300, Washington, D.C. 20009. (202)332-9110. < http://www.cspinet.org >. Publishes *Nutrition Action Newsletter.*

National Nutritional Foods Association. 1220 19th Street NW, Washington, D.C. 20036. (202)223-0101. < http://www.nnfa.org >.

OTHER

USDA Food and Nutrition Information Center. < http://www.nal.usda.gov/fnic >.

Douglas Dupler

Nystagmus

Definition

Rhythmic, oscillating motions of the eyes are called nystagmus. The to-and-fro motion is generally involuntary. Vertical nystagmus occurs much less frequently than horizontal nystagmus and is often, but not necessarily, a sign of serious brain damage. Nystagmus can be a normal physiological response or a result of a pathologic problem.

Description

The eyes play a critical role in maintaining balance. They are directly connected to other organs of equilibrium, most important of which is the inner ear. Paired structures called the semicircular canals deep in the skull behind the ears sense motion and relay that information to balance control centers in the brain. The eyes send visual information to the same centers. A third set of sensors consists of nerve endings all over the body, particularly in joints, that detect position. All this information is integrated to allow the body to navigate in space and gravity.

It is possible to fool this system or to overload it with information so that it malfunctions. A spinning ride at the amusement park is a good way to overload it with information. The system has adapted to the spinning, expects it to go on forever, and carries that momentum for some time after it is over. Nystagmus is the lingering adjustment of the eyes to tracking the world as it revolves around them.

Nystagmus can be classified depending upon the type of motion of the eyes. In pendular nystagmus the speed of motion of the eyes is the same in both directions. In jerk nystagmus there is a slow and fast phase. The eyes move slowly in one direction and then seem to jerk back in the other direction.

Nystagmus can be present at birth (congenital) or acquired later on in life. A certain type of acquired nystagmus, called spasmus nutans, includes a head tilt and head bobbing and generally occurs between four to 12 months of age. It may last a few months to a few years, but generally goes away by itself.

Railway nystagmus is a physiological type of nystagmus. It happens when someone is on a moving train (thus the term railway) and is watching a stationary object which appears to be going by. The eyes slowly follow the object and then quickly jerk back to start over. Railway nystagmus (also called optokinetic nystagmus) is a type of jerk nystagmus. This phenomenon can be used to check vision in infants. Nystagmus can also be induced by fooling the semicircular canals. Caloric stimulation refers to a medical method of testing their connections to the brain, and therefore to the eyes. Cold or warm water flushed into the ear canal will generate motion signals from the inner ear. The eyes will respond to this signal with nystagmus if the pathways are intact.

Causes and symptoms

There are many causes of nystagmus. Nystagmus may be present at birth. It may be a result of the lack of development of normal binocular fixation early on in life. This can occur if there is a cataract at birth or a problem is some other part of the visual system. Some other conditions that nystagmus may be associated with include:

- Albinism. This condition is caused by a decrease in pigmentation and may affect the eyes.

- Disorders of the eyes. This may include optic atrophy, color blindness, very high nearsightedness (**myopia**) or severe **astigmatism**, or opacities in the structures of the eyes.

- Acute **labyrinthitis**. This is an inflammation in the inner ear. The patient may have **dizziness** (vertigo), nausea and **vomiting**, and nystagmus.

- Brain lesions. Disease in many parts of the brain can result in nystagmus.

- Alcohol and drugs. Alcohol and some medications (e.g., anti-epilepsy medications) can induce or exaggerate nystagmus.

• Multiple sclerosis. A disease of the central nervous system.

Diagnosis

Nystagmus is a sign, not a disease. If abnormal, it indicates a problem in one of the systems controlling it. An ophthalmologist and/or neuro-ophthalmologist should be consulted.

Treatment

There is one kind of nystagmus that seems to occur harmlessly by itself. The condition, benign positional vertigo, produces vertigo and nystagmus when the head is moved in certain directions. It can arise spontaneously or after a concussion. Motion sickness medicines sometimes help. But the reaction will dissipate if continuously evoked. Each morning a patient is asked to produce the symptom by moving his or her head around until it no longer happens. This prevents it from returning for several hours or the entire day.

Prisms, contact lenses, eyeglasses, or eye muscle surgery are some possible treatments. These therapies may reduce the nystagmus but may not alleviate it. Again, because nystagmus may be a symptom, it is important to determine the cause.

Resources

ORGANIZATIONS

American Academy of Ophthalmology. 655 Beach Street, P.O. Box 7424, San Francisco, CA 94120-7424. <http://www.eyenet.org>.

American Optometric Association. 243 North Lindbergh Blvd., St. Louis, MO 63141. (314) 991-4100. <http://www.aoanet.org>.

J. Ricker Polsdorfer, MD

Obesity

Definition

Obesity is an abnormal accumulation of body fat, usually 20% or more over an individual's ideal body weight. Obesity is associated with increased risk of illness, disability, and **death**.

The branch of medicine that deals with the study and treatment of obesity is known as bariatrics. As obesity has become a major health problem in the United States, bariatrics has become a separate medical and surgical specialty.

Description

Obesity traditionally has been defined as a weight at least 20% above the weight corresponding to the lowest death rate for individuals of a specific height, gender, and age (ideal weight). Twenty to forty percent over ideal weight is considered mildly obese; 40–100% over ideal weight is considered moderately obese; and 100% over ideal weight is considered severely, or morbidly, obese. More recent guidelines for obesity use a measurement called BMI (body mass index) which is the individual's weight multiplied by 703 and then divided by twice the height in inches. BMI of 25.9–29 is considered overweight; BMI over 30 is considered obese. Measurements and comparisons of waist and hip circumference can also provide some information regarding risk factors associated with weight. The higher the ratio, the greater the chance for weight-associated complications. Calipers can be used to measure skin-fold thickness to determine whether tissue is muscle (lean) or adipose tissue (fat).

Much concern has been generated about the increasing incidence of obesity among Americans. Some studies have noted an increase from 12% to 18% occurring between 1991 and 1998. Other studies have actually estimated that a full 50% of all Americans are overweight. The World Health Organization terms obesity a worldwide epidemic, and the diseases which can occur due to obesity are becoming increasingly prevalent.

Excessive weight can result in many serious, potentially life-threatening health problems, including **hypertension**, Type II **diabetes mellitus** (non-insulin dependent diabetes), increased risk for coronary disease, increased unexplained **heart attack**, hyperlipidemia, **infertility**, and a higher prevalence of colon, prostate, endometrial, and, possibly, **breast cancer**. Approximately 300,000 deaths a year are attributed to obesity, prompting leaders in public health, such as former Surgeon General C. Everett Koop, M.D., to label obesity "the second leading cause of preventable deaths in the United States."

Causes and symptoms

The mechanism for excessive weight gain is clear—more calories are consumed than the body burns, and the excess calories are stored as fat (adipose) tissue. However, the exact cause is not as clear and likely arises from a complex combination of factors. Genetic factors significantly influence how the body regulates the appetite and the rate at which it turns food into energy (metabolic rate). Studies of adoptees confirm this relationship—the majority of adoptees followed a pattern of weight gain that more closely resembled that of their birth parents than their adoptive parents. A genetic predisposition to weight gain, however, does not automatically mean that a person will be obese. Eating habits and patterns of physical activity also play a significant role in the amount of weight a person gains. Recent studies have indicated that the amount of fat in a person's diet may have a greater impact on weight than the number of calories it contains. Carbohydrates like cereals, breads, fruits, and vegetables and protein (fish, lean meat, turkey breast, skim milk) are converted to fuel almost as soon as they are consumed.

Height And Weight Goals

Men

Height	Small Frame	Medium Frame	Large Frame
5'2" 5'3" 5'4"	128–134 lbs. 130–136 132–138	131–141 lbs. 133–143 135–145	138–150 lbs. 140–153 142–153
5'5" 5'6" 5'7"	134–140 136–142 138–145	137–148 139–151 142–154	144–160 146–164 149–168
5'8" 5'9" 5'10"	140–148 142–151 144–154	145–157 148–160 151–163	152–172 155–176 158–180
5'11" 6'0" 6'1"	146–157 159–160 152–164	154–166 157–170 160–174	161–184 164–188 168–192
6'2" 6'3" 6'4"	155–168 158–172 162–176	164–178 167–182 171–187	172–197 176–202 181–207

Women

Height	Small Frame	Medium Frame	Large Frame
4'10" 4'11" 5'0"	102–111 lbs. 103–113 104–115	109–121 lbs. 111–123 113–126	118–131 lbs. 120–134 112–137
5'1" 5'2" 5'3"	106–118 108–121 111–124	115–129 118–132 121–135	125–140 128–143 131–147
5'4" 5'5" 5'6"	114–127 117–130 120–133	124–141 127–141 130–144	137–151 137–155 140–159
5'7" 5'8" 5'9"	123–136 126–139 129–142	133–147 136–150 139–153	143–163 146–167 149–170
5'10" 5'11" 6'0"	132–145 135–148 138–151	142–156 145–159 148–162	152–176 155–176 158–179

Most fat calories are immediately stored in fat cells, which add to the body's weight and girth as they expand and multiply. A sedentary lifestyle, particularly prevalent in affluent societies, such as in the United States, can contribute to weight gain. Psychological factors, such as depression and low self-esteem may, in some cases, also play a role in weight gain.

At what stage of life a person becomes obese can affect his or her ability to lose weight. In childhood, excess calories are converted into new fat cells (hyperplastic obesity), while excess calories consumed in adulthood only serve to expand existing fat cells (hypertrophic obesity). Since dieting and **exercise** can only reduce the size of fat cells, not eliminate them, persons who were obese as children can have great difficulty losing weight, since they may have up to five times as many fat cells as someone who became overweight as an adult.

Obesity can also be a side effect of certain disorders and conditions, including:

- Cushing's syndrome, a disorder involving the excessive release of the hormone cortisol
- hypothyroidism, a condition caused by an underactive thyroid gland
- neurologic disturbances, such as damage to the hypothalamus, a structure located deep within the brain that helps regulate appetite
- consumption of such drugs as steroids, antipsychotic medications, or antidepressants

The major symptoms of obesity are excessive weight gain and the presence of large amounts of fatty tissue. Obesity can also give rise to several secondary conditions, including:

- arthritis and other orthopedic problems, such as lower back pain
- hernias
- heartburn
- adult-onset asthma
- gum disease
- high cholesterol levels
- gallstones
- high blood pressure
- menstrual irregularities or cessation of menstruation (amenorhhea)
- decreased fertility, and **pregnancy** complications
- shortness of breath that can be incapacitating
- sleep apnea and sleeping disorders
- skin disorders arising from the bacterial breakdown of sweat and cellular material in thick folds of skin or from increased friction between folds
- emotional and social problems

Diagnosis

Diagnosis of obesity is made by observation and by comparing the patient's weight to ideal weight charts. Many doctors and obesity researchers refer to the body mass index (BMI), which uses a height-weight relationship to calculate an individual's ideal weight and personal risk of developing obesity-related health problems. Physicians may also obtain direct measurements of an individual's body fat content by using calipers to measure skin-fold thickness at the back of the upper arm and other sites. The most accurate means of measuring body fat content involves immersing a person in water and measuring relative displacement; however, this method is very impractical and is usually only used in scientific studies requiring very specific assessments. Women whose body fat exceeds 30% and men whose body fat exceeds 25% are generally considered obese.

Doctors may also note how a person carries excess weight on his or her body. Studies have shown that this factor may indicate whether or not an individual has a predisposition to develop certain diseases or conditions that may accompany obesity. "Apple-shaped" individuals who store most of their weight around the waist and abdomen are at greater risk for **cancer**, heart disease, **stroke**, and diabetes than "pear-shaped" people whose extra pounds settle primarily in their hips and thighs.

Treatment

Treatment of obesity depends primarily on how overweight a person is and his or her overall health. However, to be successful, any treatment must affect life-long behavioral changes rather than short-term weight loss. "Yo-yo" dieting, in which weight is repeatedly lost and regained, has been shown to increase a person's likelihood of developing fatal health problems than if the weight had been lost gradually or not lost at all. Behavior-focused treatment should concentrate on:

- What and how much a person eats. This aspect may involve keeping a food diary and developing a better understanding of the nutritional value and fat content of foods. It may also involve changing grocery-shopping habits (e.g., buying only what is on a prepared list and only going on a certain day), timing of meals (to prevent feelings of hunger, a person may plan frequent, small meals), and actually slowing down the rate at which a person eats.

- How a person responds to food. This may involve understanding what psychological issues underlie a person's eating habits. For example, one person may binge eat when under **stress**, while another may always use food as a reward. In recognizing these psychological triggers, an individual can develop alternate coping mechanisms that do not focus on food.

- How they spend their time. Making activity and exercise an integrated part of everyday life is a key to achieving and maintaining weight loss. Starting slowly and building endurance keeps individuals from becoming discouraged. Varying routines and trying new activities also keeps interest high.

For most individuals who are mildly obese, these behavior modifications entail life-style changes they can make independently while being supervised by a family physician. Other mildly obese persons may seek the help of a commercial weight-loss program (e.g., Weight Watchers). The effectiveness of these programs is difficult to assess, since programs vary widely, drop-out rates are high, and few employ members of the medical community. However, programs that emphasize realistic goals, gradual progress, sensible eating, and exercise can be very helpful and are recommended by many doctors. Programs that promise instant weight loss or feature severely restricted **diets** are not effective and, in some cases, can be dangerous.

For individuals who are moderately obese, medically supervised behavior modification and weight loss are required. While doctors will put most moderately obese patients on a balanced, low-calorie diet (1200–1500 calories a day), they may recommend that certain individuals follow a very-low-calorie liquid protein diet (400–700 calories) for as long as three months. This therapy, however, should not be confused with commercial liquid protein diets or commercial weight-loss shakes and drinks. Doctors tailor these diets to specific patients, monitor patients carefully, and use them for only a short period of time. In addition to reducing the amount and type of calories consumed by the patient, doctors will recommend professional therapists or psychiatrists who can help the individual effectively change his or her behavior in regard to eating.

For individuals who are severely obese, dietary changes and behavior modification may be accompanied by surgery to reduce or bypass portions of the stomach or small intestine. Although **obesity surgery** is less risky as of 2003 because of recent innovations in equipment and surgical technique, it is still performed only on patients for whom other strategies have failed and whose obesity seriously threatens their health. Other surgical procedures are not recommended, including **liposuction**, a purely cosmetic procedure in which a suction device is used to remove fat from beneath the skin, and **jaw wiring**, which can damage gums and teeth and cause painful **muscle spasms**.

Appetite-suppressant drugs are sometimes prescribed to aid in weight loss. These drugs work by increasing levels of serotonin or catecholamine, which are brain chemicals that control feelings of fullness. Appetite suppressants, though, are not considered truly effective, since most of the weight lost while taking them is usually regained after stopping them. Also, suppressants containing amphetamines can be

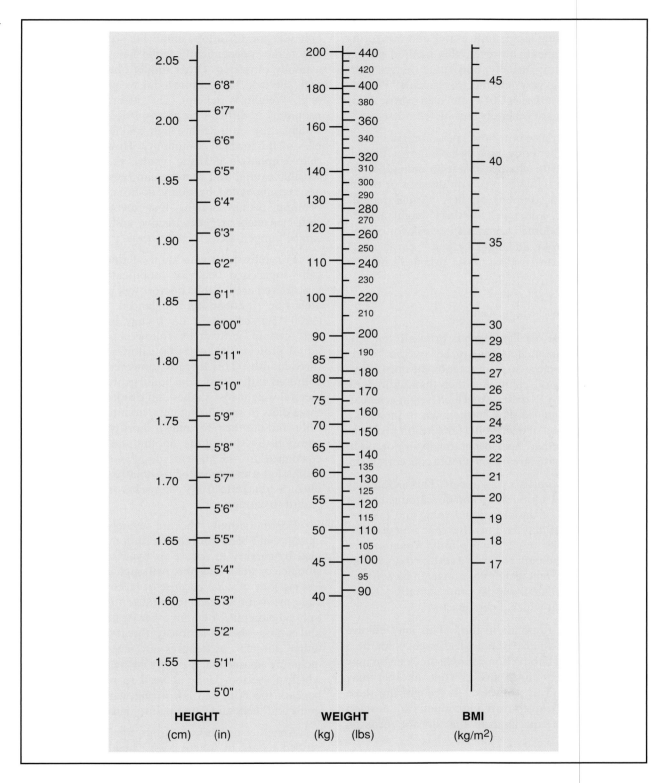

Body/mass index can be calculated by locating your height and weight on the chart and drawing a diagonal line between the two. Where the line crosses over the third bar is the approximate BMI. *(Illustration by Argosy Inc.)*

potentially abused by patients. While most of the immediate side-effects of these drugs are harmless, the long-term effects of these drugs, in many cases, are unknown. Two drugs, dexfenfluramine hydrochloride (Redux) and fenfluramine (Pondimin) as well as a combination fenfluramine-phentermine (Fen/Phen) drug, were taken off the market when they were shown to cause potentially fatal heart defects. In November 1997, the United States Food and Drug Administration (FDA) approved a new weight-loss drug, sibutramine (Meridia). Available only with a doctor's prescription, Meridia can significantly elevate blood pressure and cause **dry mouth**, **headache**, **constipation**, and **insomnia**. This medication should not be used by patients with a history of congestive **heart failure**, heart disease, stroke, or uncontrolled high blood pressure.

Other weight-loss medications available with a doctor's prescription include:

• diethylpropion (Tenuate, Tenuate dospan)

• mazindol (Mazanor, Sanorex)

• phendimetrazine (Bontril, Plegine, Prelu-2, X-Trozine)

• phentermine (Adipex-P, Fastin, Ionamin, Oby-trim)

Phenylpropanolamine (Acutrim, Dextarim) is the only nonprescription weight-loss drug approved by the FDA These over-the-counter diet aids can boost weight loss by 5%. Combined with diet and exercise and used only with a doctor's approval, prescription anti-obesity medications enable some patients to lose 10% more weight than they otherwise would. Most patients regain lost weight after discontinuing use of either prescription medications or nonprescription weight-loss products.

Prescription medications or over-the-counter weight-loss products can cause:

• constipation

• dry mouth

• headache

• irritability

• **nausea**

• nervousness

• sweating

None of them should be used by patients taking monoamine oxidase inhibitors (MAO inhibitors).

Doctors sometimes prescribe fluoxetine (Prozac), an antidepressant that can increase weight loss by about 10%. Weight loss may be temporary and side effects of this medication include **diarrhea**, **fatigue**, insomnia, nausea, and thirst. Weight-loss drugs

currently being developed or tested include ones that can prevent fat absorption or digestion; reduce the desire for food and prompt the body to burn calories more quickly; and regulate the activity of substances that control eating habits and stimulate overeating.

Alternative treatment

The Chinese herb ephedra (*Ephedra sinica*), combined with **caffeine**, exercise, and a low-fat diet in physician-supervised weight-loss programs, can cause at least a temporary increase in weight loss. However, the large doses of ephedra required to achieve the desired result can also cause:

• anxiety

• heart **arrhythmias**

• heart attack

• high blood pressure

• insomnia

• irritability

• nervousness

• seizures

• strokes

• death

Ephedra should not be used by anyone with a history of diabetes, heart disease, or thyroid problems. In fact, an article that appeared in the *Journal of the American Medical Association* in early 2003 advised against the use of ephedra.

Diuretic herbs, which increase urine production, can cause short-term weight loss but cannot help patients achieve lasting weight control. The body responds to heightened urine output by increasing thirst to replace lost fluids, and patients who use **diuretics** for an extended period of time eventually start retaining water again anyway. In moderate doses, psyllium, a mucilaginous herb available in bulk-forming **laxatives** like Metamucil, absorbs fluid and makes patients feel as if they have eaten enough. Red peppers and mustard help patients lose weight more quickly by accelerating the metabolic rate. They also make people more thirsty, so they crave water instead of food. Walnuts contain serotonin, the brain chemical that tells the body it has eaten enough. Dandelion (*Taraxacum officinale*) can raise metabolism and counter a desire for sugary foods.

Acupressure and **acupuncture** can also suppress food cravings. Visualization and **meditation** can create and reinforce a positive self-image that enhances the patient's determination to lose weight. By improving physical strength, mental concentration, and emotional serenity, **yoga** can provide the same benefits. Also, patients who play soft, slow music during meals often find that they eat less food but enjoy it more.

Getting the correct ratios of protein, carbohydrates, and good-quality fats can help in weight loss via enhancement of the metabolism. Support groups that are informed about healthy, nutritious, and balanced diets can offer an individual the support he or she needs to maintain this type of eating regimen.

Prognosis

As many as 85% of dieters who do not exercise on a regular basis regain their lost weight within two years. In five years, the figure rises to 90%. Repeatedly losing and regaining weight (yo yo dieting) encourages the body to store fat and may increase a patient's risk of developing heart disease. The primary factor in achieving and maintaining weight loss is a life-long commitment to regular exercise and sensible eating habits.

Prevention

Obesity experts suggest that a key to preventing excess weight gain is monitoring fat consumption rather than counting calories, and the National Cholesterol Education Program maintains that only 30% of calories should be derived from fat. Only one-third of those calories should be contained in saturated fats (the kind of fat found in high concentrations in meat, poultry, and dairy products). Because most people eat more than they think they do, keeping a detailed food diary is a useful way to assess eating habits. Eating three balanced, moderate-portion meals a day—with the main meal at mid-day—is a more effective way to prevent obesity than **fasting** or crash diets. Exercise increases the metabolic rate by creating muscle, which burns more calories than fat. When regular exercise is combined with regular, healthful meals, calories continue to burn at an accelerated rate for several hours. Finally, encouraging healthful habits in children is a key to preventing childhood obesity and the health problems that follow in adulthood.

New directions in obesity treatment

The rapid rise in the incidence of obesity in the United States since 1990 has prompted researchers to look for new treatments. One approach involves the application of antidiabetes drugs to the treatment of

KEY TERMS

Adipose tissue—Fat tissue.

Appetite suppressant—Drug that decreases feelings of hunger. Most work by increasing levels of serotonin or catecholamine, chemicals in the brain that control appetite.

Bariatrics—The branch of medicine that deals with the prevention and treatment of obesity and related disorders.

Ghrelin—A recently discovered peptide hormone secreted by cells in the lining of the stomach. Ghrelin is important in appetite regulation and maintaining the body's energy balance.

Hyperlipidemia—Abnormally high levels of lipids in blood plasma.

Hyperplastic obesity—Excessive weight gain in childhood, characterized by the creation of new fat cells.

Hypertension—High blood pressure.

Hypertrophic obesity—Excessive weight gain in adulthood, characterized by expansion of already existing fat cells.

Ideal weight—Weight corresponding to the lowest death rate for individuals of a specific height, gender, and age.

Leptin—A protein hormone that affects feeding behavior and hunger in humans. At present it is thought that obesity in humans may result in part from insensitivity to leptin.

obesity. Metformin (Glucophage), a drug that was approved by the Food and Dug Administration (FDA) in 1994 for the treatment of type 2 diabetes, shows promise in treating obesity associated with **insulin resistance**.

Another field of obesity research is the study of hormones, particularly leptin, which is produced by fat cells in the body, and ghrelin, which is secreted by cells in the lining of the stomach. Both hormones are known to affect appetite and the body's energy balance. Leptin is also related to reproductive function, while ghrelin stimulates the pituitary gland to release growth hormone. Further studies of these two hormones may lead to the development of new medications to control appetite and food intake.

A third approach to obesity treatment involves research into the social factors that encourage or reinforce weight gain in humans. Researchers are looking at such issues as the advertising and marketing of food products; media stereotypes of obesity; the development of eating disorders in adolescents and adults; and similar questions.

Resources

BOOKS

Beers, Mark H., MD, and Robert Berkow, MD, editors. "Nutritional Disorders: Obesity." Section 1, Chapter 5. In *The Merck Manual of Diagnosis and Therapy*. Whitehouse Station, NJ: Merck Research Laboratories, 2004.

Flancbaum, Louis, MD, with Erica Manfred and Deborah Biskin. *The Doctor's Guide to Weight Loss Surgery*. West Hurley, NY: Fredonia Communications, 2001.

Pi-Sunyer, F. Xavier. "Obesity." In *Cecil Textbook of Medicine*, edited by Russel L. Cecil, et al. Philadelphia, PA: W. B. Saunders Company, 2000.

PERIODICALS

Aronne, L. J., and K. R. Segal. "Weight Gain in the Treatment of Mood Disorders." *Journal of Clinical Psychiatry* 64, Supplement 8 (2003): 22–29.

Bell, S. J., and G. K. Goodrick. "A Functional Food Product for the Management of Weight." *Critical Reviews in Food Science and Nutrition* 42 (March 2002): 163–178.

Brudnak, M. A. "Weight-Loss Drugs and Supplements: Are There Safer Alternatives?" *Medical Hypotheses* 58 (January 2002): 28–33.

Colquitt, J., A. Clegg, M. Sidhu, and P. Royle. "Surgery for Morbid Obesity." *Cochrane Database Systems Review* 2003: CD003641.

Espelund, U., T. K. Hansen, H. Orskov, and J. Frystyk. "Assessment of Ghrelin." *APMIS Supplementum* 109 (2003): 140–145.

Hundal, R. S., and S. E. Inzucchi. "Metformin: New Understandings, New Uses." *Drugs* 63 (2003): 1879–1894.

Pirozzo, S., C. Summerbell, C. Cameron, and P. Glasziou. "Advice on Low-Fat Diets for Obesity (Cochrane Review)." *Cochrane Database Systems Review* 2002: CD003640.

Schurgin, S., and R. D. Siegel. "Pharmacotherapy of Obesity: An Update." *Nutrition in Clinical Care* 6 (January-April 2003): 27–37.

Shekelle, P. G., M. L. Hardy, S. C. Morton, et al. "Efficacy and Safety of Ephedra and Ephedrine for Weight Loss and Athletic Performance: A Meta-Analysis." *Journal of the American Medical Association* 289 (March 26, 2003): 1537–1545.

Tataranni, P. A. "Treatment of Obesity: Should We Target the Individual or Society?" *Current Pharmaceutical Design* 9 (2003): 1151–1163.

Veniant, M. M., and C. P. LeBel. "Leptin: From Animals to Humans." *Current Pharmaceutical Design* 9 (2003): 811–818.

ORGANIZATIONS

American Dietetic Association. (800) 877-1600. < www.eatright.org. >.

American Obesity Association (AOA). 1250 24th Street NW, Suite 300, Washington, DC 20037. (202) 776-7711 or (800) 98-OBESE. < www.obesity.org >.

American Society for Bariatric Surgery. 7328 West University Avenue, Suite F, Gainesville, FL 32607. (352) 331-4900. < www.asbs.org >.

American Society of Bariatric Physicians. 5453 East Evans Place, Denver, CO 80222-5234. (303) 770-2526. < www.asbp.org >.

HCF Nutrition Research Foundation, Inc. P.O. Box 22124, Lexington, KY 40522. (606) 276-3119.

National Institute of Diabetes and Digestive and Kidney Diseases. 31 Center Drive, USC2560, Building 31, Room 9A-04, Bethesda, MD 20892-2560. (301) 496-3583. < www.niddk.nih/gov >.

National Obesity Research Foundation. Temple University, Weiss Hall 867, Philadelphia, PA 19122.

Weight-Control Information Network. 1 Win Way, Bethesda, MD 20896-3665. (301) 951-1120. < www.navigator.tufts.edu/special/win.html >.

Rosalyn Carson-DeWitt, MD
Rebecca J. Frey, PhD

Obesity surgery

Definition

Obesity surgery is an operation that reduces or bypasses the stomach or small intestine so that severely overweight people can achieve significant and permanent weight loss.

Purpose

Obesity surgery, also called **bariatric surgery**, is performed only on severely overweight people who are more than twice their ideal weight. This level of obesity often is referred to as morbid obesity since it can result in many serious, and potentially deadly, health problems, including **hypertension**, Type II **diabetes mellitus** (non-insulin dependent diabetes), increased risk for coronary disease, increased unexplained **heart attack**, hyperlipidemia, and a higher prevalence of colon, prostate, endometrial, and, possibly, **breast cancer**. In 2003, researchers concluded that obesity surgery could cure Type II diabetes in many people who were not yet morbidly obese. Therefore, this surgery is performed on people whose risk of complications of surgery is outweighed by the need to lose weight to prevent health complications, and for whom supervised weight loss and **exercise** programs have repeatedly failed. Obesity surgery, however, does not make people thin. Most people lose about 60% of their excess weight through this treatment. Changes in diet and exercise still are required to maintain a normal weight.

The theory behind obesity surgery is that if the volume the stomach holds is reduced and the entrance into the intestine is made smaller to slow stomach emptying, or part of the small intestine is bypassed or shortened, people will not be able to consume and/ or absorb as many calories. With obesity surgery the volume of food the stomach can hold is reduced from about four cups to about 1/2 cup.

Insurers may consider obesity surgery elective surgery and not cover it under their policies. Documentation of the necessity for surgery and approval from the insurer should be sought before this operation is performed.

Precautions

Obesity surgery should not be performed on people who are less than twice their ideal weight. It also is not appropriate for people who have substance addictions or who have psychological disorders. Other considerations in choosing candidates for obesity surgery include the general health of the person and his or her willingness to comply with follow-up treatment.

Description

Obesity surgery is usually performed in a hospital by a surgeon who has experience with obesity surgery or at a center that specializes in the procedure. **General anesthesia** is used, and the operation takes 2–3 hours. The hospital stay lasts about a week.

Three procedures are currently used for obesity surgery:

- Gastric bypass surgery. Probably the most common type of obesity surgery, gastric bypass surgery has been performed in the United States for about 25 years. In this procedure, the volume of the stomach is reduced by four rows of stainless steel staples that separate the main body of the stomach from a small, newly created pouch. The pouch is attached at one end to the esophagus. At the other end is a very small opening into the small intestine. Food flows through this pouch, bypassing the main portion of the stomach and emptying slowly into the small intestine where it is absorbed.

- Vertical banding gastroplasty. In this procedure, an artificial pouch is created using staples in a different section of the stomach. Plastic mesh is sutured into part of the pouch to prevent it from dilating. In both surgeries the food enters the small intestine farther along that it would enter if exiting the stomach normally. This reduces the time available for absorption of nutrients. The procedure is normally done laparoscopically, meaning that the surgeon makes one or more small incisions in the abdomen and inserts the necessary tools and instruments through the tiny holes. He or she can view the patient's organs via an inserted camera that displays pictures on a monitor. This method makes for a faster and easier recovery than a large incision.

- Jejunoileal bypass. Now a rarely performed procedure, jejunoileal bypass involves shortening the small intestine. Because of the high occurance of serious complications involving chronic **diarrhea** and **liver disease**, it has largely been abandoned for the other, safer procedures

Preparation

After patients are carefully selected as appropriate for obesity surgery, they receive standard preoperative blood and urine tests and meet with an anesthesiologist to discuss how their health may affect the administration of anesthesia. Pre-surgery counseling is done to help patients anticipate what to expect after the operation.

Aftercare

Immediately after the operation, most patients are restricted to a liquid diet for 2–3 weeks; however, some may remain on it for up to 12 weeks. Patients then move on to a diet of pureed food for about a month, and, after about two months, most can tolerate solid food. High fat food is restricted because it is hard to digest and causes diarrhea. Patients are expected to work on changing their eating and exercise habits to assist in weight loss. Most people eat 3–4 small meals a day once they return to solid food. Eating too quickly or too much after obesity surgery can cause **nausea and vomiting** as well as intestinal "dumping," a condition in which undigested food is shunted too quickly into the small intestine, causing **pain**, diarrhea, weakness, and **dizziness**.

Risks

As in any abdominal surgery, there is always a risk of excessive bleeding, infection, and allergic reaction to anesthesia. Specific risks associated with obesity

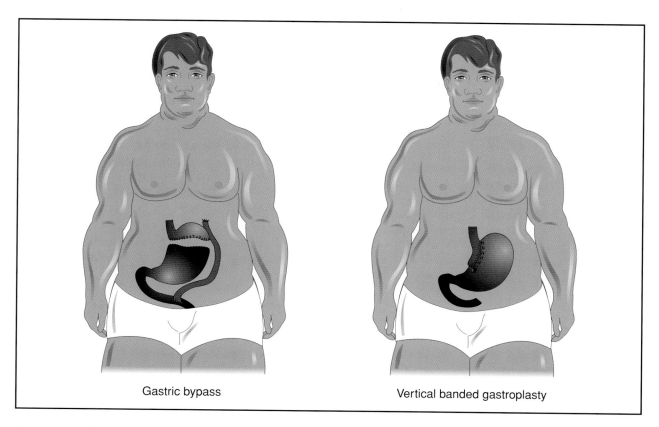

Gastric bypass

Vertical banded gastroplasty

The purpose of obesity surgery is to reduce the size of the stomach and slow the stomach emptying process by narrowing the entrance into the intestine. With this surgery, the volume of food the stomach can hold is reduced from approximately 4 cups to approximately one-half cup. There are two types of procedures used for obesity surgery: gastric bypass surgery and vertical banded gastroplasty, as shown in the illustration above. *(Illustration by Electronic Illustrators Group.)*

surgery include leaking or stretching of the pouch and loosening of the gastric staples. Although the average **death** rate associated with this procedure is less than one percent, the rate varies from center to center, ranging from 0–4%. Long-term failure rates can reach 50%, sometimes making additional surgery necessary. Other complications of obesity surgery include an intolerance to foods high in fats, **lactose intolerance**, bouts of **vomiting**, diarrhea, and intestinal discomfort

Studies on the risks of these surgeries continue. A 2003 report showed that gastric bypass surgery risk increases with age, weight and male gender. Patients age 55 and older experienced more complications than did younger patients and male patients had more life-threatening complications than female patients, particularly those who were more severely obese.

Normal results

Many people lose about 60% of the weight they need to reach their ideal weight through obesity surgery. However, surgery is not a magic weight-loss operation, and success also depends on the patient's willingness to exercise and eat low-calorie foods. A 2003 report showed that super obese patients had a lower success rate with laparoscopic vertical banding gastroplasty than those considered morbidly obese. However, the overall success rate was nearly 77% of patients carrying less than 50% excess weight four years after the procedure.

Resources

PERIODICALS

"Gastric Bypass Surgery Risk Increases with Age, Weight, and Male Gender." *Medical Devices and Surgical Technology Week* January 19, 2003: 29.
"Laparoscopic Vertical Banding Gastroplasty Safe and Effective for Morbid Obesity." *Medical Devices and Surgical Technology Week* January 19, 2003: 2.
Sadovsky, Richard. "Obesity Surgery May Cure Diabetes in Nonobese Patients." *American Family Physician* 56 (February 15, 2003): 866.

Tish Davidson, A.M.
Teresa G. Odle

Obsessive-compulsive disorder

Definition

Obsessive-compulsive disorder (OCD) is a type of anxiety disorder. **Anxiety** disorder is the experience of prolonged, excessive worry about circumstances in one's life. OCD is characterized by distressing repetitive thoughts, impulses or images that are intense, frightening, absurd, or unusual. These thoughts are followed by ritualized actions that are usually bizarre and irrational. These ritual actions, known as compulsions, help reduce anxiety caused by the individual's obsessive thoughts. Often described as the "disease of doubt," the sufferer usually knows the obsessive thoughts and compulsions are irrational but, on another level, fears they may be true.

Description

Almost one out of every 40 people will suffer from obsessive-compulsive disorder at some time in their lives. The condition is two to three times more common than either **schizophrenia** or manic depression, and strikes men and women of every ethnic group, age and social level. Because the symptoms are so distressing, sufferers often hide their fears and rituals but cannot avoid acting on them. OCD sufferers are often unable to decide if their fears are realistic and need to be acted upon.

Most people with obsessive-compulsive disorder have both obsessions and compulsions, but occasionally a person will have just one or the other. The degree to which this condition can interfere with daily living also varies. Some people are barely bothered, while others find the obsessions and compulsions to be profoundly traumatic and spend much time each day in compulsive actions.

Obsessions are intrusive, irrational thoughts that keep popping up in a person's mind, such as "my hands are dirty, I must wash them again." Typical obsessions include fears of dirt, germs, contamination, and violent or aggressive impulses. Other obsessions include feeling responsible for others' safety, or an irrational fear of hitting a pedestrian with a car. Additional obsessions can involve excessive religious feelings or intrusive sexual thoughts. The patient may need to confess frequently to a religious counselor or may fear acting out the strong sexual thoughts in a hostile way. People with obsessive-compulsive disorder may have an intense preoccupation with order and symmetry, or be unable to throw anything out.

Compulsions usually involve repetitive rituals such as excessive washing (especially handwashing or bathing), cleaning, checking and touching, counting, arranging or hoarding. As the person performs these acts, he may feel temporarily better, but there is no long-lasting sense of satisfaction or completion after the act is performed. Often, a person with obsessive-compulsive disorder believes that if the ritual is not performed, something dreadful will happen. While these compulsions may temporarily ease **stress**, short-term comfort is purchased at a heavy price—time spent repeating compulsive actions and a long-term interference with life.

The difference between OCD and other compulsive behavior is that while people who have problems with gambling, overeating or with **substance abuse** may appear to be compulsive, these activities also provide pleasure to some degree. The compulsions of OCD, on the other hand, are never pleasurable.

OCD may be related to some other conditions, such as the continual urge to pull out body hair (trichotillomania) fear of having a serious disease (**hypochondriasis**) or preoccupation with imagined defects in personal appearance disorder (body dysmorphia). Some people with OCD also have **Tourette syndrome**, a condition featuring tics and unwanted vocalizations (such as swearing). OCD is often linked with depression and other anxiety disorders.

Causes and symptoms

While no one knows for sure, research suggests that the tendency to develop obsessive-compulsive disorder is inherited. There are several theories behind the cause of OCD. Some experts believe that OCD is related to a chemical imbalance within the brain that causes a communication problem between the front part of the brain (frontal lobe) and deeper parts of the brain responsible for the repetitive behavior. Research has shown that the orbital cortex located on the underside of the brain's frontal lobe is overactive in OCD patients. This may be one reason for the feeling of alarm that pushes the patient into compulsive, repetitive actions. It is possible that people with OCD experience overactivity deep within the brain that causes the cells to get "stuck," much like a jammed transmission in a car damages the gears. This could lead to the development of rigid thinking and repetitive movements common to the disorder. The fact that drugs which boost the levels of serotonin, a brain messenger substance linked to emotion and many different anxiety disorders, in the brain can reduce OCD symptoms may indicate that to some degree OCD is related to levels of serotonin in the brain.

Recently, scientists have identified an intriguing link between childhood episodes of strep throat and the development of OCD. It appears that in some vulnerable children, strep antibodies attack a certain part of the brain. Antibodies are cells that the body produces to fight specific diseases. That attack results in the development of excessive washing or germ **phobias**. A phobia is a strong but irrational fear. In this instance the phobia is fear of disease germs present on commonly handled objects. These symptoms would normally disappear over time, but some children who have repeated infections may develop full-blown OCD. Treatment with **antibiotics** has resulted in lessening of the OCD symptoms in some of these children.

If one person in a family has obsessive-compulsive disorder, there is a 25% chance that another immediate family member has the condition. It also appears that stress and psychological factors may worsen symptoms, which usually begin during adolescence or early adulthood.

Diagnosis

People with obsessive-compulsive disorder feel ashamed of their problem and often try to hide their symptoms. They avoid seeking treatment. Because they can be very good at keeping their problem from friends and family, many sufferers do not get the help they need until the behaviors are deeply ingrained habits and hard to change. As a result, the condition is often misdiagnosed or underdiagnosed. All too often, it can take more than a decade between the onset of symptoms and proper diagnosis and treatment.

While scientists seem to agree that OCD is related to a disruption in serotonin levels, there is no blood test for the condition. Instead, doctors diagnose OCD after evaluating a person's symptoms and history.

Treatment

Obsessive-compulsive disorder can be effectively treated by a combination of **cognitive-behavioral therapy** and medication that regulates the brain's serotonin levels. Drugs that are approved to treat obsessive-compulsive disorder include fluoxetine (Prozac), fluvoxamine (Luvox), paroxetine (Paxil), and sertraline (Zoloft), all selective serotonin reuptake inhibitors (SSRIs) that affect the level of serotonin in the brain. Older drugs include the antidepressant clomipramine (Anafranil), a widely-studied drug in the treatment of OCD, but one that carries a greater risk of side effects. Drugs should be taken for at least 12 weeks before deciding whether or not they are effective.

Cognitive-behavioral therapy (CBT) teaches patients how to confront their fears and obsessive thoughts by making the effort to endure or wait out the activities that usually cause anxiety without compulsively performing the calming rituals. Eventually their anxiety decreases. People who are able to alter their thought patterns in this way can lessen their preoccupation with the compulsive rituals. At the same time, the patient is encouraged to refocus attention elsewhere, such as on a hobby.

In a few severe cases where patients have not responded to medication or behavioral therapy, brain surgery may be tried as a way of relieving the unwanted symptoms. Surgery can help up to a third of patients with the most severe form of OCD. The most common operation involves removing a section of the brain called the cingulate cortex. The serious side effects of this surgery for some patients include seizures, personality changes and less ability to plan.

Alternative treatment

Because OCD sometimes responds to **SSRI** antidepressants, a botanical medicine called St. John's wort (*Hypericum perforatum*) might have some beneficial effect as well, according to herbalists. Known popularly as "Nature's Prozac," **St. John's wort** is prescribed by herbalists for the treatment of anxiety and depression. They believe that this herb affects brain levels of serotonin in the same way that SSRI antidepressants do. Herbalists recommend a dose of 300 mg., three times per day. In about one out of 400 people, St. John's wort (like Prozac) may initially increase the level of anxiety. Homeopathic constitutional therapy can help rebalance the patient's mental, emotional, and physical well-being, allowing the behaviors of OCD to abate over time.

Prognosis

Obsessive-compulsive disorder is a chronic disease that, if untreated, can last for decades, fluctuating from mild to severe and worsening with age. When treated by a combination of drugs and behavioral therapy, some patients go into complete remission. Unfortunately, not all patients have such a good response. About 20% of people cannot find relief with either drugs or behavioral therapy. Hospitalization may be required in some cases.

Despite the crippling nature of the symptoms, many successful doctors, lawyers, business people, performers and entertainers function well in society despite their condition. Nevertheless, the emotional and financial cost of obsessive-compulsive disorder can be quite high.

KEY TERMS

Anxiety disorder—This is the experience of prolonged, excessive worry about circumstances in one's life. It disrupts daily life.

Cognitive-behavior therapy—A form of psychotherapy that seeks to modify behavior by manipulating the environment to change the patient's response.

Compulsion—A rigid behavior that is repeated over and over each day.

Obsession—A recurring, distressing idea, thought or impulse that feels "foreign" or alien to the individual.

Selective serotonin reuptake inhibitors (SSRIs)—A class of antidepressants that work by blocking the reabsorption of serotonin in brain cells, raising the level of the chemical in the brain. SSRIs include Prozac, Zoloft, Luvex, and Paxil.

Serotonin—One of three major neurotransmitters found in the brain that is related to emotion, and is linked to the development of depression and obsessive-compulsive disorder.

Resources

ORGANIZATIONS

Anxiety Disorders Association of America. 11900 Park Lawn Drive, Ste. 100, Rockville, MD 20852. (800) 545-7367. < http://www.adaa.org >.

National Alliance for the Mentally Ill (NAMI). Colonial Place Three, 2107 Wilson Blvd., Ste. 300, Arlington, VA 22201-3042. (800) 950-6264. < http://www.nami.org >.

National Anxiety Foundation. 3135 Custer Dr., Lexington, KY 40517. (606) 272-7166. < http://www.lexington-on-line.com/naf.html >.

Obsessive-Compulsive Anonymous. P.O. Box 215, New Hyde Park, NY 11040. (516) 741-4901. < west24th@aol.com > < http://members.aol.com/west24th/index.html >.

Obsessive-Compulsive Foundation. P.O. Box 70, Milford, CT 06460. (203) 874-3843. < JPHS28A@Prodigy.com > < http://pages.prodigy.com/alwillen/ocf.html >.

Carol A. Turkington

Obsessive compulsive personality disorder *see* **Personality disorders**

Obstetric sonogram *see* **Pelvic ultrasound**

Obstetrical emergencies

Definition

Obstetrical emergencies are life-threatening medical conditions that occur in **pregnancy** or during or after labor and delivery.

Description

There are a number of illnesses and disorders of pregnancy that can threaten the well-being of both mother and child. Obstetrical emergencies may also occur during active labor, and after delivery (postpartum).

Obstetrical emergencies of pregnancy

ECTOPIC PREGNANCY. An ectopic, or tubal, pregnancy occurs when the fertilized egg implants itself in the fallopian tube rather than the uterine wall. If the pregnancy is not terminated at an early stage, the fallopian tube will rupture, causing internal hemorrhaging and potentially resulting in permanent infertility.

PLACENTAL ABRUPTION. Also called *abruptio placenta*, placental abruption occurs when the placenta separates from the uterus prematurely, causing bleeding and contractions. If over 50% of the placenta separates, both the fetus and mother are at risk.

PLACENTA PREVIA. When the placenta attaches to the mouth of the uterus and partially or completely blocks the cervix, the position is termed *placenta previa* (or low-lying placenta). **Placenta previa** can result in premature bleeding and possible postpartum hemorrhage.

PREECLAMPSIA/ECLAMPSIA. Preeclampsia (toxemia), or pregnancy-induced high blood pressure, causes severe edema (swelling due to water retention) and can impair kidney and liver function. The condition occurs in approximately 5% of all United States pregnancies. If it progresses to **eclampsia**, toxemia is potentially fatal for mother and child.

PREMATURE RUPTURE OF MEMBRANES (PROM). Premature rupture of membranes is the breaking of the bag of waters (amniotic fluid) before contractions or labor begins. The situation is only considered an emergency if the break occurs before thirty-seven weeks and results in significant leakage of amniotic fluid and/or infection of the amniotic sac.

Obstetrical emergencies during labor and delivery

AMNIOTIC FLUID EMBOLISM. A rare but frequently fatal complication of labor, this condition occurs when amniotic fluid embolizes from the amniotic sac and through the veins of the uterus and into the circulatory system of the mother. The fetal cells present in the fluid then block or clog the pulmonary artery, resulting in **heart attack**. This complication can also happen during pregnancy, but usually occurs in the presence of strong contractions.

INVERSION OR RUPTURE OF UTERUS. During labor, a weak spot in the uterus (such as a scar or a uterine wall that is thinned by a multiple pregnancy) may tear, resulting in a uterine rupture. In certain circumstances, a portion of the placenta may stay attached to the wall and will pull the uterus out with it during delivery. This is called uterine inversion.

PLACENTA ACCRETA. *Placenta accreta* occurs when the placenta is implanted too deeply into the uterine wall, and will not detach during the late stages of **childbirth**, resulting in uncontrolled bleeding.

PROLAPSED UMBILICAL CORD. A prolapse of the umbilical cord occurs when the cord is pushed down into the cervix or vagina. If the cord becomes compressed, the oxygen supply to the fetus could be diminished, resulting in brain damage or possible **death**.

SHOULDER DYSTOCIA. Shoulder dystocia occurs when the baby's shoulder(s) becomes wedged in the birth canal after the head has been delivered.

Obstetrical emergencies postpartum

POSTPARTUM HEMORRHAGE OR INFECTION. Severe bleeding or uterine infection occurring after delivery is a serious, potentially fatal situation.

Causes and symptoms

Obstetrical emergencies can be caused by a number of factors, including **stress**, trauma, genetics, and other variables. In some cases, past medical history, including previous pregnancies and deliveries, may help an obstetrician anticipate the possibility of complications.

Signs and symptoms of an obstetrical emergency include, but are not limited to:

- Diminished fetal activity. In the late third trimester, fewer than ten movements in a two hour period may indicate that the fetus is in distress.

- Abnormal bleeding. During pregnancy, brown or white to pink vaginal discharge is normal, bright red blood or blood containing large clots is not. After delivery, continual blood loss of over 500 ml indicates hemorrhage.

- Leaking amniotic fluid. Amniotic fluid is straw-colored and may easily be confused with urine leakage, but can be differentiated by its slightly sweet odor.

- Severe abdominal **pain**. Stomach or lower back pain can indicate preeclampsia or an undiagnosed ectopic pregnancy. Postpartum stomach pain can be a sign of infection or hemorrhage.

- Contractions. Regular contractions before 37 weeks of gestation can signal the onset of preterm labor due to obstetrical complications.

- Abrupt and rapid increase in blood pressure. Hypertension is one of the first signs of toxemia.

- Edema. Sudden and significant swelling of hands and feet caused by fluid retention from toxemia.

- Unpleasant smelling vaginal discharge. A thick, malodorous discharge from the vagina can indicate a postpartum infection.

- **Fever**. Fever may indicate an active infection.

- Loss of consciousness. **Shock** due to blood loss (hemorrhage) or amniotic **embolism** can precipitate a loss of consciousness in the mother.

- Blurred vision and headaches. Vision problems and **headache** are possible symptoms of preeclampsia.

Diagnosis

Diagnosis of an obstetrical emergency typically takes place in a hospital or other urgent care facility. A specialist will take the patient's medical history and perform a pelvic and general physical examination. The mother's vital signs are taken, and if preeclampsia is suspected, blood pressure may be monitored over a period of time. The fetal heartbeat is assessed with a doppler stethoscope, and diagnostic blood and urine tests of the mother may also be performed, including laboratory analysis for protein and/or bacterial infection. An **abdominal ultrasound** may aid in the diagnosis of any condition that involves a malpositioned placenta, such as placenta previa or placenta abruption.

In cases where an obstetrical complication is suspected, a fetal heart monitor is positioned externally on the mother's abdomen. If the fetal heart rate is erratic or weak, or if it does not respond to movement, the fetus may be in distress. A biophysical profile (BPP) may also be performed to evaluate the health of the fetus. The BPP uses data from an ultrasound examination to analyze the fetus size, movement, heart rate, and surrounding amniotic fluid.

If the mother's membranes have ruptured and her cervix is partially dilated, an internal fetal scalp electrode can be inserted through the vagina to assess heart rate. A fetal oximetry monitor that measures the oxygen saturation levels of the fetus may also be attached to the scalp.

Treatment

Obstetrical emergencies of pregnancy

ECTOPIC PREGNANCY. Treatment of an **ectopic pregnancy** is laparoscopic surgical removal of the fertilized ovum. If the fallopian tube has burst or been damaged, further surgery will be necessary.

PLACENTAL ABRUPTION. In mild cases of **placental abruption**, bed rest may prevent further separation of the placenta and stem bleeding. If a significant abruption (over 50%) occurs, the fetus may have to be delivered immediately and a blood **transfusion** may be required.

PLACENTA PREVIA. Hospitalization or highly restricted at-home bed rest is usually recommended if placenta previa is diagnosed after the twentieth week of pregnancy. If the fetus is at least 36 weeks old and the lungs are mature, a **cesarean section** is performed to deliver the baby.

PREECLAMPSIA/ECLAMPSIA. Treatment of preeclampsia depends upon the age of the fetus and the acuteness of the condition. A woman near full term who has only mild toxemia may have labor induced to deliver the child as soon as possible. Severe preeclampsia in a woman near term also calls for immediate delivery of the child, as this is the only known cure for the condition. However, if the fetus is under 28 weeks, the mother may be hospitalized and steroids may be administered to try to hasten lung development in the fetus. If the life of the mother or fetus appears to be in danger, the baby is delivered immediately, usually by cesarean section.

PREMATURE RUPTURE OF MEMBRANES (PROM). If PROM occurs before 37 weeks and/or results in significant leakage of amniotic fluid, a course of intravenous **antibiotics** is started. A culture of the cervix may be taken to analyze for the presence of bacterial infection. If the fetus is close to term, labor is typically induced if contractions do not start within 24 hours of rupture.

Obstetrical emergencies during labor and delivery

AMNIOTIC FLUID EMBOLISM. The stress of contractions can cause this complication, which has a high mortality rate. Administering steroids to the mother and delivering the fetus as soon as possible is the standard treatment.

INVERSION OR RUPTURE OF UTERUS. An inverted uterus is either manually or surgical replaced to the proper position. A ruptured uterus is repaired if possible, although if the damage is extreme, a **hysterectomy** (removal of the uterus) may be performed. A blood transfusion may be required in either case if hemorrhaging occurs.

PLACENTA ACCRETA. Women who experience placenta accreta will typically need to have their placenta surgically removed after delivery. Hysterectomy is necessary in some cases.

PROLAPSED UMBILICAL CORD. Saline may be infused into the vagina to relieve the compression. If the cord has prolapsed out the vaginal opening, it may be replaced, but immediate delivery by cesarean section is usually indicated.

Obstetrical emergencies postpartum

POSTPARTUM HEMORRHAGE OR INFECTION. The source of the hemorrhage is determined, and blood transfusion and IV fluids are given as necessary. Oxytocic drugs may be administered to encourage contraction of the uterus. Retained placenta is a frequent cause of persistent bleeding, and surgical removal of the remaining fragments (curettage) may be required. Surgical repair of lacerations to the birth canal or uterus may be required. Drugs that encourage coagulation (clotting) of the blood may be administered to stem the bleeding. Infrequently, hysterectomy is required.

In cases of infection, a course of intravenous antibiotics is prescribed. Most postpartum infections occur in the endometrium, or lining of the uterus, and may be also caused by a piece of retained placenta. If this is the case, it will also require surgical removal.

SHOULDER DYSTOCIA. The mother is usually positioned with her knees to her chest, known as the McRoberts maneuver, in an effort to free the child's shoulder. An **episiotomy** is also performed to widen the vaginal opening. If the shoulder cannot be dislodged from the pelvis, the baby's clavicle (collarbone) may have to be broken to complete the delivery before a lack of oxygen causes brain damage to the infant.

KEY TERMS

Amniotic fluid—The liquid in the placental sac that cushions the fetus and regulates temperature in the placental environment. Amniotic fluid also contains fetal cells.

Cesarean section—The surgical delivery of a fetus through an incision in the uterus.

Embolism—Blood vessel obstruction by a blood clot or other substance (i.e., air, cell matter).

Episiotomy—Incision of the perineum, the area between the vulva and the anus, to assist delivery and avoid severe tearing of the perineum.

Laparoscopic—A minimally-invasive surgical or diagnostic procedure that uses a flexible endoscope (laparoscope) to view and operate on structures in the abdomen.

Postpartum—After childbirth.

Prognosis

If a fetus is close to full-term (37 weeks) and the complication is detected early enough, the prognosis is usually good for mother and child. With advances in neonatal care, approximately 85% of infants weighing less than 3 lbs 5 oz survive, and these infants are being delivered at 28 weeks and younger. However, preterm infants have a greater chance of serious medical problems, and developmental disabilities occur in 25–50%. They also have a higher incidence of learning disorders, and are four to six times more likely to be diagnosed with attention-deficit hyperactivity disorder (**ADHD**).

Prevention

Proper prenatal care is the best prevention for obstetrical emergencies. When complications of pregnancy do arise, pregnant women who see their OB/GYN on a regular basis are more likely to get an early diagnosis, and with it, the best chance for fast and effective treatment. In addition, eating right and taking prenatal **vitamins** and supplements as recommended by a physician will also contribute to the health of both mother and child.

Resources

PERIODICALS

Chamberlain, Geoffrey, and Phillip Steer. "Obstetric Emergencies." *British Medical Journal*. 318, no.7194 (May 1999): 1342.

ORGANIZATIONS

National Institute of Child Health and Human Development (NICHD) Clearinghouse. Bldg 31, Room 2A32, MSC 2425, 31 Center Drive, Bethesda, MD 20892-2425. (800) 370-2943. < http://www.nichd.nih.gov/publications/health.htm >.

Paula Anne Ford-Martin

Occupational asthma

Definition

Occupational **asthma** is a form of lung disease in which the breathing passages shrink, swell, or become inflamed or congested as a result of exposure to irritants in the workplace.

Description

As many as 15% of all cases of asthma may be related to on-the-job exposure to:

- animal hair
- dander
- dust composed of bacteria, protein, or organic matter like cereal, grains, cotton, and flax
- fumes created by metal soldering
- insulation and packaging materials
- mites and other insects
- paints

Hundreds of different types of jobs involve exposure to substances that could trigger occupational asthma, but only a small fraction of people who do such work develop this disorder. Occupational asthma is most apt to affect workers who have personal or family histories of allergies or asthma, or who are often required to handle or breathe dust or fumes created by especially irritating material.

Causes and symptoms

Although occupational asthma is not new, today, more than 240 causes of occupational asthma have been identified. It was probably first recorded in 1713 when one of the fathers of occupational health, Bernadina Ramazzini said bakers and textile workers had problems with coughing **shortness of breath**, hoarseness and asthma. Even short-term exposure to low levels of one or more irritating substances can cause

ALICE HAMILTON (1869–1970)

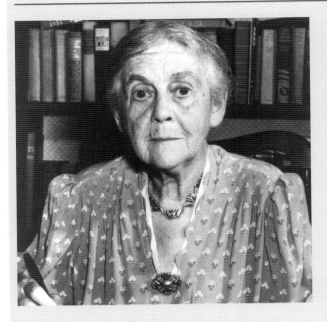

(AP/Wide World Photos. Reproduced by permission.)

Alice Hamilton was born on February 27, 1869, in New York City, the second of five children born to Montgomery Hamilton, a wholesale grocer, and Gertrude (Pond) Hamilton. She earned a medical degree from the University of Michigan in 1893, without having completed an undergraduate degree and taking surprisingly few science courses. Realizing that she wanted to pursue research rather than medical practice, Hamilton went on to do further studies both in the United States and abroad: from 1895–1896 at Leipzig and Munich; 1896–1897 at Johns Hopkins; and 1902 in Paris at the Pasteur Institute. In 1897 she accepted a post as professor of pathology at the Women's Medical College at Northwestern University in Chicago.

In Chicago Hamilton became a resident of Hull House, the pioneering settlement designed to give care and advice to the poor of Chicago. Here, under the influence of Jane Addams, the founder of Hull House, Hamilton saw the effects of poverty up close, leading her to a lifelong career focused on industrial medicine.

Alice Hamilton was a pioneer in correcting the medical problems caused by industrialization, awakening the country in the early twentieth century to the dangers of industrial poisons and hazardous working conditions. Through her untiring efforts, toxic substances in the lead, mining, painting, pottery, and rayon industries were exposed and legislation passed to protect workers. She was also a champion of worker's compensation laws, and was instrumental in bringing about this type of legislation in the state of Illinois. A medical doctor and researcher, she was the first woman of faculty status at Harvard University, and was a consultant on governmental commissions, both domestic and foreign.

Occupations Associated With Asthma

Animal Handling
Bakeries
Health Care
Jewelry Making
Laboratory Work
Manufacturing Detergents
Nickel Plating
Soldering
Snow Crab and Egg Processing
Tanneries

---

a very sensitive person to develop symptoms of occupational asthma. A person who has occupational asthma has one or more symptoms, including coughing, shortness of breath, tightness in the chest, and **wheezing**. Symptoms may appear less than 24 hours after the person is first exposed to the irritant or develop two or three years later.

At first, symptoms appear while the person is at work or several hours after the end of the workday. Symptoms disappear or diminish when the person spends time away from the workplace and return or intensify when exposure is renewed.

As the condition becomes more advanced, symptoms sometimes occur even when the person is not in the workplace. Symptoms may also develop in response to minor sources of lung irritation.

Diagnosis

An allergist, occupational medicine specialist, or a doctor who treats lung disease performs a thorough **physical examination** and takes a medical history that explores:

- the kind of work the patient has done
- the types of exposures the patient may have experienced
- what symptoms the patient has had
- when, how often, and how severely symptoms have occurred

Performed before and after work, pulmonary function tests can show how job-related exposures affect the airway. Laboratory analysis of blood and sputum may confirm a diagnosis of workplace asthma. To pinpoint the cause more precisely, the doctor may ask the patient to inhale specific substances and monitor the body's response to them. This is called a challenge test.

Treatment

The most effective treatment for occupational asthma is to reduce or eliminate exposure to symptom-producing substances.

Medication may be prescribed for workers who can not prevent occasional exposure. Leukotriene modifiers (montelukast and zafirlukast) are new drugs that help manage asthma. They work by counteracting leukotrienes, which are substances released by white blood cells in the lung that cause the air passages to constrict and promote mucus secretion. Leukotriene modifiers also fight off some forms of **rhinitis**, an added bonus for people with asthma. Medication, physical therapy, and breathing aids may be needed to relieve symptoms of advanced occupational asthma involving airway damage.

A patient who has occupational asthma should learn what causes symptoms and how to control them, and what to do when an asthma attack occurs.

Because asthma symptoms and the substances that provoke them can change, a patient who has occupational asthma should be closely monitored by a family physician, allergist, or doctor who specializes in occupational medicine or lung disease.

Prognosis

Occupational can be reversible. However, continued exposure to the symptom-producing substance can cause permanent lung damage. Follow-up studies of people with occupational asthma show that some cannot be protected from the exposure or are forced to change jobs, lose their jobs, or have worse prospects for future jobs based on their **allergies** and asthma.

In time, occupational asthma can cause asthma-like symptoms to occur when the patient is exposed to tobacco smoke, household dust, and other ordinary irritants.

Smoking aggravates symptoms of occupational asthma. Patients who eliminate workplace exposure and stop smoking are more apt to recover fully than those who change jobs but continue to smoke.

Prevention

Industries and environments where employees have a heightened exposure to substances known to cause occupational asthma can take measures to diminish or eliminate the amount of pollution in the atmosphere or decrease the number of exposed workers.

Regular medical screening of workers in these environments may enable doctors to diagnose occupational asthma before permanent lung damage takes place.

Resources

PERIODICALS

"Allergic to Work? Occupational Asthma Accounts for Up to 18 Million Lost Working Days a Year and Affects Thousand of Workers." *The Safety & Health Practitioner* September 2004: 38–41.

Solomon, Gina, Elizabeth H. Humphreys, and Mark D. Miller. "Asthma and the Environment: Connecting the Dots: What Role Do Environmental Exposures Play in the Rising Prevalence and Severity of Asthma?" *Contemporary Pediatrics* August 2004: 73–81.

"What's New in: Asthma and Allergic Rhinitis." *Pulse* September 20, 2004: 50.

ORGANIZATIONS

American College of Allergy, Asthma and Immunology. 85 West Algonquin Road, Suite 550, Arlington Heights, IL 60005. (847) 427-1200.

Maureen Haggerty
Teresa G. Odle

Occupational therapy *see* **Rehabilitation**

Ocular myopathy *see* **Ophthalmoplegia**

Ocular rosacea *see* **Rosacea**

Ofloxacin *see* **Fluoroquinolones**

Ohio Valley disease *see* **Histoplasmosis**

Oligomenorrhea

Definition

Medical dictionaries define oligomenorrhea as infrequent or very light menstruation. But physicians typically apply a narrower definition, restricting the diagnosis of oligomenorrhea to women whose periods were regularly established before they developed problems with infrequent flow. With oligomenorrhea, menstrual periods occur at intervals of greater than 35 days, with only four to nine periods in a year.

Description

True oligomenorrhea can not occur until menstrual periods have been established. In the United States, 97.5% of women have begun normal menstrual cycles by age 16. The complete absence of menstruation, whether menstrual periods never start or whether they stop after having been established, is called **amenorrhea**. Oligomenorrhea can become amenorrhea if menstruation stops for six months or more.

It is quite common for women at the beginning and end of their reproductive lives to miss or have irregular periods. This is normal and is usually the result of imperfect coordination between the hypothalamus, the pituitary gland, and the ovaries. For no apparent reason, a few women menstruate (with ovulation occurring) on a regular schedule as infrequently as once every two months. For them that schedule is normal and not a cause for concern.

Women with **polycystic ovary syndrome** (PCOS) are also likely to suffer from oligomenorrhea. PCOS is a condition in which the ovaries become filled with small cysts. Women with PCOS show menstrual irregularities that range from oligomenorrhea and amenorrhea on the one hand to very heavy, irregular periods on the other. The condition affects about 6% of premenopausal women and is related to excess androgen production.

Other physical and emotional factors also cause a woman to miss periods. These include:

- emotional **stress**
- chronic illness
- poor **nutrition**
- eating disorders such as **anorexia nervosa**
- excessive **exercise**
- estrogen-secreting tumors
- illicit use of anabolic steriod drugs to enhance athletic performance

Professional ballet dancers, gymnasts, and ice skaters are especially at risk for oligomenorrhea because they combine strenuous physical activity with a diet intended to keep their weight down. Menstrual irregularities are now known to be one of the three disorders comprising the so-called "female athlete triad," the other disorders being disordered eating and **osteoporosis**. The triad was first formally named at the annual meeting of the American College of Sports Medicine in 1993, but doctors were aware of the combination of bone mineral loss, stress **fractures**, eating disorders, and participation in women's sports for several decades before the triad was named. Women's coaches have become increasingly aware of the problem since the early 1990s, and are encouraging female athletes to seek medical advice.

Causes and symptoms

Symptoms of oligomenorrhea include:

- menstrual periods at intervals of more than 35 days
- irregular menstrual periods with unpredictable flow
- some women with oligomenorrhea may have difficulty conceiving.

Oligomenorrhea that occurs in adolescents is often caused by immaturity or lack of synchronization between the hypothalamus, pituitary gland, and ovaries. The hypothalamus is part of the brain that controls body temperature, cellular metabolism, and basic functions such as eating, sleeping, and reproduction. It secretes hormones that regulate the pituitary gland.

The pituitary gland is then stimulated to produce hormones that affect growth and reproduction. At the beginning and end of a woman's reproductive life, some of these hormone messages may not be synchronized, causing menstrual irregularities.

In PCOS, oligomenorrhea is probably caused by inappropriate levels of both female and male hormones. Male hormones are produced in small quantities by all women, but in women with PCOS, levels of male hormone (androgens) are slightly higher than in other women. More recently, however, some researchers are hypothesizing that the ovaries of women with PCOS are abnormal in other respects. In 2003, a group of researchers in London reported that there are fundamental differences between the development of egg follicles in normal ovaries and follicle development in the ovaries of women with PCOS.

In athletes, models, actresses, dancers, and women with anorexia nervosa, oligomenorrhea occurs because the ratio of body fat to weight drops too low.

Diagnosis

History and physical examination

Diagnosis of oligomenorrhea begins with the patient informing the doctor about infrequent periods. The doctor will ask for a detailed description of the problem and take a history of how long it has existed and any patterns the patient has observed. A woman can assist the doctor in diagnosing the cause of oligomenorrhea by keeping a record of the time, frequency, length, and quantity of bleeding. She should also tell the doctor about any recent illnesses, including long-standing conditions like **diabetes mellitus**. The doctor may also inquire about the patient's diet, exercise patterns, sexual activity, contraceptive use, current medications, or past surgical procedures.

The doctor will then perform a **physical examination** to evaluate the patient's weight in proportion to her height, to check for signs of normal sexual development, to make sure the heart rhythm and other vital signs are normal, and to palpate (feel) the thyroid gland for evidence of swelling.

In the case of female athletes, the doctor may need to establish a relationship of trust with the patient before asking about such matters as diet, practice and workout schedules, and the use of such drugs as steroids or ephedrine. The presence of stress fractures in young women should be investigated. In some cases, the doctor may give the patients the Eating Disorder Inventory (EDI) or a similar screening questionnaire to help determine whether the patient is at risk for developing anorexia or bulimia.

Laboratory tests

After taking the woman's history, the gynecologist or family practitioner does a pelvic examination and **Pap test**. To rule out specific causes of oligomenorrhea, the doctor may also do a **pregnancy** test and blood tests to check the level of thyroid hormone. Based on the initial test results, the doctor may want to do tests to determine the level of other hormones that play a role in reproduction.

As of 2003, more sensitive monoclonal assays have been developed for measuring hormone levels in the blood serum of women with PCOS, thus allowing earlier and more accurate diagnosis.

Imaging studies

In some cases the doctor may order an ultrasound study of the pelvic region to check for anatomical abnormalities, or x rays or a bone scan to check for bone fractures. In a few cases the doctor may order an MRI to rule out tumors affecting the hypothalamus or pituitary gland.

Treatment

Treatment of oligomenorrhea depends on the cause. In adolescents and women near **menopause**, oligomenorrhea usually needs no treatment. For some athletes, changes in training routines and eating habits may be enough to return the woman to a regular menstrual cycle.

Most patients suffering from oligomenorrhea are treated with birth control pills. Other women, including those with PCOS, are treated with hormones. Prescribed hormones depend on which particular hormones are deficient or out of balance. When oligomenorrhea is associated with an eating disorder or the female athlete triad, the underlying condition must be treated. Consultation with a psychiatrist and nutritionist is usually necessary to manage an eating disorder. Female athletes may require physical therapy or **rehabilitation** as well.

Alternative treatment

As with conventional medicial treatments, alternative treatments are based on the cause of the condition. If a hormonal imbalance is revealed by laboratory testing, hormone replacements that are more "natural" for the body (including tri-estrogen and natural progesterone) are recommended. Glandular therapy can assist in bringing about a balance in the glands involved in the reproductive cycle, including the hypothalmus, pituitary, thyroid, ovarian, and adrenal glands. Since homeopathy and **acupuncture** work on deep, energetic levels to rebalance the body, these two modalities may be helpful in treating oligomenorrhea. Western and Chinese herbal medicines also can be very effective. Herbs used to treat oligomenorrhea include dong quai (*Angelica sinensis*), black cohosh (*Cimicifuga racemosa*), and chaste tree (*Vitex agnus-castus*). Herbal preparations used to bring on the menstrual period are known as emmenagogues. For some women, **meditation, guided imagery**, and visualization can play a key role in the treatment of oligomenorrhea by relieving emotional stress.

Diet and adequate nutrition, including adequate protein, essential fatty acids, whole grains, and fresh fruits and vegetables, are important for every woman, especially if deficiencies are present or if she regularly exercises very strenuously. Female athletes at the high school or college level should consult a nutritionist to make sure that they are eating a well-balanced diet

KEY TERMS

Anorexia nervosa—A disorder of the mind and body in which people starve themselves in a desire to be thin, despite being of normal or below normal body weight for their size and age.

Cyst—An abnormal sac containing fluid or semi-solid material.

Emmenagogue—A medication or herbal preparation given to bring on a woman's menstrual period.

Female athlete triad—A combination of disorders frequently found in female athletes that includes disordered eating, osteoporosis, and oligo- or amenorrhea. The triad was first officially named in 1993.

Osteoporosis—The excessive loss of calcium from the bones, causing the bones to become fragile and break easily. Women who are not menstruating are especially vulnerable to this condition because estrogen, a hormone that protects bones against calcium loss, decreases drastically after menopause.

that is adequate to maintain a healthy weight for their height. Girls participating in dance or in sports that emphasize weight control or a slender body type (gymnastics, track and field, swimming, and cheerleading) are at higher risk of developing eating disorders than those that are involved in such sports as softball, weight lifting, or basketball. In some cases the athlete may be given calcium or vitamin D supplements to lower the risk of osteoporosis.

Many women, including those with PCOS, are successfully treated with hormones for oligomenorrhea. They have more frequent periods and begin ovulating during their menstrual cycle, restoring their fertility.

For women who do not respond to hormones or who continue to have an underlying condition that causes oligomenorrhea, the outlook is less positive. Women who have oligomenorrhea may have difficulty conceiving children and may receive fertility drugs. The absence of adequate estrogen increases risk for bone loss (osteoporosis) and cardiovascular disease. Women who do not have regular periods also are more likely to develop uterine **cancer**. Oligomenorrhea can become amenorrhea at any time, increasing the chance of having these complications.

Prevention

Oligomenorrhea is preventable only in women whose low body fat to weight ratio is keeping them from maintaining a regular menstrual cycle. Adequate nutrition and a less vigorous training schedules will normally prevent oligomenorrhea. When oligomenorrhea is caused by hormonal factors, it is not preventable, but it is often treatable.

Resources

BOOKS

American Psychiatric Association. *Diagnostic and Statistical Manual of Mental Disorders.* 4th ed., revised. Washington, D.C.: American Psychiatric Association, 2000.

Beers, Mark H., MD, and Robert Berkow, MD, editors. "Menstrual Abnormalities and Abnormal Uterine Bleeding." Section 18, Chapter 235 In *The Merck Manual of Diagnosis and Therapy.* Whitehouse Station, NJ: Merck Research Laboratories, 2004.

Pelletier, Kenneth R., MD. *The Best Alternative Medicine,* Part II, "CAM Therapies for Specific Conditions: Menstrual Symptoms, Menopause, and PMS." New York: Simon & Schuster, 2002.

PERIODICALS

Barrow, Boone, MD. "Female Athlete Triad." *eMedicine* June 17, 2004. < http://www.emedicine.com/sports/ topic163.htm > .

Chandran, Latha, MBBS, MPH. "Menstruation Disorders." *eMedicine* August 9, 2004. < http://www.emedicine.com/ ped/topic2781.htm > .

Hopkinson, R. A., and J. Lock. "Athletics, Perfectionism, and Disordered Eating." *Eating and Weight Disorders* 9 (June 2004): 99–106.

Klentrou, P., and M. Plyley. "Onset of Puberty, Menstrual Frequency, and Body Fat in Elite Rhythmic Gymnasts Compared with Normal Controls." *British Journal of Sports Medicine* 37 (December 2003): 490–494.

Milsom, S. R., M. C. Sowter, M. A. Carter, et al. "LH Levels in Women with Polycystic Ovarian Syndrome: Have Modern Assays Made Them Irrelevant?" *BJOG* 110 (August 2003): 760–764.

Nelson, Lawrence M., MD, Vladimir Bakalov, MD, and Carmen Pastor, MD. "Amenorrhea." *eMedicine* August 9, 2004. < http://www.emedicine.com/med/ topic117.htm > .

Suliman, A. M., T. P. Smith, J. Gibney, and T. J. McKenna. "Frequent Misdiagnosis and Mismanagement of Hyperprolactinemic Patients Before the Introduction of Macroprolactin Screening: Application of a New Strict Laboratory Definition of Macroprolactinemia." *Clinical Chemistry* 49 (September 2003): 1504–1509.

Webber, L. J., S. Stubbs, J. Stark, et al. "Formation and Early Development of Follicles in the Polycystic Ovary." *Lancet* 362 (September 27, 2003): 1017–1021.

ORGANIZATIONS

American Academy of Child and Adolescent Psychiatry. 3615 Wisconsin Avenue, NW, Washington, DC 20016-3007. (202) 966-7300. Fax: (202) 966-2891. < http://www. aacap.org >.

American College of Sports Medicine (ACSM). 401 West Michigan Street, Indianapolis, IN 46202-3233. (317) 637-9200. Fax: (317) 634-7817. < http:// www.acsm.org >.

Polycystic Ovarian Syndrome Association. P.O. Box 80517, Portland, OR 7280. (877) 775-7267. < http://www. pcosupport.org >.

OTHER

Clinical Research Bulletin. vol. 1, no. 14. < http://www. herbsinfo.com >.

Tish Davidson, A.M.
Rebecca J. Frey, Ph.D.

Omega-3 Fatty Acids

Definition

Essential to human health, omega-3 fatty acids are a form of polyunsaturated fats that are not made by the body and must be obtained from a person's food.

Purpose

Eating foods rich in omega-3 fatty acids is part of a healthy diet and helps people maintain their health.

Description

In recent years, a great deal of attention has been placed on the value of eating a low fat diet. In some cases, people have taken this advice to the extreme by adopting a diet that is far too low in fat or, worse yet, a diet that has no fat at all. But the truth is that not all fat is bad. Although it is true that trans and saturated fats, which are found in high amounts in red meat, butter, whole milk, and some prepackaged foods, have been shown to raise a person's total cholesterol, polyunsaturated fats can actually play a part in keeping cholesterol low. Two especially good fats are the omega-3 fatty acids and the omega-6 fatty acids, which are polyunsaturated.

Two types of omega-3 fatty acids are eicosapentaenoic acid (EPA) and docosahexanoic acid (DHA), which are found mainly in oily cold-water fish, such as tuna, salmon, trout, herring, sardines, bass, swordfish, and mackerel. With the exception of seaweed, most plants do not contain EPA or DHA. However, alpha-linolenic acid (ALA), which is another kind of omega-3 fatty acid, is found in dark green leafy vegetables, flaxseed oil, fish oil, and canola oil, as well as nuts and beans, such as walnuts and soybeans. Enzymes in a person's body can convert ALA to EPA and DHA, which are the two kinds of omega-3 fatty acids easily utilized by the body.

Many experts agree that it is important to maintain a healthy balance between omega-3 fatty acids and omega-6 fatty acids. As Dr. Penny Kris-Etherton and her colleagues reported in their article published in the *American Journal of Nutrition* an over consumption of omega-6 fatty acids has resulted in an unhealthy dietary shift in the American diet. The authors point out that what used to be a 1:1 ratio between omega-3 and omega-6 fatty acids is now estimated to be a 10:1 ratio. This poses a problem, researchers say, because consuming some of the beneficial effects gained from omega-3 fatty acids are negated by an over consumption of omega-6 fatty acids. For example, omega-3 fatty acids have anti-inflammatory properties, whereas omega-6 fatty acids tend to promote inflammation. Cereals, whole grain bread, margarine, and vegetable oils, such as corn, peanut, and sunflower oil, are examples of omega-6 fatty acids. In addition, people consume a lot of omega-6 fatty acid simply by eating the meat of animals that were fed grain rich in omega-6. Some experts suggest that eating one to four times more omega-6 fatty acids than omega-3 fatty acids is a reasonable ratio. In other words, as dietitians often say, the key to a healthy diet is moderation and balance.

The health benefits of omega-3 fatty acids

There is strong evidence that omega-3 fatty acids protect a person against **atherosclerosis** and therefore against heart disease and **stroke**, as well as abnormal heart rhythms that cause **sudden cardiac death**, and possibly **autoimmune disorders**, such as lupus and **rheumatoid arthritis**. In fact, Drs. Dean Ornish and Mehmet Oz, renowned heart physicians, said in a 2002 article published in *O Magazine* that the benefits derived from consuming the proper daily dose of omega-3 fatty acids may help to reduce sudden cardiac **death** by as much as 50%. In fact, in an article published by *American Family Physician*, Dr. Maggie Covington, a clinical assistant professor at the University of Maryland, also emphasized the value of omega-3 fatty acids with regard to cardiovascular health and referred to one of the largest clinical trials to date, the GISSI-Prevenzione Trial, to illustrate her point. In the study, 11,324 patients with coronary heart disease were divided into four groups: one group received 300 mg of vitamin E, one group received 850 mg of omega-3 fatty acids, one group received the vitamin E and fatty acids, and one group served as the control group. After a little more than three years, "the group given omega-3 fatty acids only had a 45% reduction in sudden death and a 20% reduction in all-cause mortality," as stated by Dr. Covington.

According to the American Heart Association (AHA), the ways in which omega-3 fatty acids may reduce cardiovascular disease are still being studied. However, the AHA indicates that research as shown that omega-3 fatty acids:

- decrease the risk of arrthythmias, which can lead to sudden cardiac death
- decrease triglyceride levels
- decrease the growth rate of atherosclerotic plaque
- lower blood pressure slightly

In fact, numerous studies show that a diet rich in omega-3 fatty acids not only lowers bad cholesterol, known as LDL, but also lowers triglycerides, the fatty material that circulates in the blood. Interestingly, researchers have found that the cholesterol levels of Inuit Eskimos tend to be quite good, despite the fact that they have a high fat diet. The reason for this, research has found, is that their diet is high in fatty fish, which is loaded with omega-3 fatty acids. The same has often been said about the typical Mediterranean-style diet.

Said to reduce joint inflammation, omega-3 fatty acid supplements have been the focus of many studies attempting to validate its effectiveness in treating rheumatoid arthritis. According to a large body of research in the area, omega-3 fatty acid supplements are clearly effective in reducing the symptoms associated with rheumatoid arthritis, such as joint tenderness and stiffness. In some cases, a reduction in the amount of medication needed by rheumatoid arthritis patients has been noted.

More research needs to be done to substantiate the effectiveness of omega-3 fatty acids in treating eating disorders, attention deficit disorder, and depression. Some studies have indicated, for example, that children with behavioral problems and attention deficit disorder have lower than normal amounts of omega-3 fatty acids in their bodies. However, until there is more data in these very important areas of research, a conservative approach should be taken, especially when making changes to a child's diet. Parents should to talk to their child's pediatrician to ascertain if adding more omega-3 fatty acids to their child's diet is appropriate. In addition, parents should take special care to avoid feeding their children fish high in mercury. A food list containing items rich in omega-3 fatty acids can be obtained from a licensed dietitian.

Mercury levels and concerns about safety

A great deal of media attention has been focused on the high mercury levels found in some types of fish. People concerned about fish consumption and mercury levels can review public releases on the subject issued by the U. S. Food and Drug Administration and the Environmental Protection Agency. Special precautions exist for children and pregnant or breast-feeding women. They are advised to avoid shark, mackerel, swordfish, and tilefish. However, both the U.S. Food and Drug Administration and the Environmental Protection Agency emphasis the importance of dietary fish. Fish, they caution, should not be eliminated from the diet. In fact, Robert Oh, M.D., stated in his 2005 article, which was published in *The Journal of the American Board of Family Practice* "with the potential health benefits of fish, women of childbearing age should be encouraged to eat 1 to 2 low-mercury fish meals per week."

Contaminants and concerns about safety

Other concerns regarding fish safety have also been reported. In 2004, Hites and colleagues assessed organic contaminants in salmon in an article published in *Science*. Their conclusion that farmed salmon had higher concentrations of polychlorinated biphenyls than wild salmon prompted public concerns and a response from the American Cancer Society. Farmed fish in Europe was found to have higher levels of mercury than farmed salmon in North and South America; however, the American Cancer Society reminded the public that the "levels of toxins Hites and his colleagues found in the farmed salmon were still below what the U.S. Food and Drug Administration, which regulates food, considers hazardous." The American Cancer Society still continues to promote a healthy, varied diet, which includes fish as a food source.

Recommended dosage

The AHA recommends that people eat two servings of fish, such as tuna or salmon, at least twice a week. A person with coronary heart disease, according to the AHA, should consume 1 gram of omega-3 fatty acids daily through food intake, most preferably through the consumption of fatty fish. The AHA also states that "people with elevated triglycerides may need 2 to 4 grams of EPA and DHA per day provided as a supplement," which is available in liquid or capsule form. Ground or cracked flaxseed can easily be incorporated into a person's diet by sprinkling it over salads, soup, and cereal.

Sources differ, but here are some general examples:

- 3 ounces of pickled herring = 1.2 grams of omega-3 fatty acids

- 3 ounces of salmon = 1.3 grams of omega-3 fatty acids

- 3 ounces of halibut = 1.0 grams of omega-3 fatty acids

- 3 ounces of mackerel = 1.6 grams of omega-3 fatty acids

- 1 1/2 teaspoons of flaxseeds = 3 grams of omega-3 fatty acids

Precautions

In early 2004, the U.S. Food and Drug Administration along with the the Environmental Protection Agency issued a statement that women who are or may be pregnant, as well as breastfeeding mothers and children, should avoid eating some types of fish thought to contain high levels of mercury. Fish that typically contain high levels of mercury are shark, swordfish, and mackerel, whereas shrimp, canned light tuna, salmon, and catfish are generally thought to have low levels of mercury. Because many people engage in fishing as a hobby, women should be sure before they eat any fish caught by friends and family that the local stream or lake is considered low in mercury.

Conflicting information exists whether it is safe for patients with **macular degeneration** to take omega-3 fatty acids in supplement form. Until more data becomes available, it is better for people with macular degeneration to receive their omega-3 fatty acids from the food they eat.

Side effects

Fish oil supplements can cause **diarrhea** and gas. Also, the fish oil capsules tend to have a fishy aftertaste.

Interactions

Although there are no significant **drug interactions** associated with eating foods containing omega-3 fatty acids, patients who are being treated with blood-thinning medications should not take omega-3 fatty acid supplements without seeking the advice of their physicians. Excessive bleeding could result. For the same reason, some patients who plan to take more than 3 grams of omega-3 fatty acids in supplement form should first seek the approval of their physicians.

Resources

PERIODICALS

Albert, C. M., Hennekens, C. H., O'Donnell, C. J., et al. "Fish consumption and risk of sudden cardiac death." *Journal of the American Medical Association* 279 (1998): 23–28.

Covington, M. B. "Omega-3 fatty acids." *American Family Physician* 70 (2004): 133–140.

Harris, W. S. "N-3 fatty acids and serum lipoproteins: human studies." *American Journal of Clinical Nutrition* 65 (1997): 1645–1654.

Hites, R. A., Foran, J. A., Carpenter, D. O., et al. "Global assessment of organic contaminants in farmed salmon." *Science* 303 (1997): 226–229.

Kris-Etherton, P. M., Harris, W. S., Appel, L. J., and American Heart Association Nutrition Committee. "Fish consumption, fish oil, omega-3 fatty acids, and cardiovascular disease." *Circulation* 106 (2003): 2747–2757.

Kris-Etherton, P. M., Taylor, D. S., Yu-Poth, S., et al. "Polyunsaturated fatty acids in the food chain in the United States. " *American Journal of Clinical Nutrition* 71 (2000): 1795–1885.

Oh, R. "Practical applications of fish oil (omega-3 fatty acids) in primary." *The Journal of the American Board of Family Practice* 18 (2005): 28–36.

Ornish, Dean, and Oz, Mehmet. "Caution: Strong at Heart." *O: The Oprah Magazine* November 2002:163–168.

ORGANIZATION

American Cancer Society. "Is Salmon Safe?" *American Cancer Society* 28 Jan 2004 American Cancer Society. 24 Feb 2005 < http://www.cancer.org/ >.

American Heart Association. "American Heart Association Recommendation: Fish and Omega-3 Fatty Acids." *American Heart Association* 2005 American Heart Association. 22 Feb 2005 < http://www.americanheart.org/ >.

Health and Age. "Omega-3 Fatty Acids." *Health and Age* 2005 [cited 22 Feb 2005]. < http://www.healthandage.com/html/res/com/ConsSupplements/Omega3FattyAcidscs.html >.

Kris-Etherton, P. M., Harris, W. S., Appel, L. J., and American Heart Association Nutrition Committee. "American Heart Association Statement: New Guidelines Focus on Fish, Fish Oil, Omega-3 Fatty Acids." *American Heart Association* 18 November 2002 American Heart Association. 22 Feb 2005 < http://www.americanheart.org/ >.

U.S. Food and Drug Administration. "What You Need to Know About Mercury in Fish and Shellfish." *U.S. Food and Drug Administration.* March 2004 U.S. Food and Drug Administration. 22 Feb 2005 < http://www.cfsan.fda.gov/~dms/admehg3.html >.

Lee Ann Paradise

Omeprazole *see* **Antiulcer drugs**

Omphalocele *see* **Abdominal wall defects**

Onchocerciasis *see* **Filariasis**

Onychomycosis

Definition

Onychomycosis is a fungal infection of the fingernails or toenails. The actual infection is of the bed of the nail and of the plate under the surface of the nail.

Description

Onychomycosis is the most common of all diseases of the nails in adults. In North America, the incidence falls roughly between 2–13%. The incidence of onychomycosis is also greater in older adults, and up to 90% of the elderly may be affected. Men are more commonly infected than women.

Individuals who are especially susceptible include those with chronic diseases such as diabetes and circulatory problems and those with diseases that suppress the immune system. Other risk factors include a family history, previous trauma to the nails, warm climate, and occlusive or tight footwear.

Causes and symptoms

Onychomycosis is caused by three types of fungi, called dermatophytes, yeasts, and nondermatophyte molds. Fungi are simple parasitic plant organisms that do not need sunlight to grow. Toenails are especially susceptible because fungi prefer dark damp places. Swimming pools, locker rooms, and showers typically harbor fungi. Chronic diseases such as diabetes, problems with the circulatory system, or immune deficiency disease are risk factors. A history of athlete's foot and excess perspiration are also risk factors.

Onychomycosis can be present for years without causing **pain** or disturbing symptoms. Typically, the nail becomes thicker and changes to a yellowish-brown. Foul smelling debris may collect under the nail. The infection can spread to the surrounding nails and even the skin.

Diagnosis

To make a diagnosis of onychomycosis, the clinician must collect a specimen of the nail in which infection is suspected. A clipping is taken from the nail plate, and a sample of the debris from underneath the nail bed is also taken, usually with a sharp curette. Debris from the nail surface may also be taken. These will be sent for microscopic analysis to a laboratory, as well as cultured to determine what types of fungus are growing there.

Treatment

Onychomycosis is very difficult and sometimes impossible to treat, and therapy is often long-term. Therapy consists of topical treatments that are applied directly to the nails, as well as two systemic drugs, griseofulvin and ketoconazole. Topical therapy is reserved for only the mildest cases. The use of griseofulvin and ketoconazole is problematic, and there are typically high relapse rates of 50–85%. In addition, treatment must be continued for a long duration (10–18 months for toenails), with monthly laboratory monitoring for several side effects, including liver toxicity. Individuals taking these medications must also abstain from alcohol consumption.

In the past few years, newer oral antifungal agents have been developed, and include itraconazole (Sporanox), terbinafine (Lamisil), and fluconazole (Diflucan). These agents, when taken orally for as little as 12 weeks, bring about better cure rates and fewer side effects than either griseofulvin or ketoconazole. The most common side effect is stomach upset. Patients taking oral antifungal therapy must have a complete **blood count** and liver enzyme workup every four to six weeks. Terbinafine in particular has markedly less toxicity to the liver, one of the more severe side effects of the older agents, griseofulvin and ketoconazole.

Treatment should be continued until microscopic exam or culture shows no more fungal infection. Nails may, however, continue to look damaged even after a clinical cure is achieved. Nails may take up to a full year to return to normal. If the nail growth slows or stops, additional doses of antifungal therapy should be taken.

Nail **debridement** is another treatment option, but it is considered by many to be primitive compared with topical or systemic treatment. Clinicians perform nail debridement in their offices. The nail is cut and then thinned using surgical tools or chemicals, and then the loose debris under the nail is removed. The procedure is painless, and often improves the appearance of the nails immediately. In addition, it helps whatever medication being used to penetrate the newly thinned nail. Patients with very thickened nails will sometimes undergo chemical removal of a nail. A combination of oral, topical, and surgical removal can increase the chances of curing the infection.

Alternative treatment

For controlling onychomycosis, as opposed to curing it, some experts advocate using Lotrimin cream, available over the counter. The cream should be thoroughly rubbed into the nail daily in order to control the infection.

In general, **nutrition** may also play a role in promoting good nail health and thus preventing nail disease. Adequate protein and **minerals**, in the form of nuts, seeds, whole grains, legumes, fresh vegetables, and fish, should be consumed. Sugars, alcohol, and **caffeine** should be avoided. Certain supplements may also be beneficial, including vitamin A (10,000 IU per day), zinc (15–30 mg per day), iron (ferrous glycinate 100 mg per day, vitamin B$_{12}$ (1,000 mcg per day), and essential fatty acids in the form of flax, borage, or evening primrose oil (1,000–1,5000 mg twice daily).

Herbal remedies may also relieve some of the symptoms of onychomycosis. A combination of cone-flower, oregano, spilanthes, usnea, Oregon grape root, and myrrh can be used as a tincture (20 drops four times daily).

Undiluted grapefruit seed extract and tea tree oil are also said to be beneficial when applied topically to the infected nails.

Prognosis

Onychomycosis is typically quite difficult to cure completely. Even if a clinical cure is achieved after long therapy with either topical or oral drugs, normal regrowth takes four to six months in the fingernails, and eight to 12 months in the toenails, which grow more slowly. Relapse is common, and often, the nail or nail bed is permanently damaged. For toenails infected with onychomycosis, terbinafine seems to offer the highest cure rate (35–50%). Itraconazole cure rates typically range from 25–40%, and those with fluconazole, which was recently approved in the United States, have not been documented by long-term trials

Prevention

Keeping the feet clean and dry, and washing with soap and water and drying thoroughly are important preventive steps to take to prevent onychomycosis. Other preventive measures include keeping the nails cut short and wearing shower shoes whenever walking or showering in public places. Daily changes of shoes, socks, or hosiery are also helpful. Excessively tight hose or shoes promote moisture, which in turn, provides a wonderful environment for onychomycotic infections. To prevent this, individuals should wear only socks made of synthetic fibers, which can absorb moisture more quickly than those made of cotton or wools. Manicure and pedicure tools should be disinfected after each use. Finally, nail polish should not be applied to nails that are infected, as this causes the water or moisture that collects under the surface of the nail to not evaporate and be trapped.

Resources

PERIODICALS

Harrell T. K., et al. "Onychomycosis: Improved Cure Rates withItraconazole and Terbinafine." *Journal of the American Board of Family Practitioners* July-August 2001: 268- 73.

Scher Robert K. "Novel Treatment Strategies for Superficial Mycoses." *Journal of the American Academy of Dermatology* 1999.

ORGANIZATIONS

American Academy of Dermatology. 930 N. Meacham Road, PO Box 4014, Schaumburg, IL 60168-4014. (847) 330-0230. Fax: (847) 330-0050. <http://www.aad.org>.

OTHER

<http://www.emedicine.com/derm/topic200.htm>.
<http://www.nailfungus.org/about.html>.

Liz Meszaros

Oophorectomy

Definition

Oophorectomy is the surgical removal of one or both ovaries. It is also called ovariectomy or ovarian ablation. If one ovary is removed, a woman may continue to menstruate and have children. If both ovaries are removed, menstruation stops and a woman loses the ability to have children.

Purpose

Oophorectomy is performed to:

- remove cancerous ovaries
- remove the source of estrogen that stimulates some cancers
- remove large **ovarian cysts** in women with polycystic ovarian syndrome (PCOS)
- excise an abscess
- treat **endometriosis**
- lower the risk of an ectopic **pregnancy**
- lower the risk of **cancer** in a woman with a family history of ovarian or **breast cancer**

In an oophorectomy, one or a portion of one ovary may be removed or both ovaries may be removed. When oophorectomy is done to treat **ovarian cancer** or other spreading cancers, both ovaries are always removed. This is called a bilateral oophorectomy. Oophorectomies are sometimes performed on premenopausal women who have estrogen-sensitive breast cancer in an effort to remove the main source of estrogen from their bodies. This procedure has become less common than it was in the 1990s. Today, **chemotherapy** drugs are available that alter the production of estrogen and tamoxifen blocks any of the effects any remaining estrogen may have on cancer cells.

In younger women with low-grade or early-stage ovarian tumors who have not yet completed their families, the surgeon may perform a unilateral oophorectomy. This approach is called fertility-saving or fertility-sparing surgery. Women who are appropriate candidates for this type of oophorectomy do not have higher rates of cancer recurrence than women who have both ovaries removed.

Until the 1980s, women over age 40 having hysterectomies (surgical removal of the uterus) routinely had healthy ovaries and fallopian tubes removed at the same time. This operation is called a bilateral **salpingo-oophorectomy**. Many physicians reasoned that a woman over 40 was approaching **menopause** and soon her ovaries would stop secreting estrogen and releasing eggs. Removing the ovaries would eliminate the risk of ovarian cancer and only accelerate menopause by a few years.

In the 1990s, the thinking about routine oophorectomy began to change. The risk of ovarian cancer in women who have no family history of the disease is less than 1%. Meanwhile, removing the ovaries increases the risk of cardiovascular disease and accelerates **osteoporosis** unless a woman takes prescribed hormone replacements. In addition, other studies indicate that a bilateral oophorectomy increases a woman's risk of developing **thyroid cancer**. Women with mild endometriosis can often be successfully treated with birth control pills or other hormone medications without having to undergo surgery.

Under certain circumstances, oophorectomy may still be the treatment of choice to prevent breast and ovarian cancer in certain high-risk women. A study done at the University of Pennsylvania and released in 2000 showed that healthy women who carried the BRCA1 or BRCA2 genetic mutations that predisposed them to breast cancer had their risk of breast cancer drop from 80% to 19% when their ovaries were removed before age 40. Women between the ages of 40 and 50 showed less risk reduction, and there was no significant reduction of breast cancer risk in women over age 50.

Overall, ovarian cancer still ranks low on a woman's list of health concerns: It accounts for only 4% of all cancers in women. But the lifetime risk for developing ovarian cancer in women who have mutations in BRCA1 is significantly increased over the general population and may cause an ovarian cancer risk of 30% by age 60. For women at increased risk, oophorectomy may be considered after the age of 35 if childbearing is complete.

The value of ovary removal in preventing both breast and ovarian cancer has been documented. However, there are disagreements within the medical community about when and at what age this treatment should be offered. Preventative oophorectomy, called preventative bilateral oophorectomy (PBO), is not always covered by insurance. One study conducted in 2000 at the University of California at San Francisco found that only 20% of insurers paid for PBO. Another 25% had a policy against paying for the operation, and the remaining 55% said that they would decide about payment on an individual basis.

Precautions

There are situations in which oophorectomy is a medically wise choice for women who have a family history of breast or ovarian cancer. However, women with healthy ovaries who are undergoing **hysterectomy** for reasons other than cancer should discuss with their doctors the benefits and disadvantages of having their ovaries removed at the time of the hysterectomy. It is important for women to ask questions about the long-term risks of a bilateral oophorectomy; one study published in 2003 reported that many women awaiting surgery felt that they did not have adequate information about their treatment options and were unaware of the possible long-term consequences to health.

Description

Oophorectomy is done under **general anesthesia**. It is performed through the same type of incision, either vertical or horizontal, as an abdominal hysterectomy. Horizontal incisions leave a less noticeable scar, but vertical incisions give the surgeon a better view of the abdominal cavity.

After the incision is made, the abdominal muscles are pulled apart, not cut, so that the surgeon can see the ovaries. Then the ovaries, and often the fallopian tubes, are removed.

Oophorectomy can sometimes be done with a laparoscopic procedure. With this surgery, a tube containing a tiny lens and light source is inserted through a small incision in the navel. A camera can be attached that allows the surgeon to see the abdominal cavity on a video monitor. When the ovaries are detached, they are removed though a small incision at the top of the vagina. The ovaries can also be cut into smaller sections and removed.

The advantages of abdominal incision are that the ovaries can be removed even if a woman has many **adhesions** from previous surgery. The surgeon gets a good view of the abdominal cavity and can check the surrounding tissue for disease. A vertical abdominal incision is mandatory if cancer is suspected. The disadvantages are that bleeding is more likely to be a complication of this type of operation. The operation is more painful than a laparoscopic operation and the recovery period is longer. A woman can expect to be in the hospital two to five days and will need three to six weeks to return to normal activities.

Preparation

Before surgery, the doctor will order blood and urine tests, and any additional tests such as ultrasound or x rays to help the surgeon visualize the woman's condition. The woman may also meet with the anesthesiologist to evaluate any special conditions that might affect the administration of anesthesia. A colon preparation may be done, if extensive surgery is anticipated.

On the evening before the operation, the woman should eat a light dinner, then take nothing by mouth, including water or other liquids, after midnight.

Aftercare

After surgery a woman will feel some discomfort. The degree of discomfort varies and is generally greatest with abdominal incisions, because the abdominal muscles must be stretched out of the way so that the surgeon can reach the ovaries.

When both ovaries are removed, women who do not have cancer are started on **hormone replacement therapy** to ease the symptoms of menopause that occur because estrogen produced by the ovaries is no longer present. If even part of one ovary remains, it will produce enough estrogen that a woman will continue to menstruate, unless her uterus was removed in a hysterectomy. **Antibiotics** are given to reduce the risk of post-surgery infection.

Return to normal activities takes anywhere from two to six weeks, depending on the type of surgery. When women have cancer, chemotherapy or radiation are often given in addition to surgery. Some women have emotional trauma following an oophorectomy, and can benefit from counseling and support groups.

Risks

Oophorectomy is a relatively safe operation, although, like all major surgery, it does carry some risks. These include unanticipated reaction to anesthesia, internal bleeding, **blood clots**, accidental damage to other organs, and post-surgery infection.

Complications after an oophorectomy include changes in sex drive, hot flashes, and other symptoms of menopause if both ovaries are removed. Women who have both ovaries removed and who do not take estrogen replacement therapy run an increased risk for cardiovascular disease and osteoporosis. Women with a history of psychological and emotional problems before an oophorectomy are more likely to experience psychological difficulties after the operation.

Normal results

If the surgery is successful, the ovaries will be removed without complication, and the underlying problem resolved. In the case of cancer, all the cancer will be removed.

Abnormal results

Complications may arise if the surgeon finds that cancer has spread to other places in the abdomen. If the cancer cannot be removed by surgery, it must be treated with chemotherapy and radiation.

KEY TERMS

Cyst—An abnormal sac containing fluid or semi-solid material.

Ectopic pregnancy—A pregnancy that develops when a fertilized egg implants outside the uterus, usually in the Fallopian tubes, but sometimes in the ovary itself.

Endometriosis—A benign condition that occurs when cells from the lining of the uterus begin growing outside the uterus.

Fallopian tubes—Slender tubes that carry ova from the ovaries to the uterus.

Hysterectomy—Surgical removal of the uterus.

Osteoporosis—The excessive loss of calcium from the bones, causing the bones to become fragile and break easily.

Polycystic ovarian syndrome (PCOS)—A condition in which the eggs are not released from the ovaries and instead form multiple cysts.

Ovarian remnant syndrome is a complication that results in about 18% of women who have had an oophorectomy for severe endometriosis. The syndrome is characterized by chronic pelvic **pain** and/or a pelvic mass; it is treated by further surgery to remove the remaining ovarian tissue.

Resources

BOOKS

Beers, Mark H., MD, and Robert Berkow, MD, editors. "Endometriosis." Section 18, Chapter 239. In *The Merck Manual of Diagnosis and Therapy*. Whitehouse Station, NJ: Merck Research Laboratories, 2004.

Beers, Mark H., MD, and Robert Berkow, MD, editors. "Ovarian Cancer." Section 18, Chapter 241. In *The Merck Manual of Diagnosis and Therapy*. Whitehouse Station, NJ: Merck Research Laboratories, 2004.

Pelletier, Kenneth R., MD. *The Best Alternative Medicine*, Part II, "CAM Therapies for Specific Conditions: Cancer." New York: Simon & Schuster, 2002.

PERIODICALS

Abu-Rafeh, B., G. A. Vilos, and M. Misra. "Frequency and Laparoscopic Management of Ovarian Remnant Syndrome." *Journal of the American Association of Gynecologic Laparoscopists* 10 (February 2003): 33–37.

Ayhan, A., H. Celik, C. Tskiran, et al. "Oncologic and Reproductive Outcome After Fertility-Saving Surgery in Ovarian Cancer" *European Journal of Gynaecological Oncology* 24 (March 2003): 223–232.

Bhavnani, V., and A. Clarke. "Women Awaiting Hysterectomy: A Qualitative Study of Issues Involved in Decisions About Oophorectomy." *BJOG* 110 (February 2003): 168–174.

Bleiker, E. M., D. E. Hahn, and N. K. Aaronson. "Psychosocial Issues in Cancer Genetics—Current Status and Future Directions." *Acta Oncologica* 42 (2003): 276–286.

de Carvalho, M., J. Jenkins, M. Nehrebecky, and L. Lahl. "The Role of Estrogens in BRCA1/2 Mutation Carriers: Reflections on the Past, Issues for the Future." *Cancer Nursing* 26 (December 2003): 421–430.

Itoh, H., A. Ishihara, H. Koita, et al. "Ovarian Pregnancy: Report of Four Cases and Review of the Literature." *Pathology International* 53 (November 2003): 806–809.

Lane, G. "Prophylactic Oophorectomy: Why and When?" *Journal of the British Menopause Society* 9 (December 2003): 156–160.

Sainsbury, R. "Ovarian Ablation as a Treatment for Breast Cancer." *Surgical Oncology* 12 (December 2003): 241–250.

ORGANIZATIONS

American Cancer Society. 1599 Clifton Road NE, Atlanta, GA 30329. (800)ACS-2345. < http://www.cancer.org >.

American College of Obstetricians and Gynecologists (ACOG). 409 12th Street, SW, P. O. Box 96920, Washington, DC 20090-6920. < http://www.acog.org >.

National Cancer Institute (NCI). Public Inquiries Office, Suite 3036A, 6116 Executive Blvd., MSC 8322, Bethesda, MD 20892-8322. (800) 4-CANCER. < http://www.nci.nih.gov >.

OTHER

Ovarian Cancer Home Page, National Cancer Institute. < http://www.nci.nih.gov/cancer_information/ cancer_type/ovarian/ >.

Tish Davidson, A.M.
Rebecca J. Frey, Ph.D.

Open fracture reduction *see* **Fracture repair**

Ophthalmic antibiotics *see* **Antibiotics, ophthalmic**

Ophthalmoplegia

Definition

Ophthalmoplegia is a **paralysis** or weakness of one or more of the muscles that control eye movement. The condition can be caused by any of several neurologic disorders. It may be myopathic, meaning that the muscles controlling eye movement are directly involved, or neurogenic, meaning that the nerve pathways controlling eye muscles are affected. Diseases associated with ophthalmoplegia are ocular myopathy, which affects muscles, and internuclear ophthalmoplegia, a disorder caused by **multiple sclerosis**, a disease which affects nerves.

Description

Because the eyes do not move together in ophthalmoplegia, patients may complain of double vision. Double vision is especially troublesome if the ophthalmoplegia comes on suddenly or affects each eye differently. Because ophthalmoplegia is caused by another, underlying disease, it is often associated with other neurologic symptoms, including limb weakness, lack of coordination, and **numbness**.

Causes and symptoms

Ocular myopathy is also known as mitochondrial encephalomyelopathy with ophthalmoplegia or progressive external ophthalmoplegia. Because it is so often associated with diseases affecting many levels of the neurologic system, it is often referred to as "ophthalmoplegia plus." The main feature is progressive limitation of eye movements, usually with drooping of the eyelids (**ptosis**). Ptosis may occur years before other symptoms of ophthalmoplegia. Because both eyes are equally involved and because ability to move the eyes lessens gradually over the course of years, double vision is rare. On examination, the eyelids may appear thin. This disease usually begins in childhood or adolescence but may start later.

When ophthalmoplegia is caused by muscle degeneration (myopathic), muscle biopsy, in which a small piece of muscle is surgically removed and examined microscopically, will find characteristic abnormal muscle fibers called ragged red fibers. In this form of ophthalmoplegia, the patient may experience weakness of the face, the muscles involved in swallowing, the neck, or the limbs.

Progressive external ophthalmoplegia is sometimes associated with specific neurologic syndromes. These syndromes include familial forms of spastic paraplegia, spinocerebellar disorders, or sensorimotor **peripheral neuropathy**. Kearns-Sayre syndrome causes ophthalmoplegia along with loss of pigment in the retina, the light-sensitive membrane lining the eye. In addition, the disease may cause **heart block** that must be corrected with a pacemaker, increased protein in the cerebrospinal fluid, and a progressively disabling lack of muscular coordination (cerebellar syndrome). Symptoms of the disease appear before age 15.

Some of the progressive external ophthalmoplegia syndromes are unusual in that inheritance is controlled by DNA in the mitochondria. The mitochondria are rod-shaped structures within a cell that convert food to usable energy. Most inherited diseases are passed on by DNA in the cell nucleus, the core that contains the hereditary material. Mitochondrial inheritance tends to be passed on by the mother. Other forms of progressive external ophthalmoplegia are not inherited but occur sporadically with no clear family history. It is not known why some forms are neurogenic and others are myopathic. In the forms inherited through mitochondrial DNA, it is not known which gene product is affected.

Internuclear ophthalmoplegia in multiple sclerosis is caused by damage to a bundle of fibers in the brainstem called the medial longitudinal fasciculus. In this syndrome, the eye on the same side as the damaged medial longitudinal fasciculus is unable to look outward (that is, the left eye cannot look left). The other eye exhibits jerking movements (**nystagmus**) when the patient tries to look left. Internuclear ophthalmoplegia may be seen rarely without multiple sclerosis in patients with certain types of **cancer** or with Chiari type II malformation.

Eye **movement disorders** and ophthalmoplegia can also be seen with **progressive supranuclear palsy**, thyroid disease, **diabetes mellitus**, brainstem tumors, migraine, basilar artery **stroke**, pituitary stroke, **myasthenia gravis**, **muscular dystrophy**, and the Fisher variant of **Guillain-Barré syndrome**. A tumor or aneurysm in the cavernous sinus, located behind the eyes, can cause painful ophthalmoplegia. Painful ophthalmoplegia can also be caused by an inflammatory process in the same area, called Tolosa-Hunt syndrome.

Diagnosis

The patient's medical and family history and the examination findings will usually help differentiate the various syndromes associated with ophthalmoplegia. In addition, each syndrome is associated with characteristic features, such as nystagmus or ptosis. All patients with progressive external ophthalmoplegia should have a muscle biopsy to look for ragged red fibers or changes suggesting muscular dystrophy. A sample should be sent for analysis of mitochondrial DNA. Electromyogram (EMG), measurement of electrical activity in the muscle, helps diagnose myopathy.

Computed tomography scan (CT scan) or **magnetic resonance imaging** (MRI) scans of the brain may be needed to rule out **brain tumor**, stroke, aneurysm, or multiple sclerosis. When multiple sclerosis is suspected, evoked potential testing of nerve response may also be helpful. Analysis of cerebrospinal fluid may show changes characteristic of multiple sclerosis or Kearns-Sayre syndrome. Other tests that may be helpful in Kearns-Sayre include electrocardiogram (measuring electrical activity of the heart muscles), retinal examination, and a hearing test (audiogram). For possible myasthenia gravis, the Tensilon (edrophonium) test should be done. Tests should also be done to measure activity of the cell-surface receptors for acetylcholine, a chemical that helps pass electrical impulses along nerve cells in the muscles. Thyroid disease and diabetes mellitus should be excluded by appropriate blood work.

Treatment

There are no specific cures for ocular myopathy or progressive external ophthalmoplegia. Vitamin E therapy has been used to treat Kearns-Sayre syndrome. Coenzyme Q (ubiquinone), a naturally occurring substance similar to vitamin K, is widely used to treat other forms of progressive external ophthalmoplegia, but the degree of success varies. Specific treatments are available for multiple sclerosis, myasthenia gravis, diabetes mellitus, and thyroid disease. Symptoms of ophthalmoplegia can be relieved by mechanical treatment. Surgical procedures can lift drooping eyelids or a patch over one eye can be used to relieve double vision. Because there is no blink response, a surgically lifted eyelid exposes the cornea of the eye so that it may become dry or be scratched. These complications must be avoided by using artificial tears and wearing eyepatches at night. In Kearns-Sayre syndrome, a pacemaker may be needed.

Prognosis

The prognosis of progressive external ophthalmoplegia depends on the associated neurological problems; in particular, whether there is severe limb weakness or cerebellar symptoms that may be mild or disabling. As with most chronic neurologic diseases, mortality increases with disability. Progressive external ophthalmoplegia itself is not a life-threatening condition. Kearns-Sayre syndrome is disabling, probably shortens the life span, and few if any patients have children. Overall life expectancy for multiple sclerosis patients is seven years less than normal; **death** rates are higher for women than for men.

Prevention

There is no way to prevent ophthalmoplegia.

Resources

ORGANIZATIONS

American Academy of Neurology. 1080 Montreal Ave., St. Paul, MN 55116. (612) 695-1940. < http:// www.aan. com >.

Laurie Barclay, MD

Ophthalmoscopic examination *see* **Eye examination**

Opiate withdrawal *see* **Withdrawal syndromes**

Opioid analgesics *see* **Analgesics, opioid**

Oppositional defiant disorder

Definition

Oppositional defiant disorder (ODD) is defined by the *Diagnostic and Statistical Manual of Mental Disorders*, fourth edition (DSM-IV), as a recurring pattern of negative, hostile, disobedient, and defiant behavior in a child or adolescent, lasting for at least six months without serious violation of the basic rights of others. The incidence of ODD in the American population varies somewhat according to the sample studied; DSM-IV gives the rate as between 2–16% while the American Academy of Child and Adolescent Psychiatry (AACAP) gives a figure of 5%–15%, and a researcher at a children's hospital gives a rate of 6–10%.

Description

In order to meet DSM-IV criteria for ODD, the behavior disturbances must cause clinically significant problems in social, school, or work functioning. The course of oppositional defiant disorder varies among patients. In males, the disorder is more common among those who had problem temperaments or high motor activity in the preschool years. During the school years, patients may have low self-esteem, changing moods, and a low frustration tolerance. Patients may swear and use alcohol, tobacco, or illicit drugs at an early age. There are frequent conflicts with parents, teachers, and peers.

Children with this disorder show their negative and defiant behaviors by being persistently stubborn and resisting directions. They may be unwilling to compromise, give in, or negotiate with adults. Patients may deliberately or persistently test limits, ignore orders, argue, and fail to accept blame for misdeeds. Hostility is directed at adults or peers and is shown by verbal aggression or deliberately annoying others.

Causes and symptoms

Oppositional defiant disorder is more common in boys than girls before **puberty**; the disorder typically begins by age eight. After puberty the male:female ratio is about 1:1. Although the specific causes of the disorder are unknown, parents who are overly concerned with power and control may cause an eruption to occur. Symptoms often appear at home, but over time may appear in other settings as well. Usually the disorder occurs gradually over months or years. Several theories about the causes of oppositional defiant disorder are being investigated. Oppositional defiant disorder may be related to:

- the child's temperament and the family's response to that temperament
- an inherited predisposition to the disorder in some families
- marital discord or violence between husband and wife
- frequent or multiple geographical moves
- a neurological cause, like a head injury
- a chemical imbalance in the brain (especially with the brain chemical serotonin)

Oppositional defiant disorder appears to be more common in families where at least one parent has a history of a mood disorder, **conduct disorder, attention deficit/hyperactivity disorder,** antisocial personality disorder, or a substance-related disorder. Additionally, some studies suggest that mothers with a depressive disorder are more likely to have children with oppositional behavior. However, it is unclear to what extent the mother's depression results from or causes oppositional behavior in children.

Symptoms include a pattern of negative, hostile, and defiant behavior lasting at least six months. During this time four or more specific behaviors must be present. These behaviors include the child who:

- often loses his/her temper
- often argues with adults
- often actively defies or refuses to comply with adults' requests or rules
- often deliberately annoys people
- often blames others for his/her mistakes or misbehavior
- is often touchy or easily annoyed by others
- is often angry and resentful
- is often spiteful or vindictive
- misbehaves
- swears or uses obscene language
- has a low opinion of him/herself

The diagnosis of oppositional defiant disorder is not made if the symptoms occur exclusively in psychotic or **mood disorders**. Criteria are not met for conduct disorder, and, if the child is 18 years old or older, criteria are not met for antisocial personality disorder. In other words, a child with oppositional defiant disorder does not show serious aggressive behaviors or exhibit the physical cruelty that is common in other disorders.

Additional problems may be present, including:

- learning problems
- a depressed mood
- hyperactivity (although attention deficit/hyperactivity disorder must be ruled out)
- substance **abuse** or dependence
- dramatic and erratic behavior

The patient with oppositional defiant disorder is moody, easily frustrated, and may abuse drugs.

Diagnosis

While psychological testing may be needed, the doctor must examine and talk with the child, talk with the parents, and review the medical history. Diagnosis is complicated because oppositional defiant disorder rarely travels alone. Children with attention/deficit hyperactive disorder will also have oppositional defiant disorder 50% of the time. Children with depression/anxiety will have oppositional defiant disorder 10–29% of the time. Because all of the features of this disorder are usually present in conduct disorder, oppositional defiant disorder is not diagnosed if the criteria are met for conduct disorder.

A diagnosis of oppositional defiant disorder should be considered only if the behaviors occur more frequently and have more serious consequences than is typically observed in other children of a similar developmental stage. Further, the behavior must lead to significant impairment in social, school, or work functioning.

As of 2004 a new evaluation scale known as the Oppositional Defiant Behavior Inventory (ODBI) has been developed as an aid to diagnosis. The ODBI appears to meet accepted standards of reliability and validity.

Treatment

Treatment of oppositional defiant disorder usually consists of group, individual and/or family therapy, and education. Of these, individual therapy is the most common. Therapy can provide a consistent daily schedule, support, consistent rules, discipline, and limits. It can also help train patients to get along with others and modify behaviors. Therapy can occur in residential, day treatment, or medical settings. Additionally, having a healthy role model as an example is important for the patient.

Parent management training focuses on teaching the parents specific and more effective techniques for handling the child's opposition and defiance. Research has shown that parent management training is more effective than **family therapy**. One variation of parent management training known as Parent-Child Interaction Therapy (PCIT) appears to be helpful over the long term; a group of Australian researchers reported in 2004 that families who were given a course of PCIT maintained their gains two years after the program ended.

As of the early 2000s, elementary school teachers are being trained to deal more effectively with classroom disruptions caused by children with ODD. The long-term effectiveness of these interventions, however, will require further study.

Whether involved in therapy or working on this disorder at home, the patient must work with his or her parents' guidance to make the fullest possible recovery. According to the New York Hospital/Cornell Medical Center, the patients must:

- use self timeouts
- identify what increases anxiety
- talk about feelings instead of acting on them
- find and use ways to calm themselves
- frequently remind themselves of their goals
- get involved in tasks and physical activities that provide a healthy outlet for energy
- learn how to talk with others
- develop a predictable, consistent, daily schedule of activity
- develop ways to obtain pleasure and feel good
- learn how to get along with other people
- find ways to limit stimulation
- learn to admit mistakes in a matter-of-fact way

Stimulant medication is used only when oppositional defiant disorder coexists with attention deficit/hyperactivity disorder. Currently, no research is currently available on the use of other psychiatric medications in the treatment of oppositional defiant disorder.

Prognosis

The outcome varies. In some children the disorder evolves into a conduct disorder or a mood disorder. Later in life, oppositional defiant disorder can develop into passive aggressive personality disorder or antisocial personality disorder. Some children respond well to treatment and some do not. Generally, with treatment, reasonable adjustment in social settings and in the workplace can be made in adulthood.

KEY TERMS

Attention deficit/hyperactivity disorder—A persistent pattern of inattention, hyperactivity and/or impulsiveness; the pattern is more frequent and severe than is typically observed in people at a similar level of development.

Conduct disorder—A repetitive and persistent pattern of behavior in which the basic rights of others are violated or major age-appropriate rules of society are broken.

Resources

BOOKS

American Psychiatric Association. *Diagnostic and Statistical Manual of Mental Disorders.* 4th ed., revised. Washington, D.C.: American Psychiatric Association, 2000.

PERIODICALS

Harada, Y., K. Saitoh, J. Iida, et al. "The Reliability and Validity of the Oppositional Defiant Behavior Inventory." *European Child and Adolescent Psychiatry* 13 (June 2004): 185–190.

Nixon, R. D., L. Sweeney, D. B. Erickson, and S. W. Touyz. "Parent-Child Interaction Therapy: One- and Two-Year Follow-Up of Standard and Abbreviated Treatments for Oppositional Preschoolers." *Journal of Abnormal Child Psychology* 32 (June 2004): 263–271.

Tynan, W. Douglas, PhD. "Oppositional Defiant Disorder." *eMedicine* November 2, 2003. < http://www.emedicine.com/ped/topic2791.htm >.

van Leer, P. A., B. O. Muthen, R. M. van der Sar, and A. A. Crijnen. "Preventing Disruptive Behavior in Elementary Schoolchildren: Impact of a Universal Classroom-Based Intervention." *Journal of Consulting and Clinical Psychology* 72 (June 2004): 467–478.

ORGANIZATIONS

American Academy of Child and Adolescent Psychiatry (AACAP). 3615 Wisconsin Avenue, NW, Washington, DC 20016-3007. (202) 966-7300. Fax: (202) 966-2891. < http://www.aacap.org >.

American Psychiatric Association. 1400 K Street, NW, Washington, DC 20005. < http://www.psych.org >.

Families Anonymous. Westchester County, Westchester, NY. (212) 354-8525.

OTHER

American Academy of Child and Adolescent Psychiatry (AACAP). *Children with Oppositional Defiant Disorder.* AACAP Facts for Families #72. Washington, DC: AACAP, 2000.

David James Doermann
Rebecca Frey, PhD

Optic atrophy

Definition

Optic atrophy can be defined as damage to the optic nerve resulting in a degeneration or destruction of the optic nerve. Optic atrophy may also be referred to as optic nerve head pallor because of the pale appearance of the optic nerve head as seen at the back of the eye. Possible causes of optic atrophy include:

optic neuritis, Leber's hereditary optic atrophy, toxic or nutritional optic neuropathy, **glaucoma**, vascular disorders, trauma, and other systemic disorders.

Description

The process of vision involves light entering the eye and triggering chemical changes in the retina, a pigmented layer lining the back of the eye. Nerve impulses created by this process travel to the brain via the optic nerve. Using a hand-held instrument called an ophthalmoscope, the doctor can see the optic nerve head (optic disc) which is the part of the optic nerve that enters at the back of the eyeball. In optic atrophy, the disc is pale and has fewer blood vessels than normal.

Causes and symptoms

Symptoms of optic atrophy are a change in the optic disc and a decrease in visual function. This change in visual function can be a decrease in sharpness and clarity of vision (visual acuity) or decreases in side (peripheral) vision. Color vision and contrast sensitivity can also be affected.

There are many possible causes of optic atrophy. The causes can range from trauma to systemic disorders. Some possible causes of optic atrophy include:

- Optic neuritis. Optic neuritis is an inflammation of the optic nerve. It may be associated with eye **pain** worsened by eye movement. It is more common in young to middle-aged women. Some patients with optic neuritis may develop **multiple sclerosis** later on in life.

- Leber's hereditary optic neuropathy. This is a disease of young men (late teens, early 20s), characterized by an onset over a few weeks of painless, severe, central visual loss in one eye, followed weeks or months later by the same process in the other eye. At first the optic disc may be slightly swollen, but eventually there is optic atrophy. The visual loss is generally permanent. This condition is hereditary. If a patient knows that Leber's runs in the family, **genetic counseling** should be considered.

- Toxic optic neuropathy. Nutritional deficiencies and poisons can be associated with gradual vision loss and optic atrophy, or with sudden vision loss and optic disc swelling. Toxic and nutritional optic neuropathies are uncommon in the United States, but took on epidemic proportions in Cuba in 1992–1993. The most common toxic optic neuropathy is known as tobacco-alcohol **amblyopia**, thought to be caused by exposure to cyanide from tobacco **smoking**, and by low levels of vitamin B_{12} because of poor **nutrition** and poor absorption associated with drinking alcohol.

Other possible toxins included ethambutol, methyl alcohol (moonshine), ethylene glycol (antifreeze), cyanide, lead, and carbon monoxide. Certain medications have also been implicated. Nutritional optic neuropathy may be caused by deficiencies of protein, or of the B **vitamins** and folate, associated with **starvation**, malabsorption, or **alcoholism**.

- Glaucoma. Glaucoma may be caused by an increase of pressure inside the eye. This increased pressure may eventually affect the optic nerve if left untreated.

- Compressive optic neuropathy. This is the result of a tumor or other lesion putting pressure on the optic nerve. Another possible cause is enlargement of muscles involved in eye movement seen in **hyperthyroidism** (Graves' disease).

- Retinitis pigmentosa. This is a hereditary ocular disorder.

- Syphilis. Left untreated, this disease may result in optic atrophy.

Diagnosis

Diagnosis involves recognizing the characteristic changes in the optic disc with an ophthalmoscope, and measuring visual acuity, usually with an eye chart. Visual field testing can test peripheral vision. Color vision and contrast sensitivity can also be tested. Family history is important in the diagnosis of inherited conditions. Exposure to poisons, drugs, and even medications should be determined. Suspected **poisoning** can be confirmed through blood and urine analysis, as can vitamin deficiency.

Brain **magnetic resonance imaging** (MRI) may show a tumor or other structure putting pressure on the optic nerve, or may show plaques characteristic of multiple sclerosis, which is frequently associated with optic neuritis. However, similar MRI lesions may appear in Leber's hereditary optic neuropathy. Mitochondrial DNA testing can be done on a blood sample, and can identify the mutation responsible for Leber's.

Visual evoked potentials (VEP), which measure speed of conduction over the nerve pathways involved in sight, may detect abnormalities in the clinically unaffected eye in early cases of Leber's. Fluorescein **angiography** gives more detail about blood vessels in the retina.

Treatment

Treatment of optic neuritis with steroids is controversial. As of mid-1998, there is no known treatment for Leber's hereditary optic neuropathy.

KEY TERMS

Atrophy—A destruction or dying of cells, tissues, or organs.

Cerebellar—Involving the part of the brain (cerebellum), which controls walking, balance, and coordination.

Mitochondia—A structure in the cell responsible for producing energy. A defect in the DNA in the mitochondria is involved in Leber's optic neuropathy.

Neuritis—An inflammation of the nerves.

Neuropathy—A disturbance of the nerves, not caused by an inflammation. For example, the cause may be toxins, or unknown.

Treatment of other causes of optic atrophy varies depending upon the underlying disease.

Prognosis

Many patients with optic neuritis eventually develop multiple sclerosis. Most patients have a gradual recovery of vision after a single episode of optic neuritis, even without treatment. Prognosis for visual improvement in Leber's hereditary optic neuropathy is poor, with the specific rate highly dependent on which mitochondrial DNA mutation is present. If the cause of toxic or nutritional deficiency optic neuropathy can be found and treated early, such as stopping smoking and taking vitamins in tobacco-alcohol amblyopia, vision generally returns to near normal over several months' time. However, visual loss is often permanent in cases of long-standing toxic or nutritional deficiency optic neuropathy.

Prevention

People noticing a decrease in vision (central and/or side vision) should ask their eye care practitioner for a check up. Patients should also go for regular vision exams. Patients should ask their doctor how often that should be, as certain conditons may warrant more frequent exams. Early detection of inflammations or other problems lessens the chance of developing optic atrophy.

As of mid 1998, there are no preventive measures that can definitely abort Leber's hereditary optic neuropathy in those genetically at risk, or in those at risk based on earlier involvement of one eye. However, some doctors recommend that their patients take vitamin C, vitamin E, coenzyme Q_{10}, or other anti-oxidants, and that they avoid the use of tobacco or alcohol. Patients should ask their doctors about the use of vitamins. Avoiding toxin exposure and nutritional deficiency should prevent toxic or nutritional deficiency optic neuropathy.

Resources

ORGANIZATIONS

American Academy of Neurology. 1080 Montreal Ave., St. Paul, MN 55116. (612) 695-1940. < http://www.aan .com > .

Prevent Blindness America. 500 East Remington Road, Schaumburg, IL 60173. (800) 331-2020. < http://www .preventblindness.org > .

Laurie Barclay, MD

Optic neuritis

Definition

Optic neuritis is a vision disorder characterized by inflammation of the optic nerve.

Description

Optic neuritis occurs when the optic nerve, the pathway that transmits visual information to the brain, becomes inflamed and the myelin sheath that surrounds the nerve is destroyed (a process known as demyelination). It typically occurs in one eye at a time (70%), and the resulting vision loss is rapid and progressive, but only temporary. Thirty percent of patients experience occurrence in both eyes. Optic neuritis tends to afflict young adults with an average age in their 30s. Seventy-five percent of patients with optic neuritis are women.

Nerve damage that occurs in the section of the optic nerve located behind the eyeball, is called *retrobulbar neuritis*, and is most often associated with multiple sclerosis. Optic nerve inflammation and **edema** (swelling) caused by intracranial pressure at the place where the nerve enters the eyeball is termed *papillitis*.

Causes and symptoms

Symptoms of optic neuritis include one or more of the following:

- blurred or dimmed vision
- blind spots, particularly with central vision
- pain with eye movement
- headache
- sudden color blindness
- impaired night vision
- impaired contrast sensitivity

Optic neuritis is most commonly associated with **multiple sclerosis** (MS). Other causes include viral or fungal infections, encephalomyelitis, autoimmune diseases, or pressure on the nerve from tumors or vascular diseases (i.e., temporal arteritis). Some toxins, such as methanol and lead, can also damage the optic nerve, as can long-term abuse of alcohol and tobacco. Patients with non-MS related optic neuritis are usually immunocompromised in some way.

Diagnosis

An ophthalmologist, a physician trained in diseases of the eye, will typically make a diagnosis of optic neuritis. A complete visual exam, including a visual acuity test, color vision test, and examination of the retina and optic disc with an ophthalmoscope, will be performed. Clinical signs such as impaired pupil response may be apparent during an eye exam, but in some cases the eye may appear normal. A medical history will also be performed to determine if exposure to toxins such as lead may have caused the optic neuritis.

Further diagnostic testing such as **magnetic resonance imaging** (MRI) may be necessary to confirm a diagnosis of optic neuritis. An MRI can also reveal signs of multiple sclerosis.

Treatment

Treatment of optic neuritis depends on the underlying cause of the condition. Vision loss resulting from a viral condition usually resolves itself once the virus is treated, and optic neuritis resulting from toxin damage may improve once the source of the toxin is removed.

A course of intravenous **corticosteroids** (steroids) followed by oral steroids has been found to be helpful in restoring vision quickly to patients with MS-related episodes of optic neuritis, but its efficacy in preventing relapse is debatable. The Optic Neuritis Treatment Trial (ONTT) has shown that IV steroids may be effective in reducing the onset of MS for up to two years, but further studies are necessary. Oral prednisone has been found to increase the likelihood of

KEY TERMS

Atrophy—Cell wasting or death.

Multiple sclerosis—An autoimmune disease of the central nervous system characterized by damage to the myelin sheath that covers nerves.

Temporal arteritis—Also known as giant cell arteritis. Inflammation of the large arteries located in the temples which is marked by the presence of giant cells and symptoms of headache and facial pain.

Visual acuity test—An eye examination that determines sharpness of vision, typically performed by identifying objects and/or letters on an eye chart.

recurrent episodes of optic neuritis, and is not recommended for treating the disorder.

Prognosis

The vision loss associated with optic neuritis is usually temporary. Spontaneous remission occurs in two to eight weeks. Sixty-five to eighty percent of patients can expect 20/30 or better vision after recovery. Long-term prognosis depends on the underlying cause of the condition. If a viral infection has triggered the episode, it frequently resolves itself with no after effects. If optic neuritis is associated with multiple sclerosis, future episodes are not uncommon. Thirty-three percent of optic neuritis cases recur within five years. Each recurrence results in less recovery and worsening vision. There is a strong association between optic neuritis and MS. In those without multiple sclerosis, half who experience an episode of vision loss related to optic neuritis will develop the disease within 15 years.

Prevention

Regular annual eye exams are critical to maintaining healthy vision. Early treatment of vision problems can prevent permanent optic nerve damage (atrophy).

Resources

BOOKS

Leitman, Mark. *Manual for Eye Examination and Diagnosis.* 5th ed. Boston: Blackwell Science, 2001.

PERIODICALS

Cohen, Joyce Render, et al. "Living with Low Vision." *Inside MS* 1 (2001): 46.

ORGANIZATIONS

Prevent Blindness America. 500 East Remington Road, Schaumburg, IL 60173. (800) 331-2020. < http://www .prevent-blindness.org >.

Paula Anne Ford-Martin

Oral cancer *see* **Head and neck cancer**

Oral cholecystography *see* **Gallbladder x rays**

Oral contraceptives

Definition

Oral contraceptives are medicines taken by mouth to help prevent **pregnancy**. They are also known as the Pill, OCs, or birth control pills.

Purpose

Oral contraceptives, also known as birth control pills, contain artificially made forms of two hormones produced naturally in the body. These hormones, estrogen and progestin, regulate a woman's menstrual cycle. When taken in the proper amounts, following a specific schedule, oral contraceptives are very effective in preventing pregnancy. Studies show that less than one of every one hundred women who use oral contraceptives correctly becomes pregnant during the first year of use.

These pills have several effects that help prevent pregnancy. For pregnancy to occur, an egg must become mature inside a woman's ovary, be released, and travel to the fallopian tube. A male sperm must also reach the fallopian tube, where it fertilizes the egg. Then the fertilized egg must travel to the woman's uterus (womb), where it lodges in the uterus lining and develops into a fetus. The main way that oral contraceptives prevent pregnancy is by keeping an egg from ripening fully. Eggs that do not ripen fully cannot be fertilized. In addition, birth control pills thicken mucus in the woman's body through which the sperm has to swim. This makes it more difficult for the sperm to reach the egg. Oral contraceptives also change the uterine lining so that a fertilized egg cannot lodge there to develop.

Birth control pills may cause good or bad side effects. For example, a woman's menstrual periods are regular and usually lighter when she is taking oral contraceptives, and the pills may reduce the risk of **ovarian cysts**, breast lumps, **pelvic inflammatory disease**, and other medical problems. However, taking birth control pills increases the risk of **heart attack**, **stroke**, and **blood clots** in certain women. Serious side effects such as these are more likely in women over 35 years of age who smoke cigarettes and in those with specific health problems such as high blood pressure, diabetes, or a history of breast or uterine **cancer**. A woman who wants to use oral contraceptives should ask her physician for the latest information on the risks and benefits of all types of birth control and should consider her age, health, and medical history when deciding what to use.

Precautions

No form of birth control (except not having sex) is 100% effective. However, oral contraceptives can be highly effective when used properly. Discuss the options with a health care professional.

Oral contraceptives do not protect against **AIDS** or other sexually transmitted diseases. For protection against such diseases, use a latex **condom**.

Oral contraceptives are not effective immediately after a woman begins taking them. Physicians recommend using other forms of birth control for the first 1–3 weeks. Follow the instructions of the physician who prescribed the medicine.

Smoking cigarettes while taking oral contraceptives greatly increases the risk of serious side effects. *Women who take oral contraceptives should not smoke cigarettes.*

Seeing a physician regularly while taking this medicine is very important. The physician will note unwanted side effects. Follow his or her advice on how often you should be seen.

Anyone taking oral contraceptives should be sure to tell the health care professional in charge before having any surgical or dental procedures, laboratory tests, or emergency treatment.

This medicine may increase sensitivity to sunlight. Women using oral contraceptives should avoid too much sun exposure and should not use tanning beds, tanning booths, or sunlamps until they know how the medicine affects them. Some women taking oral contraceptives may get brown splotches on exposed areas of their skin. These usually go away over time after the women stop taking birth control pills.

Oral contraceptives may cause the gums to become tender and swollen or to bleed. Careful brushing and flossing, gum massage, and regular cleaning may help prevent this problem. Check with a physician or dentist if gum problems develop.

Women who have certain medical conditions or who are taking certain other medicines may have problems if they take oral contraceptives. Before taking these drugs, be sure to let the physician know about any of these conditions:

ALLERGIES. Anyone who has had unusual reactions to estrogens or progestins in the past should let her physician know before taking oral contraceptives. The physician should also be told about any allergies to foods, dyes, preservatives, or other substances.

PREGNANCY. Women who become pregnant or think they may have become pregnant while taking birth control pills should stop taking them immediately and check with their physicians. Women who want to start taking oral contraceptives again after pregnancy should not refill their old prescriptions without checking with their physicians. The physician may need to change the prescription.

BREASTFEEDING. Women who are breastfeeding should check with their physicians before using oral contraceptives. The hormones in the pills may reduce the amount of breast milk and may cause other problems in breastfeeding. They may also cause **jaundice** and enlarged breasts in nursing babies whose mothers take the medicine.

OTHER MEDICAL CONDITIONS. Oral contraceptives may improve or worsen some medical conditions. The possibility that they may make a condition worse does not necessarily mean they cannot be used. In some cases, women may need only to be tested or followed more closely for medical problems while using oral contraceptives. Before using oral contraceptives, women with any of these medical problems should make sure their physicians are aware of their conditions:

- Female conditions such as menstrual problems, **endometriosis**, or fibroid tumors of the uterus. Birth control pills usually make these problems better, but may sometimes make them worse or more difficult to diagnose.

- Heart or circulation problems; recent or past blood clots or stroke. Women who already have these problems may be at greater risk of developing blood clots or circulation problems if they use oral contraceptives. However, healthy women who do not smoke may lower their risk of circulation problems and heart disease by taking the pills.

- Breast cysts, lumps, or other noncancerous breast problems. Oral contraceptives generally protect against these conditions, but physicians may recommend more frequent breast exams for women taking the pills.

- **Breast cancer** or other cancer (now or in the past, or family history). Oral contraceptives may make some existing cancers worse. Women with a family history of breast cancer may need more frequent screening for the disease if they decide to take birth control pills.

- Migraine headaches. This condition may improve or may get worse with the use of birth control pills.

- Diabetes. Blood sugar levels may increase slightly when oral contraceptives are used. Usually this increase is not enough to affect the amount of diabetes medicine needed. However, blood sugar will need to be monitored closely while taking oral contraceptives.

- Depression. This condition may worsen in women who already have it or may (rarely) occur again in women who were depressed in the past.

- Gallbladder disease, **gallstones**, high blood cholesterol, or chorea gravidarum (a nervous disorder). Oral contraceptives may make these conditions worse.

- Epilepsy, high blood pressure, heart or circulation problems. By increasing fluid build-up, oral contraceptives may make these conditions worse.

Description

Oral contraceptives (birth control pills) come in a wide range of estrogen-progestin combinations. The pills in use today contain much lower doses of estrogen than those available in the past, and this change has reduced the likelihood of serious side effects. Some pills contain only progestin. These are prescribed mainly for women who need to avoid estrogens and may not be as effective in preventing pregnancy as the estrogen-progestin combinations.

These medicines come in tablet form, in containers designed to help women keep track of which tablet to take each day. The tablets are different colors, indicating amounts of hormones they contain. Some may contain no hormones at all. These are included simply to help women stay in the habit of taking a pill every day, as the hormone combination needs to be taken only on certain days of the menstrual cycle. Keeping the tablets in their original container and taking them exactly on schedule is very important. They will not be as effective if they are taken in the wrong order or if doses are missed.

Oral contraceptives are available only with a physician's prescription. Some commonly used brands are Demulen, Desogen, Loestrin, Lo/Ovral, Nordette, Ortho-Novum, Ortho-Tri-Cyclen, Estrostep, Orthocept, Alesse, Levlite and Ovcon.

The dose schedule depends on the type of oral contraceptive. The two basic schedules are a 21-day schedule and a 28-day schedule. On the 21-day schedule, take one tablet a day for 21 days, then skip 7 days and repeat the cycle. On the 28-day schedule, take one tablet a day for 28 days; then repeat the cycle. Be sure to carefully follow the instructions provided with the medicine. For additional information or explanations, check with the physician who prescribed the medicine or the pharmacist who filled the prescription.

Taking doses more than 24 hours apart may increase the chance of side effects or pregnancy. Try to take the medicine at the same time every day. Take care not to run out of pills. If possible, keep an extra month's supply on hand and replace it every month with the most recently filled prescription.

Try not to miss a dose, as this increases the risk of pregnancy. If a dose is missed, follow the package directions or check with the physician who prescribed the medicine for instructions. It may be necessary to use another form of birth control for some time after missing a dose.

Taking this medicine with food or at bedtime will help prevent **nausea**, a side effect that sometimes occurs during the first few weeks. This side effect usually goes away as the body adjusts to the medicine.

Taking oral contraceptives may have several benefits outside of their ability to prevent pregnancy. Research indicates that with 10 to 12 years of oral contraceptive use, a woman's risk of ovarian cancer is reduced by up to 80 %. There may also be an approximate 50% decrease in the rate of endometrial cancers in women. One other well-known, noncontraceptive benefit of oral contraceptives is an improvement in **acne**. The combination oral contraceptive ethinyl estradiol/norgestimate has been approved by the Food and Drug Administration for the treatment of acne. Another positive effect of oral contraceptive use is improvement in abnormal uterine bleeding. Older women may also benefit from using oral contraceptives, because the pills can increase bone mass as women enter their menopausal years, when **osteoporosis** is a growing concern.

Oral contraceptives may also be used on an emergency basis as a means of preventing pregnancy in women who have had unprotected intercourse. Two products specifically designed for this purpose are Preven and Plan B. In 2001, the American College of Obstetricians and Gynecologists (ACOG) recommended that emergency oral contraceptives be available as an over-the-counter medicine. The Food and

Drug Administration, however, has not yet approved any measures that would allow this to happen.

Risks

Taking oral contraceptives with certain other drugs may affect the way the drugs work or may increase the chance of side effects.

Side Effects

Serious side effects are rare in healthy women who do not smoke cigarettes. In women with certain health problems, however, oral contraceptives may cause problems such as **liver cancer**, noncancerous liver tumors, blood clots, or stroke. Health care professionals can help women weigh the benefits of being protected against unwanted pregnancy against the risks of possible health problems.

The most common minor side effects are nausea; **vomiting**; abdominal cramping or bloating; breast **pain**, tenderness or swelling; swollen ankles or feet; tiredness; and acne. These problems usually go away as the body adjusts to the drug and do not need medical attention unless they continue or they interfere with normal activities.

Other side effects should be brought to the attention of the physician who prescribed the medicine. Check with the physician as soon as possible if any of the following side effects occur:

- menstrual changes, such as lighter periods or missed periods, longer periods, or bleeding or spotting between periods
- headaches
- vaginal infection, **itching**, or irritation
- increased blood pressure

Women who have any of the following symptoms should get emergency help right away. These symptoms may be signs of blood clots:

- sudden changes in vision, speech, breathing, or coordination
- severe or sudden **headache**
- coughing up blood
- sudden, severe, or continuing pain in the abdomen or stomach
- pain in the chest, groin, or leg (especially in the calf)
- weakness, **numbness**, or pain in an arm or leg

Oral contraceptives may continue to affect the menstrual cycle for some time after a woman stops taking them. Women who miss periods for several months after stopping this medicine should check with their physicians.

Other rare side effects may occur. Anyone who has unusual symptoms while taking oral contraceptives should get in touch with her physician.

Interactions

Oral contraceptives may interact with a number of other medicines. When this happens, the effects of one or both of the drugs may change or the risk of side effects may be greater. Anyone who takes oral contraceptives should let the physician know all other medicines she is taking and should ask whether the possible interactions can interfere with drug therapy.

These drugs may make oral contraceptives less effective in preventing pregnancy. Anyone who takes these drugs should use an additional birth control method for the entire cycle in which the medicine is used:

- ampicillin
- penicillin V
- rifampin (Rifadin)
- tetracyclines
- griseofulvin (Gris-PEG, Fulvicin)
- corticosteroids
- barbiturates
- carbamazepine (Tegretol)
- phenytoin (Dilantin)
- primidone (Mysoline)
- ritonavir (Norvir)

In addition, taking these medicines with oral contraceptives may increase the risk of side effects or interfere with the medicine's effects:

- theophylline–effects of this medicine may increase, along with the chance of unwanted side effects
- cyclosporine–effects of this medicine may increase, along with the chance of unwanted side effects
- troleandomycin (TAO)–chance of liver problems may increase. Effectiveness of oral contraceptive may also decrease, raising the risk of pregnancy

The list above does not include every drug that may interact with oral contraceptives. Be sure to check with a physician or pharmacist before combining oral contraceptives with any other prescription or nonprescription (over-the-counter) medicine.

As with any medication, the benefits and risks should be discussed with a physician.

KEY TERMS

Cyst—An abnormal sac or enclosed cavity in the body, filled with liquid or partially solid material.

Endometriosis—A condition in which tissue like that normally found in the lining of the uterus is present outside the uterus. The condition often causes pain and bleeding.

Fallopian tube—One of a pair of slender tubes that extend from each ovary to the uterus. Eggs pass through the fallopian tubes to reach the uterus.

Fetus—A developing baby inside the womb.

Fibroid tumor—A noncancerous tumor formed of fibrous tissue.

Hormone—A substance that is produced in one part of the body, then travels through the bloodstream to another part of the body where it has its effect.

Jaundice—Yellowing of the eyes and skin due to the build up of a bile pigment (bilirubin) in the blood.

Migraine—A throbbing headache that usually affects only one side of the head. Nausea, vomiting, increased sensitivity to light, and other symptoms often accompany migraine.

Mucus—Thick fluid produced by the moist membranes that line many body cavities and structures.

Ovary—A reproductive organ in females that produces eggs and hormones.

Pelvic inflammatory disease—Inflammation of the female reproductive tract, caused by any of several microorganisms. Symptoms include severe abdominal pain, high fever, and vaginal discharge. Severe cases can result in sterility. Also called PID.

Uterus—A hollow organ in a female in which a fetus develops until birth.

Resources

BOOKS

Beers, Mark H., and Robert Berkow, editors. *The Merck Manual of Diagnosis and Therapy.* 17th ed. Whitehouse Station, NJ: Merck and Company, Inc., 1999.

PERIODICALS

"Current Perspectives on OC Formulations." *Family Practice News* January 15, 2001: 2.

"Physician Group Supports Safety, Availability of Over-the-Counter Emergency Option." *Medical Letter on the CDC and FDA* March 18, 2001.

OTHER

Medline Plus Health Information, U.S. National Library of Medicine. < http://www.nlm.nih.gov/medlineplus >.

Deanna M. Swartout-Corbeil, R.N.

Oral herpes *see* **Cold sore**

Oral hygiene

Definition

Oral hygiene is the practice of keeping the mouth clean and healthy by brushing and flossing to prevent **tooth decay** and gum disease.

Purpose

The purpose of oral hygiene is to prevent the build-up of plaque, the sticky film of bacteria and food that forms on the teeth. Plaque adheres to the crevices and fissures of the teeth and generates acids that, when not removed on a regular basis, slowly eat away, or decay, the protective enamel surface of the teeth, causing holes (cavities) to form. Plaque also irritates gums and can lead to gum disease (**periodontal disease**) and tooth loss. Toothbrushing and flossing remove plaque from teeth, and antiseptic mouthwashes kill some of the bacteria that help form plaque. Fluoride—in toothpaste, drinking water, or dental treatments—also helps to protect teeth by binding with enamel to make it stronger. In addition to such daily oral care, regular visits to the dentist promote oral health. Preventative services that he or she can perform include fluoride treatments, sealant application, and scaling (scraping off the hardened plaque, called tartar). The dentist can also perform such diagnostic services as x-ray imaging and oral **cancer** screening as well as such treatment services as fillings, crowns, and bridges.

Precautions

Maintaining oral hygiene should be a lifelong habit. An infant's gums and, later, teeth should be kept clean by wiping them with a moist cloth or a soft toothbrush. However, only a very small amount (the size of a pea) of toothpaste containing fluoride should be used since too much fluoride may be toxic to infants.

An adult who has partial or full dentures should also maintain good oral hygiene. Bridges and dentures must be kept clean to prevent gum disease. Dentures should be relined and adjusted by a dentist as necessary to maintain proper fit so the gums do not become red, swollen, and tender.

Brushing and flossing should be performed thoroughly but not too vigorously. Rough mechanical action may irritate or damage sensitive oral tissues. Sore or bleeding gums may be experienced for the first few days after flossing is begun. However, bleeding continuing beyond one week should be brought to the attention of a dentist. As a general rule, any sore or abnormal condition that does not disappear after 10 days should be examined by a dentist.

Description

Brushing

Brushing should be performed with a toothbrush and a fluoride toothpaste at least twice a day and preferably after every meal and snack. Effective brushing must clean each outer tooth surface, inner tooth surface, and the flat chewing surfaces of the back teeth. To clean the outer and inner surfaces, the toothbrush should be held at a 45-degree angle against the gums and moved back and forth in short strokes (no more than one toothwidth distance). To clean the inside surfaces of the front teeth, the toothbrush should be held vertically and the bristles at the tip (called the toe of the brush) moved gently up and down against each tooth. To clean the chewing surfaces of the large back teeth, the brush should be held flat and moved back and forth. Finally, the tongue should also be brushed using a back-to-front sweeping motion to remove food particles and bacteria that may sour the breath.

Toothbrushes wear out and should be replaced every three months. Consumers should look for toothbrushes with soft, nylon, rounded bristles in a size and shape that allows them to reach all tooth surfaces easily.

Holding a toothbrush may be difficult for people with limited use of their hands. The toothbrush handle may be modified by inserting it into a rubber ball for easier gripping.

Flossing

Flossing once a day helps prevent gum disease by removing food particles and plaque at and below the gumline as well as between teeth. To begin, most of an 18-in (45-cm) strand of floss is wrapped around the third finger of one hand. A 1-in (2.5-cm) section is then grasped firmly between the thumb and forefinger of each hand. The floss is eased between two teeth and worked gently up and down several times with a rubbing motion. At the gumline, the floss is curved first around one tooth and then the other with gentle sliding into the space between the tooth and gum. After each tooth contact is cleaned, a fresh section of floss is unwrapped from one hand as the used section of floss is wrapped around the third finger of the opposite hand. Flossing proceeds between all teeth and behind the last teeth. Flossing should also be performed around the abutment (support) teeth of a bridge and under any artificial teeth using a device called a floss threader.

Dental floss comes in many varieties (waxed, unwaxed, flavored, tape) and may be chosen on personal preference. For people who have difficulty handling floss, floss holders and other types of interdental (between the teeth) cleaning aids, such as brushes and picks, are available.

Risks

Negative consequences arise from improper or infrequent brushing and flossing. The five major oral health problems are plaque, tartar, gingivitis, periodontitis, and tooth decay.

Plaque is a soft, sticky, colorless bacterial film that grows on the hard, rough surfaces of teeth. These bacteria use the sugar and starch from food particles in the mouth to produce acid. Left to accumulate, this acid destroys the outer enamel of the tooth, irritates the gums to the point of bleeding, and produces foul breath. Plaque starts forming again on teeth four to 12 hours after brushing, so brushing a minimum of twice a day is necessary for adequate oral hygiene.

When plaque is not regularly removed by brushing and flossing, it hardens into a yellow or brown mineral deposit called tartar or calculus. This formation is crusty and provides additional rough surfaces for the growth of plaque. When tartar forms below the gumline, it can lead to periodontal (gum) disease.

Gingivitis is an early form of periodontal disease, characterized by inflammation of the gums with painless bleeding during brushing and flossing. This common condition is reversible with proper dental care but if left untreated, it will progress into a more serious periodontal disease, periodontitis.

Periodontitis is a gum disease that destroys the structures supporting the teeth, including bone. Without support, the teeth will loosen and may fall out or have to be removed. To diagnose periodontitis, a dentist looks for gums that are red, swollen, bleeding, and shrinking away from the teeth, leaving widening spaces between teeth and exposed root surfaces vulnerable to decay.

Tooth decay, also called dental caries or cavities, is a common dental problem that results when the acid produced by plaque bacteria destroys the outer surface of a tooth. A dentist will remove the decay and fill the cavity with an appropriate dental material to restore and protect the tooth; left untreated, the decay will expand, destroying the entire tooth and causing significant pain.

Normal results

With proper brushing and flossing, oral hygiene may be maintained and oral health problems may be avoided. Older adults may no longer assume that they will lose all of their teeth in their lifetime. Regular oral care preserves speech and eating functions, thus prolonging the quality of life.

Resources

ORGANIZATIONS

American Dental Association. 211 E. Chicago Ave., Chicago, IL 60611. (312) 440-2500. < http://www.ada.org >.

American Dental Hygienists' Association. 444 North Michigan Ave., Chicago, IL 60611. (800) 847-6718.

OTHER

Healthtouch Online Page. < http://www.healthtouch.com >.

Bethany Thivierge

Oral hypoglycemics *see* **Antidiabetic drugs**

Orbital and periorbital cellulitis

Definition

Periorbital **cellulitis** is an inflammation and infection of the eyelid and the skin surrounding the eye. Orbital cellulitis affects the eye socket (orbit) as well as the skin closest to it.

Description

Inside the eyelid is a septum. The septum divides the eyelid into outer and inner areas. This orbital septum helps prevent the spread of infection to the eye socket. Periorbital and orbital cellulitis are more common in children than in adults. Periorbital cellulitis, which accounts for 85–90% of all ocular cellulitis, usually occurs in children under the age of five. Responsible for the remaining 10–15% of these infections, orbital cellulitis is most common in children over the age of five.

These conditions usually begin with swelling or inflammation of one eye. Infection spreads rapidly and can cause serious problems that affect the eye or the whole body.

Causes and symptoms

Orbital and periorbital cellulitis are usually caused by infection of the sinuses near the nose. Insect bites or injuries that break the skin cause about one-third of these cellulitis infections. Orbital and periorbital cellulitis may also occur in people with a history of dental infections.

The blood of about 33 of every 100 patients with orbital or periorbital cellulitis contains bacteria known to cause:

- acute ear infections
- inflammation of the epiglottis (the cartilage flap that covers the opening of the windpipe during swallowing)
- **meningitis** (inflammation of the membranes that enclose and protect the brain)
- pneumonia
- sinus infection.

People with periorbital cellulitis will have swollen, painful lids and redness, but probably no **fever**. About one child in five has a runny nose, and 20% have conjunctivitis. **Conjunctivitis**, also called pinkeye, is an inflammation of the mucous membrane that lines the eyelid and covers the front white part of the eye. It can be caused by allergy, irritation, or bacterial or viral infection.

As well as a swollen lid, other symptoms of orbital cellulitis include:

- bulging or displacement of the eyeball (proptosis)
- Chemosis (swelling of the mucous membrane of the eyeball and eyelid as a result of infection, injury, or systemic disorders like anemia or **kidney disease**)
- diminished ability to see clearly
- eye **pain**
- fever
- paralysis of nerves that control eye movements (**ophthalmoplegia**)

Diagnosis

An eye doctor may use special instruments to open a swollen lid in order to:

- examine the position of the eyeball
- evaluate eye movement
- test the patient's vision.

If the source of infection is not apparent, the position of the eyeball may suggest its location. **Computed tomography scans** (CT scans) can indicate which sinuses and bones are involved or whether abscesses have developed.

Treatment

A child who has orbital or periorbital cellulitis should be hospitalized without delay. Antibiotics are used to stop the spread of infection and prevent damage to the optic nerve, which transmits visual images to the brain.

Symptoms of optic-nerve damage or infection that has spread to sinus cavities close to the brain include:

- very limited ability to move the eye
- impaired response of the pupil to light and other stimulus
- loss of visual acuity
- papilledema (swelling of the optic disk—where the optic nerve enters the eye)

One or both eyes may be affected, and eye sockets or sinus cavities may have to be drained. These surgical procedures should be performed by an ophthalmologist or otolaryngologist.

Prognosis

If diagnosed promptly and treated with **antibiotics**, most orbital and periorbital cellulitis can be cured. These conditions are serious and need prompt treatment.

Infections that spread beyond the eye socket can cause:

- abscesses in the brain or in the protective membranes that enclose it
- bacterial meningitis
- blood clots
- vision loss

Resources

ORGANIZATIONS

American Academy of Ophthalmology. 655 Beach Street, P.O. Box 7424, San Francisco, CA 94120-7424. < http://www.eyenet.org >.
American Optometric Association. 243 North Lindbergh Blvd., St. Louis, MO 63141. (314) 991-4100. < http://www.aoanet.org >.

Maureen Haggerty

Orchiectomy *see* **Testicular surgery**

Orchiopexy *see* **Testicular surgery**

Orchitis

Definition

Orchitis is an inflammation of the testis, accompanied by swelling, **pain**, **fever**, and a sensation of heaviness in the affected area.

Description

Viral **mumps** is the most common cause of orchitis. Bacterial infections associated with the disorder are **tuberculosis**, **syphilis**, **gonorrhea**, and chlamydia. A mechanical injury to the groin area may also cause orchitis. Fifteen to twenty-five percent of males past the age of **puberty** with mumps develop orchitis. Epididymo-orchitis (inflammation of both testes and part of the spermatic duct) is the most common bacterial type of Orchitis. This form of the condition occurs most often in sexually active males fifteen years and older, and in men over 45 with enlarged prostates.

Causes and symptoms

The people most susceptible to orchitis are those with inadequate mumps inoculation and, in the case of sexually transmitted orchitis, those who practice unsafe sex or have a history of sexually transmitted disease. Inadequate protection of the groin area during contact sports or other potentially harmful physical activities may result in injury leading to orchitis. Symptoms of orchitis include swelling of one or both testicles, tenderness in the groin area, fever, **headache**, and **nausea**. Symptoms may also include bloody discharge from the penis, and pain during urination, intercourse, or ejaculation.

Diagnosis

In most cases, Orchitis can be diagnosed by an urologist, general practitioner, or emergency room physician. Diagnosis is usually based on the results of a **physical examination** and patient history. Other testing may include a **urinalysis** and **urine culture**, screening for chlamydia and gonorrhea, ultrasound imaging, or blood tests.

Treatment

Elevation and support of the scrotum, and the application of cold packs to the groin area give some relief from the pain of orchitis. Medication for pain such as codeine and meperidine may be given. Only the symptoms of viral mumps orchitis are treated. **Antibiotics** are used to alleviate orchitis that is bacterial in origin. Sexually transmitted orchitis (especially when resultant from chlamydia or gonorrhea) is often treated with the antibiotic Ceftriaxone in conjunction with azithromycin or doxycycline.

Alternative treatment

For relief from swelling, the drinking of dandelion tea is recommended in **traditional Chinese medicine** (TCM). Another traditional Chinese treatment for swelling is the application of a poultice of ground dandelion and aloe to the affected area. Homeopathic remedies to reduce swelling include apis mel, belladonna, and pulsatilla. Consult a homeopathic physician before taking or administering these remedies to ensure safe and correct dosage.

Prognosis

Orchitis is usually unilateral and lasts between one and two weeks. Atrophy of the scrotum occurs in 60% of orchitis cases. However, hormonal function is not affected and resulting sterility is rare from mumps.

KEY TERMS

Atrophy—A wasting away or withering.

Epididymo-orchitis—Inflammation of both the testes and a part of the spermatic duct system.

Unilateral—Affecting only one side.

Prevention

Keeping mumps inoculations current and diligently practicing safe sex are the best ways to prevent orchitis from occurring. For males involved in contact sports or other potentially harmful physical activities, the wearing of a protective cup over the genitals will help guard against mechanical injuries that could lead to orchitis.

Resources

PERIODICALS

Rodriguez, Rod. "Acute Scrotum Due to Epididymo-Orchitis in Male Children." *Impotence & Male Health Weekly Plus* February 1999.

OTHER

Mycyck, Mark, MD. "Orchitis from Emergency Medicine/ Genitourinary." *Emedicine, Instant Access to the Minds of Medicine.* February 2001. < http://www.emedicine. com/emerg/topic344.htm >.

Mary Jane Tenerelli, MS

Organophosphates *see* **Insecticide poisoning**

Oriental sore *see* **Leishmaniasis**

Ornithosis *see* **Parrot fever**

Oroya fever *see* **Bartonellosis**

Orthopedic surgery

Definition

Orthopedic (sometimes spelled orthopaedic) surgery is surgery performed by a medical specialist, such as an orthopedist or orthopedic surgeon, trained to deal with problems that develop in the bones, joints, and ligaments of the human body.

Purpose

Orthopedic surgery corrects problems that arise in the skeleton and its attachments, the ligaments and tendons. It may also deal with some problems of the nervous system, such as those that arise from injury of the spine. These problems can occur at birth, through injury, or as the result of **aging**. They may be acute, as in injury, or chronic, as in many aging-related problems.

Orthopedics comes from two Greek words, *ortho*, meaning straight and *pais,* meaning child. Originally orthopedic surgeons dealt with bone deformities in children, using braces to straighten the child's bones. With the development of anesthesia and an understanding of the importance of aseptic technique in surgery, orthopedic surgeons extended their role to include surgery involving the bones and related nerves and connective tissue.

The terms orthopedic surgeon and orthopedist are used interchangeably today to indicate a medical doctor with special certification in orthopedics.

Many orthopedic surgeons maintain a general practice, while some specialize in one particular aspect of orthopedics, such as hand surgery, joint replacements, or disorders of the spine. Orthopedics treats both acute and chronic disorders. Some orthopedists specialize in trauma medicine and can be found in emergency rooms and trauma centers treating injuries. Others find their work overlapping with plastic surgeons, geriatric specialists, pediatricians, or podiatrists (**foot care** specialists). A rapidly growing area of orthopedics is sports medicine, and many sports medicine doctors are board certified orthopedists.

Precautions

Choosing an orthopedist is an important step in obtaining appropriate treatment. Patients looking for a qualified orthopedist should inquire if they are "board certified" by their accrediting organization.

Description

The range of treatments done by orthopedists is enormous. It can cover anything from **traction** to **amputation**, hand reconstruction to spinal fusion or joint replacements. They also treat broken bones, **strains** and **sprains**, and **dislocations**. Some specific procedures done by orthopedic surgeons are listed as separate entries in this book, including **arthroplasty**, **arthroscopic surgery**, **bone grafting**, **fasciotomy**, **fracture repair**, **kneecap removal**, and traction.

In general orthopedists are attached to a hospital, medical center, trauma center, or free-standing surgical center where they work closely with a surgical team including an anesthesiologist and surgical nurse. Orthopedic surgery can be performed under general, regional, or **local anesthesia**.

Much of the work of the surgeon involves adding foreign material to the body in the form of screws, wires, pins, tongs, and prosthetics to hold damaged bones in their proper alignment or to replace damaged bone or connective tissue. Great improvements have been made in the development of artificial limbs and joints, and in the materials available to repair damage to bones and connective tissue. As developments occur in the fields of metallurgy and plastics, changes will take place in orthopedic surgery that will allow the surgeon to more nearly duplicate the natural functions of the bones, joints, and ligaments, and to more accurately restore damaged parts to their original range of motion.

Preparation

Patients are usually referred to an orthopedic surgeon by a general physical or family doctor. Prior to any surgery, the patient undergoes extensive testing to determine the proper corrective procedure. Tests may include x rays, **computed tomography scans** (CT scans), **magnetic resonance imaging** (MRI), myelograms, diagnostic arthroplasty, and blood tests. The orthopedist will determine the history of the disorder and any treatments that were tried previously. A period of rest to the injured part may be recommended before surgery is prescribed.

Patients undergo standard blood and urine tests before surgery and, for major surgery, may be given an electrocardiogram or other diagnostic tests prior to the operation. Patients may choose to give some of their own blood to be held in reserve for their use in major surgery, such as knee replacement, where heavy bleeding is common.

Aftercare

Rehabilitation from orthopedic injuries can be a long, arduous task. The doctor will work closely with physical therapists to assure that the patient is receiving treatment that will enhance the range of motion and return function to the affected part.

Risks

As with any surgery, there is always the risk of excessive bleeding, infection, and allergic reaction to anesthesia. Risks specifically associated with orthopedic surgery include inflammation at the site where foreign material (pins, prosthesis) is introduced into the body, infection as the result of surgery, and damage to nerves or to the spinal cord.

Normal results

Thousands of people have successful orthopedic surgery each year to recover from injuries or restore lost function. The degree of success in individual recoveries depends on the age and general health of the patient, the medical problem being treated, and the patient's willingness to comply with rehabilitative therapy after the surgery.

Resources

ORGANIZATIONS

American Academy of Orthopaedic Surgeons. 6300 North River Road, Rosemont, IL 60018-4262. (800) 823-8125. < http://www.AAOS.org >.

American Osteopathic Board of Orthopedic Surgery. < http://www.netincom.com/aobos/about.html >.

OTHER

Orthogate. < http://owl.orthogate.org/ >.

Tish Davidson, A.M.

Orthopedic x rays *see* **Bone x rays**

Orthostatic hypotension

Definition

Orthostatic **hypotension** is an abnormal decrease in blood pressure when a person stands up. This may lead to **fainting**.

Description

When a person stands upright, a certain amount of blood normally pools in the veins of the ankles and legs. This pooling means that there is slightly less blood for the heart to pump and causes a drop in blood pressure. Usually, the body responds to this drop so quickly, a person is unaware of the change. The brain tells the blood vessels to constrict so they have less capacity to carry blood, and at the same time tells the heart to beat faster and harder. These responses last for a very brief time. If the body's response to a change in vertical position is slow or absent, the result is orthostatic hypotension. It is not a true disease, but the inability to regulate blood pressure quickly.

Causes and symptoms

Orthostatic hypotension has many possible causes. The most common cause is medications used to treat other conditions. **Diuretics** reduce the amount of fluid in the body which reduces the volume of blood. Medicines used to expand the blood vessels increase the vessel's ability to carry blood and so lower blood pressure.

If there is a severe loss of body fluid from **vomiting**, **diarrhea**, untreated diabetes, or even excessive sweating, blood volume will be reduced enough to lower blood pressure. Severe bleeding can also result in orthostatic hypotension.

Any disease or **spinal cord injury** that damages the nerves which control blood vessel diameter can cause orthostatic hypotension.

Symptoms of orthostatic hypotension include faintness, **dizziness**, confusion, or blurry vision, when standing up quickly. An excessive loss of blood pressure can cause a person to pass out.

Diagnosis

When a person experiences any of the symptoms above, a physician can confirm orthostatic hypotension if the person's blood pressure falls significantly on standing up and returns to normal when lying down. The physician will then look for the cause of the condition.

Treatment

When the cause of orthostatic hypotension is related to medication, it is often possible to treat it by reducing dosage or changing the prescription.

If it is caused by low blood volume, an increase in fluid intake and retention will solve the problem.

Medications designed to keep blood pressure from falling can be used when they will not interfere with other medical problems.

When orthostatic hypotension cannot be treated, the symptoms can be significantly reduced by remembering to stand up slowly or by wearing elastic stockings.

Prognosis

The prognosis for people who have orthostatic hypotension depends on the underlying cause of the problem.

Prevention

There is no way to prevent orthostatic hypotension, since it is usually the result of another medical condition.

Resources

ORGANIZATIONS

National Heart, Lung and Blood Institute. P.O. Box 30105, Bethesda, MD 20824-0105. (301) 251-1222. < http:// www.nhlbi.nih.gov >.

National Organization for Rare Disorders. P.O. Box 8923, New Fairfield, CT 06812-8923. (800) 999-6673. < http://www.rarediseases.org >.

Dorothy Elinor Stonely

Orthotopic transplantation *see* **Liver transplantation**

Osgood-Schlatter disease *see* **Osteochondroses**

Osteitis deformans *see* **Paget's disease of bone**

Osteoarthritis

Definition

Osteoarthritis (OA), which is also known as osteoarthrosis or degenerative joint disease (DJD), is a progressive disorder of the joints caused by gradual loss of cartilage and resulting in the development of bony spurs and cysts at the margins of the joints. The name osteoarthritis comes from three Greek words meaning bone, joint, and inflammation.

Description

OA is one of the most common causes of disability due to limitations of joint movement, particularly in people over 50. It is estimated that 2% of the United States population under the age of 45 suffers from osteoarthritis; this figure rises to 30% of persons between 45 and 64, and 63–85% in those over 65. About 90% of the American population will have some features of OA in their weight-bearing joints by age 40. Men tend to develop OA at earlier ages than women.

OA occurs most commonly after 40 years of age and typically develops gradually over a period of years. Patients with OA may have joint **pain** on only one side of the body and it primarily affects the knees, hands, hips, feet, and spine.

Causes and symptoms

Osteoarthritis results from deterioration or loss of the cartilage that acts as a protective cushion between bones, particularly in weight-bearing joints such as the knees and hips. As the cartilage is worn away, the bone forms spurs, areas of abnormal hardening, and fluid-filled pockets in the marrow known as subchondral cysts. As the disorder progresses, pain results from deformation of the bones and fluid accumulation in the joints. The pain is relieved by rest and made worse by moving the joint or placing weight on it. In early OA, the pain is minor and may take the form of mild stiffness in the morning. In the later stages of OA, inflammation develops; the patient may experience pain even when the joint is not being used; and he or she may suffer permanent loss of the normal range of motion in that joint.

Until the late 1980s, OA was regarded as an inevitable part of **aging**, caused by simple "wear and tear" on the joints. This view has been replaced by recent research into cartilage formation. OA is now considered to be the end result of several different factors contributing to cartilage damage, and is classified as either primary or secondary.

Primary osteoarthritis

Primary OA results from abnormal stresses on weight-bearing joints or normal stresses operating on weakened joints. Primary OA most frequently affects the finger joints, the hips and knees, the cervical and lumbar spine, and the big toe. The enlargements of the finger joints that occur in OA are referred to as Heberden's and Bouchard's nodes. Some gene mutations appear to be associated with OA. **Obesity** also increases the pressure on the weight-bearing joints of the body. Finally, as the body ages, there is a reduction in the ability of cartilage to repair itself. In addition to these factors, some researchers have theorized that primary OA may be triggered by enzyme disturbances, bone disease, or liver dysfunction.

Secondary osteoarthritis

Secondary OA results from chronic or sudden injury to a joint. It can occur in any joint. Secondary OA is associated with the following factors:

- trauma, including sports injuries
- repetitive **stress** injuries associated with certain occupations (like the performing arts, construction or assembly line work, computer keyboard operation, etc.)
- repeated episodes of **gout** or septic arthritis
- poor posture or bone alignment caused by developmental abnormalities
- metabolic disorders

Diagnosis

History and physical examination

The two most important diagnostic clues in the patient's history are the pattern of joint involvement and the presence or absence of **fever**, rash, or other symptoms outside the joints. As part of the physical examination, the doctor will touch and move the patient's joint to evaluate swelling, limitations on the range of motion, pain on movement, and crepitus (a cracking or grinding sound heard during joint movement).

Diagnostic imaging

There is no laboratory test that is specific for osteoarthritis. Treatment is usually based on the results of diagnostic imaging. In patients with OA, x-rays may indicate narrowed joint spaces, abnormal density of the bone, and the presence of subchondral cysts or bone spurs. The patient's symptoms, however, do not always correlate with x-ray findings. Magnetic resonance imaging (MRI) and computed tomography scans (CT scans) can be used to determine more precisely the location and extent of cartilage damage.

Treatment

Treatment of OA patients is tailored to the needs of each individual. Patients vary widely in the location

of the joints involved, the rate of progression, the severity of symptoms, the degree of disability, and responses to specific forms of treatment. Most treatment programs include several forms of therapy.

Patient education and psychotherapy

Patient education is an important part of OA treatment because of the highly individual nature of the disorder and its potential impacts on the patient's life. Patients who are depressed because of changes in employment or recreation usually benefit from counseling. The patient's family should be involved in discussions of coping, household reorganization, and other aspects of the patient's disease and treatment regimen.

Medications

Patients with mild OA may be treated only with pain relievers such as **acetaminophen** (Tylenol). Most patients with OA, however, are given **nonsteroidal anti-inflammatory drugs,** or NSAIDs. These include compounds such as ibuprofen (Motrin, Advil), ketoprofen (Orudis), and flurbiprofen (Ansaid). The NSAIDs have the advantage of relieving inflammation as well as pain. They also have potentially dangerous side effects, including stomach ulcers, sensitivity to sun exposure, kidney disturbances, and nervousness or depression.

Some OA patients are treated with **corticosteroids** injected directly into the joints to reduce inflammation and slow the development of Heberden's nodes. Injections should not be regarded as a first-choice treatment and should be given only two or three times a year.

Most recently, a new class of NSAIDs, known as the cyclo-oxygenase-2 (COX-2) inhibitors have been studied and approved for the treatment of OA. These **COX-2 inhibitors** work to block the enzyme COX-2, which stimulates inflammatory responses in the body. They work to decrease both the inflammation and joint pain of OA, but without the high risk of gastrointestinal ulcers and bleeding seen with the traditional NSAIDs. This is due to the fact that they do not block COX-1, which is another enzyme that has protective effects on the stomach lining. The COX-2 inhibitors included celecoxib (Celebrex) and rofecoxib (Vioxx). Celecoxib is taken once or twice daily, and rofecoxib once daily.

Physical therapy

Patients with OA are encouraged to **exercise** as a way of keeping joint cartilage lubricated. Exercises that increase balance, flexibility, and range of motion

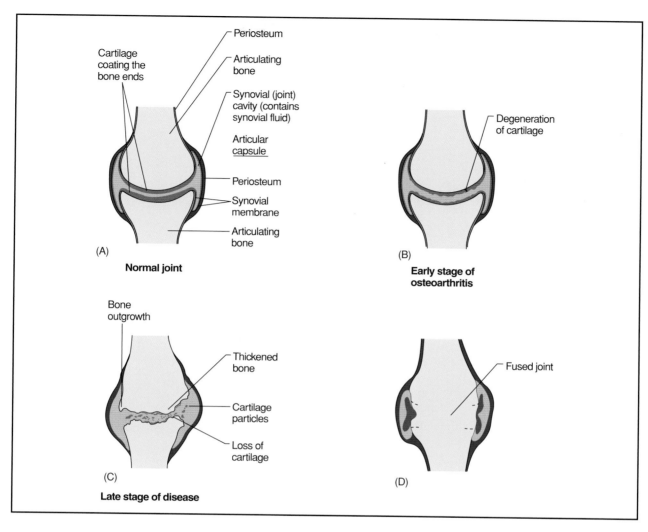

The progression of osteoarthritis. *(Illustration by Hans & Cassady.)*

are recommended for OA patients. These may include walking, swimming and other water exercises, **yoga** and other stretching exercises, or isometric exercises.

Physical therapy may also include massage, moist hot packs, or soaking in a hot tub.

Surgery

Surgical treatment of osteoarthritis may include the replacement of a damaged joint with an artificial part or appliance; surgical fusion of spinal bones; scraping or removal of damaged bone from the joint; or the removal of a piece of bone in order to realign the bone.

Protective measures

Depending on the location of the affected joint, patients with OA may be advised to use neck braces or collars, crutches, canes, hip braces, knee supports, bed boards, or elevated chair and toilet seats. They are also advised to avoid unnecessary knee bending, stair climbing, or lifting of heavy objects.

New treatments

Since 1997, several new methods of treatment for OA have been investigated. Although they are still being developed and tested, they appear to hold promise. They include:

• Disease-modifying drugs. These compounds may be useful in assisting the body to form new cartilage or improve its repair of existing cartilage.

• Hyaluronic acid. Injections of this substance may help to lubricate and protect cartilage, thereby promoting flexibility and reduced pain. These agents include hyaluronan (Hyalgan) and hylan G-F20 (Synvisc).

- Cartilage transplantation. This technique is presently used in Sweden.

Alternative treatment

Diet

Food intolerance can be a contributing factor in OA, although this is more significant in rheumatoid arthritis. Dietary suggestions that may be helpful for people with OA include emphasizing high-fiber, complex-carbohydrate foods, while minimizing fats. Plants in the Solanaceae family, such as tomatoes, eggplant, and potatoes, should be avoided, as should refined and processed foods. Foods that are high in bioflavonoids (berries as well as red, orange, and purple fruits and vegetables) should be eaten often.

Nutritional supplements

In the past several years, a combination of glucosamine and chondroitin sulfate has been proposed as a dietary supplement that helps the body maintain and repair cartilage. Studies conducted in Europe have shown the effectiveness of this treatment in many cases. These substances are nontoxic and do not require prescriptions. Other supplements that may be helpful in the treatment of OA include the antioxidant **vitamins** and **minerals** (vitamins A, C, E, selenium, and zinc) and the B vitamins, especially vitamins B_6 and B_5.

Naturopathy

Naturopathic treatment for OA includes hydrotherapy, diathermy (deep-heat therapy), **nutritional supplements**, and botanical preparations, including yucca, devil's claw (*Harpagophytum procumbens*), and hawthorn (*Crataegus laevigata*) berries.

Traditional Chinese medicine (TCM)

Practitioners of Chinese medicine treat arthritis with suction cups, massage, moxibustion (warming an area of skin by burning a herbal wick a slight distance above the skin), the application of herbal poultices, and internal doses of Chinese herbal formulas.

Other alternatives

Recently, several alternative treatments for OA have received considerable attention and study. These include:

- transcutaneous **electrical nerve stimulation** (TENS)
- magnet therapy

KEY TERMS

Bouchard's nodes—Swelling of the middle joint of the finger.

Cartilage—Elastic connective tissue that covers and protects the ends of bones.

Heberden's nodes—Swelling or deformation of the finger joints closest to the fingertips.

Primary osteoarthritis—OA that results from hereditary factors or stresses on weight-bearing joints.

Secondary osteoarthritis—OA that develops following joint surgery, trauma, or repetitive joint injury.

Subchondral cysts—Fluid-filled sacs that form inside the marrow at the ends of bones as part of the development of OA.

- therapeutic touch
- acupuncture
- yoga

Prognosis

OA is a progressive disorder without a permanent cure. In some patients, the rate of progression can be slowed by weight loss, appropriate exercise, surgical treatment, and the use of alternative therapies.

Resources

PERIODICALS

Berger, R. G. "Intelligent Use of NSAIDs: Where Do We Stand." *Expert Opinions in Pharmacotherapy* 1, no. 2 (January 2001): 19-30.

Brandt, K. D. "The Role of Analgesics in the Management of Osteoarthritis." *American Journal of Therapeutics* March 2000: 75-90.

Little, C. V., and T. Parsons. "Herbal Therapy for Treating Osteoarthritis." *Cochrane Database System Review* 2001: 1.

Pavelka, K. "Treatment of Pain in Osteoarthritis." *European Journal of Pain* 2000: 23-30.

Schnitzer, T. J. "Osteoarthritis Management: The Role of Cyclooxygenase-2-selective Inhibitors." *Clinical Therapeutics* March 2001: 313-26.

Towheed, T. E., et al. "Glucosamine Therapy for Treating Osteoarthritis." *Cochrane Database System Review* 2001: 1.

Liz Meszaros

Osteoarthrosis *see* **Osteoarthritis**

Osteochondroses

Definition

Osteochondroses is a group of diseases of children and adolescents in which localized tissue death (necrosis) occurs, usually followed by full regeneration of healthy bone tissue. The singular term is osteochondrosis.

Description

During the years of rapid bone growth, blood supply to the growing ends of bones (epiphyses) may become insufficient resulting in necrotic bone, usually near joints. The term avascular necrosis is used to describe osteochondrosis. Since bone is normally undergoing a continuous rebuilding process, the necrotic areas are most often self-repaired over a period of weeks or months.

Osteochondrosis can affect different areas of the body and is often categorized by one of three locations: articular, non-articular, and physeal.

Physeal osteochondrosis is known as Scheuermann's disease. It occurs in the spine at the intervertebral joints (physes), especially in the chest (thoracic) region.

Articular disease occurs at the joints (articulations). One of the more common forms is Legg-Calvé-Perthes disease, occurring at the hip. Other forms include Köhler's disease (foot), Freiberg's disease (second toe), and Panner's disease (elbow). Freiberg's disease is the one type of osteochondrosis that is more common in females than in males. All others affect the sexes equally.

Non-articular osteochondrosis occurs at any other skeletal location. For instance, Osgood-Schlatter disease of the tibia (the large inner bone of the leg between the knee and ankle) is relatively common.

Osteochondritis dissecans is a form of osteochondrosis in which loose bone fragments may form in a joint.

Causes and symptoms

Many theories have been advanced to account for osteochondrosis, but none has proven fully satisfactory. **Stress** and **ischemia** (reduced blood supply) are two of the most commonly mentioned factors. Athletic young children are often affected when they overstress their developing limbs with a particular repetitive motion. Many cases are idiopathic, meaning that no specific cause is known.

The most common symptom for most types of osteochondrosis is simply **pain** at the affected joint, especially when pressure is applied. Locking of a joint or limited range of motion at a joint can also occur.

Scheuermann's disease can lead to serious **kyphosis** (hunchback condition) due to erosion of the vertebral bodies. Usually, however, the kyphosis is mild, causing no further symptoms and requiring no special treatment.

Diagnosis

Diagnosis can be confirmed by x-ray findings.

Treatment

Conservative treatment is usually attempted first. In many cases, simply resting the affected body part for a period of days or weeks will bring relief. A cast may be applied if needed to prevent movement of a joint.

Surgical intervention may be needed in some cases of osteochondritis dissecans to remove abnormal bone fragments in a joint.

Prognosis

Accurate prediction of the outcome for individual patients is difficult with osteochondrosis. Some patients will heal spontaneously. Others will heal with little treatment other than keeping weight or stress off the affected limb. The earlier the age of onset, the better the prospects for full recovery. Surgical intervention is often successful in osteochondritis dissecans.

Prevention

No preventive measures are known.

Resources

BOOKS

Eilert, Robert E., and Gaia Geogopoulos. "Orthopedics." In *Current Pediatric Diagnosis and Treatment*, edited by W. W. Hay, Jr., et al. Stamford: Appleton & Lange, 1997.

Victor Leipzig, PhD

Osteogenesis imperfecta

Definition

Osteogenesis imperfecta (OI) is a group of genetic diseases of collagen in which the bones are formed improperly, making them fragile and prone to breaking.

Description

Collagen is a fibrous protein material. It serves as the structural foundation of skin, bone, cartilage, and ligaments. In osteogenesis imperfecta, the collagen produced is abnormal and disorganized. This results in a number of abnormalities throughout the body, the most notable being fragile, easily broken bones.

There are four forms of OI, Types I through IV. Of these, Type II is the most severe, and is usually fatal within a short time after birth. Types I, III, and IV have some overlapping and some distinctive symptoms, particularly weak bones.

Evidence suggests that OI results from abnormalities in the collagen gene COL1A1 or COL1A2, and possibly abnormalities in other genes. In OI Type I, II, and III, the gene map locus is 17q21.31-q22, 7q22.1, and in OI Type IV, the gene map locus is 17q21.31-q22.

In OI, the genetic abnormality causes one of two things to occur. It may direct cells to make an altered collagen protein and the presence of this altered collagen causes OI Type II, III, or IV. Alternately, the dominant altered gene may fail to direct cells to make any collagen protein. Although some collagen is produced by instructions from the normal gene, an overall decrease in the total amount of collagen produced results in OI Type I.

A child with only one parent who is a carrier of a single altered copy of the gene has no chance of actually having the disease, but a 50% chance of being a carrier.

If both parents have OI caused by an autosomal dominant gene change, there is a 75% chance that the child will inherit one or both OI genes. In other words, there is a 25% chance the child will inherit only the mother's OI gene (and the father's unaffected gene), a 25% chance the child will inherit only the father's OI gene (and the mother's unaffected gene), and a 25% chance the child will inherit both parents' OI genes. Because this situation has been uncommon, the outcome of a child inheriting two OI genes is hard to predict. It is likely that the child would have a severe, possibly lethal, form of the disorder.

About 25% of children with OI are born into a family with no history of the disorder. This occurs when the gene spontaneously mutates in either the sperm or the egg before the child's conception. No triggers for this type of mutation are known. This is called a new dominant mutation. The child has a 50% chance of passing the disorder on to his or her children. In most cases, when a family with no history of OI has a child with OI, they are not at greater risk than the general population for having a second child with OI, and unaffected siblings of a person with OI are at no greater risk of having children with OI than the general population.

In studies of families into which infants with OI Type II were born, most of the babies had a new dominant mutation in a collagen gene. In some of these families, however, more than one infant was born with OI. Previously, researchers had seen this recurrence as evidence of recessive inheritance of this form of OI. More recently, however, researchers have concluded that the rare recurrence of OI to a couple with a child with autosomal dominant OI is more likely due to gonadal mosaicism. Instead of mutation occurring in an individual sperm or egg, it occurs in a percentage of the cells that give rise to a parent's multiple sperm or eggs. This mutation, present in a percentage of his or her reproductive cells, can result in more than one affected child without affecting the parent with the disorder. An estimated 2%–4% of families into which an infant with OI Type II is born are at risk of having another affected child because of gonadal mosaicism.

Demographics

OI affects equal numbers of males and females. It occurs in about one of every 20,000 births.

Causes and symptoms

OI is usually inherited as an autosomal dominant condition. In autosomal dominant inheritance, a single abnormal gene on one of the autosomal chromosomes (one of the first 22 "non-sex" chromosomes) from either parent can cause the disease. One of the parents will have the disease (since it is dominant) and is the carrier. Only one parent needs to be a carrier in order for the child to inherit the disease. A child who has one parent with the disease has a 50% chance of also having the disease.

Type I

This is the most common and mildest type. Among the common features of Type I are the following:

- bones are predisposed to fracture, with most fractures occurring before **puberty**; people with OI type I typically have about 20–40 **fractures** before puberty.

- stature is normal or near-normal

- joints are loose and muscle tone is low

- usually sclera (whites of the eyes) have blue, purple, or gray tint
- face shape is triangular
- tendency toward **scoliosis** (a curvature of the spine)
- bone deformity is absent or minimal
- dentinogenesis imperfecta may occur, causing brittle teeth
- hearing loss is a possible symptom, often beginning in early 20s or 30s
- structure of collagen is normal, but the amount is less than normal

Type II

Sometimes called the lethal form, Type II is the most severe form of OI. Among the common features of Type II are the following:

- frequently, OI Type II is lethal at or shortly after birth, often as a result of respiratory problems
- fractures are numerous and bone deformity is severe
- stature is small with underdeveloped lungs
- collagen is formed improperly

Type III

Among the common features of Type III are the following:

- bones fracture easily (fractures are often present at birth, and x rays may reveal healed fractures that occurred before birth; people with OI Type III may have more than 100 fractures before puberty)
- stature is significantly shorter than normal
- sclera (whites of the eyes) have blue, purple, or gray tint
- joints are loose and muscle development is poor in arms and legs
- rib cage is barrel-shaped
- face shape is triangular
- scoliosis (a curvature of the spine) is present
- respiratory problems are possible
- bones are deformed and deformity is often severe
- dentinogenesis imperfecta may occur, causing brittle teeth
- hearing loss is possible
- collagen is formed improperly

Type IV

OI Type IV falls between Type I and Type III in severity. Among the common features of Type IV are the following:

- bones fracture easily, with most fractures occurring before puberty
- stature is shorter than average
- sclera (whites of the eyes) are normal in color, appearing white or near-white
- bone deformity is mild to moderate
- scoliosis (curvature of the spine) is likely
- rib cage is barrel-shaped
- face is triangular in shape
- dentinogenesis imperfecta may occur, causing brittle teeth
- hearing loss is possible
- collagen is formed improperly

Diagnosis

It is often possible to diagnose OI solely on clinical features and x-ray findings. Collagen or DNA tests may help confirm a diagnosis of OI. These tests generally require several weeks before results are known. Approximately 10–15% of individuals with mild OI who have collagen testing, and approximately 5% of those who have genetic testing, test negative for OI despite having the disorder.

Diagnosis is usually suspected when a baby has bone fractures after having suffered no apparent injury. Another indication is small, irregular, isolated bones in the sutures between the bones of the skull (wormian bones). Sometimes the bluish sclera serves as a diagnostic clue. Unfortunately, because of the unusual nature of the fractures occurring in a baby who cannot yet move, some parents have been accused of **child abuse** before the actual diagnosis of osteogenesis imperfecta was reached.

Prenatal diagnosis

Testing is available to assist in prenatal diagnosis. Women with OI who become pregnant, or women who conceive a child with a man who has OI, may wish to explore prenatal diagnosis. Because of the relatively small risk (2–4%) of recurrence of OI Type II in a family, families may opt for ultrasound studies to determine if a developing fetus has the disorder.

Ultrasound is the least invasive procedure for prenatal diagnosis, and carries the least risk. Using ultrasound, a doctor can examine the fetus's skeleton for bowing of the leg or arm bones, fractures, shortening, or other bone abnormalities that may indicate OI. Different forms of OI may be detected by ultrasound in the second trimester. The reality is that when it occurs as a new dominant mutation, it is found inadvertently on ultrasound, and it may be difficult to know the diagnosis until after delivery since other genetic conditions can cause bowing and/or fractures prenatally.

Chorionic villus sampling is a procedure to obtain chorionic villi tissue for testing. Examination of fetal collagen proteins in the tissue can reveal information about the quantitative or qualitative collagen defects that leads to OI. When a parent has OI, it is necessary for the affected parent to have the results of his or her own collagen test available. Chorionic villus sampling can be performed at 10–12 weeks of **pregnancy**.

Amniocentesis is a procedure that involves inserting a thin needle into the uterus, into the amniotic sac, and withdrawing a small amount of amniotic fluid. DNA can be extracted from the fetal cells contained in the amniotic fluid and tested for the specific mutation known to cause OI in that family. This technique is useful only when the mutation causing OI in a particular family has been identified through previous **genetic testing** of affected family members, including previous pregnancies involving a baby with OI. Amniocentesis is performed at 16–18 weeks of pregnancy.

Treatment

There are no treatments available to cure OI, nor to prevent most of its complications. Most treatments are aimed at treating the fractures and bone deformities caused by OI. Splints, casts, braces, and rods are all used. Rodding refers to a surgical procedure in which a metal rod is implanted within a bone (usually the long bones of the thigh and leg). This is done when bowing or repeated fractures of these bones has interfered with a child's ability to begin to walk.

Other treatments include **hearing aids** and early capping of teeth. Patients may require the use of a walker or wheelchair. Pain may be treated with a variety of medications. **Exercise** is encouraged as a means to promote muscle and bone strength. Swimming is a form of exercise that puts a minimal amount of strain on muscles, joints, and bones. Walking is encouraged for those who are able.

Smoking, excessive alcohol and **caffeine** consumption, and steroid medications may deplete bone and exacerbate bone fragility.

KEY TERMS

Collagen—The main supportive protein of cartilage, connective tissue, tendon, skin, and bone.

Ligament—A type of connective tissue that connects bones or cartilage and provides support and strength to joints.

Mutation—A permanent change in the genetic material that may alter a trait or characteristic of an individual, or manifest as disease, and can be transmitted to offspring.

Sclera—The tough white membrane that forms the outer layer of the eyeball.

Scoliosis—An abnormal, side-to-side curvature of the spine.

Alternative treatment such as **acupuncture**, naturopathic therapies, hypnosis, relaxation training, visual imagery, and **biofeedback** have all been used to try to decrease the constant **pain** of fractures.

Prognosis

Lifespan for people with OI Type I, III, and IV is not generally shortened. The prognosis for people with these types of OI is quite variable, depending on the severity of the disorder and the number and severity of the fractures and bony deformities.

Fifty percent of all babies with OI Type II are stillborn. The rest of these babies usually die within a very short time after birth. In recent years, some people with Type II have lived into young adulthood.

Resources

PERIODICALS

Kocher, M. S., and J. R. Kasser. "Orthopaedic aspects of child abuse." *Journal of the American Academy of Orthopedic Surgery* 8 (January-February 2000): 10 + .

Niyibizi, C., et al. "Potential of gene therapy for treating osteogenesis imperfecta." *Clinical Orthopedics* 379 (October 2000): S126 + .

Smith, R. "Severe osteogenesis imperfecta: new therapeutic options?" *British Medical Journal* 322 (January 13, 2001): 63 + .

Wacaster, Priscilla. "Osteogenesis Imperfecta." *Exceptional Parent* 30 (April 2000): 94 + .

ORGANIZATIONS

Children's Brittle Bone Foundation. 7701 95th St., Pleasant Prairie, WI 53158. (847) 433-498. < http:// www.cbbf.org >.

OTHER

"Osteogenesis Imperfecta." *National Institutes of Health Osteoporosis and Related Bone Diseases–National Resource Center.* < http://www.osteo.org/oi.html >.

Jennifer F. Wilson, MS

Osteogenic sarcoma *see* **Sarcomas**

Osteomalacia *see* **Vitamin D deficiency**

Osteomyelitis

Definition

Osteomyelitis refers to a bone infection, almost always caused by a bacteria. Over time, the result can be destruction of the bone itself.

Description

Bone infections may occur at any age. Certain conditions increase the risk of developing such an infection, including sickle cell anemia, injury, the presence of a foreign body (such as a bullet or a screw placed to hold together a broken bone), intravenous drug use (such as heroin), diabetes, **kidney dialysis**, surgical procedures to bony areas, untreated infections of tissue near a bone (for example, extreme cases of untreated sinus infections have led to osteomyelitis of the bones of the skull).

Causes and symptoms

Staphylococcus aureus, a bacterium, is the most common organism involved in osteomyelitis. Other types of organisms include the mycobacterium which causes **tuberculosis**, a type of Salmonella bacteria in patients with sickle cell anemia, *Pseudomonas aeurginosa* in drug addicts, and organisms which usually reside in the gastrointestinal tract in the elderly. Extremely rarely, the viruses which cause **chickenpox** and **smallpox** have been found to cause a viral osteomyelitis.

There are two main ways that infecting bacteria find their way to bone, resulting in the development of osteomyelitis. These include:

- Spread via the bloodstream; 95% of these types of infections are due to *Staphylococcus aureus*. In this situation, the bacteria travels through the bloodstream to reach the bone. In children, the most likely site of infection is within one of the long bones, particularly the thigh bone (femur), one of the bones of the lower leg (tibia), or the bone of the upper arm (humerus). This is because in children these bones have particularly extensive blood circulation, making them more susceptible to invasion by bacteria. Different patterns of blood circulation in adults make the long bones less well-served by the circulatory system. These bones are therefore unlikely to develop osteomyelitis in adult patients. Instead, the bones of the spine (vertebrae) receive a lot of blood flow. Therefore, osteomyelitis in adults is most likely to affect a vertebra. Drug addicts may have osteomyelitis in the pubic bone or clavicle.

- Spread from adjacent infected soft tissue; about 50% of all such cases are infected by *Staphylococcus aureus*. This often occurs in cases where recent surgery or injury has result in a soft tissue infection. The bacteria can then spread to nearby bone, resulting in osteomyelitis. Patients with diabetes are particularly susceptible to this source of osteomyelitis. The diabetes interferes with both nerve sensation and good blood flow to the feet. Diabetic patients are therefore prone to developing poorly healing **wounds** to their feet, which can then spread to bone, causing osteomyelitis.

Acute osteomyelitis refers to an infection which develops and peaks over a relatively short period of time. In children, acute osteomyelitis usually presents itself as **pain** in the affected bone, tenderness to pressure over the infected area, **fever** and chills. Patients who develop osteomyelitis, due to spread from a nearby area of soft tissue infection, may only note poor healing of the original wound or infection.

Adult patients with osteomyelitis of the spine usually have a longer period of dull, aching pain in the back, and no fever. Some patients note pain in the chest, abdomen, arm, or leg. This occurs when the inflammation in the spine causes pressure on a nerve root serving one of these other areas. The lower back is the most common location for osteomyelitis. When caused by tuberculosis, osteomyelitis usually affects the thoracic spine (that section of the spine running approximately from the base of the neck down to where the ribs stop).

When osteomyelitis is not properly treated, a chronic (long-term) type of infection may occur. In this case, the infection may wax and wane indefinitely, despite treatment during its active phases. An abnormal opening in the skin overlaying the area of bone infection (called a sinus tract) may occasionally drain pus. This type of smoldering infection may also result in areas of dead bone, called sequestra. These areas occur when the infection interferes with blood flow to a particular part of the bone. Such sequestra lack cells called osteocytes, which in normal bone are continuously involved in the process of producing bony material.

Diagnosis

Diagnosis of osteomyelitis involves several procedures. Blood is usually drawn and tested to demonstrate an increased number of the infection-fighting white blood cells (particularly elevated in children with acute osteomyelitis). Blood is also cultured in a laboratory, a process which allows any bacteria present to multiply. A specimen from the culture is then specially treated, and examined under a microscope to try to identify the causative bacteria.

Injection of certain radioactive elements into the bloodstream, followed by a series of x-ray pictures, called a scan (radionuclide scanning), will reveal areas of bone inflammation. Another type of scan used to diagnose osteomyelitis is called **magnetic resonance imaging**, or MRI

When pockets of pus are available, or overlaying soft tissue infection exists, these can serve as sources for samples which can be cultured to allow identification of bacteria present. A long, sharp needle can be used to obtain a specimen of bone (biopsy), which can then be tested to attempt to identify any bacteria present.

Treatment

Antibiotics are medications used to kill bacteria. These medications are usually given through a needle in a vein (intravenously) for at least part of the time. In children, these antibiotics can be given by mouth after initial treatment by vein. In adults, four to six weeks of intravenous antibiotic treatment is usually recommended, along with bed-rest for part or all of that time. Occasionally, a patient will have such extensive ostemyelitis that surgery will be required to drain any pockets of pus, and to clean the infected area.

Alternative treatment

General recommendations for the treatment of infections include increasing vitamin supplements, such as **vitamins** A and C. Liquid garlic extract is sometimes suggested. **Guided imagery** can help induce relaxation and improve pain, both of which are considered to improve healing. Herbs such as **echinacea** (*Echinacea* spp.), goldenseal (*Hydrastis canadensis*), Siberian ginseng (*Eleutherococcus senticosus*), and

---

KEY TERMS

Abscess—A pus-filled pocket of infection.

Femur—The thighbone.

Humerus—The bone of the upper arm.

Thoracic—Pertaining to the area bounded by the rib cage.

Tibia—One of the two bones of the lower leg.

---

myrrh (*Commiphora molmol*) are all suggested for infections. Juice therapists recommend drinking combinations of carrot, celery, beet, and cantaloupe juices. A variety of homeopathic remedies may be helpful, especially those used to counter inflammation.

Prognosis

Prognosis varies depending on how quickly an infection is identified, and what other underlying conditions exist to complicate the infection. With quick, appropriate treatment, only about 5% of all cases of acute osteomyelitis will eventually become chronic osteomyelitis. Patients with chronic osteomyelitis may require antibiotics periodically for the rest of their lives.

Prevention

About the only way to have any impact on the development of osteomyelitis involves excellent care of any wounds or injuries.

Resources

PERIODICALS

Calhoun, Jason H., et al. "Osteomyelitis: Diagnosis, Staging, Management." *Patient Care* 32 (January 30, 1998): 93 + .

Rosalyn Carson-DeWitt, MD

Osteopathic medicine *see* **Osteopathy**

Osteopathy

Definition

Osteopathy is a system and philosophy of health care that separated from traditional (allopathic) medical practice about a century ago. It places emphasis on the musculoskeletal system, hence the name—osteo refers to bone and path refers to disease. Osteopaths also believe strongly in the healing power of the body and do their best to facilitate that strength. During this century, the disciplines of osteopathy and allopathic medicine have been converging.

Purpose

Osteopathy shares many of the same goals as traditional medicine, but places greater emphasis on the relationship between the organs and the musculoskeletal system as well as on treating the whole individual rather than just the disease.

Precautions

Pain is the chief reason patients seek musculoskeletal treatment. Pain is a symptom, not a disease by itself. Of critical importance is first to determine the cause of the pain. Cancers, brain or spinal cord disease, and many other causes may be lying beneath this symptom. Once it is clear that the pain is originating in the musculoskeletal system, treatment that includes manipulation is appropriate.

Description

History

Osteopathy was founded in the 1890s by Dr. Andrew Taylor, who believed that the musculoskeletal system was central to health. The primacy of the musculoskeletal system is also fundamental to **chiropractic**, a related health discipline. The original theory behind both approaches presumed that energy flowing through the nervous system is influenced by the supporting structure that encase and protect it—the skull and vertebral column. A defect in the musculoskeletal system was believed to alter the flow of this energy and cause disease. Correcting the defect cured the disease. Defects were thought to be misalignments—parts out of place by tiny distances. Treating misalignments became a matter of restoring the parts to their natural arrangement by adjusting them.

As medical science advanced, defining causes of disease and discovering cures, schools of osteopathy adopted modern science, incorporated it into their curriculum, and redefined their original theory of disease in light of these discoveries. Near the middle of the 20th century the equivalance of medical education between osteopathy and allopathic medicine was recognized, and the D.O. degree (Doctor of Osteopathy) was granted official parity with the M.D. (Doctor of Medicine) degree. Physicians could adopt either set of initials.

However, osteopaths have continued their emphasis on the musculoskeletal system and their traditional focus on "whole person" medicine. As of 1998, osteopaths constitute 5.5% of American physicians, approximately 45,000. They provide 100 million patient visits a year. From its origins in the United States, osteopathy has spread to countries all over the world.

Practice

Osteopaths, chiropractors, and physical therapists are the experts in manipulations (adjustments). The place of manipulation in medical care is far from settled, but millions of patients find relief from it. Particularly backs, but also necks, command most of the attention of the musculoskeletal community. This community includes orthopedic surgeons, osteopaths, general and family physicians, orthopedic physicians, chiropractors, physical therapists, massage therapists, specialists in orthotics and prosthetics, and even some dentists and podiatrists. Many types of headaches also originate in the musculoskeletal system. Studies comparing different methods of treating musculoskeletal back, head, and neck pain have not reached a consensus, in spite of the huge numbers of people that suffer from it.

The theory behind manipulation focuses on joints, mostly those of the vertebrae and ribs. Some believe there is a very slight offset of the joint members—a subluxation. Others believe there is a vacuum lock of the joint surfaces, similar to two suction cups stuck together. Such a condition would squeeze joint lubricant out and produce abrasion of the joint surfaces with movement. Another theory focuses on weakness of the ligaments that support the joint, allowing it freedom to get into trouble. Everyone agrees that the result produces pain, that pain produces **muscle spasms and cramps**, which further aggravates the pain.

Some, but not all, practitioners in this field believe that the skull bones can also be manipulated. The skull is, in fact, several bones that are all moveable in infants. Whether they can be moved in adults is controversial. Other practitioners manipulate peripheral joints to relieve arthritis and similar afflictions.

Manipulation returns the joint to its normal configuration. There are several approaches. Techniques vary among practitioners more than between disciplines. Muscle relaxation of some degree is often required for the manipulation to be successful. This

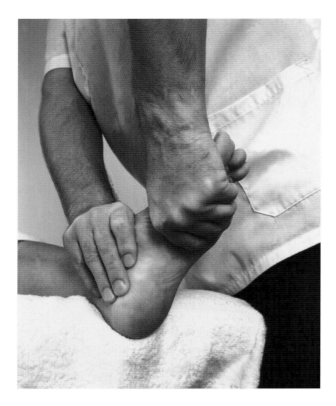

Osteopathic physician demonstrating the articulation of a foot. *(Photo Researchers, Inc. Reproduced by permission.)*

can be done with heat or medication. Muscles can also be induced to relax by gentle but persistent stretching. The manipulation is most often done by a short, fast motion called a thrust, precisely in the right direction. A satisfying "pop" is evidence of success. Others prefer steady force until relaxation permits movement.

Return of the joint to its normal status may be only the first step in treating these disorders. There is a reason for the initial event. It may be a fall, a stumble, or a mild impact, in which case the manipulation is a cure. On the other hand, there may be a postural misalignment (such as a short leg), a limp, or a stretched ligament that permits the joint to slip back into dysfunction. Tension, as well as pain, for emotional reasons causes muscles to tighten. If the pain has been present for any length of time, there will also be muscle deterioration. The osteopathic approach to the whole person takes all these factors into account in returning the patient to a state of health.

Other repairs may be needed. A short leg is thought by some to be a subluxation in the pelvis that may be manipulated back into position. Other short legs may require a lift in one shoe. Long-standing pain requires additional methods of physical therapy

to rehabilitate muscles, correct posture, and extinguish habits that arose to compensate for the pain. Medications that relieve muscle spasm and pain are usually part of the treatment. Psychological problems may need attention and medication.

Risks

Manipulation has rarely caused problems. Once in a while too forceful a thrust has damaged structures in the neck and caused serious problems. The most common adverse event, though, is misdiagnosis. Cancers have been missed; surgical back disease has been ignored until spinal nerves have been permanently damaged.

Normal results

Many patients find that one or a series of manipulations cures long-standing pain. Other patients need repeated treatments. Some do not respond at all. It is always a good idea to reassess any treatment that is not producing the expected results.

Resources

ORGANIZATIONS

American Association of Colleges of Osteopathic Medicine. 5550 Friendship Blvd., Suite 310, Chevy Chase, MD 20815-7231. (301) 968-4100. < http://www.aacom.org >.

American Osteopathic Association. < osteomed@wwa.com > < http://www.am-osteo-assn.org >.

J. Ricker Polsdorfer, MD

Osteopetroses

Definition

Osteopetrosis (plural osteopetroses) is a rare hereditary disorder that makes bones increase in both density and fragility. A potentially fatal condition that can deform bone structure and distort the appearance, osteopetrosis is also called chalk bones, ivory bones, or marble bones.

Description

Osteopetrosis occurs when bones are spongy or porous, or new bone is repeatedly added to calcified cartilage (hardened connective tissue).

Bone density begins to increase at birth or earlier, but symptoms may not become evident until adulthood. In mild cases, bone density increases at gradual, irregular intervals until full adult height is attained. Some bones are not affected.

More severe osteopetrosis progresses at a rapid pace and destroys bone structure. This condition involves bones throughout the body, but the lower jaw is never affected.

Types of osteopetroses

In early-onset osteopetrosis ends of the long bones of the arms and legs appear clubbed (widened and thickened) at birth, and bone density continues to increase sporadically or without pause. Early-onset osteopetroses can be a fatal condition, resulting in **death** before the age of two.

Malignant infantile osteopetrosis is most often discovered by the time a baby is a few months old. One-third of all malignant infantile osteopetroses cases result in death before the age of 10.

Intermediate osteopetrosis generally appears in children under 10. This condition, usually less severe than early-onset or malignant infantile osteopetrosis, is not life-threatening.

Symptoms of adult or delayed-onset osteopetrosis may not become evident until the child becomes a teenager or adult.

Relatively common in many parts of the world, Albers-Schönberg disease is a mild form of this condition. People who have this disease are born with normal bone structure. Bone density increases as they age but does not affect appearance, health, intelligence, or life span.

Causes and symptoms

Osteopetrosis is the result of a genetic defect that causes the body to add new bone more rapidly than existing bone disintegrates.

When fibrous or bony tissue invades bone marrow and displaces red blood cells, the patient may develop anemia. Infection results when excess bone impairs the immune system, and hemorrhage can occur when platelet production is disrupted. When the skeleton grows so thick that nerves are unable to pass between bones, the patient may have a **stroke** or become blind or deaf.

Other symptoms associated with osteopetrosis include:

- bones that break easily and do not heal properly
- bruising
- convulsions
- enlargement of the liver, lymph glands, or spleen
- failure to thrive (delayed growth, weight gain, and development)
- hydrocephalus (fluid on the brain)
- macrocephaly (abnormal enlargement of the head)
- paralysis or loss of control of muscles in the face or eyes

Diagnosis

Osteopetrosis is usually diagnosed when x rays reveal abnormalities or increases in bone density. **Bone biopsy** can confirm the presence of osteopetrosis, but additional tests may be needed to distinguish one type of the disorder from another.

Treatment

High doses of vitamin D can stimulate cells responsible for disintegration of old bone and significantly alleviate symptoms of severe disease. Experimental interferon gamma 1-b therapy has been shown to reduce the risk of infection experienced by patients who are severely ill.

When bone overgrowth deforms the shape of the skull, surgery may be required to relieve pressure on the brain. Orthodontic treatment is sometimes necessary to correct **malocclusion** (a condition that shifts the position of the teeth and makes closing the mouth impossible).

Professional counseling can help patients cope with the emotional aspects of deformed features.

Bone marrow transplants (BMT) have cured some cases of early-onset and malignant infantile osteopetrosis. Because 30–60% of children who undergo BMT do not survive, this procedure is rarely performed.

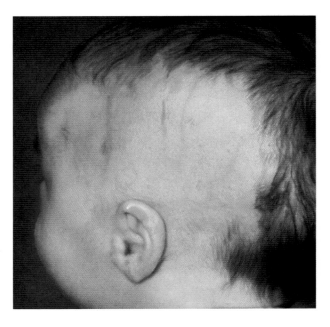

This infant has osteopetrosis, a condition which thickens and hardens the bone. *(Custom Medical Stock Photo. Reproduced by permission.)*

Prognosis

The severity of anemia seems to determine the course of an individual's osteopetrosis. When pronounced symptoms are present at the time of birth, the child's condition deteriorates rapidly. Death usually occurs within two years. When mild or moderate disease develops in older children or adults and symptoms can be controlled, the patient is likely to survive.

Resources

ORGANIZATIONS

Osteoporosis and Related Bone Diseases-National Resource Center. 1150 17th S. NW, Ste. 500, Washington, DC 20036. (800) 624-2663.

Maureen Haggerty

Osteoporosis

Definition

The word osteoporosis literally means "porous bones." It occurs when bones lose an excessive amount of their protein and mineral content, particularly calcium. Over time, bone mass, and therefore bone strength, is decreased. As a result, bones become fragile and break easily. Even a sneeze or a sudden movement may be enough to break a bone in someone with severe osteoporosis.

Description

Osteoporosis is a serious public health problem. Some 44 million people in the United States are at risk for this potentially debilitating disease, which is responsible for 1.5 million **fractures** (broken bones) annually. These fractures, which are often the first sign of the disease, can affect any bone, but the most common locations are the hip, spine, and wrist. Breaks in the hip and spine are of special concern because they almost always require hospitalization and major surgery, and may lead to other serious consequences, including permanent disability and even **death**.

To understand osteoporosis, it is helpful to understand the basics of bone formation. Bone is living tissue that is constantly being renewed in a two-stage process (resorption and formation) that occurs throughout life. In the resorption stage, old bone is broken down and removed by cells called osteoclasts. In the formation stage, cells called osteoblasts build new bone to replace the old. During childhood and early adulthood, more bone is produced than removed, reaching its maximum mass and strength by the mid-30s. After that, bone is lost at a faster pace than it is formed, so the amount of bone in the skeleton begins to slowly decline. Most cases of osteoporosis occur as an acceleration of this normal **aging** process, which is referred to as primary osteoporosis. The condition also can be caused by other disease processes or prolonged use of certain medications that result in bone loss. If so, this is called secondary osteoporosis.

Osteoporosis occurs most often in older people and in women after **menopause**. It affects nearly half of men and women over the age of 75. Women are about five times more likely than men to develop the disease. They have smaller, thinner bones than men to begin with, and they lose bone mass more rapidly after menopause (usually around age 50), when they stop producing a bone-protecting hormone called estrogen. In the five to seven years following menopause, women can lose about 20% of their bone mass. By age 65 or 70, though, men and women lose bone mass at the same rate. As an increasing number of men reach an older age, there is more awareness that osteoporosis is an important health issue for them as well. In fact, a 2003 report noted that one in every eight men over age 50 will suffer a hip fracture as a result of osteoporosis.

Causes and symptoms

A number of factors increase the risk of developing osteoporosis. They include:

- Age. Osteoporosis is more likely as people grow older and their bones lose tissue.

- Gender. Women are smaller and start out with less bone. They also lose bone tissue more rapidly as they age. While women commonly lose 30–50% of their bone mass over their lifetimes, men lose only 20–33%.

- Race. Caucasian and Asian women are most at risk for the disease, but African American and Hispanic women can get it too.

- Figure type. Women with small bones and those who are thin are more liable to have osteoporosis.

- Early menopause. Women who stop menstruating early because of heredity, surgery or lots of physical **exercise** may lose large amounts of bone tissue early in life. Conditions such as anorexia and bulimia also may lead to early menopause and osteoporosis.

- Lifestyle. People who smoke or drink too much, or do not get enough exercise have an increased chance of osteoporosis.

- Diet. Those who do not get enough calcium or protein may be more likely to have osteoporosis. That is why people who constantly diet are more prone to the disease.

- Genetics. Research in Europe reported in 2003 that variations of a gene on chromosome 20 might make some postmenopausal women more likely to have osteoporosis. Studies were continuing on how to identify the gene and use information from the research to prevent osteoporosis in carriers.

Osteoporosis is often called the "silent" disease, because bone loss occurs without symptoms. People often do not know they have the disease until a bone breaks, frequently in a minor fall that would not normally cause a fracture. A common occurrence is compression fractures of the spine. These can happen even after a seemingly normal activity, such as bending or twisting to pick up a light object. The fractures can cause severe back **pain**, but sometimes go unnoticed—either way, the vertebrae collapse down on themselves, and the person actually loses height. The hunchback appearance of many elderly women, sometimes called "dowager's" hump or "widow's" hump, is due to this effect of osteoporosis on the vertebrae.

Diagnosis

Certain types of doctors may have more training and experience than others in diagnosing and treating people with osteoporosis. These include a geriatrician, who specializes in treating the aged; an endocrinologist, who specializes in treating diseases of the body's endocrine system (glands and hormones); and an orthopedic surgeon, who treats fractures such as those caused by osteoporosis.

Before making a diagnosis of osteoporosis, the doctor usually takes a complete medical history, conducts a physical exam, and orders x rays, as well as blood and urine tests, to rule out other diseases that cause loss of bone mass. The doctor also may recommend a **bone density test**. This is the only way to know for certain if osteoporosis is present. It also can show how far the disease has progressed.

Several diagnostic tools are available to measure bone density. The ordinary x ray is one, though it is the least accurate for early detection of osteoporosis, because it does not reveal bone loss until the disease is advanced and most of the damage has already been done. Two other tools that are more likely to catch osteoporosis at an early stage are **computed tomography scans** (CT scans) and machines called densitometers, which are designed specifically to measure bone density.

The CT scan, which takes a large number of x rays of the same spot from different angles, is an accurate test, but uses higher levels of radiation than other methods. The most accurate and advanced of the densitometers uses a technique called DEXA (dual energy x-ray absorptiometry). With the DEXA scan, a double x-ray beam takes pictures of the spine, hip, or entire body. It takes about 20 minutes to do, is painless, and exposes the patient to only a small amount of radiation—about one-fiftieth that of a **chest x ray**.

Doctors do not routinely recommend the test, partly because access to densitometers is still not widely available. People should talk to their doctors about their risk factors for osteoporosis and if, and when, they should get the test. Ideally, women should have bone density measured at menopause, and periodically afterward, depending on the condition of their bones. Men should be tested around age 65. Men and women with additional risk factors, such as those who take certain medications, may need to be tested earlier.

Treatment

There are a number of good treatments for primary osteoporosis, most of them medications.

Two medications, alendronate and calcitonin (in nose spray form), have been approved by the Food and Drug Administration (FDA). They provide people who have osteoporosis with a variety of choices for treatment. For people with secondary osteoporosis, treatment may focus on curing the underlying disease.

Drugs

For many women who have gone through menopause, the treatment of choice for osteoporosis has been **hormone replacement therapy** (HRT), also called estrogen replacement therapy. Many women choose HRT when they undergo menopause to alleviate symptoms such as hot flashes, but hormones increase a woman's supply of estrogen, which helps build new bone, while preventing further bone loss. A 2002 report from a large clinical trial called the Women's Health Initiative helped verify HRT's positive effects in preventing osteoporosis in postmenopausal women.

However, the WHI also revealed several risks with taking combined HRT (estrogen and progesterone). In fact, the trial was stopped early because the incidence of invasive **breast cancer** in women on HRT passed a threshold that was considered too risky for the benefits they were receiving. The study also found that the women on combined hormone therapy were at increased risk for coronary heart disease and **stroke**. Whether or not a woman takes hormones and for how long is a decision she should make carefully with her doctor. Women should talk to their doctors about personal risks for osteoporosis, as well as their risks for heart disease and breast **cancer**.

Since estrogen may no longer be recommended for prevention of osteoporosis, selective use of alendronate and calcitonin are possible alternatives. Alendronate and calcitonin both stop bone loss, help build bone, and decrease fracture risk by as much as 50%. Alendronate (sold under the name Fosamax) is the first nonhormonal medication for osteoporosis ever approved by the FDA. It attaches itself to bone that has been targeted by bone-eating osteoclasts, protecting the bone from these cells. Osteoclasts help the body break down old bone tissue.

Calcitonin is a hormone that has been used as an injection for many years. A new version is on the market as a nasal spray. It too slows down bone-eating osteoclasts.

Side effects of these drugs are minimal, but calcitonin builds bone by only 1.5% a year, which may not be enough for some women to recover the bone they lose. Fosamax has proven safe in large, multi-year studies, but not much is known about the effects of

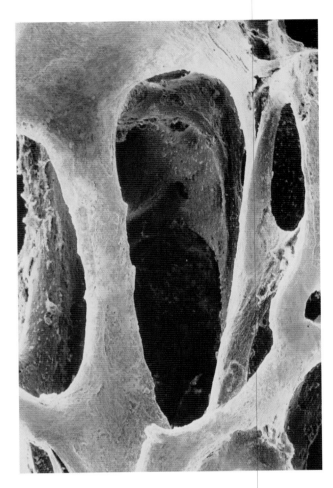

A scanning electron microscopy (SEM) image of cancellous (spongy) bone from an osteoporosis patient. Osteoporosis is characterized by increased brittleness of the bones and a greater risk of fractures. This is reflected here in the thin appearance of the bony network of the cancellous bone that forms the core of the body's long bones. (Photograph by Professor P. Motta, Photo Researchers, Inc. Reproduced by permission.)

its long-term use. Several medications under study include other bisphosphonates that slow bone breakdown (like alendronate), sodium fluoride, vitamin D metabolites, and selective estrogen receptor modulators. Some of these treatments are already being used in other countries, but have not yet been approved by the FDA for use in the United States.

In early 2003, a report announced that the FDA had recently approved the first drug that could form bone in osteoporosis patients. The drug is a form of the human parathyroid hormone called teriparatide. It shows promise for those patients at highest risk for fracture from the disease. There are some patients who cannot use the drug, so all considering the new treatment must check with their physician and may need to undergo bone densitometry scans or other testing.

Surgery

Unfortunately, much of the treatment for osteoporosis is for fractures that result from advanced stages of the disease. For complicated fractures, such as broken hips, hospitalization and a surgical procedure are required. In hip replacement surgery, the broken hip is removed and replaced with a new hip made of plastic, or metal and plastic. Though the surgery itself is usually successful, complications of the hip fracture can be serious. Those individuals have a 5–20% greater risk of dying within the first year following the injury than do others in their age group. A large percentage of those who survive are unable to return to their previous level of activity, and many move self-care to a supervised living situation or nursing home. That is why getting early treatment and taking steps to reduce bone loss are vital.

Alternative treatment

Alternative treatments for osteoporosis focus on maintaining or building strong bones. A healthy diet low in fats and animal products and containing whole grains, fresh fruits and vegetables, and calcium-rich foods (such as dairy products, dark-green leafy vegetables, sardines, salmon, and almonds), along with **nutritional supplements** (such as calcium, magnesium, and vitamin D), and weight-bearing exercises are important components of both conventional prevention and treatment strategies and alternative approaches to the disease. In addition, alternative practitioners recommend a variety of botanical medicines or herbal supplements. Herbal supplements designed to help slow bone loss emphasize the use of calcium-containing plants, such as horsetail (*Equisetum arvense*), oat straw (*Avena sativa*), alfalfa (*Medicago sativa*), licorice (*Glycyrrhiza galbra*), marsh mallow (*Althaea officinalis*), and yellow dock (*Rumex crispus*). Homeopathic remedies focus on treatments believed to help the body absorb calcium. These remedies are likely to include such substances as *Calcarea carbonica* (calcium carbonate) or silica. In **traditional Chinese medicine**, practitioners recommend herbs thought to slow or prevent bone loss, including dong quai (*Angelica sinensis*) and Asian ginseng (*Panax ginseng*). Natural hormone therapy, using plant estrogens (from soybeans) or progesterone (from wild yams), may be recommended for women who cannot or choose not to take synthetic hormones.

Prognosis

There is no cure for osteoporosis, but it can be controlled. Most people who have osteoporosis fare well once they receive treatment. The medicines available now build bone, protect against bone loss, and halt the progress of this disease.

Prevention

Building strong bones, especially before the age of 35, and maintaining a healthy lifestyle are the best ways to prevent osteoporosis. To build as much bone mass as early as possible in life, and to help slow the rate of bone loss later in life, doctors advise:

Getting calcium from foods

Experts recommend 1,500 milligrams (mg) of calcium per day for adolescents, pregnant or breast-feeding women, older adults (over 65), and post-menopausal women not using hormone replacement therapy. All others should get 1,000 mg per day. Foods are the best source for this important mineral. Milk, cheese, and yogurt have the highest amounts. Other foods that are high in calcium are green leafy vegetables, tofu, shellfish, Brazil nuts, sardines, and almonds.

Taking calcium supplements

Many people, especially those who do not like or can not eat dairy foods, do not get enough calcium in their **diets** and may need calcium supplements. Supplements vary in the amount of calcium they contain. Those with calcium carbonate have the most amount of useful calcium. Supplements should be taken with meals and accompanied by six to eight glasses of water a day.

Getting vitamin D

Vitamin D helps the body absorb calcium. People can get vitamin D from sunshine with a quick (15–20 minute) walk each day or from foods such as liver, fish oil, and vitamin-D fortified milk. During the winter months it may be necessary to take supplements. Four hundred mg daily is usually the recommended amount.

Avoiding smoking and alcohol

Smoking reduces bone mass, as does heavy drinking. Avoiding smoking and limiting alcoholic drinks to no more than two per day reduces risks. An alcoholic drink is one-and-a-half ounces of hard liquor, 12 ounces of beer, or five ounces of wine.

KEY TERMS

Alendronate—A nonhormonal drug used to treat osteoporosis in postmenopausal women.

Anticonvulsants—Drugs used to control seizures, such as in epilepsy.

Biphosphonates—Compounds (like alendronate) that slow bone loss and increase bone density.

Calcitonin—A hormonal drug used to treat post-menopausal osteoporosis

Estrogen—A female hormone that also keeps bones strong. After menopause, a woman may take hormonal drugs with estrogen to prevent bone loss.

Glucocorticoids—Any of a group of hormones (like cortisone) that influence many body functions and are widely used in medicine, such as for treatment of rheumatoid arthritis inflammation.

Hormone replacement therapy (HRT)—Also called estrogen replacement therapy, this controversial treatment is used to relieve the discomforts of menopause. Estrogen and another female hormone, progesterone, are usually taken together to replace the estrogen no longer made by the body.

Menopause—The ending of a woman's menstrual cycle, when production of bone-protecting estrogen decreases.

Osteoblasts—Cells in the body that build new bone tissue.

Osteoclasts—Cells that break down and remove old bone tissue.

Selective estrogen receptor modulator—A hormonal preparation that offers the beneficial effects of hormone replacement therapy without the increased risk of breast and uterine cancer associated with HRT.

Exercise

Exercising regularly builds and strengthens bones. Weight-bearing exercises—where bones and muscles work against gravity—are best. These include aerobics, dancing, jogging, stair climbing, tennis, walking, and lifting weights. People who have osteoporosis may want to attempt gentle exercise, such as walking, rather than jogging or fast-paced aerobics, which increase the chance of falling. Exercising three to four times per week for 20–30 minutes each time helps.

Resources

PERIODICALS

Doering, Paul L. "Treatment of Menopause Post-WHI: What Now?" *Drug Topics* April 21, 2003: 85.

Elliott, William T. "HRT, Estrogen, and Postmenopausal Women: Year-old WHI Study Continues to Raise Questions." *Critical Care Alert* July 2003: 1.

LoBuono, Charlotte. "New Osteoporosis Drug is First to Form Bone." *Drug Topics* January 6, 2003: 24.

"More Men at Osteoporosis Risk than Commonly Believed." *Tufts University Health and Nutrition Letter* August 2003: 8.

Nelson, Heidi D. "Postmenopausal Osteoporosis and Estrogen." *American Family Physician* August 15, 2003: 606.

"Osteoporosis Gene Identified." *Diagnostics and Imaging Week* March 13, 2003 4.

"Three Out of Four Women Currently Taking Prescriptions for Osteoporosis Are Not Receiving Full Treatment, According to Recent Data from a National Physician Audit." *Drug Cost Management Report* January 2003: 11.

Barbara Boughton
Teresa G. Odle

Osteosarcoma *see* **Sarcomas**

Ostomy

Definition

A surgical procedure creating an opening in the body for the discharge of body wastes.

Purpose

Certain diseases of the bowel or urinary tract involve removing all or part of the intestine or bladder. This creates a need for an alternate way for feces or urine to leave the body. An opening is surgically created in the abdomen for body wastes to pass through. The surgical procedure is called an ostomy. The opening that is created at the end of the bowel or ureter is called a stoma, which is pulled through the abdominal wall.

Description

Different types of ostomy are performed depending on how much and what part of the intestines or bladder is removed.

The three most common types of ostomies are:

- **colostomy**
- ileostomy
- urostomy

Colostomy

A colostomy is a when a small portion of the colon (large intestine) is brought to the surface of the abdominal wall to allow stool to be eliminated. A colostomy may be temporary or permanent. A permanent colostomy usually involves the loss of the rectum.

A colostomy might be performed due to cancer, diverticulitis, imperforate anus, **Hirschsprung's disease**, or trauma to the affected area.

Ileostomy

An ileostomy is an opening created in the small intestine to bypass the colon for stool elimination. The end of the ileum, which is the lowest part of the small intestine, is brought through the abdominal wall to form a stoma.

Ileoanal reservoir surgery is an alternative to a permanent ileostomy. It requires two surgical procedures. The first removes the colon and rectum and a temporary ileostomy is created. The second procedure creates an internal pouch from a portion of the small intestine to hold stool. This is then attached to the anus. Since the muscle of the rectum is left in place, there is control over bowel movements.

An ileostomy might be performed due to ulcerative colitis, Crohn's disease, or familial polyposis.

Urostomy

A urostomy is a surgical procedure that diverts urine away from a diseased or defective bladder. Among several methods to create the urostomy, the most common method is called an ileal or cecal conduit. Either a section at the end of the small intestine (ileum) or at the beginning of the large intestine (cecum) is relocated surgically to form a stoma for urine to pass out of the body. Other common names for this procedure are ileal loop or colon conduit.

A urostomy may be performed due to **bladder cancer**, spinal cord injuries, malfunction of the bladder, and **birth defects** such as spina bifida.

Since colostomy, ileostomy, and usotomy bypass the sphincter muscle there is no voluntary control over bowel movements and an external pouch must be worn to catch the discharge.

Preparation

Aftercare

The skin around the stoma, called the peristomal skin, must be protected from direct contact with discharge. The discharge can be irritating to the stoma since it is very high in digestive enzymes. The peristomal skin should be cleansed with plain soap and rinsed with water at each change of the pouch.

The stoma can change in size due to weight gain/loss or several other situations. To ensure proper fit of discharge pouch the stoma should be measured each time supplies are purchased.

Risks

People with ostomies can be prone to certain types of skin infections. Skin irritations or rashes around the stoma may be caused by leakage from around the pouch due to an improperly fitted pouch. Correctly fitting the pouch and carefully cleaning the skin around the stoma after each change are the best ways of preventing skin irritation.

Urinary tract infections are common among people who have urostomies. Preventative measures include drinking plenty of fluids, emptying the pouch regularly and using a pouch with an anti-reflux valve to prohibit the discharge from moving back into the stoma.

Normal results

Most ostomy pouches are inconspicuous and can be worn under almost any kind of clothing. There are typically no restrictions of activity, sport, or travel with an ostomy. Certain contact sports would warrant special protection for the stoma.

After recovery from surgery, most people with ostomies can resume a balanced diet.

Ostomy surgery does not generally interfere with a person's sexual or reproductive capacities.

Abnormal results

After an ileostomy, water and electrolyte loss may occur. It may be necessary to drink a significant amount of fluid or fruit juice each day to prevent **dehydration**.

After any type of ostomy surgery digestion and absorbtion of medications may also be affected.

High-fiber foods can cause blockages in the ileum, especially after surgery. Chewing food well helps

KEY TERMS

Crohn's disease—A chronic inflammatory disease, primarily involving the small and large intestine, but which can affect other parts of the digestive system as well.

Diverticulitis—Inflammation of the diverticula (small outpouchings) along the wall of the colon, the large intestine.

Familial polyposis—An inherited condition in which several hundred polyps develop in the colon and rectum.

Hirschsprung disease—Hirschsprung disease is a congenital abnormality (birth defect) of the bowel in which there is absence of the ganglia (nerves) in the wall of the bowel. Nerves are missing starting at the anus and extending a variable distance up the bowel. This results in megacolon (massive enlargement of the bowel) above the point where the nerves are missing. (The nerves are needed to assist in the natural movement of the muscles in the lining of the bowels that move bowel contents through.)

Ileum—The lowest part of the small intestine, located beyond the duodenum and jejunum, just before the large intestine (the colon).

Imperforate anus—A congenital malformation (a birth defect) in which the rectum is a blind alley (a cul-de-sac) and there is no anus.

Spina bifida—A birth defect (a congenital malformation) in which there is a bony defect in the vertebral column so that part of the spinal cord, which is normally protected within the vertebral column, is exposed. People with spina bifida can suffer from bladder and bowel incontinence, cognitive (learning) problems and limited mobility.

break fiber into smaller pieces and makes it less likely to accumulate at a narrow point in the bowel. Drinking plenty of fluids can also help.

Resources

ORGANIZATIONS

Crohn's & Colitis Foundation of America, Inc. 386 Park Avenue South 17th Floor, New York, NY 10016-8804. (800) 932-2423 or (212) 685-3440.

International Foundation for Functional Gastrointestinal Disorders. P.O. Box 17864, Milwaukee, WI 53217. (414) 964-1799.

National Digestive Diseases Clearinghouse. 2 Information Way, Bethesda, MD 20892-3570. < http://www.niddk.nih.gov/ >.

United Ostomy Association. 19772 MacArthur Boulevard, Suite 200 Irvine, CA 92612-2405. (800) 826-0826 or (949) 660-8624.

Gary Gilles

Otitis externa

Definition

Otitis externa refers to an infection of the ear canal, the tube leading from the outside opening of the ear in towards the ear drum.

Description

The external ear canal is a tube approximately 1 in (2.5 cm) in length. It runs from the outside opening of the ear to the start of the middle ear, designated by the ear drum or tympanic membrane. The canal is partly cartilage and partly bone. In early childhood, the first two-thirds of the canal is made of cartilage, and the last one-third is made of bone. By late childhood, and lasting throughout all of adulthood, this proportion is reversed, so that the first one-third is cartilage, and the last two-thirds is bone. The lining of the ear canal is skin, which is attached directly to the covering of the bone. Glands within the skin of the canal produce a waxy substance called cerumen (popularly called earwax). Cerumen is designed to protect the ear canal, repel water, and keep the ear canal too acidic to allow bacteria to grow.

Causes and symptoms

Bacteria, fungi, and viruses have all been implicated in causing ear infections called otitis externa. The most common cause of otitis externa is bacterial infection. The usual offenders include *Pseudomonas aeruginosa*, *Enterobacter aerogenes*, *Proteus mirabilis*, *Klebsiella pneumoniae*, *Staphylococcus epidermidis*, and bacteria of the family called Streptococci. Occasionally, fungi may cause otitis externa. These include *Candida* and *Aspergillus*. Two types of viruses, called herpesvirus hominis and varicella-zoster virus, have also been identified as causing otitis externa.

Otitis externa occurs most often in the summer months, when people are frequenting swimming pools and lakes. Continually exposing the ear canal to moisture may cause significant loss of cerumen. The delicate skin of the ear canal, unprotected by cerumen, retains moisture and becomes irritated. Without cerumen, the ear canal stops being appropriately acidic, which allows bacteria the opportunity to multiply. Thus, the warm, moist, dark environment of the ear canal becomes a breeding ground for bacteria.

Other conditions predisposing to otitis externa include the use of cotton swabs to clean the ear canals. This pushes cerumen and normal skin debris back into the ear canal, instead of allowing the ear canal's normal cleaning mechanism to work, which would ordinarily move accumulations of cerumen and debris out of the ear. Also, putting other items into the ear can scratch the canal, making it more susceptible to infection.

The first symptom of otitis externa is often **itching** of the ear canal. Eventually, the ear begins to feel extremely painful. Any touch, movement, or pressure on the outside structure of the ear (auricle) may cause quite severe **pain**. This is because of the way in which the skin lining the ear canal is directly attached to the covering of the underlying bone. If the canal is sufficiently swollen, hearing may become muffled. The canal may appear swollen and red, and there may be evidence of greenish-yellow pus.

In severe cases, otitis externa may have an accompanying **fever**. Often, this indicates that the outside ear structure (auricle) has become infected as well. It will become red and swollen, and there may be enlarged and tender lymph nodes in front of, or behind, the auricle.

A serious and life-threatening otitis externa is called malignant otitis externa. This is an infection which most commonly affects patients who have diabetes, especially the elderly. It can also occur in other patients who have weakened immune systems. In malignant otitis externa, a patient has usually had minor symptoms of otitis externa for some months, with pain and drainage. The causative bacteria is usually *Pseudomonas aeruginosa*. In malignant otitis externa, this bacteria spreads from the external canal into all of the nearby tissues, including the bones of the skull. Swelling and destruction of these tissues may lead to damage of certain nerves, resulting in spasms of the jaw muscles or paralysis of the facial muscles. Other, more severe, complications of this very destructive infection include meningitis (swelling and infection of the coverings of the spinal cord and brain), brain infection, or **brain abscess** (the development of a pocket of infection with pus).

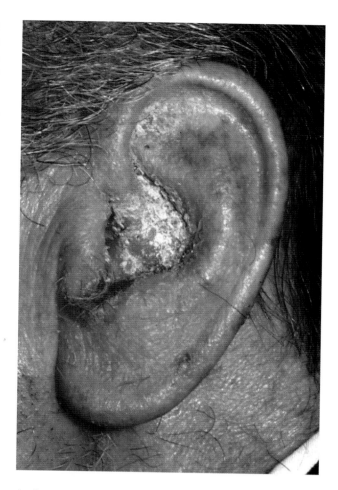

A close-up image of the ear of an elderly man suffering from non-infectious otitis externa. The skin in the ear canal and outer ear is scaly. *(Photograph by Dr. P. Marazzi, Custom Medical Stock Photo. Reproduced by permission.)*

Diagnosis

Diagnosis of uncomplicated otitis externa is usually quite simple. The symptoms alone, of ear pain worsened by any touch to the auricle, are characteristic of otitis externa. Attempts to examine the ear canal will usually reveal redness and swelling. It may be impossible (due to pain and swelling) to see much of the ear canal, but this inability itself is diagnostic.

If there is any confusion about the types of organisms causing otitis externa, the canal can be gently swabbed to obtain a specimen. The organisms present in the specimen can then be cultured (allowed to multiply) in a laboratory, and then viewed under a microscope to allow identification of the causative organisms.

If the rare disease malignant otitis externa is suspected, **computed tomography scan** (CT scan) or magnetic resonance imaging (MRI) scans will be performed to determine how widely the infection has spread within bone and tissue. A swab of the external canal will not necessarily reveal the actual causative organism, so some other tissue sample (biopsy) will need to be obtained. The CT or MRI will help the practitioner decide where the most severe focus of infection is located, in order to guide the choice of a biopsy site.

Treatment

Antibiotics which can be applied directly to the skin of the ear canal (**topical antibiotics**) are usually excellent for treatment of otitis externa. These are often combined in a preparation which includes a steroid medication. The steroid helps cut down on the inflammation and swelling within the ear canal. Some practitioners prefer to insert a cotton wick into the ear canal, leaving it there for about 48 hours. The medications are applied directly to the wick, enough times per day to allow the wick to remain continuously saturated. After the wick is removed, the medications are then put directly into the ear canal three to four times each day.

In malignant otitis externa, antibiotics will almost always need to be given through a needle in the vein (intravenously or IV). If the CT or MRI scan reveals that the infection has spread extensively, these IV antibiotics will need to be continued for six to eight weeks. If the infection is in an earlier stage, two weeks of IV antibiotics can be followed by six weeks of antibiotics by mouth.

Prognosis

The prognosis is excellent for otitis externa. It is usually easily treated, although it may tend to recur in certain susceptible individuals. Left untreated, malignant otitis externa may spread sufficiently to cause **death**.

Prevention

Keeping the ear dry is an important aspect of prevention of otitis externa. Several drops of a mixture of alcohol and acetic acid can be put into the ear canal after swimming to insure that it dries adequately.

The most serious complications of malignant otitis externa can be avoided by careful attention to early symptoms of ear pain and drainage from the ear canal. Patients with conditions that put them at higher risk for this infection (diabetes, conditions

KEY TERMS

Auricle—The external structure of the ear.

Biopsy—The removal and examination, usually under a microscope, of tissue from the living body. Used for diagnosis.

Cerumen—Earwax.

which weakened the immune system) should always report new symptoms immediately.

Resources

ORGANIZATIONS

American Academy of Otolaryngology-Head and Neck Surgery, Inc. One Prince St., Alexandria VA 22314-3357. (703) 836-4444. < http://www.entnet.org >.

Rosalyn Carson-DeWitt, MD

Otitis media

Definition

Otitis media is an infection of the middle ear space, behind the eardrum (tympanic membrane). It is characterized by **pain**, **dizziness**, and partial loss of hearing.

Description

A little knowledge of the basic anatomy of the middle ear will be helpful for understanding the development of otitis media. The external ear canal is that tube which leads from the outside opening of the ear to the structure called the tympanic membrane. Behind the tympanic membrane is the space called the middle ear. Within the middle ear are three tiny bones, called ossicles. Sound (in the form of vibration) causes movement in the eardrum, and then the ossicles. The ossicles transmit the sound to a structure within the inner ear, which sends it to the brain for processing.

The nasopharynx is that passageway behind the nose which takes inhaled air into the breathing tubes leading to the lungs. The eustachian tube is a canal which runs between the middle ear and the nasopharynx. One of the functions of the eustachian tube is to keep the air pressure in the middle ear equal to that outside. This allows the eardrum and ossicles to vibrate appropriately, so that hearing is normal.

By age three, almost 85% of all children will have had otitis media at least once. Babies and children between the ages of six months and six years are most likely to develop otitis media. Children at higher risk factors for otitis media include boys, children from poor families, Native Americans, Native Alaskans, children born with **cleft palate** or other defects of the structures of the head and face, and children with **Down syndrome**. Exposure to cigarette smoke significantly increases the risk of otitis media as well as other problems affecting the respiratory system. Also, children who enter daycare at an early age have more upper respiratory infections (URIs or colds), and thus more cases of otitis media. The most usual times of year for otitis media to strike are in winter and early spring (the same times URIs are most common).

Otitis media is an important problem, because it often results in fluid accumulation within the middle ear (effusion). The effusion can last for weeks to months. Effusion within the middle ear can cause significant hearing impairment. When such hearing impairment occurs in a young child, it may interfere with the development of normal speech.

In adults, acute otitis media can lead to such complications as **paralysis** of the facial nerves. Recovery from these complications may take from two weeks to as long as three months.

Causes and symptoms

The first precondition for the development of acute otitis media is exposure to an organism capable of causing the infection. Otitis media can be caused by either viruses or bacteria. Virus infections account for about 15% of cases. The three most common bacterial pathogens are *Streptococcus pneumoniae*, *Haemophilus influenzae*, or *Moraxella catarrhalis*. As of 2003, about 75% of ear infections caused by *S. pneumoniae* are reported to be penicillin-resistant.

Otitis media may also be caused by other disease organisms, including *Bordetella pertussis*, the causative agent of **whooping cough**, and *Pneumocystis carinii*, which often causes opportunistic infections in patients with **AIDS**.

There are other factors which make the development of an ear infection more likely. Because the eustachian tube has a more horizontal orientation and is considerably shorter in early childhood, material from the nasopharynx (including infection-causing

organisms) is better able to reach the middle ear. Children also have a lot of lymph tissue (commonly called the adenoids) in the area of the eustachian tube. These adenoids may enlarge with repeated respiratory tract infections (colds), ultimately blocking the eustachian tubes. When the eustachian tube is blocked, the middle ear is more likely to fill with fluid. This fluid, then, increases the risk of infection, and the risk of **hearing loss** and delayed speech development.

Most cases of acute otitis media occur during the course of a URI. Symptoms include fever, ear pain, and problems with hearing. Babies may have difficulty feeding. When significant fluid is present within the middle ear, pain may increase depending on position. Lying down may cause an increase in painful pressure within the middle ear, so that babies may fuss if not held upright. If the fluid build-up behind the eardrum is sufficient, the eardrum may develop a hole (perforate), causing bloody fluid or greenish-yellow pus to drip from the ear. Although pain may be significant leading up to such a perforation, the pain is usually relieved by the reduction of pressure brought on by a perforation.

Recent advances in gene mapping have led to the discovery of genetic factors that increase a child's susceptibility to otitis media. Researchers are hoping to develop molecular diagnostic assays that will help to identify children at risk for severe ear infections.

Diagnosis

Diagnosis is usually made simply by looking at the eardrum through a special lighted instrument called an otoscope. The eardrum will appear red and swollen, and may appear either abnormally drawn inward, or bulging outward. Under normal conditions, the ossicles create a particular pattern on the eardrum, referred to as "landmarks." These landmarks may be obscured. Normally, the light from the otoscope reflects off of the eardrum in a characteristic fashion. This is called the "cone of light." In an infection, this cone of light may be shifted or absent.

A special attachment to the otoscope allows a puff of air to be blown lightly into the ear. Normally, this should cause movement of the eardrum. In an infection, or when there is fluid behind the eardrum, this movement may be decreased or absent.

If fluid or pus is draining from the ear, it can be collected. This sample can then be processed in a laboratory to allow any organisms present to multiply sufficiently (cultured) to permit the organisms to be viewed under a microscope and identified.

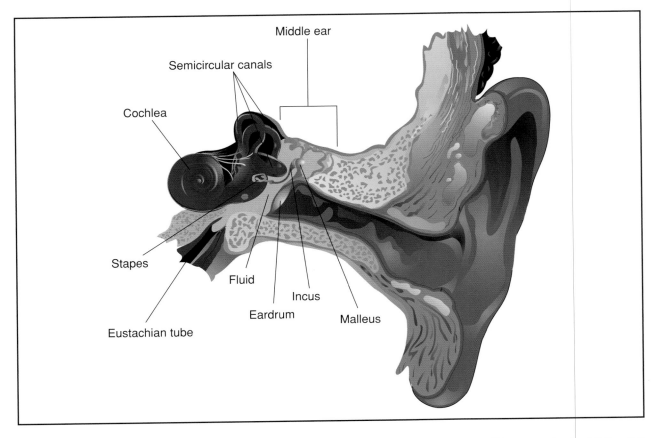

Otitis media is an ear infection in which fluid accumulates within the middle ear. A common condition occurring in childhood, it is estimated that 85% of all American children will develop otitis media at least once. *(Illustration by Electronic Illustrators Group.)*

Treatment

Medications

Antibiotics are the treatment of choice for acute otitis media (AOM). Different antibiotics are used depending on the type of bacteria most likely to be causing the infection. This decision involves knowledge of the types of antibiotics that have worked on other ear infections occurring within a particular community at a particular time. Options include sulfa-based antibiotics, as well as a variety of **penicillins**, **cephalosporins**, and others. The patient's sensitivity to certain medications, as well as previously demonstrated resistant strains, also contributes to the choice of antibiotic. As of 2003, an 0.3% topical solution of ofloxacin has been recommended as a more effective medication than other oral or **topical antibiotics**.

Some controversy exists regarding whether overuse of antibiotics is actually contributing to the development of bacteria, which may evolve and become able to avoid being killed by antibiotics. Research is being done to try to help determine whether there may be some ear infections that will clear up without antibiotic treatment. In the meantime, the classic treatment of an ear infection continues to involve a seven to 10-day course of antibiotic medication.

Some medical practitioners prescribe the use of special nosedrops, **decongestants**, or **antihistamines** to improve the functioning of the eustachian tube.

Whether or not antibiotics are used, such pain relievers as Tylenol or Motrin can be very helpful in reducing the pain and inflammation associated with otitis media.

Surgery

In a few rare cases, a surgical perforation to drain the middle ear of pus may be performed. This procedure is called a **myringotomy**. The hole created by the myringotomy generally heals itself in about a week.

In 2002 a new minimally invasive procedure was introduced that uses a laser to perform the myringotomy. It can be performed in the doctor's office and heals more rapidly than the standard myringotomy.

Although some doctors have recommended removing the adenoids to prevent recurrent otitis media in young children, recent studies indicate that surgical removal of the adenoids does not appear to offer any advantages over a myringotomy as a preventive measure.

Alternative treatment

Some practitioners believe that **food allergies** may increase the risk of ear infections, and they suggest eliminating suspected food allergens from the diet. The top food allergens are wheat, dairy products, corn, peanuts, citrus fruits, and eggs. Elimination of sugar and sugar products can allow the immune system to work more effectively. A number of herbal treatments have been recommended, including ear drops made with goldenseal (*Hydrastis canadensis*), mullein (*Verbascum thapsus*), **St. John's wort** (*Hypericum perforatum*), and echinacea (*Echinacea* spp.). Among the herbs often recommended for oral treatment of otitis media are **echinacea** and cleavers (*Galium aparine*), or black cohosh (*Cimicifuga racemosa*) and ginkgo (*Ginkgo biloba*). Homeopathic remedies that may be prescribed include aconite (*Acontium napellus*), *Ferrum phosphoricum,* belladonna, chamomile, *Lycopodium,* pulsatilla (*Pulsatilla nigricans*), or silica. **Craniosacral therapy** uses gentle manipulation of the bones of the skull to relieve pressure and improve eustachian tube function.

Prognosis

With treatment, the prognosis for acute otitis media is very good. However, long-lasting accumulations of fluid within the middle ear are a risk both for difficulties with hearing and speech, and for the repeated development of ear infections. Furthermore, without treatment, otitis media can lead to an infection within the nearby mastoid bone, called **mastoiditis**.

Prevention

Although otitis media seems somewhat inevitable in childhood, some measures can be taken to decrease the chance of repeated infections and fluid accumulation. Breastfeeding provides some protection against URIs, which in turn protects against the development of otitis media. If a child is bottle-fed, parents should be advised to feed him or her upright, rather than allowing the baby to lie down with the bottle. General good hygiene practices (especially handwashing) help to decrease the number of upper respiratory infections in a household or daycare center.

The use of pacifiers should be avoided or limited. They may act as fomites, particularly in a daycare setting. In children who are more susceptible to otitis media, pacifier use can increase by as much as 50% the number of ear infections experienced.

Two vaccines can prevent otitis media associated with certain strains of bacteria. One is designed to prevent **meningitis** and other diseases, including otitis media, that result from infection with *Haemophilus influenzae* type B. Another is a vaccine against *Streptococcus pneumoniae*, a very common cause of otitis media. Children who are at high risk or have had severe or chronic infections may be good candidates for these vaccines; in fact, a recent consensus report among pediatricians recommended routine administration of the pneumococcal conjugate vaccine to children younger than two years, as well as those at high risk for AOM. Parents should consult a health care provider concerning the advisability of this treatment.

Another vaccine that appears to lower the risk of AOM in children is the intranasal vaccine that was recently introduced for preventing **influenza**. Although the flu vaccine was not developed to prevent AOM directly, one team of researchers found that children who were given the vaccine before the start of flu season were 43% less likely to develop AOM than children who were not vaccinated.

As of early 2003, there is no vaccine effective against *M. catarrhalis*. Researchers are working on developing such a vaccine, as well as a tribacterial vaccine that would be effective against all three pathogens that commonly cause otitis media.

A nutrition-based approach to preventive treatment is undergoing clinical trials as of late 2002. This treatment involves giving children a dietary supplement of lemon-flavored cod liver oil plus a multivitamin formula containing selenium. The pilot study found that children receiving the supplement had fewer cases of otitis media, and that those who did develop it recovered with a shorter course of antibiotic treatment than children who were not receiving the supplement.

After a child has completed treatment for otitis media, a return visit to the practitioner should be scheduled. This visit should occur after the

KEY TERMS

Adenoid—A collection of lymph tissue located in the nasopharynx.

Effusion—A collection of fluid which has leaked out into some body cavity or tissue.

Eustachian tube—A small tube which runs between the middle ear space and the nasopharynx.

Fomite—An inanimate object that can transmit infectious organisms.

Myringotomy—A surgical procedure performed to drain an infected middle ear. A newer type of myringotomy uses a laser instead of a scalpel.

Nasopharynx—The part of the airway into which the nose leads.

Ossicles—Tiny bones located within the middle ear which are responsible for conveying the vibrations of sound through to the inner ear.

Perforation—A hole.

Topical—Referring to a medication applied to the skin or outward surface of the body. Ear drops are one type of topical medication.

antibiotic has been completed, and allows the practitioner to evaluate the patient for the persistent presence of fluid within the middle ear. In children who have a problem with recurrent otitis media, a small daily dose of an antibiotic may prevent repeated full attacks of otitis media. In children who have persistent fluid, a procedure to place tiny tubes within the eardrum may help equalize pressure between the middle ear and the outside, thus preventing further fluid accumulation.

Resources

BOOKS

Pelletier, Kenneth R., MD. *The Best Alternative Medicine, Part I: Chiropractic and Osteopathy.* New York: Simon & Schuster, 2002.

PERIODICALS

Abes, G., N. Espallardo, M. Tong, et al. "A Systematic Review of the Effectiveness of Ofloxacin Otic Solution for the Treatment of Suppurative Otitis Media." *ORL* 65 (March-April 2003): 106–116.

Bucknam, J. A., and P. C. Weber. "Laser Assisted Myringotomy for Otitis Media with Effusion in Children." *ORL-Head and Neck Nursing* 20 (Summer 2002): 11-13.

Cripps, A. W., and J. Kyd. "Bacterial Otitis Media: Current Vaccine Development Strategies." *Immunology and Cell Biology* 81 (February 2003): 46–51.

Decherd, M. E., R. W. Deskin, J. L. Rowen, and M. B. Brindley. "*Bordetella pertussis* Causing Otitis Media: A Case Report." *Laryngoscope* 113 (February 2003): 226–227.

Goodwin, J. H., and J. C. Post. "The Genetics of Otitis Media." *Current Allergy and Asthma Reports* 2 (July 2002): 304-308.

Hoberman, A., C. D. Marchant, S. L. Kaplan, and S. Feldman. "Treatment of Acute Otitis Media Consensus Recommendations." *Clinical Pediatrics* 41 (July-August 2002): 373-390.

Linday, L. A., J. N. Dolitsky, R. D. Shindledecker, and C. E. Pippinger. "Lemon-Flavored Cod Liver Oil and a Multivitamin-Mineral Supplement for the Secondary Prevention of Otitis Media in Young Children: Pilot Research." *Annals of Otology, Rhinology, and Laryngology* 111 (July 2002): 642-652.

Marchisio, P., R. Cavagna, B. Maspes, et al. "Efficacy of Intranasal Virosomal Influenza Vaccine in the Prevention of Recurrent Acute Otitis Media in Children." *Clinical Infectious Diseases* 35 (July 15, 2002): 168-174.

Mattila, P. S., V. P. Joki-Erkkila, T. Kilpi, et al. "Prevention of Otitis Media by Adenoidectomy in Children Younger Than 2 Years." *Archives of Otolaryngology— Head and Neck Surgery* 129 (February 2003): 163–168.

Menger, D. J., and R. G. van den Berg. "*Pneumocystis carinii* Infection of the Middle Ear and External Auditory Canal. Report of a Case and Review of the Literature." *ORL* 65 (January-February 2003): 49–51.

Redaelli de Zinis, L. O., P. Gamba, and C. Balzanelli. "Acute Otitis Media and Facial Nerve Paralysis in Adults." *Otology and Neurotology* 24 (January 2003): 113–117.

Weiner, R., and P. J. Collison. "Middle Ear Pathogens in Otitis-Prone Children." *South Dakota Journal of Medicine* 56 (March 2003): 103–107.

ORGANIZATIONS

American Academy of Otolaryngology, Head and Neck Surgery, Inc. One Prince Street, Alexandria, VA 22314-3357. (703) 836-4444.

American Academy of Pediatrics (AAP). 141 Northwest Point Boulevard, Elk Grove Village, IL 60007. (847) 434-4000. <www.aap.org>.

American Osteopathic Association (AOA). 142 East Ontario Street, Chicago, IL 60611. (800) 621- 1773. <www.aoa-net.org>.

Rosalyn Carson-DeWitt, MD
Rebecca J. Frey, PhD

Otosclerosis

Definition

Otosclerosis is an excessive growth in the bones of the middle ear which interferes with the transmission of sound.

Description

The middle ear consists of the eardrum and a chamber which contains three bones called the hammer, the anvil, and the stirrup (or stapes). Sound waves passing through the ear cause the ear drum to vibrate. This vibration is transmitted to the inner ear by the three bones. In the inner ear, the vibrations are changed into impulses which are carried by the nerves, to the brain. If excessive bone growth interferes with the stapes ability to vibrate and transmit sound waves, hearing loss will result.

Otosclerosis is classified as a conductive disorder because it involves the bones of the ear, which conduct the sound to the nerve. If a person has **hearing loss** classified as neural, the nerve conducting the impulses to the brain is involved.

Otosclerosis is a common hereditary condition. About 10% of the caucasion population has some form of otosclerosis, however, it is rare among other ethnic backgrounds. Women are more likely than men to suffer from otosclerosis. It is the most common cause of conductive hearing loss between the ages of 15–50, but if the bony growth affects only the hammer or anvil, there are no symptoms and the condition goes undetected. Disease affecting the stapes is also associated with progressive hearing loss.

Causes and symptoms

Otosclerosis is hereditary. Acquired illness and accidents have no relationship to its development.

The primary symptom of otosclerosis is loss of hearing. In addition, many people experience **tinnitus** (noice originating inside the ear). The amount of tinnitus is not necessarily related to the kind or severity of hearing loss.

Diagnosis

Hearing loss due to otosclerosis is usually first noticed in the late teens or early twenties. Hearing loss usually occurs in the low frequencies first, followed by high frequencies, then middle frequencies. Extensive hearing tests will confirm the diagnosis.

Treatment

People with otosclerosis often benefit from a properly fitted hearing aid.

The surgical replacement of the stapes has become a common procedure to improve conductive hearing problems. During this operation, called a **stapedectomy**, the stapes is removed and replaced with an artificial device. The operation is performed under **local anesthesia** and is usually an outpatient procedure. Surgery is done on only one ear at a time, with a one year wait between procedures. The degree of hearing improvement reaches its maximum about four months after the surgery. Over 80% of these procedures successfully improve or restore hearing.

Prognosis

People with otosclerosis almost never become totally deaf, and will usually be able to hear with a hearing aid or with surgery plus a hearing aid. In older people, the tendency for additional hearing loss is diminished due to the hardening of the bones.

Prevention

Otosclerosis cannot be prevented.

Resources

ORGANIZATIONS

American Tinnitus Association. P.O. Box 5, Portland, OR 97207. (503) 248-9985. < tinnitus@ata.org >.

National Association of the Deaf. 814 Thayer Ave., Silver Spring, MD, 20910. (301) 587-1788. < http:// nad.policy.net >.

NIDCD Hereditary Hearing Impairment Resource Registry. c/o Boys Town National Research Hospital. 555 N. 30th St., Omaha NE 68131. (800) 320-1171.

Self Help for Hard of Hearing People, Inc. 7800 Wisconsin Ave., Bethesda, MD 20814. (301) 657-2248. < http://www.shhh.org >.

Dorothy Elinor Stonely

Otoscopic examination *see* **Ear exam with an otoscope**

Ototoxicity

Definition

Ototoxicity is damage to the hearing or balance functions of the ear by drugs or chemicals.

Description

Ototoxicity is drug or chemical damage to the inner ear. This section of the ear contains both the hearing mechanism and the vestibulocochlear nerve, the nerve that sends hearing and balance information to the brain. Because of this, ototoxic drugs may cause lack of hearing, and loss of sense of balance.

The extent of ototoxicity varies with the drug, the dose, and other conditions. In some cases, there is full recovery after the drug has been discontinued. In other cases, the extent of damage is limited, and may even be too small to be noticed. This may occur in high-frequency **hearing loss**, where the damage to the ear makes it difficult to hear high pitched musical notes, but does not affect the ability to hear the spoken word, or carry on a conversation. In extreme cases, there may be permanent and complete deafness.

Although ototoxicity is undesirable, the ear damage can actually be used to help people with **Ménière's disease.** This is a disease of no known cause that is marked by sudden episodes of **dizziness** and vertigo. Other symptoms include a feeling of "fullness" in the ears, roaring in the ears, and ringing in the ears. While most people with this condition can be controlled with medication, about 10% require surgery. However, use of some ototoxic drugs can actually improve this condition, while causing less damage to the hearing mechanism than traditional treatments.

Causes and symptoms

Many drugs can cause ototoxicity.

Antibiotics

- amikacin (Amikin)
- streptomycin
- neomycin
- gentamicin (Garamycin)
- erythromycin (E-Mycin, Eryc)
- kanamycin (Kantrex)
- tobramycin (Nebcin)
- netilmycin (Netromycin)
- vancomycin (Vancocin)

Anti-cancer drugs

- cisplatin (Platinol AQ)
- bleomycin (Blenoxane)
- vincristine (Oncovin)

Diuretics

- acetazolamide (Diamox)
- furosemide (Lasix)
- bumetanide (Bumex)
- ethacrynic acid (Edecrine)

A number of other drugs and chemicals may also cause ototoxicity. **Aspirin** overdose causes ringing in the ears. The **antimalarial drugs** quinine and chloroquine may also cause ear damage. Among the environmental chemicals that can cause ear damage are tin, lead, mercury, carbon monoxide, and carbon disulfide. This list is not complete, and many other drugs and chemicals, such as industrial solvents, may cause ear problems.

Diagnosis

Ototoxicity often goes undiagnosed. This occurs when the hearing loss is slight, or when it is restricted to the higher frequencies. Patients may notice a change in their hearing, but it may not be significant enough to report.

In other cases, the loss of hearing may be very significant, or the ototoxicity may take the form of ringing in the ears, or other sensations.

When physicians are administering medications that are known to cause hearing loss, it is often recommended that the patient receive regular hearing tests. By monitoring hearing on a regular basis, it may be possible to discontinue the medication, or reduce the dose so that no further damage is done.

Ototoxicity that causes loss of balance may be even more difficult to diagnose. These changes may take place gradually, over time, and may be confused with the effects of the condition the drugs are meant to treat. If ototoxicity is suspected, balance tests are available, including a platform balance test, and a rotary chair. These, and other tests, determine how a patient responds to motion and changes in body position.

Treatment

There are no current treatments to reverse the effects of ototoxicity.

People who suffer permanent hearing loss may elect to use hearing aids, or, when appropriate, receive a cochlear implant. For those who have balance problems, physical therapy may often be helpful. Physical therapists can help people with balance problems learn to rely more on vision and the sensations from muscles to achieve balance.

Prognosis

The prognosis depends on the drugs that caused the ototoxicity, and their dose.

The aminoglycoside **antibiotics**, gentamicin, kanamycin, netilmycin and tobramycin all cause hearing loss to varying degrees. These drugs may be used to treat life-threatening infections that are resistant to other classes of drugs, and so there may be no choice but to use them. Careful dosing can minimize, but not eliminate the risk. It is estimated that the chances of recovery are 10-15%. The hearing loss usually begins at the higher frequencies, and is usually not recognized immediately.

Erythromycin may cause hearing loss that affects all frequencies. This hearing loss usually reverses itself over time.

Aspirin and the **non-steroidal anti-inflammatory drugs** (NSAIDS) may cause ringing in the ears (**tinnitus**). This stops when the drug is discontinued.

The **diuretics** may cause a hearing loss with a rapid onset. This will usually, but not always, reverse itself when the drugs are stopped.

In some cases, the prognosis is not really clear. Vancomycin appears to cause hearing loss, but this may only occur when vancomycin is used at the same time as other ototoxic drugs, such as gentamicin or erythromycin.

Prevention

Since most ototoxicity occurs when the harmful drugs are used in high doses, careful dose calculations are the best method of prevention. Sometimes it is possible to replace the ototoxic drugs with drugs that have less severe adverse effects.

Resources

BOOKS

Ototoxicity: Basic Science and Clinical Application. New York: New York Academy of Sciences, June 1999.

KEY TERMS

Antibiotic—Drugs that kill or inhibit the growth of bacteria.

Cochlea—A division of the inner ear.

Diuretic—A drug that increases water loss through increased urination.

Ménière's disease—A disorder of the membranous labyrinth of the inner ear that is marked by recurrent attacks of dizziness, tinnitus, and deafness—also called Ménière's syndrome. It is named after Prosper Ménière (1799–1862), a French physician who was among the first people to study diseases of the ear, nose, and throat.

Tinnitus—Ringing sounds in the ears.

ORGANIZATIONS

Deafness Research Foundation. 1225 I St. NW, No. 500, Washington, DC 20005.

Ear Research Foundation. 1901 Floyd St., Sarasota, FL 34239-2909.

National Institute on Deafness and Other Communication Disorders. NIH Bldg. 10, Rm. 5C-306 9000, Rockville Park, Bethesda, MD 20892.

Samuel D. Uretsky, PharmD

Ova & parasites collection *see* **Stool O & P test**

Ovarian cancer

Definition

Ovarian **cancer** is cancer of the ovaries, the egg-releasing and hormone-producing organs of the female reproductive tract. Cancerous, or malignant, cells divide and multiply in an abnormal fashion.

Description

The ovaries are small, almond-shaped organs, located in the pelvic region, one on either side of the uterus. When a woman is in her childbearing years, the ovaries alternate to produce and release an egg each month during the menstrual cycle. The released egg is picked up by the adjacent fallopian tube, and continues down toward the uterus. The ovaries also produce and secrete the female hormones estrogen and progesterone, which regulate the menstrual cycle and pregnancy, as well as support the development of the secondary female sexual characteristics (breasts, body shape, and body hair). During **pregnancy** and when women take certain medications, such as **oral contraceptives**, the ovaries are given a rest from their usual monthly duties.

Types of ovarian cancers

Ninety percent of all ovarian cancers develop in the cells lining the surface, or epithelium, of the ovaries and so are called epithelial cell tumors. About 15% of epithelial cancers are considered low malignant potential or LMP tumors. These tumors occur more often in younger women, and are more likely to be caught early, so prognosis is good.

Germ cell tumors develop in the egg-producing cells of the ovary, and comprise about 5% of ovarian tumors. These tumors are usually found in teenage girls or young women. The prognosis is good if found early, but as with other ovarian cancers, early detection is difficult.

Primary peritoneal carcinoma (PPC) is a cancer of the peritoneum, the lining of the abdominal cavity where the internal organs are located. Although it is a distinct disease, it is linked with ovarian cancer. This is because the ovarian and peritoneal cells have the same embryonic origin. This means that the very early cells of the embryo that will ultimately develop into the ovaries and the peritoneum share a common origin. The term "primary" means that the cancer started first in the peritoneum, as opposed to the cancer starting in the ovary and then moving, or metastasizing, into the peritoneum.

Ovarian cancer can develop at any age, but is most likely to occur in women who are 50 years or older. More than half the cases are among women who are aged 65 years and older. Industrialized countries have the highest incidence of ovarian cancer. Native American and Caucasian women, especially Caucasians of Ashkenazi Jewish descent, are at somewhat higher risk; Hispanic, African-American, and Asian women are at a slightly lower risk. The risk of developing the disease increases with age. Ovarian cancer is the fifth most common cancer among women in the United States, and the second most common gynecologic cancer. It accounts for 4% of all cancers in women. However, because of poor early detection, the **death** rate for ovarian cancer is higher than for that of any other cancer among women. About 1 in 70 women in the United States will

eventually develop ovarian cancer, and 1 in 100 will die from it. The American Cancer Society estimates that 26,000 new cases of ovarian cancer will be diagnosed in the United States in 2004, and that 16,000 women will die from the disease.

Only 50% of the women who are diagnosed with ovarian cancer will survive five years after initial diagnosis. This is due to the cancer being at an advanced stage at the time of diagnosis. With early detection, however, survival at five years post diagnosis may be 95%.

Causes and symptoms

Causes

The actual cause of ovarian cancer remains unknown, but several factors are known to increase one's chances of developing the disease. These are called risk factors. Women at a higher risk than average of developing ovarian cancer include women who:

- have never been pregnant or had children,
- are Caucasian, especially of Northern European or Ashkenazi Jewish descent,
- are over 50 (half of all diagnosed cases are in women over 65),
- have a family history of breast, ovarian, endometrial (uterine), prostate, or colon cancer,
- have had breast cancer,
- have a first-degree relative (mother, daughter, sister) who has had ovarian cancer. (The risk is greater if two or more first-degree relatives had the disease. Having a grandmother, aunt or cousin with ovarian cancer also puts a woman at higher-than-average risk.)
- have the genetic mutation BRCA1 or BRCA2. (Not all women with these genetic breast cancer mutations will develop ovarian cancer. By age 70, a woman who has the BRCA1 mutation carries about a 40–60% risk of developing ovarian cancer. Women with the genetic mutation BRCA2 have a 15% increased risk of developing ovarian cancer. However, heredity only plays a role in about 5–10% of cases of ovarian cancer.)

Women who have a strong familial history may benefit from genetic counseling to better understand their risk factors.

In addition to the above risk factors, the following factors appear to play a role in affecting a women's chances of developing ovarian cancer.

Reproduction and hormones. Early menstruation (before age 12) and late **menopause** seem to put women at a higher risk for ovarian cancer. This appears to be because the longer, or more often, a woman ovulates, the higher her risk for ovarian cancer. As mentioned above, women who were never pregnant have a higher risk of developing the disease than women with one or more pregnancies. It is not yet clear from research studies whether a pregnancy that ends in **miscarriage** or **stillbirth** lowers the risk factor to the same degree as the number of term pregnancies. The use of post-menopausal estrogen supplementation for 10 years or more may double a woman's risk of ovarian cancer. Short-term use does not seem to alter one's risk factor.

Infertility drug-stimulated ovulation. Research studies have reported mixed findings on this issue. It appears that women who take medications to stimulate ovulation, yet do not become pregnant, are at higher risk of developing ovarian cancer. Women who do become pregnant after taking fertility drugs do not appear to be at higher risk. One study reported that the use of the fertility drug clomiphene citrate for more than a year increased the risk of developing LMP tumors. LMP tumors respond better to treatment than other ovarian tumors.

Talc. The use of talcum powder in the genital area has been implicated in ovarian cancer in many studies. It may be because talc contains particles of asbestos, a known carcinogen. Female workers exposed to asbestos had a higher-than-normal risk of developing ovarian cancer. Genital deodorant sprays may also present an increased risk. Not all studies have brought consistent results.

Fat. A high-fat diet has been reported in some studies to increase the risk of developing ovarian cancer. In one study the risk level increased with every 10 grams of saturated fat added to the diet. This may be because of its effect on estrogen production.

Symptoms

Most of the literature on ovarian cancer states that there are usually no early warning symptoms for the disease. Ovarian cancer is often referred to as a silent killer, because women either are unaware of having it, or have symptoms that are not accurately diagnosed until the disease is in an advanced state. However, a November 2000 study reported in the medical journal *Cancer* analyzed more than 1,700 questionnaires completed by women with stage III and stage IV ovarian cancer. The researchers found that 95% of the women reported having had early symptoms that they brought to their doctors. Most symptoms were somewhat vague and either abdominal or gastrointestinal in nature, and consequently were either not properly diagnosed or were recognized

as being ovarian in nature only after a significant length of time had passed.

The following symptoms are warning signs of ovarian cancer, but could also be due to other causes. Symptoms that persist for two to three weeks, or symptoms that are unusual for the particular woman should be evaluated by a doctor right away.

- digestive symptoms, such as gas, **indigestion**, **constipation**, or a feeling of fullness after a light meal
- bloating, distention or cramping
- abdominal or low-back discomfort
- pelvic pressure or frequent urination
- unexplained changes in bowel habits
- **nausea** or **vomiting**
- **pain** or swelling in the abdomen
- loss of appetite
- **fatigue**
- unexplained weight gain or loss
- pain during intercourse
- vaginal bleeding in post-menopausal women

Diagnosis

In the best-case scenario a woman is diagnosed with ovarian cancer while it is still contained in just one ovary. Early detection can bring five-year survival to near 95%. Unfortunately, about 75% of women (3 out of 4) have advanced ovarian cancer at the time of diagnosis. (Advanced cancer is at stage III or stage IV when it has already spread to other organs.) Five-year survival for women with stage IV ovarian cancer may be less than 5%.

Diagnostic tests and techniques

If ovarian cancer is suspected, several of the following tests and examinations will be necessary to make a diagnosis:

- a complete medical history to assess all the risk factors
- a thorough bi-manual pelvic examination
- CA-125 assay
- one or more various imaging procedures
- a lower GI series, or **barium enema**
- diagnostic laparoscopy

BI-MANUAL PELVIC EXAMINATION. The exam should include feeling the following organs for any abnormalities in shape or size: the ovaries, fallopian tubes, uterus, vagina, bladder, and rectum. Because the ovaries are located deep within the pelvic area, it is unlikely that a manual exam will pick up an abnormality while the cancer is still localized. However, a full examination provides the practitioner with a more complete picture. An enlarged ovary does not confirm cancer, as the ovary may be large because of a cyst or **endometriosis**. While women should have an annual **Pap test**, this test screens for cervical cancer. Cancerous ovarian cells, however, might be detected on the slide. Effectiveness of using Pap smears for ovarian cancer detection is about 10-30%.

CA-125 ASSAY. This is a blood test to determine the level of CA-125, a tumor marker. A tumor marker is a measurable protein-based substance given off by the tumor. A series of CA-125 tests may be done to see if the amount of the marker in the blood is staying stable, increasing or decreasing. A rising CA-125 level usually indicates cancer, while a stable or declining value is more characteristic of a cyst. The CA-125 level should never be used alone to diagnose ovarian cancer. It is elevated in about 80% of women with ovarian cancer, but in 20% of cases is not. In addition, it could be elevated because of a non-ovarian cancer, or it can be elevated with non-malignant gynecologic conditions, such as endometriosis or **ectopic pregnancy**. During menstruation the CA-125 level may be elevated, so the test is best done when the woman is not in her menses.

IMAGING. There are several different imaging techniques used in ovarian cancer evaluation. A fluid-filled structure such as a cyst creates a different image than does a solid structure, such as a tumor. An ultrasound uses high-frequency sound waves that create a visual pattern of echoes of the structures at which they are aimed. It is painless, and is the same technique used to check the developing fetus in the womb. Ultrasound may be done externally through the abdomen and lower pelvic area, or with a transvaginal probe.

Other painless imaging techniques are computed tomography (CT) and **magnetic resonance imaging** (MRI). Color Doppler analysis provides additional contrast and accuracy in distinguishing masses. It remains unclear whether Doppler is effective in reducing the high number of false-positives with transvaginal ultrasonography. These imaging techniques allow better visualization of the internal organs and can detect abnormalities without having to perform surgery.

LOWER GI SERIES. A lower GI series, or barium enema, uses a series of x rays to highlight the colon and rectum. To provide contrast, the patient drinks a chalky liquid containing barium. This test might be done to see if the cancer had spread to these areas.

DIAGNOSTIC LAPAROSCOPY. This technique uses a thin hollow lighted instrument inserted through a small incision in the skin near the belly button to visualize the organs inside of the abdominal cavity. If the ovary is believed to be malignant, the entire ovary is removed (**oophorectomy**) and its tissue sent for evaluation to the pathologist, even though only a small piece of the tissue is needed for evaluation. If cancer is present, great care must be taken not to cause the rupture of the malignant tumor, as this would cause spreading of the cancer to adjacent organs. If the cancer is completely contained in the ovary, its removal functions also as the treatment. If the cancer has spread or is suspected to have spread, then a saline solution may be instilled into the cavity and then drawn out again. This technique is called peritoneal lavage. The aspirated fluid will be evaluated for the presence of cancer cells. If peritoneal fluid is present, called **ascites**, a sample of this will also be drawn and examined for malignant cells. If cancer cells are present in the peritoneum, then treatment will be directed at the abdominal cavity as well.

RESEARCH AND NEW DIAGNOSTIC TESTS. Many cancer researchers recognize the urgency of developing a new diagnostic test for ovarian cancer that is both sensitive and reliable. Some experts in the field look to proteomics, which is the large-scale identification and analysis of all the proteins in an organism or organ, to lead eventually to the development of a useful new test for ovarian cancer.

A group of researchers in Canada reported in 2003 that human kallikrein gene 14 (KLK14) might serve as a new biomarker for ovarian cancer. Kallikreins are a group of compounds that help to split up complex protein molecules into smaller units; prostate-specific antigen, or PSA, is a kallikrein. Early results of tests for KLK14 indicate that about 65% of women known to have ovarian cancer have elevated levels of this kallikrein.

Treatment

Clinical staging

Staging is the term used to determine if the cancer is localized or has spread, and if so, how far and to where. Staging helps define the cancer, and will determine the course of suggested treatment. Staging involves examining any tissue samples that have been taken from the ovary, nearby lymph nodes, as well as

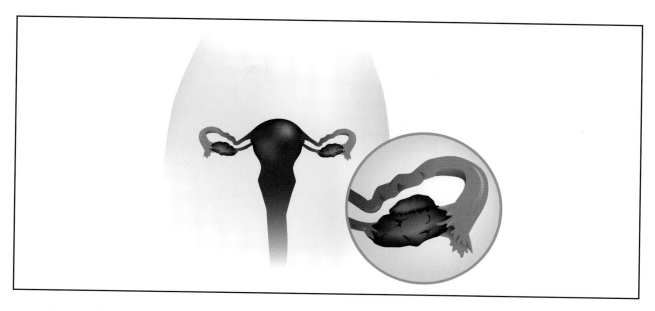

A stage I tumor of the ovary. *(Illustration by Argosy Inc.)*

from any nearby organs or structures where metastasis was suspected. This may include the diaphragm, lungs, stomach, intestines and omentum (the tissue covering internal organs), and any fluid as described above.

The National Cancer Institute Stages for ovarian cancer are:

- Stage I: Cancer is confined to one or both ovaries.

- Stage II: Cancer is found in one or both ovaries and/ or has spread to the uterus, fallopian tubes, and/or other body parts within the pelvic cavity.

- Stage III: Cancer is found in one or both ovaries and has spread to lymph nodes or other body parts within the abdominal cavity, such as the surfaces of the liver or intestines.

- Stage IV: Cancer is found in one or both ovaries and has spread to other organs such as the liver or lung.

The individual stages are also further broken down in detail, such as Ia, Ib, etc. Accurate staging is important for several reasons. Treatment plans are based on staging, in part because of trying to duplicate the best results achieved in prior research trials. When staging is inconsistent, it becomes more difficult to know how different research studies compare, so the results themselves cannot be relied upon.

Treatment offered will primarily depend on the stage of the cancer and the woman's age. It is always appropriate to consider getting a second opinion, especially when treatment involves surgery, **chemotherapy**, and possible radiation. Before the patient makes her decision as to which course of treatment to take, she should feel that she has the information necessary with which to make an informed decision. The diagnostic tools mentioned above are used to determine the course of treatment. However, the treatment plan may need to be revised if the surgeon sees that the tumor has spread beyond the scope of what was seen during diagnostic tests.

Surgery

Surgery is done to remove as much of the tumor as possible (called tissue debulking), utilizing chemotherapy and/or radiation to target cancer cells that have remained in the body, without jeopardizing the woman's health. This can be hard to balance once the cancer has spread. Removal of the ovary is called oophorectomy, and removal of both ovaries is called bilateral oophorectomy. Unless it is very clear that the cancer has not spread, the fallopian tubes are usually removed as well (**salpingo-oophorectomy**). Removal of the uterus is called **hysterectomy**.

If the woman is very young, all attempts will be made to spare the uterus. It is crucial that a woman discuss with her surgeon her childbearing plans prior to surgery. Unfortunately, ovarian cancer spreads easily and often swiftly throughout the reproductive tract. It may be necessary to remove all reproductive organs as well as part of the lining of the peritoneum to provide the woman with the best possible chance of long-term survival. Fertility-sparing surgery can be successful if the ovarian cancer is caught very early.

Side effects of the surgery will depend on the extent of the surgery, but may include pain and temporary difficulty with bladder and bowel function, as well as reaction to the loss of hormones produced by the organs removed. A hormone replacement patch may be applied to the woman's skin in the recovery room to help with the transition. An emotional side effect may be the feeling of loss stemming from the removal of reproductive organs.

Chemotherapy

Chemotherapy is used to target cells that have traveled to other organs, and throughout the body via the lymphatic system or the blood stream. Chemotherapy drugs are designed to kill cancer cells, but may also be harmful to healthy cells as well. Chemotherapy may be administered through a vein in the arm (intravenous, IV), may be taken in tablet form, and/or may be given through a thin tube called a catheter directly into the abdominal cavity (intraperitoneal). IV and oral chemotherapy drugs travel throughout the body; intraperitoneal chemotherapy is localized in the abdominal cavity.

Side effects of chemotherapy can vary greatly depending on the drugs used. Currently, chemotherapy drugs are often used in combinations to treat advanced ovarian cancer, and usually the combination includes a platinum-based drug (such as cisplatin) with a taxol agent, such as paclitaxel. Some of the combinations used or being studied include: carboplatin/paclitaxel, cisplatin/paclitaxel, cisplatin/topotecan, and cisplatin/carboplatin. As new drugs are evaluated and developed, the goal is always for maximum effectiveness with minimum side effects. Side effects include **nausea and vomiting**, **diarrhea**, decreased appetite and resulting weight loss, fatigue, headaches, loss of hair, and **numbness and tingling** in the hands or feet. Managing these side effects is an important part of cancer treatment.

After the full course of chemotherapy has been given, the surgeon may perform a "second look" surgery to examine the abdominal cavity again to evaluate the success of treatment.

Radiation

Radiation uses high-energy, highly focused x rays to target very specific areas of cancer. This is done using a machine that generates an external beam. Very careful measurements are taken so that the targeted area can be as focused and small as possible. Another form of radiation uses a radioactive liquid that is administered into the abdominal cavity in the same fashion as intraperitoneal chemotherapy. Radiation is usually given on a daily Monday though Friday schedule and for several weeks continuously. Radiation is not painful, but side effects can include skin damage at the area exposed to the external beam, and extreme fatigue. The fatigue may hit suddenly in the third week or so of treatment, and may take a while to recover even after treatments have terminated. Other side effects may include nausea, vomiting, diarrhea, loss of appetite, weight loss and urinary difficulties. For patients with incurable ovarian cancer, radiation may be used to shrink tumor masses to provide pain relief and improve quality of life.

Once the full course of treatment has been undertaken, it is important to have regular follow-up care to monitor for any long-term side effects as well as for future relapse or metastases.

Alternative treatment

The term alternative therapy refers to therapy utilized instead of conventional treatment. By definition, these treatments have not been scientifically proven or investigated as thoroughly and by the same standards as conventional treatments. The terms complementary or integrative therapies denote practices used in conjunction with conventional treatment. Regardless of the therapies chosen, it is key for patients to inform their doctors of any alternative or complementary therapies being used or considered. (Some alternative and complementary therapies adversely affect the effectiveness of conventional treatments.) Some common complementary and alternative medicine techniques and therapies include:

- prayer and faith healing
- **meditation**
- mind/body techniques such as support groups, visualization, guided imagery and hypnosis
- energy work such as **therapeutic touch** and Reiki
- **Acupuncture** and Chinese herbal medicine
- body work such as **yoga**, massage and **t'ai chi**
- **vitamins** and herbal supplements
- diets such as **vegetarianism** and macrobiotic

Mind/body techniques along with meditation, prayer, yoga, T'ai Chi and acupuncture have been shown to reduce **stress** levels, and the relaxation provided may help boost the body's immune system. The effectiveness of other complementary and alternative treatments is being studied by the National Institutes of Health's National Center for Complementary and

Alternative Medicine (NCCAM). For a current list of the research studies occurring, results of recent studies, or publications available, patients can visit the NCCAM web site or call at (888) 644-6226.

Some programs for treatment of ovarian cancer integrate alternative or complementary treatments with conventional surgery or chemotherapy. As of early 2003, the University of Kansas Medical Center is conducting a study of the effectiveness of adding four well-known antioxidants (vitamins A, C, E, and beta-carotene) to standard chemotherapy regimens for ovarian cancer.

Prognosis

Prognosis for ovarian cancer depends greatly on the stage at which it is first diagnosed. While stage I cancer may have a 95% success rate, stages III and IV may have a survival rate of 17-30% at five years post-diagnosis. Early detection remains an elusive, yet hopeful, goal of research. Also, clinical trials are addressing new drug and treatment combinations to prolong survival in women with more advanced disease. Learning one's family history may assist in early detection, and genetic studies may clarify who is at greater risk for the disease.

Research studies are usually designed to compare a new treatment method against the standard method, or the effectiveness of a drug against a placebo (an inert substance that would be expected to have no effect on the outcome). Since the research is experimental in nature, there are no guarantees about the outcome. New drugs being used may have harmful, unknown side effects. Some people participate to help further knowledge about their disease. For others, the study may provide a possible treatment that is not yet available otherwise. If one participates in a study and is in the group receiving the standard care or the placebo, and the treatment group gets clear benefit, it may be possible to receive the experimental treatment once one's original participation role is over. Participants will have to meet certain criteria before being admitted into the study. It is important to fully understand one's role in the study, and weigh the potential risks versus benefits when deciding whether or not to participate.

Prevention

Since the cause of ovarian cancer is not known, it is not possible to fully prevent the disease. However, there are ways to reduce one's risks of developing the disease.

KEY TERMS

Biomarker—A biochemical substance that can be detected in blood samples and indicates the presence of a cancerous tumor.

Gynecologic oncologist—A physician specializing in the treatment of cancers of the female reproductive tract.

Kallikrein—Any of a group of compounds in the body known as serine endopeptidases that help to break down proteins into smaller units. Prostate-specific antigen belongs to this group of chemicals. A recently discovered kallikrein may be useful as a biomarker for ovarian cancer.

Lymphatic system—A connected network of nodes, or glands, that carry lymph throughout the body. Lymph is a fluid that contains the infection-fighting white blood cells that form part of the body's immune system. Because the network goes throughout the body, cancer cells that enter the lymphatic system can travel to and be deposited at any point into the tissues and organs and form new tumors there.

Paclitaxel—A drug derived from the common yew tree (*Taxus baccata*) that is the mainstay of chemotherapy for ovarian cancer.

Pathologist—The pathologist is a doctor specializing in determining the presence and type of disease by looking at cells and tissue samples.

Decrease ovulation. Pregnancy gives a break from ovulation, and multiple pregnancies appear to further reduce the risk of ovarian cancer. The research is not clear as to whether the pregnancy must result in a term delivery to have full benefit. Women who breastfeed their children also have a lower risk of developing the disease. Since oral contraceptives suppress ovulation, women who take birth control pills (BCPs), even for as little as 3 to 6 months have a lower incidence of the disease. It appears that the longer a woman takes BCPs, the lower her risk for ovarian cancer. Also, this benefit may last for up to 15 years after a woman has stopped taking them. However, since BCPs alter a woman's hormonal status, her risk for other hormonally related cancers may change. For this reason it is very important to discuss all the risks and benefits with one's health care provider.

Genetic testing. Tests are available which can help to determine whether a woman who has a family history of breast, endometrial, or ovarian cancer has inherited the mutated BRCA gene that predisposes her to these cancers. If the woman tests positive for the mutation, then she may be able to choose to have her ovaries removed. Even without testing for the mutated gene, some women with strong family histories of ovarian cancer may consider having their ovaries removed as a preventative measure (prophylactic oophorectomy). This procedure diminishes but does not completely remove the risk of cancer, as some women may still develop primary peritoneal carcinoma after oophorectomy.

Surgery. Procedures such as **tubal ligation** (in which the fallopian tubes are blocked or cut off) and hysterectomy (in which the uterus is removed) appear to reduce the risk of ovarian cancer. However, any removal of the reproductive tract organs has surgical as well as hormonal side effects.

Screening. There are no definitive tests or screening procedures to detect ovarian cancer in its early stages, although a blood test for early detection of asymptomatic ovarian cancer is under development as of early 2003. Women at high risk should consult with their physicians about regular screenings, which may include **transvaginal ultrasound** and the blood test for the CA-125 protein.

The American Cancer Society recommends annual pelvic examinations for all women after age 40, in order to increase the chances of early detection of ovarian cancer.

Resources

BOOKS

Beers, Mark H., MD, and Robert Berkow, MD, editors. "Ovarian Cancer." Section 18, Chapter 241. In *The Merck Manual of Diagnosis and Therapy*. Whitehouse Station, NJ: Merck Research Laboratories, 2004.

Pelletier, Kenneth R., MD. *The Best Alternative Medicine*, Part II, "CAM Therapies for Specific Conditions: Cancer." New York: Simon & Schuster, 2002.

Runowicz, Carolyn D., Jeanne A. Petrek, and Ted S. Gansler. *American Cancer Society: Women and Cancer*. New York: Villard Books/Random House, 1999.

Teeley, Peter, and Philip Bashe. *The Complete Cancer Survival Guide*. New York: Doubleday, 2000.

PERIODICALS

Almadrones, L. A. "Treatment Advances in Ovarian Cancer." *Cancer Nursing* 26, Supplement 6 (December 2003): 16S–20S.

Ayhan, A., H. Celik, C. Taskiran, et al. "Oncologic and Reproductive Outcome after Fertility-Saving Surgery in Ovarian Cancer." *European Journal of Gynaecological Oncology* (March 2003): 223–232.

Balat, O., and M. G. Ugur. "Prolonged Stabilization of Platinum/Paclitaxel-Refractory Ovarian Cancer with Topotecan: A Case Report and Review of the Literature." *Clinical and Experimental Obstetrics and Gynecology* 30 (February 2003): 151–152.

Borgono, C. A., L. Grass, A. Soosaipillai, et al. "Human Kallikrein 14: A New Potential Biomarker for Ovarian and Breast Cancer." *Cancer Research* 63 (December 15, 2003): 9032–9041.

Drisko, J. A., J. Chapman, and V. J. Hunter. "The Use of Antioxidant Therapies During Chemotherapy." *Gynecologic Oncology* 88 (March 2003): 434–439.

Kohn, E. C., G. B. Mills, and L. Liotta. "Promising Directions for the Diagnosis and Management of Gynecological Cancers." *International Journal of Gynaecology and Obstetrics* 83, Supplement 1 (October 2003): 203–209.

McCorkle, R., J. Pasacreta, and S. T. Tang. "The Silent Killer: Psychological Issues in Ovarian Cancer." *Holistic Nursing Practice* 17 (November-December 2003): 300–308.

O'Rourke, J., and S. M. Mahon. "A Comprehensive Look at the Early Detection of Ovarian Cancer." *Clinical Journal of Oncology Nursing* 7 (January-February 2003): 41–47.

Ray-Coquard, I., T. Bachelot, J. P. Guastalla, et al. "Epirubicin and Paclitaxel (EPI-TAX Regimen) for Advanced Ovarian Cancer After Failure of Platinum-Containing Regimens." *Gynecologic Oncology* 88 (March 2003): 351–357.

See, H. T., J. J. Kavanagh, W. Hu, and R. C. Bast. "Targeted Therapy for Epithelial Ovarian Cancer: Current Status and Future Prospects." *International Journal of Gynecological Cancer* 13 (November-December 2003): 701–734.

ORGANIZATIONS

American Cancer Society. (800) ACS-2345. < http:// www.cancer.org >.

Cancer Research Institute. 681 Fifth Avenue, New York, NY 10022. (800) 992-2623. < http:// www.cancerresearch.org >.

National Cancer Institute. Building 31, Room 10A31, 31 Center Drive, MSC 2580, Bethesda, MD 20892-2580. (301) 435-3848. < http://www.nci.nih.gov >.

National Center for Complementary and Alternative Medicine. NCCAM Clearinghouse, P.O. Box 8218, Silver Spring, MD 20907-8218. (888) 644-6226. < http://nccam.nih.gov >.

Oncolink at the University of Pennsylvania. < http:// www.oncolink.upenn.edu >.

Women's Cancer Network. c/o Gynecologic Cancer Foundation, 401 N. Michigan Avenue, Chicago, IL 60611. (312) 644-6610. < http://www.wcn.org >.

OTHER

Ovarian Cancer Home Page, National Cancer Institute. < http://www.nci.nih.gov/cancer_information/ cancer_type/ovarian/ >.

"Ovarian Cancer." *OncoLink: University of Pennsylvania Cancer Center*. July 5, 2001. [cited July 6, 2001]. < http://cancer.med.upenn.edu/specialty/gyn_onc/ovarian/ >.

Esther Csapo Rastegari, R.N., B.S.N., Ed.M.
Rebecca J. Frey, PhD

Ovarian cysts

Definition

Ovarian cysts are sacs containing fluid or semi-solid material that develop in or on the surface of an ovary.

Description

Ovarian cysts are common and the vast majority are harmless. Because they cause symptoms that may be the same as ovarian tumors that may be cancerous, ovarian cysts should always be checked out. The most common types of ovarian cysts are follicular and corpus luteum, which are related to the menstrual cycle. Follicular cysts occur when the cyst-like follicle on the ovary in which the egg develops does not burst and release the egg. They are usually small and harmless, disappearing within two to three menstrual cycles. Corpus luteum cysts occur when the corpus luteum—a small, yellow body that secretes hormones—does not dissolve after the egg is released. They usually disappear in a few weeks but can grow to more than 4 in (10 cm) in diameter and may twist the ovary.

Ovarian cysts can develop at any time in a female's life from infancy to **puberty** to menopause, including during **pregnancy**. Follicular cysts occur frequently during the years when a woman is menstruating, and are nonexistent in postmenopausal women or any woman who is not ovulating. Corpus luteum cysts occur occasionally during the menstrual years and during early pregnancy. (Dermoid cysts, which may contain hair, teeth, or skin derived from the outer layer of cells of an embryo, are also occasionally found in the ovary.)

Causes and symptoms

Causes

Follicular cysts are caused by the formation of too much fluid around a developing egg. Corpus luteum cysts are caused by excessive accumulation of blood during the menstrual cycle, hormone therapy, or other types of ovarian tumors.

There is also a condition known as **polycystic ovary syndrome** (PCOS) in which the eggs and follicles are not released from the ovaries and instead form multiple cysts. **Obesity** is linked to this condition, as 50% of women with PCOS are also obese. Hormonal imbalances play a major role in this condition, including high levels of the hormone androgen and low levels of progesterone, the female hormone necessary for egg release. High levels of insulin, the hormone that regulates blood sugar, are often found in women with PCOS. PCOS is also characterized by irregular menstrual periods, **infertility**, and **hirsutism** (excessive hair growth on the body and face). Although PCOS was formerly thought to be an adult-onset condition, more recent research indicates that it begins in childhood, possibly even during fetal development.

PCOS is also known to run in families, which suggests that genetic factors contribute to its development. As of 2002, the specific gene or genes responsible for PCOS have not yet been identified; however, several groups of researchers in different countries have been investigating genetic variations associated with increased risk of type 2 diabetes in order to determine whether the same genetic variations may be involved in PCOS.

In adolescent girls, ovarian cysts may be associated with a genetic disorder known as McCune-Albright syndrome, which is characterized by abnormal bone growth, discoloration of the skin, and early onset of puberty. The ovarian cysts are responsible for the early sexual maturation.

As of early 2003, McCune-Albright syndrome is known to be associated with mutations in the GNAS1 gene. The mutation is sporadic, which means that it occurs during the child's development in the womb and that the syndrome is not inherited.

Symptoms

Many ovarian cysts have no symptoms. When the growth is large or there are multiple cysts, the patient may experience any of the following symptoms:

- Fullness or heaviness in the abdomen.

- Pressure on the rectum or bladder.

- Pelvic **pain** that is a constant dull ache and may spread to the lower back and thighs, occurs shortly before the beginning or end of menstruation, or occurs during intercourse.

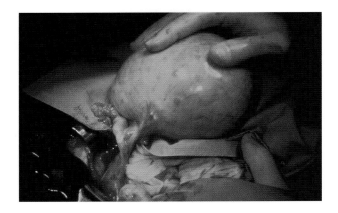

An ovarian cyst is being surgically removed from a 25-year-old female patient. *(Photograph by Art Siegel, Custom Medical Stock Photo. Reproduced by permission.)*

Diagnosis

Non-symptomatic ovarian cysts are often felt by a doctor examining the ovaries during a routine **pelvic exam**. Symptomatic ovarian cysts are diagnosed through a pelvic exam and ultrasound. Ultrasonography is a painless test that uses a hand-held wand to send and receive sound waves to create images of the ovaries on a computer screen. The images are photographed for later analysis. It takes about 15 minutes and is usually done in a hospital or a physician's office.

Ovarian cysts can be diagnosed in female fetuses by transabdominal ultrasound during the mother's pregnancy.

Treatment

Watchful waiting

Many follicular and corpus luteum cysts require no treatment and disappear on their own. Often the physician will wait and re-examine the patient in four to six weeks before taking any action. Follicular cysts do not require treatment, but birth control pills may be taken if the cysts interfere with the patient's daily activities.

Most uncomplicated ovarian cysts in female infants resolve on their own shortly after delivery. Complicated cysts are treated by **laparoscopy** or laparotomy after the baby is born.

Medications

McCune-Albright syndrome is treated with testolactone (Teslac), an anti-estrogen drug that corrects the hormonal imbalance caused by the ovarian cysts.

Long-term management of PCOS has been complicated in the past by lack of a clear understanding of the causes of the disorder. Most commonly, hormonal therapy has been recommended, including estrogen and progesterone and such other hormone-regulating drugs as ganirelix (Antagon). Birth control pills have also been prescribed by doctors to regulate the menstrual cycle and to shrink functional cysts.

More recent studies have shown that increasing sensitivity to insulin in women with PCOS leads to improvement in both the hormonal and metabolic symptoms of the disorder. As of 2002, this sensitivity is increased by either weight loss and **exercise** programs or by medications. Metformin (Glucophage), a drug originally developed to treat type 2 diabetes, has been shown to be effective in reducing the symptoms of hyperandrogenism as well as **insulin resistance** in women with PCOS.

Another strategy that is being tried with PCOS is administration of flutamide (Eulexin), a drug normally used to treat **prostate cancer** in men. Preliminary results indicate that the antiandrogenic effects of flutamide benefit patients with PCOS by increasing blood flow to the uterus and ovaries.

Surgery

Surgery is usually indicated for patients who have not reached puberty and have an ovarian mass and in postmenopausal patients. Surgery is also indicated if the growth is larger than 4 in (10 cm), complex, growing, persistent, solid and irregularly shaped, on both ovaries, or causes pain or other symptoms. Ovarian cysts are curable with surgery but often recur without it.

Surgical options include removal of the cyst or removal of one or both ovaries. More than 90% of benign ovarian cysts can be removed using laparoscopy, a minimally invasive outpatient procedure. In laparoscopic **cystectomy**, the patient receives a general or local anesthetic, then a small incision is made in the abdomen. The laparoscope is inserted into the incision and the cyst or the entire ovary is removed. Laparoscopic cystectomy enables the patient to return to normal activities within two weeks. Surgical cystectomy to remove cysts and/or ovaries is performed under general anesthesia in a hospital and requires a stay of five to seven days. After an incision is made in the abdomen, the muscles are separated and the membrane surrounding the abdominal cavity (peritoneum) is opened. Blood vessels to the ovaries are clamped and tied. The cyst is located and removed. The peritoneum is closed, and the abdominal muscles and skin

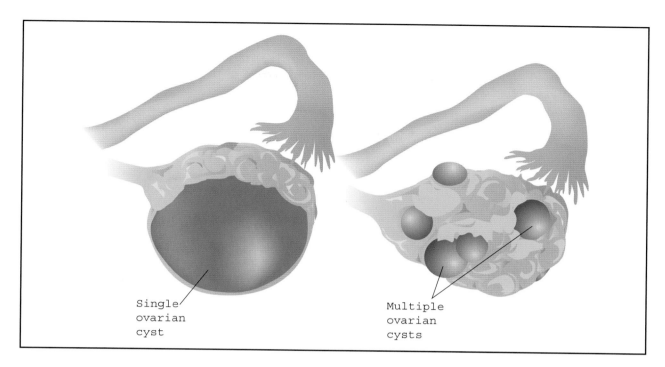

Single ovarian cyst

Multiple ovarian cysts

(Illustration by Argosy Inc.)

are closed with sutures or clips. Recovery takes four weeks.

A surgical procedure known as ovarian wedge resection appears to improve fertility in women with PCOS who have not responded to drug treatments. In an ovarian wedge resection, the surgeon removes a portion of the polycystic ovary in order to induce ovulation.

Alternative treatment

Alternative treatments for ovarian problems—herbal therapies, **nutrition** and diet, and homeopathy—should be used to supplement, not replace, conventional treatment. General herbal tonics for female reproductive organs that can be taken in tea or tincture (an alcohol-based herbal extract) form include blue cohosh (*Caulophylum thalictroides*) and false unicorn root (*Chamaelirium luteum*). Recommendations to help prevent and treat ovarian cysts include a vegan diet (no dairy or animal products) that includes beets, carrots, dark-green leafy vegetables, and lemons; anitoxidant supplements including zinc and **vitamins** A, E, and C; as well as black currant oil, borage oil, and evening primrose oil (*Oenothera biennis*) supplements. Homeopathic treatments—tablets, powders, and liquids prepared from plant, mineral, and animal extracts—may also be

effective in treating ovarian cysts. Castor oil packs can help reduce inflammation. Hydrotherapy applied to the abdomen can help prevent rupture of the cyst and assist its reabsorption.

Prognosis

The prognosis for non-cancerous ovarian cysts is excellent.

Prevention

Ovarian cysts cannot be prevented.

Resources

BOOKS

Beers, Mark H., MD, and Robert Berkow, MD, editors. "Pelvic Pain." Section 18, Chapter 237. In *The Merck Manual of Diagnosis and Therapy*. Whitehouse Station, NJ: Merck Research Laboratories, 2004.

Beers, Mark H., MD, and Robert Berkow, MD., editors. "Physical Conditions in Adolescence." Section 19, Chapter 275. In *The Merck Manual of Diagnosis and Therapy*. Whitehouse Station, NJ: Merck Research Laboratories, 2004.

Beers, Mark H., MD, and Robert Berkow, MD, editors. "Pregnancy Complicated by Disease: Disorders Requiring Surgery." Section 18, Chapter 251. In *The*

Merck Manual of Diagnosis and Therapy. Whitehouse Station, NJ: Merck Research Laboratories, 2004.

PERIODICALS

Ajossa, S., S. Guerriero, A. M. Paoletti, et al. "The Antiandrogenic Effect of Flutamide Improves Uterine Perfusion in Women with Polycystic Ovary Syndrome." *Fertility and Sterility* 77 (June 2002): 1136–1140.

de Sanctis, C., R. Lala, P. Matarazzo, et al. "Pubertal Development in Patients with McCune-Albright Syndrome or Pseudohypoparathyroidism." *Journal of Pediatric Endocrinology and Metabolism* 16, Supplement 2 (March 2003): 293–296.

Ehrmann, D. A., P. E. Schwarz, M. Hara, et al. "Relationship of Calpain-10 Genotype to Phenotypic Features of Polycystic Ovary Syndrome." *Journal of Clinical Endocrinology and Metabolism* 87 (April 2002): 1669–1673.

Elkind-Hirsch, K. E., B. W. Webster, C. P. Brown, and M. W. Vernon. "Concurrent Ganirelix and Follitropin Beta Therapy is an Effective and Safe Regimen for Ovulation Induction in Women with Polycystic Ovary Syndrome." *Fertility and Sterility* 79 (March 2003): 603–607.

Franks, S. "Adult Polycystic Ovary Syndrome Begins in Childhood." *Best Practice and Research: Clinical Endocrinology and Metabolism* 16 (June 2002): 263–272.

Kazerooni, T., and M. Dehghan-Kooshkghazi. "Effects of Metformin Therapy on Hyperandrogenism in Women with Polycystic Ovarian Syndrome." *Gynecological Endocrinology* 17 (February 2003): 51–56.

Legro, R. S. "Polycystic Ovary Syndrome. Long-Term Sequelae and Management." *Minerva ginecologica* 54 (April 2002): 97–114.

Marx, T. L., and A. E. Mehta. "Polycystic Ovary Syndrome: Pathogenesis and Treatment Over the Short and Long Term." *Cleveland Clinic Journal of Medicine* 70 (January 2003): 31–33, 36–41, 45.

Mittermayer, C., W. Blaicher, D. Grassauer, et al. "Fetal Ovarian Cysts: Development and Neonatal Outcome." *Ultraschall in der Medizin* 24 (February 2003): 21–26.

Ovalle, F., and R. Azziz. "Insulin Resistance, Polycystic Ovary Syndrome, and Type 2 Diabetes Mellitus." *Fertility and Sterility* 77 (June 2002): 1095–1105.

Vankova, M., J. Vrbikova, M. Hill, et al. "Association of Insulin Gene VNTR Polymorphism with Polycystic Ovary Syndrome." *Annual of the New York Academy of Sciences* 967 (June 2002): 558–565.

Yildirim, M., V. Noyan, M. Bulent Tiras, et al. "Ovarian Wedge Resection by Minilaparatomy in Infertile Patients with Polycystic Ovarian Syndrome: A New Technique." *European Journal of Obstetrics, Gynecology, and Reproductive Biology* 107 (March 26, 2003): 85–87.

ORGANIZATIONS

American College of Obstetricians and Gynecologists (ACOG). 409 12th Street, SW, P. O. Box 96920, Washington, DC 20090-6920. < http:// www.acog.org >.

The Health Resource. 209 Katherine Drive. Conway, AR 72032. (501) 329-5272.

Polycystic Ovarian Syndrome Association. P. O. Box 80517, Portland, OR 97280. (877) 775-PCOS. < www.pcosupport.org >.

Lori De Milto
Rebecca J. Frey, PhD

Ovarian torsion

Definition

Ovarian torsion is the twisting of the ovary due to the influence of another condition or disease. This results in extreme lower abdominal **pain**.

Description

Ovarian torsion occurs infrequently only in females. In can occur in women of all ages, but most women that experience this are younger. Approximately 70-75% of cases occur in women under 30 years old. About 20% of all reported cases are in pregnant women. It is the fifth most common gynecological emergency which can include surgical intervention.

Ovarian torsion usually arises in only one ovary at a time. They can occur in either normal or enlarged ovaries and fallopian tubes, and occasionally they develop in both.

Causes and symptoms

There are a variety of conditions that can cause torsion of the ovary ranging from changes in normal ovaries to congenital and developmental abnormalities or even a disease that affects the tube or ovary. Normal ovaries that experience spasms or changes in the blood vessels in the mesosalpinx can become twisted. For example, if the veins in the mesosalpinx become congested, the ovaries will undergo torsion.

Developmental abnormalities of the fallopian tube such as extremely longer-than-normal tubes or a missing mesosalpinx will cause ovarian torsion. Diseases such as **ovarian cysts** or fibromas, tumor of the ovary or tubes, and trauma to either the ovaries or the tubes will also cause ovarian torsion.

The characteristic symptom of ovarian torsion is the sudden onset of extreme lower abdominal pain that radiates to the back, side and thigh. **Nausea**, **vomiting**, **diarrhea**, and **constipation** can accompany the pain. The patient may also experience tenderness in the lower abdominal area, a mild **fever** and tachycardia.

Diagnosis

The diagnosis of ovarian torsions usually occurs in an emergency room due to the suddenness of extreme pain. Emergency room physicians may consult with another physician specializing in obstetrics and gynecology. Since 20% of ovarian torsions occur in pregnant women, physicians will order a **pregnancy** test. Visualization with an ultrasound and CT scan (computed tomography) will help pinpoint the ovarian structures and allow physicians to diagnose. Diagnosis is often confirmed through **laparoscopy**.

Treatment

Ovarian torsions need to be repaired. This is done through surgery, and for less severe cases laparoscopic

---

KEY TERMS

Congenital—condition present at birth

Laparoscopy—endoscope used to observe structures in the abdomen

Mesosalpinx—a ligament connected to the fallopian tube

Ovary—female reproductive gland that contains the ova (eggs)

Tachycardia—rapidly beating heart

Torsion—the action of twisting

---

surgery is used. Medications such as NSAIDs are given to control pain.

Prognosis

If ovarian torsions are diagnosed and treated early, then the prognosis is favorable. However, if diagnosis is delayed, the torsions can worsen and cut off arterial blood flow into and venous blood flow out of the ovary. This results in necrosis (death) of the ovarian tissue. Delayed diagnosis can also result in problems when trying to conceive due to infertility.

Prevention

Currently, there are no known methods for prevention of ovarian torsion.

Sally C. McFarlane-Parrott

Ovary and fallopian tube removal *see* **Salpingo-oophorectomy**

Ovary removal *see* **Oophorectomy**

Overactive bladder

Definition

Overactive bladder is the leakage of large amounts of urine at unexpected times, including during sleep.

Description

People who lose urine for no apparent reason while suddenly feeling the need or urge to urinate may have overactive bladder. The condition effects 17 million Americans. The most common cause of overactive bladder is inappropriate bladder contractions. Medical professionals describe such a bladder as "unstable," "spastic," or "overactive." A doctor might call the condition "reflex incontinence" if it results from overactive nerves controlling the bladder. Having an overactive bladder can mean that the bladder empties during sleep, after drinking a small amount of water, or when touching water or hearing it running (as when someone else is taking a shower or washing dishes). Involuntary actions of bladder muscles can occur because of damage to the nerves of the bladder, to the nervous system (spinal cord and brain), or to muscles themselves. **Multiple sclerosis**, Parkinson's disease, **Alzheimer's disease**, **stroke**, brain tumors, and injury—including injury that occurs during surgery—all can harm bladder nerves or muscles.

Causes and symptoms

People with overactive bladder lose urine as soon as they feel a strong need to go to the bathroom. People with overactive bladder may leak urine:

- When they can not get to the bathroom quickly enough

- When they drink even a small amount of liquid, or when they hear or touch running water

People with overactive bladder may also go to the bathroom very often; for example, every two hours during the day and night. They may even wet the bed.

Diagnosis

To diagnose the problem, a doctor will first ask about symptoms and medical history. Other obvious factors that can help define the problem include straining and discomfort, use of drugs, recent surgery, and illness. If the patient's medical history does not define the problem, it will at least suggest which tests are needed. The doctor will physically examine the patient for signs of medical conditions causing the overactive bladder, such as tumors that block the urinary tract, stool impaction, and poor reflexes or sensations, which may be evidence of a nerve-related cause. Overactive bladder is often treated by general or family practitioners but the patient may be referred to a urologist, who specializes in the urinary tract, or a urogynecologist, who focuses on urological problems in women.

Common tests used to diagnose overactive bladder include:

- Blood tests to examine blood for levels of various chemicals

- Cystoscopy to look for abnormalities in the bladder and lower urinary tract. It works by inserting a small tube into the bladder that has a telescope for the doctor to look through

- Post-void residual (PVR) measurement to see how much urine is left in the bladder after urinating by placing a small soft tube into the bladder or by using ultrasound (sound waves)

- Urinalysis to examine urine for signs of infection, blood, or other abnormalities

- Urodynamic testing to examine bladder and urethral sphincter function (may involve inserting a small tube into the bladder; x rays also can be used to see the bladder)

Treatment

Medications can reduce many types of leakage. Some drugs inhibit contractions of an overactive bladder. Others, such as *solifenacin succinate* (Vesicare), relax muscles, leading to more complete bladder emptying during urination. Some drugs tighten muscles at the bladder neck and urethra, preventing leakage. Among the drugs used are *oxybutynin* (Ditropan XL), 5-30 mg daily; *solifenacin* (Vesicare), 5-10 mg a day; *darifenacin* (Enablex), 3.75-15 mg daily; and *tolterodine* (Detrol), 2-4 mg daily. A one-month supply of these drugs costs $90-125. Some medications, especially hormones such as estrogen, are believed to cause muscles involved in urination to function normally. Some of these medications can produce harmful side effects if used for long periods. In particular, estrogen therapy has been associated with an increased risk for cancers of the breast and the lining of the uterus. Patients should talk to their doctor about the risks and benefits of long-term use of medications.

Alternative treatment

Adjusting dietary habits and avoiding acidic and spicy foods, alcohol, **caffeine**, and other bladder irritants can help to prevent urinary leaking. Eat recommended amounts of whole grains, fruits, and vegetables to avoid **constipation**. **Bladder training**, used to treat urge incontinence, can also be a useful treatment tool. The technique involves placing a patient on a toileting schedule. The time interval between urination is then gradually increased until an acceptable time period between bathroom breaks is consistently achieved.

Biofeedback techniques can teach overactive bladder patients to control the urge to urinate.

KEY TERMS

Alzheimer's disease—A degenerative disorder that affects the brain and causes dementia, especially late in life.

Biofeedback—The use of monitoring devices that display information about the operation of a bodily function, for example, heart rate or blood pressure, that is not normally consciously controlled.

Cystoscopy—The use of a narrow tubular instrument that is passed through the urethra to examine the interior of the urethra and the urinary bladder.

Estrogen—Any of several steroid hormones, produced mainly in the ovaries, that stimulate estrus and the development of female secondary sexual characteristics.

Multiple sclerosis—A serious progressive disease of the central nervous system.

Parkinson's disease—An incurable nervous disorder marked by the symptoms of trembling hands, lifeless face, monotone voice, and a slow, shuffling walk.

Sphincter—A circular band of muscle that surrounds an opening or passage in the body and narrows or closes the opening by contracting.

Urethal—Referring to the tube in humans that carries urine from the bladder out of the body.

Urogynecologist—A physician that deals with women's health, especially with the health of women's reproductive organs and urinary tract.

Urologist—A physician who deals with the study and treatment of disorders of the urinary tract in women and the urogenital system in men.

Biofeedback uses sensors to monitor temperature and muscle contractions in the vagina to help overactive bladder patients learn to increase their control over the pelvic muscles.

An infusion, or tea, of horsetail *(Equisetum arvense)*, agrimony *(Agrimonia eupatoria)*, and sweet sumach *(Rhus aromatica)* may be prescribed by an herbalist or naturopath to an overactive bladder. These herbs are natural astringents, and encourage toning of the digestive and urinary tracts. Other herbs, such as urtica, or stinging nettle *(Urtica urens)*, plantain *(Plantago major)*, or maize *(Zea mays)* may be helpful. Homeopathic remedies may include pulsatilla and causticum. Chinese herbalists might recommend golden lock tea, a mixture of several herbs that helps the body retain fluids.

Prognosis

With proper treatment, the prognosis for controlling the disorder is very good. There is no cure for overactive bladder.

Prevention

There are no known preventative measures for overactive bladder.

Resources

BOOKS

Ellsworth, Pamela. *100 Q & A About Overactive Bladder and Urinary Incontinence.* Boston: Jones and Bartlett Publishers, 2005.

Newman, Diane K., and Alan J. Wein. *Overcoming Overactive Bladder: Your Complete Self-Care Guide.* Oakland, CA: New Harbinger Publications, 2004.

PERIODICALS

Perry, Patrick. "On Tour With Debbie Reynolds: The Feisty and Fit Actress Speaks Out About an All-Too-Common Problem—Overactive Bladder." *Saturday Evening Post* (January-February 2003): 26-27.

Radley, Stephen, and Maggi Saunders. "Sex and the Overactive Bladder: Stephen Radley and Maggi Saunders Discuss the Treatment of Patients With an Overactive Bladder in Primary Care." *Primary Health Care* (October 2004): 13-14.

Weiss, Barry D. "Selecting Medications for the Treatment of Urinary Incontinence." *American Family Physician* (January 15, 2005): 315.

Zepf, Bill. "Diagnosis and Management of Overactive Bladder." *American Family Physician* (October 1, 2004): 1386.

ORGANIZATIONS

National Bladder Foundation. P.O. Box 1095, Ridgefield, CT 06877. (877) 252-3337. debsla@aol.com. http://www.bladder.org.

Ken R. Wells

Overhydration

Definition

Overhydration, also called water excess or water intoxication, is a condition in which the body contains too much water.

Description

Overhydration occurs when the body takes in more water than it excretes and its normal sodium level is diluted. This can result in digestive problems, behavioral changes, brain damage, seizures, or **coma**. An adult whose heart, kidneys, and pituitary gland are functioning properly would have to drink more than two gallons of water a day to develop water intoxication. This condition is most common in patients whose kidney function is impaired and may occur when doctors, nurses, or other healthcare professionals administer greater amounts of water-producing fluids and medications than the patient's body can excrete. Overhydration is the most common electrolyte imbalance in hospitals, occurring in about 2% of all patients.

Infants seem to be at greater risk for developing overhydration. The Centers for Disease Control and Prevention has declared that babies are especially susceptible to oral overhydration during the first month of life, when the kidneys' filtering mechanism is too immature to excrete fluid as rapidly as older infants do. Breast milk or formula provide all the fluids a healthy baby needs. Water should be given slowly, sparingly, and only during extremely hot weather. Overhydration, which has been cited as a hazard of infant swimming lessons, occurs whenever a baby drinks too much water, excretes too little fluid, or consumes and retains too much water.

Causes and symptoms

Drinking too much water rarely causes overhydration when the body's systems are working normally. People with heart, kidney, or **liver disease** are more likely to develop overhydration because their kidneys are unable to excrete water normally. It may be necessary for people with these disorders to restrict the amount of water they drink and/or adjust the amount of salt in their diets.

Since the brain is the organ most susceptible to overhydration, a change in behavior is usually the first symptom of water intoxication. The patient may become confused, drowsy, or inattentive. Shouting and **delirium** are common. Other symptoms of overhydration may include blurred vision, **muscle cramps** and twitching, **paralysis** on one side of the body, poor coordination, nausea and **vomiting**, rapid breathing, sudden weight gain, and weakness. The patient's complexion is normal or flushed. Blood pressure is sometimes higher than normal, but elevations may not be noticed even when the degree of water intoxication is serious.

Overhydration can cause acidosis (a condition in which blood and body tissues have an abnormally high acid content), anemia, **cyanosis** (a condition that occurs when oxygen levels in the blood drop sharply), hemorrhage, and **shock**. The brain is the organ most vulnerable to the effects of overhydration. If excess fluid levels accumulate gradually, the brain may be able to adapt to them and the patient will have only a few symptoms. If the condition develops rapidly, confusion, seizures, and coma are likely to occur.

Risk factors

Chronic illness, **malnutrition**, a tendency to retain water, and kidney diseases and disorders increase the likelihood of becoming overhydrated. Infants and the elderly seem to be at increased risk for overhydration, as are people with certain mental disorders or **alcoholism**.

Diagnosis

Before treatment can begin, a doctor must determine whether a patient's symptoms are due to overhydration, in which excess water is found within and outside cells, or excess blood volume, in which high sodium levels prevent the body from storing excess water inside the cells. Overhydration is characterized by excess water both within and around the body's cells, while excess blood volume occurs when the body has too much sodium and can not move water to reservoirs within the cells. In cases of overhydration, symptoms of fluid accumulation do not usually occur. On the other hand, in cases of excess blood volume, fluid tends to accumulate around cells in the lower legs, abdomen, and chest. Overhydration can occur alone or in conjunction with excess blood volume, and differentiating between these two conditions may be difficult.

Treatment

Mild overhydration can generally be corrected by following a doctor's instructions to limit fluid intake. In more serious cases, **diuretics** may be prescribed to increase urination, although these drugs tend to be most effective in the treatment of excess blood volume. Identifying and treating any underlying condition (such as impaired heart or kidney function) is a priority, and fluid restrictions are a critical component of every treatment plan.

In patients with severe neurologic symptoms, fluid imbalances must be corrected without delay. A powerful diuretic and fluids to restore normal sodium concentrations are administered rapidly at first. When the patient has absorbed 50% of the therapeutic substances, blood levels are measured. Therapy is continued at a more moderate pace in order to prevent brain damage as a result of sudden changes in blood chemistry.

Prognosis

Mild water intoxication is usually corrected by drinking less than a quart of water a day for several days. Untreated water intoxication can be fatal, but this outcome is quite rare.

Resources

BOOKS

McPhee, Stephen, et al., editors. *Current Medical Diagnosisand Treatment, 1998.* 37th ed. Stamford: Appleton & Lange, 1997.

Maureen Haggerty

Oxycodo *see* **Analgesics, opioid**

Oxygen inhalation therapy *see* **Oxygen/ozone therapy**

Oxygen/ozone therapy

Definition

Oxygen/ozone therapy is a term that describes a number of different practices in which oxygen, ozone, or hydrogen peroxide are administered via gas or water to kill disease microorganisms, improve cellular function, and promote the healing of damaged tissues. The rationale behind bio-oxidative therapies, as they are sometimes known, is the notion that as long as the body's needs for antioxidants are met, the use of certain oxidative substances will stimulate the movement of oxygen atoms from the bloodstream to the cells. With higher levels of oxygen in the tissues, bacteria and viruses are killed along with defective tissue cells. The healthy cells survive and multiply more rapidly. The result is a stronger immune system.

Ozone itself is a form of oxygen, O_3, produced when ultraviolet light or an electric spark passes through air or oxygen. It is a toxic gas that creates free radicals, the opposite of what antioxidant **vitamins** do. Oxidation, however, is good when it occurs in harmful foreign organisms that have invaded the body. Ozone inactivates many disease bacteria and viruses.

Purpose

Oxygen and ozone therapies are thought to benefit patients in the following ways:

- stimulating white blood cell production
- killing viruses (ozone and hydrogen peroxide)
- improving the delivery of oxygen from the blood stream to the tissues of the body
- speeding up the breakdown of petrochemicals
- increasing the production of interferon and tumor necrosis factor, thus helping the body to fight infections and cancers
- increasing the efficiency of antioxidant enzymes
- increasing the flexibility and efficiency of the membranes of red blood cells
- speeding up the citric acid cycle, which in turn stimulates the body's basic metabolism

Description

Origins

The various forms of oxygen and ozone therapy have been in use since the late nineteenth century. The earliest recorded use of oxygen to treat a patient was by Dr. J. A. Fontaine in 1879. In the 1950s, hyperbaric oxygen treatment was used by cancer researchers. The term "hyperbaric" means that the oxygen is given under pressure higher than normal air pressure. Recently, oxygen therapy has also been touted as a quick purification treatment for mass-market consumers. Oxygen bars can be found in airports and large cities, and provide pure oxygen in 20-minute sessions for approximately $16. While proponents claim that breathing oxygen will purify the body, most medical doctors do not agree. What is more, oxygen can be harmful to people with severe lung diseases, and these people should never self-treat with oxygen.

Ozone has been used since 1856 to disinfect operating rooms in European hospitals, and since 1860 to purify the water supplies of several large German cities. Ozone was not, however, used to treat patients until 1915, when a German doctor named Albert Wolff began to use it to treat skin diseases. During World War I, the German Army used ozone to treat **wounds** and **anaerobic infections**. In the 1950s, several German physicians used ozone to treat **cancer** alongside mainstream therapeutic methods. It is estimated that as of the late 1990s, about 8,000 practitioners in Germany were using ozone in their practices. This figure includes medical doctors as well as naturopaths and homeopaths.

Hydrogen peroxide is familiar to most people as an over-the-counter preparation that is easily available at supermarkets as well as pharmacies, and is used as an antiseptic for cleansing minor cuts and scrapes. It was first used as an intravenous infusion in 1920 by a British physician in India, T. H. Oliver, to treat a group of 25 Indian patients who were critically ill with **pneumonia**. Oliver's patients had a mortality rate of 48%, compared to the standard mortality rate of 80% for the disease. In the 1920s, an American physician named William Koch experimented with hydrogen peroxide as a treatment for cancer. He left the United States after a legal battle with the FDA. In the early 1960s, researchers at Baylor University studied the effects of hydrogen peroxide in removing plaque from the arteries as well as its usefulness in treating cancer, but their findings were largely ignored.

Oxygen, ozone, and hydrogen peroxide are used therapeutically in a variety of different ways.

Hyperbaric oxygen therapy (HBO)

Hyperbaric oxygen therapy (HBO) involves putting the patient in a pressurized chamber in which he or she breathes pure oxygen for a period of 90 minutes to two hours. HBO may also be administered by using a tight-fitting mask, similar to the masks used for anesthesia. A nasal catheter may be used for small children.

Ozone therapy

Ozone therapy may be administered in a variety of ways.

- Intramuscular injection: A mixture of oxygen and ozone is injected into the muscles of the buttocks.

- Rectal insufflation: A mixture of oxygen and ozone is introduced into the rectum and absorbed through the intestines.

- Autohemotherapy: Between 10–15 mL of the patient's blood is removed, treated with a mixture of oxygen and ozone and reinjected into the patient.

- Intra-articular injection: Ozone-treated water is injected into the patient's joints to treat arthritis, rheumatism and other joint diseases.

- Ozonated water: Ozone is bubbled through water that is used to cleanse wounds, **burns**, and skin infections, or to treat the mouth after dental surgery.

- Ozonated oil: Ozone is bubbled through olive or safflower oil, forming a cream that is used to treat fungal infections, insect bites, **acne**, and skin problems.

- Ozone bagging: Ozone and oxygen are pumped into an airtight bag that surrounds the area to be treated, allowing the body tissues to absorb the mixture.

Hydrogen peroxide

Hydrogen peroxide may be administered intravenously in a 0.03% solution. It is infused slowly into the patient's vein over a period of one to three hours. Treatments are given about once a week for chronic illness but may be given daily for such acute illnesses as pneumonia or influenza. A course of intravenous hydrogen peroxide therapy may range from one to 20 treatments, depending on the patient's condition and the type of illness being treated. Injections of 0.03% hydrogen peroxide have also been used to treat rheumatoid and osteoarthritis. The solution is injected directly into the inflamed joint.

Hydrogen peroxide is also used externally to treat stiff joints, **psoriasis**, and fungal infections. The patient soaks for a minimum of 20 minutes in a tub of warm water to which 1 pint of 35% food-grade hydrogen peroxide (a preparation used by the food industry as a disinfectant) has been added.

Preparations

Oxygen is usually delivered to the patient as a gas; ozone as a gas mixed with oxygen or bubbled through oil or water; and hydrogen peroxide as an 0.03% solution for intravenous injection or a 35% solution for external **hydrotherapy**.

Precautions

Patients interested in oxygen/ozone therapies must consult with a physician before receiving treatment. Hyperbaric oxygen treatment should not be given to patients with untreated pneumothorax, a condition in which air or gas is present in the cavity surrounding the lungs. Patients with a history of **pneumothorax**, chest surgery, **emphysema**, middle **ear surgery**, uncontrolled high fevers, upper respiratory infections, seizures, or disorders of the red blood cells are not suitable candidates for oxygen/ozone therapy. In addition, patients should be aware that oxygen is highly flammable. If treatments are administered incorrectly or by an unskilled person, there is a risk of fire.

KEY TERMS

Autohemotherapy—A form of ozone therapy in which a small quantity of the patient's blood is withdrawn, treated with a mixture of ozone and oxygen, and reinfused into the patient.

Hydrogen peroxide—A colorless, unstable compound of hydrogen and oxygen (H_2O_2). An aqueous solution of hydrogen peroxide is used as an antiseptic and bleaching agent.

Hyperbaric oxygen therapy (HBO)—A form of oxygen therapy in which the patient breathes oxygen in a pressurized chamber.

Ozone—A form of oxygen with three atoms in its molecule (O_3), produced by an electric spark or ultraviolet light passing through air or oxygen. Ozone is used therapeutically as a disinfectant and oxidative agent.

Side effects

Typical side effects of oxygen or ozone therapy can include elevated blood pressure and ear pressure similar to that experienced while flying. Side effects may also include **headache**, **numbness** in the fingers, temporary changes in the lens of the eye, and seizures.

Research and general acceptance

Oxygen/ozone therapies are far more widely accepted in Europe than in the United States. The most intensive research in these therapies is presently being conducted in the former Soviet Union and in Cuba. In the United States, the work of the Baylor researchers was not followed up. In 2000, the Office of Alternative Medicine of the National Institutes of Health (presently the National Center for Complementary and Alternative Medicine, or NCCAM) indicated interest in conducting clinical trials of oxygen/ozone therapies; as of 2003, however, these studies have not been carried out.

Recent European research in ozone therapy includes studies in the oxygenation of resting muscles, the treatment of vascular disorders, and the relief of **pain** from herniated lumbar disks. No corresponding studies are being done in the United States as of late 2003.

Resources

PERIODICALS

Andreula, C. F., L. Simonetti, F. De Santis, et al. "Minimally Invasive Oxygen-Ozone Therapy for Lumbar Disk Herniation." *American Journal of Neuroradiology* 24 (May 2003): 996–1000.

Clavo, B., J. L. Perez, L. Lopez, et al. "Effect of Ozone Therapy on Muscle Oxygenation." *Journal of Alternative and Complementary Medicine* 9 (April 2003): 251–256.

Tylicki, L., T. Nieweglowski, B. Biedunkiewicz, et al. "The Influence of Ozonated Autohemotherapy on Oxidative Stress in Hemodialyzed Patients with Atherosclerotic Ischemia of Lower Limbs." *International Journal of Artificial Organs* 26 (April 2003): 297–303.

ORGANIZATIONS

International Bio-Oxidative Medicine Foundation (IBOMF). P.O. Box 891954. Oklahoma City, OK 73109. (405) 634-7855. Fax (405) 634-7320.

International Ozone Association, Ind. Pan American Group. 31 Strawberry Hill Ave. Stamford, CT 06902. (203) 348-3542. Fax (203) 967-4845.

NIH National Center for Complementary and Alternative Medicine (NCCAM). NCCAM Clearinghouse. P. O. Box 8218. Silver Spring, MD 20907-8218. TTY/TDY: (888) 644-6226. < http://nccam.nih.gov >.

OTHER

Oxygen Healing Therapies. < http://www.oxygen healingtherapies.com >.

Amy Cooper
Rebecca J. Frey, PhD

Oxymetazoline *see* **Decongestants**

Oxytocin *see* **Drugs used in labor**

Ozone therapy *see* **Oxygen/ozone therapy**

PAC *see* **Atrial ectopic beats**

Pacemaker implantation *see* **Pacemakers**

Pacemakers

Definition

A pacemaker is a surgically-implanted electronic device that regulates a slow or erratic heartbeat.

Purpose

Pacemakers are implanted to regulate irregular contractions of the heart (arrhythmia). They are most frequently prescribed to speed the heartbeat of patients who have a heart rate well under 60 beats per minute (severe symptomatic bradycardia). They are also used in some cases to slow a fast heart rate (tachycardia).

Precautions

The symptoms of **fatigue** and lightheadedness that are characteristic of bradycardia can also be caused by a number of other medical conditions, including anemia. Certain prescription medications can also slow the heart rate. A doctor should take a complete medical history and perform a full physical work-up to rule out all non-cardiac causes of bradycardia.

Patients with cardiac pacemakers should not undergo a magnetic resonance imaging (MRI) procedure. Devices that emit electromagnetic waves (including magnets) may alter pacemaker programming or functioning. A 1997 study found that cellular phones often interfere with pacemaker programming and cause irregular heart rhythm. However, advances in pacemaker design and materials have greatly reduced the risk of pacemaker interference from electromagnetic fields.

Description

Approximately 500,000 Americans have an implantable permanent pacemaker device. A pacemaker implantation is performed under **local anesthesia** in a hospital by a surgeon assisted by a cardiologist. An insulated wire called a lead is inserted into an incision above the collarbone and guided through a large vein into the chambers of the heart. Depending on the configuration of the pacemaker and the clinical needs of the patient, as many as three leads may be used in a pacing system. Current pacemakers have a double, or bipolar, electrode attached to the end of each lead. The electrodes deliver an electrical charge to the heart to regulate heartbeat. They are positioned on the areas of the heart that require stimulation. The leads are then attached to the pacemaker device, which is implanted under the skin of the patient's chest.

Patients undergoing surgical pacemaker implantation usually stay in the hospital overnight. Once the procedure is complete, the patient's vital signs are monitored and a **chest x ray** is taken to ensure that the pacemaker and leads are properly positioned.

Modern pacemakers have sophisticated programming capabilities and are extremely compact. The smallest weigh less than 13 grams (under half an ounce) and are the size of two stacked silver dollars. The actual pacing device contains a pulse generator, circuitry programmed to monitor heart rate and deliver stimulation, and a lithiumiodide battery. Battery life typically ranges from seven to 15 years, depending on the number of leads the pacemaker is configured with and how much energy the pacemaker uses. When a new battery is required, the unit can be exchanged in a simple outpatient procedure.

A temporary pacing system is sometimes recommended for patients who are experiencing irregular heartbeats as a result of a recent **heart attack** or other acute medical condition. The implantation procedure for the pacemaker leads is similar to that for a

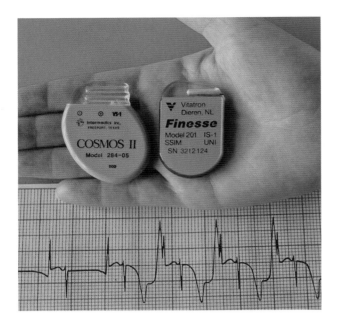

Pacemakers like these are usually implanted under the skin below the collarbone. The pacemaker is connected to the heart by a wire inserted into a major vein in the neck and guided down into the heart. *(Photograph by Eamonn McNulty, Photo Researchers, Inc. Reproduced by permission.)*

permanent pacing system, but the actual pacemaker unit housing the pulse generator remains outside the patient's body. Temporary pacing systems may be replaced with a permanent device at a later date.

Preparation

Patients being considered for pacemaker implantation will undergo a full battery of cardiac tests, including an electrocardiogram (ECG) or an electrophysiological study or both to fully evaluate the bradycardia or tachycardia.

Patients are advised to abstain from eating 6-8 hours before the surgical procedure. The patient is usually given a sedative to help him or her relax for the procedure. An intravenous (IV) line will also be inserted into a vein in the patient's arm before the procedure begins in case medication or blood products are required during the insertion.

Aftercare

Pacemaker patients should schedule a follow-up visit with their cardiologist approximately six weeks after the surgery. During this visit, the doctor will make any necessary adjustments to the settings of the pacemaker. Pacemakers are programmed externally with a handheld electromagnetic device. Pacemaker

batteries must be checked regularly. Some pacing systems allow patients to monitor battery life through a special telephone monitoring service that can read pacemaker signals.

Risks

Because pacemaker implantation is an invasive surgical procedure, internal bleeding, infection, hemorrhage, and **embolism** are all possible complications. Infection is more common in patients with temporary pacing systems. Antibiotic therapy given as a precautionary measure can reduce the risk of pacemaker infection. If infection does occur, the entire pacing system may have to be removed.

The placing of the leads and electrodes during the implantation procedure also presents certain risks for the patient. The lead or electrode could perforate the heart or cause scarring or other damage. The electrodes can also cause involuntary stimulation of nearby skeletal muscles.

A complication known as *pacemaker syndrome* develops in approximately 7% of pacemaker patients with single-chamber pacing systems. The syndrome is characterized by the low blood pressure and **dizziness** that are symptomatic of bradycardia. It can usually be corrected by the implantation of a dual-chamber pacing system.

Normal results

Pacemakers that are properly implanted and programmed can correct a patient's arrhythmia and resolve related symptoms.

Resources

ORGANIZATIONS

American Heart Association. 7320 Greenville Ave. Dallas, TX 75231. (214) 373-6300. < http://www.americanheart.org >.

Paula Anne Ford-Martin

Packed cell volume *see* **Hematocrit**

Packed red blood cell volume *see* **Hematocrit**

Paget's disease of bone

Definition

Paget's disease of bone (*osteitis deformans*) is the abnormal formation of bone tissue that results in weakened and deformed bones.

Description

Named for Sir James Paget (1814–1899), this disease affects 1–3% of people over 50 years of age, but affects over 10% of people over 80 years of age. Paget's disease can affect one or more bones in the body. Most often, the pelvis, bones in the skull, the long bones (the large bones that make up the arms and legs), and the collarbones are affected by Paget's disease. In addition, the joints between bones (the knees or elbows, for example) can develop arthritis because of this condition.

Paget's disease is characterized by changes in the normal mechanism of bone formation. Bone is a living material made by the body through the continual processes of formation and breakdown (resorption). The combination of these two actions is called remodeling and is used by the body to build bone tissue that is strong and healthy. Strong bones are formed when bone tissue is made up of plate-shaped crystals of **minerals** called hydroxyapatite. Normal wear and tear on the skeletal system is repaired throughout life

by the ongoing process of remodeling. In fact, the entire human skeleton is remodeled every five years.

Healthy bone tissue has an ordered structure that gives the bone its strength. Bones affected by Paget's disease, however, have a structure that is disorganized. This disorganized structure weakens the diseased bone and makes people suffering from this disease more likely to have fractures. These **fractures** are slow to heal.

Paget's disease of bone is most commonly found in Europe, England, Australia, New Zealand, and North America. In these areas, up to 3% of all people over 55 years of age are affected with the disease. It is interesting to note that Paget's disease is rare in Asia, possibly showing that this disease may affect some ethnic groups and geographic areas more than others.

Causes and symptoms

The cause of Paget's disease is not known. Various viruses have been suggested to be involved in this disease, but the relationship between viral infections and Paget's disease remains uncertain. There also may to be a genetic component to this disease since it may appear in more than one person within the same family.

Paget's disease usually begins without any symptoms. And, in its early stages, the symptoms that do occur are often confused with symptoms of arthritis. However, as the disease progresses, bone and joint **pain** develop. A unique feature of Paget's disease is the enlargement of areas of affected bone. This type of enlargement is clearly identifiable on an x ray.

If the bones of the skull are affected by Paget's disease, enlargement of the skull can occur and may result in a loss of hearing. When the long bones in the legs are affected, they can become bent under the body's weight because of their weakness. Little or no injury to a bone can cause fractures in the weakened bones. Fractures that occur when no traumatic injury is present are known as spontaneous fractures.

Although rare, bone **cancer** occurs in less than 1% of patients with Paget's disease. Such cancer is often accompanied by an abrupt increase in the intensity of pain at the diseased site. Unfortunately, this type of cancer has a poor prognosis; the average survival time from the onset of symptoms is generally one to three years.

Diagnosis

Paget's disease is often found when an individual is having x rays taken for medical reasons unrelated to this bone disease. A diagnosis of Paget's disease can also be made when higher than normal levels of a

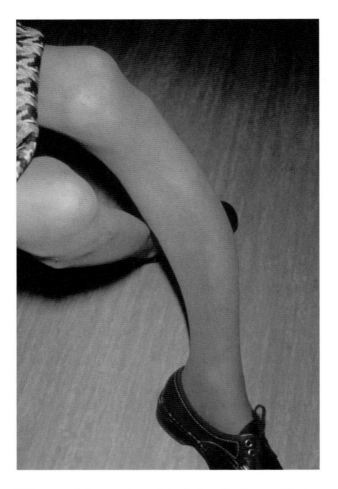

This woman's legs are bowed due to Paget's disease. *(Custom Medical Stock Photo. Reproduced by permission.)*

chemical called alkaline phosphatase are found in the blood. Alkaline phosphatase is a substance involved in the bone formation process, so if its levels are abnormally high this indicates that the balance between bone formation and resorption is upset.

Treatment

Treatment, given only when symptoms are present, consists of the following types:

Drugs

Paget's disease is most often treated with drug therapy, with bone pain lessening within weeks of starting the treatment. While non-steroidal antiinflammatory drugs can reduce bone pain, two additional categories of drugs are used to treat this disease.

HORMONE TREATMENT. Calcitonin, a hormone which is made naturally by the thyroid gland, is used

to treat Paget's disease. This chemical rapidly decreases the amount of bone breakdown or loss (resorption). After approximately two to three weeks of treatment with extra calcitonin, bone pain lessens and new bone tissue forms. Calcitonin is commonly given as daily injections for one month, followed by three injections each week for several additional months. The total dose of calcitonin given to an individual depends upon the amount of disease present and how well the individual's condition responds to the treatment.

Although calcitonin is effective in slowing the progression of Paget's disease, the favorable effects of the drug do not continue for very long once administration of the drug is stopped. In addition, some temporary side effects can occur with this drug. **Nausea** and flushing are the most common side effects and have been found in 20-30% of individuals taking calcitonin. Vomiting, diarrhea, and abdominal pain can also occur, but these effects are also temporary. A form of calcitonin taken nasally causes fewer side effects, but requires higher doses because less of the drug reaches the diseased bone.

BISPHOSPHONATES. The bisphosphonate group of drugs are drugs that bind directly to bone minerals because of their specific chemical structure. Once bound to the bone, these drugs inhibit bone loss by reducing the action of bone cells that normally degrade bone during the remodeling process. Unlike treatment with calcitonin, the positive effects of increased bone formation and reduced pain can continue for many months or even years after bisphosphonate treatment is stopped. Bisphosphonates are considered the treatment of choice for Paget's disease and are usually given for 3-6 months at a time.

Bisphosphonate drugs suitable for the treatment of Paget's disease are alendronate, clodronate, etidronate, pamidronate, risedronate, and tiludronate. The main side effects of these drugs include a flu-like reaction (pamidronate), gastrointestinal disturbances (alendronate, clodronate), and abnormal bone formation (etidronate, when taken in high doses). Risedronate is the newest of these drugs. It is about 1,000 times more potent than etidronate and 3 to 5 times more potent than alendronate. Because of the greater potency of this drug, lower doses and a shorter duration of treatment are required. This leads to fewer side effects with similar, or better, clinical results in the patient.

Surgery

Treatment of Paget's disease usually begins with drug therapy. However, various surgical treatments can also be used to treat skeletal conditions that occur in patients with Paget's disease.

KEY TERMS

Bisphosphonate—A class of drugs used to treat Paget's disease. These drugs bind to the minerals in bone tissue and lessen the amount of bone loss associated with Paget's disease.

Calcitonin—A naturally occurring hormone made by the thyroid gland that can be used as a drug to treat Paget's disease.

Remodeling—The ongoing process of bone formation and breakdown that results in healthy bone development.

In patients with severe arthritis of the hip or knee, a joint replacement operation can be beneficial. However, in addition to the malformation of bone tissue caused by this condition, there are greater numbers of blood vessels that form in the diseased bone relative to a healthy bone. This makes surgery on bones affected with Paget's disease more difficult.

Prognosis

There is no cure for Paget's disease. However, the development of potent bisphosphonate drugs like risedronate has resulted in the ability to slow the progress of the disease.

Paul A. Johnson, Ed.M.

Paget's disease of the breast

Definition

Paget's disease of the breast is a rare form of breast cancer which makes up approximately 1-4 % of all breast tumors. While sharing its name with **Paget's disease of bone**, these are two medically unrelated conditions. They are simply named after the same doctor who first described them.

Description

Paget's disease of the breast is generally associated with an underlying **breast cancer**. It is generally seen in people between the ages of 40 and 80 years. Cases in men have been identified, but they are extremely rare.

Paget's disease of the breast may also be called mammary Paget's disease (MPD). There is a much rarer form of this disease called extramammary Paget's disease (EMPD). MPD affects the breast nipple and is also called Paget's disease of the nipple. EMPD can affect the skin of the external genital tissues in both women and men, as well as the skin of the eyelids and external ear canal. MPD is believed to develop from a tumor growth within the milk ducts of the breast. EMPD may represent a spreading (metastasis) of MPD to other parts of the body.

Causes and symptoms

The cause of Paget's disease of the breast is unknown, but it is usually associated with an underlying **cancer** of the breast.

The symptoms of Paget's disease of the breast include:

- red scaly patches of skin on the nipple and sometimes also on the dark area of skin around the nipple (areola)

- crusting, bleeding, or ulceration of the skin of the affected area

- a discharge of fluid from the nipple

- a turning inward (inversion) of the nipple

In approximately 30-40 % of cases of Paget's disease of the breast, there is also a detectable lump in the breast.

Diagnosis

Paget's disease of the breast is often confused with other skin conditions, such as eczema, dermatitis, or **psoriasis**. These misdiagnoses often lead to delays in appropriate treatment. Misdiagnosis is more common when both breast are affected and no lump in the breast is detected. When only one breast is affected, or when the presence of a lump in the breast is also detected, a correct initial diagnosis is more likely to occur.

Once Paget's disease of the breast is suspected, it can be definitively confirmed by biopsy of the affected tissue. In this procedure, a small piece of the affected skin and the underlying tissue is removed and sent to a laboratory for examination under a microscope. The shape and other characteristics of the cells in the biopsied sample will allow the laboratory personnel to determine if the sample is affected with Paget's disease of the breast, or some other condition.

KEY TERMS

Metastasis—The spread of a cancer from one part of the body (where the cancer originated) to another part of the body.

Ulceration—The formation of an ulcer, a patch of tissue that is discontinuous with the surrounding tissue because the tissue within the ulcer has decayed or died and been swept away.

Topical steroid creams are usually used to treat eczema, **dermatitis**, and psoriasis. These creams will have no effect on the skin conditions caused by Paget's disease of the breast.

Treatment

Surgery is the main treatment for Paget's disease of the breast. Removal of the breast (mastectomy) may be recommended if the cancer is seen in a wide area away from the nipple or appears to be deep into the breast tissue. Breast conservation surgery, aimed at keeping as much of the breast as possible, may be recommended in cases where the disease is diagnosed early enough and the cancer has not spread far from the surface of the nipple.

Some people will require further treatment after surgery. This treatment may include radiation therapy, **chemotherapy**, or a combination of both. **Radiation therapy** involves using high-energy x rays to destroy any cancer cells that may remain after surgical removal of the primary tumor. Radiation therapy is most common after breast conservation surgery. Chemotherapy involves the use of medicinal drugs to destroy the growth of any cancer cells that may remain after removal of the primary cancer. Chemotherapy treatments are most common after **mastectomy**.

Alternative treatment

Alternative treatments for Paget's disease of the breast include: the use of cartilage from cows or sharks; a diet known as Gerson therapy; administration of the chemicals hydrazine sulfate or laetrile; and, the injection of solutions derived from the mistletoe plant.

Prognosis

The prognosis for Paget's disease of the breast depends on the underlying cancer that is causing this condition and whether or not this cancer has spread (metastasized) to other parts of the body.

Prevention

Because the cause of Paget's disease of the breast is not known, prevention of this disease is not possible. In instances where this conditions arises from other underlying cancers of the breast, it may be possible to prevent Paget's disease of the breast from occurring if the underlying cause is diagnosed and successfully treated prior to the development of Paget's disease of the breast.

Resources

BOOKS

Love, Susan M., and Karen Lindsey. *Dr. Susan Love's Breast Book*. 3rd ed. Reading, MA: Perseus Book Group, 2000.

PERIODICALS

Sheen-Chen, S.M., et al. "Paget Disease of the Breast - an EasilyOverlooked Disease?" *Journal of Surgical Oncology* 76 (April 2001): 261-5.

ORGANIZATIONS

American Cancer Society. 1599 Clifton Road NE, Atlanta, GA 30329. (800)ACS-2345. < http://www.cancer.org >.

National Alliance of Breast Cancer Organizations. 9 East 37th Street, 10th Floor, New York, NY 10016. (888) 806-2226. Fax: 212-689-1213. < http://www.nabco.org/ >.

National Breast Cancer Coalition. 1707 L Street Northwest, Suite 1060, Washington, DC 20036. (800) 622-2838. Fax: 202-265-6854. < http://www.natlbcc.org/ >.

OTHER

Paget's Disease of the Breast: The CancerBACUP Factsheet. May 12, 2001. < http://www.cancerbacup.org.uk/info/paget.htm >.

Ruth, Laura. *Paget's Disease: A Rare Form of Breast Cancer.* May 12, 2001. < http://users.cnmnetwork.com/~lrs1/paget.htm >.

Paul A. Johnson, Ed.M.

Pain

Definition

Pain is an unpleasant feeling that is conveyed to the brain by sensory neurons. The discomfort signals actual or potential injury to the body. However, pain is more than a sensation, or the physical awareness of pain; it also includes perception, the subjective interpretation of the discomfort. Perception gives information on the pain's location, intensity, and something about its nature. The various conscious and unconscious responses to both sensation and perception, including the emotional response, add further definition to the overall concept of pain.

Description

Pain arises from any number of situations. Injury is a major cause, but pain may also arise from an illness. It may accompany a psychological condition, such as depression, or may even occur in the absence of a recognizable trigger.

Acute pain

Acute pain often results from tissue damage, such as a skin burn or broken bone. Acute pain can also be associated with headaches or **muscle cramps**. This type of pain usually goes away as the injury heals or the cause of the pain (stimulus) is removed.

To understand acute pain, it is necessary to understand the nerves that support it. Nerve cells, or neurons, perform many functions in the body. Although their general purpose, providing an interface between the brain and the body, remains constant, their capabilities vary widely. Certain types of neurons are capable of transmitting a pain signal to the brain.

As a group, these pain-sensing neurons are called nociceptors, and virtually every surface and organ of the body is wired with them. The central part of these cells is located in the spine, and they send threadlike projections to every part of the body. Nociceptors are classified according to the stimulus that prompts them to transmit a pain signal. Thermoreceptive nociceptors are stimulated by temperatures that are potentially tissue damaging. Mechanoreceptive nociceptors respond to a pressure stimulus that may cause injury. Polymodal nociceptors are the most sensitive and can respond to temperature and pressure. Polymodal nociceptors also respond to chemicals released by the cells in the area from which the pain originates.

Nerve cell endings, or receptors, are at the front end of pain sensation. A stimulus at this part of the nociceptor unleashes a cascade of neurotransmitters (chemicals that transmit information within the nervous system) in the spine. Each neurotransmitter has a purpose. For example, substance P relays the pain message to nerves leading to the spinal cord and brain. These neurotransmitters may also stimulate nerves leading back to the site of the injury. This response prompts cells in the injured area to release chemicals that not only trigger an immune response, but also influence the intensity and duration of the pain.

Chronic and abnormal pain

Chronic pain refers to pain that persists after an injury heals, **cancer** pain, pain related to a persistent or degenerative disease, and long-term pain from an unidentifiable cause. It is estimated that one in three people in the United States will experience chronic pain at some point in their lives. Of these people, approximately 50 million are either partially or completely disabled.

Chronic pain may be caused by the body's response to acute pain. In the presence of continued stimulation of nociceptors, changes occur within the nervous system. Changes at the molecular level are dramatic and may include alterations in genetic transcription of neurotransmitters and receptors. These changes may also occur in the absence of an identifiable cause; one of the frustrating aspects of chronic pain is that the stimulus may be unknown. For example, the stimulus cannot be identified in as many as 85% of individuals suffering lower back pain.

Scientists have long recognized a relationship between depression and chronic pain. In 2004, a survey of California adults diagnosed with major depressive disorder revealed that more than one-half of them also suffered from chronic pain.

Other types of abnormal pain include allodynia, hyperalgesia, and phantom limb pain. These types of pain often arise from some damage to the nervous system (neuropathic). Allodynia refers to a feeling of pain in response to a normally harmless stimulus. For example, some individuals who have suffered nerve damage as a result of viral infection experience unbearable pain from just the light weight of their clothing. Hyperalgesia is somewhat related to allodynia in that the response to a painful stimulus is extreme. In this case, a mild pain stimulus, such as a pin prick, causes a maximum pain response. Phantom limb pain occurs after a limb is amputated; although an individual may be missing the limb, the nervous system continues to perceive pain originating from the area.

Causes and symptoms

Pain is the most common symptom of injury and disease, and descriptions can range in intensity from a mere ache to unbearable agony. Nociceptors have the ability to convey information to the brain that indicates the location, nature, and intensity of the pain. For example, stepping on a nail sends an information-packed message to the brain: the foot has experienced a puncture wound that hurts a lot.

Pain perception also varies depending on the location of the pain. The kinds of stimuli that cause a pain response on the skin include pricking, cutting, crushing, burning, and freezing. These same stimuli would not generate much of a response in the intestine. Intestinal pain arises from stimuli such as swelling, inflammation, and distension.

Diagnosis

Pain is considered in view of other symptoms and individual experiences. An observable injury, such as a broken bone, may be a clear indicator of the type of pain a person is suffering. Determining the specific cause of internal pain is more difficult. Other symptoms, such as fever or **nausea**, help narrow down the possibilities. In some cases, such as lower back pain, a specific cause may not be identifiable. Diagnosis of the disease causing a specific pain is further complicated by the fact that pain can be referred to (felt at) a skin site that does not seem to be connected to the site of the pain's origin. For example, pain arising from fluid accumulating at the base of the lung may be referred to the shoulder.

Since pain is a subjective experience, it may be very difficult to communicate its exact quality and intensity to other people. There are no diagnostic tests that can determine the quality or intensity of an individual's pain. Therefore, a medical examination will include a lot of questions about where the pain is located, its intensity, and its nature. Questions are also directed at what kinds of things increase or relieve the pain, how long it has lasted, and whether there are any variations in it. An individual may be asked to use a pain scale to describe the pain. One such scale assigns a number to the pain intensity; for example, 0 may indicate no pain, and 10 may indicate the worst pain the person has ever experienced. Scales are modified for infants and children to accommodate their level of comprehension.

Treatment

There are many drugs aimed at preventing or treating pain. Nonopioid **analgesics**, narcotic analgesics, anticonvulsant drugs, and **tricyclic antidepressants** work by blocking the production, release, or uptake of neurotransmitters. Drugs from different classes may be combined to handle certain types of pain.

Nonopioid analgesics include common over-the-counter medications such as **aspirin**, **acetaminophen** (Tylenol), and ibuprofen (Advil). These are most often used for minor pain, but there are some prescription-strength medications in this class.

Narcotic analgesics are only available with a doctor's prescription and are used for more severe pain, such as cancer pain. These drugs include codeine, morphine, and **methadone**. **Addiction** to these painkillers is not as common as once thought. Many people who genuinely need these drugs for pain control typically do not become addicted. However, narcotic use should be limited to patients thought to have a short life span (such as people with terminal cancer) or patients whose pain is only expected to last for a short time (such as people recovering from surgery). In August 2004, the Drug Enforcement Administration (DEA) issued new guidelines to help physicians prescribe **narcotics** appropriately without fear of being arrested for prescribing the drugs beyond the scope of their medical practice. DEA is trying to work with physicians to ensure that those who need to drugs receive them but to ensure opioids are not abused.

Anticonvulsants, as well as **antidepressant drugs**, were initially developed to treat seizures and depression, respectively. However, it was discovered that these drugs also have pain-killing applications. Furthermore, since in cases of chronic or extreme pain, it is not unusual for an individual to suffer some degree of depression; antidepressants may serve a dual role. Commonly prescribed anticonvulsants for pain include phenytoin, carbamazepine, and clonazepam. Tricyclic antidepressants include doxepin, amitriptyline, and imipramine.

Intractable (unrelenting) pain may be treated by injections directly into or near the nerve that is transmitting the pain signal. These root blocks may also be useful in determining the site of pain generation. As the underlying mechanisms of abnormal pain are uncovered, other pain medications are being developed.

Drugs are not always effective in controlling pain. Surgical methods are used as a last resort if drugs and local anesthetics fail. The least destructive surgical procedure involves implanting a device that emits electrical signals. These signals disrupt the nerve and prevent it from transmitting the pain message. However, this method may not completely control pain and is not used frequently. Other surgical techniques involve destroying or severing the nerve, but the use of this technique is limited by side effects, including unpleasant **numbness**.

Alternative treatment

Both physical and psychological aspects of pain can be dealt with through alternative treatment. Some of the most popular treatment options include **acupressure** and **acupuncture**, massage, chiropractic,

KEY TERMS

Acute pain—Pain in response to injury or another stimulus that resolves when the injury heals or the stimulus is removed.

Chronic pain—Pain that lasts beyond the term of an injury or painful stimulus. Can also refer to cancer pain, pain from a chronic or degenerative disease, and pain from an unidentified cause.

Neuron—A nerve cell.

Neurotransmitters—Chemicals within the nervous system that transmit information from or between nerve cells.

Nociceptor—A neuron that is capable of sensing pain.

Referred pain—Pain felt at a site different from the location of the injured or diseased part of the body. Referred pain is due to the fact that nerve signals from several areas of the body may "feed" the same nerve pathway leading to the spinal cord and brain.

Stimulus—A factor capable of eliciting a response in a nerve.

and relaxation techniques such as **yoga**, hypnosis, and **meditation**. Herbal therapies are gaining increased recognition as viable options; for example, capsaicin, the component that makes cayenne peppers spicy, is used in ointments to relieve the joint pain associated with arthritis. Contrast **hydrotherapy** can also be very beneficial for pain relief.

Lifestyles can be changed to incorporate a healthier diet and regular **exercise**. Regular exercise, aside from relieving **stress**, has been shown to increase endorphins, painkillers naturally produced in the body.

Prognosis

Successful pain treatment is highly dependent on successful resolution of the pain's cause. Acute pain will stop when an injury heals or when an underlying problem is treated successfully. Chronic pain and abnormal pain are more difficult to treat, and it may take longer to find a successful resolution. Some pain is intractable and will require extreme measures for relief.

Prevention

Pain is generally preventable only to the degree that the cause of the pain is preventable. For example, improved surgical procedures, such as those done

through a thin tube called a laparascope, minimize post-operative pain. Anesthesia techniques for surgeries also continuously improve. Some disease and injuries are often unavoidable. However, pain from some surgeries and other medical procedures and continuing pain are preventable through drug treatments and alternative therapies.

Resources

PERIODICALS

"Advances in Pain Management, New Focus Greatly Easing Postoperative Care." *Medical Devices & Surgical Technology Week* September 26, 2004: 260.

Finn, Robert. "More than Half of Patients With Major Depression Have Chronic Pain." *Family Practice News* October 15, 2004: 38.

"New Guidelines Set for Better Pain Treatment." *Medical Letter on the CDC & FDA* September 5, 2004: 95.

ORGANIZATIONS

American Chronic Pain Association. P.O. Box 850, Rocklin, CA 95677-0850. (916) 632-0922. < http://members.tripod.com/~widdy/ACPA.html >.

American Pain Society. 4700 W. Lake Ave., Glenview, IL 60025. (847) 375-4715. < http://www.ampainsoc.org >.

Julia Barrett
Teresa G. Odle

Pain management

Definition

Pain management encompasses pharmacological, nonpharmacological, and other approaches to prevent, reduce, or stop pain sensations.

Purpose

Pain serves as an alert to potential or actual damage to the body. The definition for damage is quite broad; pain can arise from injury as well as disease. After the message is received and interpreted, further pain can be counter-productive. Pain can have a negative impact on a person's quality of life and impede recovery from illness or injury. Unrelieved pain can become a syndrome in its own right and cause a downward spiral in a person's health and outlook. Managing pain properly facilitates recovery, prevents additional health complications, and improves an individual's quality of life.

Description

What is pain?

Before considering pain management, a review of pain definitions and mechanisms may be useful. Pain is the means by which the peripheral nervous system (PNS) warns the central nervous system (CNS) of injury or potential injury to the body. The CNS comprises the brain and spinal cord, and the PNS is composed of the nerves that stem from and lead into the CNS. The PNS includes all nerves throughout the body except the brain and spinal cord.

A pain message is transmitted to the CNS by special PNS nerve cells called nociceptors. Nociceptors are distributed throughout the body and respond to different stimuli depending on their location. For example, nociceptors that extend from the skin are stimulated by sensations such as pressure, temperature, and chemical changes.

When a nociceptor is stimulated, neurotransmitters are released within the cell. Neurotransmitters are chemicals found within the nervous system that facilitate nerve cell communication. The nociceptor transmits its signal to nerve cells within the spinal cord, which conveys the pain message to the thalamus, a specific region in the brain.

Once the brain has received and processed the pain message and coordinated an appropriate response, pain has served its purpose. The body uses natural pain killers, called endorphins, that are meant to derail further pain messages from the same source. However, these natural pain killers may not adequately dampen a continuing pain message. Also, depending on how the brain has processed the pain information, certain hormones, such as prostaglandins, may be released. These hormones enhance the pain message and play a role in immune system responses to injury, such as inflammation. Certain neurotransmitters, especially substance P and calcitonin gene-related peptide, actively enhance the pain message at the injury site and within the spinal cord.

Pain is generally divided into two categories: acute and chronic. Nociceptive pain, or the pain that is transmitted by nociceptors, is typically called acute pain. This kind of pain is associated with injury, headaches, disease, and many other conditions. It usually resolves once the condition that caused it is resolved.

Following some disorders, pain does not resolve. Even after healing or a cure has been achieved, the brain continues to perceive pain. In this situation, the pain may be considered chronic. The time limit used to define chronic pain typically ranges from three to six months, although some healthcare professionals prefer a more flexible definition, and consider chronic pain as pain that endures beyond a normal healing time. The pain associated with **cancer**, persistent and degenerative conditions, and neuropathy, or nerve damage, is included in the chronic category. Also, unremitting pain that lacks an identifiable physical cause, such as the majority of cases of **low back pain**, may be considered chronic. The underlying biochemistry of chronic pain appears to be different from regular nociceptive pain.

Some researchers have said that uninterrupted and unrelenting pain can induce changes in the spinal cord. In the past, intractable pain has been treated by severing a nerve's connection to the CNS. However, the lack of any sensory information being relayed by that nerve can cause pain transmission in the spinal cord to go into overdrive, as evidenced by the phantom limb pain experienced by amputees. Evidence is accumulating that unrelenting pain or the complete lack of nerve signals increases the number of pain receptors in the spinal cord. Nerve cells in the spinal cord may also begin secreting pain-amplifying neurotransmitters independent of actual pain signals from the body. Immune chemicals, primarily cytokines, may play a prominent role in such changes.

Scientists have long recognized a relationship between depression and chronic pain. In 2004, a survey of California adults diagnosed with major depressive disorder revealed that more than one-half of them also suffered from chronic pain.

Managing pain

Considering the different causes and types of pain, as well as its nature and intensity, management can require an interdisciplinary approach. The elements of this approach include treating the underlying cause of pain, pharmacological and nonpharmacological therapies, and some invasive (surgical) procedures.

Treating the cause of pain underpins the idea of managing it. Injuries are repaired, diseases are diagnosed, and certain encounters with pain can be anticipated and treated prophylactically (by prevention). However, there are no guarantees of immediate relief from pain. Recovery can be impeded by pain and quality of life can be damaged. Therefore, pharmacological and other therapies have developed over time to address these aspects of disease and injury.

PHARMACOLOGICAL OPTIONS. Pain-relieving drugs, otherwise called **analgesics**, include nonsteroidal anti-inflammatory drugs (NSAIDs), **acetaminophen**, **narcotics**, antidepressants, anticonvulsants, and others. NSAIDs and acetaminophen are available as over-the-counter and prescription medications, and are frequently the initial pharmacological treatment for pain. These drugs can also be used as adjuncts to the other drug therapies, which might require a doctor's prescription.

NSAIDs include **aspirin**, ibuprofen (Motrin, Advil, Nuprin), naproxen sodium (Aleve), and ketoprofen (Orudis KT). These drugs are used to treat pain from inflammation and work by blocking production of pain-enhancing neurotransmitters, such as prostaglandins. Acetaminophen is also effective against pain, but its ability to reduce inflammation is limited.

NSAIDs and acetaminophen are effective for most forms of acute (sharp, but of a short course) pain, but moderate and severe pain may require stronger medication. Narcotics handle intense pain effectively, and are used for cancer pain and acute pain that does not respond to NSAIDs and acetaminophen. Narcotics are classified as either opiates or opioids, and are available only with a doctor's prescription. Opiates include morphine and codeine, which are derived from opium, a substance naturally found in some poppy species. Opioids are synthetic drugs based on the structure of opium. This drug class includes drugs such as oxycodon, **methadone**, and meperidine (Demerol). In August 2004, the Drug Enforcement Administration (DEA) issued new guidelines to help physicians prescribe narcotics appropriately without fear of being arrested for prescribing the drugs beyond the scope of their medical practice. DEA is trying to work with physicians to ensure that those who need to drugs receive them but to ensure opioids are not abused.

Narcotics may be ineffective against some forms of chronic pain, especially since changes in the spinal cord may alter the usual pain signaling pathways. In such situations, pain can be managed with the help of with antidepressants and anticonvulsants, which are also only available with a doctor's prescription.

Although **antidepressant drugs** were developed to treat depression, it has been discovered that they are also effective in combating some chronic headaches, cancer pain, and pain associated with nerve damage. Antidepressants that have been shown to have analgesic (pain reducing) properties include amitriptyline (Elavil), trazodone (Desyrel), and imipramine (Tofranil). **Anticonvulsant drugs** share a similar background with antidepressants. Developed to treat epilepsy, certain anticonvulsants were found to relieve pain as well. Drugs such as phenytoin (Dilantin) and carbamazepine (Tegretol) are prescribed to treat the pain associated with nerve damage.

Other prescription drugs are used to treat specific types of pain or specific pain syndromes. For example, **corticosteroids** are effective against pain caused by inflammation and swelling, and sumatriptan (Imitrex) was developed to treat migraine headaches.

Drug administration depends on the drug type and the required dose. Some drugs are not absorbed very well from the stomach and must be injected or administered intravenously. Injections and intravenous administration may also be used when high doses are needed or if an individual is nauseous. Following surgery and other medical procedures, patients may have the option of controlling the pain medication themselves. By pressing a button, they can release a set dose of medication into an intravenous solution. This procedure has also been employed in other situations requiring pain management. Another mode of administration involves implanted catheters that deliver pain medication directly to the spinal cord. Delivering drugs in this way can reduce side effects and increase the effectiveness of the drug.

NONPHARMACOLOGICAL OPTIONS. Pain treatment options that do not use drugs are often used as adjuncts to, rather than replacements for, drug therapy. One of the benefits of non-drug therapies is that an individual can take a more active stance against pain. Relaxation techniques, such as **yoga** and **meditation**, are used to decrease muscle tension and reduce **stress**. Tension and stress can also be reduced through **biofeedback**, in which an individual consciously attempts to modify skin temperature, muscle tension, blood pressure, and heart rate.

Participating in normal activities and exercising can also help control pain levels. Through physical therapy, an individual learns beneficial exercises for reducing stress, strengthening muscles, and staying fit. Regular **exercise** has been linked to production of endorphins, the body's natural pain killers.

Acupuncture involves the insertion of small needles into the skin at key points. **Acupressure** uses these same key points, but involves applying pressure rather than inserting needles. Both of these methods may work by prompting the body to release endorphins. Applying heat or being massaged are very relaxing and help reduce stress. Transcutaneous electrical nerve stimulation (TENS) applies a small electric current to certain parts of nerves, potentially interrupting pain signals and inducing release of endorphins. To be effective, use of TENS should be medically supervised.

INVASIVE PROCEDURES. There are three types of invasive procedures that may be used to manage or treat pain: anatomic, augmentative, and ablative.

These procedures involve surgery, and certain guidelines should be followed before carrying out a procedure with permanent effects. First, the cause of the pain must be clearly identified. Next, surgery should be done only if noninvasive procedures are ineffective. Third, any psychological issues should be addressed. Finally, there should be a reasonable expectation of success.

Anatomic procedures involve correcting the injury or removing the cause of pain. Relatively common anatomic procedures are decompression surgeries, such as repairing a herniated disk in the lower back or relieving the nerve compression related to **carpal tunnel syndrome**. Another anatomic procedure is neurolysis, also called a nerve block, which involves destroying a portion of a peripheral nerve.

Augmentative procedures include electrical stimulation or direct application of drugs to the nerves that are transmitting the pain signals. Electrical stimulation works on the same principle as TENS. In this procedure, instead of applying the current across the skin, electrodes are implanted to stimulate peripheral nerves or nerves in the spinal cord. Augmentative procedures also include implanted drug-delivery systems. In these systems, catheters are implanted in the spine to allow direct delivery of drugs to the CNS.

Ablative procedures are characterized by severing a nerve and disconnecting it from the CNS. However, this method may not address potential alterations within the spinal cord. These changes perpetuate pain messages and do not cease even when the connection between the sensory nerve and the CNS is severed. With growing understanding of neuropathic pain and development of less invasive procedures, ablative procedures are used less frequently. However, they do have applications in select cases of **peripheral neuropathy**, cancer pain, and other disorders.

Preparation

Prior to beginning management, pain is thoroughly evaluated. Pain scales or questionnaires are used to attach an objective measure to a subjective experience. Objective measurements allow health care workers a better understanding of the pain being experienced by the patient. Evaluation also includes physical examinations and diagnostic tests to determine underlying causes. Some evaluations require assessments from several viewpoints, including neurology, psychiatry and psychology, and physical therapy. If pain is due to a medical procedure, management consists of anticipating the type and intensity of associated pain and managing it preemptively.

KEY TERMS

Acute—Referring to pain in response to injury or other stimulus that resolves when the injury heals or the stimulus is removed.

Chronic—Referring to pain that endures beyond the term of an injury or painful stimulus. Can also refer to cancer pain, pain from a chronic or degenerative disease, and pain from an unidentified cause.

CNS or central nervous system—The part of the nervous system that includes the brain and the spinal cord.

Iatrogenic—Resulting from the activity of the physician.

Neuropathy—Nerve damage.

Neurotransmitter—Chemicals within the nervous system that transmit information from or between nerve cells.

Nociceptor—A nerve cell that is capable of sensing pain and transmitting a pain signal.

Nonpharmacological—Referring to therapy that does not involve drugs.

Pharmacological—Referring to therapy that relies on drugs.

PNS or peripheral nervous system—Nerves that are outside of the brain and spinal cord.

Stimulus—A factor capable of eliciting a response in a nerve.

Risks

Owing to toxicity over the long term, some drugs can only be used for acute pain or as adjuncts in chronic pain management. NSAIDs have the well-known side effect of causing gastrointestinal bleeding, and long-term use of acetaminophen has been linked to kidney and liver damage. Other drugs, especially narcotics, have serious side effects, such as **constipation**, drowsiness, and **nausea**. Serious side effects can also accompany pharmacological therapies; mood swings, confusion, bone thinning, cataract formation, increased blood pressure, and other problems may discourage or prevent use of some analgesics.

Nonpharmacological therapies carry little or no risk. However, it is advised that individuals recovering from serious illness or injury consult with their health care providers or physical therapists before making use of adjunct therapies. Invasive procedures carry risks similar to other surgical procedures, such as infection, reaction to anesthesia, iatrogenic (injury as a result of treatment) injury, and failure.

A traditional concern about narcotics use has been the risk of promoting **addiction**. As narcotic use continues over time, the body becomes accustomed to the drug and adjusts normal functions to accommodate to its presence. Therefore, to elicit the same level of action, it is necessary to increase dosage over time. As dosage increases, an individual may become physically dependent on narcotic drugs.

However, physical dependence is different from psychological addiction. Physical dependence is characterized by discomfort if drug administration suddenly stops, while psychological addiction is characterized by an overpowering craving for the drug for reasons other than pain relief. Psychological addiction is a very real and necessary concern in some instances, but it should not interfere with a genuine need for narcotic pain relief. However, caution must be taken with people with a history of addictive behavior.

Normal results

Effective application of pain management techniques reduces or eliminates acute or chronic pain. This treatment can improve an individual's quality of life and aid in recovery from injury and disease.

Resources

PERIODICALS

Finn, Robert. "More than Half of Patients With Major Depression Have Chronic Pain." *Family Practice News* October 15, 2004: 38.

"New Guidelines Set for Better Pain Treatment." *Medical Letter on the CDC & FDA* September 5, 2004: 95.

ORGANIZATIONS

American Chronic Pain Association. P.O. Box 850, Rocklin, CA 95677-0850. (916) 632-0922. < http://members.tripod.com/~widdy/ACPA.html >.

American Pain Society. 4700 West Lake Ave., Glenview, IL 60025. (847) 375-4715. < http://www.ampainsoc.org >.

National Chronic Pain Outreach Association, Inc. P.O. Box 274, Millboro, VA 24460-9606. (540) 997-5004.

Julia Barrett
Teresa G. Odle

Pain relievers *see* **Analgesics**

Painful menstruation *see* **Dysmenorrhea**

Palliative cancer therapy *see* **Cancer therapy, palliative**

Palpitations

Definition

A sensation in which a person is aware of an irregular, hard, or rapid heartbeat.

Description

Palpitations mean that the heart is not behaving normally. It can appear to skip beats, beat rapidly, beat irregularly, or thump in the chest. Although palpitations are very common and often harmless, they can be frightening to the person, who is usually unaware of his or her heartbeat.

Palpitations can also be a sign of serious heart trouble. Palpitations that are caused by certain types of abnormal heart rhythms (**arrhythmias**) can be serious, and even fatal if left untreated. Recognizable arrhythmias are present in a small number of patients who have palpitations. Immediate medical attention should be sought for palpitations that feel like a very fast series of heartbeats, last more than two or three minutes, and are unrelated to strenuous physical activity, obvious fright, or anger. Medical attention should also be sought if palpitations are accompanied by chest **pain, dizziness, shortness of breath**, or an overall feeling of weakness.

Most people have experienced a skipped or missed heartbeat, which is really an early beat and not a skipped beat at all. After a premature heartbeat, the heart rests for an instant then beats with extra force, making the person feel as if the heart has skipped a beat. This type of palpitation is nothing to worry about unless it occurs frequently. Severe palpitations feel like a thudding or fluttering sensation in the chest. After chest pain, palpitations are the most common reason that people are referred for cardiology evaluation.

Causes and symptoms

Palpitations can be caused by **anxiety**, arrhythmias, caffeine, certain medications, **cocaine** and other amphetamines, emotional **stress**, overeating, panic, somatization, and vigorous **exercise**. There may be no other symptoms. But, anxiety, dizziness, shortness of breath, and chest pain may be signs of more severe arrhythmias.

Diagnosis

Palpitations are diagnosed through a medical history, a physical examination, an electrocardiogram

(ECG), and screening for psychiatric disorders. It is often difficult to distinguish palpitations from **panic disorder**, a common problem in which the person experiences frequent and unexplained "fight-or-flight" responses, which is the body's natural physical reaction to extreme danger or physical exertion, but without the obvious external stimulus.

To accurately diagnose palpitations, one of the irregular heartbeats must be "captured" on an EKG, which shows the heart's activity. Electrodes covered with a type of gel that conducts electrical impulses are placed on the patient's chest, arms, and legs. These electrodes send impulses of the heart's activity to a recorder, which traces them on paper. This **electrocardiography** test takes about 10 minutes and is performed in a physician's office or hospital. Because the palpitations are unlikely to occur during a standard EKG, **Holter monitoring** is often performed. In this procedure, the patient wears a small, portable tape recorder that is attached to a belt or shoulder strap and connected to electrode disks on his or her chest. The Holter monitor records the heart's rhythm during normal activities. Some medical centers are now using event recorders that the patient can carry for weeks or months. When the palpitations occur, the patient presses a button on the device, which captures the information about the palpitations for physician evaluation. Later the recording can be transmitted over the telephone line for analysis.

Treatment

Most palpitations require no treatment. Persistent palpitations can be treated with small doses of a beta blocker. **Beta blockers** are drugs that tend to lower blood pressure. They slow the heart rate and decrease the force with which the heart pumps. If the cause of the palpitations is determined to be an arrhythmia, medical or surgical treatment may be prescribed, although surgery is rarely needed.

Alternative treatment

Alternative treatments for palpitations should be used only as a complement to traditional medicine. Alternative treatments include: **aromatherapy**, Chinese herbs, herbal therapies, **homeopathic medicine**, exercise, mind/body medicine, and diet and nutrition. In aromatherapy, adding citrus oils to bath water may help with minor palpitations. Some Chinese herbs can also help, but others can worsen arrhythmias, so a qualified herbalist should be consulted. Herbal therapies such as hawthorn

(*Crataegus laevigata*) and motherwort (*Leonurus cardiaca*) can help with palpitations. Homeopathic remedies such as *Lachesis, Digitalis,* and *Aconite* (*Aconitum nnapellus*) may be used to control palpitations but should be taken only when prescribed by a homeopathic physician. Mind/body medicine such as **meditation** and **yoga** can help the person relax, eliminating or reducing palpitations caused by anxiety or stress. Reducing or eliminating tea, cola, coffee, and chocolate, and consuming adequate amounts of the **minerals** calcium, magnesium, and potassium can help reduce or eliminate palpitations.

Prognosis

Most palpitations are harmless, but some can be a sign of heart trouble, which could be fatal if left untreated.

Prevention

Palpitations not caused by arrhythmias can be prevented by reducing or eliminating anxiety and emotional stress, and reducing or eliminating consumption of tea, cola, coffee, and chocolate. Exercise can also help, but a treadmill **stress test** performed by a physician should be considered first to make sure the exercise is safe.

Resources

PERIODICALS

Mayou, Richard. "Chest Pain, Palpitations, and Panic." *Journal of Psychosomatic Research* 44 (1998): 53-70.

Lori De Milto

Panax quinquefolius see **Ginseng**

Pancreas removal *see* **Pancreatectomy**

Pancreas transplantation

Definition

Pancreas transplantation is a surgical procedure in which a diseased pancreas is replaced with a healthy pancreas that has been obtained immediately after **death** from an immunologically compatible donor.

Purpose

The pancreas secretes insulin to regulate glucose (sugar) metabolism. Failure to regulate glucose levels leads to diabetes. Over one million patients in the United States have insulin dependent (type I) **diabetes mellitus**. Successful pancreas transplantation allows the body to make and secrete its own insulin, and establishes insulin independence for these patients.

Pancreas transplantation is major surgery that requires suppression of the immune system to prevent the body from rejecting the transplanted pancreas. Immunosuppressive drugs have serious side effects. Because of these side effects, in 1996, 85% of pancreas transplants were performed simultaneously with kidney transplants, 10% after a kidney transplant, and only 5% were performed as a pancreas transplant alone.

The rationale for this is that patients will already be receiving immunosuppressive treatments for the kidney transplant, so they might as well receive the benefit of a pancreas transplant as well. Patients considering pancreas transplantation alone must decide with their doctors whether life-long treatment with immunosuppressive drugs is preferable to life-long insulin dependence.

The best candidates for pancreas transplantation are:

- between the ages of 20–40
- those who have extreme difficulty regulating their glucose levels
- those who have few secondary complications of diabetes
- those who are in good cardiovascular health.

Precautions

Many people with diabetes are not good candidates for a pancreas transplant. Others do not have tissue compatibility with the donor organ. People who are successfully controlling their diabetes with insulin

National Transplant Waiting List By Organ Type (June 2000)	
Organ Needed	**Number Waiting**
Kidney	48,349
Liver	15,987
Heart	4,139
Lung	3,695
Kidney-Pancreas	2,437
Pancreas	942
Heart-Lung	212
Intestine	137

injections are usually not considered for pancreas transplants.

Description

Once a donor pancreas is located, the patient is prepared for surgery. Since only about 1,000 pancreas transplants are performed each year in the United States, the operation usually occurs at a hospital where surgeons have special expertise in the procedure.

The surgeon makes an incision under the ribs and locates the pancreas and duodenum. The pancreas and duodenum (part of the small intestine) are removed. The new pancreas and duodenum are then connected to the patient's blood vessels.

Replacing the duodenum allows the pancreas to drain into the gastrointestinal system. The transplant can also be done creating a bladder drainage. Bladder drainage makes it easier to monitor organ rejection. Once the new pancreas is in place, the abdomen and skin are closed. This surgery is often done at the same time as kidney transplant surgery.

Preparation

After the patient and doctor have decided on a pancreas transplant, a complete immunological study is done to match the patient to a donor. All body functions are evaluated. The timing of surgery depends on the availability of a donated organ.

Aftercare

Patients receiving a pancreas transplantation are monitored closely for organ rejection, and all vital body functions are monitored also. The average hospital stay is three weeks. It takes about six months to recover from surgery. Patients will take immunosuppressive drugs for the rest of their lives.

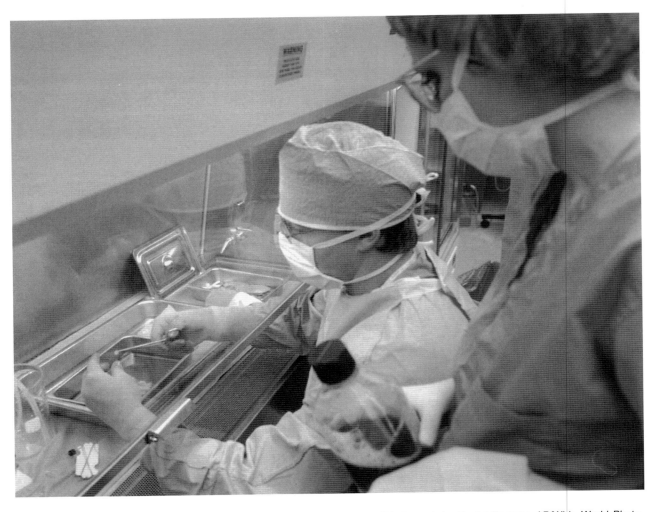

A surgeon harvests the islets of Langerhans from a donor pancreas. *(Photograph by Daniel Portnoy. AP/Wide World Photo. Reproduced by permission.)*

KEY TERMS

Duodenum—The section of the small intestine immediately after the stomach.

Risks

Diabetes and poor kidney function greatly increase the risk of complications from anesthesia during surgery. Organ rejection, excessive bleeding, and infection are other major risks associated with this surgery.

Normal results

During a nine year period from 1987 to 1996, the patient survival rate for all types of pancreas transplants (with or without associated kidney transplant) was 92% after one year and 86% after three years. In a successful transplant, the pancreas begins producing insulin, bringing the regulation of glucose back under normal body control. Natural availability of insulin prevents the development of additional damage to the kidneys and blindness associated with diabetes. Many patients report an improved quality of life.

Resources

ORGANIZATIONS

American Diabetes Association. 1701 North Beauregard Street, Alexandria, VA 22311. (800) 342-2383. < http://www.diabetes.org >.

Tish Davidson, A.M.

Pancreatectomy

Definition

Pancreatectomy is the surgical removal of the pancreas. Pancreatectomy may be total, in which case the whole organ is removed, or partial, referring to the removal of part of the pancreas.

Purpose

Pancreatectomy is the most effective treatment for **cancer** of the pancreas, an abdominal organ that secretes digestive enzymes, insulin, and other hormones. The thickest part of the pancreas near the duodenum (small intestine) is called the head, the middle part is called the body, and the thinnest part adjacent to the spleen is called the tail.

While surgical removal of tumors in the pancreas is preferred, it is only possible in the 10-15% of patients who are diagnosed early enough for a potential cure. Patients who are considered suitable for surgery usually have small tumors in the head of the pancreas (close to the duodenum, or first part of the small intestine), have **jaundice** as their initial symptom, and have no evidence of metastatic disease (spread of cancer to other sites).

Pancreatectomy is sometimes necessary when the pancreas has been severely injured by trauma, especially injury to the body and tail of the pancreas. While such surgery removes normal pancreatic tissue as well, the long-term consequences of this surgery are minimal, with virtually no effects on the production of insulin, digestive enzymes, and other hormones.

Chronic **pancreatitis** is another condition for which pancreatectomy is occasionally performed. Chronic pancreatitis—or continuing inflammation of the pancreas that results in permanent damage to this organ—can develop from long-standing, recurring episodes of acute (periodic) pancreatitis. This painful condition usually results from alcohol abuse or the presence of **gallstones**. In most patients with alcohol-induced disease, the pancreas is widely involved, therefore, surgical correction is almost impossible.

Precautions

Pancreatectomy is only performed when surgery provides a clear benefit. Patients who have tumors that are obviously not operable should be carefully excluded from consideration.

Description

Pancreatectomy sometimes entails removal of the entire pancreas, called a total pancreatectomy, but more often involves removal of part of the pancreas, which is called a subtotal pancreatectomy, or distal pancreatectomy, when the body and tail of the pancreas are removed. When the duodenum is removed along with all or part of the pancreas, the procedure is called a pancreaticoduodenectomy, which surgeons sometimes refer to as "Whipple's procedure." Pancreaticoduodenectomy is being used increasingly for treatment of a variety of malignant and benign diseases of the pancreas.

Regional lymph nodes are usually removed during pancreaticoduodenectomy. In distal pancreatectomy, the spleen may also be removed.

Preparation

Patients with symptoms of a pancreatic disorder usually undergo a number of tests before surgery is even considered. These can include ultrasonography, x-ray examinations, **computed tomography scans** (CT scan), and endoscopic retrograde cholangiopancreatography (ERCP), an x-ray imaging technique. Tests may also include **angiography**, an x-ray technique for visualizing the arteries feeding the pancreas, and needle aspiration cytology, in which cells are drawn from areas suspected to contain cancer. Such tests aid in the diagnosis of the pancreatic disorder and in the planning of the operation.

Since many patients with pancreatic cancer are undernourished, appropriate nutritional support, sometimes by **tube feedings**, may be required prior to surgery.

Some patients with pancreatic cancer deemed suitable for pancreatectomy will undergo chemotherapy and/or radiation therapy. This treatment is aimed at shrinking the tumor, which will improve the chances for successful surgical removal. Sometimes, patients who are not initially considered surgical candidates may respond so well to chemoradiation that surgical treatment becomes possible. **Radiation therapy** may also be applied during the surgery (intraoperatively) to improve the patient's chances of survival, but this treatment is not yet in routine use. Some studies have shown that intraoperative radiation therapy extends survival by several months.

Patients undergoing distal pancreatectomy that involves removal of the spleen may receive preoperative medication to decrease the risk of infection.

Aftercare

Pancreatectomy is major surgery. Therefore, extended hospitalization is usually required. Some studies report an average hospital stay of about two weeks.

Some cancer patients may also receive combined **chemotherapy** and radiation therapy after surgery. This additional treatment has been clearly shown to enhance survival from pancreatic cancer.

Removal of all or part of the pancreas can lead to a condition called pancreatic insufficiency, in which food cannot be normally processed by the body, and insulin secretion may be inadequate. These conditions can be treated with pancreatic enzyme replacement therapy, to supply digestive enzymes, and insulin injections, to supply insulin.

Risks

The mortality rate for pancreatectomy has improved in recent years to 5–10%, depending on the extent of the surgery and the experience of the surgeon. A study of 650 patients at Johns Hopkins Medical Institution, Baltimore, found that only nine patients, or 1.4%, died from complications related to surgery.

There is still, however, a fairly high risk of complications following any form of pancreatectomy. The Johns Hopkins study documented complications in 41% of cases. The most devastating complication is postoperative bleeding, which increases the mortality risk to 20-50%. In cases of postoperative bleeding, the patient may be returned to surgery to find the source of hemorrhage, or may undergo other procedures to stop the bleeding.

One of the most common complications from a pancreaticoduodenectomy is delayed gastric emptying, a condition in which food and liquids are slow to leave the stomach. This complication occurred in 19% of patients in the Johns Hopkins study. To manage this problem, many surgeons insert feeding tubes at the original operation site, through which nutrients can be fed directly into the patient's intestines. This procedure, called enteral nutrition, maintains the patient's **nutrition** if the stomach is slow to recover normal function. Certain medications, called promotility agents, can help move the nutritional contents through the gastrointestinal tract.

The other most common complication is pancreatic anastomotic leak. This is a leak in the connection that the surgeon makes between the remainder of the pancreas and the other structures in the abdomen.

Most surgeons handle the potential for this problem by assuring that there will be adequate drainage from the surgical site.

Normal results

Unfortunately, pancreatic cancer is the most lethal form of gastrointestinal malignancy. However, for a highly selective group of patients, pancreatectomy offers a chance for cure, especially when performed by experienced surgeons. The overall five-year survival rate for patients who undergo pancreatectomy for pancreatic cancer is about 10%; patients who undergo pancreaticoduodenectomy have a 4–5% survival at five years. The risk for tumor recurrence is thought to be unaffected by whether the patient undergoes a total pancreatectomy or a pancreaticoduodenectomy, but is increased when the tumor is larger than 3 cm and the cancer has spread to the lymph nodes or surrounding tissue.

After total pancreatectomy, the body loses the ability to secrete insulin, enzymes, and other substances, therefore, certain medications will be required to compensate for this. In some cases of pancreatic disease, the pancreas ceases to function normally, then total pancreatectomy may be preferable to other less radical forms of the operation.

When pancreatectomy is performed for chronic pancreatitis, the majority of patients obtain some relief from **pain**. Some studies report that one half to three quarters of patients become free of pain.

Resources

BOOKS

Bastidas, J. Augusto, and John E. Niederhuber. "The Pancreas." In *Fundamentals of Surgery*, edited by John E. Niederhuber. Stamford: Appleton & Lange, 1998.

Caroline A. Helwick

Pancreatic cancer, endocrine

Definition

Endocrine pancreatic **cancer** is a disease in which cancerous cells originate within the tissues of the pancreas that produce hormones.

Description

The pancreas is a 6-8 in (15-20 cm) long, slipper-shaped gland located in the abdomen. It lies behind the stomach, within a loop formed by the small intestine. Other nearby organs include the gallbladder, spleen, and liver. The pancreas has a wide end (head), a narrow end (tail), and a middle section (body). A healthy pancreas is important for normal food digestion and plays a critical role in the body's metabolic processes. The pancreas has two main functions, each performed by distinct types of tissue. The exocrine tissue secretes fluids into the other organs of the digestive system, while the endocrine tissue secretes substances that are circulated in the bloodstream. The exocrine pancreas makes up the vast majority of the gland; it produces pancreatic juices containing enzymes that help break down proteins and fatty food. The endocrine tissue of the pancreas makes up only 2% of the gland's total mass. It consists of small patches of cells that produce hormones (like insulin) that control how the body stores and uses nutrients. These patches are called islets (islands) of Langerhans or islet cells and are interspersed evenly throughout the pancreas. Each islet contains approximately 1,000 endocrine cells and a dense network of capillaries (tiny blood vessels), which allows immediate entry of hormones into the circulatory system.

Pancreatic tumors are classified as either exocrine or endocrine tumors depending on which type of tissue they arise from within the gland. Endocrine tumors of the pancreas are very rare, accounting for only 5% of all pancreatic cancers. The majority of endocrine pancreatic tumors are functional adenocarcinomas that overproduce a specific hormone. There are several types of islet cells and each produces its own hormone or peptide (small protein molecule). Functional endocrine tumors are named after the hormone they secrete. Insulinoma is the most common tumor of the endocrine pancreas. Patients with this disease usually develop hypoglycemia due to increased insulin production that leads to abnormally low blood sugar levels. **Gastrinoma**, a disease in which gastrin (hormone that stimulates stomach acid production) is overproduced, causes multiple ulcers in the upper gastrointestinal (GI) tract. Gastrinoma was first described in patients with a rare form of severe peptic ulcer disease known as Zollinger-Ellison syndrome (ZES). The less common glucagonoma causes mild diabetes due to excess glucagon (hormone that stimulates glucose production) secretion. Other rare islet cell tumors include vipoma (vasoactive intestinal peptide) and somatostatinoma. Nonfunctional pancreatic endocrine tumors are not associated with an excess production of any hormone and can be difficult to distinguish from exocrine pancreatic cancer. Cancers of the endocrine pancreas are relatively slow-growing compared to the more common ductal adenocarcinomas of the exocrine pancreas.

Between one and four cases of insulinoma occur per million people per year, and 90% of these tumors are benign. They occur mostly between the ages of 50 and 60 and affect men and women equally. Less than three cases of gastrinoma per million people are diagnosed each year, but it is the most common functional islet cell tumor in patients with multiple endocrine tumors, a condition known as multiple endocrine neoplasia (MEN) syndrome. Vipoma and glucagonoma are even rarer and they occur more frequently in women. Somatostatinoma is exceedingly uncommon, and less than 100 cases have been reported worldwide. Nonfunctional islet cell cancers account for approximately one-third of all cancers of the endocrine pancreas, and the majority of these are malignant.

Causes and symptoms

There are no known causes of islet cell cancer, but a small percentage of cases occur due to hereditary syndromes such as MEN. This is a condition that frequently causes more than one tumor in several endocrine glands, such as the parathyroid and pituitary, in addition to the islet cells of the pancreas. Twenty-five percent of gastrinomas and less than 10% of insulinomas occur in MEN patients. Von Hippel-Lindau (VHL) syndrome is another genetic disorder that causes multiple tumors, and 10–15% of VHL patients will develop islet cell cancer.

Symptoms vary among the different islet cell cancer types. Insulinoma causes repeated episodes of **hypoglycemia**, sweating, and **tremors**, while patients with gastrinoma have inflammation of the esophagus, epigastric **pain**, multiple ulcers, and possibly **diarrhea**. Symptoms of glucagonoma include a distinctive skin rash, inflammation of the stomach, glucose intolerance, weight loss, weakness, and anemia (less common). Patients with vipoma have episodes of profuse, watery diarrhea, even after **fasting**. Somatostatinoma causes mild diabetes, diarrhea/steatorrhea (fatty stools), weight loss, and gallbladder disease. Nonfunctional endocrine tumors frequently produce the same symptoms as cancer of the exocrine pancreas such as abdominal pain, jaundice, and weight loss.

Diagnosis

A thorough physical exam is usually performed when a patient presents with the above symptoms, however, functional endocrine tumors of the pancreas tend to be small and are not detected by palpating the abdomen. Once other illnesses such as infection are ruled out, the doctor will order a series of blood and urine tests. The functional endocrine tumors can be identified through increased levels of hormone in the bloodstream.

Functional endocrine tumors can occur in multiple sites in the pancreas and are often small (less than 1 cm), making them difficult to diagnose. Nonfunctional tumors tend to be larger, which makes them difficult to distinguish from tumors of the exocrine pancreas. Methods such as computed tomography (CT) scan and **magnetic resonance imaging (MRI)** are used to take pictures of the internal organs and allow the doctor to determine whether a tumor is present. Somatostatin receptor scintigraphy (trade name OctreoScan) is an imaging system used to localize endocrine tumors, especially gastrinomas and somatostatinomas. Endoscopic ultrasound (EUS) is a more sensitive technique that may be used if a CT scan fails to detect a tumor. Endocrine tumors usually have many blood vessels, so **angiography** may be useful in the doctor's assessment and staging of the tumor. Surgical exploration is sometimes necessary in order to locate very small tumors that occur in multiple sites. These techniques also help the doctor evaluate how far the tumor has spread. A biopsy can be taken to confirm diagnosis, but more often, doctors look at the size and local invasion of the tumor in order to plan a treatment strategy.

Treatment

Staging

The staging system for islet cell cancer is still evolving, but the tumors typically fall into three categories: cancers that arise in one location within the pancreas, cancers that arise in several locations within the pancreas, and cancers that have spread to nearby lymph nodes or to other organs in the body.

Surgery is the only curative method for islet cell cancers, and studies have shown that an aggressive surgical approach can improve survival and alleviate symptoms of the disease. As with most forms of cancer, the earlier it is diagnosed, the greater the chance for survival. With the exception of insulinoma, the majority of islet cell tumors are malignant at the time of diagnosis, and more than half are metastatic. However, surgery and **chemotherapy** have been shown to improve the outcome of patients even if they have metastatic disease. Surgery may include partial or total removal of the pancreas, and in patients with gastrinoma, the stomach may be removed as well. Streptozotocin, doxorubicin, and 5-fluorouracil (5-FU) are chemotherapeutic agents commonly used in the treatment of islet cell cancer. Patients may experience **nausea** and vomiting as well as kidney toxicity from streptozotocin, and bone marrow suppression from doxorubicin. Hormone therapy is used to relieve the symptoms of functional tumors by inhibiting excess hormone production. Other techniques may be used to block blood flow to the liver in an attempt to kill the cancer cells that have

KEY TERMS

Adenocarcinoma—A malignant tumor that arises within the tissues of a gland and retains its glandular structure.

Angiography—Diagnostic technique used to study blood vessels in a tumor.

Biopsy—Removal and microscopic examination of cells to determine whether they are cancerous.

Chemotherapy—Drug treatment administered to kill cancerous cells.

Endocrine—Refers to glands that secrete hormones circulated in the bloodstream.

Endoscopic ultrasonography (EUS)—Diagnostic imaging technique where an ultrasound probe is inserted down a patient's throat to determine if a tumor is present.

Gastrinoma—Tumor that arises from the gastrin-producing cells in the pancreas.

Insulinoma—Tumor that arises from the insulin-producing cells in the pancreas.

Islets of Langerhans—Clusters of cells in the pancreas that make up the endocrine tissue.

spread there. Abdominal pain, nausea, **vomiting** and **fever** may result from this type of treatment. Radiation has little if any role in the treatment of islet cell cancer.

Prognosis

Islet cell cancers overall have a more favorable prognosis than cancers of the exocrine pancreas, and the median survival from diagnosis is three and a half years. This is mainly due to their slow-growing nature. Insulinomas have a five-year survival rate of 80% and gastrinomas have 65%. When malignant, islet cell cancers do not generally respond well to chemotherapy, and the treatment is mainly palliative. Most patients with metastasis do not survive five years. Islet cell cancer tends to spread to the surrounding lymph nodes, stomach, small intestine, and liver.

Prevention

There are no known risk factors associated with sporadic islet cell cancer. Therefore, it is not clear how to prevent its occurrence. Individuals with MEN syndrome or VHL, however, have a genetic predisposition to developing islet cell cancer and should be screened regularly in an effort to catch the disease early.

Resources

PERIODICALS

Anderson, M.A., et. al. "Endoscopic Ultrasound is HighlyAccurate and Directs Management of Patients With Neuroendocrine Tumors of the Pancreas." *American Journal of Gastroenterology* 95, no. 9 (September 2000): 2271–7.

Hellman, Per, et. al. "Surgical Strategy for Large or Malignant Endocrine Pancreatic Tumors." *World Journal of Surgery* 24 (2000): 1353–60.

ORGANIZATIONS

National Cancer Institute. 9000 Rockville Pike, Bldg. 31, Rm.10A16, Bethesda, MD, 20892. (800) 422-6237. < http://www.nci.nih.gov >.

National Familial Pancreas Tumor Registry. The Johns Hopkins Hospital. 600 North Wolfe St., Baltimore, MD 21287-6417. (410) 377-7450.

National Organization for Rare Disorders. 100 Route 37, PO Box 8923, New Fairfield, CT 06812. (203) 746-6518. < http://www.nord-rdb.com/~orphan >.

OTHER

"Islet Cell Carcinoma." *CancerNetPDQ* May 2001. [cited July 19, 2001]. < http://www.cancernet.nci.nih.gov >.

Pancreatic Cancer Home Page. Johns Hopkins Medical Institutions. July 19, 2001. < http://www.path.jhu.edu/pancreas >.

Elizabeth Pulcini, M.Sc.

Pancreatic cancer, exocrine

Definition

Exocrine pancreatic **cancer** is a disease in which cancerous cells originate within the tissues of the pancreas that produce digestive juices.

Description

The pancreas is a 6-8 in (15-20 cm) long, slipper-shaped gland located in the abdomen. It lies behind the stomach, within a loop formed by the small intestine. Other nearby organs include the gallbladder, spleen, and liver. The pancreas has a wide end (head), a narrow end (tail), and a middle section (body). A healthy pancreas is important for normal food digestion and also plays a critical role in the body's metabolic processes. The pancreas has two main functions, and each are performed by distinct types of tissue. The exocrine tissue makes up the vast majority of the gland and secretes fluids into the other organs of the digestive system. The endocrine tissue secretes hormones (like insulin) that are circulated in the bloodstream, and these substances control how the body stores and uses nutrients. The exocrine tissue of the pancreas, comprised mostly of acinar cells and ductal cells, produces pancreatic (digestive) juices. These juices contain several enzymes that help break down proteins and fatty foods. The exocrine pancreas forms an intricate system of channels or ducts, which are tubular structures that carry pancreatic juices to the small intestine where they are used for digestion.

Pancreatic tumors are classified as either exocrine or endocrine tumors depending on which type of tissue they arise from within the gland. Ninety-five percent of pancreatic cancers occur in the tissues of the exocrine pancreas. Ductal adenocarcinomas arise in the cells that line the ducts of the exocrine pancreas and account for 80% to 90% of all tumors of the pancreas. Unless specified, nearly all reports on pancreatic cancer refer to ductal adenocarcinomas. Less common types of pancreatic exocrine tumors include acinar cell carcinoma, cystic tumors that are typically benign but may become cancerous, and papillary tumors that grow within the pancreatic ducts. Pancreatoblastoma is a very rare disease that primarily affects young children. Two-thirds of pancreatic tumors occur in the head of the pancreas, and tumor growth in this area can lead to the obstruction of the nearby common bile duct that empties bile fluid into the small intestine. When bile cannot be passed into the intestine, patients may develop yellowing of the skin and eyes (jaundice) due to the buildup of bilirubin (a component of bile) in the bloodstream. Tumor blockage of bile or pancreatic ducts may also cause digestive problems since these fluids contain critical enzymes in the digestive process. Depending on their size, pancreatic tumors may cause abdominal **pain** by pressing on the surrounding nerves. Because of its location deep within the abdomen, pancreatic cancer often remains undetected until it has spread to other organs such as the liver or lung. Pancreatic cancer tends to rapidly spread to other organs, even when the primary (original) tumor is relatively small.

Though pancreatic cancer accounts for only 3% of all cancers, it is the fifth most frequent cause of cancer deaths. In 2001, an estimated 29,200 new cases of pancreatic cancer will be diagnosed in the United States. Pancreatic cancer is primarily a disease associated with advanced age, with 80% of cases occurring between the ages of 60 and 80. Men are almost twice as likely to develop this disease than women. Countries with the highest frequencies of pancreatic cancer include the United States, New Zealand, Western European nations, and Scandinavia. The lowest occurrences of the disease are reported in India, Kuwait and Singapore. African Americans have the highest incidence of pancreatic cancer of any ethnic group worldwide. Whether this difference is due to diet or environmental factors remains unclear.

Causes and symptoms

Although the exact cause for pancreatic cancer is not known, several risk factors have been shown to increase susceptibility to this particular cancer, the greatest of which is cigarette smoking. Approximately one-third of pancreatic cancer cases occur among smokers. People who have diabetes develop pancreatic cancer twice as often as non-diabetics. Numerous studies suggest that a family history of pancreatic cancer is another strong risk factor for developing the disease, particularly if two or more relatives in the immediate family have the disease. Other risk factors include chronic (long-term) inflammation of the pancreas (**pancreatitis**), **diets** high in fat, and occupational exposure to certain chemicals such as petroleum.

Pancreatic cancer often does not produce symptoms until it reaches an advanced stage. Patients may then present with the following signs and symptoms:

- upper abdominal and/or back pain
- **jaundice**
- weight loss
- loss of appetite
- diarrhea
- weakness
- **nausea**

These symptoms may also be caused by other illnesses; therefore, it is important to consult a doctor for an accurate diagnosis.

Diagnosis

Pancreatic cancer is difficult to diagnose, especially in the absence of symptoms, and there is no current screening method for early detection. The most sophisticated techniques available often do not detect very small tumors that are localized (have not begun to spread). At advanced stages where patients show symptoms, a number of tests may be performed to confirm diagnosis and to assess the stage of the disease. Approximately half of all pancreatic cancers are metastatic (have spread to other sites) at the time of diagnosis.

The first step in diagnosing pancreatic cancer is a thorough medical history and complete physical examination. The abdomen will be palpated to check for fluid accumulation, lumps, or masses. If there are signs of jaundice, blood tests will be performed to rule out the possibility of liver diseases such as hepatitis. Urine and stool tests may be performed as well.

Non-invasive imaging tools such as computed tomography (CT) scans and magnetic resonance imaging (MRI) can be used to produce detailed pictures of the internal organs. CT is the tool most often used to diagnose pancreatic cancer, as it allows the doctor to determine if the tumor can be removed by surgery or not. It is also useful in staging a tumor by showing the extent to which the tumor has spread. During a CT scan, patients receive an intravenous injection of a contrast dye so the organs can be visualized more clearly. MRI may be performed instead of CT if a patient has an allergy to the CT contrast dye. In some cases where the tumor is impinging on blood vessels or nearby ducts, MRI may be used to generate an image of the pancreatic ducts.

If the doctor suspects pancreatic cancer and no visible masses are seen with a CT scan, a patient may undergo a combination of invasive tests to confirm the presence of a pancreatic tumor. Endoscopic ultrasound (EUS) involves the use of an ultrasound probe at the end of a long, flexible tube that is passed down the patient's throat and into the stomach. This instrument can detect a tumor mass through high frequency sound waves and echoes. EUS can be accompanied by fine needle aspiration (FNA), where a long needle, guided by the ultrasound, is inserted into the tumor mass in order to take a biopsy sample. **Endoscopic retrograde cholangiopancreatography** (ERCP) is a technique often used in patients with severe jaundice because it enables the doctor to relieve blockage of the pancreatic ducts. The doctor, guided by endoscopy and x rays, inserts a small metal or plastic stent into the duct to keep it open. During ERCP, a biopsy can be done by collecting cells from the pancreas with a small brush. The cells are then examined under the microscope by a pathologist, who determines the presence of any cancerous cells.

In some cases, a biopsy may be performed during a type of surgery called laparoscopy, which is done under **general anesthesia**. Doctors insert a small camera and instruments into the abdomen after a minor incision is made. Tissue samples are removed for examination under the microscope. This procedure allows a doctor to determine the extent to which the disease has spread and decide if the tumor can be removed by further surgery.

An **angiography** is a type of test that studies the blood vessels in and around the pancreas. This test may be done before surgery so that the doctor can determine the extent to which the tumor invades and interacts with the blood vessels within the pancreas. The test requires local anesthesia and a catheter is inserted into the patient's upper thigh. A dye is then injected into blood vessels that lead into the pancreas, and x rays are taken.

As of April 2001, doctors at major cancer research institutions such as Memorial Sloan-Kettering Cancer Center in New York are investigating CT angiography, an imaging technique that is less invasive than angiography alone. CT angiography is similar to a standard CT scan, but allows doctors to take a series of pictures of the blood vessels that support tumor growth. A dye is injected as in a CT scan (but at rapid intervals) and no catheter or **sedation** is required. A computer generates 3D images from the pictures that are taken, and the information is gathered by the surgical team who will develop an appropriate strategy if the patient's disease can be operated on.

Treatment

Staging

After cancer of the pancreas has been diagnosed, doctors typically use a TNM staging system to classify the tumor based on its size and the degree to which it has spread to other areas in the body. T indicates the size and local advancement of the primary tumor. Since cancers often invade the lymphatic system before spreading to other organs, regional lymph node involvement (N) is an important factor in staging. M indicates whether the tumor has metastasized (spread) to distant organs. In stage I, the tumor is localized to the pancreas and has not spread to surrounding lymph nodes or other organs. Stage II pancreatic cancer has spread to nearby organs such as the small intestine or bile duct, but not the surrounding lymph nodes. Stage III indicates lymph node involvement, whether the cancer has spread to nearby organs or not. Stage IVA pancreatic cancer has spread to organs near the pancreas such as the stomach, spleen, or colon. Stage IVB is a cancer that has spread to distant sites (liver, lung). If pancreatic cancer has been treated with success and then appears again in the pancreas or in other organs, it is referred to as recurrent disease.

Treatment of pancreatic cancer will depend on several factors, including the stage of the disease and the patient's age and overall health status. A combination of therapies is often employed in the treatment of this disease to improve the patient's chances for survival. Surgery is used whenever possible and is the only means by which cancer of the pancreas can be cured. However, less than 15% of pancreatic tumors can be removed by surgery. By the time the disease is diagnosed (usually at stage III), therapies such as radiation and **chemotherapy** or both are used in addition to surgery to relieve a patient's symptoms and enhance quality of life. For patients with metastatic disease, chemotherapy and radiation are used mainly as palliative (pain alleviating) treatments.

Surgery

Three types of surgery are used in the treatment of pancreatic cancer, depending on what section of the pancreas the tumor is located in. A Whipple procedure removes the head of the pancreas, part of the small intestine and some of the surrounding tissues. This procedure is most common since the majority of pancreatic cancers occur in the head of the organ. A total pancreatectomy removes the entire pancreas and the organs around it. Distal pancreatectomy removes only the body and tail of the pancreas. Chemotherapy and radiation may precede surgery (neoadjuvant therapy) or follow surgery (adjuvant therapy). Surgery is also used to relieve symptoms of pancreatic cancer by draining fluids or bypassing obstructions. Side effects from surgery can include pain, weakness, **fatigue**, and digestive problems. Some patients may develop diabetes or malabsorption as a result of partial or total removal of the pancreas.

Radiation therapy

Radiation therapy is sometimes used to shrink a tumor before surgery or to remove remaining cancer cells after surgery. Radiation may also be used to relieve pain or digestive problems caused by the tumor if it cannot be removed by surgery. External radiation therapy refers to radiation applied externally to the abdomen using a beam of high-energy x rays. High-dose intraoperative radiation therapy is sometimes used during surgery on tumors that have spread to nearby organs. Internal radiation therapy refers to the use of small radioactive seeds implanted in the tumor tissue. The seeds emit radiation over a period of time to kill tumor cells. Radiation treatment may cause side effects such as fatigue, tender or itchy skin, nausea, **vomiting**, and digestive problems.

Chemotherapy

Chemotherapeutic agents are powerful drugs that are used to kill cancer cells. They are classified according to the mechanism by which they induce cancer cell death. Multiple agents are often used to increase the chances of tumor cell death. Gemcitabine is the standard drug used to treat pancreatic cancers and can be used alone or in combination with other drugs, such as 5-flourouracil (5-FU). Other drugs are being tested in combination with gemcitabine in several ongoing clinical trials, specifically irinotecan (CPT-11) and oxaliplatin. Chemotherapy may be administered orally or intravenously in a series of doses over several weeks. During treatment, patients may experience fatigue, nausea, vomiting, hair loss, and mouth sores, depending on which drugs are used.

Biological treatments

Numerous vaccine treatments are being developed in an effort to stimulate the body's immune system into attacking cancer cells. This is also referred to as immunotherapy. Another type of biological treatment involves using a targeted monoclonal antibody to inhibit the growth of cancer cells. The antibody is thought to bind to and neutralize a protein that contributes to the growth of the cancer cells. Investigational treatments such as these may be considered by patients with metastatic disease who would like to participate in a clinical trial. Biological treatments typically cause flu-like symptoms (chills, **fever**, loss of appetite) during the treatment period.

Alternative treatment

Acupuncture or **hypnotherapy** may be used in addition to standard therapies to help relieve the pain associated with pancreatic cancer. Because of the poor prognosis associated with pancreatic cancer, some patients may try special diets with vitamin supplements, certain exercise programs, or unconventional treatments not yet approved by the FDA. Patients should always inform their doctors of any alternative treatments they are using as they could interfere with standard therapies. As of the year 2000, the National Cancer Institute (NCI) is funding phase III clinical trials of a controversial treatment for pancreatic cancer that involves the use of supplemental pancreatic enzymes (to digest cancerous cells) and coffee **enemas** (to stimulate the liver to detoxify the cancer). These theories remain unproven and the study is widely criticized in the medical community. It remains to been seen whether this method of treatment has any advantage over the standard

KEY TERMS

Acinar cell carcinoma—A malignant tumor arising from the acinar cells of the pancreas.

Angiography—Diagnostic technique used to study blood vessels in a tumor.

Biopsy—Removal and microscopic examination of cells to determine whether they are cancerous.

Cancer vaccines—A treatment that uses the patient's immune system to attack cancer cells.

Chemotherapy—Drug treatment administered to kill cancerous cells.

Ductal adenocarcinoma—A malignant tumor arising from the duct cells within a gland.

Endoscopic retrograde cholangiopancreatography (ERCP)—Diagnostic technique used to obtain a biopsy. Also a surgical method of relieving biliary obstruction caused by a tumor.

Endoscopic ultrasonography (EUS)—Diagnostic imaging technique in which an ultrasound probe is inserted down a patient's throat to determine if a tumor is present.

Exocrine—Refers to glands which secrete their products through a duct.

Laparoscopic surgery—Minimally invasive surgery in which a camera and surgical instruments are inserted through a small incision.

Pancreatectomy—Partial or total surgical removal of the pancreas.

Radiation therapy—Use of radioisotopes to kill tumor cells. Applied externally through a beam of x rays, intraoperatively (during surgery), or deposited internally by implanting radioactive seeds in tumor tissue.

Whipple procedure—Surgical removal of the head of the pancreas, part of the small intestine, and some surrounding tissue.

chemotherapeutic regimen in prolonging patient survival or improving quality of life.

Prognosis

Unfortunately, cancer of the pancreas is often fatal, and median survival from diagnosis is less than six months, while the five-year survival rate is 4%. This is mainly due to the lack of screening methods available for early detection of the disease. Yet, even when localized tumors can be removed by surgery, patient survival after five years is only 10% to 15%. These statistics demonstrate the aggressive nature of most pancreatic cancers and their tendency to recur. Pancreatic cancers tend to be resistant to radiation and chemotherapy and these modes of treatment are mainly used to relieve pain and tumor burden.

Prevention

Although the exact cause of pancreatic cancer is not known, there are certain risk factors that may increase a person's chances of developing the disease. Quitting **smoking** will certainly reduce the risk for pancreatic cancer and many other cancers. The American Cancer Society recommends a diet rich in fruits, vegetables, and dietary fiber in order to reduce the risk of pancreatic cancer. According to the NCI, workers who are exposed to petroleum and other chemicals may be at greater risk for developing the disease and should follow their employer's safety precautions. People with a family history of pancreatic cancer are at greater risk than the general population, as a small percentage of pancreatic cancers are considered hereditary.

Resources

BOOKS

Teeley, Peter, and Philip Bashe. *The Complete Cancer Survival Guide*. New York: Doubleday, 2000.

PERIODICALS

Bornman, P. C., and I. J. Beckingham. "ABC of Diseases of Liver, Pancreas, and Biliary System. Pancreatic Tumours." *British Medical Journal* 322, no. 7288 (24 March 2001): 721–3.

Haut, E., A. Abbas, and A. Schuricht. "Pancreatic Cancer: The Role of the Primary Care Physican." *Consultant* 39, no. 12 (December 1999): 3329.

Parks, R. W., and O. J. Garden. "Ensuring Early Diagnosis in Pancreatic Cancer." *Practitioner* 244, no. 1609 (April 2000): 336–8, 340–1, 343.

ORGANIZATIONS

CancerNet. National Cancer Institute, 9000 Rockville Pike, Bldg. 31, Rm.10A16, Bethesda, Maryland, 20892. (800) 422-6237. < http://wwwicic.nci.nih.gov >.

Hirshberg Foundation for Pancreatic Cancer Research. 375 Homewood Rd., Los Angeles, CA 90049. (310) 472-6310. < http://www.pancreatic.org >.

National Pancreas Foundation. PO Box 935, Wexford, PA 15090-0935. < http://www.pancreasfoundation.org >.

Pancreatic Cancer Action Network. PO Box 1010, Torrance, CA 90505. (877) 272-6226. < http://www.pancan.org >.

OTHER

Johns Hopkins Medical Institutions. July 20, 2001 < http://www.path.jhu.edu/pancreas >.

Memorial Sloan-Kettering Cancer Center. Patient Information on Pancreatic Cancer. July 20, 2001. < http://www.mskcc.org/patients_n_public/about_cancer_and_treatment/cancer_information_by_type/pancreatic_cancer/index.html >.

University of Texas MD Anderson Cancer Center. Pancreatic Tumor Study Group. July 20, 2001. < http://www.mdanderson.org/DEPARTMENTS/pancreatic/ >.

"What You Need To Know About Cancer of the Pancreas." National Cancer Institute. December 12, 2000. [cited July 20, 2001]. < http://cancernet.nci.nih.gov/wyntk_pubs/pancreas.htm >.

Lata Cherath, PhD
Elizabeth Pulcini, MSc

Pancreatitis

Definition

Pancreatitis is an inflammation of the pancreas, an organ that is important in digestion. Pancreatitis can be acute (beginning suddenly, usually with the patient recovering fully) or chronic (progressing slowly with continued, permanent injury to the pancreas).

Description

The pancreas is located in the midline of the back of the abdomen, closely associated with the liver, stomach, and duodenum (the first part of the small intestine). The pancreas is considered a gland. A gland is an organ whose primary function is to produce chemicals that pass either into the main blood circulation (called an endocrine function), or pass into another organ (called an exocrine function). The pancreas is unusual because it has both endocrine and exocrine functions. Its endocrine function produces three hormones. Two of these hormones, insulin and glucagon, are central to the processing of sugars in the diet (carbohydrate metabolism or breakdown). The third hormone produced by the endocrine cells of the pancreas affects gastrointestinal functioning. This hormone is called vasoactive intestinal polypeptide (VIP). The pancreas's exocrine function produces a variety of digestive enzymes (trypsin, chymotrypsin, lipase, and amylase, among others). These enzymes are passed into the duodenum through a channel called the pancreatic duct. In the duodenum, the enzymes begin the process of breaking down a variety of food components, including, proteins, fats, and starches.

Acute pancreatitis occurs when the pancreas suddenly becomes inflamed but improves. Patients recover fully from the disease, and in almost 90% of cases the symptoms disappear within about a week after treatment. The pancreas returns to its normal architecture and functioning after healing from the illness. After an attack of acute pancreatitis, tissue and cells of the pancreas return to normal. With chronic pancreatitis, damage to the pancreas occurs slowly over time. Symptoms may be persistent or sporadic, but the condition does not disappear and the pancreas is permanently impaired. Pancreatic tissue is damaged, and the tissue and cells function poorly.

Causes and symptoms

There are a number of causes of acute pancreatitis. The most common, however, are gallbladder disease and **alcoholism**. These two diseases are responsible for more than 80% of all hospitalizations for acute pancreatitis. Other factors in the development of pancreatitis include:

- certain drugs
- infections
- structural problems of the pancreatic duct and bile ducts (channels leading from the gallbladder to the duodenum)
- injury to the abdomen resulting in injury to the pancreas (including injuries occurring during surgery)
- abnormally high levels of circulating fats in the bloodstream
- malfunction of the parathyroid gland, with high blood levels of calcium
- complications from kidney transplants
- a hereditary tendency toward pancreatitis.

Pancreatitis caused by drugs accounts for about 5% of all cases. Some drugs that are definitely related to pancreatitis include:

- Azathioprine, 6-mercaptopurine (Imuran)
- Dideoxyinosine (Videx)
- Estrogens (birth control pills)
- Furosemide (Lasix)
- Pentamidine (NebuPent)
- Sulfonamides (Urobak, Azulfidine)
- Tetracycline

- Thiazide **diuretics** (Diuril, Enduron)
- Valproic acid (Depakote).

Some drugs that are probably related to pancreatitis include:

- Acetaminophen (Tylenol)
- Angiotensin-converting enzyme (ACE) inhibitors (Capoten, Vasotec)
- Erythromycin
- Methyldopa (Aldomet)
- Metronidazole (Flagyl, Protostat)
- Nitrofurantoin (Furadantin, Furan)
- **Nonsteroidal anti-inflammatory drugs** (NSAIDs) (Aleve, Naprosyn, Motrin)
- Salicylates (aspirin).

All of these causes of pancreatitis seem to have a similar mechanism in common. Under normal circumstances, many of the extremely potent enzymes produced by the pancreas are not active until they are passed into the duodenum, where contact with certain other chemicals allow them to function. In pancreatitis, something allows these enzymes to become prematurely activated, so that they actually begin their digestive functions within the pancreas. The pancreas, in essence, begins digesting itself. A cycle of inflammation begins, including swelling and loss of function. Digestion of the blood vessels in the pancreas results in bleeding. Other active pancreatic chemicals cause blood vessels to become leaky, and fluid begins leaking out of the normal circulation into the abdominal cavity. The activated enzymes also gain access to the bloodstream through leaky, eroded blood vessels, and begin circulating throughout the body.

Pain is a major symptom in pancreatitis. The pain is usually quite intense and steady, located in the upper right hand corner of the abdomen, and often described as "boring." This pain is also often felt all the way through to the patient's back. The patient's breathing may become quite shallow because deeper breathing tends to cause more pain. Relief of pain by sitting up and bending forward is characteristic of pancreatic pain. **Nausea and vomiting**, and abdominal swelling are all common as well. A patient will often have a slight **fever**, with an increased heart rate and low blood pressure.

Classic signs of **shock** may appear in more severely ill patients. Shock is a very serious syndrome that occurs when the volume (quantity) of fluid in the blood is very low. In shock, a patient's arms and legs become extremely cold, the blood pressure drops dangerously low, the heart rate is quite fast, and the patient may begin to experience changes in mental status.

In very severe cases of pancreatitis (called necrotizing pancreatitis), the pancreatic tissue begins to die, and bleeding increases. Due to the bleeding into the abdomen, two distinctive signs may be noted in patients with necrotizing pancreatitis. Turner's sign is a reddish-purple or greenish-brown color to the flank area (the area between the ribs and the hip bone). Cullen's sign is a bluish color around the navel.

Some of the complications of pancreatitis are due to shock. When shock occurs, all of the body's major organs are deprived of blood (and, therefore, oxygen), resulting in damage. Kidney, respiratory, and **heart failure** are serious risks of shock. The pancreatic enzymes that have begun circulating throughout the body (as well as various poisons created by the abnormal digestion of the pancreas by those enzymes) have severe effects on the major body systems. Any number of complications can occur, including damage to the heart, lungs, kidneys, lining of the gastrointestinal tract, liver, eyes, bones, and skin. As the pancreatic enzymes work on blood vessels surrounding the pancreas, and even blood vessels located at a distance, the risk of **blood clots** increases. These blood clots complicate the situation by blocking blood flow in the vessels. When blood flow is blocked, the supply of oxygen is decreased to various organs and the organ can be damaged.

The pancreas may develop additional problems, even after the pancreatitis decreases. When the entire organ becomes swollen and suffers extensive cell death (pancreatic necrosis), the pancreas becomes extremely susceptible to serious infection. A local collection of pus (called a pancreatic **abscess**) may develop several weeks after the illness subsides, and may result in increased fever and a return of pain. Another late complication of pancreatitis, occurring several weeks after the illness begins, is called a pancreatic pseudocyst. This occurs when dead pancreatic tissue, blood, white blood cells, enzymes, and fluid leaked from the circulatory system accumulate. In an attempt to enclose and organize this abnormal accumulation, a kind of wall forms from the dead tissue and the growing scar tissue in the area. Pseudocysts cause additional abdominal pain by putting pressure on and displacing pancreatic tissue (resulting in more pancreatic damage). Pseudocysts also press on other nearby structures in the gastrointestinal tract, causing more disruption of function. Pseudocysts are life-threatening when they become infected (abscess) and when they rupture. Simple rupture of a pseudocyst causes death 14% of the time. Rupture complicated by bleeding causes death 60% of the time.

As the pancreatic tissue is increasingly destroyed in chronic pancreatitis, many digestive functions become disturbed. The quantity of hormones and enzymes normally produced by the pancreas begins to seriously decrease. Decreases in the production of enzymes result in the inability to appropriately digest food. Fat digestion, in particular, is impaired. A patient's stools become greasy as fats are passed out of the body. The inability to digest and use proteins results in smaller muscles (wasting) and weakness. The inability to digest and use the nutrients in food leads to **malnutrition**, and a generally weakened condition. As the disease progresses, permanent injury to the pancreas can lead to diabetes.

Diagnosis

Diagnosis of pancreatitis can be made very early in the disease by noting high levels of pancreatic enzymes circulating in the blood (amylase and lipase). Later in the disease, and in chronic pancreatitis, these enzyme levels will no longer be elevated. Because of this fact, and because increased amylase and lipase can also occur in other diseases, the discovery of such elevations are helpful but not mandatory in the diagnosis of pancreatitis. Other abnormalities in the blood may also point to pancreatitis, including increased white blood cells (occurring with inflammation and/or infection), changes due to **dehydration** from fluid loss, and abnormalities in the blood concentration of calcium, magnesium, sodium, potassium, bicarbonate, and sugars.

X rays or ultrasound examination of the abdomen may reveal **gallstones**, perhaps responsible for blocking the pancreatic duct. The gastrointestinal tract will show signs of inactivity (**ileus**) due to the presence of pancreatitis. Chest x rays may reveal abnormalities due to air trapping from shallow breathing, or due to lung complications from the circulating pancreatic enzyme irritants. **Computed tomography scans** (CT scans) of the abdomen may reveal the inflammation and fluid accumulation of pancreatitis, and may also be useful when complications like an abscess or a pseudocyst are suspected.

In the case of chronic pancreatitis, a number of blood tests will reveal the loss of pancreatic function that occurs over time. Blood sugar (glucose) levels will rise, eventually reaching the levels present in diabetes. The levels of various pancreatic enzymes will fall, as the organ is increasingly destroyed and replaced by non-functioning scar tissue. Calcification of the pancreas can also be seen on x rays. Endoscopic retrograde cholangiopancreatography (ERCP) may be used to diagnose chronic pancreatitis in severe cases. In this procedure, the doctor uses a medical instrument fitted with a fiber-optic camera to inspect the pancreas. A magnified image of the area is shown on a television screen viewed by the doctor. Many endoscopes also allow the doctor to retrieve a small sample (biopsy) of pancreatic tissue to examine under a microscope. A contrast product may also be used for radiographic examination of the area.

Treatment

Treatment of pancreatitis involves quickly and sufficiently replacing lost fluids by giving the patient new fluids through a needle inserted in a vein (intravenous or IV fluids). These IV solutions need to contain appropriate amounts of salts, sugars, and sometimes even proteins, in order to correct the patient's disturbances in blood chemistry. Pain is treated with a variety of medications. In order to decrease pancreatic function (and decrease the discharge of more potentially harmful enzymes into the bloodstream), the patient is not allowed to eat. A thin, flexible tube (nasogastric tube) may be inserted through the patient's nose and down into his or her stomach. The nasogastric tube can empty the stomach of fluid and air, which may accumulate due to the inactivity of the gastrointestinal tract. Oxygen may need to be administered by nasal prongs or by a mask.

The patient will need careful monitoring in order to identify complications that may develop. Infections (often occurring in cases of necrotizing pancreatitis, abscesses, and pseudocysts) will require **antibiotics** through the IV. Severe necrotizing pancreatitis may require surgery to remove part of the dying pancreas. A pancreatic abscess can be drained by a needle inserted through the abdomen and into the collection of pus (percutaneous needle aspiration). If this is not sufficient, an abscess may also require surgical removal. Pancreatic pseudocysts may shrink on their own (in 25–40% of cases) or may continue to expand, requiring needle aspiration or surgery. When diagnostic exams reveal the presence of gallstones, surgery may be necessary for their removal. When a patient is extremely ill from pancreatitis, however, such surgery may need to be delayed until any infection is treated, and the patient's condition stabilizes.

Because chronic pancreatitis often includes repeated flares of acute pancreatitis, the same kinds of basic treatment are necessary. Patients cannot take solids or fluids by mouth. They receive IV replacement fluids, receive pain medication, and are monitored for complications. Treatment of chronic pancreatitis caused by alcohol consumption requires that the patient stop drinking alcohol entirely. As chronic pancreatitis continues and insulin levels drop, a patient may require insulin injections in order to be able to process sugars in his or her diet. Pancreatic enzymes can be replaced with oral medicines, and patients sometimes have to take as many as eight pills with each meal. As the pancreas is progressively destroyed, some patients stop feeling the abdominal pain that was initially so severe. Others continue to have constant abdominal pain, and may even require a surgical procedure for relief. Drugs can be used to reduce the pain, but when narcotics are used for pain relief there is danger of the patient becoming addicted.

Prognosis

A number of systems have been developed to help determine the prognosis of an individual with pancreatitis. A very basic evaluation of a patient will allow some prediction to be made based on the presence of dying pancreatic tissue (necrosis) and bleeding. When necrosis and bleeding are present, as many as 50% of patients may die.

More elaborate systems have been created to help determine the prognosis of patients with pancreatitis. The most commonly used system identifies 11 different signs (Ranson's signs) that can be used to determine the severity of the disease. The first five categories are evaluated when the patient is admitted to the hospital:

- age over 55 years
- blood sugar level over 200 mg/Dl
- serum lactic dehydrogenase over 350 IU/L (increased with increased breakdown of blood, as would occur with internal bleeding, and with heart or liver damage)
- AST over 250 mu (a measure of liver function, as well as a gauge of damage to the heart, muscle, brain, and kidney)
- white **blood count** over 16,000 u L

The next six of Ranson's signs are reviewed 48 hours after admission to the hospital. These are:

- greater than 10% decrease in **hematocrit** (a measure of red blood cell volume)
- increase in BUN greater than 5 mg/dL (blood urea nitrogen, an indicator of kidney function)
- blood calcium less than 8 mg/dL
- PaO$_2$ less than 60 mm Hg (a measure of oxygen in the blood)
- base deficit greater than 4 mEg/L (a measure of change in the normal acidity of the blood)

KEY TERMS

Abscess—A pocket of infection; pus.

Acute—Of short and sharp course. Illnesses that are acute appear quickly and can be serious or life-threatening. The illness ends and the patient usually recovers fully.

Chronic—Of long duration and slow progression. Illnesses that are chronic develop slowly over time, and do not end. Symptoms may be continual or intermittent, but the patient usually has the condition for life.

Diabetes—A disease characterized by an inability to process sugars in the diet, due to a decrease in or total absence of insulin production. May require injections of insulin before meals to aid in the metabolism of sugars.

Duodenum—The first section of the small intestine that receives partly digested material from the stomach.

Endocrine—A system of organs that produces chemicals that go into the bloodstream to reach other organs whose functioning they affect.

Enzyme—A chemical that speeds up or makes a particular chemical reaction more efficient. In the digestive system, enzymes are involved in breaking down large food molecules into smaller molecules that can be processed and utilized by the body.

Exocrine—A system of organs that produces chemicals that go through a duct (or tube) to reach other organs whose functioning they affect.

Gland—Collections of tissue that produce chemicals needed for chemical reactions elsewhere in the body.

Hormone—A chemical produced in one part of the body that travels to another part of the body in order to exert an effect.

- fluid sequestration greater than 6 L (an estimation of the quantity of fluid that has leaked out of the blood circulation and into other body spaces)

Once a doctor determines how many of Ranson's signs are present and gives the patient a score, the doctor can better predict the risk of death. The more signs present, the greater the chance of fatal complications. A patient with less than three positive Ranson's signs has a 95% survival rate. A patient with three to four positive Ranson's signs has a 80-85% survival rate.

The results of a CT scan can also be used to predict the severity of pancreatitis. Slight swelling of the pancreas indicates mild illness. Significant swelling, especially with evidence of destruction of the pancreas and/or fluid build-up in the abdominal cavity, indicates more severe illness. With severe illness, there is a worse prognosis.

Prevention

Alcoholism is essentially the only preventable cause of pancreatitis. Patients with chronic pancreatitis must stop drinking alcohol entirely. The drugs that cause or may cause pancreatitis should also be avoided.

Resources

ORGANIZATIONS

National Digestive Diseases Information Clearinghouse. 2 Information Way, Bethesda, MD 20892-3570. (800) 891-5389. <http://www.niddk.nih.gov/health/digest/nddic.htm>.

Rosalyn Carson-DeWitt, MD

Panic attack *see* **Panic disorder**

Panic disorder

Definition

A panic attack is a sudden, intense experience of fear coupled with an overwhelming feeling of danger, accompanied by physical symptoms of anxiety, such as a pounding heart, sweating, and rapid breathing. A person with panic disorder may have repeated panic attacks (at least several a month) and feel severe **anxiety** about having another attack.

Description

Each year, panic disorder affects one out of 63 Americans. While many people experience moments of anxiety, panic attacks are sudden and unprovoked, having little to do with real danger.

Panic disorder is a chronic, debilitating condition that can have a devastating impact on a person's family, work, and social life. Typically, the first attack strikes without warning. A person might be walking down the street, driving a car, or riding an escalator when suddenly panic strikes. Pounding heart, sweating palms, and an overwhelming feeling of impending doom are common features. While the attack may last

only seconds or minutes, the experience can be profoundly disturbing. A person who has had one panic attack typically worries that another one may occur at any time.

As the fear of future panic attacks deepens, the person begins to avoid situations in which panic occurred in the past. In severe cases of panic disorder, the victim refuses to leave the house for fear of having a panic attack. This fear of being in exposed places is often called **agoraphobia**.

People with untreated panic disorder may have problems getting to work or staying on the job. As the person's world narrows, untreated panic disorder can lead to depression, substance abuse, and in rare instances, **suicide**.

Causes and symptoms

Scientists are not sure what causes panic disorder, but they suspect the tendency to develop the condition can be inherited. Some experts think that people with panic disorder may have a hypersensitive nervous system that unnecessarily responds to nonexistent threats. Research suggests that people with panic disorder may not be able to make proper use of their body's normal stress-reducing chemicals.

People with panic disorder usually have their first panic attack in their 20s. Four or more of the following symptoms during panic attacks would indicate panic disorder if no medical, drug-related, neurologic, or other psychiatric disorder is found:

- pounding, skipping or palpitating heartbeat
- shortness of breath or the sensation of smothering
- dizziness or lightheadedness
- nausea or stomach problems
- chest pains or pressure
- choking sensation or a "lump in the throat"
- chills or hot flashes
- sweating
- fear of dying
- feelings of unreality or being detached
- tingling or **numbness**
- shaking and trembling
- fear of losing control or going crazy

A panic attack is often accompanied by the urge to escape, together with a feeling of certainty that **death** is imminent. Others are convinced they are about to have a **heart attack**, suffocate, lose control, or "go crazy." Once people experience a panic attack, they tend to worry so much about having another attack that they avoid the place or situation associated with the original episode.

Diagnosis

Because its physical symptoms are easily confused with other conditions, panic disorder often goes undiagnosed. A thorough **physical examination** is needed to rule out a medical condition. Because the physical symptoms are so pronounced and frightening, panic attacks can be mistaken for a heart problem. Some people experiencing a panic attack go to an emergency room and endure batteries of tests until a diagnosis is made.

Once a medical condition is ruled out, a mental health professional is the best person to diagnose panic attack and panic disorder, taking into account not just the actual episodes, but how the patient feels about the attacks, and how they affect everyday life.

Most health insurance policies include some limited amount of mental health coverage, although few completely cover outpatient mental health care.

Treatment

Most patients with panic disorder respond best to a combination of **cognitive-behavioral therapy** and medication. Cognitive-behavioral therapy usually runs from 12–15 sessions. It teaches patients:

- how to identify and alter thought patterns so as not to misconstrue bodily sensations, events, or situations as catastrophic

- how to prepare for the situations and physical symptoms that trigger a panic attack

- how to identify and change unrealistic self-talk (such as "I'm going to die!") that can worsen a panic attack

- how to calm down and learn breathing exercises to counteract the physical symptoms of panic

- how to gradually confront the frightening situation step by step until it becomes less terrifying

- how to "desensitize" themselves to their own physical sensations, such as rapid heart rate

At the same time, many people find that medications can help reduce or prevent panic attacks by changing the way certain chemicals interact in the brain. People with panic disorder usually notice whether or not the drug is effective within two months,

but most people take medication for at least six months to a year.

Several kinds of drugs can reduce or prevent panic attacks, including:

- selective serotonin reuptake inhibitor (**SSRI**) antidepressants like paroxetine (Paxil) or fluoxetine (Prozac), are approved specifically for the treatment of panic

- tricyclic antidepressants such as clomipramine (Anafranil)

- **benzodiazepines** such as alprazolam (Xanax) and clonazepam (Klonopin)

Finally, patients can make certain lifestyle changes to help keep panic at bay, such as eliminating **caffeine** and alcohol, **cocaine**, amphetamines, and **marijuana**.

Alternative treatment

One approach used in several medical centers focuses on teaching patients how to accept their fear instead of dreading it. In this method, the therapist repeatedly stimulates a person's body sensations (such as a pounding heartbeat) that can trigger fear. Eventually, the patient gets used to these sensations and learns not to be afraid of them. Patients who respond report almost complete absence of panic attacks.

A variety of other alternative therapies may be helpful in treating panic attacks. Neurolinguistic programming and **hypnotherapy** can be beneificial, since these techniques can help bring an awareness of the root cause of the attacks to the conscious mind. Herbal remedies, including lemon balm (*Melissa officinalis*), oat straw (*Avena sativa*), passionflower (*Passiflora incarnata*), and skullcap (*Scutellaria lateriflora*), may help significantly by strengthening the nervous system. Homeopathic medicine, nutritional supplementation (especially with B vitamins, magnesium, and antioxidant **vitamins**), creative visualization, guided imagery, and relaxation techniques may help some people experiencing panic attacks. Hydrotherapies, especially hot epsom salt baths or baths with essential oil of lavender (*Lavandula officinalis*), can help patients relax.

Prognosis

While there may be occasional periods of improvement, the episodes of panic rarely disappear on their own. Fortunately, panic disorder responds very well to treatment; panic attacks decrease in up

KEY TERMS

Agoraphobia—Fear of open spaces.

Benzodiazepines—A class of drugs that have a hypnotic and sedative action, used mainly as tranquilizers to control symptoms of anxiety or panic.

Cognitive-behavioral therapy—A type of psychotherapy used to treat anxiety disorders (including panic disorder) that emphasizes behavioral change together with alteration of negative thought patterns.

Selective serotonin reuptake inhibitors (SSRIs)—A class of antidepressants used to treat panic that affects mood by boosting the levels of the brain chemical serotonin.

Tricyclic antidepressants—A class of antidepressants named for their three-ring structure that increase the levels of serotonin and other brain chemicals. They are used to treat depression and anxiety disorders, but have more side effects than the newer class of antidepressants called SSRIs.

to 90% of people after 6-8 weeks of a combination of cognitive-behavioral therapy and medication.

Unfortunately, many people with panic disorder never get the help they need. If untreated, panic disorder can last for years and may become so severe that a normal life is impossible. Many people who struggle with untreated panic disorder and try to hide their symptoms end up losing their friends, family, and jobs.

Prevention

There is no way to prevent the initial onset of panic attacks. **Antidepressant drugs** or benzodiazepines can prevent future panic attacks, especially when combined with cognitive-behavioral therapy. There is some suggestion that avoiding stimulants (including caffeine, alcohol, or over-the-counter cold medicines) may help prevent attacks as well.

Resources

ORGANIZATIONS

American Psychiatric Association. 1400 K Street NW, Washington, DC 20005. (888) 357-7924. < http://www.psych.org >.

Anxiety Disorders Association of America. 11900 Park Lawn Drive, Ste. 100, Rockville, MD 20852. (800) 545-7367. < http://www.adaa.org >.

Freedom From Fear. 308 Seaview Ave., Staten Island, NY 10305. (718) 351-1717.

National Alliance for the Mentally Ill (NAMI). Colonial Place Three, 2107 Wilson Blvd., Ste. 300, Arlington, VA 22201-3042. (800) 950-6264. < http://www.nami.org >.

National Anxiety Foundation. 3135 Custer Dr., Lexington, KY 40517. (606) 272-7166. < http://www.lexington-on-line.com/naf.html >.

National Institute of Mental Health, Panic Campaign. Rm 15C-05, 5600 Fishers Lane, Rockville, MD 20857. (800) 647-2642. < http://www.nimh.nih.gov >.

National Mental Health Association. 1021 Prince St., Alexandria, VA 22314. (703) 684-7722. < http://www.nmha.org >.

OTHER

The Anxiety and Panic Internet Resource. < http://www.algy.com/anxiety >.

Anxiety Network Page. < http:// www.anxietynetwork.com >.

National Institute of Mental Health Page. < http://www.nimh.nih.gov >.

"Panic Disorder." *Internet Mental Health Page.* < http://www.mentalhealth.com >.

Carol A. Turkington

Pap test

Definition

The Pap test is a procedure in which a physician scrapes cells from the cervix or vagina to check for **cervical cancer**, vaginal **cancer**, or abnormal changes that could lead to cancer. It often is called a "Pap smear."

Purpose

The Pap test is used to detect abnormal growth of cervical cells at an early stage so that treatment can be started when the condition is easiest to treat. This microscopic analysis of cells can detect cervical cancer, precancerous changes, inflammation (vaginitis), infections, and some **sexually transmitted diseases** (STDs). The Pap test can occasionally detect endometrial (uterine) cancer or **ovarian cancer**, although it was not designed for this purpose.

Women should begin to have Pap tests at the age of 21 or within three years of becoming sexually active, whichever comes first. Young people are more likely to have multiple sex partners, which increases their risk of certain diseases that can cause cancer, such as human papillomavirus (HPV).

The American Cancer Society (ACS) updated its guidelines concerning Pap test frequency in late 2002. In brief, women should continue screening every year with regular Pap tests until age 30, every two years if using the liquid-based Pap test. Once a woman age 30 and older has had three normal results in a row, she may get screened every two to three years. A doctor may suggest more frequent screening if a woman has certain risk factors for cervical cancer. Women who have had total hysterectomies including the removal of the cervix do not need Pap tests unless the **hysterectomy** resulted from cervical cancer. Those over age 70 who have had three normal results generally do not need to continue having Pap tests under the new guidelines.

Women with certain risk factors may have yearly tests. Those at highest risk for cervical cancer are women who started having sex before age 18, those with many sex partners (especially if they did not use condoms, which protect against STDs), those who have had STDs such as **genital herpes** or **genital warts**, and those who smoke. Women older than 40 may have the test yearly, if experiencing bleeding after **menopause**. Women who have had a positive test result in the past may need screening every six months. Women who have had cervical cancer or precancer should have regular Pap smears.

Other women also benefit from the Pap test. Women over age 65 account for 25% of all cases of cervical cancer and 41% of deaths from this disease. Women over age 65 who have never had a Pap smear benefit the most from the test. Some women have the cervix left in place after hysterectomy and will continue to receive regular Pap tests. Finally, a pregnant woman should have a Pap test as part of her first prenatal examination.

The Pap smear is a screening test. It identifies women who are at increased risk of cervical dysplasia (abnormal cells) or cervical cancer. Only an examination of the cervix with a special lighted instrument (**colposcopy**) and samples of cervical tissue (biopsies) can actually diagnose these problems.

Precautions

The Pap test is usually not done during the menstrual period because of the presence of blood cells. The best time is in the middle of the menstrual cycle.

Description

The Pap test is an extremely cost-effective and beneficial exam. Cervical cancer used to be a leading cause of cancer deaths in American women, but widespread use of this diagnostic procedure reduced the **death** rate from this disease by 74% between 1955 and 1992. A 2003 study reported that the test reduces rates of invasive cervical cancer by as much as 94%. In 2003, the FDA approved a new screening test that combines DNA testing for the HPV type that causes the most cases of cervical cancer with the standard Pap test, increasing its screening value.

The Pap test, sometimes called a cervical smear, is the microscopic examination of cells scraped from both the outer cervix and the cervical canal. (The cervix is the opening between the vagina and the uterus, or womb.) It is called the "Pap" test after its developer, Dr. George N. Papanicolaou. This simple procedure is performed during a gynecologic examination and is usually covered by insurance. For those with coverage, Medicare will pay for one screening Pap smear every three years.

During the pelvic examination, an instrument called a speculum is inserted into the vagina to open it. The doctor then uses a tiny brush, or a cotton-tipped swab and a small spatula to wipe loose cells off the cervix and to scrape them from the inside of the cervix. The cells are transferred or "smeared" onto glass slides, the slides are treated to stabilize the cells, and the slides are sent to a laboratory for microscopic examination. The entire procedure is usually painless and takes five to 10 minutes at most.

The newer method called liquid-based cytology, or the liquid-based Pap test, involves spreading the cells more evenly on a slide after removing them from the sample. The liquid-based method prevents cells from drying out and becoming distorted. Studies show that liquid-based testing slightly improves cancer detection and greatly improves detection of precancers, but it costs more than the traditional Pap test. Trade names in 2003 for liquid-based Pap smears were ThinPrep and AutoCyte.

Preparation

The Pap test may show abnormal results when a woman is healthy or normal results in women with cervical abnormalities as much as 25% of the time. It may even miss up to 5% of cervical cancers. Some simple preparations may help to ensure that the results are reliable. Among the measures that may help increase test reliability are:

- avoiding sexual intercourse for two days before the test
- not using douches for two or three days before the test

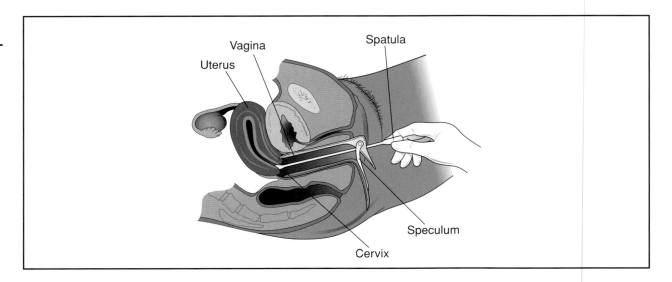

The Pap test is a procedure used to detect abnormal growth of cervical cells which may be a precursor to cancer of the cervix. It is administered by a physician who inserts a speculum into the vagina to open and separate the vaginal walls. A spatula is then inserted to scrape cells from the cervix. These cells are transferred onto glass slides for laboratory analysis. The Pap test may also identify vaginitis, some sexually transmitted diseases, and cancers of the uterus and ovaries. *(Illustration by Electronic Illustrators Group.)*

• avoiding tampons, vaginal creams, or birth control foams or jellies for two to three days before the test

• scheduling the Pap smear when not menstruating.

However, most women are not routinely advised to make any special preparations for a Pap test.

If possible, women may want to ensure that their test is performed by an experienced gynecologist, physician, or provider and sent to a reputable laboratory. The physician should be confident in the accuracy of the chosen lab.

Before the exam, the physician will take a complete sexual history to determine a woman's risk status for cervical cancer. Questions may include date and results of the last Pap test, any history of abnormal Pap tests, date of last menstrual period and any irregularity, use of hormones and birth control, family history of gynecologic disorders, and any vaginal symptoms. These topics are relevant to the interpretation of the Pap test, especially if any abnormalities are detected. Immediately before the Pap test, the woman should empty her bladder to avoid discomfort during the procedure.

Aftercare

Harmless cervical bleeding is possible immediately after the test; a woman may need to use a sanitary napkin. She should also be sure to comply with her doctor's orders for follow-up visits.

Risks

No appreciable health risks are associated with the Pap test. However, abnormal results (whether valid or due to technical error) can cause significant **anxiety**. Women may wish to have their sample double-checked, either by the same laboratory or by the new technique of computer-assisted rescreening. The Food and Drug Administration (FDA) has approved the use of AutoPap and PAPNET to doublecheck samples that have been examined by technologists. AutoPap may also be used to perform initial screening of slides, which are then checked by a technologist. Any abnormal Pap test should be followed by colposcopy, not by double checking the Pap test.

Normal results

Normal (negative) results from the laboratory exam mean that no atypical, dysplastic, or cancer cells were detected, and the cervix is normal.

Abnormal results

Terminology

Abnormal cells found on the Pap test may be described using two different grading systems. Although this can be confusing, the systems are quite similar. The Bethesda system is based on the term "squamous intraepithelial lesion" (SIL). Precancerous cells are classified as atypical squamous cells of

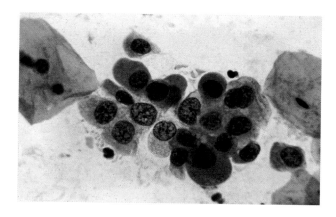

These malignant cells were taken from a woman's cervix during a Pap test. *(Photograph by Parviz M. Pour, Photo Researchers, Inc. Reproduced by permission.)*

undetermined significance, low-grade SIL, or high-grade SIL. Low-grade SIL includes mild dysplasia (abnormal cell growth) and abnormalities caused by HPV; high-grade SIL includes moderate or severe dysplasia and carcinoma in situ (cancer that has not spread beyond the cervix).

Another term that may be used is "cervical intraepithelial neoplasia" (CIN). In this classification system, mild dysplasia is called CIN I, moderate is CIN II, and severe dysplasia or carcinoma in situ is CIN III.

Regardless of terminology, it is important to remember that an abnormal (positive) result does not necessarily indicate cancer. Results may be falsely abnormal after infection or irritation of the cervix. Up to 40% of mild dysplasia reverts to normal tissue without treatment, and only 1% of mild abnormalities ever develop into cancer.

Changes of unknown cause

ASCUS or LSIL cells are found in 5%–10% of all Pap tests. The most common abnormality is atypical squamous cells of undetermined significance, which are found in 4% of all Pap tests. Sometimes these results are described further as either reactive or precancerous. Reactive changes suggest that the cervical cells are responding to inflammation, such as from a yeast infection. These women may be treated for infection and then undergo repeat Pap testing in three to six months. If those results are negative, no further treatment is necessary. This category may also include atypical "glandular" cells, which could imply a more severe type of cancer and requires repeat testing and further evaluation.

Dysplasia

The next most common finding (in about 25 of every 1,000 tests) is low-grade SIL, which includes mild dysplasia or CIN I and changes caused by HPV. Unlike cancer cells, these cells do not invade normal tissues. Women are most susceptible to cervical dysplasia between the ages of 25 and 35. Typically, dysplasia causes no symptoms, although women may experience abnormal vaginal bleeding. Because dysplasia is precancerous, it should be treated if it is moderate or severe.

Treatment of dysplasia depends on the degree of abnormality. In women with no other risk factors for cervical cancer, mild precancerous changes may be simply observed over time with repeat testing, perhaps every four to six months. This strategy works only if women are diligent about keeping later appointments. Premalignant cells may remain that way without causing cancer for five to ten years, and may never become malignant.

In women with positive results or risk factors, the gynecologist must perform colposcopy and biopsy. A colposcope is an instrument that looks like binoculars, with a light and a magnifier, used to view the cervix. Biopsy, or removal of a small piece of abnormal cervical or vaginal tissue for analysis, is usually done at the same time.

High-grade SIL (found in three of every 50 Pap tests) includes moderate to severe dysplasia or carcinoma in situ (CIN II or III). After confirmation by colposcopy and biopsy, it must be removed or destroyed to prevent further growth. Several outpatient techniques are available: conization (removal of a cone-shaped piece of tissue), **laser surgery**, **cryotherapy** (freezing), or the "loop electrosurgical excision procedure." Cure rates are nearly 100% after prompt and appropriate treatment of carcinoma in situ. Of course, frequent checkups are then necessary.

Cancer

HPV, the most common STD in the United States, may be responsible for many cervical cancers. Cancer may be manifested by unusual vaginal bleeding or discharge, bowel and bladder problems, and **pain**. Women are at greatest risk of developing cervical cancer between the ages of 30 and 40 and between the ages of 50 and 60. Most new cancers are diagnosed in women between 50 and 55. Although the likelihood of developing this disease begins to level off for Caucasian women at the age of 45, it increases steadily for African Americans for another

KEY TERMS

Carcinoma in situ—Malignant cells that are present only in the outer layer of the cervix.

Cervical intraepithelial neoplasia (CIN)—A term used to categorize degrees of dysplasia arising in the epithelium, or outer layer, of the cervix.

Dysplasia—Abnormal changes in cells.

Human papillomavirus (HPV)—The most common STD in the United States. Various types of HPV are known to cause cancer.

Neoplasia—Abnormal growth of cells, which may lead to a neoplasm, or tumor.

Squamous intraepithelial lesion (SIL)—A term used to categorize the severity of abnormal changes arising in the squamous, or outermost, layer of the cervix.

40 years. Biopsy is indicated when any abnormal growth is found on the cervix, even if the Pap test is negative.

Doctors have traditionally used **radiation therapy** and surgery to treat cervical cancer that has spread within the cervix or throughout the pelvis. In severe cases, postoperative radiation is administered to kill any remaining cancer cells, and **chemotherapy** may be used if cancer has spread to other organs. Recent studies have shown that giving chemotherapy and radiation at the same time improves a patient's chance of survival. The National Cancer Institute has urged physicians to strongly consider using both chemotherapy and radiation to treat patients with invasive cervical cancer. The survival rate at five years after treatment of early invasive cancer is 91%; rates are below 70% for more severe invasive cancer. That is why prevention, risk reduction, and frequent Pap tests are the best defense for a woman's gynecologic health.

The Pap test is a procedure used to detect abnormal growth of cervical cells which may be a precursor to cancer of the cervix. It is administered by a physician who inserts a speculum into the vagina to open and separate the vaginal walls. A spatula is then inserted to scrape cells from the cervix. These cells are transferred onto glass slides for laboratory analysis. The Pap test may also identify vaginitis, some sexually transmitted diseases, and cancers of the uterus and ovaries.

Resources

PERIODICALS

"American Cancer Society Issues New Early Detection Guidelines." *Women's Health Weekly* December 19, 2002: 12.

Law, Malcolm. "How Frequently Should Cervical Screening Be Conducted." *Important Journal of Medical Screening* (Winter 2003): 159–161.

OTHER

"Pap smear: Simple, life-saving test." April 29, 1999. April 26, 2001. [cited June 28, 2001]. < http://www.mayohealth.org/home?id = HQ01177 >.

"Pap Smears: The simple test that can save your life." January 29, 2001. April 26, 2001. [cited June 28, 2001]. < http://www.mayohealth.org/home?id = HQ01178 >.

Laura J. Ninger
Teresa G. Odle

Papanicolaou test *see* **PAP test**

Papilledema

Definition

Papilledema is a swelling of the optic nerve, at the point where this nerve joins the eye, that is caused by an increase in fluid pressure within the skull (intracranial pressure). Swelling of the optic nerve due to other causes such as infection or inflammatory disease is not called papilledema.

Description

The optic nerve is the nerve that transmits signals from the eye to the brain. Papilledema is a swelling of this nerve where it meets the eye (the optic disc) caused by an increase in intracranial pressure. Almost all cases of papilledema are bilateral (affect both eyes). Papilledema can be observed in people of any age, but is relatively uncommon in infants because the bones of the skull are not fully fused together at this age.

Causes and symptoms

Papilledema is caused by an increase in the pressure of the fluid (cerebrospinal fluid) that is present between the brain and the skull, inside the head. This increase in intracranial pressure may be caused by any of a variety of conditions within the skull, brain, or spinal cord. The most common causes of papilledema are:

- tumor of the brain, spinal cord, skull, spinal column, or optic nerve

- abscess (the accumulation of pus within a confined space)

- craniosynostosis (an abnormal closure of the bones of the skull)

- hemorrhage (bleeding)

- hydrocephalus (an accumulation of cerebrospinal fluid within the skull)

- intracranial infection (any infection within the skull such as **meningitis** and encephalitis)

- head injury

The symptoms of papilledema include:

- headaches, which are usually worse upon awakening and exacerbated by coughing, holding the breath, or other maneuvers that tend to increase intracranial pressure.

- nausea and vomiting.

- changes in vision, such as temporary and transient blurring, graying, flickering, or double vision

Diagnosis

A diagnosis of papilledema is achieved by visual examination of the eye with an ophthalmoscope. This instrument shines light through the pupil of the eye and illuminates the retina while the clinician looks through it. Eye drops to dilate the pupils are used to insure a thorough examination.

Treatment

Treatment of papilledema is generally aimed at the treatment of the underlying disorder that is causing papilledema.

Diuretic drugs combined with a weight reduction program may be useful in cases of papilledema that are caused by an abnormally high production of cerebrospinal fluid.

Corticosteroids have been shown to be effective in relieving the symptoms in some patients with papilledema caused by inflammatory disorders.

Alternative treatment

Alternative treatments for conditions that cause the occurrence of papilledema include acupuncture, aromatherapy, hydrotherapy, massage, and herbal remedies.

Prognosis

With prompt medical care to treat the underlying cause of papilledema, a person affected with papilledema will not have permanent damage to his or her eye-sight. However, prolonged papilledema can result in permanent damage to the optic nerve which could lead to blindness.

Prevention

Preventing papilledema is only possible if the underlying condition causing the papilledema can be found. Treatment of this underlying condition may prevent recurrences of papilledema.

Resources

BOOKS

Rhee, Douglas J., and Mark F. Pyfer. *The Wills Eye Manual.* 3rd ed. Philadelphia, PA: Lippincott Williams and Wilkins, 1999.

PERIODICALS

Agarwal, A. K., et al. "Papilledema." *Journal of the Indian Academy of Clinical Medicine* 1 (October-December 2000): 270-277.

ORGANIZATIONS

National Eye Institute. 2020 Vision Place, Bethesda, MD 20892-3655. (301) 496-5248. <http://www.nei.nih.gov/>.

OTHER

Giovannini, Joseph, and Georgia Chrousos. "Papilledema." *eMedicine.* May 12, 2001. <http://www.emedicine.com/OPH/topic187.htm>.

Paul A. Johnson, Ed.M.

Papillomavirus infection *see* **Genital warts**

Papule *see* **Skin lesions**

Paracentesis

Definition

Paracentesis is a procedure during which fluid from the abdomen is removed through a needle.

Purpose

There are two reasons to take fluid out of the abdomen. One is to analyze it. The other is to relieve pressure.

Liquid that accumulates in the abdomen is called ascites. Ascites seeps out of organs for several reasons related either to disease in the organ or fluid pressures that are changing.

Liver disease

All the blood flowing through the intestines passes through the liver on its way back to the heart. When progressive disease such as alcohol damage or hepatitis destroys enough liver tissue, the scarring that results shrinks the liver and constricts the blood flow. Such scarring of the liver is called **cirrhosis**. Pressure builds up in the intestinal circulation, slowing flow and pushing fluid into the tissues. Slowly the fluid accumulates in areas with the lowest pressure and greatest capacity. The free space around abdominal organs receives most of it. This space is called the peritoneal space because it is enclosed by a thin membrane called the peritoneum. The peritoneum wraps around nearly every organ in the abdomen, providing many folds and spaces for the fluid to gather.

Infections

Peritonitis is an infection of the peritoneum. Infection changes the dynamics of body fluids, causing them to seep into tissues and spaces. Peritonitis can develop in several ways. Many abdominal organs contain germs that do not belong elsewhere in the body. If they spill their contents into the peritoneum, infection is the result. The gall bladder, the stomach, any part of the intestine, and most especially the appendix–all cause peritonitis when they leak or rupture. **Tuberculosis** can infect many organs in the body; it is not confined to the lungs. Tuberculous peritonitis causes **ascites**.

Other inflammations

Peritoneal fluid is not just produced by infections. The pancreas can cause a massive sterile peritonitis when it leaks its digestive enzymes into the abdomen.

Cancer

Any **cancer** that begins in or spreads to the abdomen can leak fluid. One particular tumor of the ovary that leaks fluid, the resulting presentation of the disease, is Meigs' syndrome.

Kidney disease

Since the kidneys are intimately involved with the body's fluid balance, diseases of the kidney often cause excessive fluid to accumulate. Nephrosis and nephrotic syndrome are the general terms for diseases that cause the kidneys to retain water and provoke its movement into body tissues and spaces.

Heart failure

The ultimate source of fluid pressure in the body is the heart, which generates blood pressure. All other pressures in the body are related to blood pressure. As the heart starts to fail, blood backs up, waiting to be pumped. This increases back pressure upstream, particularly below the heart where gravity is also pulling blood away from the heart. The extra fluid from **heart failure** is first noticed in the feet and ankles, where gravitational effects are most potent. In the abdomen, the liver swells first, then it and other abdominal organs start to leak.

Pleural fluid

The other major body cavity is the chest. The tissue in the chest corresponding to the peritoneum is called the pleura, and the space contained within the pleura, between the ribs and the lungs, is called the pleural space. Fluid is often found in both cavities, and fluid from one cavity can find its way into the other.

Fluid that accumulates in the abdomen creates abnormal pressures on organs in the abdomen. Digestion is hindered; blood flow is slowed. Pressure upward on the chest compromises breathing. The kidneys function poorly in the presence of such external pressures and may even fail with tense, massive ascites.

Description

During paracentesis, special needles puncture the abdominal wall, being careful not to hit internal organs. If fluid is needed only for analysis, just a bit is removed. If pressure relief is an additional goal, many quarts may be removed. Rapid removal of large amounts of fluid can cause blood pressure to drop suddenly. For this reason, the physician will often leave a tube in place so that fluid can be removed slowly, giving the circulation time to adapt.

A related procedure called culpocentesis removes ascitic fluid from the very bottom of the abdominal cavity through the back of the vagina. This is used mostly to diagnose female genital disorders like **ectopic pregnancy** that bleed or exude fluid into the peritoneal space.

Fluid is sent to the laboratory for testing, where cancer and blood cells can be detected, infections identified, and chemical analysis can direct further investigations.

Aftercare

An adhesive bandage and perhaps a single stitch close the hole. Nothing more is required.

Risks

Risks are negligible. It is remotely possible that an organ could be punctured and bleed or that an infection could be introduced.

Normal results

A diagnosis of the cause and/or relief from accumulated fluid pressure are the expected results.

Abnormal results

Fluid will continue to accumulate until the cause is corrected. Repeat procedures may be needed.

Resources

BOOKS

Glickman, Robert M. "Abdominal Swelling and Ascites." In *Harrison's Principles of Internal Medicine*, edited by Anthony S. Fauci, et al. New York: McGraw-Hill, 1997.

J. Ricker Polsdorfer, MD

Paracoccidioidomycosis *see* **South American blastomycosis**

Paragonamiasis *see* **Fluke infections**

Paralysis

Definition

Paralysis is defined as complete loss of strength in an affected limb or muscle group.

Description

The chain of nerve cells that runs from the brain through the spinal cord out to the muscle is called the motor pathway. Normal muscle function requires intact connections all along this motor pathway. Damage at any point reduces the brain's ability to control the muscle's movements. This reduced efficiency causes weakness, also called paresis. Complete loss of communication prevents any willed movement at all. This lack of control is called paralysis. Certain inherited abnormalities in muscle cause **periodic paralysis**, in which the weakness comes and goes.

The line between weakness and paralysis is not absolute. A condition causing weakness may progress to paralysis. On the other hand, strength may be restored to a paralyzed limb. Nerve regeneration or regrowth is one way in which strength can return to a paralyzed muscle. Paralysis almost always causes a change in muscle tone. Paralyzed muscle may be flaccid, flabby, and without appreciable tone, or it may be spastic, tight, and with abnormally high tone that increases when the muscle is moved.

Paralysis may affect an individual muscle, but it usually affects an entire body region. The distribution of weakness is an important clue to the location of the nerve damage that is causing the paralysis. Words describing the distribution of paralysis use the suffix "-plegia," from the Greek word for "stroke." The types of paralysis are classified by region:

- monoplegia, affecting only one limb
- diplegia, affecting the same body region on both sides of the body (both arms, for example, or both sides of the face)
- hemiplegia, affecting one side of the body
- paraplegia, affecting both legs and the trunk
- quadriplegia, affecting all four limbs and the trunk

Causes and symptoms

Causes

The nerve damage that causes paralysis may be in the brain or spinal cord (the central nervous system) or it may be in the nerves outside the spinal cord (the peripheral nervous system). The most common causes of damage to the brain are:

- **stroke**

- tumor

- trauma (caused by a fall or a blow)

- Multiple sclerosis (a disease that destroys the protective sheath covering nerve cells)

- **cerebral palsy** (a condition caused by a defect or injury to the brain that occurs at or shortly after birth)

- metabolic disorder (a disorder that interferes with the body's ability to maintain itself)

Damage to the spinal cord is most often caused by trauma, such as a fall or a car crash. Other conditions that may damage nerves within or immediately adjacent to the spine include:

- tumor

- herniated disk (also called a ruptured or slipped disk)

- spondylosis (a disease that causes stiffness in the joints of the spine)

- rheumatoid arthritis of the spine

- neurodegenerative disease (a disease that damages nerve cells)

- multiple sclerosis

Damage to peripheral nerves may be caused by:

- trauma

- compression or entrapment (such as carpal tunnel syndrome)

- **Guillain-Barré syndrome** (a disease of the nerves that sometimes follows **fever** caused by a viral infection or immunization)

- chronic inflammatory demyelinating polyradiculoneuropathy (CIDP) (a condition that causes **pain** and swelling in the protective sheath covering nerve cells)

- radiation

- inherited demyelinating disease (a condition that destroys the protective sheath around the nerve cell)

- toxins or poisons

Symptoms

The distribution of paralysis offers important clues to the site of nerve damage. Hemiplegia is almost always caused by brain damage on the side opposite the paralysis, often from a stroke. Paraplegia occurs after injury to the lower spinal cord, and quadriplegia occurs after damage to the upper spinal cord at the level of the shoulders or higher (the nerves controlling the arms leave the spine at that level). Diplegia usually indicates brain damage, most often from cerebral palsy. Monoplegia may be caused by isolated damage to either the central or the peripheral nervous system. Weakness or paralysis that occurs only in the arms and legs may indicate demyelinating disease. Fluctuating symptoms in different parts of the body may be caused by multiple sclerosis.

Sudden paralysis is most often caused by injury or stroke. Spreading paralysis may indicate degenerative disease, inflammatory disease such as Guillain-Barré syndrome or CIDP, metabolic disorders, or inherited demyelinating disease.

Other symptoms often accompany paralysis from any cause. These symptoms may include numbness and **tingling**, pain, changes in vision, difficulties with speech, or problems with balance. **Spinal cord injury** often causes loss of function in the bladder, bowel, and sexual organs. High spinal cord injuries may cause difficulties in breathing.

Diagnosis

Careful attention should be paid to any events in the patient's history that might reveal the cause of the paralysis. The examiner should look for incidents such as falls or other traumas, exposure to toxins, recent infections or surgery, unexplained **headache**, preexisting metabolic disease, and family history of weakness or other neurologic conditions. A neurologic examination tests strength, reflexes, and sensation in the affected area and normal areas.

Imaging studies, including **computed tomography scans** (CT scans), **magnetic resonance imaging** (MRI) scans, or **myelography** may reveal the site of the injury. **Electromyography** and nerve conduction velocity tests are performed to test the function of the muscles and peripheral nerves.

Treatment

The only treatment for paralysis is to treat its underlying cause. The loss of function caused by long-term paralysis can be treated through a comprehensive **rehabilitation** program. Rehabilitation includes:

- Physical therapy. The physical therapist focuses on mobility. Physical therapy helps develop strategies to compensate for paralysis by using those muscles that still have normal function, helps maintain and build any strength and control that remain in the affected muscles, and helps maintain range of motion in the

KEY TERMS

Computed tomography (CT)—An imaging technique in which cross-sectional x rays of the body are compiled to create a three-dimensional image of the body's internal structures.

Electromyography—A test that uses electrodes to record the electrical activity of muscle. The information gathered is used to diagnose neuromuscular disorders.

Magnetic resonance imaging (MRI)—An imaging technique that uses a large circular magnet and radio waves to generate signals from atoms in the body. These signals are used to construct images of internal structures.

Myelin—The insulation covering nerve cells. Demyelinating disease causes a breakdown of myelin.

Myelography—An x-ray process that uses a dye or contrast medium injected into the space around the spine.

Nerve conduction velocity test—A test that measures the time it takes a nerve impulse to travel a specific distance over the nerve after electronic stimulation.

affected limbs to prevent muscles from shortening (contracture) and becoming deformed. If nerve regrowth is expected, physical therapy is used to retrain affected limbs during recovery. A physical therapist also suggests adaptive equipment such as braces, canes, or wheelchairs.

- Occupational therapy. The occupational therapist focuses on daily activities such as eating and bathing. Occupational therapy develops special tools and techniques that permit self-care and suggests ways to modify the home and workplace so that a patient with an impairment may live a normal life.

- Other specialties. The nature of the impairment may mean that the patient needs the services of a respiratory therapist, vocational rehabilitation counselor, social worker, speech-language pathologist, nutritionist, special education teacher, recreation therapist, or clinical psychologist.

Prognosis

The likelihood of recovery from paralysis depends on what is causing it and how much damage has been done to the nervous system.

Prevention

Prevention of paralysis depends on prevention of the underlying causes. Risk of stroke can be reduced by controlling high blood pressure and cholesterol levels. Seatbelts, air bags, and helmets reduce the risk of injury from motor vehicle accidents and falls. Good prenatal care can help prevent premature birth, which is a common cause of cerebral palsy.

Resources

BOOKS

Bradley, Walter G., et al., editors. *Neurology in Clinical Practice*. 2nd ed. Boston: Butterworth-Heinemann, 1996.

Richard Robinson

Paralysis agitans *see* **Parkinson's disease**

Paralytic shellfish poisoning *see* **Fish and shellfish poisoning**

Paranoia

Definition

Paranoia is an unfounded or exaggerated distrust of others, sometimes reaching delusional proportions. Paranoid individuals constantly suspect the motives of those around them, and believe that certain individuals, or people in general, are "out to get them."

Description

Paranoid perceptions and behavior may appear as features of a number of mental illnesses, including depression and **dementia**, but are most prominent in three types of psychological disorders: paranoid schizophrenia, delusional disorder (persecutory type), and paranoid personality disorder (PPD).

Individuals with paranoid **schizophrenia** and persecutory delusional disorder experience what is known as persecutory **delusions**: an irrational, yet unshakable, belief that someone is plotting against them. Persecutory delusions in paranoid schizophrenia are bizarre, sometimes grandiose, and often accompanied by auditory **hallucinations**. Delusions experienced by individuals with delusional disorder are more plausible than those experienced by paranoid schizophrenics; not bizarre, though still unjustified. Individuals with delusional disorder may seem offbeat or quirky rather than mentally ill, and, as such, may never seek treatment.

Persons with paranoid personality disorder tend to be self-centered, self-important, defensive, and emotionally distant. Their paranoia manifests itself in constant suspicions rather than full-blown delusions. The disorder often impedes social and personal relationships and career advancement. Some individuals with PPD are described as "litigious," as they are constantly initiating frivolous law suits. PPD is more common in men than in women, and typically begins in early adulthood.

Causes and symptoms

The exact cause of paranoia is unknown. Potential causal factors may be genetics, neurological abnormalities, changes in brain chemistry, and stress. Paranoia is also a possible side effect of drug use and **abuse** (for example, alcohol, marijuana, amphetamines, **cocaine**, PCP). Acute, or short term, paranoia may occur in some individuals overwhelmed by **stress**.

The *Diagnostic and Statistical Manual of Mental Disorders*, fourth edition (*DSM-IV*), the diagnostic standard for mental health professionals in the United States, lists the following symptoms for paranoid personality disorder:

- suspicious; unfounded suspicions; believes others are plotting against him/her

- preoccupied with unsupported doubts about friends or associates

- reluctant to confide in others due to a fear that information may be used against him/her

- reads negative meanings into innocuous remarks

- bears grudges

- perceives attacks on his/her reputation that are not clear to others, and is quick to counterattack

- maintains unfounded suspicions regarding the fidelity of a spouse or significant other

Diagnosis

Patients with paranoid symptoms should undergo a thorough physical examination and patient history to rule out possible organic causes (such as dementia) or environmental causes (such as extreme stress). If a psychological cause is suspected, a psychologist will conduct an interview with the patient and may administer one of several clinical inventories, or tests, to evaluate mental status.

KEY TERMS

Persecutory delusion—A fixed, false, and inflexible belief that others are engaging in a plot or plan to harm an individual.

Treatment

Paranoia that is symptomatic of paranoid schizophrenia, delusional disorder, or paranoid personality disorder should be treated by a psychologist and/or psychiatrist. Antipsychotic medication such as thioridazine (Mellaril), haloperidol (Haldol), chlorpromazine (Thorazine), clozapine (Clozaril), or risperidone (Risperdal) may be prescribed, and cognitive therapy or psychotherapy may be employed to help the patient cope with their paranoia and/or persecutory delusions. Antipsychotic medication, however, is of uncertain benefit to individuals with paranoid personality disorder and may pose long-term risks.

If an underlying condition, such as depression or drug abuse, is found to be triggering the paranoia, an appropriate course of medication and/or psychosocial therapy is employed to treat the primary disorder.

Prognosis

Because of the inherent mistrust felt by paranoid individuals, they often must be coerced into entering treatment. As unwilling participants, their recovery may be hampered by efforts to sabotage treatment (for example, not taking medication or not being forthcoming with a therapist), a lack of insight into their condition, or the belief that the therapist is plotting against them. Albeit with restricted lifestyles, some patients with PPD or persecutory delusional disorder continue to function in society without treatment.

Resources

ORGANIZATIONS

American Psychiatric Association. 1400 K Street NW, Washington, DC 20005. (888) 357-7924. < http://www.psych.org >.

American Psychological Association (APA). 750 First St. NE, Washington, DC 20002-4242. (202) 336-5700. < ttp://www.apa.org >.

National Alliance for the Mentally Ill (NAMI). Colonial Place Three, 2107 Wilson Blvd., Ste. 300, Arlington, VA 22201-3042. (800) 950-6264. < http://www.nami.org >.

National Institute of Mental Health. Mental Health Public Inquiries, 5600 Fishers Lane, Room 15C-05, Rockville, MD 20857. (888) 826-9438. < http:// www.nimh.nih.gov >.

Paula Anne Ford-Martin

Parapharyngeal abscess *see* **Abscess**

Paraphilias *see* **Sexual perversions**

Paraplegia *see* **Paralysis**

Parasomnia *see* **Sleep disorders**

Parathyroid gland removal *see* **Parathyroidectomy**

Parathyroid hormone test

Definition

The parathyroid hormone (PTH) test is a blood test performed to determine the serum levels of a hormone secreted by the parathyroid gland in response to low blood calcium levels. PTH works together with vitamin D to maintain healthy bones. The parathyroid glands are small paired glands located near the thyroid gland at the base of the neck.

Purpose

The PTH level is measured to evaluate the level of blood calcium. It is routinely monitored in patients with a kidney disorder called chronic renal failure (CRF). Because PTH is one of the major factors affecting calcium metabolism, the PTH test helps to distinguish nonparathyroid from parathyroid causes of too much calcium in the blood (**hypercalcemia**).

Differential diagnosis of hyperparathyroidism

PTH is also useful in the differential diagnosis of overactive parathyroid glands (hyperparathyroidism). Primary **hyperparathyroidism** is most often caused by a benign tumor in one or more of the parathyroid glands. It is rarely caused by parathyroid **cancer**. Patients with this condition have high PTH and calcium levels.

Secondary hyperparathyroidism is often seen in patients with chronic renal failure (CRF). The kidneys fail to excrete sufficient phosphate, and the parathyroid gland secretes PTH in an effort to lower calcium levels to balance the calcium-phosphate ratio. Because

of the constant stimulation of the parathyroid, CRF patients have high PTH and normal or slightly low calcium levels.

Tertiary hyperparathyroidism occurs when CRF causes a severe imbalance in the calcium-phosphate ratio, leading to very high PTH production that results in hypercalcemia. Patients with this condition have high PTH and high calcium levels.

Specific PTH assays

PTH is broken down in the body into three different molecular forms: the intact PTH molecule and several smaller fragments which include an amino acid or N-terminal, a midregion or midmolecule, and a carboxyl or C-terminal. Two tests are currently used to measure intact PTH and its terminal fragments. While both tests are used to diagnose hyper-or **hypoparathyroidism**, each test also has specific applications as well. The C-terminal PTH assay is used to diagnose the ongoing disturbances in PTH metabolism that occur with secondary and tertiary hyperparathyroidism. The assay for intact PTH and the N-terminal fragment, which are both measured at the same time, is more accurate in detecting sudden changes in the PTH level. For this reason, the N-terminal PTH assay is used to monitor a patient's response to therapy.

Precautions

Drug interactions

Some prescription drugs affect the results of PTH tests. Drugs that *increase* PTH levels include phosphates, anticonvulsants, steroids, isoniazid, lithium, and rifampin. Drugs that *decrease* PTH include cimetidine and propranolol.

Timing

PTH levels are subject to daily variation, ranging from a peak around 2:00 A.M. to a low point around 2:00 P.M. Specimens are usually drawn at 8:00 A.M. The laboratory should be notified if the patient works a night shift so that this difference in biological rhythm can be taken into account.

Other serum level tests

Due to the relationship between PTH and calcium, calcium levels should be tested at the same time as PTH. Most laboratories have established reference values to indicate what PTH level is normal for a particular calcium level. In addition, the effects of PTH on kidney function and bone strength indicate that serum calcium, phosphorus, and creatinine levels should be measured together with PTH. The **creatinine test** measures kidney function and aids in the diagnosis of parathyroid dysfunction.

Description

The PTH test is performed on a sample of the patient's blood, withdrawn from a vein into a vacuum tube. The procedure, which is called a venipuncture, takes about five minutes.

Preparation

The patient should have nothing to eat or drink from midnight of the day of the test.

Risks

Risks for this test are minimal, but may include slight bleeding from the puncture site, a small bruise or swelling in the area, or **fainting** or feeling lightheaded.

Normal results

Reference ranges for PTH tests vary somewhat depending on the laboratory, and must be interpreted in association with calcium results. The following ranges are typical:

- Intact PTH: 10–65 pg/mL
- PTH N-terminal (includes intact PTH): 8–24 pg/mL
- PTH C-terminal (includes C-terminal, intact PTH, and midmolecule): 50–330 pg/mL.

Abnormal results

When measured with serum calcium levels, abnormally *high* PTH values may indicate primary, secondary, or tertiary hyperparathyroidism, chronic renal failure, **malabsorption syndrome**, and **vitamin D deficiency**. Abnormally *low* PTH levels may indicate hypoparathyroidism, hypercalcemia, and certain malignancies.

Resources

BOOKS

Pagana, Kathleen Deska. *Mosby's Manual of Diagnostic and Laboratory Tests*. St. Louis: Mosby, Inc., 1998.

Janis O. Flores

Parathyroid scan

Definition

A parathyroid scan is sometimes called a parathyroid localization scan or parathyroid scintigraphy. This scan uses radioactive pharmaceuticals that are readily taken up by cells in the parathyroid glands to obtain an image of the glands and any abnormally active areas within them.

Purpose

The parathyroid glands, embedded in the thyroid gland in the neck, but separate from the thyroid in function, control calcium metabolism in the body. The parathyroid glands produce parathyroid hormone (PTH). PTH regulates the level of calcium in the blood.

Calcium is critical to cellular metabolism, as well as being the main component of bones. If too much PTH is secreted, the bones release calcium into the bloodstream. Over time, the bones become brittle and more likely to break. A person with levels of calcium in the blood that are too high feels tired, run down, irritable, and has difficulty sleeping. Additional signs of too much calcium in the blood are **nausea and vomiting**, frequent urination, kidney stones and bone **pain**. A parathyroid scan is administered when the parathyroid appears to be overactive and a tumor is suspected.

Precautions

Parathyroid scans are not recommended for pregnant women because of the potential harm to the developing fetus. People who have had another recent nuclear medicine procedure or an intravenous contrast test may need to wait until the earlier radioactive

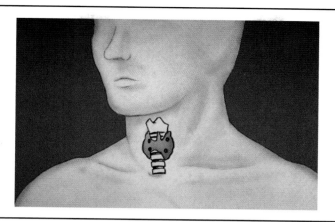

The parathyroid glands, embedded in the thyroid gland in the neck but separate from the thyroid gland in function, control calcium metabolism in the body by producing parathyroid hormone, or PTH. *(Custom Medical Stock Photo. Reproduced by permission.)*

markers have been eliminated from their system in order to obtain accurate results from the parathyroid scan.

Description

A parathyroid scan is a non-invasive procedure that uses two radiopharmaceuticals (drugs with a radioactive marker) to obtain an image of highly active areas of the parathyroid glands. The test can be done in two ways.

Immediate scan

If the test is to be performed immediately, the patient lies down on an imaging table with his head and neck extended and immobilized. The patient is injected with the first radiopharmaceutical. After waiting 20 minutes, the patient is positioned under the camera for imaging. Each image takes five minutes. It is essential that the patient remain still during imaging.

After the first image, the patient is injected with a second radiopharmaceutical, and imaging continues for another 25 minutes. Total time for the test is about one hour: injection 10 minutes, waiting period 20 minutes, and imaging 30 minutes.

Another way to do this test is as follows. After the first images are acquired, the patient returns two hours later for additional images. Time for this procedure totals about three hours: injection 10 minutes, waiting period two hours and 20 minutes, and imaging 30 minutes.

Delayed scan

In a delayed parathyroid scan, the patient is asked to swallow capsules containing the first

radiopharmaceutical. The patient returns after a four hour waiting period, and the initial image is made. Then the patient is injected with the second radiopharmaceutical. Imaging continues for another 25 minutes. The total time is about four hours and 40 minutes: waiting period four hours, injection 10 minutes, and imaging 30 minutes.

Preparation

No special preparations are necessary for this test. It is not necessary to fast or maintain a special diet. The patient should wear comfortable clothing and no metal jewelry around the neck.

Aftercare

The patient should not feel any adverse effects of the test and can resume normal activities immediately.

Risks

The only risk associated with this test is to the fetus of a pregnant woman.

Normal results

Normal results will show no unusual activity in the parathyroid glands.

Abnormal results

A concentration of radioactive materials in the parathyroid gland beyond background levels suggests excessive activity and the presence of a tumor. False positive results sometimes result from the presence of multinodular **goiter**, neoplasm, or cysts. False positive tests are tests that interpret the results as abnormal when this is not true.

Resources

OTHER

"Parathyroid Scan." *HealthGate Page.* June 13, 1998. < http://www.healthgate.com >.

Tish Davidson, A.M.

Parathyroidectomy

Definition

Parathyroidectomy is the removal of one or more of the parathyroid glands. The parathyroid glands are usually four in number, although the exact number may vary from three to seven. They are located in the neck in front of the Adam's apple and are closely linked to the thyroid gland. The parathyroid glands regulate the balance of calcium in the body.

Purpose

Parathyroidectomy is usually done to treat **hyperparathyroidism** (abnormal over-functioning of the parathyroid glands).

Precautions

Parathyroidectomy should only be done when other non-operative methods have failed to control the patient's hyperparathyroidism.

Description

Parathyroidectomy is an operation done most commonly by a general surgeon, or occasionally by an otolaryngologist, in the operating room of a hospital. The operation begins when the anesthesiologist anesthetizes or puts the patient to sleep. The surgeon makes an incision in the front of the neck where a tight-fitting necklace would rest. All of the parathyroid glands are identified. The surgeon then identifies the gland or glands with the disease and confirms the diagnosis by sending a piece of the gland(s) to the pathology department for immediate microscopic examination. The glands are then removed and the incision is closed and a dressing is placed over the incision.

Patients generally stay overnight in the hospital after completion of the operation and may remain for one or two additional days. These procedures are reimbursed by insurance companies. Surgeon's fees typically range from $1,000–$2,000. Anesthesiologists charge for their services based on the medical status of the patient and the length of the operative procedure. Hospitals charge for use of the operating suite, equipment, lab and diagnostic tests, and medications.

Preparation

Prior to the operation, the diagnosis of hyperparathyroidism should be confirmed using lab tests. Occasionally, physicians order **computed tomography scans** (CT scans), ultrasound exams, and/or **magnetic resonance imaging** (MRI) tests to determine the total number of parathyroid glands and their location prior to the procedure.

Aftercare

The incision should be watched for signs of infection. In general, no specific wound care is required.

The level of calcium in the body should be monitored during the first 48 hours after the operation by obtaining frequent blood samples for laboratory analysis.

Risks

The major risk of parathyroidectomy is injury to the recurrent laryngeal nerve (a nerve that lies very near the parathyroid glands and serves the larynx or voice box). If this nerve is injured, the voice may become hoarse or weak.

Occasionally, too much parathyroid tissue is removed, and the patient may develop hypoparathyroidism (under-functioning of the parathyroid glands). If this occurs, the patient will require daily calcium supplements.

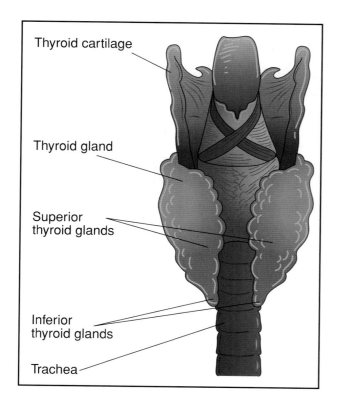

- Thyroid cartilage
- Thyroid gland
- Superior thyroid glands
- Inferior thyroid glands
- Trachea

Parathyroidectomy refers to the surgical removal of one or more of the parathyroid glands due to hyperparathyroidism (an abnormal over-functioning of the parathyroid glands). It is usually done after other non-operative methods have failed to control or correct this condition. *(Illustration by Electronic Illustrators Group.)*

Sometimes not all of the parathyroid glands are found in the initial operation. A fifth or sixth gland may be located in an aberrant location such as the chest (ectopic parathroid). If this occurs, the patient's hyperparathyroidism may not be corrected, and a second procedure may be required to find the other gland(s).

Hematoma formation (collection of blood under the incision) is a possible complication of any operative procedure. However, in procedures that involve the neck it is of particular concern, because a rapidly enlarging hematoma can obstruct the airway.

Infection of the surgical incision may occur, as with any operative procedure, but this is not common.

Normal results

Most patients require only two or three days of hospitalization to recover from the operation. They usually can resume most of their normal activities within one to two weeks.

Resources

OTHER

"Parathyroidectomy." *ThriveOnline.*
< http://thriveonline.oxygen.com >.

Mary Jeanne Krob, MD, FACS

Paratyphoid fever

Definition

Paratyphoid **fever**, which is sometimes called *Salmonella paratyphi* infection, is a serious contagious disease caused by a gram-negative bacterium. It is also grouped together with **typhoid fever** under the name enteric fever.

Description

Enteric fever is increasingly rare in the United States. Of the 500 cases reported in an average year, about 60% are infections acquired during travel in Mexico, India, or South America.

Paratyphoid fever has three stages: an early stage marked by high fever; a toxic stage with abdominal **pain** and intestinal symptoms, and a long period of recovery from fever (defervescence). In adults, these three phases may cover a period of four to six weeks; in children, they are shorter and may cover 10 days to two weeks. During the toxic stage there is a 1–10% chance of intestinal perforation or hemorrhage.

Causes and symptoms

Paratyphoid fever is caused by any of three strains of *Salmonella paratyphi*: *S. paratyphi A*; *S. schottmuelleri* (also called *S. paratyphi C*); or *S. hirschfeldii* (also called *S. paratyphi B*). It can be transmitted from animals or animal products to humans or from person to person. The incubation period is one to two weeks but is often shorter in children. Symptom onset may be gradual in adults but is often sudden in children.

Paratyphoid fever is marked by high fever, **headache**, loss of appetite, **vomiting**, and **constipation** or **diarrhea**. The patient typically develops an enlarged spleen. About 30% of patients have rose spots on the front of the chest during the first week of illness. The rose spots develop into small hemorrhages that may be hard to see in African or Native Americans.

Patients with intestinal complications have symptoms resembling those of **appendicitis**: intense cramping pain with soreness in the right lower quadrant of the abdomen.

Diagnosis

The diagnosis is usually made on the basis of a history of recent travel and culturing the paratyphoid organism. Because the disease is unusual in the United States, the doctor may not consider paratyphoid in the diagnosis unless the patient has the classic symptoms of an enlarged spleen and rose spots. The doctor will need to rule out other diseases with high fevers, including typhus, **brucellosis**, **tularemia** (rabbit fever), psittacosis (**parrot fever**), mononucleosis, and Kawasaki syndrome. *S. paratyphi* is easily cultured from samples of blood, stool, urine, or bone marrow.

Treatment

Medications

Paratyphoid fever is treated with **antibiotics** over a two- to three-week period with trimethoprim-sulfamethoxazole (Bactrim, Septra); amoxicillin (Amoxil, Novamoxin); and ampicillin (Amcill). Third-generation **cephalosporins** (ceftriaxone [Rocephin], cefotaxime [Claforan], or cefixime [Suprax]) or chloramphenicol (Chloromycetin) may be given if the specific strain is resistant to other antibiotics.

Surgery

Patients with intestinal perforation or hemorrhage may need surgery if the infection cannot be controlled by antibiotics.

KEY TERMS

Defervescence—Return to normal body temperature after high fever.

Enteric fever—A term that is sometimes used for either typhoid or paratyphoid fever.

Rose spots—Small slightly raised reddish pimples that are a distinguishing feature of typhoid or paratyphoid infection.

Supportive care

Patients with paratyphoid fever need careful monitoring for signs of complications as well as bed rest and nutritional support. Patients with severe infections may require fluid replacement or blood transfusions.

Prognosis

Most patients with paratyphoid fever recover completely, although intestinal complications can result in **death**. With early treatment, the mortality rate is less than 1%.

Prevention

Immunization

Vaccination against paratyphoid fever is not necessary within the United States but is recommended for travel to countries with high rates of enteric fever.

Hygienic measures

Travelers in countries with high rates of paratyphoid fever should be careful to wash hands before eating and to avoid meat, egg, or poultry dishes unless they have been thoroughly cooked.

Resources

BOOKS

Fauci, Anthony S., et al., editors. *Harrison's Principles of Internal Medicine*. New York: McGraw-Hill, 1997.

Rebecca J. Frey, PhD

Paresthesias *see* **Numbness and tingling**

Parkinson disease

Definition

Parkinson disease (PD) is a progressive movement disorder marked by **tremors**, rigidity, slow movements (bradykinesia), and posture instability. It occurs when cells in one of the movement-control centers of the brain begin to die for unknown reasons. PD was first noted by British physician James Parkinson in the early 1800s.

Description

Usually beginning in a person's late fifties or early sixties, Parkinson disease causes a progressive decline in movement control, affecting the ability to control initiation, speed, and smoothness of motion. Symptoms of PD are seen in up to 15% of those ages 65–74, and almost 30% of those ages 75–84.

Most cases of PD are sporadic. This means that there is a spontaneous and permanent change in nucleotide sequences (the building blocks of genes). Sporadic mutations also involve unknown environmental factors in combination with genetic defects. The abnormal gene (mutated gene) will form an altered end-product or protein. This will cause abnormalities in specific areas in the body where the protein is used. Some evidence suggests that the disease is transmitted by autosomal dominant inheritance. This implies that an affected parent has a 50% chance of transmitting the disease to any child. This type of inheritance is not commonly observed. The most recent evidence is linking PD with a gene that codes for a protein called alpha-synuclein. Further research is attempting to fully understand the relationship with this protein and nerve cell degeneration.

PD affects approximately 500,000 people in the United States, both men and women, with as many as 50,000 new cases each year.

Causes and symptoms

The immediate cause of PD is degeneration of brain cells in the area known as the substantia nigra, one of the movement control centers of the brain. Damage to this area leads to the cluster of symptoms known as "parkinsonism." In PD, degenerating brain cells contain Lewy bodies, which help identify the disease. The cell death leading to parkinsonism may be caused by a number of conditions, including infection, trauma, and **poisoning**. Some drugs given for **psychosis**, such as haloperidol (Haldol) or chlorpromazine (thorazine), may cause parkinsonism. When no cause for nigral cell degeneration can be found, the disorder is called idiopathic parkinsonism, or Parkinson disease. Parkinsonism may be seen in other degenerative conditions, known as the "parkinsonism plus" syndromes, such as **progressive supranuclear palsy**.

The substantia nigra, or "black substance," is one of the principal movement control centers in the brain. By releasing the neurotransmitter known as dopamine, it helps to refine movement patterns throughout the body. The dopamine released by nerve cells of substantia nigra stimulates another brain region, the corpus striatum. Without enough dopamine, the corpus striatum cannot control its targets, and so on down the line. Ultimately, the movement patterns of walking, writing, reaching for objects, and other basic programs cannot operate properly, and the symptoms of parkinsonism are the result.

There are some known toxins that can cause parkinsonism, most notoriously a chemical called MPTP, found as an impurity in some illegal drugs. Parkinsonian symptoms appear within hours of ingestion, and are permanent. MPTP may exert its effects through generation of toxic molecular fragments called free radicals, and reducing free radicals has been a target of several experimental treatments for PD using antioxidants.

It is possible that early exposure to some as-yet-unidentified environmental toxin or virus leads to undetected nigral cell death, and PD then manifests as normal age-related decline brings the number of functioning nigral cells below the threshold needed for normal movement. It is also possible that, for genetic reasons, some people are simply born with fewer cells in their substantia nigra than others, and they develop PD as a consequence of normal decline.

Symptoms

The identifying symptoms of PD include:

- Tremors, usually beginning in the hands, often occuring on one side before the other. The classic tremor of PD is called a "pill-rolling tremor," because the movement resembles rolling a pill between the thumb and forefinger. This tremor occurs at a frequency of about three per second.

- Slow movements (bradykinesia) occur, which may involve slowing down or stopping in the middle of familiar tasks such as walking, eating, or shaving. This may include freezing in place during movements (akinesia).

- Muscle rigidity or stiffness, occuring with jerky movements replacing smooth motion.
- Postural instability or balance difficulty occurs. This may lead to a rapid, shuffling gait (festination) to prevent falling.
- In most cases, there is a "masked face," with little facial expression and decreased eye-blinking.

In addition, a wide range of other symptoms may often be seen, some beginning earlier than others:

- depression
- speech changes, including rapid speech without inflection changes
- problems with sleep, including restlessness and nightmares
- emotional changes, including fear, irritability, and insecurity
- incontinence
- **constipation**
- handwriting changes, with letters becoming smaller across the page (micrographia)
- progressive problems with intellectual function (**dementia**)

Diagnosis

The diagnosis of Parkinson disease involves a careful medical history and a neurological exam to look for characteristic symptoms. There are no definitive tests for PD, although a variety of lab tests may be done to rule out other causes of symptoms, especially if only some of the identifying symptoms are present. Tests for other causes of parkinsonism may include brain scans, blood tests, lumbar puncture, and x rays.

Treatment

There is no cure for Parkinson disease. Most drugs treat the symptoms of the disease only, although one drug, selegiline (Eldepryl), may slow degeneration of the substantia nigra.

Exercise, nutrition, and physical therapy

Regular, moderate **exercise** has been shown to improve motor function without an increase in medication for a person with PD. Exercise helps maintain range of motion in stiff muscles, improve circulation, and stimulate appetite. An exercise program designed by a physical therapist has the best chance of meeting the specific needs of the person with PD. A physical therapist may also suggest strategies for balance compensation and techniques to stimulate movement during slowdowns or freezes.

Good **nutrition** is important to maintenance of general health. A person with PD may lose some interest in food, especially if depressed, and may have **nausea** from the disease or from medications, especially those known as dopamine agonists. Slow movements may make it difficult to eat quickly, and delayed gastric emptying may lead to a feeling of fullness without having eaten much. Increasing fiber in the diet can improve constipation, soft foods can reduce the amount of needed chewing, and a prokinetic drug such as cisapride (Propulsid) can increase the movement of food through the digestive system.

People with PD may need to limit the amount of protein in their **diets**. The main drug used to treat PD, L-dopa, is an amino acid, and is absorbed by the digestive system by the same transporters that pick up other amino acids broken down from proteins in the diet. Limiting protein, under the direction of the physician or a nutritionist, can improve the absorption of L-dopa.

No evidence indicates that vitamin or mineral supplements can have any effect on the disease other than in the improvement of the patient's general health. No antioxidants used to date have shown promise as a treatment except for selegiline, an MAO-B inhibitor which is discussed in the Drugs section. A large, carefully controlled study of vitamin E demonstrated that it could not halt disease progression.

Drugs

The pharmacological treatment of Parkinson disease is complex. While there are a large number of drugs that can be effective, their effectiveness varies with the patient, disease progression, and the length of time the drug has been used. Dose-related side effects may preclude using the most effective dose, or require the introduction of a new drug to counteract them. There are five classes of drugs currently used to treat PD.

DRUGS THAT REPLACE DOPAMINE. One drug that helps replace dopamine, levodopa (L-dopa), is the single most effective treatment for the symptoms of PD. L-dopa is a derivative of dopamine, and is converted into dopamine by the brain. It may be started when symptoms begin, or when they become serious enough to interfere with work or daily living.

L-dopa therapy usually remains effective for five years or longer. Following this, many patients develop motor fluctuations, including peak-dose "dyskinesias" (abnormal movements such as tics, twisting, or restlessness), rapid loss of response after dosing (known as the "on-off" phenomenon), and unpredictable drug response. Higher doses are usually tried, but may lead to an increase in dyskinesias. In addition, side effects of L-dopa include **nausea and vomiting**, and low blood pressure upon standing (**orthostatic hypotension**), which can cause **dizziness**. These effects usually lessen after several weeks of therapy.

ENZYME INHIBITORS. Dopamine is broken down by several enzyme systems in the brain and elsewhere in the body, and blocking these enzymes is a key strategy to prolonging the effect of dopamine. The two most commonly prescribed forms of L-dopa contain a drug to inhibit the amino acid decarboxylase (an AADC inhibitor), one type of enzyme that breaks down dopamine. These combination drugs are Sinemet (L-dopa plus carbidopa) and Madopar (L-dopa plus benzaseride). Controlled-release formulations also aid in prolonging the effective interval of an L-dopa dose.

The enzyme monoamine oxidase B (MAO-B) inhibitor selegiline may be given as add-on therapy for L-dopa. Research indicates selegiline may have a neuroprotective effect, sparing nigral cells from damage by free radicals. Because of this, and the fact that it has few side effects, it is also frequently prescribed early in the disease before L-dopa is begun. Entacapone and tolcapone, two inhibitors of another enzyme system called catechol-o-methyl transferase (COMT), may soon reach the market as early studies suggest that they effectively treat PD symptoms with fewer motor fluctuations and decreased daily L-dopa requirements.

DOPAMINE AGONISTS. Dopamine works by stimulating receptors on the surface of corpus striatum cells. Drugs that also stimulate these cells are called dopamine agonists, or DAs. DAs may be used before L-dopa therapy, or added on to avoid requirements for higher L-dopa doses late in the disease. DAs available in the United States as of early 1998, include bromocriptine (Permax, Parlodel), pergolide (Permax), and pramipexole (Mirapex). Two more, cabergoline (Dostinex) and ropinirole (Requip), are expected to be approved soon. Other dopamine agonists in use elsewhere include lisuride (Dopergine) and apomorphine. Side effects of all the DAs are similar to those of dopamine, plus confusion and **hallucinations** at higher doses.

ANTICHOLINERGIC DRUGS. Anticholinergics maintain dopamine balance as levels decrease. However, the side effects of anticholinergics (**dry mouth**, constipation, confusion, and blurred vision) are usually

too severe in older patients or in patients with dementia. In addition, anticholinergics rarely work for very long. They are often prescribed for younger patients who have predominant shaking. Trihexyphenidyl (Artane) is the drug most commonly prescribed.

DRUGS WHOSE MODE OF ACTION IS UNCERTAIN. Amantadine (Symmetrel) is sometimes used as an early therapy before L-dopa is begun, and as an add-on later in the disease. Its anti-parkinsonian effects are mild, and are not seen in many patients. Clozapine (Clozaril) is effective especially against psychiatric symptoms of late PD, including psychosis and hallucinations.

Surgery

Two surgical procedures are used for treatment of PD that cannot be controlled adequately with drug therapy. In PD, a brain structure called the globus pallidus (GPi) receives excess stimulation from the corpus striatum. In a pallidotomy, the GPi is destroyed by heat, delivered by long thin needles inserted under anesthesia. Electrical stimulation of the GPi is another way to reduce its action. In this procedure, fine electrodes are inserted to deliver the stimulation, which may be adjusted or turned off as the response dictates. Other regions of the brain may also be stimulated by electrodes inserted elsewhere. In most patients, these procedures lead to significant improvement for some motor symptoms, including peak-dose dyskinesias. This allows the patient to receive more L-dopa, since these dyskinesias are usually what causes an upper limit on the L-dopa dose.

A third procedure, transplant of fetal nigral cells, is still highly experimental. Its benefits to date have been modest, although improvements in technique and patient selection are likely to change that.

Alternative treatment

Currently, the best treatments for PD involve the use of conventional drugs such as levodopa. Alternative therapies, including **acupuncture**, massage, and **yoga**, can help relieve some symptoms of the disease and loosen tight muscles. Alternative practitioners have also applied herbal and dietary therapies, including amino acid supplementation, antioxidant (**vitamins** A, C, E, selenium, and zinc) therapy, B vitamin supplementation, and calcium and magnesium supplementation, to the treatment of PD. Anyone using these therapies in conjunction with conventional drugs should check with their doctor to

KEY TERMS

AADC inhibitors—Drugs that block the amino acid decarboxylase; one type of enzyme that breaks down dopamine. Also called DC inhibitors, they include carbidopa and benserazide.

Akinesia—A loss of the ability to move; freezing in place.

Bradykinesia—Extremely slow movement.

COMT inhibitors—Drugs that block catechol-o-methyl transferase, an enzyme that breaks down dopamine. COMT inhibitors include entacapone and tolcapone.

Dopamine—A neurochemical made in the brain that is involved in many brain activities, including movement and emotion.

Dyskinesia—Impaired ability to make voluntary movements.

MAO-B inhibitors—Inhibitors of the enzyme monoamine oxidase B. MAO-B helps break down dopamine; inhibiting it prolongs the action of dopamine in the brain. Selegiline is an MAO-B inhibitor.

Orthostatic hypotension—A sudden decrease in blood pressure upon sitting up or standing. May be a side effect of several types of drugs.

Substantia nigra—One of the movement control centers of the brain.

avoid the possibility of adverse interactions. For example, vitamin B_6 (either as a supplement or from foods such as whole grains, bananas, beef, fish, liver, and potatoes) can interfere with the action of L-dopa when the drug is taken without carbidopa.

Prognosis

Despite medical treatment, the symptoms of Parkinson disease worsen over time, and become less responsive to drug therapy. Late-stage psychiatric symptoms are often the most troubling, including difficulty sleeping, nightmares, intellectual impairment (dementia), hallucinations, and loss of contact with reality (psychosis).

Prevention

There is no known way to prevent Parkinson disease.

Resources

ORGANIZATIONS

National Parkinson Foundation. 1501 NW Ninth Ave., Bob Hope Road, Miami, FL 33136. < http://www.parkinson.org >.
Parkinson Disease Foundation. 710 West 168th St., New York, NY 10032. (800) 457-6676. < http://www.apdaparkinson.com >.
Worldwide Education and Awareness for Movement Disorders. One Gustave Levy Place, New York, NY 10029. (800) 437-MOV2. < http://www.wemove.org >.

OTHER

AWAKENINGS. < http://www.parkinsonsdisease.com >.

Laith Farid Gulli, M.D.

Parkinsonism *see* **Parkinson disease**
Parotid gland removal *see* **Parotidectomy**
Parotid gland scan *see* **Salivary gland scan**

Parotidectomy

Definition

Parotidectomy is the removal of the parotid gland, a salivary gland near the ear.

Purpose

The main purpose of parotidectomy is to remove cancerous tumors in the parotid gland. A number of tumors can develop in the parotid gland. Many of these are tumors that have spread from other areas of the body, entering the parotid gland by way of the lymphatic system. Among the tumors seen in the parotid gland are lymphoma, melanoma, and squamous cell carcinoma.

Description

The parotid gland is the largest of the salivary glands. There are two parotid glands, one on each side of the face. They lie just in front of the ears and a duct runs from each to the inside of the cheek. Each parotid gland has several lobes. Surgery is recommend as part of the treatment for all cancers in the parotid gland. Superficial or localized parotidectomy is recommended by some authorities, unless a lipoma or Warthin's tumor is present. One of the advantages to this approach is that nerves to facial muscles are left intact. Many facial nerves run through the same area as the parotid gland and can be damaged during more complete parotidectomies. Most authorities recommend total parotidectomy, especially if **cancer** is found in both the superficial and deep lobes of the parotid gland. If the tumor has spread to involve the facial nerve, the operation is expanded to include parts of bone behind the ear (mastoid) to remove as much tumor as possible. Some authorities recommend post-surgery radiation as follow-up treatment for cancer.

Aftercare

After surgery, the patient will remain in the hospital for one to three days. The site of incision will be watched closely for signs of infection and heavy bleeding (hemorrhage). The incision site should be kept clean and dry until it is completely healed. The patient should not wash their hair until the stitches have been removed. If the patient has difficulty smiling, winking, or drinking fluids, the physician should be contacted immediately. These are signs of facial nerve damage.

Risks

There are a number of complications that follow parotidectomy. Facial nerve **paralysis** after minor surgery should be minimal. During surgery, it is possible to repair cut nerves. After major surgery, a graft is attempted to restore nerve function to facial muscles. Salivary fistulas can occur when saliva collects in the incision site or drains through the incision. Reoccurrence of cancer is the single most important consideration for patients who have undergone parotidectomy. Long term survival rates are largely dependent on the tumor types and the stage of tumor development at the time of the operation.

Other risks include **blood clots** (hematoma) and infection. The most common long-term complication of parotidectomy is redness and sweating in the cheek, known as Frey's syndrome. Rarely, paralysis may extend throughout all the branches of the facial nervous system.

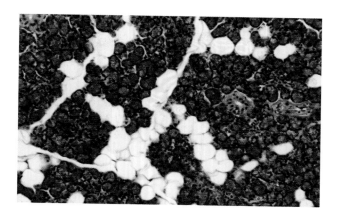

A micrograph of a normal human parotid gland. One of the salivary glands, the parotid consists of acini arranged in lobes. This image shows a junction between several lobes; the clear spaces represent the interlobular connective tissue. The masses of secretory cells produce a watery secretion which is passed to the intralobular. *(Photograph by Astrid and Hanns-Frieder Michler, Custom Medical Stock Photo. Reproduced by permission.)*

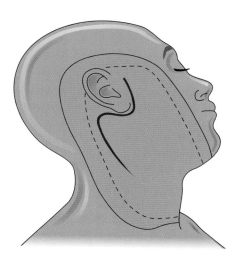

Parotidectomy is a surgical procedure performed to remove cancerous tumors in the parotid gland, a salivary gland near the ear. Among the tumors seen in the parotid gland are lymphoma, melanoma, and squamous cell carcinoma. The illustration above shows the facial incision sites for this procedure. *(Illustration by Electronic Illustrators Group.)*

Resources

BOOKS

Bentz, M. L. *Pediatric Plastic Surgery.* Stamford: Appleton & Lange, 1998.

Mary K. Fyke

Parotitis, epidemic *see* **Mumps**

Paroxetine *see* **Selective serotonin reuptake inhibitors**

Paroxysmal atrial tachycardia

Definition

A period of very rapid and regular heart beats that begins and ends abruptly. The heart rate is usually between 160 and 200 beats per minute. This condition is also known as paroxysmal supraventricular tachycardia.

Description

The term paroxysmal means that the event begins suddenly, without warning and ends abruptly. Atrial tachycardia means that the upper chambers of the heart are beating abnormally fast. Paroxysmal atrial tachycardia can occur without any heart disease being present. It is usually more annoying than dangerous.

Causes and symptoms

Paroxysmal atrial tachycardia may be caused by several different things. The fast rate may be triggered by a premature atrial beat that sends an impulse along an abnormal electrical path to the ventricles. Other causes stem from **anxiety**, stimulants, overactive thyroid, and in some women, the onset of menstruation.

Though seldom life-threatening, paroxysmal atrial tachycardia produces annoying symptoms which can include lightheadedness, chest pain, palpitations, anxiety, sweating, and shortness of breath.

Diagnosis

Diagnosis is not always easy, because the event is usually over by the time the patient sees a doctor. A careful description of the episode will aid the doctor in his diagnosis. If the rapid heart rate is still occurring, an electrocardiograph (ECG) will show the condition. If the event is over, physicians often recommend a period of ambulatory electrocardiographic monitoring (called Holter monitoring) to confirm the diagnosis.

Treatment

The doctor may suggest that during an episode of paroxysmal atrial tachycardia the following practice may help. Briefly hold the nose and mouth closed and breathe out, or by bearing down, as though straining at a bowel movement. The doctor may try to stop the episode by gently massaging an area in the neck called the carotid sinus.

If these conservative measures do not work, an injection of the drug verapamil or adenosine should stop the episode quickly.

In rare cases, the drugs do not work and electrical shock (**cardioversion**) may be necessary, particularly if serious symptoms are also present with the tachycardia.

Prognosis

Paroxysmal atrial tachycardia is not a disease, and is seldom life-threatening. The episodes are usually more unpleasant than they are dangerous, and the prognosis is generally good.

Prevention

Frequent episodes are usually cause for medication. In rare cases, the doctor may recommend a procedure called **catheter ablation**, which will remove (or ablate) the precise area of the heart responsible for triggering the fast heart rate.

In a catheter ablation procedure, the doctor will place a special catheter against the area of the heart responsible for the problem. Radio-frequency energy is then passed to the tip of the catheter, so that it heats up and destroys the target area. Catheter ablation is considered a non-surgical technique.

Resources

ORGANIZATIONS

American Heart Association. 7320 Greenville Ave., Dallas, TX 75231. (214) 373-6300. < http://www.americanheart.org >.

Dorothy Elinor Stonely

Paroxysmal supraventricular tachycardia *see* **Paroxysmal atrial tachycardia**

Parrot fever

Definition

Parrot **fever** is a rare infectious disease that causes **pneumonia** in humans. It is transmitted from pet birds or poultry. The illness is caused by a chlamydia, which is a type of intracellular parasite closely related to bacteria. Parrot fever is also called chlamydiosis, psittacosis, or ornithosis.

Description

Parrot fever, which is referred to as avian psittacosis when it infects birds, is caused by *Chlamydia psittaci*. Pet birds in the parrot family, including parrots, parakeets, macaws, and cockatiels, are the most common carriers of the infection. Other birds that may also spread *C. psittaci* include pigeons, doves, mynah birds, and turkeys. Birds that are carrying the organism may appear healthy, but can shed it in their feces. The symptoms of avian psittacosis include inactivity, loss of appetite and ruffled feathers, **diarrhea**, runny eyes and nasal discharge, and green or yellow-green urine. Sick birds can be treated with **antibiotics** by a veterinarian.

C. psittaci is usually spread from birds to humans through exposure to infected bird feces during cage cleaning or by handling infected birds. In humans, parrot fever can range in severity from minor flu-like symptoms to severe and life-threatening pneumonia.

Causes and symptoms

Parrot fever is usually transmitted by inhaling dust from dried bird droppings or by handling infected birds. Humans can also spread the disease by person-to-person contact, but that is very rare. The symptoms usually develop within five to 14 days of exposure and include fever, **headache**, chills, loss of appetite, **cough**, and tiredness. In the most severe cases of parrot fever, the patient develops pneumonia. People who work in pet shops or who keep pet birds are the most likely to become infected.

Diagnosis

Only 100–200 cases of parrot fever are reported each year in the United States. It is possible, however, that the illness is more common since it is easily confused with other types of influenza or pneumonia. Doctors are most likely to consider a diagnosis of parrot fever if the patient has a recent history of exposure to birds. The diagnosis can be confirmed by blood

---

KEY TERMS

Avian chlamydiosis—An illness in pet birds and poultry caused by *Chlamydia psittaci*. It is also known as parrot fever in birds.

Chlamydia psittaci—An organism related to bacteria that infects some types of birds and can be transmitted to humans to cause parrot fever.

Chlamydiosis, psittacosis, or ornithosis—Other names for parrot fever in humans.

---

tests for antibodies, usually complement fixation or immunofluorescence tests. The organism is difficult to culture. A **chest x ray** may also be used to diagnose the pneumonia caused by *C. psittaci*.

Treatment

Psittacosis is treated with an antibiotic, usually tetracycline (Achromycin, Sumycin); doxycycline (Doxy, Vibramycin); or erythromycin (Eryc, Ilotycin). Oral medication is typically prescribed for at least 10–14 days. Severely ill patients may be given intravenous antibiotics for the first few days of therapy.

Prognosis

The prognosis for recovery is excellent; with antibiotic treatment, more than 99% of patients with parrot fever will recover. Severe infections, however, may be fatal to the elderly, untreated persons, and persons with weak immune systems.

Prevention

As of 1998, there is no vaccine that is effective against parrot fever. Birds that are imported into the country as pets should be quarantined to ensure that they are not infected before they can be sold. Health authorities recommend that breeders and importers feed imported birds a special blend of feed mixed with antibiotics for 45 days to ensure that any *C. psittaci* organisms are destroyed. In addition, bird cages and food and water bowls should be cleaned daily.

Resources

ORGANIZATIONS

Centers for Disease Control and Prevention. 1600 Clifton Rd., NE, Atlanta, GA 30333. (800) 311-3435, (404) 639-3311. <http://www.cdc.gov>.

OTHER

"Psittacosis (Parrot Fever; Ornithosis)." *ThriveOnline.*
< http://thriveonline.oxygen.com >.

Altha Roberts Edgren

Partial birth abortion *see* **Abortion, partial birth**

Partial thromboplastin time

Definition

The partial thromboplastin time (PTT) test is a blood test that is done to investigate bleeding disorders and to monitor patients taking an anticlotting drug (heparin).

Purpose

Diagnosis

Blood clotting (coagulation) depends on the action of substances in the blood called clotting factors. Measuring the partial thromboplastin time helps to assess which specific clotting factors may be missing or defective.

Monitoring

Certain surgical procedures and diseases cause **blood clots** to form within blood vessels. Heparin is used to treat these clots. The PTT test can be used to monitor the effect of heparin on a patient's coagulation system.

Precautions

Certain medications besides heparin can affect the results of the PPT test. These include **antihistamines**, vitamin C (ascorbic acid), **aspirin**, and chlorpromazine (Thorazine).

Description

When a body tissue is injured and begins to bleed, it starts a sequence of clotting factor activities called the coagulation cascade, which leads to the formation of a blood clot. The cascade has three pathways: extrinsic, intrinsic, and common. Many of the thirteen known clotting factors in human blood are shared by both pathways; several are found in only one. The PTT test evaluates the factors found in the intrinsic and common pathways. It is usually done in combination with other tests, such as the prothrombin test, which evaluate the factors of the extrinsic pathway. The combination of tests narrows the list of possible missing or defective factors.

Heparin prevents clotting by blocking certain factors in the intrinsic pathway. The PTT test allows a doctor to check that there is enough heparin in the blood to prevent clotting, but not so much as to cause bleeding. The test is done before the first dose of heparin or whenever the dosage level is changed; and again when the heparin has reached a constant level in the blood. The PTT test is repeated at scheduled intervals.

The PTT test uses blood to which a chemical has been added to prevent clotting before the test begins. About 5 mL of blood are drawn from a vein in the patient's inner elbow region. Collection of the sample takes only a few minutes. The blood is spun in a centrifuge, which separates the pale yellow liquid part of blood (plasma) from the cells. Calcium and activating substances are added to the plasma to start the intrinsic pathway of the coagulation cascade. The partial thromboplastin time is the time it takes for a clot to form, measured in seconds.

The test can be done without activators, but they are usually added to shorten the clotting time, making the test more useful for monitoring heparin levels. When activators are used, the test is called activated partial thromboplastin time or APTT.

Test results can be obtained in less than one hour. The test is usually covered by insurance.

Preparation

The doctor should check to see if the patient is taking any of the medications that may influence the test results. If the patient is on heparin therapy, the blood sample is drawn one hour before the next dose of heparin.

Aftercare

Aftercare includes routine care of the puncture site. In addition, patients on heparin therapy must be watched for signs of spontaneous bleeding. The patient should not be left alone until the doctor or nurse is sure that bleeding has stopped. Patients should also be advised to watch for bleeding gums, bruising easily, and other signs of clotting problems; to avoid activities that might cause minor cuts or **bruises**; and to avoid using aspirin.

KEY TERMS

Activated partial thromboplastin time—Partial thromboplastin time test that uses activators to shorten the clotting time, making it more useful for heparin monitoring.

Clotting factors—Substances in the blood that act in sequence to stop bleeding by forming a clot.

Coagulation—The process of blood clotting.

Coagulation cascade—The sequence of biochemical activities, involving clotting factors, that stop bleeding by forming a clot.

Common pathway—The pathway that results from the merging of the extrinsic and intrinsic pathways. The common pathway includes the final steps before a clot is formed.

Extrinsic pathway—One of three pathways in the coagulation cascade.

Heparin—A medication that prevents blood clots.

Intrinsic pathway—One of three pathways in the coagulation cascade.

Partial thromboplastin time—A test that checks the clotting factors of the intrinsic pathway.

Plasma—The fluid part of blood, as distinguished from blood cells.

Risks

The patient may develop a bruise or swelling around the puncture site, which can be treated with moist warm compresses. People with coagulation problems may bleed for a longer period than normal.

Normal results

Normal results vary based on the method and activators used. Normal APTT results are usually between 25–40 seconds; PTT results are between 60–70 seconds. APTT results for a patient on heparin should be 1.5–2.5 times normal values. An APTT longer than 100 seconds indicates spontaneous bleeding.

Abnormal results

Increased levels in a person with a bleeding disorder indicate a clotting factor may be missing or defective. Further tests are done to identify the factor involved. **Liver disease** decreases production of factors, increasing the PTT.

Low levels in a patient on heparin indicate too little heparin is in the blood to prevent clots. High levels indicate too much heparin is present, placing the person at risk of excessive bleeding.

Resources

PERIODICALS

Berry, Brian R., and Stephen Nantel. "Heparin Therapy: Current Regimens and Principles of Monitoring." *Postgraduate Medicine* 99 (June 1996): 64-76.

Nancy J. Nordenson

Paruresis

Definition

The inability to urinate in the presence of others.

Description

Paruresis, also known as shy or bashful bladder, is the inability or difficulty to urinate in the presence of other people, when under time pressure, or on vehicles such as trains or airplanes. Urination is normal when those constraints or factors are absent, typically when in the bathroom at home. Research suggests up to 17 million Americans, 3.25 million Canadians, and 51 million Europeans suffer from the social **anxiety** disorder. Paruresis ranges in intensity from mild, in which the person can urinate in public facilities under certain circumstances, to severe, in which the person can only urinate when alone at home. The condition almost exclusively affects males although it can occur in females.

Paruresis can be socially disabling and can often completely take over a person's life. Examples include avoiding travel, social functions, and sports arenas. Just as serious are the psychological consequences, such as depression, and anxiety. Job choices and career decisions are often adversely affected. People with the condition often avoid jobs where there is mandatory drug testing done by the supervised collection of a urine sample.

Causes and symptoms

Paruretics (people who suffer from paruresis) commonly refer to three triggers that influence them when in public restrooms. For the typical paruretic, these triggers must be removed, or the person must try another toilet, for urination to occur on a particular occasion. First, the condition occurs much more frequently when strangers are present in the restroom as opposed to friends or relatives. Second, proximity plays a role in the problem. Proximity for the paruretic is both physical, involving the relative closeness of others in or near the restroom, and psychological, involving the need for privacy. The most frequent complaint about physical stimuli in public facilities is the absence of suitable partitions and doors on urinals or stalls. Third, temporary psychological states, especially anxiety, anger, and fear can interfere with urination.

Diagnosis

The condition is diagnosed on the basis of the sufferer's account of their symptoms. In severe cases, sufferers can waste considerable time waiting for everyone else to leave the toilet before they can urinate, and might totally avoid urinating in public toilets. The condition is usually self-diagnosed when any or all of the three main triggers of paruresis are present and the condition is chronic.

Treatment

The most well documented current treatment is based upon **cognitive-behavioral therapy**, of which the aim is to reorganize the "abnormal" emotional schemes arising from the anxiety generating elements that trigger this problem. This can be done individually in a self-help situation, in a support group, or through psychotherapy with a psychologist or psychiatrist.

Therapy includes three separate but linked components:

- Cognitive—An attempt to modify the abnormal thoughts and ideas around the object of anxiety, such as the thought, "When I use a toilet, everybody looks at me and wonders what I'm doing."

- Behavioral—Step by step desensitization by very gradual exposure to the feared situation, the aim being to achieve a series of small successes, and thus reassure the subconscious mind that it is "safe" to urinate in a situation that previously led to panic and failure. This can be thought of as relearning urination in a social situation.

- Relaxation—Learning techniques that facilitate relaxation, both mental and physical, such as sphincter relaxation exercises.

Drug treatments, usually with medications used to treat benign prostate hyperplasia (BPH), an enlargement of the prostate gland, such as *terazosin* (Hytrin), *tamsulosin* (Flomax), and *alfuzosin* (Uroxatral) are the subject of much debate and usually produce poor results.

KEY TERMS

Benign prostate hyperplasia (BPH)—Enlargement of the prostate gland.

Psychotherapy—The treatment of mental disorders by psychological methods, usually by a psychiatrist or psychologist.

Sphincter—A circular band of muscle that surrounds an opening or passage in the body and narrows or closes the opening by contracting.

Urethra—The tube in humans that carries urine from the bladder out of the body.

Alternative treatment

One possible alternative medicine treatment is **saw palmetto**, used to treat urinary problems in men with BPH, an enlargement of the prostate gland. BPH results in a swelling of the prostate gland that obstructs the urethra. This causes painful urination, reduced urine flow, difficulty starting or stopping the flow, dribbling after urination, and more frequent nighttime urination. A typical dose is 320 mg per day of standardized extract. It may take up to four weeks of use before beneficial effects are seen.

Prognosis

Most people who suffer from the condition never seek help or treatment. Many never even discuss the problem with anyone. But anecdotal evidence suggests that those who do seek help have a good success rate at overcoming their fear or anxiety over time, sometimes a year or longer.

Prevention

There is no known way to prevent a person from developing paruresis. Anecdotal evidence suggests it often does not occur until around the age of **puberty**. One suggestion for prevention is to condition children from an early age to urinate in public restrooms.

Resources

PERIODICALS

Landers, Peter. "Looking for Relief: Shy Bladder Syndrome is Widespread; But in Many Cases it Can Be Treated Successfully." *The Wall Street Journal* (April 22, 2003): R5.

Siwolop, Sana. "For Some, Drug Tests Are Almost Impossible." *The New York Times* (April 14, 2002): NJ1.

ORGANIZATIONS

International Paruresis Association. P.O. Box 65111, Baltimore, MD 21209. (800) 247-3864. info@paruresis.org. http://www.paruresis.org.

OTHER

June 11, 2001. WebMD*The Secret Social Phobia.* http://my.webmd.com/content/Article/14/1674_51491.htm. (Accessed March 31, 2005).

Ken R. Wells

Parvovirus B19 infection *see* **Fifth disease**

Pasteurellosis *see* **Animal bite infections**

Patau syndrome

Definition

Patau syndrome, also called trisomy 13, is a congenital (present at birth) disorder associated with the presence of an extra copy of chromosome 13. The extra chromosome 13 causes numerous physical and mental abnormalities, especially heart defects. Patau syndrome is named for Dr. Klaus Patau, who reported the syndrome and its association with trisomy in 1960. It is sometimes called Bartholin-Patau syndrome, named in part for Thomas Bartholin, a French physician who described an infant with the syndrome in 1656.

Description

Children normally inherit 23 chromosomes from each parent, for a total of 46 chromosomes. A typical human being has 46 chromosomes: 22 pairs of non-sex linked chromosomes and one pair of sex-linked chromosomes, that determine that child's sex. Sometimes a child may end up with more than 46 chromosomes because of problems with the father's sperm or the mother's egg; or, because of mutations that occurred after the sperm and the egg fused to form the embryo (conception).

Normally, there are two copies of each of the 23 chromosomes: one from each parent. A condition called trisomy occurs when three, instead of two, copies of a chromosome are present in a developing human embryo. An extra copy of a particular chromosome can come either from the egg or sperm, or because of mutations that occur after conception.

The best-known trisomy-related disorder is **Down syndrome** (trisomy 21), in which the developing embryo has an extra copy of chromosome 21. Patau syndrome is trisomy 13, in which the developing embryo has three copies of chromosome 13.

An extra copy of chromosome 13 is not the only cause of Patau syndrome. Other changes in chromosome 13, such as mispositioning (translocation), can also result in the characteristics classified as Patau syndrome. In these cases, an error occurs that causes a portion of chromosome 13 to be exchanged for a portion of another chromosome. There is no production of extra chromosomes, but a portion of each affected chromosome is "misplaced" (translocated) to another chromosome.

Patau syndrome causes serious physical and mental abnormalities including: heart defects; incomplete brain development; such unusual facial features as a sloping forehead, a smaller than average head (microcephaly), small or missing eyes, low-set ears, and **cleft palate** or hare lip; extra fingers and toes (**polydactyly**); abnormal genitalia; spinal defects; seizures; gastrointestinal hernias, particularly at the navel (omphalocele); and mental retardation. Due to the severity of these conditions, fewer than 20% of those affected with Patau syndrome survive beyond infancy. Most infants with the syndrome die within the first three months of life; the average life expectancy of the survivors is about 10 years.

Genetic profile

When an extra copy (trisomy) of a chromosome is made, it may either be a total trisomy (in which an extra copy of the entire chromosome is made), or partial trisomy (in which only one part of the chromosome is made an extra time).

In most cases of trisomy, errors in chromosome duplication occur at conception because of problems with the egg or the sperm that are coming together to produce an offspring. In these cases, every cell in the body of the offspring has an extra copy of the affected chromosome. However, errors in chromosome duplication may also occur during the rapid cell division that takes place immediately after conception. In these cases, only some cells of the body have the extra chromosome error. The condition in which only some of the cells in the body have the extra chromosome is called mosaicism.

Seventy-five to 80 percent of the cases of Patau syndrome are caused by a trisomy of chromosome 13. Some of these cases are the result of a total trisomy, while others are the result of a partial trisomy. Partial trisomy generally causes less severe physical symptoms than full trisomy. Ten percent of these cases are of the mosaic type, in which only some of the body's cells have the extra chromosome. The physical symptoms of the mosaic form of Patau syndrome depends on the number and type of cells that carry the trisomy.

Most cases of trisomy are not passed on from one generation to the next. Usually they result from a malfunction in the cell division (mitosis) that occurs after conception. At least 75% of the cases of Patau syndrome are caused by errors in chromosome replication that occur after conception. The remaining 25% are caused by the inheritance of translocations of chromosome 13 with other chromosomes within the parental chromosomes. In these cases, a portion of another chromosome switches places with a portion of chromosome 13. This leads to errors in the genes on both chromosome 13 and the chromosome from which the translocated portion originated.

Patau syndrome occurs in approximately one in 8,000–12,000 live births in the United States. In many cases, spontaneous abortion (**miscarriage**) occurs and the fetus does not survive to term. In other cases, the affected individual is stillborn. As appears to be the case in all trisonomies, the risks of Patau syndrome seem to increase with the mother's age, particularly if she is over 30 when pregnant. Male and female children are equally affected, and the syndrome occurs in all races and ethnic groups. Females with Patau syndrome, however, have a better chance of surviving past infancy than males.

Causes and symptoms

The severity and symptoms of Patau syndrome vary with the type of chromosomal anomaly, from extremely serious conditions to nearly normal appearance and functioning.

Full trisomy 13, which is present in the majority of the cases, results in the most severe and numerous internal and external abnormalities. Commonly, the forebrain fails to divide into lobes or hemispheres (holoprosencephaly) and the entire head is unusually small (microcephaly). The spinal cord may protrude through a defect in the vertebrae of the spinal column (myelomeningocele). Children who survive infancy have profound **mental retardation** and may experience seizures. In a few rare cases Patau syndrome may coexist with Klinefelter's syndrome or other chromosomal abnormalities.

Incomplete development of the optic (sight) and olfactory (smell) nerves often accompany the brain defects described above. The eyes may be unusually small (**microphthalmia**) or one eye may be absent (**anophthalmia**). The eyes are sometimes set close together (hypotelorism) or even fused into a single structure. Incomplete development of any structures in the eye (coloboma) or failure of the retina to develop properly (retinal dysplasia) will also produce vision problems. Patau syndrome affected individuals may be born either partially or totally deaf and many are subject to recurring ear infections.

The facial features of many Patau syndrome-affected individuals appear flattened. The ears are generally malformed and lowset. Frequently, a child with trisomy 13 has a **cleft lip**, a cleft palate, or both. Other physical characteristics include loose folds of skin at the back of the neck, extra fingers or toes (polydactyly), permanently flexed (closed) fingers (camptodactyly), noticeably prominent heels, "rocker-bottom foot," and missing ribs. Genital malformations are common in individuals affected with Patau syndrome and include undescended testicles (cryptorchidism), an abnormally developed scrotum, and ambiguous genitalia in males, or an abnormally formed uterus (bicornuate uterus) in females.

In nearly all cases, Patau syndrome affected infants have respiratory difficulties and heart defects, including atrial and ventricular septal defects (holes between chambers of the heart); malformed ducts that cause abnormal direction of blood flow (patent ductus arteriosus); holes in the valves of the lungs and the heart (pulmonary and aortic valves); and misplacement of the heart in the right, rather than the left, side of the chest (dextrocardia). The kidneys and gastrointestinal system may also be affected with cysts similar to those seen in **polycystic kidney disease**. These defects are frequently severe and life-threatening.

Partial trisomy of the distal segment of chromosome 13 results in generally less severe, but still serious, symptoms and a distinctive facial appearance including a short upturned nose, a longer than usual area between the nose and upper lip (philtrum), bushy eyebrows, and tumors made up of blood capillaries on the forehead (frontal capillary hemangiomata). Partial trisomy of the proximal segment of chromosome 13 is much less likely to be fatal and has been associated with a variety of facial features including a large nose, a short upper lip, and a receding jaw. Both forms of partial trisomy also result in severe mental retardation.

Beyond one month of age, other symptoms that are seen in individuals with Patau syndrome are:

feeding difficulties and **constipation**, reflux disease, slow growth rates, curvature of the spine (**scoliosis**), irritability, sensitivity to sunlight, low muscle tone, high blood pressure, sinus infections, urinary tract infections, and ear and eye infections.

Diagnosis

Patau syndrome is detectable during **pregnancy** through the use of ultrasound imaging, **amniocentesis**, and **chorionic villus sampling** (CVS). At birth, the newborn's numerous malformations indicate a possible chromosomal abnormality. Trisomy 13 is confirmed by examining the infant's chromosomal pattern through karyotyping or another procedure. Karyotyping involves the separation and isolation of the chromosomes present in cells taken from an individual. These cells are generally extracted from cells found in a blood sample. The 22 non-sex linked chromosomes are identified by size, from largest to smallest, as chromosomes 1 through 22. The sex-determining chromosomes are also identified. The diagnosis of Patau syndrome is confirmed by the presence of three, rather than the normal two, copies of the thirteenth largest chromosome.

A newer method of diagnosing trisomies that has the advantages of speed and lower cost is the quantitative fluorescent PCR (QF-PCR) assay. QF-PCR testing allows a doctor to determine the presence of a chromosomal abnormality within 24 hours with a very high degree of accuracy.

Treatment

Some infants born with Patau syndrome have severe and incurable birth defects. However, children with better prognoses require medical treatment to correct structural abnormalities and associated complications. For feeding problems, special formulas, positions, and techniques may be used. Tube feeding or the placement of a gastric tube (**gastrostomy**) may be required. Structural abnormalities such as cleft lip and cleft palate can be corrected through surgery. Special diets, hearing aids, and vision aids can be used to mitigate the symptoms of Patau syndrome. Physical therapy, speech therapy, and other types of developmental therapy will help the child reach his or her potential.

Since the translocation form of Patau syndrome is genetically transmitted, **genetic counseling** for the parents should be part of the management of the disease.

KEY TERMS

Amniocentesis—A procedure performed at 16–18 weeks of pregnancy in which a needle is inserted through a woman's abdomen into her uterus to draw out a small sample of the amniotic fluid from around the baby. Either the fluid itself or cells from the fluid can be used for a variety of tests to obtain information about genetic disorders and other medical conditions in the fetus.

Chorionic villus sampling (CVS)—A procedure used for prenatal diagnosis at 10–12 weeks gestation. Under ultrasound guidance a needle is inserted either through the mother's vagina or abdominal wall and a sample of cells is collected from around the fetus. These cells are then tested for chromosome abnormalities or other genetic diseases.

Chromosome—A microscopic thread-like structure found within each cell of the body consisting of a complex of proteins and DNA. Humans have 46 chromosomes arranged into 23 pairs. Changes in either the total number of chromosomes or their shape and size (structure) may lead to physical or mental abnormalities.

Karyotyping—A laboratory procedure in which chromosomes are separated from cells, stained, and arranged so that their structure can be studied under the microscope.

Mosaicism—A genetic condition resulting from a mutation, crossing over, or nondisjunction of chromosomes during cell division, causing a variation in the number of chromosomes in the cells.

Translocation—The transfer of one part of a chromosome to another chromosome during cell division. A balanced translocation occurs when pieces from two different chromosomes exchange places without loss or gain of any chromosome material. An unbalanced translocation involves the unequal loss or gain of genetic information between two chromosomes.

Trisomy—The condition of having three identical chromosomes instead of the normal two in a cell.

Ultrasound—An imaging technique that uses sound waves to help visualize internal structures in the body.

Prognosis

Approximately 45% of trisomy 13 babies die within their first month of life; up to 70% in the first six months; and over 70% by one year of age. Survival to adulthood is very rare. Only one adult is known to have survived to age 33.

Most survivors have profound mental and physical disabilities; however, the capacity for learning in children with Patau syndrome varies from case to case. Older children may be able to walk with or without a walker. They may also be able to understand words and phrases, follow simple commands, use a few words or signs, and recognize and interact with others.

Resources

BOOKS

Beers, Mark H., MD, and Robert Berkow, MD, editors. "Congenital Anomalies." Section 19, Chapter 261. In *The Merck Manual of Diagnosis and Therapy.* Whitehouse Station, NJ: Merck Research Laboratories, 2004.

PERIODICALS

Best, Robert G., PhD., and James Stallworth, MD. "Patau Syndrome." *eMedicine* November 21, 2002. < http:// www.emedicine.com/ped/topic1745.htm > .

Cirigliano, V., G. Voglino, M. P. Canadas, et al. "Rapid Prenatal Diagnosis of Common Chromosome Aneuploidies by QF-PCR. Assessment on 18,000 Consecutive Clinical Samples." *Molecular Human Reproduction* 10 (November 2004): 839–846.

Mann, K., C. Donaghue, S. P. Fox, et al. "Strategies for the Rapid Prenatal Diagnosis of Chromosome Aneuploidy." *European Journal of Human Genetics* 12 (November 2004): 907–915.

Oyler, M., B. W. Long, and L. A. Cox. "Sonographic Markers Used to Detect Frequent Trisomies." *Radiologic Technology* 76 (September-October 2004): 13–18.

Rossino, R., and A. L. Nucaro. "Prenatal Diagnosis of a Double Trisomy 48, XXY, + 13: Klinefelter and Patau Syndromes." *American Journal of Medical Genetics, Part A* 132A (December 15, 2004): 342.

ORGANIZATIONS

National Organization for Rare Disorders (NORD). 55 Kenosia Avenue, P. O. Box 1968, Danbury, CT 06813-1968. (203) 744-0100. Fax: (203) 798-2291. < http://www.rarediseases.org >.

Rainbows Down Under—A Trisomy 18 and Trisomy 13 Resource. SOFT Australia, 198 Oak Rd., Kirrawee, NSW 2232. Australia 02-9521-6039. < http://members.optushome.com.au/karens >.

Support Organization for Trisomy 18, 13, and Related Disorders (SOFT). 2982 South Union St., Rochester, NY 14624. (800) 716-SOFT. < http://www.trisomy.org >.

OTHER

Pediatric Database (PEDBASE) Homepage. February 9, 2001. < http://www.icondata.com/health/pedbase/ files/TRISOMY1.HTM >.

"Trisomy 13." *WebMD* February 9, 2001. < http:// my.webmd.com/content/asset/ adam_disease_trisomy_13 >.

Paul A. Johnson, Ed.M.
Rebecca J. Frey, Ph.D.

Patent ductus arteriosus

Definition

Patent ductus arteriosus (PDA) is a heart defect that occurs when the ductus arteriosus (the temporary fetal blood vessel that connects the aorta and the pulmonary artery) does not close at birth.

Description

The ductus arteriosus is a temporary fetal blood vessel that connects the aorta and the pulmonary artery before birth. The ductus arteriosus should be present and open before birth while the fetus is developing in the uterus. Since oxygen and nutrients are received from the placenta and the umbilical cord instead of the lungs, the ductus arteriosus acts as a "short cut" that allows blood to bypass the deflated lungs and go straight out to the body. After birth, when the lungs are needed to add oxygen to the blood, the ductus arteriosus normally closes. The closure of the ductus arteriosus ensures that blood goes to the lungs to pick up oxygen before going out to the body. Closure of the ductus arteriosus usually occurs at birth as levels of certain chemicals, called prostagladins, change and the lungs fill with air. If the ductus arteriosus closes correctly, the blood pumped from the heart goes to the lungs, back into the heart, and then out to the body through the aorta. The blood returning from the lungs and moving out of the aorta carries oxygen to the cells of the body.

In some infants, the ductus arteriosus remains open (or patent) and the resulting heart defect is known as patent ductus arteriosus. In most cases, a small PDA does not result in physical symptoms. If the PDA is larger, health complications may occur.

In an average individual's body, the power of blood being pumped by the heart and other forces leads to a certain level of pressure between the heart and lungs.

The pressure between the heart and lungs of an individual affected by PDA causes some of the oxygenated blood that should go out to the body (through the aorta) to return back through the PDA into the pulmonary artery. The pulmonary artery takes the blood immediately back to the lungs. The recycling of the already oxygenated blood forces the heart to work harder as it tries to supply enough oxygenated blood to the body. In this case, usually the left side of the heart grows larger as it works harder and must contain all of the extra blood moving back into the heart. This is know as a left-to-right or aortic-pulmonary shunt.

As noted, the size of the PDA determines how much harder the heart has to work and how much bigger the heart becomes. If the PDA is large, the bottom left side of the heart is forced to pump twice as much blood because it must supply enough blood to recycle back to the lungs and move out to the body. As the heart responds to the increased demands for more oxygenated blood by pumping harder, the pulmonary artery has to change in size and shape in order to adapt to the increased amount and force of the blood. In some cases, the increase in size and shape changes the pressure in the pulmonary artery and lungs. If the pressure in the lungs is higher than that of the heart and body, blood returning to the heart will take the short cut back into the aorta from the pulmonary artery through the PDA instead of going to the lungs. This backward flowing of blood does not carry much oxygen. If blood without much oxygen is being delivered to the body, the legs and toes will turn blue or cyanotic. This is called a shunt reversal.

When a PDA results in a large amount of blood being cycled in the wrong order, either through a left-to-right shunt or shunt reversal, the overworked, enlarged heart may stop working (congestive **heart failure**) and the lungs can become filled with too much fluid (**pulmonary edema**). At this time, there is also an increased risk for a bacterial infection that can inflame the lining of the heart (**endocarditis**). These three complications are very serious.

PDA is a very common heart defect. Though an exact incidence of PDA is difficult to determine, one review in 1990 found that approximately 8% of live births were found to be affected by PDA. PDA can occur in full-term infants, but it seen most frequently in preterm infants, infants born at a high altitude, and babies whose mothers were affected by the German measles (**rubella**) during pregnancy. PDA is two to three times more common in females than males. PDA occurs in individuals of every ethnic origin and does not occur more frequently in any one country or ethnic population.

Causes and symptoms

PDA can be a result of an environmental exposure before birth, inheriting a specific changed or mutated gene or genes, a symptom of a genetic syndrome, or be caused by a combination of genetic and environmental factors (multifactorial).

Environmental exposures that can increase the chance for a baby to be affected by PDA include fetal exposure to rubella before birth, preterm delivery, and birth at a high altitude location.

PDA can be an inherited condition running in families as isolated PDA or part of a genetic syndrome. In either case, there are specific gene changes or mutations which lead to a defect in the elastic tissue forming the walls of the ductus arteriosus. The genes causing isolated PDA have not been identified, but it is known that PDA can be inherited through a family in an autosomal dominant pattern or an autosomal recessive pattern.

Every person has approximately 30,000 genes, which tell our bodies how to grow and develop correctly. Each gene is present in pairs since one is inherited from our mother, and one is inherited from our father. In an autosomal dominant condition, only one specific changed or mutated copy of the gene for PDA is necessary for a person to have PDA. If a parent has an autosomal dominant form of PDA, there is a 50% chance for each child to have the same or similar condition.

PDA can also be inherited in an autosomal recessive manner. A recessive condition occurs when a child receives two changed or mutated copies of the gene for a particular condition, such as PDA (one copy from each parent). Individuals with a single changed or mutated copy of a gene for a recessive condition, are known as "carriers," and have no health problems related to the condition. In fact, each of us carries between five and 10 genes for harmful, recessive conditions. However, when two people who each carry a changed or mutated copy of the same gene for a recessive condition meet, there is a chance, with each **pregnancy**, for the child to inherit the two changed or mutated copies from each parent. In this case, the child would have PDA. For two known carriers, there is a 25% risk with each child to have a child with PDA, a 50% chance to have a child who is a carrier, and a 25% chance to have a child who is neither affected nor a carrier.

Most cases of PDA occur as the result of multifactorial inheritance which is caused by the combination of genetic factors and environmental factors. The

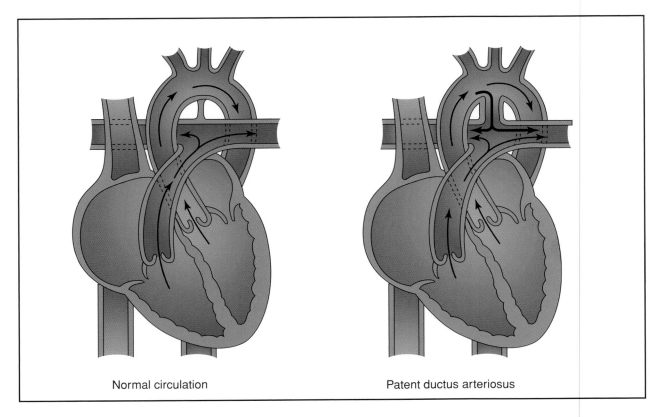

Normal circulation

Patent ductus arteriosus

Patent ductus arteriosus (PDA) is the failure of the ductus arteriosus to close after birth, allowing blood to inappropriately flow from the aorta into the pulmonary artery. *(Illustration by Electronic Illustrators Group.)*

combined factors lead to isolated defects in the elastic tissue forming the walls of the ductus arteriosus. Family studies can provide different recurrence risks depending on the family member affected by multifactorial PDA. If an individual is affected by isolated, multifactorial PDA, they have a 2–4% chance of having a child affected by PDA. If a couple has one child with isolated, multifactorial PDA, there is a 3% chance that another of their children could be affected by PDA. If a couple has two children affected by isolated, multifactorial PDA, there is a 10–25% chance that they could have another child affected by PDA.

Unless a specific pattern of inheritance, preterm delivery, or known exposure is found through the examination of a detailed pregnancy and family history, the multifactorial family studies are used to estimated the possible risk of recurrence of PDA in a family.

The main sign of PDA is a constant heart murmur that sounds like the hum of a refrigerator or other machinery. This murmur is usually heard by the doctor using a stethoscope. Otherwise, there are no specific symptoms of PDA, unless the ductus arteriosus size is large. Children and adults with a large ductus arteriosus can show difficulty in breathing during moderate physical exercise, an enlarged heart, and failure to gain weight. In some cases, heart failure and pulmonary congestion can indicate a PDA.

Diagnosis

Diagnosis is most often made by detecting the characteristic "machinery" heart murmur heard by a doctor through a stethoscope. Tests such as a chest x ray, echocardiograph, and ECG are used to support the initial diagnosis. Other indications of PDA include failure to gain weight, frequent chest infections, heavy breathing during mild physical exertion, congestive heart failure, and pulmonary **edema**. Prenatal ultrasounds are unable to detect PDA because the heart defect does not occur until the time of birth.

Treatment

The treatment and management of PDA depends upon the size of the PDA and symptoms being

KEY TERMS

Aorta—The main artery located above the heart which pumps oxygenated blood out into the body. Many congenital heart defects affect the aorta.

Catheterization—The process of inserting a hollow tube into a body cavity or blood vessel.

Ductus arteriosus—The temporary channel or blood vessel between the aorta and pulmonary artery in the fetus.

Echocardiograph—A record of the internal structures of the heart obtained from beams of ultrasonic waves directed through the wall of the chest.

Electrocardiogram (ECG, EKG)—A test used to measure electrical impulses coming from the heart in order to gain information about its structure or function.

Endocarditis—A dangerous infection of the heart valves caused by certain bacteria.

Oxygenated blood—Blood carrying oxygen through the body.

Pulmonary artery—An artery that carries blood from the heart to the lungs.

Pulmonary edema—A problem caused when fluid backs up into the veins of the lungs. Increased pressure in these veins forces fluid out of the vein and into the air spaces (alveoli). This interferes with the exchange of oxygen and carbon dioxide in the alveoli.

and frequently occurs without complications. Proper treatment allows children and adults to lead normal lives.

Resources

BOOKS

Jaworski, Anna Marie, editor. *The Heart of a Mother.* Temple, Texas: Baby Hearts Press, 1999.

ORGANIZATIONS

CHASER (Congenital Heart Anomalies Support, Education, and Resources). 2112 North Wilkins Rd., Swanton, OH 43558. (419) 825-5575. < http://www.csun.edu/~hfmth006/chaser >.

Kids with Heart. 1578 Careful Dr., Green Bay, WI 54304. (800) 538-5390. < http://www.execpc.com/~kdswhrt >.

OTHER

Berger, Sheri. The Congenital Heart Defects Resource Page. January 6, 2000. < http://www.csun.edu/ ~hfmth006/chaser/ >.

"Congenital Cardiovascular Disease." *American Heart Association* 2000. < http://www.americanheart.org/ Heart_and_Stroke_A_Z_Guide/conghd.html >.

"Heart Disorders." *Family Village.* March 24, 2000. < http://www.familyvillage.wisc.edu/index.html >.

Dawn A. Jacob

PCV *see* **Hematocrit**

Pediculosis *see* **Lice infestation**

Pedophilia *see* **Sexual perversions**

Pellagra

Definition

Pellagra is a disorder brought on by a deficiency of the nutrient called niacin or nicotinic acid, one of the B-complex **vitamins**.

Description

Nicotinic acid plays a crucial role in the cellular process called respiration. Respiration is the process by which nutrients (specifically sugar, or glucose) and oxygen are taken in, chemical reactions take place, energy is produced and stored, and carbon dioxide and wastes are given off. This process is absolutely central to basic cell functioning, and thus the functioning of the body as a whole.

Niacin is a B vitamin found in such foods as yeast, liver, meat, fish, whole-grain cereals and breads, and

experienced by the affected individual. In some cases, a PDA can correct itself in the first months of life. In preterm infants experiencing symptoms, the first step in correcting a PDA is treatment through medications such as indomethacin. In preterm infants whose PDA is not closed through medication, full term infants affected by PDA, and adults, surgery is an option for closing the ductus arteriosus. In 2000 and 2001, medicine has developed and reviewed alternatives to surgical closure such as interventional **cardiac catheterization** and video-assisted thorascopic surgical repair. A cardiologist can help individuals determine the best method for treatment based on their physical symptoms and medical history.

Prognosis

Adults and children can survive with a small opening remaining in the ductus arteriosus. Treatment, including surgery, of a larger PDA is usually successful legumes. Niacin can also be produced within the body from the essential amino acid called tryptophan. Dietary requirements for niacin depend on the age, gender, size, and activity level of the individual. Niacin requirements range from 5 mg in infants up to 20 mg in certain adults.

Causes and symptoms

Pellagra can be either primary or secondary. Primary pellagra results when the diet is extremely deficient in niacin-rich foods. A classic example occurs in geographic locations where Indian corn (maize) is the dietary staple. Maize does contain niacin, but in a form which cannot be absorbed from the intestine (except when it has been treated with alkali, as happens in the preparation of tortillas). People who rely on maize as their major food source often develop pellagra. Pellagra can also occur when a hospitalized patient, unable to eat for a very prolonged period of time, is given fluids devoid of vitamins through a needle in the vein (intravenous or IV fluids).

Secondary pellagra occurs when adequate quantities of niacin are present in the diet, but other diseases or conditions interfere with its absorption and/or processing. This is seen in various diseases that cause prolonged **diarrhea**, with **cirrhosis** of the liver and **alcoholism**, with long-term use of the anti-tuberculosis drug called isoniazid, in patients with malignant carcinoid tumor, and in patients suffering from **Hartnup disease** (an inherited disorder which results in disordered absorption of amino acids from the intestine and kidney).

Pellagra causes a variety of symptoms affecting the skin; mucous membranes (moist linings of the mouth, organs, etc.); central nervous system (including the brain and nerves); and the gastrointestinal system. The classic collection of symptoms includes redness and swelling of the mouth and tongue, diarrhea, skin rash, and abnormal mental functioning, including memory loss. While early patients may simply have a light skin rash, over time the skin becomes increasingly thickened, pigmented, and may slough off in places. Areas of the skin may become prone to bacterial infection. The mouth and tongue, and sometimes the vagina, become increasingly thick, swollen, and red. Abdominal **pain** and bloating occur, with **nausea and vomiting**, and bloody diarrhea to follow. Initial mental changes appear as inability to sleep (**insomnia**), **fatigue**, and a sense of disconnectedness (apathy). These mental changes progress to memory loss, confusion, depression, and **hallucinations** (in which the individual sees sights or hears sounds that

> ## KEY TERMS
>
> **Niacinamide**—A form of niacin, which is usually used as a dietary supplement for people with insufficient niacin.
>
> **Respiration**—Respiration is the process by which nutrients (specifically sugar, or glucose) and oxygen are taken in to a cell; chemical reactions take place; energy is produce and stored; and carbon dioxide and wastes are given off.

do not really exist). The most severe states include stiffness of the arms and legs, with resistance to attempts to move the limbs; variations in level of consciousness; and the development of involuntary sucking and grasping motions. This collection of symptoms is called "encephalopathic syndrome."

Diagnosis

Diagnosis is purely based on the patient's collection of symptoms, together with information regarding the patient's diet. When this information points to niacin deficiency, replacement is started, and the diagnosis is then partly made by evaluating the patient's response to increased amounts of niacin. There are no chemical tests available to definitively diagnose pellagra.

Treatment

Treatment of pellagra usually involves supplementing the individual's diet with a form of niacin called niacinamide (niacin itself in pure supplementation form causes a number of unpleasant side effects, including sensations of **itching**, burning, and flushing). The niacinamide can be given by mouth (orally) or by injection (when diarrhea would interfere with its absorption). The usual oral dosage is 300–500 mg each day; the usual dosage of an injection is 100–250 mg, administered two to three times each day. When pellagra has progressed to the point of the encephalopathic syndrome, a patient will require 1,000 mg of niacinamide orally, and 100–250 mg of niacinamide by injection. Once the symptoms of pellagra have subsided, a maintenance dose of niacin can be calculated, along with attempting (where possible) to make appropriate changes in the diet. Because many B-complex vitamin deficiencies occur simultaneously, patients will usually require the administration of other B-complex vitamins as well.

Prognosis

Untreated pellagra will continue progressing over the course of several years, and is ultimately fatal. Often, **death** is due to complications from infections, massive **malnutrition** brought on by continuous diarrhea, blood loss due to bleeding from the gastrointestinal tract, or severe encephalopathic syndrome.

Prevention

Prevention of pellagra is completely possible; what is required is either a diet adequate in niacin-rich foods, or appropriate supplementation. However, in many geographic locations in the world such foods are unavailable to the general population, and pellagra becomes an unavoidable complication of poverty.

Resources

ORGANIZATIONS

American Dietetic Association, 216 W. Jackson Blvd., Chicago, IL 60606-6995. (800) 745-0775. < http://www.eatright.org/cdr.html >.

Rosalyn Carson-DeWitt, MD

Pelvic endoscopy *see* **Laparoscopy**

Pelvic exam

Definition

A pelvic examination is a routine procedure used to assess the well being of the female patients' lower genito-urinary tract. This is done as part of a usual health screening and prevention tool, and is an element of the total health care for the female patient.

Purpose

Pelvic exams are useful as a screening tool for sexually transmitted diseases such as **gonorrhea**, chlamydia, **genital warts**, herpes, and **syphilis**. In addition, exams detect some forms of **cancer** that may affect the genitalia. By analyzing the cervical region with a Papanicolaou or Pap smear, clinicians are able to look for signs of **cervical cancer**. The American Cancer Society and the American College of Obstetricians and Gynecologists recommend pelvic exams with **Pap tests** for women starting at age 18. It is also recommended that exams start earlier if the teenager requests oral **contraception**. Pap smears

should continue once yearly for three years and at the physicians discretion following this time. Various groups differ in opinions on when to discontinue screening for cervical cancer, however, the United States Preventative Services Task Force recommends screening continue until age 65 if the patient has not had previous abnormal results. Women who have undergone a total **hysterectomy** for reasons other than cervical cancer do not need to be screened.

Precautions

Pelvic examinations are safe procedures, thus no precautions are necessary.

Description

The first part of the examination involves visual inspection and palpation of the external genitalia. The examiner will note the characteristics of the labia majora, labia minora, clitoris, urethral orifice, and the Skene's and Bartholin's glands. In addition, the perineum and anus will be checked. The clinician will be examining these areas for any indication of swelling, inflammation, abnormal discharge, polyps, abnormal odor, or other lesions.

The next part involves examining the internal genitalia. The examiner will first insert a gloved finger into the vagina in order to palpate the cervix. Next an instrument called a speculum is inserted. This device is made of plastic or metal and used to open the vaginal cavity in order for the examiner to be able to view the vaginal walls and cervix. Any lesions, bleeding, or abnormal discharge can be visualized with the speculum in place. If indicated, a Pap smear will then be performed. With the speculum still in place, the examiner gently scrapes the patient's cervix with a wooden or plastic spatula as well as a cylindrical-type brush. The spatula collects cells from the outer surface of the cervix, while the brush is used to collect cells from the inner-cervix. The collected cells are then spread on a glass slide, sprayed with a fixative, and sent to a laboratory for analysis. The examiner may then insert a cotton or Dacron swab into the cervix. This will be held in place for 10–30 seconds and when withdrawn spread on a plastic plate or into a tube containing a reagent for the specimen. This procedure may be repeated again with the anus. Such swab tests are used to check for gonorrhea and chlamydia, or bacterial vaginitis, which is a bacterial infection resulting in inflammation of the vagina.

Following the Pap smear is the bimanual examination during which the examiner will place an index

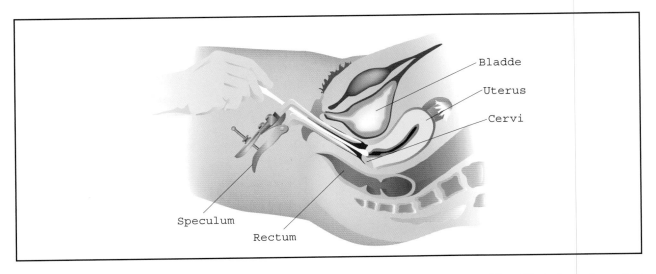

Bladde

Uterus

Cervi

Speculum

Rectum

During a pelvic exam, cells from the cervix are scraped on a spatula and are tested for abnormalities. *(Illustration by Argosy Inc.)*

and middle finger into the vagina to first examine the vaginal walls for any irregularities or tenderness. The cervix will then be palpated in order to note its shape, consistency, mobility, and any tenderness. The examiner will then place his or her other hand on the abdomen and gently push down while pushing the cervix up. This is done to assess the size and shape of the uterus, and also to note any tenderness or abnormal lesions. During this time, the ovaries are also checked for any masses, or tenderness.

The last part of the pelvic exam is the rectovaginal examination. This allows the clinician to better examine the pelvic organs and structures. The examiner will place their index finger into the vagina and a lubricated, gloved middle finger against the anus. During this part, the patient may feel an urgency to have a bowel movement. However, this is a natural feeling and a bowel movement will not occur. The patient will then be asked to strain down in order for the anal sphincter to relax. As relaxation occurs the examiner will insert the middle finger into the rectum, enabling the position and shape of the uterus to be better assessed. In addition, any masses or tenderness can be evaluated at this point. The anal canal and rectum can also be examined for any polyps, or other lesions at this time. After the rectovaginal exam, the patient will be allowed clean off any excess lubricant and get dressed. The examiner will then discuss the procedure and any findings with the patient.

Preparation

Pelvic exams require the patient to void prior to starting, as a full bladder can add to discomfort and

make palpation difficult for the examiner. Even though some tests cannot be done on a menstruating patient, an examination can still be performed. Any tampons should be removed prior to the exam. Douching is not recommended before an exam due to the hazard of washing away cells that are needed for examination. If a Pap smear is to be done, the patients should also refrain from sexual intercourse or using vaginal suppositories for 24 to 48 hours prior to the exam. The patient will be asked to undress and put on a gown. The examiner will instruct the patient to lie on the examination table on her back and may assist her in putting her feet in stirrups. The buttocks are then slid to the edge of the table in order for a full view of the area to be examined.

Aftercare

Even with the invasiveness of this procedure, the patient should be able to immediately resume normal daily activities.

Risks

Other than minor discomfort, there are no risks associated with a routine pelvic examination.

Normal results

No significant findings by the examiner indicate a normal pelvic examination. The external and internal genitalia will be free of any lesions or abnormal discharge. The Pap smear will not reveal cervical dysplasia or abnormal tissue development, and there will not

KEY TERMS

Bacterial vaginitis—This is the term for inflammation of the vagina due to a bacterial infection.

Bartholin's glands—These glands are embedded in the vestibule of the vagina and function to maintain moisture.

Cervical dysplasia—Dysplasia is the abnormal growth of the epithelial cells. This is what a Pap smear will detect in the cervix.

Colposcopy—This procedure is done when a Pap smear reveals abnormal results. With an endoscope placed through the vagina and into the cervix, a physician can determine exactly where lesions of the cervix are.

Hematoma—Hematomas are masses of blood (or clotted blood) that accumulate in tissues and may result from trauma.

Myoma—These are benign (non-malignant) tumors of the uterus.

Papanicolaou or Pap smear—This is a screening test for cancer of the cervix. Cells are scraped from the cervix, smeared on a glass plate, and sent to a laboratory to examine for any abnormal cells or dysplasia. This test may also detect other cells seen in certain vaginal infections.

Skene's glands—These are the glands of the female urethra.

Speculum—A speculum is an instrument that is used during the internal genitalia examination. It can be made of plastic or metal and is used to open up the vaginal cavity in order for the examiner to view the walls of the vagina and the cervix.

Urethral meatus—This is the external opening of the urethra.

be any abnormal masses or tenderness upon palpation.

Abnormal results

The examiner may discover abnormal lesions during the course of the exam that may require additional tests. Ulcerations, bumps, sores, blisters, or vesicles on the external genitalia may be signs of a sexually transmitted disease. Some of the **sexually transmitted diseases** that may cause lesions to the external genitalia include venereal warts, syphilis, and **genital herpes**. Gonorrhea or chlamydia may also cause inflammation to the urethral meatus or the external opening of the urethra. These, in addition to bacterial infections, can also cause inflammation of the Skene's glands, Bartholin's glands, and vulva. Infections may result in an irritating discharge. Discharge may also be noted in yeast infections. Other abnormal findings of the external genitalia include carcinomas, vulvar tumors, or hematomas. Hematomas are masses of accumulated blood that appears as a bluish swelling of the labium that may occur following trauma to this area. Examination of the internal genitalia may reveal similar findings in regards to sexually transmitted diseases and carcinomas. Cervical abnormalities can also be found and may include lacerations, infections, ulcers, cysts, and polyps. All of these will require further evaluation in order to determine the underlying cause.

Since Pap smears screen for cervical cancer, abnormal results require special attention. Due to the incidence of false-positives or false-negatives, the test may be repeated or the physician may choose to have the patient undergo a **colposcopy**. This procedure uses an endoscope and will examine the vagina and cervix in more depth. This will identify 100% of lesions present. A biopsy may then be taken of the lesion in order to determine the exact type of abnormality. Several new techniques are now available that improve the accuracy of the Pap smear including automated analysis machines. Bimanual and rectovaginal exams may reveal abnormalities of the uterus or other pelvic structures. One commonly encountered finding is a myoma, which is a benign uterine tumor. In addition, the uterus may be positioned abnormally by being angled too far forward or backward. Ovarian cysts and tumors, as well as some disorders of the fallopian tubes, can be findings of these two exams.

Resources

BOOKS

DeGowin, Richard L., and Donald D. Brown. *DeGowin's Diagnostic Examination*. 7th ed. New York: McGraw-Hill, 2000.

Johnson, Bruce E., et al. *Women's Health Care Handbook*. 2nd ed. Philadelphia: Hanley and Belfus, Inc., 2000.

Seidel, Henry M., et al. *Mosby's Guide to Physical Examination*. 4th ed. St. Louis: Mosby Inc., 1999.

PERIODICALS

Russo, Joseph F. "Controversies in the Management of Abnormal Pap Smears." *Current Opinion in Obstetrics and Gynecology* 12 (Oct. 2000): 339.

Sawya, George F., et al. "Current Approaches to Cervical-Cancer Screening." *New England Journal of Medicine* 344 (May 2001): 1603.

Stewart, Felicia H., et al. "Clinical Breast and Pelvic Examination Requirements for Hormonal Contraception: Current Practice vs. Evidence." *Journal of the American Medical Association* 285 (May 2001): 2232.

OTHER

"Screening for Cervical Cancer." 2001. < http://my.webmd.com/content/article/1680.50756 >.

Laith Farid Gulli, M.D.
Robert Ramirez, B.S.

Pelvic fracture

Definition

A pelvic fracture is a break in one or more bones of the pelvis.

Description

The pelvis is a butterfly-shaped group of bones located at the base of the spine. The pelvis consists of the pubis, ilium, and ischium bones (among others) held together by tough ligaments. With a cavity in its center, the pelvis forms one major ring and two smaller rings of bone that support and protect internal organs such as the bladder, intestines, and rectum. In women, the pelvis also surrounds the uterus and vagina. The pelvis is wider and has a larger cavity in females than in males because it must accommodate **childbirth**.

Fractures of the pelvis are uncommon, accounting for only 0.3–6% of all fractures. Pelvic rings often break in more than one place. Pelvic fractures range widely in severity. Disruption of the major ring is usually a severe injury while disruption of a minor ring is often not serious. A mild fracture (for example, one that occurs due to the impact of jogging) may heal in several weeks without surgery. However, a serious pelvic fracture can be a life-threatening event requiring emergency medical care and lengthy **rehabilitation**. The latter type of injury may involve damage to nearby internal organs.

Pelvic fractures are classified as stable or unstable, and as open or closed. A stable fracture is one in which the pelvis remains stable and involves one break-point in the pelvic ring with minimal hemorrhage. An unstable fracture is one in which the pelvis is unstable with two or more break-points in the pelvic ring with moderate to severe hemorrhage. All types of pelvic fractures are further divided into "open" or "closed," depending on whether open skin **wounds** are present or not in the lower abdomen.

Causes and symptoms

Most pelvic fractures occur during high-speed accidents (such as car or motorcycle crashes) or falls from great heights. The greater the force, the greater the opportunity for a severe fracture. Pelvic fractures can also occur spontaneously or after minor falls in people with bone-weakening diseases such as **osteoporosis**. Less commonly, pelvic fractures may occur during athletic activities such as football, hockey, skiing, and long-distance running.

The primary symptom of a pelvic fracture is **pain** in the groin, hip, or lower back, which may worsen when walking or moving the legs. Other symptoms may include abdominal pain; numbness/tingling in the groin or legs; bleeding from the vagina, urethra (urine tube), or rectum; difficulty urinating; and difficulty walking or standing. A stress fracture that occurs while jogging may cause pain in the thigh or buttock.

Diagnosis

A pelvic fracture is typically diagnosed by an emergency physician looking for bone tenderness, limitations of movement, difficulty walking, and any loss of nerve function in the lower part of the body. In addition, the physician looks for signs of injury to nearby organs of the intestinal or genitourinary systems. This search may include checking the rectum, vagina, and urethra for signs of bleeding. The physician will order a plain x ray of the pelvis; this will usually detect the presence of a fracture. Blood and urine tests may also be done. A computed tomography (CT) scan will be performed in complicated cases. Depending on the severity of the fracture, other imaging procedures may be required as well, such as contrasting studies involving the injection of a radioactive dye; the pictures can be used to evaluate organs and structures in the pelvic area, such as the urethra, bladder, and blood vessels.

Treatment

In the case of a potentially serious pelvic fracture (such as that occurring after an accident or high fall), emergency assistance should be summoned. The person with the injury should be covered with a blanket or jacket (to maintain body heat), and should not be moved by non-trained personnel, especially if there is severe pain or signs of possible nerve injury.

KEY TERMS

Fracture—A break in a bone.

Computed tomography (CT) scan—An imaging procedure that produces a series of thin x-ray slices of internal body organs or structures.

Orthopedist—A doctor who specializes in disorders of the musculoskeletal system.

Osteoporosis—A decrease in the amount of bone mass, leading to fractures.

Shock—A condition of profound physiological disturbance characterized by failure of the circulatory system to maintain adequate blood supply to vital organs.

Stress fracture—A crack in a bone (usually the result of overuse).

Treatment depends on the severity of the injury. In the case of a minor fracture, treatment may consist of bed rest and over-the-counter (OTC) or prescription pain killers. Physical therapy, the use of crutches, and surgery may also be recommended. Healing can take anywhere from a few weeks to several months.

Severe injuries to the pelvis (such as those involving more than one break) can be life threatening, resulting in **shock**, extensive internal bleeding, and damage to internal organs. In these situations, the immediate goal is to control the bleeding and stabilize the injured person's condition. Resuscitation procedures may be required as well as large amounts of intravenous fluids and blood transfusions if internal bleeding is present. These injuries often require extensive surgery as well as lengthy rehabilitation.

Alternative treatment

To speed up the healing process, some practitioners of alternative medicine recommend magnetic field therapy, hydrogen peroxide therapy, calcium, vitamin D, vitamin B complex, and zinc.

Prognosis

The prognosis for minor pelvic fractures is excellent, with most people gaining full mobility in a matter of weeks or months. Severe pelvic fractures can be fatal due to internal bleeding or damage to nearby organs, or result in chronic pain and physical disabilities.

Prevention

People with bone-weakening conditions such as osteoporosis or **cancer**, or tendencies to fall are more vulnerable to bone fractures. They should follow their treatment regimens and make use of canes and other walking aids as well as safety devices in the home (bars, non skidding mats) and avoid climbing up, even on a small stool.

Resources

PERIODICALS

Korovessis, P., et al. "Medium- and long-term results of open reduction and internal fixation for unstable pelvic ring fractures."*Orthopedics* November 2000: 1165-71.

Malavaud, B., et al. "Evaluation of male sexual function after pelvic trauma by the International Index of Erectile Function." *Urology* June 2000: 842-6.

ORGANIZATIONS

American Academy of Orthopaedic Surgeons. 6300 North River Road, Rosemont, IL 60018-4262. (800) 346-AAOS. < http://www.aaos.org >.

Greg Annussek

Pelvic gynecologic sonogram *see* **Pelvic ultrasound**

Pelvic inflammatory disease

Definition

Pelvic inflammatory disease (PID) is a term used to describe any infection in the lower female reproductive tract that spreads to the upper female reproductive tract. The lower female genital tract consists of the vagina and the cervix. The upper female genital tract consists of the body of the uterus, the fallopian or uterine tubes, and the ovaries.

Description

PID is the most common and the most serious consequence of infection with **sexually transmitted diseases** (STD) in women. Over one million cases of PID are diagnosed annually in the United States, and it is the most common cause for hospitalization of reproductive-age women. Sexually active women aged 15–25 are at highest risk for developing PID. The disease can also occur, although less frequently, in women having monogamous sexual relationships.

The most serious consequences of PID are increased risk of infertility and ectopic pregnancy.

To understand PID, it is helpful to understand the basics of inflammation. Inflammation is the body's response to disease-causing (pathogenic) microorganisms. The affected body part may swell due to accumulation of fluid in the tissue or may become reddened due to an excessive accumulation of blood. A discharge (pus) may be produced that consists of white blood cells and dead tissue. Following inflammation, scar tissue may form by the proliferation of scar-forming cells and is called fibrosis. **Adhesions** of fibrous tissue form and cause organs or parts of organs to stick together.

PID may be used synonymously with the following terms:

- salpingitis (Inflammation of the fallopian tubes)

- endometritis (Inflammation of the inside lining of the body of the uterus)

- tubo-ovarian abscesses (Abscesses in the tubes and ovaries)

- pelvic **peritonitis** (Inflammation inside of the abdominal cavity surrounding the female reproductive organs)

Causes and symptoms

A number of factors affect the risk of developing PID. They include:

- Age. The incidence of PID is very high in younger women and decreases as a woman ages.

- Race. The incidence of PID is 8–10 times higher in nonwhites than in whites.

- Socioeconomic status. The higher incidence of PID in women of lower socioeconomic status is due in part to a woman's lack of education and awareness of health and disease and her accessibility to medical care.

- Contraception. Induced abortion, use of an **IUD**, non-use of barrier contraceptives such as condoms, and frequent douching are all associated with a higher risk of developing PID.

- Lifestyle. High risk behaviors, such as drug and alcohol **abuse**, early age of first intercourse, number of sexual partners, and **smoking** all are associated with a higher risk of developing PID.

- Types of sexual practices. Intercourse during menses and frequent intercourse may offer more opportunities for the admission of pathogenic organisms to the inside of the uterus.

- Disease. Sixty to 75% of cases of PID are associated with STDs. A prior episode of PID increases the chances of developing subsequent infections.

The two major causes of STDs are the organisms *Neisseria gonorrhoeae* and *Chlamydia trachomatis.* The main symptom of *N. gonorrheae* infection (**gonorrhea**) is a vaginal discharge of mucus and pus. Sometimes bacteria from the colon normally in the vaginal cavity may travel upward to infect the upper female genital organs, facilitated by the infection with gonorrhea. Infections with *C. trachomatis* and other nongonoccal organisms are more likely to have mild or no symptoms.

Normally, the cervix produces mucus which acts as a barrier to prevent disease-causing microorganisms, called pathogens, from entering the uterus and moving upward to the tubes and ovaries. This barrier may be breached in two ways. A sexually transmitted pathogen, usually a single organism, invades the lining cells, alters them, and gains entry. Another way for organisms to gain entry happens when trauma or alteration to the cervix occurs. **Childbirth**, spontaneous or induced abortion, or use of an intrauterine contraceptive device (IUD) are all conditions that may alter or weaken the normal lining cells, making them susceptible to infection, usually by several organisms. During menstruation, the cervix widens and may allow pathogens entry into the uterine cavity.

Recent evidence suggests that **bacterial vaginosis** (BV), a bacterial infection of the vagina, may be associated with PID. BV results from the alteration of the balance of normal organisms in the vagina, by douching, for example. While the balance is altered, conditions are formed that favor the overgrowth of anaerobic bacteria, which thrive in the absence of free oxygen. A copious discharge is usually present. Should some trauma occur in the presence of anaerobic bacteria, such as menses, abortion, intercourse, or childbirth, these organisms may gain entrance to the upper genital organs.

The most common symptom of PID is pelvic pain. However, many women with PID have symptoms so mild that they may be unaware that an infection exists.

In acute salpingitis, a common form of PID, swelling of the fallopian tubes may cause tenderness on **physical examination. Fever** may be present. Abscesses may develop in the tubes, ovaries, or in the surrounding pelvic cavity. Infectious discharge may leak into the peritoneal cavity and cause peritonitis, or abscesses may rupture causing a life-threatening surgical emergency.

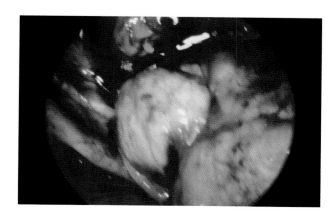

Laparoscopic view of pelvic inflammatory disease. *(Custom Medical Stock Photo. Reproduced by permission.)*

Chronic salpingitis may follow an acute attack. Subsequent to inflammation, scarring and resulting adhesions may result in chronic **pain** and irregular menses. Due to blockage of the tubes by scar tissue, women with chronic salpingitis are at high risk of having an **ectopic pregnancy**. The fertilized ovum is unable to travel down the fallopian tube to the uterus and implants itself in the tube, on the ovary, or in the peritoneal cavity. This condition can also be a life-threatening surgical emergency.

IUD

IUD usage has been strongly associated with the development of PID. Bacteria may be introduced to the uterine cavity while the IUD is being inserted or may travel up the tail of the IUD from the cervix into the uterus. Uterine tissue in association with the IUD shows areas of inflammation that may increase its susceptibility to pathogens.

Susceptibility to STDs

Susceptibility to STDs involves many factors, some of which are not known. The ability of the organism to produce disease and the circumstances that place the organism in the right place at a time when a trauma or alteration to the lining cells has occurred are factors. The individual's own immune response also helps to determine whether infection occurs.

Diagnosis

If PID is suspected, the physician will take a complete medical history and perform an internal pelvic examination. Other diseases that may cause pelvic pain, such as **appendicitis** and **endometriosis**, must be ruled out. If pelvic examination reveals tenderness or pain in that region, or tenderness on movement of the cervix, these are good physical signs that PID is present.

Specific diagnosis of PID is difficult to make because the upper pelvic organs are hard to reach for samplings. The physician may take samples directly from the cervix to identify the organisms that may be responsible for infection. Two blood tests may help to establish the existence of an inflammatory process. A positive **C-reactive protein** (CRP) and an elevated erythrocyte sedimentation rate (ESR) indicate the presence of inflammation. The physician may take fluid from the cavity surrounding the ovaries called the *cul de sac*; this fluid may be examined directly for bacteria or may be used for culture. Diagnosis of PID may also be done using a laparoscope, but **laparoscopy** is expensive, and it is an invasive procedure that carries some risk for the patient.

Treatment

The goals of treatment are to reduce or eliminate the clinical symptoms and abnormal physical findings, to get rid of the microorganisms, and to prevent long term consequences such as infertility and the possibility of ectopic **pregnancy**. If acute salpingitis is suspected, treatment with antibiotics should begin immediately. Early intervention is crucial to keep the fallopian tubes undamaged. The patient is usually treated with at least two broad spectrum **antibiotics** that can kill both *N. gonorrhoeae* and *C. trachomatis* plus other types of bacteria that may have the potential to cause infection. Hospitalization may be required to ensure compliance. Treatment for chronic PID may involve **hysterectomy**, which may be helpful in some cases.

If a woman is diagnosed with PID, she should see that her sexual partner is also treated to prevent the possibility of reinfection.

Alternative treatment

Alternative therapy should be complementary to antibiotic therapy. For pain relief, an experienced practitioner may apply castor oil packs, or use **acupressure** or **acupuncture**. Some herbs, such as *Echinacea* (*Echinacea* spp.) and calendula (*Calendula officinalis*) are believed to have antimicrobial activity and may be taken to augment the action of prescribed antibiotics. General tonic herbs, as well as good **nutrition** and rest, are important in recovery and strengthening after an episode of PID. Blue cohosh

(*Caulophyllum thalictroides*) and false unicorn root (*Chamaelirium luteum*) are recommended as tonics for the general well-being of the female genital tract.

Prognosis

PID can be cured if the initial infection is treated immediately. If infection is not recognized, as frequently happens, the process of tissue destruction and scarring that results from inflammation of the tubes results in irreversible changes in the tube structure that cannot be restored to normal. Subsequent bouts of PID increase a woman's risks manyfold. Thirty to forty percent of cases of female **infertility** are due to acute salpingitis.

With modern antibiotic therapy, **death** from PID is almost nonexistent. In rare instances, death may occur from the rupture of tubo-ovarian abscesses and the resulting infection in the abdominal cavity. One recent study has linked infertility, a consequence of PID, with a higher risk of **ovarian cancer**.

Prevention

The prevention of PID is a direct result of the prevention and prompt recognition and treatment of STDs or of any suspected infection involving the female genital tract. The main symptom of infection is an abnormal discharge. To distinguish an abnormal discharge from the mild fluctuations of normal discharge associated with the menstrual cycle takes vigilance and self-awareness. Sexually active women must be able to detect symptoms of lower genital tract disease. Ideally these women will be able to have a frank dialogue regarding their sexual history, risks for PID, and treatment options with their physicians. Also, these women should have open discussions with their sexual partners regarding disclosure of significant symptoms of possible infection.

Lifestyle changes should be geared to preventing the transfer of organisms when the body's delicate lining cells are unprotected or compromised. Barrier contraceptives, such as condoms, diaphragms, and cervical caps should be used. Women in monogamous relationships should use barrier contraceptives during menses and take their physician's advice regarding intercourse following abortion, childbirth, or biopsy procedures.

Resources

BOOKS

Landers, D. V., and R. L. Sweet, editors. *Pelvic Inflammatory Disease*. New York: Springer, 1997.

Karen J. Wells

Pelvic relaxation

Definition

Pelvic relaxation is a weakening of the supportive muscles and ligaments of the pelvic floor. This condition, which affects women and is usually caused by **childbirth**, **aging**, and problems with support, causes the pelvic floor to sag and press into the wall of the vagina.

Description

The pelvic floor normally holds the uterus and the bladder in position above the vagina. When the pelvic floor becomes stretched and damaged, these organs can sag into the vagina, sometimes bulging out through the vaginal opening. A sagging uterus is referred to as a uterine prolapse, pelvic floor **hernia**, or pudendal hernia. A sagging bladder is referred to as a bladder prolapse, or cystocele. Other organs, such as the rectum and intestine, can also sag into the vagina as a result of a weakened pelvic floor.

Causes and symptoms

Childbirth increases the risk of pelvic relaxation. Other causes include **constipation**, a chronic **cough**, **obesity**, and heavy lifting. Some women develop the condition after **menopause**, when the body loses the estrogen that helps maintain muscle tone. Mild pelvic relaxation may cause no symptoms. More severe pelvic relaxation can cause the following symptoms:

- an aching sensation in the vagina, lower abdomen, groin or lower back
- heaviness or pressure in the vaginal area, as if something is about to "fall out" of the vagina
- bladder control problems that worsen with heavy lifting, coughing, or sneezing
- frequent urinary tract infections
- difficulty having a bowel movement

Diagnosis

A thorough **pelvic exam** can help diagnose pelvic relaxation, as can tests of bladder function.

Treatment

Exercises called Kegel exercises can strengthen pelvic floor muscles and lessen the symptoms of pelvic relaxation. These exercises involve squeezing the muscles that stop the flow of urine. The pelvic floor can also be strengthened by estrogen supplements. Physicians sometimes prescribe the insertion of a supportive ring-shaped device called a pessary into the vagina, to prevent the uterus and bladder from pressing into the vagina. Sometimes surgery is recommended to repair a sagging bladder or uterus, and sometimes surgical removal of the uterus (**hysterectomy**) is recommended. Patients are often advised to adhere to a high-fiber diet to reduce the strain of bowel movements, maintain a moderate weight, and avoid activities that strain the pelvic floor. They are sometimes prescribed medications to help control urination and prevent leakage.

KEY TERMS

Cystocele—Bulging of the bladder into the vagina.

Cystourethrocele—Bulging of the bladder neck into the vagina.

Enterocele—Bulging of the intestine into the upper part of the vagina.

Kegel exercises—Pelvic muscle exercises that strengthen bladder and bowel control.

Pessary—A device inserted into the vagina to support sagging organs.

Rectocele—Bulging of the rectum into the vaginal wall.

Uterine prolapse—Bulging of the uterus into the vagina.

Vaginal prolapse—Bulging of the top of the vagina into the lower vagina or outside the opening of the vagina.

Prognosis

Mild cases of pelvic relaxation can sometimes be reversed through Kegel exercises, while severe cases usually do not respond to **exercise** or estrogen therapy, but usually require pessary support or surgery.

Prevention

To limit **stress** on the pelvic support system, women are advised to maintain a normal body weight, limit heavy lifting, and avoid unnecessary straining to have bowel movements.

Resources

ORGANIZATIONS

American College of Obstetricians and Gynecologists. 409 12th St., S.W., P.O. Box 96920, Washington, DC 20090-6920. <http://www.acog.org>.

American Foundation for Urologic Disease. 1128 North Charles Street, Baltimore, MD 21201. (800) 242-2383. <http://www.afud.org>.

National Association For Continence. P.O. Box 8310, Spartanburg, SC 29305-8310. (800) BLADDER. <http://www.nafc.org>.

National Kidney and Urologic Diseases Information Clearinghouse. 3 Information Way, Bethesda, MD, 20892. NIH Publication No. 97-4195. (800) 891-5390. <http://www.niddk.nih.gov/health/kidney/nkudic.htm>.

Ann Quigley

Pelvic ultrasound

Definition

Pelvic ultrasound is a procedure where harmless, high-frequency sound waves are projected into the abdomen. These waves reflect off of the internal structures and create shadowy black and white pictures on a display screen.

Purpose

Ultrasound is performed routinely during **pregnancy**. Early in the pregnancy (at about seven weeks), it might be used to determine the size of the uterus or the fetus, to detect multiple or **ectopic pregnancy**, to confirm that the fetus is alive (or viable), or to confirm the due date. Toward the middle of the pregnancy (at about 16–20 weeks), ultrasound may be used to confirm fetal growth, to reveal defects in the anatomy of the fetus, and to check the placenta. Toward the end of pregnancy, it may be used to evaluate fetal size, position, growth, or to check the placenta. Doctors may use ultrasound during diagnostic procedures like **amniocentesis** and **chorionic villus sampling**. Both of these tests use long needles inserted through the mother's abdomen into the uterus or placenta to gather cells. Ultrasound can also be used in men or women to examine other internal organs, such as the liver, gallbladder, kidney, and heart. The procedure can be useful in detecting cysts, tumors, and cancer of the uterus, ovaries, and breasts.

Precautions

There are no special precautions recommended before an ultrasound examination. Unlike x rays, ultrasound does not produce any harmful radiation and does not pose a risk to the mother or the fetus. While many woman have an ultrasound as part of their prenatal care, there may be no medical need to perform the procedure.

Description

Ultrasound examinations can be done in a doctor's office, clinic, or hospital setting. Typically, the pregnant woman will lie on an examination table with her abdomen exposed. Gel or oil is applied to the area. The doctor or technician will move a handheld scanner (called a transducer) over the abdomen. The transducer emits high-frequency sound waves (usually in the range of 3.5–7.0 megahertz) into the abdomen. The waves are reflected back to the transducer and the wave patterns are shown as an image on a display screen. An ultrasound scan reveals the shapes, densities, and even movements of organs and tissues. Although the pictures transmitted by an ultrasound scan appear gray and grainy, a trained technician can identify the fetus within the uterus, monitor its heartbeat, and sometimes determine its sex. Using computerized tools, the technician can measure various structures shown on the screen. For example, the length of the upper thigh bone (femur) or the distance between the two sides of the skull can indicate the age of the fetus.

Ultrasound technology has been used safely in medical settings for over 30 years, and several significant improvements have been made to the procedure. A specially designed transducer probe can be placed in the vagina to provide better ultrasound images. This transvaginal or endovaginal scan is particularly useful in early pregnancy or in cases where ectopic pregnancy is suspected. Doppler ultrasound uses enhanced sound waves to monitor subtle events, like the flow of fetal blood through the heart and arteries. Color imaging is a recent addition to ultrasound technology. With this process, color can be assigned to the various shades of gray for better visualization of subtle tissue details. A new technology under development is three-dimensional ultrasound, which has the potential for detecting even very subtle fetal defects.

Preparation

Before undergoing a pelvic ultrasound, a woman may be asked to drink several glasses of water and to avoid urinating for about one hour before the examination. When the bladder is full, the uterus and fetus are easier to see. A lubricating gel or mineral oil may be applied to the area to make moving the transducer easier.

Aftercare

The lubricating jelly or oil applied to the abdomen is wiped off at the end of the procedure. After an ultrasound examination, a patient can immediately resume normal activities.

Risks

There are no known risks, to either the mother or the fetus, associated with the use of ultrasound.

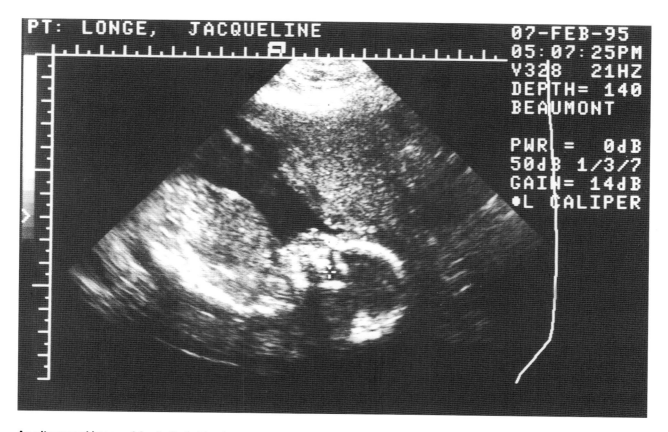

PT: LONGE, JACQUELINE
07-FEB-95
05:07:25PM
V328 21HZ
DEPTH= 140
BEAUMONT

PWR = 0dB
50dB 1/3/7
GAIN= 14dB
●L CALIPER

An ultrasound image of Anabelle Ashlyn Longe at 20 weeks. *(Courtesy of Jacqueline Longe.)*

KEY TERMS

Amniocentesis—A procedure where a needle is inserted through the pregnant mother's abdomen and into the uterus to draw off some of the amniotic fluid surrounding the fetus.

Chorionic villus sampling—A procedure where a needle is inserted into the placenta to draw off some of the placenta's inner wall cells surrounding the fetus.

Ectopic pregnancy—A pregnancy where the fertilized egg becomes implanted somewhere other than in the uterus. A tubal pregnancy is when the fertilized egg implants in the fallopian tube.

Fetus—A term for an unborn baby, usually from the end of week eight to the moment of birth.

Placenta—The organ that allows interchange between the fetus and the mother. Blood from the fetus and the mother do not directly mix, but the thin placental membrane allows the fetus to absorb nutrients and oxygen from the mother. Waste products from the fetus can exit through the placenta.

Ultrasonography—Another term for ultrasound.

Normal results

The reliability of ultrasound readings depends on the skill of the technician or doctor performing the scan. Patients should be aware that fetal abnormalities cannot be detected with 100% accuracy using ultrasound. A normal ultrasound result does not necessarily guarantee that the fetus will be normal.

Abnormal results

Ultrasound examinations in obstetrics may detect abnormalities or defects in the fetus. This information may reveal that the fetus cannot survive on its own after birth or that it will require extensive treatment or care. Some surgical procedures can be performed to correct defects while the fetus is still in the uterus. Parents faced with information regarding possible **birth defects** may require counseling to consider their choice to either continue or end the pregnancy.

The diagnostic use of ultrasound may reveal the presence of cysts, tumors, or **cancer** in internal organs.

Resources

ORGANIZATIONS

American Institute of Ultrasound in Medicine. 14750 Sweitzer Lane, Suite 100, Laurel, MD 20707-5906. (800) 638-5352. < http://www.aium.org >.

Altha Roberts Edgren

Penicillin V *see* **Penicillins**

Penicillins

Definition

Penicillins are medicines that kill bacteria or prevent their growth.

Purpose

Penicillins are **antibiotics** (medicines used to treat infections caused by microorganisms). There are several types of penicillins, each used to treat different kinds of infections, such as skin infections, dental infections, ear infections, respiratory tract infections, urinary tract infections, **gonorrhea**, and other infections caused by bacteria. These drugs will *not* work for colds, flu, and other infections caused by viruses.

Description

Examples of penicillins are penicillin V (Beepen-VK, Pen-Vee K, V-cillin K, Veetids) and amoxicillin (Amoxil, Polymox, Trimox, Wymox). Penicillins are sometimes combined with other ingredients called beta-lactamase inhibitors, which protect the penicillin from bacterial enzymes that may destroy it before it can do its work. The drug Augmentin, for example, contains a combination of amoxicillin and a beta-lactamase inhibitor, clavulanic acid.

Penicillins are available only with a physician's prescription. They are sold in capsule, tablet (regular and chewable), liquid, and injectable forms.

Recommended dosage

The recommended dosage depends on the type of penicillin, the strength of the medicine, and the medical problem for which it is being taken. Check with the physician who prescribed the drug or the pharmacist who filled the prescription for the correct dosage.

Always take penicillins exactly as directed. Never take larger, smaller, more frequent, or less frequent doses. To make sure the infection clears up completely, take the medicine for as long as it has been prescribed. Do not stop taking the drug just because symptoms begin to improve. This is important with all types of infections, but it is especially important with "strep" infections, which can lead to serious heart problems if they are not cleared up completely.

Take this medicine only for the infection for which it was prescribed. Different kinds of penicillins cannot be substituted for one another. Do not save some of the medicine to use on future infections. It may not be the right treatment for other kinds of infections, even if the symptoms are the same.

Penicillins work best when they are at constant levels in the blood. To help keep levels constant, take the medicine in doses spaced evenly through the day and night. Do not miss any doses.

Some penicillins, notably penicillin V, should be taken on an empty stomach, but others may be taken with food. Check package directions or ask the physician or pharmacist for instructions on how to take the medicine.

Precautions

Symptoms should begin to improve within a few days of beginning to take this medicine. If they do not, or if they get worse, check with the physician who prescribed the medicine.

Penicillins may cause **diarrhea**. Certain diarrhea medicines may make the problem worse. Check with a physician before using any diarrhea medicine to treat diarrhea caused by taking penicillin. If diarrhea is severe, check with a physician as soon as possible. This could be a sign of a serious side effect.

Penicillins may change the results of some medical tests. Before having medical tests, patients who are taking penicillin should be sure to let the physician in charge know that they are taking this medicine.

Special conditions

People with certain medical conditions or who are taking certain other medicines can have problems if they take penicillins. Before taking these drugs, be sure to let the physician know about any of these conditions:

ALLERGIES. People who have hay **fever, asthma,** eczema, or other general **allergies** (or who have had such allergies in the past) may be more likely to have severe reactions to penicillins. They should be sure their health care provider knows about their allergies.

Anyone who has had unusual reactions to penicillins or **cephalosporins** in the past should let his or her physician know before taking the drugs again. The physician should also be told about any allergies to foods, dyes, preservatives, or other substances.

LOW-SODIUM DIET. Some penicillin medicines contain large enough amounts of sodium to cause problems for people on low-sodium **diets**. Anyone on such a diet should make sure that the physician treating the infection knows about the special diet.

DIABETES. Penicillins may cause false positive results on urine sugar tests for diabetes. People with diabetes should check with their physicians to see if they need to change their diet or the doses of their diabetes medicine.

PHENYLKETONURIA. Some formulations of Augmentin contain phenylalanine. People with **phenylketonuria** (PKU) should consult a physician before taking this medicine.

OTHER MEDICAL CONDITIONS. Before using penicillins, people with any of these medical problems should make sure their physicians are aware of their conditions:

- bleeding problems
- congestive **heart failure**
- **cystic fibrosis**
- kidney disease
- mononucleosis ("mono")
- stomach or intestinal problems, especially ulcerative colitis

USE OF CERTAIN MEDICINES. Taking penicillins with certain other drugs may affect the way the drugs work or may increase the chance of side effects.

Side effects

The most common side effects are mild diarrhea, headache, vaginal **itching** and discharge, sore mouth or tongue, or white patches in the mouth or on the tongue. These problems usually go away as the body adjusts to the drug and do not require medical treatment unless they continue or they are bothersome.

More serious side effects are not common, but may occur. If any of the following side effects occur, get emergency medical help immediately:

- breathing problems, such as **shortness of breath** or fast or irregular breathing
- fever
- sudden lightheadedness or faintness

KEY TERMS

Enzyme—A type of protein that brings about or speeds up chemical reactions.

Microorganism—An organism that is too small to be seen with the naked eye.

Mononucleosis—An infectious disease with symptoms that include severe fatigue, fever, sore throat, and swollen lymph nodes in the neck and armpits. Also called "mono."

- joint **pain**
- skin rash, **hives**, itching, or red, scaly skin
- swelling or puffiness in the face

Other rare side effects may occur. Anyone who has unusual symptoms after taking penicillin should get in touch with his or her physician.

Interactions

Birth control pills may not work properly when taken at the same time as penicillin. To prevent **pregnancy**, use additional methods of birth control while taking penicillin, such as latex condoms or spermicide.

Penicillins may interact with many other medicines. When this happens, the effects of one or both of the drugs may change or the risk of side effects may be greater. Anyone who takes penicillin should let the physician know all other medicines he or she is taking. Among the drugs that may interact with penicillins are:

- Acetaminophen (Tylenol) and other medicines that relieve pain and inflammation
- medicine for overactive thyroid
- male hormones (androgens)
- female hormones (estrogens)
- other antibiotics
- blood thinners
- Disulfiram (Antabuse), used to treat alcohol **abuse**
- antiseizure medicines such as Depakote and Depakene
- blood pressure drugs such as Capoten, Monopril, and Lotensin

The list above does not include every drug that may interact with penicillins. Be sure to check with a physician or pharmacist before combining penicillins with any other prescription or nonprescription (over-the-counter) medicine.

Nancy Ross-Flanigan

Penile cancer

Definition

Penile **cancer** is the growth of malignant cells on the external skin and in the tissues of the penis.

Description

Penile cancer is a disease in which cancerous cells appear on the penis. If left untreated, this cancer can grow and spread from the penis to the lymph nodes in the groin and eventually to other parts of the body.

Demographics

Penile cancer is a rare form of cancer that develops in about one out of 100,000 men per year in the United States. Penile cancer is more common in other parts of the world, particularly Africa and Asia. In Uganda, penile cancer is the most common form of cancer for men.

Causes and symptoms

The cause of penile cancer is unknown. The most common symptoms of penile cancer are:

- a tender spot, an open sore, or a wart-like lump on the penis
- unusual liquid discharges from the penis
- pain or bleeding in the genital area

Diagnosis

In order to diagnose penile cancer, the doctor examines the patient's penis for lumps or other abnormalities. A tissue sample, or biopsy, may be ordered to distinguish cancerous cells from **syphilis** and penile **warts**. If the results confirm a diagnosis of cancer, additional tests are done to determine whether the disease has spread to other parts of the body.

Treatment

In Stage I penile cancer, malignant cells are found only on the surface of the head (glans) and on the foreskin of the penis. If the cancer is limited to the foreskin, treatment may involve wide local excision and **circumcision**. Wide local excision is a form of surgery that removes only cancer cells and a small amount of normal tissue adjacent to them. Circumcision is removal of the foreskin.

If the Stage I cancer is only on the glans, treatment may involve the use of a fluorouracil cream (Adrucil, Efudex), and/or microsurgery. Microsurgery removes cancerous tissue and the smallest possible amount of normal tissue. During microsurgery, the doctor uses a special instrument that provides a comprehensive view of the area where cancer cells are located and makes it possible to determine that all malignant cells have been removed.

In Stage II, the penile cancer has spread to the surface of the glans, tissues beneath the surface, and the shaft of the penis. The treatment recommended may be **amputation** of all or part of the penis (total or partial penectomy). If the disease is diagnosed early enough, surgeons are often able to preserve enough of the organ for urination and sexual activity. Treatment may also include microsurgery and external **radiation therapy**, in which a machine provides radiation to the affected area. **Laser surgery** is an experimental treatment for Stage II cancers. Laser surgery uses an intense precisely focused beam of light to dissolve or burn away cancer cells.

In Stage III, malignant cells have spread to lymph nodes in the groin, where they cause swelling. The recommended treatment may include amputation of the penis and removal of the lymph nodes on both sides. Radiation therapy may also be suggested. More advanced disease requires systemic treatments using drugs (**chemotherapy**). In chemotherapy, medicines are administered intravenously or taken by mouth. These drugs enter the bloodstream and kill cancer cells that have spread to any part of the body.

In Stage IV, the disease has spread throughout the penis and lymph nodes in the groin, or has traveled to other parts of the body. Treatments are similar to that for Stage III cancer.

Recurrent penile cancer is disease that recurs in the penis or develops in another part of the body after treatment has eradicated the original cancer cells.

Cure rates are high for cancers diagnosed in Stage I or II, but much lower for Stages III and IV, by which time cancer cells have spread to the lymph nodes.

Alternative treatment

In addition to the treatments previously described, biological therapy is another treatment that is currently being studied. Biological therapy is a type of treatment that is sometimes called biological response modifier (BRM) therapy. It uses natural or artificial substances to boost, focus, or reinforce the body's disease-fighting resources.

Prevention

Conditions which increase a person's chance of getting penile cancer include:

• infection with **genital warts** (human papillomavirus, or HPV)

• a skin disease called psoriasis

• a condition called **phimosis**, in which the foreskin becomes difficult to retract

• other conditions that result in repeated irritation of the penis.

• a history of smoking.

There appears to be a connection between development of the disease and lack of personal hygiene. Failure to regularly and thoroughly cleanse the part of the penis covered by the foreskin increases the risk of developing the disease. Penile cancer is also more common in uncircumcised men.

Resources

ORGANIZATIONS

American Cancer Society. 1599 Clifton Road NE, Atlanta, GA 30329. (800) ACS-2345. < http://www.cancer.org >.

Cancer Group Institute. 17620 9th Ave. NE, North Miami Beach, FL 33162. (305) 493-1980. < http://www.cancergroup.com >.

OTHER

CancerNet: Penile Cancer. March 25, 2001. [cited June 28, 2001]. < http://www.cancernet.nci.nih.gov/cancer_types/penile_cancer.shtml >.

Maureen Haggerty
Paul A. Johnson, Ed.M.

Penile implant surgery *see* **Penile prostheses**

Penile prostheses

Definition

Penile prostheses are semirigid or inflatable devices that are implanted into penises to alleviate **impotence**.

Purpose

The penis is composed of one channel for urine and semen and three compartments with tough, fibrous walls containing "erectile tissue." With appropriate stimulation, the blood vessels that lead out of these compartments constrict, trapping blood. Blood pressure fills and hardens the compartments producing an erection of sufficient firmness to perform sexual intercourse. Additional stimulation leads to ejaculation, where semen is pumped out of the urethra. When this system fails, impotence (failure to create and maintain an erection) occurs.

Impotence can be caused by a number of conditions, including diabetes, **spinal cord injury**, prolonged drug **abuse**, and removal of a prostate gland. If the medical condition is irreversible, a penile prosthesis may be considered. Patients whose impotence is caused by psychological problems are not recommended for implant surgery.

Description

Penile implant surgery is conducted on patients who have exhausted all other areas of treatment. The semirigid device consists of two rods that are easier and less expensive to implant than the inflatable cylinders. Once implanted, the semirigid device needs no follow-up adjustments, however it produces a penis which constantly remains semi-erect. The inflatable

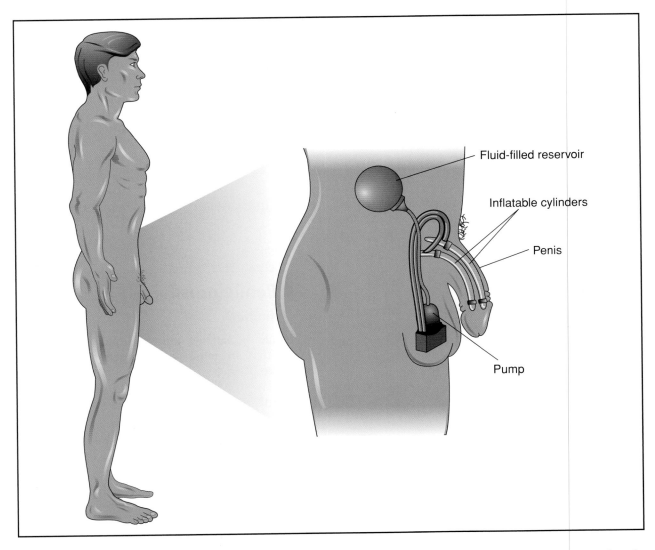

The inflatable implant is a common penile prosthesis. This device connects through a tube to a flexible fluid reservoir and a pump. The pump is shaped like a testicle and inserted in the scrotum. When the pump is squeezed, the fluid is forced into the inflatable cylinders implanted inside the penis, producing an erection. *(Illustration by Electronic Illustrators Group.)*

cylinders produce a more natural effect. The patient is able to simulate an erection by using a pump located in the scrotum.

With the patient asleep under **general anesthesia**, the device is inserted into the erectile tissue of the penis through an incision in the fibrous wall. In order to implant the pump for the inflatable implant, incisions are made in the abdomen and the perineum (area between the anus and the genitals). A fluid reservoir is inserted into the groin and the pump is placed in the scrotum. The cylinders, reservoir, and pump are connected by tubes and tested before the incisions are closed.

Preparation

Surgery always requires an adequately informed patient, both as to risks and benefits. In this case, the sexual partner should also be involved in the discussion. Prior to surgery, antibacterial cleansing occurs and the surrounding areas are shaved.

Aftercare

To minimize swelling, ice packs are applied to the penis for the first 24 hours following surgery. The incision sites are cleansed daily to prevent infection. **Pain** relievers may be taken.

KEY TERMS

General anesthesia—Deep sleep induced by a combination of medicines that allows surgery to be performed.

Genital—Sexual organ.

Perineum—Area between the anus and genitals.

Scrotum—The external pouch containing the male reproductive glands (testes) and part of the spermatic cord.

Risks

With any implant, there is a slightly greater risk of infection. The implant may irritate the penis and cause continuous pain. The inflatable prosthesis may need follow-up surgery to repair leaks in the reservoir or to reconnect the tubing.

Resources

BOOKS

Jordan, Gerald H., et al. "Surgery of the Penis and Urethra." In *Campbell's Urology,* edited by Patrick C. Walsh, et al. Philadelphia: W. B. Saunders Co., 1998.

J. Ricker Polsdorfer, MD

Pentoxifylline *see* **Blood-viscosity reducing drugs**

Peptic ulcer disease *see* **Heliobacteriosis**

Percutaneous renal biopsy *see* **Kidney biopsy**

Percutaneous transhepatic cholangiography

Definition

Percutaneous transhepatic cholangiography (PTHC) is an x-ray test used to identify obstructions either in the liver or bile ducts that slow or stop the flow of bile from the liver to the digestive system.

Purpose

Because the liver and bile ducts are not normally seen on x rays, the doctor injects the liver with a special dye that will show up on the resulting picture. This dye distributes evenly to fill the whole liver drainage system. If the dye does not distribute evenly, this is indicative of a blockage, which may be caused by a gallstone or a tumor in the liver, bile ducts, or pancreas.

Precautions

Patients should report allergic reactions to:

- anesthetics
- dyes used in medical tests
- iodine
- shellfish

PTHC should not be performed on anyone who has **cholangitis** (inflammation of the bile duct), massive **ascites**, a severe allergy to iodine, or a serious uncorrectable or uncontrollable bleeding disorder. Patients who have diabetes should inform their doctor.

Description

PTHC is performed in a hospital, doctor's office, or outpatient surgical or x-ray facility. The patient lies on a movable x-ray table and is given a local anesthetic. The patient will be told to hold his or her breath, and a doctor, nurse, or laboratory technician will inject a special dye into the liver as the patient exhales.

The patient may feel a twinge when the needle penetrates the liver, a pressure or fullness, or brief discomfort in the upper right side of the back. Hands and feet may become numb during the 30–60 minute procedure.

The x-ray table will be rotated several times during the test, and the patient helped to assume a variety of positions. A special x-ray machine called a fluoroscope will track the dye's movement through the bile ducts and show whether the fluid is moving freely or if its passage is obstructed.

PTHC costs about $1,600. The test may have to be repeated if the patient moves while x rays are being taken.

Preparation

An intravenous antibiotic may be given every 4–6 hours during the 24 hours before the test. The patient will be told to fast overnight. Having an empty stomach is a safety measure in case of complications, such as bleeding, that might require emergency repair surgery. Medications such as **aspirin**, or **non-steroidal**

KEY TERMS

Ascites—Abnormal accumulation of fluid in the abdomen.

Bile ducts—Tubes that carry bile, a thick yellowish-green fluid that is made by the liver, stored in the gallbladder, and helps the body digest fats.

Cholangitis—Inflammation of the bile duct.

Fluoroscope—An x-ray machine that projects images of organs.

Granulomatous disease—Characterized by growth of tiny blood vessels and connective tissue.

Jaundice—Disease that causes bile to accumulate in the blood, causing the skin and whites of the eyes to turn yellow. Obstructive jaundice is caused by blockage of bile ducts, while non-obstructive jaundice is caused by disease or infection of the liver.

anti-inflammatory drugs that thin the blood, should be stopped three–seven days prior to taking the PRHC test. Patients may also be given a sedative a few minutes before the test begins.

Aftercare

A nurse will monitor the patient's vital signs and watch for:

- itching
- flushing
- nausea and vomiting
- sweating
- excessive flow of saliva
- possible serious allergic reactions to contrast dye

The patient should stay in bed for at least six hours after the test, lying on the right side to prevent bleeding from the injection site. The patient may resume normal eating habits and gradually resume normal activities. The doctor should be informed right away if **pain** develops in the right abdomen or shoulder or in case of **fever**, **dizziness**, or a change in stool color to black or red.

Risks

Septicemia (blood **poisoning**) and bile **peritonitis** (a potentially fatal infection or inflammation of the membrane covering the walls of the abdomen) are rare but serious complications of this procedure. Dye occasionally leaks from the liver into the abdomen, and there is a slight risk of bleeding or infection.

Normal results

Normal x rays show dye evenly distributed throughout the bile ducts. **Obesity**, gas, and failure to fast can affect test results.

Abnormal results

Enlargement of bile ducts may indicate:

- obstructive or non-obstructive **jaundice**
- cholelithiasis (gallstones)
- hepatitis (inflammation of the liver)
- cirrhosis (chronic liver disease)
- granulomatous disease
- pancreatic cancer
- bile duct or gallbladder cancers

Resources

BOOKS

Komaroff, A. L. *The Harvard Medical School Family Health Guide.* New York: Simon & Schuster, 1999.

PERIODICALS

Cieszanowski, A., et al. "Imaging Techniques in Patients with Biliary Obstruction." *Medical Science Monitor* 6 (November-December 2000): 1197-202.

OTHER

Percutaneous Transhepatic Cholangiography. < http:// 207.25.144.143/health/Library/medtests/ >.
Percutaneous Transhepatic Cholangiography (PTHC). < http://www.uhs.org/frames/health/test/ test3554.htm >.
Test Universe Site: Percutaneous Transhepatic Cholangiography. < http://www.testuniverse.com/ mdx/MDX-3055.html >.

Maureen Haggerty

Perforated eardrum

Definition

A perforated eardrum exists when there is a hole or rupture in the eardrum, the thin membrane that separates the outer ear canal from the middle ear. A perforated eardrum may cause temporary **hearing loss** and occasional discharge.

Description

The eardrum (tympanic membrane) is a thin wall that separates the outer ear from the middle ear, vibrating when sound waves strike the membrane. The middle ear is connected to the nose by the Eustachian tube.

In addition to conducting sound, the eardrum also protects the middle ear from bacteria. When it is perforated, bacteria can more easily get into this part of the ear, causing ear infections.

In general, the larger the hole in the eardrum, the greater the temporary loss of hearing. The location of the perforation also affects the degree of hearing loss. Severe hearing loss may follow a skull fracture that disrupts the bones in the middle ear. Eardrum perforation caused by a loud noise may result in ringing in the ear (**tinnitus**), in addition to a temporary hearing loss. Over time, this hearing loss improves and the ringing usually fades in a few days.

Causes and symptoms

The eardrum can become damaged by a direct injury. It is possible to perforate the eardrum:

• with a cotton-tipped swab or another foreign object
• by hitting the ear with an open hand
• after a skull fracture
• after a loud explosion or other loud noise

In addition, an ear infection can rupture the eardrum as pressure within the middle ear rises when fluid builds up. If the eardrum is punctured by pressure from an ear infection, there may be infected or bloody drainage from the ear.

Rarely, a small hole may remain in the eardrum after a pressure-equalizing tube falls out or is removed by a doctor.

Symptoms include an earache or **pain** in the ear, which may be severe, or a sudden decrease in ear pain, followed by ear drainage of clear, bloody, or pus-filled fluid, hearing loss, or ear noise/buzzing.

Diagnosis

A doctor can diagnose a perforated eardrum by direct inspection with an otoscope. Hearing tests may reveal a hearing loss.

Treatment

A perforated eardrum usually heals by itself within two months. **Antibiotics** may be given to

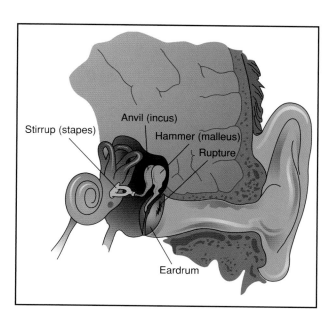

Stirrup (stapes)
Anvil (incus)
Hammer (malleus)
Rupture
Eardrum

A perforated eardrum is caused by a hole or rupture in the eardrum, the thin membrane that separates the outer ear canal from the middle ear. It may result in temporary hearing loss and occasional discharge. *(Illustration by Electronic Illustrators Group.)*

KEY TERMS

Eustachian tube—The air duct that connects the area behind the nose to the middle ear.

Otoscope—An instrument used to examine the ear, to inspect the outer ear canal and the eardrum, and to detect diseases in the middle ear.

---

prevent infection or to treat an existing ear infection. Painkillers can relieve any ear pain.

Sometimes, a paper patch is placed over the eardrum until the membrane heals. Three or four patches may be needed before the perforation closes completely. If the eardrum does not heal on its own, surgical repair (tympanoplasty) may be necessary.

The ear should be kept clean and dry while the eardrum heals; patients should insert cotton balls into the ear when showering or shampooing to block any water from getting into the ear. Pain in the ear may be eased by applying warm compresses.

Prognosis

While a perforated eardrum may be uncomfortable, it usually heals on its own. Any hearing loss that accompanies the perforation is usually temporary.

Prevention

A perforated eardrum can be prevented by avoiding insertion of any object into the ear to clean it. If a foreign object becomes lodged in the ear, only a doctor should try to remove it.

Promptly treating all ear infections is another way to guard against a ruptured eardrum.

Resources

ORGANIZATIONS

American Academy of Otolaryngology-Head and Neck Surgery, Inc. One Prince St., Alexandria VA 22314-3357. (703) 836-4444. < http://www.entnet.org >.
Better Hearing Institute. 515 King Street, Suite 420, Alexandria, VA 22314. (703) 684-3391.

Carol A. Turkington

Perforated septum

Definition

A perforated septum is a hole in the nasal septum, the vertical plane of tissue that separates the nostrils.

Description

The nasal septum is a thin structure in the middle of the nose. In front, it is cartilage, further back it is bone. On either side, it is covered with mucus membranes. The cartilage depends upon the blood vessels in the mucus membranes on either side for its **nutrition**. If that blood supply is shut off, the cartilage dies, producing a hole or perforation.

Causes and symptoms

There are several causes of a perforated septum.

- Wearing ornaments in the nose. To hang an ornament from the middle of the nose requires that the tissue directly in front of the septal cartilage be pierced or perforated.
- Sniffing **cocaine**. Cocaine is a potent vasoconstrictor, which means that it causes small blood vessels to

close. It is used in nose surgery because it shrinks mucus membranes, permitting better visualization and access into the nose. Used continuously, tissues are deprived of blood and die. The nasal septum is the most vulnerable to this effect of sniffing cocaine.

- Getting the septum cauterized. Nosebleeds usually come from the front part of the nasal septum, which is rich in blood vessels. Uncontrolled repeated bleeding from these vessels may require cautery–burning the vessels with electricity or chemicals to close them off. Injudicious cautery of both sides of the septum has in the past led to death of tissue and consequent perforation.

- More and more people are having **cosmetic surgery** done on their nose. The procedure, called **rhinoplasty**, occasionally damages the septum's blood supply.

- Contracting certain diseases. Several diseases—typhoid, **syphilis**, **systemic lupus erythematosus**, and tuberculosis—can infect this tissue and destroy it.

- Being exposed to harmful vapors. Toxic air pollutant-like acid fumes, phosphorus, and copper vapor—and sometimes even cortisone sprays—can destroy nasal tissue.

Perforation is not serious. It causes irritation, mostly complaints of dryness and crusting. Sometimes air blowing past it whistles. Picking at the crusts can cause bleeding.

Treatment

Surgical repair is not difficult. The surgeon may devise a plastic button that fits exactly into the defect and stays in place like a collar button.

Alternative treatment

Saline nasal sprays may be sufficient to control symptoms and prevent the need for surgery.

Prevention

Nosebleeds from the septum can usually be controlled with pinching. Vaginal estrogen cream has also been used successfully to toughen the blood vessels.

Resources

BOOKS

Ballenger, John Jacob. *Disorders of the Nose, Throat, Ear, Head, and Neck.* Philadelphia: Lea & Febiger, 1991.

J. Ricker Polsdorfer, MD

Pericardiocentesis

Definition

Pericardiocentesis is the removal by needle of pericardial fluid from the sac surrounding the heart for diagnostic or therapeutic purposes.

Purpose

The pericardium, the sac (or membrane) that surrounds the heart muscle, normally contains a small amount of fluid that cushions and lubricates the heart as the heart expands and contracts. When too much fluid gathers in the pericardial cavity, the space between the pericardium and the outer layers of the heart, a condition known as pericardial effusion occurs. Abnormal amounts of fluid may result from:

- **pericarditis** (caused by infection, inflammation)
- trauma (producing blood in the pericardial sac)
- surgery or other invasive procedures performed on the heart
- **cancer** (producing malignant effusions)
- myocardial infarction, congestive heart failure
- renal failure

Possible causes of pericarditis include chest trauma, systemic infection (bacterial, viral, or fungal), myocardial infarction (**heart attack**), or **tuberculosis**. When pericarditis is suspected, pericardiocentesis may be advisable in order to obtain a fluid sample for laboratory analysis to identify the underlying cause of the condition.

Pericardiocentesis is also used in emergency situations to remove excessive accumulations of blood or fluid from the pericardial sac, such as with **cardiac tamponade**. When fluid builds up too rapidly or excessively in the pericardial cavity, the resulting compression on the heart impairs the pumping action of the vascular system. Cardiac tamponade is a life-threatening condition that requires immediate treatment.

Precautions

Whenever possible, an echocardiogram (ultrasound test) should be performed to confirm the presence of the pericardial effusion and to guide the pericardiocentesis needle during the procedure. Because of the risk of accidental puncture to major arteries or organs in pericardiocentesis, surgical drainage may be a preferred treatment option for pericardial effusion in non-emergency situations.

Description

The patient's vital signs are monitored throughout the procedure, and an ECG tracing is continuously run. If time allows, **sedation** is administered, the puncture site is cleaned with an antiseptic iodine solution, and a local anesthetic is injected into the skin to numb the area. The patient is instructed to remain still. The physician performing pericardiocentesis will insert a syringe with an attached cardiac needle slowly into the chest wall until the needle tip reaches the pericardial sac. The patient may experience a sensation of pressure as the needle enters the membrane. When the needle is in the correct position, the physician will aspirate, or withdraw, fluid from the pericardial sac.

When the procedure is performed for diagnostic purposes, the fluid will be collected into specimen tubes for laboratory analysis. If the pericardiocentesis is performed to treat a cardiac tamponade or other significant fluid build-up, a pericardial catheter may be attached to the needle to allow for continuous drainage.

After the cardiac needle is removed, pressure is applied to the puncture site for approximately five minutes, and the site is then bandaged.

Preparation

Prior to pericardiocentesis, the test procedure is explained to the patient, along with the risks and possible complications involved, and the patient is asked to sign an informed consent form. If the patient is incapacitated, the same steps are followed with a family member.

No special diet or **fasting** is required for the test. After the patient changes into a hospital gown, an intravenous line is inserted into a vein in the arm. The IV will be used to administer sedation, and any required medications or blood products. Leads for an electrocardiogram (ECG) tracing are attached to the patient's right and left arms and legs, and the fifth lead is attached to the cardiac needle used for the procedure. The patient is instructed to lie flat on the table, with the upper body elevated to a 60 degree angle.

KEY TERMS

Cardiac tamponade—Compression and restriction of the heart that occurs when the pericardium fills with blood or fluid. This increase in pressure outside the heart interferes with heart function and can result in shock and/or death.

Catheter—A long, thin, flexible tube used to drain or administer fluids.

Echocardiogram—An imaging test using high-frequency sound waves to obtain pictures of the heart and surrounding tissues.

Electrocardiogram—A cardiac test that measures the electrical activity of the heart.

Myocardium—The middle layer of the heart wall.

Pericardium—A double membranous sac that envelops and protects the heart.

Aftercare

The site of the puncture and any drainage catheter should be checked regularly for signs of infection such as redness and swelling. Blood pressure and pulse are also monitored following the procedure. Patients who experience continued bleeding or abnormal swelling of the puncture site, sudden **dizziness**, difficulty breathing, or chest pains in the days following a pericardiocentesis procedure should seek immediate medical attention.

Risks

Pericardiocentesis is an invasive procedure, and infection of the puncture site or pericardium is always a risk. Possible complications include perforation of a major artery, lung, or liver. The myocardium, the outer muscle layer of the heart, could also be damaged if the cardiac needle is inserted too deeply.

Normal results

Normal pericardial fluid is clear to straw-colored in appearance with no bacteria, blood, cancer cells or pathogens. There is typically a minimal amount of the fluid (10–50 ml) in the pericardial cavity.

Abnormal results

A large volume of pericardial fluid (over 50 ml) indicates the presence of pericardial effusion. Laboratory analysis of the fluid can aid in the diagnosis of the cause of pericarditis. The presence of an infectious organism such as *staphylococcus aureus* is a sign of bacterial pericarditis. Excessive protein is present in cases of **systemic lupus erythematosus** or myocardial infarction (heart attack). An elevated white **blood count** may point to a fungal infection. If the patient has a hemorrhage, a cardiac rupture, or cancer, there may be blood in the pericardial fluid.

Resources

BOOKS

Weinstock, Doris et al. eds. "Body system Tests: Cardiovascular System." In *Illustrated Guide to Diagnostic Tests, 2nd edition.* Springhouse, PA: Springhouse Corporation, 1998.

ORGANIZATION

The American Heart Association. National Center. 7272 Greenville Avenue, Dallas, Texas 75231. (800) AHA-USA 1. < http://www.americanheart.org >.

Paula Anne Ford-Martin

Pericarditis

Definition

Pericarditis is an inflammation of the two layers of the thin, sac-like membrane that surrounds the heart. This membrane is called the pericardium, so the term pericarditis means inflammation of the pericardium.

Description

Pericarditis is fairly common. It affects approximately one in 1,000 people. The most common form is caused by infection with a virus. People in their 20s and 30s who have had a recent upper respiratory infection are most likely to be affected, along with men aged 20–50. One out of every four people who have had pericarditis will get it again, but after two years these relapses are less likely.

Causes and symptoms

The viruses that cause pericarditis include those that cause **influenza**, **polio**, and **rubella** (German **measles**). In children, the most common viruses that cause pericarditis are the adenovirus and the cocksackievirus (which is most likely to affect children during warmer weather).

Although pericarditis is usually caused by a virus, it also can be caused by an injury to the heart or it can follow a **heart attack**. It may also be caused by certain inflammatory diseases such as **rheumatoid arthritis** or systemic lupus erythematosus. Bacteria, fungi, parasites, **tuberculosis**, **cancer** or kidney failure may also affect the pericardium. Sometimes the cause is unknown.

There are several forms of pericarditis, depending on the cause.

Acute pericarditis

This is caused by infection with a virus, bacteria, or fungus—usually in the lungs and upper respiratory tract. This form of the disease causes a sharp, severe **pain** that starts in the region of the breastbone. If the pericarditis is caused by a bacteria, it is called bacterial or purulent pericarditis.

Cardiac tamponade

Sometimes fluid collects between the heart and the pericardium. This is called pericardial effusion, and may lead to a condition called cardiac tamponade. When the fluid accumulates, it can squeeze the heart and prevent it from filling with blood. This keeps the rest of the body from getting the necessary supply of oxygen and can cause dangerously low blood pressure. A **cardiac tamponade** can happen when the chest is injured during surgery, radiation therapy, or an accident. Cardiac tamponade is a serious medical emergency and must be treated immediately.

Constrictive pericarditis

When the pericardium is scarred or thickened, the heart has difficulty contracting. This is because the pericardium has shrunken or tightened around the heart, constricting the muscle's heart movement. This usually occurs as a result of tuberculosis, which now is rarely found in the United States, except in immigrant, **AIDS**, and prison populations.

Symptoms of pericarditis

Symptoms likely to be associated with pericarditis include:

- rapid breathing
- breathlessness
- dry **cough**
- fever and chills
- weakness
- broken blood vessels (hemorrhages) in the mucus membrane of the eyes, the back, the chest, fingers, and toes
- feelings of anxiety

- A sharp or dull pain that starts in the front of the chest under the breastbone and radiates to the left side of the neck, upper abdomen, and left shoulder the pain is less intense when the patient sits up or leans forward and worsens when lying down; it may worsen with a deep breath, like pleurisy, which may accompany pericarditis

In cardiac tamponade, neck veins may be swollen and blood pressure may be very low.

Diagnosis

The heart of a person with pericarditis is likely to produce a grating sound (friction rub) when heard through a stethoscope. This sound occurs because the roughened pericardium surfaces are rubbing against each other.

The following tests will also help diagnose pericarditis and what is causing it:

- electrocardiograph (ECG) and echocardiogram to distinguish between pericarditis and a heart attack.
- x ray to show the traditional "water bottle" shadow around the heart that is often seen in pericarditis where there is a sufficient fluid build up.
- computed tomography scan (CT scan) of the chest.
- heart catheterization to view the heart's chambers and valves.
- **pericardiocentesis** to test for viruses, bacteria, fungus, cancer, and tuberculosis.
- blood tests such as LDH and CPK to measure cardiac enzymes and distinguish between a heart attack and pericarditis, as well as a complete blood count (CBC) to look for infection.

Treatment

Since most pericarditis is caused by a virus and will heal naturally, there is no specific, curative treatment. Ordinary **antibiotics** do not work against viruses. Pericarditis that comes from a virus usually clears up in two weeks to three months. Medications may be used to reduce inflammation, however. They include **nonsteroidal anti-inflammatory drugs** (NSAIDs), such as ibuprofen and aspirin. **Corticosteroids** are helpful if the pericarditis was caused by a heart attack or **systemic lupus erythematosus**. **Analgesics** (painkillers such as **aspirin** or **acetaminophen**) also may be given.

If the pericarditis recurs, removal of all or part of the pericardium (pericardiectomy) may be necessary. In the case of constrictive pericarditis, the pericardiectomy may be necessary to remove the stiffened

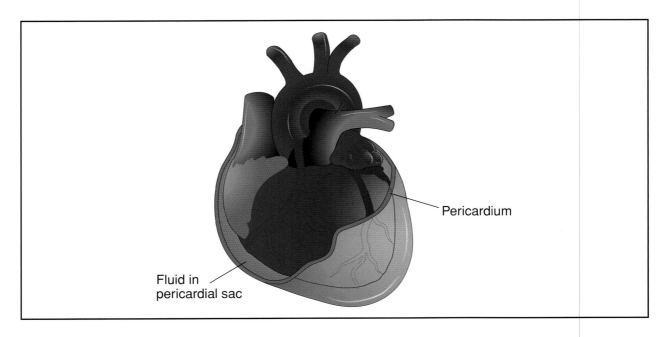

Pericardium

Fluid in
pericardial sac

Cardiac tamponade occurs when fluid collects in the pericardial sac between the heart and the surrounding pericardium. A medical emergency, cardiac tamponade deprives the body of oxygen and requires immediate treatment. *(Illustration by Electronic Illustrators Group.)*

KEY TERMS

Computed tomography (CT) scan—A CT scan uses x rays to scan the body from many angles. A computer compiles the x rays into a picture of the area being studied. The images are viewed on a monitor and printed-out.

Echocardiogram—An echocardiogram bounces sound waves off the heart to create a picture of its chambers and valves.

Electrocardiogram (ECG)—An ECG is a test to measure electrical activity in the heart.

Heart catheterization—A heart catheterization is used to view the heart's chamber and valves. A tube (catheter) is inserted into an artery, usually in the groin. A dye is then put into the artery through the tube. The dye makes its way to the heart to create an image of the heart on x-ray film. The image is photographed and stored for further examination.

Pericardiocentesis—Pericardiocentesis is a procedure used to test for viruses, bacteria, and fungus. The physician puts a small tube through the skin, directly into the pericardial sac, and withdraws fluid. The fluid then is tested for viruses, bacteria, and fungus.

Pericardium—The pericardium is the thin, sac-like membrane that surrounds the heart. It has two layers: the serous pericardium and the fibrous pericardium.

---

parts of the pericardium that are preventing the heart from beating correctly.

If a cardiac tamponade is present, it may be necessary to drain excess fluid from the pericardium. Pericardiocentesis, the same procedure used for testing, will be used to withdraw the fluid.

For most people, home care with rest and medications to relieve pain are sufficient. A warm heating pad or compress also may help relieve pain. Sitting in an upright position and bending forward helps relieve discomfort. A person with pericarditis may also be kept in bed, with the head of the bed elevated to reduce the heart's need to work hard as it pumps blood. Along with painkillers and antibiotics, diuretic drugs ("water pills") to reduce fluids may also be used judiciously.

Prognosis

Prognosis is good. Most people recover within three weeks to several months and do not need any additional treatment.

Prevention

There is no way to prevent pericarditis, but a healthy lifestyle with proper **nutrition** and **exercise** will help keep the body's immune system strong and more likely to fight off invading microorganisms.

Resources

ORGANIZATIONS

American Heart Association. 7320 Greenville Ave. Dallas, TX 75231. (214) 373-6300 or (800) 242-8721. inquire@heart.org. <http://www.americanheart.org>.

National Heart, Lung and Blood Institute. P.O. Box 30105, Bethesda, MD 20824-0105. (301) 251-1222. <http://www.nhlbi.nih.gov>.

Christine Kuehn Kelly

Perinatal infection

Definition

An infection caused by a bacteria or virus that can be passed from a mother to her baby during **pregnancy** or delivery is called a perinatal infection.

Description

Perinatal infections include bacterial or viral illnesses that can be passed from a mother to her baby either while the baby is still in the uterus, during the delivery process, or shortly after birth. Maternal infection can, in some cases, cause complications at birth. The mother may or may not experience active symptoms of the infection during the pregnancy. The most serious and most common perinatal infections, and the impact of these diseases on the mother and infant, are discussed below in alphabetical order. It is important to note that men can become infected and can transmit many of these infections to other women. The sexual partners of women who have these infections also should seek medical treatment.

Causes and symptoms

Chlamydia

Chlamydia trachomatis is the most common bacterial sexually transmitted disease in the United States, causing more than 4 million infections each year. The majority of women with chlamydial infection experience no obvious symptoms. The infection affects the reproductive tract and causes pelvic inflammatory disease, **infertility**, and ectopic pregnancy (the fertilized egg implants somewhere other than in the uterus). This infection can cause premature rupture of the membranes and early labor. It can be passed to the infant during delivery and can cause ophthalmia neonatorum (an eye infection) within the first month of

life and **pneumonia** within one to three months of age. Symptoms of **chlamydial pneumonia** are a repetitive **cough** and rapid breathing. **Wheezing** is rare and the infant does not develop a **fever**.

Cytomegalovirus

Cytomegalovirus (CMV) is a common virus in the herpes virus family. It is found in saliva, urine, and other body fluids and can be spread through sexual contact or other more casual forms of physical contact like kissing. In adults, CMV may cause mild symptoms of swollen lymph glands, fever, and **fatigue**. Many people who carry the virus experience no symptoms at all. Infants can become infected with CMV while still in the uterus if the mother becomes infected or develops a recurrence of the infection during pregnancy. Most infants exposed to CMV before birth develop normally and do not show any symptoms. As many as 6,000 infants who were exposed to CMV before birth are born with serious complications each year. CMV interferes with normal fetal development and can cause mental retardation, blindness, deafness, or epilepsy in these infants.

Genital herpes

Genital herpes, which is usually caused by herpes simplex virus type 2 (HSV-2), is a sexually transmitted disease that causes painful sores on the genitals. Women who have their first outbreak of genital herpes during pregnancy are at high risk of miscarriage or delivering a low birth weight baby. The infection can be passed to the infant at the time of delivery if the mother has an active sore. The most serious risk to the infant is the possibility of developing HSV-2 **encephalitis**, an inflammation of the brain, with symptoms of irritability and poor feeding.

Hepatitis B

Hepatitis B is a contagious virus that causes liver damage and is a leading cause of chronic **liver disease** and cirrhosis. Approximately 20,000 infants are born each year to mothers who test positive for the hepatitis B virus. These infants are at high risk for developing hepatitis B infection through exposure to their mothers blood during delivery.

Human immunodeficiency virus (HIV)

Human **immunodeficiency** virus (HIV) is a serious, contagious virus that causes acquired immunodeficiency syndrome (**AIDS**). About one-fourth of pregnant women with HIV pass the infection on to their newborn infants. An infant with HIV usually develops AIDS and dies before the age of two.

Human papillomavirus

Human papillomavirus (HPV) is a sexually transmitted disease that causes **genital warts** and can increase the risk of developing some cancers. HPV appears to be transferred from the mother to the infant during the birth process.

Rubella (German measles)

Rubella is a virus that causes German **measles**, an illness that includes rash, fever, and symptoms of an upper respiratory tract infection. Most people are exposed to rubella during childhood and develop antibodies to the virus so they will never get it again. Rubella infection during early pregnancy can pass through the placenta to the developing infant and cause serious **birth defects** including heart abnormalities, mental retardation, blindness, and deafness.

Streptococcus

Group B streptococcus (GBS) infection is the most common bacterial cause of infection and **death** in newborn infants. Although rates have declined in the United States since the introduction of **antibiotics** to at-risk women during labor in the 1980s, about 1,600 cases and 80 newborn deaths still occur each year. In women, GBS can cause vaginitis and urinary tract infections. Both infections can cause premature birth and the bacteria can be transferred to the infant in the uterus or during delivery. GBS causes pneumonia, **meningitis**, and other serious infections in infants.

Syphilis

Syphilis is a sexually transmitted bacterial infection that can be transferred from a mother to an infant through the placenta before birth. Up to 50% of infants born to mothers with syphilis will be premature, stillborn, or will die shortly after birth. Infected infants may have severe birth defects. Those infants who survive infancy may develop symptoms of syphilis up to two years later.

Diagnosis

Chlamydia

Chlamydial bacteria can be diagnosed by taking a cotton swab sample of the cervix and vagina during the third trimester of the pregnancy. Chlamydial cell cultures take three to seven days to grow but many laboratories are not equipped to run the tests necessary to confirm the diagnosis.

Cytomegalovirus

Past or recent infection with CMV can be identified by antibody tests and CMV can be grown from body fluids.

Genital herpes

The appearance of a genital sore is enough to suspect an outbreak of genital herpes. The sore can be cultured and tested to confirm that HSV-2 is present.

Hepatitis B

A blood test can be used to screen pregnant women for the hepatitis B surface antigen (HBsAg) in prenatal health programs.

Human immunodeficiency virus (HIV)

HIV can be detected using a blood test and is part of most prenatal screening programs.

Human papillomavirus

HPV causes the growth of **warts** in the genital area. The wart tissue can be removed with a scalpel and tested to determine what type of HPV virus caused the infection.

Rubella (German measles)

Pregnant women are usually tested for antibodies to rubella, which would indicate that they have been previously exposed to the virus and therefore would not develop infection during pregnancy if exposed.

Streptococcus

GBS can be detected by a vaginal or rectal swab culture, and sometimes from a **urine culture**. Blood tests can be used to confirm GBS infection in infants who exhibit symptoms.

Syphilis

Pregnant women are usually tested for syphilis as part of the prenatal screening.

Treatment

Chlamydia

Pregnant women can be treated during the third trimester with oral erythromycin, for seven–14 days depending on the dose used. Newborn infants can be treated with erythromycin liquid for 10–14 days at a dosage determined by their body weight.

Cytomegalovirus

No drugs or vaccines are currently available for prevention or treatment of CMV.

Genital herpes

The **antiviral drugs** acyclovir or famciclovir can be administered to the mother during pregnancy. Little is known about the risks of these drugs to the fetus, however, the risk of birth defects does not seem to be any higher than for women who do not take these medications. Infants with suspected HSV-2 can be treated with acyclovir. Delivery of the infant by **cesarean section** is recommended if the mother has an active case of genital herpes.

Hepatitis B

Infants born to mothers who test positive to the HBsAg test should be treated with hepatitis B immune globulin at birth to give them immediate protection against developing hepatitis B. These infants, as well as all infants, should also receive a series of three hepatitis B vaccine injections as part of their routine immunizations.

Human immunodeficiency virus (HIV)

Recent studies have shown that prenatal care and HIV testing before delivery are major opportunities to prevent perinatal HIV infection. Pregnant women with HIV should be treated as early in the pregnancy as possible with zidovudine (AZT). Other newer drugs designed to treat HIV/AIDS also may be used during pregnancy with the knowledge that these drugs may have unknown effects on the infant. The risks and benefits of such treatments need to be discussed. Infants born with HIV should receive aggressive drug treatment to prevent development of AIDS.

Human papillomavirus

Genital warts are very difficult to treat and frequently recur even after treatment. They can be removed by **cryotherapy** (freezing), laser or electrocauterization (burning), or surgical excision (cutting) of the warts. Some medications (imiquimod 5% cream, podophyllin, trichloroacetic acid or topical 5-fluorouracil) can be applied to help dissolve genital warts. Cesarean delivery rather than vaginal delivery seems to reduce the risk of transmission of HPV from mothers to infants.

Rubella (German measles)

No treatment is available. Some health care providers may recommend giving the mother an injection of immune globulin (to boost the immune system to fight off the virus) if she is exposed to rubella early in the pregnancy. However, no evidence to support the use of these injections exists. Exposure to rubella early in pregnancy poses a high risk that the infant will have serious birth defects. Termination of the pregnancy may be considered. Women who have not been previously exposed to rubella will usually be vaccinated immediately after the first pregnancy to protect infants of future pregnancies.

Streptococcus

Pregnant women diagnosed with GBS late in the pregnancy should be treated with antibiotics injected intravenously to prevent **premature labor**. In 2003, the Centers for Disease Control and Prevention (CDC) issued revised guidelines for preventing perinatal GBS disease. They began recommending that women not only be tested as soon as they learn of their pregnancy, but again at 35 to 37 weeks gestation. The CDC also recommended updated **prophylaxis** regimens for women with penicillin **allergies**, as well as new guidelines for patients with threatened preterm deliveries and other new recommendations. If transmission of GBS to the newborn infant already is suspected or if the baby develops symptoms of infection, infants often are treated with antibiotics.

Syphilis

Antibiotic therapy, usually penicillin, given early in the pregnancy can be used to treat the infection and may prevent transmission to the infant.

Prognosis

Chlamydia

Without treatment, the most serious consequences of chlamydial infection are related to complications of premature delivery. Treatment of the mother with antibiotics during the third trimester can prevent premature delivery and the transfer of the infection to the baby. Infants treated with antibiotics for eye infection or pneumonia generally recover.

Cytomegalovirus

The chance for recovery after exposure to CMV is very good for both the mother and the infant. Exposure to CMV can be serious and even life threatening for mothers and infants whose immune systems are compromised, for example those receiving **chemotherapy** or who have HIV/AIDS. Those infants who develop birth defects after CMV exposure may have serious, lifelong complications.

Genital herpes

Once a woman or infant is infected, outbreaks of genital herpes sores can recur at any point during their lifetimes.

Hepatitis B

Infants treated at birth with immune globulin and the series of vaccinations will be protected from development of hepatitis B infection. Infants infected with hepatitis B develop a chronic, mild form of hepatitis and are at increased risk for developing liver disease.

Human immunodeficiency virus (HIV)

Treatment with AZT during pregnancy significantly reduces the chance that the infant will be infected with HIV from the mother.

Human papillomavirus

Once infected with HPV, there is a lifelong risk of developing warts and an increased risk of some cancers.

Rubella (German measles)

Infants exposed to rubella virus in the uterus are at high risk for severe birth defects including heart defects, blindness, and deafness.

Streptococcus

Infection of the urinary tract or genital tract of pregnant women can cause premature birth. Infants infected with GBS can develop serious, life-threatening infections.

Syphilis

Premature birth, birth defects, or the development of serious syphilis symptoms is likely to occur in untreated pregnant women.

Prevention

Use of a barrier method of contraceptive (**condom**) can prevent transmission of some of the infections. Intravenous drug use and sexual intercourse with infected partners increases the risks of exposure to most of these infections. Pregnant women can be tested for many of the bacterial or viral infections described; however, effective treatment may not be available to protect the infant. New studies show that a woman's nutritional status may contribute to her ability to fight off infections, particularly in cases of **malnutrition**. Proper prenatal care may improve outcomes and prevent some infections.

Resources

PERIODICALS

Goldenberg, Robert L. "The Plausibility of Micronutrient Deficiency in Relationship to Perinatal Infection." *The Journal of Nutrition* May 2003: 1645S.

Morantz, Carrie A. "CDC Updates Guidelines for Prevention of Perinatal Group B Streptococcal Disease." *American Family Physician* March 1, 2003: 1121.

Peters, Vicki, et al. "Missed Opportunities for Perinatal HIV Prevention Among HIV-exposed Infants Born 1996–2000, Pediatric Spectrum of HIV Disease Cohort." *Pediatrics* May 2003: S1186.

Altha Roberts Edgren
Teresa G. Odle

Periodic paralysis

Definition

Periodic **paralysis** (PP) is the name for several rare, inherited muscle disorders marked by temporary weakness, especially following rest, sleep, or exercise.

Description

Periodic paralysis disorders are genetic disorders that affect muscle strength. There are two major forms, hypokalemic and hyperkalemic, each caused by defects in different genes.

In hypokalemic PP, the level of potassium in the blood falls in the early stages of a paralytic attack, while in hyperkalemic PP, it rises slightly or is normal. (The root of both words, "kali," refers to potassium.) Hyperkalemic PP is also called potassium-sensitive PP.

Causes and symptoms

Causes

Both forms of PP are caused by inheritance of defective genes. Both genes are dominant, meaning that only one copy of the defective gene is needed for a person to develop the disease. A parent with the gene has a 50% chance of passing it along to each offspring, and the likelihood of passing it on is unaffected by the results of previous pregnancies.

The gene for hypokalemic PP is present equally in both sexes, but leads to noticeable symptoms more often in men than in women. The normal gene is responsible for a muscle protein controlling the flow of calcium during muscle contraction.

The gene for hyperkalemic PP affects virtually all who inherit it, with no difference in male-vs.-female expression. The normal gene is responsible for a muscle protein controlling the flow of sodium during muscle contraction.

Symptoms

The attacks of weakness in hypokalemic PP usually begin in late childhood or early adolescence and often become less frequent during middle age. The majority of patients develop symptoms before age 16. Since they begin in the school years, the symptoms of hypokalemic PP are often first seen during physical education classes or after-school sports, and may be mistaken for laziness, or lack of interest on the part of the child.

Attacks are most commonly brought on by:

- strenuous **exercise** followed by a short period of rest
- large meals, especially ones rich in carbohydrates or salt
- emotional **stress**
- alcohol use
- infection
- **pregnancy**

The weakness from a particular attack may last from several hours to as long as several days, and may be localized to a particular limb, or might involve the entire body.

The attacks of weakness of hyperkalemic PP usually begin in infancy or early childhood, and may become less severe later in life. As in the hypokalemic form, attacks are brought on by stress, pregnancy, and exercise followed by rest. In contrast, though, hyperkalemic attacks are not associated with a heavy meal but rather with missing a meal, with high potassium intake, or use of glucocorticoid drugs such as prednisone. (Glucocorticoids are a group of steroids that regulate metabolism and affect muscle tone.)

Weakness usually lasts less than three hours, and often persists for only several minutes. The attacks are usually less severe, but more frequent, than those of the hypokalemic form. Weakness usually progresses from the lower limbs to the upper, and may involve the facial muscles as well.

Diagnosis

Diagnosis of either form of PP begins with a careful medical history and a complete physical and neurological exam. A family medical history may reveal other affected relatives. Blood and urine tests done at the onset of an attack show whether there are elevated or depressed levels of potassium. Electrical tests of muscle and a muscle biopsy show characteristic changes.

Challenge tests, to aid in diagnosis, differ for the two forms. In hypokalemic PP, an attack of weakness can be brought on by administration of glucose and insulin, with exercise if necessary. An attack of hyperkalemic PP can be induced with administration of potassium after exercise during **fasting**. These tests are potentially hazardous and require careful monitoring.

Genetic tests are available at some research centers and are usually recommended for patients with a known family history. However, the number of

---

KEY TERMS

Gene—A biologic unit of heredity transmitted from parents to offspring.

---

different possible mutations leading to each form is too great to allow a single comprehensive test for either form, thus limiting the usefulness of **genetic testing**.

Treatment

Severe respiratory weakness from hypokalemic PP may require intensive care to ensure adequate ventilation. Potassium chloride may be given by mouth or intravenously to normalize blood levels.

Attacks requiring treatment are much less common in hyperkalemic PP. Glucose and insulin may be prescribed. Eating carbohydrates may also relieve attacks.

Prognosis

Most patients learn to prevent their attacks well enough that no significant deterioration in the quality of life occurs. Strenuous exercise must be avoided, however. Attacks often lessen in severity and frequency during middle age. Frequent or severe attacks increase the likelihood of permanent residual weakness, a risk in both forms of periodic paralysis.

Prevention

There is no way to prevent the occurrence of either disease in a person with the gene for the disease. The likelihood of an attack of either form of PP may be lessened by avoiding the triggers (the events or combinations of circumstances which cause an attack) for each.

Hypokalemic PP attacks may be prevented with use of acetazolamide (or another carbonic anhydrase inhibitor drug) or a diuretic to help retain potassium in the bloodstream. These attacks may also be prevented by avoiding such triggers as salty food, large meals, a high-carbohydrate diet, and strenuous exercise.

Attacks of hyperkalemic PP may be prevented with frequent small meals high in carbohydrates, and the avoidance of foods high in potassium such as orange juice or bananas. Acetazolamide or thiazide (a diuretic) may be prescribed.

Resources

ORGANIZATIONS

Muscular Dystrophy Association. 3300 East Sunrise Drive, Tucson, AZ 85718. (800) 572-1717. < http:// www.mdausa.org >.

Periodic Paralysis Association. 5225 Canyon Crest Drive #71-351, Riverside, CA 92507. (909) 781-4401. < http:// www.periodicparalysis.org >.

Richard Robinson

Periodontal disease

Definition

Periodontal diseases are a group of diseases that affect the tissues that support and anchor the teeth. Left untreated, periodontal disease results in the destruction of the gums, alveolar bone (the part of the jaws where the teeth arise), and the outer layer of the tooth root.

Description

Periodontal disease is usually seen as a chronic inflammatory disease. An acute infection of the periodontal tissue may occur, but is not usually reported to the dentist. The tissues that are involved in periodontal diseases are the gums, which include the gingiva, periodontal ligament, cementum, and alveolar bone. The gingiva is a pink-colored mucus membrane that covers parts of the teeth and the alveolar bone. The periodontal ligament is the main part of the gums. The cementum is a calcified structure that covers the lower parts of the teeth. The alveolar bone is a set of ridges from the jaw bones (maxillary and mandible) in which the teeth are embedded. The main area involved in periodontal disease is the gingival sulcus, a pocket between the teeth and the gums. Several distinct forms of periodontal disease are known. These are gingivitis, acute necrotizing ulcerative gingivitis, adult periodontitis, and localized juvenile periodontitis. Although periodontal disease is thought to be widespread, serious cases of periodontitis are not common. Gingivitis is also one of the early signs of leukemia in some children.

Gingivitis

Gingivitis is an inflammation of the outermost soft tissue of the gums. The gingivae become red and inflamed, loose their normal shape, and bleed easily. Gingivitis may remain a chronic disease for years without affecting other periodontal tissues. Chronic gingivitis may lead to a deepening of the gingival sulcus. Acute necrotizing ulcerative gingivitis is mainly seen in young adults. This form of gingivitis is characterized by painful, bleeding gums, and death (necrosis) and erosion of gingival tissue between the teeth. It is thought that stress, malnutrition, **fatigue**, and poor oral hygiene are among the causes for acute necrotizing ulcerative gingivitis.

Adult periodontitis

Adult periodontitis is the most serious form of the periodontal diseases. It involves the gingiva, periodontal ligament, and alveolar bone. A deep periodontal pocket forms between the teeth, the cementum, and the gums. Plaque, calculus, and debris from food and other sources collect in the pocket. Without treatment, the periodontal ligament can be destroyed and resorption of the alveolar bone occurs. This allows the teeth to move more freely and eventually results in the loss of teeth. Most cases of adult periodontitis are chronic, but some cases occur in episodes or periods of tissue destruction.

Localized juvenile periodontitis

Localized juvenile periodontitis is a less common form of periodontal disease and is seen mainly in young people. Primarily, localized juvenile periodontitis affects the molars and incisors. Among the distinctions that separate this form of periodontitis are the low incidence of bacteria in the periodontal pocket, minimal plaque formation, and mild inflammation.

Herpetic gingivostomatitis

Herpes infection of the gums and other parts of the mouth is called herpetic gingivostomatitis and is frequently grouped with periodontal diseases. The infected areas of the gums turn red in color and have whitish herpetic lesions. There are two principal differences between this form of periodontal diseases and most other forms. Herpetic gingivostomatitis is caused by a virus, Herpes simplex, not by bacteria, and the viral infection tends to heal by itself in approximately two weeks. Also, herpetic gingivostomatitis is infectious to other people who come in contact with the herpes lesions or saliva that contains virus from the lesion.

Pericoronitis

Pericoronitis is a condition found in children who are in the process of producing molar teeth. The

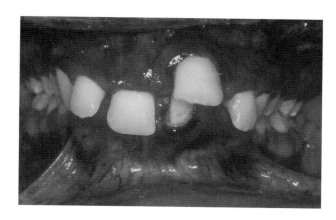

An extreme case of juvenile periodontitis. *(Custom Medical Stock Photo. Reproduced by permission.)*

disease is seen more frequently in the lower molar teeth. As the molar emerges, a flap of gum still covers the tooth. The flap of gum traps bacteria and food, leading to a mild irritation. If the upper molar fully emerges before the lower one, it may bite down on the flap during chewing. This can increase the irritation of the flap and lead to an infection. In bad cases, the infection can spread to the neck and cheeks.

Desquamative gingivitis

Desquamative gingivitis occurs mainly in postmenopausal women. The cause of the disease is not understood. The outer layers of the gums slough off, leaving raw tissue and exposed nerves.

Trench mouth

Trench mouth is an acute, necrotizing (causing tissue death), ulcerating (causing open sores) form of gingivitis. It causes **pain** in the affected gums. **Fever** and fatigue are usually present also. Trench mouth, also known as Vincent's disease, is a complication of mild cases of gingivitis. Frequently, poor **oral hygiene** is the main cause. **Stress**, an unbalanced diet, or lack of sleep are frequent cofactors in the development of trench mouth. This form of periodontal disease is more common in people who smoke. The term "trench mouth" was created in World War I, when the disease was common in soldiers who lived in the trenches. Symptoms of trench mouth appear suddenly. The initial symptoms include painful gums and foul breath. Gum tissue between teeth becomes infected and dies, and starts to disappear. Often, what appears to be remaining gum is dead tissue. Usually, the gums bleed easily, especially when chewing. The pain can increase to the point where eating and swallowing become difficult. Inflammation or infection from

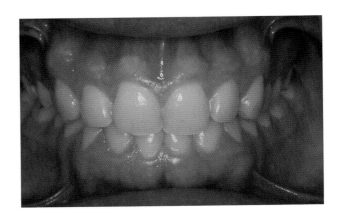

Gingivitis, an inflammation of the gums, is a common periodontal disease. *(Photograph by Edward H. Gill, Custom Medical Stock Photo. Reproduced by permission.)*

trench mouth can spread to nearby tissues of the face and neck.

Periodontitis

Periodontitis is a condition in which gingivitis has extended down around the tooth and into the supporting bone structure. Periodontitis is also called pyorrhea. Plaque and tarter buildup sometimes lead to the formation of large pockets between the gums and teeth. When this happens, anaerobic bacteria grow in the pockets. The pockets eventually extend down around the roots of the teeth where the bacteria cause damage to the bone structure supporting the teeth. The teeth become loose and tooth loss can result. Some medical conditions are associated with an increased likelihood of developing periodontitis. These diseases include diabetes, **Down syndrome**, Cohn's disease, **AIDS**, and any disease that reduces the number of white blood cells in the body for extended periods of time.

Causes and symptoms

Several factors play a role in the development of periodontal disease. The most important are age and oral hygiene. The number and type of bacteria present on the gingival tissues also play a role in the development of periodontal diseases. The presence of certain species of bacteria in large enough numbers in the gingival pocket and related areas correlates with the development of periodontal disease. Also, removal of the bacteria correlates with reduction or elimination of disease. In most cases of periodontal disease, the bacteria remain in the periodontal pocket and do not invade surrounding tissue.

The mechanisms by which bacteria in the periodontal pocket cause tissue destruction in the surrounding region are not fully understood. Several bacterial products that diffuse through tissue are thought to play a role in disease formation. Bacterial endotoxin is a toxin produced by some bacteria that can kill cells. Studies show that the amount of endotoxin present correlates with the severity of periodontal disease. Other bacterial products include proteolytic enzymes, molecules that digest protein found in cells, thereby causing cell destruction. The immune response has also been implicated in tissue destruction. As part of the normal immune response, white blood cells enter regions of inflammation to destroy bacteria. In the process of destroying bacteria, periodontal tissue is also destroyed.

Gingivitis usually results from inadequate oral hygiene. Proper brushing of the teeth and flossing decreases plaque buildup. The bacteria responsible for causing gingivitis reside in the plaque. Plaque is a sticky film that is largely made from bacteria. Tartar is plaque that has hardened. Plaque can turn into tartar in as little as three days if not brushed off. Tartar is difficult to remove by brushing. Gingivitis can be aggravated by hormones, and sometimes becomes temporarily worse during **pregnancy**, **puberty**, and when the patient is taking birth control pills. Interestingly, some drugs used to treat other conditions can cause an overgrowth of the gingival tissue that can result in gingivitis because plaque builds up more easily. Drugs associated with this condition are phenytoin, used to treat seizures; cyclosporin, given to organ transplant patients to reduce the likelihood of organ rejection; and calcium blockers, used to treat several different heart conditions. **Scurvy**, a vitamin C deficiency, and **pellagra**, a niacin deficiency, can also lead to bleeding gums and gingivitis.

The initial symptoms of periodontitis are bleeding and inflamed gums, and **bad breath**. Periodontitis follows cases of gingivitis, which may not be severe enough to cause a patient to seek dental help. Although the symptoms of periodontitis are also seen in other forms of periodontal diseases, the key characteristic in periodontitis is a large pocket that forms between the teeth and gums. Another characteristic of periodontitis is that pain usually does not develop until late in the disease, when a tooth loosens or an **abscess** forms.

Diagnosis

Diagnosis is made by observation of infected gums. Usually, a dentist is the person to diagnose

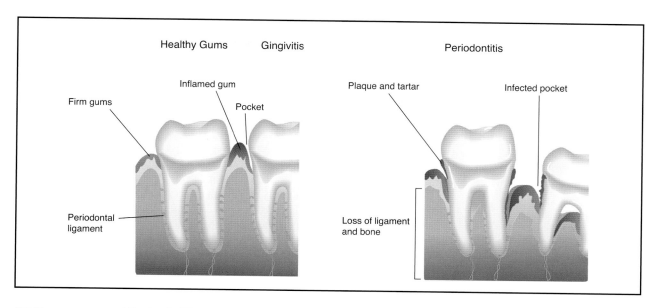

Healthy gums support the teeth. When gingivitis goes untreated, the gums become weak and pockets form around the teeth. Plaque and tartar build up in the pockets, the gum recedes, and periodontitis occurs. *(Illustration by Argosy Inc.)*

KEY TERMS

Anaerobic bacteria—Microorganisms that grow in the absence of oxygen.

Inflammation—A painful redness and swelling of an area of tissue in response to infection or injury.

---

and characterize the various types of periodontal disease. In cases such as acute herpetic gingivostomatitis, there are characteristic herpetic lesions. Many of the periodontal diseases are distinguished based on the severity of the infection and the number and type of tissues involved.

Diagnosis of periodontitis includes measuring the size of the pockets formed between the gums and teeth. Normal gingival pockets are shallow. If periodontal disease is severe, jaw bone loss will be detected in x-ray images of the teeth. If too much bone is lost, the teeth become loose and can change position. This will also be seen in x-ray images.

Treatment

Tartar can only be removed by professional dental treatment. Following treatment, periodontal tissues usually heal quickly. Gingivitis caused by vitamin deficiencies is treated by administering the needed vitamin. There are no useful drugs to treat herpetic

gingivostomatitis. Because of the pain associated with the herpes lesions, patients may not brush their teeth while the lesions are present. Herpes lesions heal by themselves without treatment. After the herpetic lesions have disappeared, the gums usually return to normal if good oral hygiene is resumed. Pericoronitis is treated by removing debris under the flap of gum covering the molar. This operation is usually performed by a dentist. Surgery is used to remove molars that are not likely to form properly.

Treatment for trench mouth starts with a complete cleaning of the teeth, removal of all plaque, tartar, and dead tissue on the gums. For the first few days after cleaning, the patient uses hydrogen peroxide mouth washes instead of brushing. After cleaning, the gum tissue will be very raw and rinsing minimizes damage to the gums that might be caused by the toothbrush. For the first few days, the patient should visit the dentist daily for checkups and then every second or third day for the next two weeks. Occasionally, antibiotic treatment is used to supplement dental cleaning of the teeth and gums. Surgery may be needed if the damage to the gums is extensive and they do not heal properly.

Treatment of periodontitis requires professional dental care. The pockets around the teeth must be cleaned, and all tartar and plaque removed. In periodontitis, tartar and plaque can extend far down the tooth root. Normal dental hygiene, brushing and flossing, cannot reach deep enough to be effective in treating periodontitis. In cases where pockets are very deep (more than 0.25 in [0.64 cm] deep), surgery is required to clean the pocket. This is performed in a dental office. Sections of gum that are not likely to reattach to the teeth may be removed to promote healing by healthy sections of gum. Abscesses are treated with a combination of **antibiotics** and surgery. The antibiotics may be delivered directly to the infected gum and bone tissues to ensure that high concentrations of the antibiotic reach the infected area. Abscess infections, especially of bone, are difficult to treat and require long term antibiotic treatments to prevent a reoccurrence of infection.

Prognosis

Periodontal diseases can be easily treated. The gums usually heal and resume their normal shape and function. In cases where they do not, prostheses or surgery can restore most of the support for proper functioning of the teeth.

Prevention

Most forms of periodontal disease can be prevented with good dental hygiene. Daily use of a toothbrush and flossing is sufficient to prevent most cases of periodontal disease. Tartar control toothpastes help prevent tartar formation, but do not remove tartar once it has formed.

Resources

BOOKS

Gorbach, S. L., J. G. Bartlett, and N. R. Blacklow. *Infectious Diseases.* 2nd ed. Philadelphia: W. B. Saunders Co.,1998.

John T. Lohr, PhD

Periodontitis *see* **Periodontal disease**

Periorbital cellulitis *see* **Orbital and periorbital cellulitis**

Peripheral arterial disease *see* **Peripheral vascular disease**

Peripheral neuritis *see* **Peripheral neuropathy**

Peripheral neuropathy

Definition

The term peripheral neuropathy encompasses a wide range of disorders in which the nerves outside of the brain and spinal cord—peripheral nerves—have been damaged. Peripheral neuropathy may also be referred to as peripheral neuritis, or if many nerves are involved, the terms polyneuropathy or polyneuritis may be used.

Description

Peripheral neuropathy is a widespread disorder, and there are many underlying causes. Some of these causes are common, such as diabetes, and others are extremely rare, such as acrylamide **poisoning** and certain inherited disorders. The most common worldwide cause of peripheral neuropathy is leprosy. Leprosy is caused by the bacterium *Mycobacterium leprae*, which attacks the peripheral nerves of affected people. According to statistics gathered by the World Health Organization, an estimated 1.15 million people have **leprosy** worldwide.

Leprosy is extremely rare in the United States, where diabetes is the most commonly known cause of peripheral neuropathy. It has been estimated that more than 17 million people in the United States and Europe have diabetes-related polyneuropathy. Many neuropathies are idiopathic, meaning that no known cause can be found. The most common of the inherited peripheral neuropathies in the United States is **Charcot-Marie-Tooth disease**, which affects approximately 125,000 persons.

Another of the better known peripheral neuropathies is **Guillain-Barré syndrome**, which arises from complications associated with viral illnesses, such as cytomegalovirus, Epstein-Barr virus, and human **immunodeficiency** virus (HIV), or bacterial infection, including *Campylobacter jejuni* and **Lyme disease**. The worldwide incidence rate is approximately 1.7 cases per 100,000 people annually. Other well-known causes of peripheral neuropathies include chronic **alcoholism**, infection of the varicella-zoster virus, **botulism**, and poliomyelitis. Peripheral neuropathy may develop as a primary symptom, or it may be due to another disease. For example, peripheral neuropathy is only one symptom of diseases such as amyloid neuropathy, certain cancers, or inherited neurologic disorders. Such diseases may affect the peripheral nervous system (PNS) and the central nervous system (CNS), as well as other body tissues.

To understand peripheral neuropathy and its underlying causes, it may be helpful to review the structures and arrangement of the PNS.

Nerve cells and nerves

Nerve cells are the basic building block of the nervous system. In the PNS, nerve cells can be threadlike–their width is microscopic, but their length can be measured in feet. The long, spidery extensions of nerve cells are called axons. When a nerve cell is stimulated, by touch or pain, for example, the message is carried along the axon, and neurotransmitters are released within the cell. Neurotransmitters are chemicals within the nervous system that direct nerve cell communication.

Certain nerve cell axons, such as the ones in the PNS, are covered with a substance called myelin. The myelin sheath may be compared to the plastic coating on electrical wires–it is there both to protect the cells and to prevent interference with the signals being transmitted. Protection is also given by Schwann cells, special cells within the nervous system that wrap around both myelinated and unmyelinated axons. The effect is similar to beads threaded on a necklace.

Nerve cell axons leading to the same areas of the body may be bundled together into nerves. Continuing the comparison to electrical wires, nerves may be compared to an electrical cord–the individual components are coated in their own sheaths and then encased together inside a larger protective covering.

Peripheral nervous system

The nervous system is classified into two parts: the CNS and the PNS. The CNS is made up of the brain and the spinal cord, and the PNS is composed of the nerves that lead to or branch off from the CNS.

The peripheral nerves handle a diverse array of functions in the body. This diversity is reflected in the major divisions of the PNS–the afferent and the efferent divisions. The afferent division is in charge of sending sensory information from the body to the CNS. When afferent nerve cell endings, called receptors, are stimulated, they release neurotransmitters. These neurotransmitters relay a signal to the brain, which interprets it and reacts by releasing other neurotransmitters.

Some of the neurotransmitters released by the brain are directed at the efferent division of the PNS. The efferent nerves control voluntary movements, such as moving the arms and legs, and involuntary movements, such as making the heart pump blood. The nerves controlling voluntary movements are called motor nerves, and the nerves controlling involuntary actions are referred to as autonomic nerves. The afferent and efferent divisions continually interact with each other. For example, if a person were to touch a hot stove, the receptors in the skin would transmit a message of heat and **pain** through the sensory nerves to the brain. The message would be processed in the brain and a reaction, such as pulling back the hand, would be transmitted via a motor nerve.

Neuropathy

NERVE DAMAGE. When an individual has a peripheral neuropathy, nerves of the PNS have been damaged. Nerve damage can arise from a number of causes, such as disease, physical injury, poisoning, or malnutrition. These agents may affect either afferent or efferent nerves. Depending on the cause of damage, the nerve cell axon, its protective myelin sheath, or both may be injured or destroyed.

CLASSIFICATION. There are hundreds of peripheral neuropathies. Reflecting the scope of PNS activity, symptoms may involve sensory, motor, or autonomic functions. To aid in diagnosis and treatment, the symptoms are classified into principal neuropathic syndromes based on the type of affected nerves and how long symptoms have been developing. Acute development refers to symptoms that have appeared within days, and subacute refers to those that have evolved over a number of weeks. Early chronic symptoms are those that take months to a few years to develop, and late chronic symptoms have been present for several years.

The classification system is composed of six principal neuropathic syndromes, which are subdivided into more specific categories. By narrowing down the possible diagnoses in this way, specific medical tests can be used more efficiently and effectively. The six syndromes and a few associated causes are listed below:

- Acute motor **paralysis**, accompanied by variable problems with sensory and autonomic functions. Neuropathies associated with this syndrome are mainly accompanied by motor nerve problems, but the sensory and autonomic nerves may also be involved. Associated disorders include Guillain-Barré syndrome, diphtheritic polyneuropathy, and porphyritic neuropathy.

- Subacute sensorimotor paralysis. The term sensorimotor refers to neuropathies that are mainly characterized by sensory symptoms, but also have a minor component of motor nerve problems. Poisoning with heavy metals (e.g., lead, mercury, and arsenic), chemicals, or drugs are linked to this syndrome. Diabetes, Lyme disease, and **malnutrition** are also possible causes.

- Chronic sensorimotor paralysis. Physical symptoms may resemble those in the above syndrome, but the time scale of symptom development is extended. This syndrome encompasses neuropathies arising from cancers, diabetes, leprosy, inherited neurologic and metabolic disorders, and **hypothyroidism**.

- Neuropathy associated with mitochondrial diseases. Mitochondria are organelles–structures within cells–responsible for handling a cell's energy requirements. If the mitochondria are damaged or destroyed, the cell's energy requirements are not met and it can die.

- Recurrent or relapsing polyneuropathy. This syndrome covers neuropathies that affect several nerves and may come and go, such as Guillain-Barré syndrome, porphyria, and chronic inflammatory demyelinating polyneuropathy.

- Mononeuropathy or plexopathy. Nerve damage associated with this syndrome is limited to a single nerve or a few closely associated nerves. Neuropathies related to physical injury to the nerve, such as **carpal tunnel syndrome** and **sciatica**, are included in this syndrome.

Causes and symptoms

Typical symptoms of neuropathy are related to the type of affected nerve. If a sensory nerve is damaged, common symptoms include **numbness**, **tingling** in the area, a prickling sensation, or pain. Pain associated with neuropathy can be quite intense and may be described as cutting, stabbing, crushing, or burning. In some cases, a nonpainful stimulus may be perceived as excruciating or pain may be felt even in the absence of a stimulus. Damage to a motor nerve is usually indicated by weakness in the affected area. If the problem with the motor nerve has continued over a length of time, muscle shrinkage (atrophy) or lack of muscle tone may be noticeable. Autonomic nerve damage is most noticeable when an individual stands upright and experiences problems such as lightheadedness or changes in blood pressure. Other indicators of autonomic nerve damage are lack of sweat, tears, and saliva; **constipation**; urinary retention; and impotence. In some cases, heart beat irregularities and respiratory problems can develop.

Symptoms may appear over days, weeks, months, or years. Their duration and the ultimate outcome of the neuropathy are linked to the cause of the nerve damage. Potential causes include diseases, physical injuries, poisoning, and malnutrition or alcohol **abuse**. In some cases, neuropathy is not the primary disorder, but a symptom of an underlying disease.

Disease

Diseases that cause peripheral neuropathies may either be acquired or inherited; in some cases, it is difficult to make that distinction. The diabetes-peripheral neuropathy link has been well established. A typical pattern of diabetes-associated neuropathic symptoms includes sensory effects that first begin in the feet. The associated pain or pins-and-needles, burning, crawling, or prickling sensations form a typical "stocking" distribution in the feet and lower legs. Other diabetic neuropathies affect the autonomic nerves and have potentially fatal cardiovascular complications.

Several other metabolic diseases have a strong association with peripheral neuropathy. Uremia, or **chronic kidney failure**, carries a 10–90% risk of eventually developing neuropathy, and there may be an association between liver failure and peripheral neuropathy. Accumulation of lipids inside blood vessels (**atherosclerosis**) can choke-off blood supply to certain peripheral nerves. Without oxygen and nutrients, the nerves slowly die. Mild polyneuropathy may develop in persons with low thyroid hormone levels. Individuals with abnormally enlarged skeletal extremities (acromegaly), caused by an overabundance of growth hormone, may also develop mild polyneuropathy.

Neuropathy can also result from severe vasculitides, a group of disorders in which blood vessels are inflamed. When the blood vessels are inflamed or damaged, blood supply to the nerve can be affected, injuring the nerve.

Both viral and bacterial infections have been implicated in peripheral neuropathy. Leprosy is caused by the bacteria *M. leprae*, which directly attack sensory nerves. Other bacterial illness may set the stage for an immune-mediated attack on the nerves. For example, one theory about Guillain-Barré syndrome involves complications following infection with *Campylobacter jejuni*, a bacterium commonly associated with **food poisoning**. This bacterium carries a protein that closely resembles components of myelin. The immune system launches an attack against the bacteria; but, according to the theory, the immune system confuses the myelin with the bacteria in some cases and attacks the myelin sheath as well. The underlying cause of neuropathy associated with Lyme disease is unknown; the bacteria may either promote an immune-mediated attack on the nerve or inflict damage directly.

Infection with certain viruses is associated with extremely painful sensory neuropathies. A primary example of such a neuropathy is caused by **shingles**. After a case of **chickenpox**, the causative virus, varicella-zoster virus, becomes inactive in sensory nerves. Years later, the virus may be reactivated. Once reactivated, it attacks and destroys axons. Infection with HIV is also associated with peripheral neuropathy, but the type of neuropathy that develops can vary. Some HIV-linked neuropathies are noted for myelin destruction rather than axonal degradation. Also, HIV infection is frequently accompanied by other infections, both bacterial and viral, that are associated with neuropathy.

Several types of peripheral neuropathies are associated with inherited disorders. These inherited disorders may primarily involve the nervous system, or the effects on the nervous system may be secondary to an inherited metabolic disorder. Inherited neuropathies can fall into several of the principal syndromes, because symptoms may be sensory, motor, or autonomic. The inheritance patterns also vary, depending on the specific disorder. The development of inherited disorders is typically drawn out over several years and may herald a degenerative condition–that is, a condition that becomes progressively worse over time. Even among specific disorders, there may be a degree of variability in inheritance patterns and symptoms. For example, Charcot-Marie-Tooth disease is usually inherited as an autosomal dominant disorder, but it can be autosomal recessive or, in rare cases, linked to the X chromosome. Its estimated frequency is approximately one in 2,500 people. Age of onset and sensory nerve involvement can vary between cases. The main symptom is a degeneration of the motor nerves in legs and arms, and resultant muscle atrophy. Other inherited neuropathies have a distinctly metabolic component. For example, in familial amyloid polyneuropathies, protein components that make up the myelin are constructed and deposited incorrectly.

Physical injury

Accidental falls and mishaps during sports and recreational activities are common causes of physical injuries that can result in peripheral neuropathy. The common types of injuries in these situations occur from placing too much pressure on the nerve, exceeding the nerve's capacity to stretch, blocking adequate blood supply of oxygen and nutrients to the nerve, and tearing the nerve. Pain may not always be immediately noticeable, and obvious signs of damage may take a while to develop.

These injuries usually affect one nerve or a group of closely associated nerves. For example, a common injury encountered in contact sports such as football is

the "burner," or "stinger," syndrome. Typically, a stinger is caused by overstretching the main nerves that span from the neck into the arm. Immediate symptoms are numbness, tingling, and pain that travels down the arm, lasting only a minute or two. A single incident of a stinger is not dangerous, but recurrences can eventually cause permanent motor and sensory loss.

Poisoning

The poisons, or toxins, that cause peripheral neuropathy include drugs, industrial chemicals, and environmental toxins. Neuropathy that is caused by drugs usually involves sensory nerves on both sides of the body, particularly in the hands and feet, and pain is a common symptom. Neuropathy is an unusual side effect of medications; therefore, most people can use these drugs safely. A few of the drugs that have been linked with peripheral neuropathy include metronidazole, an antibiotic; phenytoin, an anticonvulsant; and simvastatin, a cholesterol-lowering medication.

Certain industrial chemicals have been shown to be poisonous to nerves (neurotoxic) following work-related exposures. Chemicals such as acrylamide, allyl chloride, and carbon disulfide have all been strongly linked to development of peripheral neuropathy. Organic compounds, such as N-hexane and toluene, are also encountered in work-related settings, as well as in glue-sniffing and solvent abuse. Either route of exposure can produce severe sensorimotor neuropathy that develops rapidly.

Heavy metals are the third group of toxins that cause peripheral neuropathy. Lead, arsenic, thallium, and mercury usually are not toxic in their elemental form, but rather as components in organic or inorganic compounds. The types of metal-induced neuropathies vary widely. Arsenic poisoning may mimic Guillain-Barré syndrome; lead affects motor nerves more than sensory nerves; thallium produces painful sensorimotor neuropathy; and the effects of mercury are seen in both the CNS and PNS.

Malnutrition and alcohol abuse

Burning, stabbing pains and numbness in the feet, and sometimes in the hands, are distinguishing features of alcoholic neuropathy. The level of alcohol consumption associated with this variety of peripheral neuropathy has been estimated as approximately 3 L of beer or 300 mL of liquor daily for three years. However, it is unclear whether alcohol alone is responsible for the neuropathic symptoms, because chronic alcoholism is strongly associated with malnutrition.

Malnutrition refers to an extreme lack of nutrients in the diet. It is unknown precisely which nutrient deficiencies cause peripheral neuropathies in alcoholics and famine and **starvation** patients, but it is suspected that the B **vitamins** have a significant role. For example, thiamine (vitamin B_1) deficiency is the cause of **beriberi**, a neuropathic disease characterized by **heart failure** and painful polyneuropathy of sensory nerves. **Vitamin E deficiency** seems to have a role in both CNS and PNS neuropathy.

Diagnosis

Clinical symptoms can indicate peripheral neuropathy, but an exact diagnosis requires a combination of medical history, medical tests, and possibly a process of exclusion. Certain symptoms can suggest a diagnosis, but more information is commonly needed. For example, painful, burning feet may be a symptom of alcohol abuse, diabetes, HIV infection, or an underlying malignant tumor, among other causes. Without further details, effective treatment would be difficult.

During a **physical examination**, an individual is asked to describe the symptoms very carefully. Detailed information about the location, nature, and duration of symptoms can help exclude some causes or even pinpoint the actual problem. The person's medical history may also provide clues as to the cause, because certain diseases and medications are linked to specific peripheral neuropathies. A medical history should also include information about diseases that run in the family, because some peripheral neuropathies are genetically linked. Information about hobbies, recreational activities, alcohol consumption, and work place activities can uncover possible injuries or exposures to poisonous substances.

The physical examination also includes blood tests, such as those that check levels of glucose and creatinine to detect diabetes and kidney problems, respectively. A **blood count** is also done to determine levels of different blood cell types. Iron, vitamin B_{12}, and other factors may be measured as well, to rule out malnutrition. More specific tests, such as an assay for heavy metals or poisonous substances, or tests to detect **vasculitis**, are not typically done unless there is reason to suspect a particular cause.

An individual with neuropathy may be sent to a doctor that specializes in nervous system disorders (neurologist). By considering the results of the physical examination and observations of the referring doctor, the neurologist may be able to narrow down the possible diagnoses. Additional tests, such as nerve conduction studies and **electromyography**, which tests muscle reactions, can confirm that nerve damage has occurred and may also be able to indicate the nature of the damage. For example, some neuropathies are characterized by destruction of the myelin. This type of damage is shown by slowed nerve conduction. If the axon itself has suffered damage, the nerve conduction may be slowed, but it will also be diminished in strength. Electromyography adds further information by measuring nerve conduction and muscle response, which determines whether the symptoms are due to a neuropathy or to a muscle disorder.

In approximately 10% of peripheral neuropathy cases, a nerve biopsy may be helpful. In this test, a small part of the nerve is surgically removed and examined under a microscope. This procedure is usually the most helpful in confirming a suspected diagnosis, rather than as a diagnostic procedure by itself.

Treatment

Treat the cause

Attacking the underlying cause of the neuropathy can prevent further nerve damage and may allow for a better recovery. For example, in cases of bacterial infection such as leprosy or Lyme disease, **antibiotics** may be given to destroy the infectious bacteria. Viral infections are more difficult to treat, because antibiotics are not effective against them. Neuropathies associated with drugs, chemicals, and toxins are treated in part by stopping exposure to the damaging agent. Chemicals such as ethylenediaminetetraacetic acid (EDTA) are used to help the body concentrate and excrete some toxins. Diabetic neuropathies may be treated by gaining better control of blood sugar levels, but chronic kidney failure may require dialysis or even kidney transplant to prevent or reduce nerve damage. In some cases, such as compression injury or tumors, surgery may be considered to relieve pressure on a nerve.

In a crisis situation, as in the onset of Guillain-Barré syndrome, plasma exchange, intravenous immunoglobulin, and steroids may be given. Intubation, in which a tube is inserted into the trachea to maintain an open airway, and ventilation may be required to support the respiratory system. Treatment may focus more on symptom management than on combating the underlying cause, at least until a definitive diagnosis has been made.

Supportive care and long-term therapy

Some peripheral neuropathies cannot be resolved or require time for resolution. In these cases,

KEY TERMS

Afferent—Refers to peripheral nerves that transmit signals to the spinal cord and the brain. These nerves carry out sensory function.

Autonomic—Refers to peripheral nerves that carry signals from the brain and that control involuntary actions in the body, such as the beating of the heart.

Autosomal dominant or autosomal recessive—Refers to the inheritance pattern of a gene on a chromosome other than X or Y. Genes are inherited in pairs–one gene from each parent. However, the inheritance may not be equal, and one gene may overshadow the other in determining the final form of the encoded characteristic. The gene that overshadows the other is called the dominant gene; the overshadowed gene is the recessive one.

Axon—A long, threadlike projection that is part of a nerve cell.

Central nervous system (CNS)—The part of the nervous system that includes the brain and the spinal cord.

Efferent—Refers to peripheral nerves that carry signals away from the brain and spinal cord. These nerves carry out motor and autonomic functions.

Electromyography—A medical test that assesses nerve signals and muscle reactions. It can determine

if there is a disorder with the nerve or if the muscle is not capable of responding.

Inheritance pattern—Refers to dominant or recessive inheritance.

Motor—Refers to peripheral nerves that control voluntary movements, such as moving the arms and legs.

Myelin—The protective coating on axons.

Nerve biopsy—A medical test in which a small portion of a damaged nerve is surgically removed and examined under a microscope.

Nerve conduction—The speed and strength of a signal being transmitted by nerve cells. Testing these factors can reveal the nature of nerve injury, such as damage to nerve cells or to the protective myelin sheath.

Neurotransmitter—Chemicals within the nervous system that transmit information from or between nerve cells.

Peripheral nervous system (PNS)—Nerves that are outside of the brain and spinal cord.

Sensory—Refers to peripheral nerves that transmit information from the senses to the brain.

long-term monitoring and supportive care is necessary. Medical tests may be repeated to chart the progress of the neuropathy. If autonomic nerve involvement is a concern, regular monitoring of the cardiovascular system may be carried out.

Because pain is associated with many of the neuropathies, a pain management plan may need to be mapped out, especially if the pain becomes chronic. As in any chronic disease, **narcotics** are best avoided. Agents that may be helpful in neuropathic pain include amitriptyline, carbamazepine, and capsaicin cream. Physical therapy and physician-directed exercises can help maintain or improve function. In cases in which motor nerves are affected, braces and other supportive equipment can aid an individual's ability to move about.

Prognosis

The outcome for peripheral neuropathy depends heavily on the cause. Peripheral neuropathy ranges from a reversible problem to a potentially fatal complication. In the best cases, a damaged nerve

regenerates. Nerve cells cannot be replaced if they are killed, but they are capable of recovering from damage. The extent of recovery is tied to the extent of the damage and a person's age and general health status. Recovery can take weeks to years, because neurons grow very slowly. Full recovery may not be possible and it may also not be possible to determine the prognosis at the outset.

If the neuropathy is a degenerative condition, such as Charcot-Marie-Tooth disease, an individual's condition will become worse. There may be periods of time when the disease seems to reach a plateau, but cures have not yet been discovered for many of these degenerative diseases. Therefore, continued symptoms, potentially worsening to disabilities are to be expected.

A few peripheral neuropathies are eventually fatal. Fatalities have been associated with some cases of **diphtheria**, botulism, and others. Some diseases associated with neuropathy may also be fatal, but the ultimate cause of **death** is not necessarily related to the neuropathy, such as with **cancer**.

Prevention

Peripheral neuropathies are preventable only to the extent that the underlying causes are preventable. Steps that a person can take to prevent potential problems include vaccines against diseases that cause neuropathy, such as **polio** and diphtheria. Treatment for physical injuries in a timely manner can help prevent permanent or worsening damage to nerves. Precautions when using certain chemicals and drugs are well advised in order to prevent exposure to neurotoxic agents. Control of chronic diseases such as diabetes may also reduce the chances of developing peripheral neuropathy.

Although not a preventive measure, genetic screening can serve as an early warning for potential problems. Genetic screening is available for some inherited conditions, but not all. In some cases, presence of a particular gene may not mean that a person will necessarily develop the disease, because there may be environmental and other components involved.

Resources

ORGANIZATIONS

American Diabetes Association. 1701 North Beauregard Street, Alexandria, VA 22311. (800) 342-2383. < http://www.diabetes.org >.

Myelin Project Headquarters. Suite 225, 2001 Pennsylvania Ave., N.W., Washington, D.C. 20006-1850. (202) 452-8994. < http://www.myelin.org >.

Neuropathy Association. 60 E. 42nd St., Suite 942, New York, NY 10165. (800) 247-6968. < http://www.neuropathy.org/association.html >.

Julia Barrett

Peripheral vascular disease

Definition

Peripheral vascular disease is a narrowing of blood vessels that restricts blood flow. It mostly occurs in the legs, but is sometimes seen in the arms.

Description

Peripheral vascular disease includes a group of diseases in which blood vessels become restricted or blocked. Typically, the patient has peripheral vascular disease from **atherosclerosis**. Atherosclerosis is a disease in which fatty plaques form in the inside walls of blood vessels. Other processes, such as **blood clots**, further restrict blood flow in the blood vessels. Both veins and arteries may be affected, but the disease is usually arterial. All the symptoms and consequences of peripheral vascular disease are related to restricted blood flow. Peripheral vascular disease is a progressive disease that can lead to **gangrene** of the affected area. Peripheral vascular disease may also occur suddenly if an **embolism** occurs or when a blot clot rapidly develops in a blood vessel already restricted by an atherosclerotic plaque, and the blood flow is quickly cut off.

Causes and symptoms

There are many causes of peripheral vascular disease. One major risk factor is **smoking** cigarettes. Other diseases predispose patients to develop peripheral vascular disease. These include diabetes, Buerger's disease, hypertension, and Raynaud's disease. The main symptom is **pain** in the affected area. Early symptoms include an achy, tired sensation in the affected muscles. Since this disease is seen mainly in the legs, these sensations usually occur when walking. The symptoms may disappear when resting. As the disease becomes worse, symptoms occur even during light exertion and, eventually, occur all the time, even at rest. In the severe stages of the disease the leg and foot may be cold to the touch and will feel numb. The skin may become dry and scaly. If the leg is even slightly injured, ulcers may form because, without a good blood supply, proper healing can not take place. At the most severe stage of the disease, when the blood flow is greatly restricted, gangrene can develop in those areas lacking blood supply. In some cases, peripheral vascular disease occurs suddenly. This happens when an embolism rapidly blocks blood flow to a blood vessel. The patient will experience a sharp pain. followed by a loss of sensation in the affected area. The limb will become cold and numb, and loose color or turn bluish.

Diagnosis

Peripheral vascular disease can be diagnosed by comparing blood pressures taken above and below the point of pain. The area below the pain (downstream from the obstruction) will have a much lower or undetectable blood pressure reading. Doppler ultrasonography and **angiography** can also be used to diagnose and define this disease.

Treatment

If the person is a smoker, they should stop smoking immediately. **Exercise** is essential to treating this disease. The patient should walk until pain appears, rest until the pain disappears, and then resume walking. The amount of walking a patient can do should increase gradually as the symptoms improve. Ideally, the patient should walk 30–60 minutes per day. Infections in the affected area should be treated promptly. Surgery may be required to attempt to treat clogged blood vessels. Limbs with gangrene must be amputated to prevent the **death** of the patient.

Prognosis

The prognosis depends on the underlying disease and the stage at which peripheral vascular disease is discovered. Removal of risk factors, such as smoking, should be done immediately. In many cases, peripheral vascular disease can be treated successfully but coexisting cardiovascular problems may ultimately prove to be fatal.

Resources

BOOKS

Alexander, R. W., R. C. Schlant, and V. Fuster, editors. *The Heart*. 9th ed. New York: McGraw-Hill, 1998.

John T. Lohr, PhD

Peritoneal dialysis *see* **Dialysis, kidney**

Peritoneal endoscopy *see* **Laparoscopy**

Peritoneal fluid analysis *see* **Paracentesis**

▌ Peritonitis

Definition

Peritonitis is an inflammation of the membrane which lines the inside of the abdomen and all of the internal organs. This membrane is called the peritoneum.

Description

Peritonitis may be primary (meaning that it occurs spontaneously, and not as the result of some other medical problem) or secondary (meaning that it results from some other condition). It is most often due to infection by bacteria, but may also be due to some kind of a chemical irritant (such as spillage of acid from the stomach, bile from the gall bladder and biliary tract, or enzymes from the pancreas during the illness called **pancreatitis**). Peritonitis has even been seen in patients who develop a reaction to the cornstarch used to powder gloves worn during surgery. Peritonitis with no evidence of bacteria, chemical irritant, or foreign body has occurred in such diseases as systemic lupus erythematosus, porphyria, and **familial Mediterranean fever**. When the peritoneum is contaminated by blood, the blood can both irritate the peritoneum and serve as a source of bacteria to cause an infection. Blood may leak into the abdomen due to a burst tubal **pregnancy**, an injury, or bleeding after surgery.

Causes and symptoms

Primary peritonitis usually occurs in people who have an accumulation of fluid in their abdomens (**ascites**). Ascites is a common complication of severe cirrhosis of the liver (a disease in which the liver grows increasingly scarred and dysfunctional). The fluid that accumulates creates a good environment for the growth of bacteria.

Secondary peritonitis most commonly occurs when some other medical condition causes bacteria to spill into the abdominal cavity. Bacteria are normal residents of a healthy intestine, but they should have no way to escape and enter the abdomen, where they could cause an infection. Bacteria can infect the peritoneum due to conditions in which a hole (perforation) develops in the stomach (due to an ulcer eating its way through the stomach wall) or intestine (due to a large number of causes, including a ruptured appendix or a ruptured diverticulum). Bacteria can infect the peritoneum due to a severe case of pelvic inflammatory disease (a massive infection of the female organs, including the uterus and fallopian tubes). Bacteria can also escape into the abdominal cavity due to an injury that causes the intestine to burst, or an injury to an internal organ which bleeds into the abdominal cavity.

Symptoms of peritonitis include **fever** and abdominal pain. An acutely ill patient usually tries to lie very still, because any amount of movement causes excruciating **pain**. Often, the patient lies with the knees bent, to decrease strain on the tender peritoneum. There is often **nausea** and vomiting. The usual sounds made by

KEY TERMS

Ascites—An accumulation of fluid within the abdominal cavity.

Cirrhosis—A progressive liver disease in which the liver grows increasingly more scarred. The presence of scar tissue then interferes with liver function.

Diverticulum—An outpouching of the intestine.

Laparotomy—An open operation on the abdomen.

Pancreatitis—An inflammation of the pancreas.

Perforation—A hole.

Peritoneum—The membrane that lines the inside of the abdominal cavity, and all of the internal organs.

the active intestine and heard during examination with a stethoscope will be absent, because the intestine usually stops functioning. The abdomen may be rigid and boardlike. Accumulations of fluid will be notable in primary peritonitis due to ascites. Other signs and symptoms of the underlying cause of secondary peritonitis may be present.

Diagnosis

A diagnosis of peritonitis is usually based on symptoms. Discovering the underlying reason for the peritonitis, however, may require some work. A blood sample will be drawn in order to determine the white blood cell count. Because white blood cells are produced by the body in an effort to combat foreign invaders, the white blood cell count will be elevated in the case of an infection. A long, thin needle can be used to take a sample of fluid from the abdomen in an effort to diagnose primary peritonitis. The types of immune cells present are usually characteristic in this form of peritonitis. X-ray films may be taken if there is some suspicion that a perforation exists. In the case of a perforation, air will have escaped into the abdomen and will be visible on the picture. When a cause for peritonitis cannot be found, an open exploratory operation on the abdomen (laparotomy) is considered to be a crucial diagnostic procedure, and at the same time provides the opportunity to begin treatment.

Treatment

Treatment depends on the source of the peritonitis, but an emergency laparotomy is usually performed. Any perforated or damaged organ is usually repaired at this time. If a clear diagnosis of **pelvic inflammatory disease** or pancreatitis can be made, however, surgery is not usually performed. Peritonitis from any cause is treated with antibiotics given through a needle in the vein, along with fluids to prevent **dehydration**.

Prognosis

Prognosis for untreated peritonitis is poor, usually resulting in **death**. With treatment, the prognosis is variable, dependent on the underlying cause.

Prevention

There is no way to prevent peritonitis, since the diseases it accompanies are usually not under the voluntary control of an individual. However, prompt treatment can prevent complications.

Resources

BOOKS

Isselbacher, Kurt J., and Alan Epstein. "Diverticular, Vascular,and Other Disorders of the Intestine and Peritoneum." In *Harrison's Principles of Internal Medicine*, edited by Anthony S. Fauci, et al. New York: McGraw-Hill,1997.

Rosalyn Carson-DeWitt, MD

Permanent pacemakers *see* **Pacemakers**

Pernicious anemia

Definition

Pernicious anemia is a disease in which the red blood cells are abnormally formed, due to an inability to absorb vitamin B_{12}. True pernicious anemia refers specifically to a disorder of atrophied parietal cells leading to absent intrinsic factor, resulting in an inability to absorb B_{12}.

Description

Vitamin B_{12}, or cobalamin, plays an important role in the development of red blood cells. It is found in significant quantities in liver, meats, milk and milk products, and legumes. During the course of the digestion of foods containing B_{12}, the B_{12} becomes attached to a substance called intrinsic factor. Intrinsic factor is produced by parietal cells that line the stomach. The B_{12}-intrinsic factor complex then enters the intestine, where the vitamin is absorbed into the bloodstream. In fact, B_{12} can only be absorbed when it is attached to intrinsic factor.

In pernicious anemia, the parietal cells stop producing intrinsic factor. The intestine is then completely unable to absorb B_{12}. So, the vitamin passes out of the body as waste. Although the body has significant amounts of stored B_{12}, this will eventually be used up. At this point, the symptoms of pernicious anemia will develop.

Pernicious anemia is most common among people from northern Europe and among African Americans. It is far less frequently seen among people from southern Europe and Asia. Pernicious anemia occurs in equal numbers in both men and women. Most patients with pernicious anemia are older, usually over 60. Occasionally, a child will have an inherited condition that results in defective intrinsic factor. Pernicious anemia seems to run in families, so that anyone with a relative diagnosed with the disease has a greater likelihood of developing it as well.

Causes and symptoms

Intrinsic factor is produced by specialized cells within the stomach called parietal cells. When these parietal cells shrink in size (atrophy), they produce less and less intrinsic factor. Eventually, the parietal cells stop functioning altogether. Other important products of parietal cells are also lessened, including stomach acid, and an enzyme involved in the digestion of proteins.

People with pernicious anemia seem to have a greater chance of having certain other conditions. These conditions include **autoimmune disorders**, particularly those affecting the thyroid, parathyroid, and adrenals. It is thought that the immune system, already out of control in these diseases, incorrectly becomes directed against the parietal cells. Ultimately, the parietal cells seem to be destroyed by the actions of the immune system.

As noted, true pernicious anemia refers specifically to a disorder of atrophied parietal cells leading to absent intrinsic factor, resulting in an inability to absorb B_{12}. However, there are other related conditions that result in decreased absorption of B_{12}. These conditions cause the same types of symptoms as true pernicious anemia. Other conditions that interfere with either the production of intrinsic factor, or the

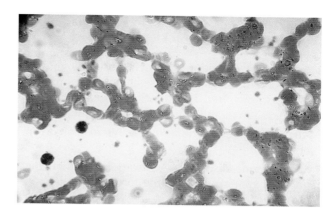

A smear of red blood cells indicating folic acid (vitamin B_{12}) deficiency. (Custom Medical Stock Photo. Reproduced by permission.)

body's use of B_{12}, include conditions that require surgical removal of the stomach, or poisonings with corrosive substances which destroy the lining of the stomach. Certain structural defects of the intestinal system can result in an overgrowth of normal bacteria. These bacteria then absorb B_{12} themselves, for use in their own growth. Intestinal worms (especially one called fish tapeworm) may also use B_{12}, resulting in anemia. Various conditions that affect the first part of the intestine (the ileum), from which B_{12} is absorbed, can also cause anemia due to B_{12} deficiency. These ilium-related disorders include tropical sprue, Whipple's disease, **Crohn's disease**, **tuberculosis**, and the Zollinger-Ellison syndrome.

Symptoms of pernicious anemia and decreased B_{12} affect three systems of the body: the system that is involved in the formation of blood cells (hematopoietic system); the gastrointestinal system; and the nervous system.

The hematopoietic system is harmed because B_{12} is required for the proper formation of red blood cells. Without B_{12}, red blood cell production is greatly reduced. Those red blood cells that are produced are abnormally large and abnormal in shape. Because red blood cells are responsible for carrying oxygen around the body, decreased numbers (termed anemia) result in a number of symptoms, including **fatigue**, **dizziness**, ringing in the ears, pale or yellowish skin, fast heart rate, enlarged heart with an abnormal heart sound (murmur) evident on examination, and chest **pain**.

Symptoms that affect the gastrointestinal system include a sore and brightly red tongue, loss of appetite, weight loss, **diarrhea**, and abdominal cramping.

The nervous system is severely affected when pernicious anemia goes untreated. Symptoms include **numbness**, **tingling**, or burning in the arms, legs, hands, and feet; muscle weakness; difficulty and loss of balance while walking; changes in reflexes; irritability, confusion, and depression.

Diagnosis

Diagnosis of pernicious anemia is suggested when a blood test reveals abnormally large red blood cells. Many of these will also be abnormally shaped. The earliest, least mature forms of red blood cells (reticulocytes) will also be low in number. White blood cells and platelets may also be decreased in number. Measurements of the quantity of B_{12} circulating in the bloodstream will be low.

Once these determinations are made, it will be important to diagnose the cause of the anemia. True pernicious anemia means that the parietal cells of the stomach are atrophied, resulting in decreased production of intrinsic factor. This diagnosis is made by the Schilling test. In this test, a patient is given radioactive B_{12} under two different sets of conditions: once alone,

and once attached to intrinsic factor. Normally, large amounts of B_{12} are absorbed through the intestine, then circulate through the blood, and enter the kidneys, where a certain amount of B_{12} is then passed out in the urine. When a patient has pernicious anemia, the dose of B_{12} given by itself will not be absorbed by the intestine, so it will not pass into the urine. Therefore, levels of B_{12} in the urine will be low. When the B_{12} is given along with intrinsic factor, the intestine is able to absorb the vitamin. Urine levels of B_{12} will therefore be higher.

Treatment

Treatment of pernicious anemia requires the administration of lifelong injections of B_{12}. Vitamin B_{12} given by injection enters the bloodstream directly, and does not require intrinsic factor. At first, injections may need to be given several times a week, in order to build up adequate stores of the vitamin. After this, the injections can be given on a monthly basis. Other substances required for blood cell production may also need to be given, iron and vitamin C.

Prognosis

Prognosis is generally good for patients with pernicious anemia. Many of the symptoms improve within just a few days of beginning treatment, although some of the nervous system symptoms may take up to 18 months to improve. Occasionally, when diagnosis and treatment have been delayed for a long time, some of the nervous system symptoms may be permanent.

Because an increased risk of **stomach cancer** has been noted in patients with pernicious anemia, careful monitoring is necessary, even when all the symptoms of the original disorder have improved.

Resources

BOOKS

Babior, Bernard M., and H. Franklin Bunn. "Megaloblastic Anemias." In *Harrison's Principles of Internal Medicine*, edited by Anthony S. Fauci, et al. New York: McGraw-Hill, 1997.

PERIODICALS

Toh, Ban-Hock, et al. "Pernicious Anemia." *The New England Journal of Medicine* 337, no. 20 (November 13, 1997): 52+.

Rosalyn Carson-DeWitt, MD

Peroneal muscular atrophy *see* **Charcot-Marie-Tooth disease**

Peroxisomal disorders

Definition

Peroxisomal disorders are a group of congenital (existing from birth) diseases characterized by the absence of normal peroxisomes in the cells of the body. Peroxisomes are special parts (organelles) within a cell that contain enzymes responsible for critical cellular processes, including oxidation of fatty acids, biosynthesis of membrane phospholipids (plasmalogens), cholesterol, and bile acids, conversion of amino acids into glucose, reduction of hydrogen peroxide by catalase, and prevention of excess synthesis of oxalate (which can form crystals with calcium, resulting in **kidney stones**). Peroxisomal disorders are subdivided into two major categories. The first are disorders resulting from a failure to form intact, normal peroxisomes, resulting in multiple metabolic abnormalities, which are referred to as peroxisome biogenesis disorders (PBD) or as generalized peroxisomal disorders. The second category includes those disorders resulting from the deficiency of a single peroxisomal enzyme. There are about 25 peroxisomal disorders known, although the number of diseases that are considered to be separate, distinct peroxisomal disorders varies among researchers and health care practitioners.

Description

A cell can contain several hundred peroxisomes, which are round or oval bodies with diameters of about 0.5 micron, that contain proteins that function as enzymes in metabolic processes. By definition, a peroxisome must contain catalase, which is an enzyme that breaks down hydrogen peroxide.

Approximately 50 different biochemical reactions occur entirely or partially within a peroxisome. Some of the processes are anabolic, or constructive, resulting in the synthesis of essential biochemical compounds, including bile acids, cholesterol, plasmalogens, and docosahexanoic acid (DHA), which is a long chain fatty acid that is a component of complex lipids, including the membranes of the central nervous system. Other reactions are catabolic, or destructive, and lead to the destruction of some fatty acids, including very long chain fatty acids (VLCFAs, fatty acids with more than 22 carbon atoms in their chains), phytanic acid, pipecolic acid, and the prostoglandins. The peroxisome is involved in breaking down VLCFAs to lengths that the body can use or get rid of.

When VLCFAs accumulate due to abnormal functioning of the peroxisomes, they are disruptive to the structure and stability of certain cells, especially those associated with the central nervous system and the myelin sheath, which is the fatty covering of nerve fibers. The peroxisomal disorders that include effects on the growth of the myelin sheath are considered to be part of a group of genetic disorders referred to as leukodystrophies. While metachromatic leukodystrophy (MLD) usually has its onset in infants or juveniles, there have been reports of its onset in young adults.

There are many other metabolic deficiencies that can occur in those who have peroxisomal disorders, which result in other types of detrimental effects, and together result in the abnormalities associated with the peroxisomal disorders. Unfortunately, it is not known how these abnormalities, and combinations of abnormalities, cause the disabilities seen in those afflicted with the disease.

Peroxisomal disorders form a heterogeneous disease group, with different degrees of severity. Included in the group referred to as PBD are:

- Zellweger syndrome (ZS), which is usually fatal within the first year of life,

- neonatal **adrenoleukodystrophy** (NALD), which is usually fatal within the first 10 years,

- infantile Refsum disease (IRD), which is not as devastating as ZS and NALD, as the children with this disorder with time and patience can develop some degree of motor, cognitive, and communication skills, although **death** generally occurs during the second decade of life.

- rhizomelic chondrodysplasia punctata (RCDP), which in its most severe form is fatal within the first year or two of life. However, survival into the teens has been known to occur. It is characterized by shortening of the proximal limbs (i.e., the legs from knee to foot, and the arms from elbow to hand).

- Zellweger-like syndrome, which is fatal in infancy, and is known to be a defect of three particular enzymes.

The differences among these disorders are continuous, with overlap between abnormalities. The range of disease abnormalities may be a result of a corresponding range of peroxisome failure; that is, in severe cases of ZS, the failure is nearly complete, while in IRD, there is some degree of peroxisome activity.

In peroxisomal single-enzyme disorders, the peroxisome is intact and functioning, but there is a defect in only one enzymatic process, with only one corresponding biochemical abnormality. However, these disorders can be as severe as those in which peroxisomal activity is nearly or completely absent.

X-linked adrenoleukodystrophy (X-ALD) is the most common of the peroxisomal disorders, affecting about one in 20,000 males. It is estimated that there are about 1,400 people in the United States with the disorder. In X–ALD there is a deficiency in the enzyme that breaks down VLCFAs, which then accumulate in the myelin and adrenal glands. Onset of X-ALD-related neurological symptoms occurs at about five–12 years of age, with death occurring within one to 10 years after onset of symptoms. In addition to physical abnormalities seen in other types of peroxisomal disorders, common symptoms of X-ALD also include behavioral changes such as abnormal withdrawal or aggression, poor memory, **dementia**, and poor academic performance. Other symptoms are muscle weakness and difficulties with hearing, speech, and vision. As the disease progresses, muscle tone deteriorates, swallowing becomes difficult and the patient becomes comatose. Unless treated with a diet that includes Lorenzo's oil, the disease will result in **paralysis**, **hearing loss**, blindness, **vegetative state**, and death. There are also milder forms of X-ALD: an adult onset ALD that typically begins between the ages of 21 and 35, and a form that is occasionally seen in women who are carriers of the disorder. In addition to X-ALD, there are at least 10 other single-enzyme peroxisomal disorders, each with its own specific abnormalities.

Causes and symptoms

Most peroxisomal disorders are inherited autosomal recessive diseases, with X-ALD as an exception. They occur in all countries, among all races and ethnic groups. They are extremely rare, with frequencies reported at one in 30,000 to one in 150,000, although these numbers are only estimates.

In general, developmental delay, **mental retardation**, and vision and hearing impairment are common in those who have these disorders. Acquisition of speech appears to be especially difficult, and because of the reduced communication abilities, **autism** is common in those who live longer. Peroxisomal disorder patients have decreased muscle tone (hypotonia), which in the most severe cases is generalized, while in less severe cases, is usually restricted to the neck and trunk muscles. Sometimes this lack of control is only noticeable by a curved back in the sitting position. Head control and independent sitting is delayed, with most patients unable to walk independently.

Failure to thrive is a common characteristic of patients with peroxisomal disorder, along with an enlarged liver, abnormalities in liver enzyme function, and loss of fats in stools (steatorrhea).

Peroxisomal disorders are also associated with facial abnormalities, including high forehead, frontal bossing (swelling), small face, low set ears, and slanted eyes. These characteristics may not be prominent in some children, and are especially difficult to identify in an infant.

Diagnosis

Since hearing and vision deficiencies may be difficult to identify in infants, peroxisomal disorders are usually detected by observations of failure to thrive, hypotonia, mental retardation, widely open fontanel, abnormalities in liver enzymes, and an enlarged liver. If peroxisomal disorders are suspected, blood plasma assays for VLCFAs, phytanic acid, and pipecolic acid are conducted. Additional tests include plasmalogen biosynthesis potential.

Treatment

For many of the peroxisomal disorders, there is no standard course of treatment, with supportive treatment strategies focusing on alleviation of complications and symptoms. In general, most treatments that are attempted are dietary, whereby attempts are made to artificially correct biochemical abnormalities associated with the disorders. Therapies include supplementation of the diet with antioxidant **vitamins**, or limitation of intake of fatty acids, especially VLCFAs.

Another area of dietary therapy that is being investigated is the supplementation of the diet with pure DHA, given as early in life as possible, in conjunction with a normal well-balanced diet. Some results have indicated that if given soon enough during development, DHA therapy may prevent some of the devastating consequences of peroxisomal disorders, including brain damage and the loss of vision.

Other treatment strategies include addition of important missing chemicals. For example, in disorders where there is faulty adrenal function, replacement adrenal hormone therapy is used.

Any dietary changes should be monitored biochemically to determine if the supplements are having their desired effects and are not causing additional adverse effects.

Bone marrow transplants may be used to treat X-ALD, and can be effective if done early in the course of the childhood form of the disease.

Physical and psychological therapies are important for all types of peroxisomal disorders.

KEY TERMS

Autosomal recessive inheritance—Two copies of an altered gene located on one of the autosomes must be present for an individual to be affected with the trait or condition determined by that gene:

- an affected individual (homozygote) has two parents who are unaffected but each parent carries the altered gene (heterozygote).

- the risk of two heterozygotes, or carriers, having an affected child is 25%, one in four, for each child that they have; similarly, there is a three in four chance that each child will not be affected.

- males and females are at equal risk for being affected.

- two affected individuals usually produce children, all of whom are affected as well.

Autosome—A chromosome not involved in sex determination.

Fontanel—One of the membranous intervals between the uncompleted angles of the parietal and neighboring bones of a fetal or young skull; so called because it exhibits a rhythmical pulsation.

Metabolic—Relating to the chemical changes in living cells.

Organelle—Specialized structure within a cell, which is separated from the rest of the cell by a membrane composed of lipids and proteins, where chemical and metabolic functions take place.

Alternative treatment

Patients with peroxisomal disorders, and particularly X-ALD, have been treated with a mixture of glycerol trioleate-glycerol trieucate (4:1 by volume), prepared from olive and rapeseed oils, and referred to as Lorenzo's oil (developed by parents of a son, Lorenzo, who had X-ALD, whose story was documented in the 1992 movie, *Lorenzo's Oil*), to decrease the levels of VLCFA. Other **diets** that have been tried include dietary supplementation with plasmalogen precursors to increase plasmalogen levels and with cholic acid to normalize bile acids. However, there has been only limited success demonstrated with the use of these treatments. More research is needed to determine the long-term safety and effectiveness of these treatment strategies.

Prognosis

Peroxisomal disorders range from life-threatening to cases in which people may function with some degree of mental and motor retardation. As of 2001, there was not yet a cure. Enzyme replacement therapies, including enzyme infusion, transplantation, and **gene therapy**, may hold promise for future advances in the treatment of these disorders. Research is being conducted to increase scientific understanding of these disorders and to find ways to prevent, treat, and cure them.

Prevention

Unfortunately not enough is yet known about these diseases to develop comprehensive strategies for prevention. **Genetic counseling** is recommended for known or suspected carriers. As genes are identified that result in the disorders, **genetic testing** is being developed to identify carriers, who then can manage their reproduction to avoid the possibility of children being born with these deficiencies. As the genetic bases for the disorders are defined, prenatal diagnosis and identification of carriers will be facilitated. For example, for X-ALD, diagnosis can be made from cultured skin fibroblasts or amniotic fluid cells. This allows prenatal diagnosis and carrier identification in 90% of those affected. More recently it has been shown that biochemical diagnosis can be performed through chorionic villi biopsy, a procedure performed very early in the first trimester of **pregnancy**.

Animal models of ZS and X-ADL have been developed and are providing researchers with methods to define pathogenic mechanisms and to evaluate new therapies.

Resources

PERIODICALS

Gallo, S., et al. "Late Onset MLD With Normal Nerve Conduction Associated With Two Novel Missense Mutations in the ASA Gene." *Journal of Neurology, Neurosurgery, and Psychiatry* April 2004: 655–658.

Martinez, Manuela. "The Fundamental and Practice of Docosahexanoic Acid Therapy in Peroxisomal Disorders." *Current Opinion in Clinical Nutrition and Metabolic Care* 3 (2000): 101–108.

Martinez, M., E. Vazquez, M. T. Garcia Silva, J. Manzanares, J. M. Bertran, F. Castello, and I. Mougan. "Therapeutic Effects of Docosahexanoic Acid in Patients with Generalized Peroxisomal Disorders." *American Journal of Clinical Nutrition* 71 (2000): 376s–385s.

Moser, Hugo W. "Molecular Genetics of Peroxisomal Disorders." *Frontiers in Bioscience* 5 (March 1, 2001): 298–306.

Raymond, G. V. "Peroxisomal Disorders." *Current Opinion in Pediatrics* 11 (December 1999): 572–576.

ORGANIZATIONS

National Institute of Neurological Disorders and Stroke, NIH Neurological Institute. P.O. Box 5801 Bethesda, MD 20824. (800) 352-9424. < http://www.ninds.nih.gov/index.htm >.

National Organization for Rare Disorders. *P.O. Box 8923, New Fairfield, CT 06812- 8923.*

OTHER

The Peroxisome Website. < http://www.peroxisome.org >.

Judith Sims
Teresa G. Odle

Persantine-thallium heart scan *see* **Thallium heart scan**

Personality disorders

Definition

Personality disorders are a group of mental disturbances defined by the fourth edition, text revision (2000) of the *Diagnostic and Statistical Manual of Mental Disorders* (*DSM-IV*) as "enduring pattern[s] of inner experience and behavior" that are sufficiently rigid and deep-seated to bring a person into repeated conflicts with his or her social and occupational environment. *DSM-IV* specifies that these dysfunctional patterns must be regarded as nonconforming or deviant by the person's culture, and cause significant emotional **pain** and/or difficulties in relationships and occupational performance. In addition, the patient usually sees the disorder as being consistent with his or her self-image (ego-syntonic) and may blame others for his or her social, educational, or work-related problems.

Description

To meet the diagnosis of personality disorder, which is sometimes called character disorder, the patient's problematic behaviors must appear in two or more of the following areas:

- perception and interpretation of the self and other people
- intensity and duration of feelings and their appropriateness to situations
- relationships with others
- ability to control impulses

Personality disorders have their onset in late adolescence or early adulthood. Doctors rarely give a diagnosis of personality disorder to children on the grounds that children's personalities are still in the process of formation and may change considerably by the time they are in their late teens. In retrospect, however, many individuals with personality disorders could be judged to have shown evidence of the problems in childhood.

It is difficult to give close estimates of the percentage of the population that has personality disorders. Patients with certain personality disorders, including antisocial and borderline disorders, are more likely to get into trouble with the law or otherwise attract attention than are patients whose disorders chiefly affect their capacity for intimacy. On the other hand, some patients, such as those with narcissistic or obsessive-compulsive personality disorders, may be outwardly successful because their symptoms are useful within their particular occupations. It has, however, been estimated that about 15% of the general population of the United States has a personality disorder, with higher rates in poor or troubled neighborhoods. The rate of personality disorders among patients in psychiatric treatment is between 30% and 50%. It is possible for patients to have a so-called dual diagnosis; for example, they may have more than one personality disorder, or a personality disorder together with a substance-abuse problem.

By contrast, *DSM-IV* classifies personality disorders into three clusters based on symptom similarities:

- Cluster A (paranoid, schizoid, schizotypal): Patients appear odd or eccentric to others.
- Cluster B (antisocial, borderline, histrionic, narcissistic): Patients appear overly emotional, unstable, or self-dramatizing to others.
- Cluster C (avoidant, dependent, obsessive-compulsive): Patients appear tense and anxiety-ridden to others.

The *DSM-IV* clustering system does not mean that all patients can be fitted neatly into one of the three clusters. It is possible for patients to have symptoms of more than one personality disorder or to have symptoms from different clusters.

Some psychiatrists maintain that the DSM-IV classification is inadequate and should be expanded to include three additional categories: passive-aggressive personality disorder, characterized by a need to control or punish others through frustrating them or sabotaging plans; cyclothymic personality disorder, characterized by intense mood swings alternating between high spirits and moroseness or gloom; and depressive personality disorder, characterized by a negative and pessimistic approach to life.

Since the criteria for personality disorders include friction or conflict between the patient and his or her social environment, these syndromes are open to redefinition as societies change. Successive editions of *DSM* have tried to be sensitive to cultural differences, including changes over time, when defining personality disorders. One category that had been proposed for *DSM-III-R,* self-defeating personality disorder, was excluded from *DSM-IV* on the grounds that its definition reflected prejudice against women. *DSM-IV* recommends that doctors take a patient's background, especially recent immigration, into account before deciding that he or she has a personality disorder. One criticism that has been made of the general category of personality disorder is that it is based on Western notions of individual uniqueness. Its applicability to people from cultures with different definitions of human personhood is thus open to question. Furthermore, even within a culture, it can be difficult to define the limits of "normalcy."

The personality disorders defined by *DSM-IV* are as follows:

Paranoid

Patients with paranoid personality disorder are characterized by suspiciousness and a belief that others are out to harm or cheat them. They have problems with intimacy and may join cults or groups with paranoid belief systems. Some are litigious, bringing lawsuits against those they believe have wronged them. Although not ordinarily delusional, these patients may develop psychotic symptoms under severe **stress**. It is estimated that 0.5–2.5% of the general population meet the criteria for paranoid personality disorder.

Schizoid

Schizoid patients are perceived by others as "loners" without close family relationships or social contacts. Indeed, they are aloof and really do prefer to be alone. They may appear cold to others because they rarely display strong emotions. They may, however, be successful in occupations that do not require personal interaction. About 2% of the general population has this disorder. It is slightly more common in men than in women.

Schizotypal

Patients diagnosed as schizotypal are often considered odd or eccentric because they pay little attention to their clothing and sometimes have peculiar speech mannerisms. They are socially isolated and uncomfortable in parties or other social gatherings. In addition, people with schizotypal personality disorder often have oddities of thought, including "magical" beliefs or peculiar ideas (for example, a belief in telepathy or UFOs) that are outside of their cultural norms. It is thought that 3% of the general population has schizotypal personality disorder. It is slightly more common in males. Schizotypal disorder should not be confused with **schizophrenia**, although there is some evidence that the disorders are genetically related.

Antisocial

Patients with antisocial personality disorder are sometimes referred to as sociopaths or psychopaths. They are characterized by lying, manipulativeness, and a selfish disregard for the rights of others; some may act impulsively. People with antisocial personality disorder are frequently chemically dependent and sexually promiscuous. It is estimated that 3% of males in the general population and 1% of females have antisocial personality disorder.

Borderline

Patients with borderline personality disorder (BPD) are highly unstable, with wide mood swings, a history of intense but stormy relationships, impulsive behavior, and confusion about career goals, personal values, or sexual orientation. These often highly conflictual ideas may correspond to an even deeper confusion about their sense of self (identity). People with BPD frequently cut or burn themselves, or threaten or attempt **suicide**. Many of these patients have histories of severe childhood **abuse** or neglect. About 2% of the general population have BPD; 75% of these patients are female.

Histrionic

Patients diagnosed with this disorder impress others as overly emotional, overly dramatic, and hungry for attention. They may be flirtatious or seductive as a way of drawing attention to themselves, yet they are emotionally shallow. Histrionic patients often live in a romantic fantasy world and are easily bored with routine. About 2–3% of the population is thought to have this disorder. Although historically the disorder has been more associated with women in clinical settings, there may be bias toward diagnosing women with the histrionic personality disorder.

Narcissistic

Narcissistic patients are characterized by self-importance, a craving for admiration, and exploitative attitudes toward others. They have unrealistically inflated views of their talents and accomplishments, and may become extremely angry if they are criticized or outshone by others. Narcissists may be professionally successful but rarely have long-lasting intimate relationships. Fewer than 1% of the population has this disorder; about 75% of those diagnosed with it are male.

Avoidant

Patients with avoidant personality disorder are fearful of rejection and shy away from situations or occupations that might expose their supposed inadequacy. They may reject opportunities to develop close relationships because of their fears of criticism or humiliation. Patients with this personality disorder are often diagnosed with dependent personality disorder as well. Many also fit the criteria for social phobia. Between 0.5–1.0% of the population have avoidant personality disorder.

Dependent

Dependent patients are afraid of being on their own and typically develop submissive or compliant behaviors in order to avoid displeasing people. They are afraid to question authority and often ask others for guidance or direction. Dependent personality disorder is diagnosed more often in women, but it has been suggested that this finding reflects social pressures on women to conform to gender stereotyping or bias on the part of clinicians.

Obsessive-compulsive

Patients diagnosed with this disorder are preoccupied with keeping order, attaining perfection, and maintaining mental and interpersonal control. They may spend a great deal of time adhering to plans, schedules, or rules from which they will not deviate, even at the expense of openness, flexibility, and efficiency. These patients are often unable to relax and may become "workaholics." They may have problems in employment as well as in intimate relationships because they are very stiff and formal, and insist on doing everything their way. About 1% of the population has obsessive-compulsive personality disorder; the male/female ratio is about 2:1.

Causes and symptoms

Personality disorders are thought to result from a bad interface, so to speak, between a child's temperament and character on one hand and his or her family environment on the other. Temperament can be defined as a person's innate or biologically shaped basic disposition. Human infants vary in their sensitivity to light or noise, their level of physical activity, their adaptability to schedules, and similar traits. Even such traits as **shyness** or novelty-seeking may be at least in part determined by the biology of the brain and the genes one inherits.

Character is defined as the set of attitudes and behavior patterns that the individual acquires or learns over time. It includes such personal qualities as work and study habits, moral convictions, neatness or cleanliness, and consideration of others. Since children must learn to adapt to their specific families, they may develop personality disorders in the course of struggling to survive psychologically in disturbed or stressful families. For example, nervous or high-strung parents might be unhappy with a baby who is very active and try to restrain him or her at every opportunity. The child might then develop an avoidant personality disorder as the outcome of coping with constant frustration and parental disapproval. As another example, **child abuse** is believed to play a role in shaping borderline personality disorder. One reason that some therapists use the term developmental damage instead of personality disorder is that it takes the presumed source of the person's problems into account.

Some patients with personality disorders come from families that appear to be stable and healthy. It has been suggested that these patients are biologically hypersensitive to normal family stress levels. Levels of the brain chemical (neurotransmitter) dopamine may influence a person's level of novelty-seeking, and serotonin levels may influence aggression.

Other factors that have been cited as affecting children's personality development are the mass media and social or group **hysteria**, particularly after the events of September 11, 2001. Cases of so-called mass sociogenic illness have been identified, in which a group of children began to vomit or have other physical symptoms brought on in response to an imaginary threat. In two such cases, the children were reacting to the suggestion that toxic fumes were spreading through their school. Some authors believe that overly frequent or age-inappropriate discussions of terrorist attacks or bioterrorism may make children more susceptible to sociogenic illness as well as other distortions of personality.

Diagnosis

Diagnosis of personality disorders is complicated by the fact that affected persons rarely seek help until they are in serious trouble or until their families (or the law) pressure them to get treatment. The reason for this slowness is that the problematic traits are so deeply entrenched that they seem normal (ego-syntonic) to the patient. Diagnosis of a personality disorder depends in part on the patient's age. Although personality disorders originate during the childhood years, they are considered adult disorders. Some patients, in fact, are not diagnosed until late in life because their symptoms had been modified by the demands of their job or by marriage. After retirement or the spouse's **death**, however, these patients' personality disorders become fully apparent. In general, however, if the onset of the patient's problem is in mid- or late-life, the doctor will rule out **substance abuse** or personality change caused by medical or neurological problems before considering the diagnosis of a personality disorder. It is unusual for people to develop personality disorders "out of the blue" in mid-life.

There are no tests that can provide a definitive diagnosis of personality disorder. Most doctors will evaluate a patient on the basis of several sources of information collected over a period of time in order to determine how long the patient has been having difficulties, how many areas of life are affected, and how severe the dysfunction is. These sources of information may include:

Interviews

The doctor may schedule two or three interviews with the patient, spaced over several weeks or months, in order to rule out an adjustment disorder caused by job loss, **bereavement**, or a similar problem. An office interview allows the doctor to form an impression of the patient's overall personality as well as obtain information about his or her occupation and family. During the interview, the doctor will note the patient's appearance, tone of voice, body language, eye contact, and other important non-verbal signals, as well as the content of the conversation. In some cases, the doctor may contact other people (family members, employers, close friends) who know the patient well in order to assess the accuracy of the patient's perception of his or her difficulties. It is quite common for people with personality disorders to have distorted views of their situations or to be unaware of the impact of their behavior on others.

Psychologic testing

Doctors use psychologic testing to help in the diagnosis of a personality disorder. Most of these tests require interpretation by a professional with specialized training. Doctors usually refer patients to a clinical psychologist for this type of test.

PERSONALITY INVENTORIES. Personality inventories are tests with true/false or yes/no answers that can be used to compare the patient's scores with those of people with known personality distortions. The single most commonly used test of this type is the Minnesota Multiphasic Personality Inventory, or MMPI. Another test that is often used is the Millon Clinical Multiaxial Inventory, or MCMI.

PROJECTIVE TESTS. Projective tests are unstructured. Unstructured means that instead of giving one-word answers to questions, the patient is asked to talk at some length about a picture that the psychologist has shown him or her, or to supply an ending for the beginning of a story. Projective tests allow the clinician to assess the patient's patterns of thinking, fantasies, worries or anxieties, moral concerns, values, and habits. Common projective tests include the Rorschach, in which the patient responds to a set of ten inkblots; and the Thematic Apperception Test (TAT), in which the patient is shown drawings of people in different situations and then tells a story about the picture.

Treatment

At one time psychiatrists thought that personality disorders did not respond very well to treatment. This opinion was derived from the notion that human personality is fixed for life once it has been molded in childhood, and from the belief among people with personality disorders that their own views and behaviors are correct, and that others are the ones at fault. More recently, however, doctors have recognized that humans can continue to grow and change throughout life. Most patients with personality disorders are now considered to be treatable, although the degree of improvement may vary. The type of treatment recommended depends on the personality characteristics associated with the specific disorder.

Hospitalization

Inpatient treatment is rarely required for patients with personality disorders, with two major exceptions: borderline patients who are threatening suicide or suffering from drug or alcohol withdrawal; and patients with paranoid personality disorder who are having psychotic symptoms.

Psychotherapy

Psychoanalytic psychotherapy is suggested for patients who can benefit from insight-oriented treatment. These patients typically include those with dependent, obsessive-compulsive, and avoidant personality disorders. Doctors usually recommend individual psychotherapy for narcissistic and borderline patients, but often refer these patients to therapists with specialized training in these disorders. Psychotherapeutic treatment for personality disorders may take as long as three to five years.

Insight-oriented approaches are not recommended for patients with paranoid or antisocial personality disorders. These patients are likely to resent the therapist and see him or her as trying to control or dominate them.

Supportive therapy is regarded as the most helpful form of psychotherapy for patients with schizoid personality disorder.

Cognitive-behavioral therapy

Cognitive-behavioral approaches are often recommended for patients with avoidant or dependent personality disorders. Patients in these groups typically have mistaken beliefs about their competence or likableness. These assumptions can be successfully challenged by cognitive-behavioral methods. More recently, Aaron Beck and his coworkers have successfully extended their approach to cognitive therapy to all ten personality disorders as defined by DSM-IV.

Group therapy

Group therapy is frequently useful for patients with schizoid or avoidant personality disorders because it helps them to break out of their social isolation. It has also been recommended for patients with histrionic and antisocial personality disorders. These patients tend to act out, and pressure from peers in group treatment can motivate them to change. Because patients with antisocial personality disorder can destabilize groups that include people with other disorders, it is usually best if these people meet exclusively with others who have APD (in homogeneous groups).

Family therapy

Family therapy may be suggested for patients whose personality disorders cause serious problems for members of their families. It is also sometimes recommended for borderline patients from overinvolved or possessive families.

Medications

Medications may be prescribed for patients with specific personality disorders. The type of medication depends on the disorder. In general, however, patients with personality disorders are helped only moderately by medications.

ANTIPSYCHOTIC DRUGS. Antipsychotic drugs, such as haloperidol (Haldol), may be given to patients with paranoid personality disorder if they are having brief psychotic episodes. Patients with borderline or schizotypal personality disorder are sometimes given antipsychotic drugs in low doses; however, the efficacy of these drugs in treating personality disorder is less clear than in schizophrenia.

MOOD STABILIZERS. Carbamazepine (Tegretol) is a drug that is commonly used to treat seizures, but is also helpful for borderline patients with rage outbursts and similar behavioral problems. Lithium and valproate may also be used as mood stabilizers, especially among people with borderline personality disorder.

ANTIDEPRESSANTS AND ANTI-ANXIETY MEDICATIONS. Medications in these categories are sometimes prescribed for patients with schizoid personality disorder to help them manage **anxiety** symptoms while they are in psychotherapy. Antidepressants are also commonly used to treat people with borderline personality disorder.

Treatment with medications is not recommended for patients with avoidant, histrionic, dependent, or narcissistic personality disorders. The use of potentially addictive medications should be avoided in people with borderline or antisocial personality disorders. However, some avoidant patients who also have social phobia may benefit from monoamine oxidase inhibitors (MAO inhibitors), a particular class of antidepressant.

Prognosis

The prognosis for recovery depends in part on the specific disorder. Although some patients improve as they grow older and have positive experiences in life, personality disorders are generally life-long disturbances with periods of worsening (exacerbations) and periods of improvement (remissions). Others, particularly schizoid patients, have better prognoses if they are given appropriate treatment. Beck and his coworkers estimate that effective cognitive therapy with patients with personality disorders takes two to three years on average. Patients with paranoid personality disorder are at some risk for developing delusional disorders or schizophrenia.

The personality disorders with the poorest prognoses are the antisocial and the borderline. Borderline patients are at high risk for developing substance abuse disorders or bulimia. About 80% of

KEY TERMS

Character—An individual's set of emotional, cognitive, and behavioral patterns learned and accumulated over time.

Character disorder—Another name for personality disorder.

Cognitive therapy—A form of psychotherapy that focuses on changing people's patterns of emotional reaction by correcting distorted patterns of thinking and perception.

Developmental damage—A term that some therapists prefer to personality disorder, on the grounds that it is more respectful of the patient's capacity for growth and change.

Ego-syntonic—Consistent with one's sense of self, as opposed to ego-alien or dystonic (foreign to one's sense of self). Ego-syntonic traits typify patients with personality disorders.

Neuroleptic—Another name for older antipsychotic medications, such as haloperidol. The term does not apply to such newer atypical agents as clozapine (Clozaril).

Personality—The organized pattern of behaviors and attitudes that makes a human being distinctive. Personality is formed by the ongoing interaction of temperament, character, and environment.

Projective tests—Psychological tests that probe into personality by obtaining open-ended responses to such materials as pictures or stories. Projective tests are often used to evaluate patients with personality disorders.

Rorschach test—A well-known projective test that requires the patient to describe what he or she sees in each of 10 inkblots. It is named for the Swiss psychiatrist who invented it.

Temperament—A person's natural or genetically determined disposition.

children at risk. High-risk groups include abused children, children from troubled families, children with close relatives diagnosed with personality disorders, children of substance abusers, and children who grow up in cults or extremist political groups.

Resources

BOOKS

American Psychiatric Association. *Diagnostic and Statistical Manual of Mental Disorders.* 4th ed., revised. Washington, D.C.: American Psychiatric Association, 2000.

Beck, Aaron T., Arthur Freeman, Denise D. Davis, et al. *Cognitive Therapy of Personality Disorders.* 2nd ed. New York: The Guilford Press, 2004.

Beers, Mark H., MD, and Robert Berkow, MD., editors. "Personality Disorders." In *The Merck Manual of Diagnosis and Therapy.* Whitehouse Station, NJ: Merck Research Laboratories, 2004.

PERIODICALS

Battle, C. L., M. T. Shea, D. M. Johnson, et al. "Childhood Maltreatment Associated with Adult Personality Disorders: Findings from the Collaborative Longitudinal Personality Disorders Study." *Journal of Personality Disorders* 18 (April 2004): 193–211.

Bienenfeld, David, MD. "Personality Disorders." *eMedicine* August 18, 2004. < http://www.emedicine.com/med/topic3472.htm >.

Doyle, C. R., J. Akhtar, R. Mrvos, and E. P. Krenzelok. "Mass Sociogenic Illness—Real and Imaginary." *Veterinary and Human Toxicology* 46 (April 2004): 93–95.

Gutheil, T. G. "Suicide, Suicide Litigation, and Borderline Personality Disorder." *Journal of Personality Disorders* 18 (June 2004): 248–256.

Jordan, A. "The Role of Media in Children's Development: An Ecological Perspective." *Journal of Developmental and Behavioral Pediatrics* 25 (June 2004): 196–206.

ORGANIZATIONS

American Academy of Child and Adolescent Psychiatry (AACAP). 3615 Wisconsin Avenue, NW, Washington, DC 20016-3007. (202) 966-7300. Fax: (202) 966-2891. < http://www.aacap.org >.

American Psychiatric Association (APA). 1400 K Street, NW, Washington, DC 20005. < http://www.psych.org >.

National Institute of Mental Health (NIMH). 6001 Executive Boulevard, Room 8184, MSC 9663, Bethesda, MD 20892-9663. (301) 443-4513. < http://www.nimh.nih.gov >.

Rebecca J. Frey, PhD

hospitalized borderline patients attempt suicide at some point during treatment, and about 5% succeed in committing suicide. Borderline patients are also the most likely to sue their mental health professional for malpractice.

Prevention

The most effective preventive strategy for personality disorders is early identification and treatment of

Perthes disease *see* **Osteochondroses**

Pertussis *see* **Whooping cough**

Pervasive developmental disorders

Definition

Pervasive developmental disorders include five different conditions: Asperger's syndrome, autistic disorder, childhood disintegrative disorder (CDD), pervasive developmental disorder not otherwise specified (PDDNOS), and Rett's syndrome. They are grouped together because of the similarities between them. The three most common shared problems involve communication skills, motor skills, and social skills. Since there are no clear diagnostic boundaries separating these conditions it is sometimes difficult to distinguish one from the other for diagnostic purposes.

Asperger's syndrome, autistic disorder, and childhood disintegrative disorder are four to five times more common in boys, and Rett's syndrome has been diagnosed primarily in girls. All of these disorders are rare.

Description

Asperger's syndrome

Children afflicted with Asperger's syndrome exhibit difficulties in social relationships and communication. They are reluctant to make eye contact, do not respond to social or emotional contacts, do not initiate play activities with peers, and do not give or receive attention or affection. To receive this diagnosis the individual must demonstrate normal development of language, thinking and coping skills. Due to an impaired coordination of muscle movements, they appear to be clumsy. They usually become deeply involved in very few interests, which tend to occupy most of their time and attention.

Autistic disorder

Autistic disorder is frequently evident within the first year of life, and must be diagnosed before age three. It is associated with moderate **mental retardation** in three out of four cases. These children do not want to be held, rocked, cuddled or played with. They are unresponsive to affection, show no interest in peers or adults and have few interests. Other traits include avoidance of eye contact, an expressionless face and the use of gestures to express needs. Their actions are repetitive, routine and restricted. Rocking, hand and arm flapping, unusual hand and finger movements, and attachment to objects rather than pets and people

are common. Speech, play, and other behaviors are repetitive and without imagination. They tend to be overactive, aggressive, and self-injurious. They are often highly sensitive to touch, noise, and smells and do not like changes in routine. **Autism** and several disorders classified with it have increased significantly in recent years so that they now are diagnosed more often in children than **spina bifida**, **cancer**, or **Down syndrome**. This may be due partly to improved recognition and diagnosis.

Childhood disintegrative disorder

Childhood disintegrative disorder is also called Heller's disease and most often develops between two and ten years of age. Children with CDD develop normally until two to three years of age and then begin to disintegrate rapidly. Signs and symptoms include deterioration of the ability to use and understand language to the point where they are unable to carry on a conversation. This is accompanied by loss of control of the bladder and bowels. Any interest or ability to play and engage in social activities is lost. The behaviors are nearly identical with those that are characteristic of autistic disorder. However, childhood disintegrative disorder becomes evident later in life and results in developmental regression, or loss of previously attained skills, whereas autistic disorder can be detected as early as the first month of life and results in a failure to progress.

Pervasive developmental disorder not otherwise specified

The term pervasive developmental disorder not otherwise specified (PDDNOS) is also referred to as atypical personality development, atypical PDD, or atypical autism. Individuals with this disorder share some of the same signs and symptoms of autism or other conditions under the category of pervasive developmental disorders, but do not meet all of the criteria for diagnosis for any of the four syndromes included in this group of diseases. Because the children diagnosed with PDDNOS do not all exhibit the same combination of characteristics, it is difficult to do research on this disorder, but the limited evidence available suggests that patients are seen by medical professionals later in life than is the case for autistic children, and they are less likely to have intellectual deficits.

Rett's syndrome

Rett's syndrome was first described in 1966 and is found almost exclusively in girls. It is a disease in which cells in the brain experience difficulty in communicating with each other. At the same time the growth of the head falls behind the growth of the body so that these children are usually mentally retarded. These conditions are accompanied by deficits in movement (motor) skills and a loss of interest in social activities.

The course of the illness has been divided into four stages. In stage one the child develops normally for six to 18 months. In stage two, development slows down and stops. Stage three is characterized by a loss of the speech and motor skills already acquired. Typically this happens between nine months and three years of age. Stage four begins with a return to learning that will continue across the lifespan, but at a very slow rate. Problems with coordination and walking are likely to continue and even worsen. Other conditions that can occur with Rett's syndrome are convulsions, **constipation**, breathing problems, impaired circulation in the feet and legs, and difficulty chewing or swallowing.

Causes and symptoms

The causes of these disorders are unknown although brain structure abnormalities, genetic mutation, and alterations in brain function are believed to play a role. Still, no single brain abnormality or location has been connected to a cause. In 2004, scientists reported finding the gene mutation (on gene MECP2) that is present in 80% of people affected with Rett's syndrome. In 2004, comprehensive review of research on twins revealed that interactions between multiple genes may play a role in the cause of autism. A number of neurological conditions, such as convulsions, are commonly found to accompany these disorders.

Diagnosis

The diagnosis of pervasive developmental disorder is made by medical specialists based on a thorough examination of the patient, including observing behavior and gathering information from parents and caregivers. Because many symptoms are common to more than one condition, distinctions between conditions must be carefully made. The following summary describes the distinction between three common disorders.

PDDNOS:

• impairment of two-way social interaction

• Repetitive and predictable behavior patterns and activities

Autism:

• all listed for PDDNOS

• severe impairment in communication

• abnormal social interaction and use of language for social communication or imaginative play before age of three

• not better accounted for by another psychiatric order

Asperger's disorder:

• all listed for PDDNOS

• clinically significant impairment in social, occupational, or other areas of functioning

• no general delay in language

• no delay in cognitive development, self-help skills, or adaptive behavior

• not better accounted for by another pervasive developmental disorder or schizophrenia

Rett's syndrome:

• a period of normal development between 6–18 months

• normal head circumference at birth, followed by a slowing of head growth

• retardation

• repetitive hand movements

CDD:

• normal development for at least two years

• loss of skills in at least two of the following areas: language, social skills, bowel or bladder control, play, movement skills

• abnormal functioning in at least two of the following areas: social interaction, communication, behavior patterns

• not better accounted for by another PDD or mental illness

Treatment

Treatment for children with pervasive developmental disorders is limited. Those who can be enrolled in educational programs will need a highly structured learning environment, a teacher-student ratio of not more than 1:2, and a high level of parental involvement that provides consistent care at home. Psychotherapy and social skills training can prove helpful to some. There is no specific medication available for treating the core symptoms of any of these disorders, though research is promising. Some psychiatric medications may be helpful in controlling particular behavior difficulties, such as agitation, mood instability, and self-injury. Music, massage, and **hydrotherapy** may exert a calming effect on behavior. Treatment may also include physical and occupational therapy.

Prognosis

In general, the prognosis in all of these conditions is tied to the severity of the illness.

The prognosis for Asperger's syndrome is more hopeful than that for other diseases in this cluster. These children are likely to grow up to be functional independent adults, but will always have problems with social relationships. They are also at greater risk for developing serious mental illness than the general population.

The prognosis for autistic disorder is not as good, although great strides have been made in recent years in its treatment. The higher the patient's IQ (intelligence quotient) and ability to communicate, the better the prognosis. However, many patients will always need some level of custodial care. In the past, most of these individuals were confined to institutions, but many are now able to live in group homes or supervised apartments. The prognosis for childhood disintegrative disorder is even less favorable. These children will require intensive and long-term care. Children diagnosed with PDDNOS have a better prognosis because their initial symptoms are usually milder, IQ scores are higher, and language development is stronger.

Prevention

The causes of pervasive developmental disorders are not understood, although research efforts are getting closer to understanding the problem. Until the causes are discovered, it will remain impossible to prevent these conditions.

Resources

PERIODICALS

"MECP2 Open Reading Framd Defines Protein Linked to Rett Syndrome." *Biotech Week* June 9, 2004: 300.
Muhle, Rebecca, Stephanie V. Trentacoste, and Isabelle Rapin. "The Genetics of Autism." *Pediatrics* May 2004: 1389–1391.

ORGANIZATIONS

Autism Society of America. 7910 Woodmont Avenue, Suite 300, Bethesda, Maryland 20814-3067. (800) 328-8476. < http://www.autism-society.org >.
International Rett Syndrome Association. 9121 Piscataway Road, Suite 2B, Clinton, MD 20735. (800) 818-7388. < http://www.rettsyndrome.org >.
Learning Disabilities Association of America. 4156 Library Road, Pittsburg, PA 15234. (412) 341-1515. < http://www.ldanatl.org >.
National Organization for Rare Disorders. P.O. Box 8923, New Fairfield, CT 06812-8923. (800) 999-6673. < http://www.rarediseases.org >.

OTHER

Boyle, Thomas D. "Diagnosing Autism and Other Pervasive Personality Disorders." *INJersye.com Page*. < http://www.injersey.com >.
"Childhood Disintegrative Disorder." *HealthAnswers.com*. < http://www.healthanswers.com/database/ami/converted/001535.html >.
"Information on Childhood Disintegrative Disorder." *Yale-New Haven Medical Center Page*. < http://info.med.yale.edu >.
The International Rett Syndrome Association. 9121 Piscataway Road, Suite 2B, Clinton, MD 20735. (800) 818-7388 < http://www.rettsyndrome.org >.
Koenig, Kathy. "Frequently Asked Questions." *Yale-New Haven Medical Center Page*. < http://info.med.yale.edu >.

Donald G. Barstow, RN
Teresa G. Odle

PET scan *see* **Positron emission tomography (PET)**

Pet therapy

Definition

Animal-assisted therapy (AAT), also known as pet therapy, utilizes trained animals and handlers to

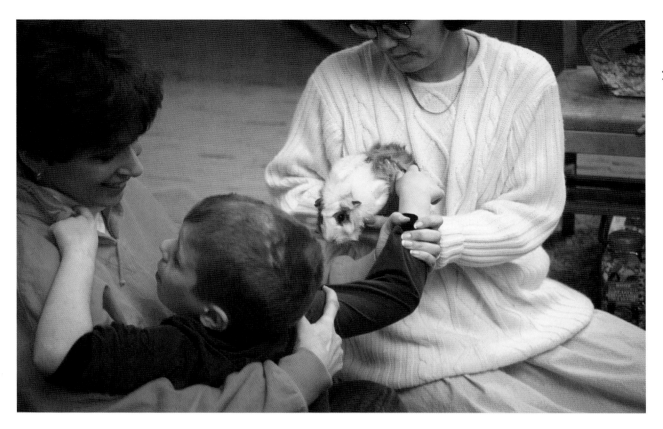

This autistic child is encouraged to interact with the guinea pig in an effort to improve his social interaction. *(Helen B. Senisi. Photo Researchers, Inc. Reproduced by permission.)*

achieve specific physical, social, cognitive, and emotional goals with patients.

Purpose

Studies have shown that physical contact with a pet can lower high blood pressure, and improve survival rates for **heart attack** victims. There is also evidence that petting an animal can cause endorphins to be released. Endorphins are chemicals in the body that suppress the **pain** response. These are benefits that can be enjoyed from pet ownership, as well as from visiting therapeutic animals.

Many skills can be learned or improved with the assistance of a therapy animal. Patient rehabilitation can be encouraged by such activities as walking or running with a dog, or throwing objects for the animal to retrieve. Fine motor skills may be developed by petting, grooming, or feeding the animal. Patient communication is encouraged by the response of the animal to either verbal or physical commands. Activities such as writing or talking about the therapy animals or past pets also develop cognitive skills and

communication. Creative inclusion of an animal in the life or therapy of a patient can make a major difference in the patient's comfort, progress, and recovery.

Description

Origins

The enjoyment of animals as companions dates back many centuries, perhaps even to prehistoric times. The first known therapeutic use of animals started in Gheel, Belgium in the ninth century. In this town, learning to care for farm animals has long been an important part of an assisted living program designed for people with disabilities.

Some of the earliest uses of animal-assisted healing in the United States were for psychiatric patients. The presence of the therapy animals produced a beneficial effect on both children and adults with mental health issues. It is only in the last few decades that AAT has been more formally applied in a variety of therapeutic settings, including schools and prisons, as well as hospitals, hospices, nursing homes, and outpatient care programs.

The way in which AAT is undertaken depends on the needs and abilities of the individual patient. Dogs are the most common visiting therapy animals, but cats, horses, birds, rabbits, and other domestic pets can be used as long as they are appropriately screened and trained.

For patients who are confined, small animals can be brought to the bed if the patient is willing and is not allergic to the animal. A therapeutic plan may include a simple interaction aimed at improving communication and small motor skills, or a demonstration with educational content to engage the patient cognitively.

If the patient is able to walk or move around, more options are available. Patients can walk small animals outside, or learn how to care for farm animals. Both of these activities develop confidence and motor abilities. Horseback riding has recently gained great therapeutic popularity. It offers an opportunity to work on balance, trunk control, and other skills. Many patients who walk with difficulty, or not at all, get great emotional benefit from interacting with and controlling a large animal.

One advantage of having volunteers provide this service is that cost and insurance are not at issue.

Precautions

AAT does not involve just any pet interacting with a patient. Standards for the training of the volunteers and their animals are crucial in order to promote a safe, positive experience for the patient. Trained volunteers will understand how to work with other medical professionals to set goals for the patient and keep records of progress. Animals that have been appropriately trained are well socialized to people, other animals, and medical equipment. They are not distracted by the food and odors that may be present in the therapy environment and will not chew inappropriate objects or mark territory.

Animals participating in AAT should be covered by some form of liability insurance.

Research and general acceptance

While the research evidence supporting the efficacy of AAT is slim, the anecdotal support is vast. Although it may not be given much credence by medical personnel as a therapy with the potential to assist the progress of the patients, some institutions do at least allow it as something that will uplift the patients or distract them from their discomforts.

Resources

ORGANIZATIONS

Delta Society. < http://www.deltasociety.org >.

Judith Turner

Peyronie's disease

Definition

Peyronie's disease is a condition characterized by a bent penis.

Description

The cause of Peyronie's disease is unknown and the disease is often difficult to treat. For some reason, a thick scar develops in the penis and bends it. Almost a third of patients with Peyronie's disease also have similar contracting **scars** on their hands, a disease called Dupuytren's contractures. Some cases are associated with diabetes, and others appear after prostate surgery. Because prostate surgery always requires a catheter in the bladder, there is some suspicion that catheters can cause the scarring. However, many cases of Peyronie's disease arise without any use of a catheter. There is also a congenital form of penile deviation, again with no known cause. Most of the scars are located in the mid-line, therefore most of the angulations are either up or down.

Causes and symptoms

Peyronie's disease occurs in about 1% of men, most of them between 45–60 years old. Although there is no good research data to back it up, the suspicion exists that Peyronie's disease is the result of injury. If not a catheter, then sudden, forceful bending

KEY TERMS

Catheter—A flexible tube placed into a body vessel or cavity.

Congenital—Present at birth.

Plastic surgery—The restoring and reshaping of the skin and its appendages to improve their function and appearance.

Prostate—A gland that surrounds the outlet to the male bladder.

Prosthesis—Artificial substitute for a body part.

during sexual intercourse could easily tear the supporting tissues and lead to scarring.

The symptom is bending of an erect penis, sometimes with **pain**. It often interferes with sexual intercourse. Erectile failure associated with the angulation often precedes it.

Treatment

Attempts have been made to reduce the angulation with injections of cortisone-like drugs directly into the scar, but they are rarely successful. Surgery seems to be the better answer. After the scar is removed, plastic repair of the penis is attempted, often with a graft of tissue from somewhere else on the body. The Nesbit procedure is one of the more successful methods of doing this. The other surgical approach is to implant a penile prosthesis that overcomes the angulation mechanically. Results with these procedures are reported to be 60–80% satisfactory, including the return of orgasm.

Prognosis

Sometimes the condition disappears spontaneously. A careful look for other causes of impotence should be done before surgery.

Resources

BOOKS

Jordan, Gerald H., et al. "Surgery of the Penis and Urethra." In *Campbell's Urology*, edited by Patrick C. Walsh, et al. Philadelphia: W. B. Saunders Co., 1998.

J. Ricker Polsdorfer, MD

Pharmacogenetics

Definition

Pharmacogenetics is the study of how the actions of and reactions to drugs vary with the patient's genes.

Description

Genes are the portions of chromosomes that determine many of the traits in every living thing. In humans, genes influence race, hair and eye color, gender, height, weight, aspects of behavior, and even the likelihood of developing certain diseases. Although some traits are a combination of genetics and environment, researchers are still discovering new ways in which people are affected by their genes.

Pharmacogenetics is the study of how people respond to drug therapy. Although this science is still new, there have been many useful discoveries. It has long been known that genes influence the risk of developing certain diseases, or that genes could determine traits such as hair and eye color. Genes can also alter the risk of developing different diseases. It has long been known that people of African descent were more likely to have sickle cell anemia than people of other races. People of Armenian, Arab, and Turkish heritage are more prone to familiar Mediterranean **fever** than people of other nationalities. More recently, discoveries have shown that genes can determine other aspects of each individual, down to the level of the enzymes produced in the liver. Since these enzymes determine how quickly a drug is removed from the body, they can make major differences in the way people respond to drugs. Some of the most basic work concerns the way race and gender influence drug reactions—and race and gender are genetically determined.

Women often respond differently than men to drugs at the same dose levels. For example, women are more likely to have a good response to the **antidepressant drugs** that act as serotonin specific reuptake inhibitors (SSRIs, the group that includes Prozac and Paxil) than they are to the older group of **tricyclic antidepressants** (the group that includes Elavil and Tofranil). Women have a greater response to some narcotic **pain** reliving drugs than do men, but get less relief from some non-narcotic pain medications. Women may show a greater response to some steroid hormones than men do, but have a lower level of response to some anti-anxiety medications than men.

Race may also affect the way people respond to some medications. In this case, race implies specific genetic factors that are generally, but not always, found among members of specific ethnic groups. For example, the angiotensin II inhibitor enalopril (Vasotec), which is used to lower blood pressure, works better in Caucasians than in Blacks. Carvedilol (Coreg), a beta-adrenergic blocking agent that is also used to lower blood pressure, is more effective than other drugs in the same class when used to treat Black patients. Black patients with **heart failure** appear to respond better to a combination of hydralazine and isosorbide than do Caucasian patients using the same medication.

More specific research has identified individual genes than may influence drugs response, without relying on group information such as gender and race. Specific genes have been identified that may determine how patients will respond to specific drugs. For example, some genes may determine whether people will get pain relief from codeine, or how well they will respond to drugs used to treat **cancer**.

Causes and symptoms

Genes alter responses to drugs because the genes influence many parts of the body iteself. One of the simplest examples is the gene that influences body weight. Since many drugs are soluble in body fat, people with large amounts of fat will have these drug deposited into their fat stores. This means that there are lower levels of the drug that can reach the actual organs on which they work.

In the case of gender responses to antidepressants, women show greater response to serotonin specific antidepressants because women naturally have lower levels of serotonin than men do. This makes women more likely to develop a type of depression marked by low serotonin levels, but it also means that women will respond better to replacement of serotonin.

Because people of the same race carry similar genes, studies based on race were the earliest types of pharmacogenetic studies. One study evaluated the levels of alcohol dehydrogenase in people of different nationalities. This is an enzyme involved in the metabolism of alcohol. When people with high levels of this enzyme, or people in whom the enzyme acts more rapidly than in other people, drink alcohol, they are subject to facial flushing and slowing of the heartbeat. The activity of this enzyme is determined by genetics, and different levels can be seen in different races because these people belong to the same gene pools.

Among Asiatic people, 85% have high levels of this enzyme, compared to 20% of Swiss people, and only 5–10% of British people.

Another trait that is influenced by genes is a liver enzyme, CYP2D6. This enzyme metabolizes some drugs, convert them to a form that can be removed from the body. Genes determine the level of this enzyme in the liver. People with low levels of CYP2D6 will metabolize drugs slowly. Slow metabolism means the drugs will act for a longer period of time. Slow metabolizers reaspond to smaller doses of medications that are eliminated by this enzyme, while fast metabolizers, people who have a lot of the enzyme, will need larger drug doses to get the same effects. At the same time, low levels of CYP2D6 means that people taking the drugs that are metabolized by this enzyme will have higher drug levels, and are more likely to have unwanted side effects.

Another enzyme that can be important in drug dosing is called 2C9, and this enzyme is responsible for metabolizing the anticoagulant drug warfarin (Coumadin). Most people take warfarin in a dose of about 5 milligrams a day, but people who have low levels of 2C9 normally require a dose of only 1–5 milligrams a week.

Yet another mechanism of drug activity is the presence or absence of a specific drug receptor site. Drugs act by binding to specific chemicals, receptor sites, within body cells. Genes may help determine how many of these cells there are. The action of the widely used antipsychotic drug haloperidol (Haldol) depends on its ability to bind to the dopamine (D2) receptor site. The number of these sites are determined by genetics. In one study, 63% of patients whose genes caused a large number of these receptor sites had a response to treatment with haloperidol, while only about 29% of patients with a smaller number of dopamine (D2) receptor sites did well on the drug.

Other genetic studies indicate that genes may affect how people respond to foods as well as to drugs. An Australian study of **osteoporosis** (softening of the bones that often occurs in elderly people), reported that separate genes may affect response to vitamin D, calcium, and estrogens.

Implications

Although the study is still new, pharmacogenetics promises to offer great benefits in drug effectiveness and safety.

At the present time, most drug treatment is done by trial and error. Physicians prescribe medication, and the patient tries the drug. The drug may work,

KEY TERMS

Enzyme—Proteins produced by living cells that help produce specific biochemical reactions in the body.

Metabolism—The process by which foods and drugs are broken down for use and removal from the body.

Sickle cell anemia—A severe, inheritable disease, most common among people of African descent, marked by deformation and destruction of red blood cells, and by adherence of blood cells to the walls of blood vessels.

or it may not. It may cause adverse effects, or it may be safe. If the drug does not work, the dose is increased. If it causes harmful or unpleasant effects, a new drug is tried until, finally, the right drug is found. In some cases this procedure may take weeks or even months.

In other cases, drugs are carefully tested, and appear to be safe and effective. Only after they are approved for general use are reports of serious adverse effects that did not appear in the initial studies documented. This can occur if there is a rare gene that affects the way in which the drug acts, or the way in which the drug is metabolized.

With increasing understanding of how genes determine the way people respond to drugs, it will be possible to select drugs and doses based on a greater understanding of each individual patient. This promises more effective drug therapy, with greater safety and fewer treatment failures.

Physicians may be able to compare the person's genetic make-up with the properties of specific drugs, and make informed decisions about which drug in a group will work most effectively or most safely.

Resources

BOOKS

From Genome to Therapy: Integrating New Technologies with Drug Development. New York: John Wiley, 2000.

PERIODICALS

"A DNA tragedy." *Fortune* October 30, 2000.
"Screening for genes." *Newsweek* February 8, 1999.

ORGANIZATIONS

National Institute of General Medical Sciences. Division of Pharmacology, Physiology, and Biological Chemistry. 45 Center Dr., MSC 6200 Bethesda, MD 20892-6200.

University of California, Los Angeles Harbor-UCLA Medical Center Research and Education Institute 1124 W Carson St., B-4 South Torrance, CA 90502.

Samuel D. Uretsky, PharmD

Pharyngeal pouch *see* **Esophageal pouches**

Pharyngitis *see* **Sore throat**

Phenelzine *see* **Monoamine oxidase inhibitors**

Phenobarbital *see* **Barbiturates**

Phenol *see* **Antiseptics**

Phenolphthalein *see* **Laxatives**

Phenylalaninemia *see* **Phenylketonuria**

Phenylketonuria

Definition

Phenylketonuria (PKU) can be defined as a rare metabolic disorder caused by a deficiency in the production of the hepatic (liver) enzyme phenylalanine hydroxylase (PAH). PKU is the most serious form of a class of diseases referred to as "hyperphenylalaninemia," all of which involve above normal (elevated) levels of phenylalanine in the blood. The primary symptom of untreated PKU, **mental retardation**, is the result of consuming foods that contain the amino acid phenylalanine, which is toxic to brain tissue.

PKU is an inherited, autosomal recessive disorder. It is the most common genetic disease involving "amino acid metabolism." PKU is incurable, but early, effective treatment can prevent the development of serious mental incapacity.

Description

PKU is a disease caused by the liver's inability to produce a particular type of PAH enzyme. This enzyme converts (metabolizes) the amino acid called phenylalanine into another amino acid, tyrosine. This is the only role of PAH in the body. A lack of PAH results in the buildup of abnormally high phenylalanine concentrations (or levels) in the blood and brain. Above normal levels of phenylalanine are toxic to the cells that make up the nervous system and causes irreversible abnormalities in brain structure and function in PKU patients. Phenylalanine is a type of teratogen. Teratogens are any substance or organism that can cause **birth defects** in a developing fetus.

The liver is the body's chief protein processing center. Proteins are one of the major food nutrients. They are generally very large molecules composed of strings of smaller building blocks or molecules called amino acids. About twenty amino acids exist in nature. The body breaks down proteins from food into individual amino acids and then reassembles them into "human" proteins. Proteins are needed for growth and repair of cells and tissues, and are the key components of enzymes, antibodies, and other essential substances.

PKU affects on the human nervous system

The extensive network of nerves in the brain and the rest of the nervous system are made up of nerve cells. Nerve cells have specialized extensions called dendrites and axons. Stimulating a nerve cell triggers nerve impulses, or signals, that speed down the axon. These nerve impulses then stimulate the end of an axon to release chemicals called "neurotransmitters" that spread out and communicate with the dendrites of neighboring nerve cells.

Many nerve cells have long, wire-like axons that are covered by an insulating layer called the myelin sheath. This covering helps speed nerve impulses along the axon. In untreated PKU patients, abnormally high phenylalanine levels in the blood and brain can produce nerve cells with "deformed" axons and dendrites, and cause imperfections in the myelin sheath referred to as hypomyelination and demyelination. This loss of myelin can "short circuit" nerve impulses (messages) and interrupt cell communication. A number of brain scan studies also indicate a degeneration of the "white matter" in the brains of older patients who have not maintained adequate dietary control.

PKU can also affect the production of one of the major neurotransmitters in the brain, called dopamine. The brain makes dopamine from the amino acid tyrosine. PKU patients who do not consume enough tyrosine in their diet cannot produce sufficient amounts of dopamine. Low dopamine levels in the brain disrupt normal communication between nerve cells, which results in impaired cognitive (mental) function.

Some preliminary research suggests that nerve cells of PKU patients also have difficulty absorbing tyrosine. This abnormality may explain why many PKU patients who receive sufficient dietary tyrosine still experience some form of learning disability.

Behavior and academic performance

IQ (intelligence quotient) tests provide a measure of cognitive function. The IQ of PKU patients is generally lower than the IQ of their healthy peers. Students with PKU often find academic tasks difficult and must struggle harder to succeed than their non-PKU peers. They may require special tutoring and need to repeat some of their courses. Even patients undergoing treatment programs may experience problems with typical academic tasks as math, reading, and spelling. Visual perception, visual-motor skills, and critical thinking skills can also be affected. Ten years of age seems to be an important milestone for PKU patients. After age 10, variations in a patient's diet seems to have less influence on their IQ development.

People with PKU tend to avoid contact with others, appear anxious and show signs of depression. However, some patients may be much more expressive and tend to have hyperactive, talkative, and impulsive personalities. It is also interesting to note that people with PKU are less likely to display such "antisocial" habits as lying, teasing, and active disobedience. It should be emphasized that current research findings are still quite preliminary and more extensive research is needed to clearly show how abnormal phenylalanine levels in the blood and brain might affect behavior and academic performance.

One in fifty individuals in the United States have inherited a gene for PKU. About five million Americans are PKU carriers. About one in 15,000 babies test positive for PKU in the United States. Studies indicate that the incidence of this disease in Caucasian and Native American populations is higher than in African-American, Hispanic, and Asian populations.

Causes and symptoms

PKU symptoms are caused by alterations or "mutations" in the genetic code for the PAH enzyme. Mutations in the PAH gene prevent the liver from producing adequate levels of the PAH enzyme needed to break down phenylalanine. The PAH gene and its PKU mutations are found on chromosome 12 in the human genome. In more detail, PKU mutations can involve many different types of changes, such as deletions and insertions, in the DNA of the gene that codes for the PAH enzyme.

PKU is described as an inherited, autosomal recessive disorder. The term autosomal means that the gene for PKU is not located on either the X or Y sex chromosome. The normal PAH gene is dominant to recessive PKU mutations. A recessive genetic trait, such as PKU, is one that is expressed—or shows up— only when two copies are inherited (one from each parent).

A person with one normal and one PKU gene is called a carrier. A carrier does not display any symptoms of the disease because their liver produces normal quantities of the PAH enzyme. However, PKU carriers can pass the PKU genetic mutation onto their children. Two carrier parents have a 25% chance of producing a baby with PKU symptoms, and a 50% chance having a baby that is a carrier for the disease. Although PKU conforms to these basic genetic patterns of inheritance, the actual expression, or phenotype, of the disease is not strictly an "either/or" situation. This is because there are at least 400 different types of PKU mutations. Although some PKU mutations cause rather mild forms of the disease, others can initiate much more severe symptoms in untreated individuals. The more severe the PKU mutation, the greater the effect on cognitive development and performance (mental ability).

Untreated PKU patients develop a broad range of symptoms related to severely impaired cognitive function, sometimes referred to as mental retardation. Other symptoms can include extreme patterns of behavior, delayed speech development, seizures, a characteristic body odor, and light body pigmentation. The light pigmentation is due to a lack of melanin, which normally colors the hair, skin and eyes. Melanin is made from the amino acid tyrosine, which is lacking in untreated cases of PKU. Physiologically, PKU patients show high levels of phenylalanine and low levels of tyrosine in the blood. Babies do not show any visible symptoms of the disease for the first few months of life. However, typical PKU symptoms usually do show up by a baby's first birthday.

Diagnosis

The primary diagnostic test for PKU is the measurement of phenylalanine levels in a drop of blood taken from the heel of a newborn baby's foot. This screening procedure is referred to as the Guthrie test (Guthrie bacterial inhibition assay). In this test, PKU is confirmed by the appearance of bacteria growing around high concentrations of phenylalanine in the blood spot. PKU testing was introduced in the early 1960s and is the largest genetic screening program in the United States. It is required by law in all 50 states. Early diagnosis is critical. It ensures early the treatment PKU babies need to develop normally and avoid the ravages of PKU.

The American Academy of Pediatrics recommends that this test should be performed on infants between 24 hours and seven days after birth. The preferred time for testing is after the baby's first feeding. If the initial PKU test produces a positive result, then follow-up tests are performed to confirm the diagnosis and to determine if the elevated phenylalanine levels may be caused by some medical condition other than PKU. Treatment for PKU is recommended for babies that show a blood phenylalanine level of 7–10 mg/dL or higher for more than a few consecutive days. Another, more accurate test procedure for PKU measures the ratio (comparison) of the amount of phenylalanine to the amount of tyrosine in the blood.

Newer diagnostic procedures (called mutation analysis and genotype determination) can actually identify the specific types of PAH gene mutations inherited by PKU infants. Large-scale studies have helped to clarify how various mutations affect the ability of patients to process phenylalanine. This information can help doctors develop more effective customized treatment plans for each of their PKU patients.

Treatment

The severity of the PKU symptoms experienced by people with this disease is determined by both lifestyle as well as genetic factors. In the early 1950s, researchers first demonstrated that phenylalanine-restricted **diets** could eliminate most of the typical PKU symptoms—except for mental retardation. Today, dietary therapy (also called **nutrition** therapy) is the most common form of treatment for PKU patients. PKU patients who receive early and consistent dietary therapy can develop fairly normal mental capacity to within about five IQ points of their healthy peers. By comparison, untreated PKU patients generally have IQ scores below 50.

Infants with PKU should be put on a specialized diet as soon as they are diagnosed to avoid progressive brain damage and other problems caused by an accumulation of phenylalanine in the body. A PKU diet helps patients maintain very low blood levels of phenylalanine by restricting the intake of natural foods that contain this amino acid. Even breast milk is a problem for PKU babies. Special PKU dietary mixtures or formulas are usually obtained from medical clinics or pharmacies.

Phenylalanine is actually an essential amino acid. This means that it has to be obtained from food because the body cannot produce this substance on its own. Typical diets prescribed for PKU patients provide very small amounts of phenylalanine and higher quantities of other amino acids, including tyrosine. The amount of allowable phenylalanine can be increased slightly as a child becomes older.

In addition, PKU diets include all the nutrients normally required for good health and normal growth, such as carbohydrates, fats, **vitamins**, and **minerals**. High protein foods like meat, fish, chicken, eggs, nuts, beans, milk, and other dairy products are banned from PKU diets. Small amounts of moderate protein foods (such as grains and potatoes) and low protein foods (some fruits and vegetables, low protein breads and pastas) are allowed. Sugar-free foods, such as diet soda, which contain the artificial sweetener aspartame, are also prohibited foods for PKU patients. That is because aspartame contains the amino acid phenylalanine.

Ideally, school-age children with PKU should be taught to assume responsibility for managing their diet, recording food intake, and for performing simple blood tests to monitor their phenylalanine levels. Blood tests should be done in the early morning when phenylalanine levels are highest. Infants and young children require more frequent blood tests than older children and adults. The amount of natural foods allowed in a diet could be adjusted to ensure that the level of phenylalanine in the blood is kept within a safe range—two to 6 mg/dL before 12 years of age and 2–15 mg/dL for PKU patients over 12 years old.

A specialized PKU diet can cause abnormal fluctuations in tyrosine levels throughout the day. Thus, some health professionals recommend adding time released tyrosine that can provide a more constant supply of this amino acid to the body. It should be noted that some PKU patients show signs of learning disabilities even with a special diet containing extra tyrosine. Research studies suggests that these PKU patients may not be able to process tyrosine normally.

For PKU caregivers, providing a diet that is appealing as well as healthy and nutritious is a constant challenge. Many PKU patients, especially teenagers, find it difficult to stick to the relatively bland PKU diet for extended periods of time. Some older patients decide to go off their diet plan simply because they feel healthy. However, many patients who abandon careful nutritional management develop cognitive problems, such as difficulties remembering, maintaining focus, and paying attention. Many PKU health professionals contend that all PKU patients should adhere to a strictly controlled diet for life.

One promising line of PKU research involves the synthesis (manufacturing) of a new type of enzyme that can break down phenylalanine in food consumed by the patient. This medication would be taken orally and could prevent the absorption of digested phenylalanine into the patient's bloodstream.

In general, medical researchers express concern about the great variation in treatment programs currently available to PKU patients around the world. They have highlighted the urgent need for new, consistent international standards for proper management of PKU patients, which should emphasize comprehensive psychological as well as physiological monitoring and assessment.

PKU and Pregnancy

Women with PKU must be especially careful with their diets if they want to have children. They should ensure that phenylalanine blood levels are under control before conception and throughout her **pregnancy**. Mothers with elevated (higher than normal) phenylalanine levels are high risk for having babies with significant birth defects, such as microencephaly (smaller than normal head size), and **congenital heart disease** (abnormal heart structure and function), stunted growth, mental retardation, and psychomotor (coordination) difficulties. This condition is referred to as maternal PKU and can even affect babies who do not have the PKU disease.

Prognosis

Early newborn screening, careful monitoring, and a life-long strict dietary management can help PKU patients to live normal, healthy, and long lives.

Resources

BOOKS

Brust, John C. M. *The Practice Of Neural Science: From Synapses To Symptoms.* New York: McGraw-Hill, 2000.

Gilroy, John. *Basic Neurology.* 3rd ed. New York: McGraw-Hill, 2000.

Ratey, John J. *A User's Guide To The Brain: Perception, Attention, And The Four Theaters Of The Brain.* 1st ed. New York: Pantheon Books, 2001.

Weiner, William J., and Christopher G. Goetz, editors. *Neurology For The Non-Neurologist.* 4th ed. Philadelphia: Lippincott, Williams & Wilkins, 1999.

PERIODICALS

Burgard, P. "Development of intelligence in early treated phenylketonuria." *European Journal of Pediatrics* 159, Supplement 2 (October 2000): S74–9.

Chang, Pi-Nian, Robert M. Gray, and Lisa Lehn O'Brien. "Review: Patterns of academic achievement among patients treated early with phenylketonuria." *European Journal of Pediatrics* 159, no.14 (2000): S96–9.

KEY TERMS

Amino acid—Organic compounds that form the building blocks of protein. There are 20 types of amino acids (eight are "essential amino acids" which the body cannot make and must therefore be obtained from food).

Axon—Skinny, wire-like extension of nerve cells.

Enzyme—A protein that catalyzes a biochemical reaction or change without changing its own structure or function.

Gene—A building block of inheritance, which contains the instructions for the production of a particular protein, and is made up of a molecular sequence found on a section of DNA. Each gene is found on a precise location on a chromosome.

Genetic disease—A disease that is (partly or completely) the result of the abnormal function or expression of a gene; a disease caused by the inheritance and expression of a genetic mutation.

IQ—Abbreviation for Intelligence Quotient. Compares an individual's mental age to his/her true or chronological age and multiplies that ratio by 100.

Metabolism—The total combination of all of the chemical processes that occur within cells and tissues of a living body.

Mutation—A permanent change in the genetic material that may alter a trait or characteristic of an individual, or manifest as disease, and can be transmitted to offspring.

Myelin—A fatty sheath surrounding nerves in the peripheral nervous system, which help them conduct impulses more quickly.

Nervous system—The complete network of nerves, sense organs, and brain in the body.

Phenylalanine—An essential amino acid that must be obtained from food since the human body cannot manufacture it.

Protein—Important building blocks of the body, composed of amino acids, involved in the formation of body structures and controlling the basic functions of the human body.

Recessive—Genetic trait expressed only when present on both members of a pair of chromosomes, one inherited from each parent.

Eastman, J.W., J.E. Sherwin, R. Wong, C.L. Liao, R.J. Currier, F. Lorey, and G. Cunningham. "Use of the phenylalanine:tyrosine ratio to test newborns for phenylketonuria in a large public health screening programme." *Journal of Medical Screening* 7, no. 3 (2000): 131–5.

MacDonald, A. "Diet and compliance in phenylketonuria." *European Journal of Pediatrics* 159, Supplement 2 (October 2000): S136–41.

Smith, Isabel, and Julie Knowles. "Behaviour in early treated phenylketonuria: a systematic review." *European Journal of Pediatrics* 159, no. 14 (2000): S89–93.

Stemerdink, B.A., A.F. Kalverboer, J.J. van der Meere, M.W. van der Molen, J. Huisman, L.W. de Jong, F.M. Slijper, P.H. Verkerk, and F.J. van Spronsen. "Behaviour and school achievement in patients with early and continuously treated phenylketonuria." *Journal of Inherited Metabolic Disorders* 23, no. 6 (2000): 548–62.

van Spronsen, F.J.F., M.M. van Rijn, J. Bekhof, R. Koch, and P.G. Smit. "Phenylketonuria: tyrosine supplementation in phenylalanine-restricted diets." *American Journal of Clinical Nutrition* 73, no. 2 (2001): 153–7.

Wappner, Rebecca, Sechin Cho, Richard A. Kronmal, Virginia Schuett, and Margretta Reed Seashore. "Management of Phenylketonuria for Optimal Outcome: A Review of Guidelines for Phenylketonuria Management and a Report of Surveys of Parents, Patients, and Clinic Directors." *Pediatrics* 104, no. 6 (December 1999): e68.

ORGANIZATIONS

American Academy of Allergy, Asthma & Immunology. 611 E. Wells St, Milwaukee, WI 53202. (414) 272-6071. Fax: (414) 272-6070. < http://www.aaaai.org/default.stm >.

Centers for Disease Control. GDP Office, 4770 Buford Highway NE, Atlanta, GA 30341-3724. (770) 488-3235. < http://www.cdc.gov/genetics >.

Children's PKU Network. 1520 State St., Suite 111, San Diego, CA 92101-2930. (619) 233-3202. Fax: (619) 233 0838. pkunetwork@aol.com.

March of Dimes Birth Defects Foundation. 1275 Mamaroneck Ave., White Plains, NY 10605. (888) 663-4637. resourcecenter@modimes.org. < http://www.modimes.org >.

National PKU News. Virginia Schuett, editor/dietician. 6869 Woodlawn Avenue NE #116, Seattle, WA 98115-5469. (206) 525-8140. Fax: (206) 525-5023. < http://www.pkunews.org >.

University of Washington PKU Clinic. CHDD, Box 357920, University of Washington, Seattle, WA. (206) 685-3015. Within Washington State: (877) 685-3015. Clinic Coordinator: vam@u.washington.edu. < http://depts.-washington.edu/pku/contact.html. >.

OTHER

Allergy and Asthma Network. Mothers of Asthmatics, Inc. 2751 Prosperity Ave., Suite 150, Fairfax, VA 22031. (800) 878-4403. Fax: (703)573-7794.

Consensus Development Conference on Phenylketonuria (PKU): Screening and Management, October 16–18,

2000. < http://odp.od.nih.gov/consensus/news/upcoming/pku/pku_info.htm#overview >.

Genetics and Public Health in the 21st Century. Using Genetic Information to Improve Health and Prevent Disease. < http://www.cdc.gov/genetics/_archive/publications/Table >.

Marshall G. Letcher, MA

Phenylpropanolamine *see* **Decongestants**

Phenytoin *see* **Anticonvulsant drugs**

Pheochromocytoma

Definition

Pheochromocytoma is a tumor of special cells (called chromaffin cells), most often found in the middle of the adrenal gland.

Description

Because pheochromocytomas arise from chromaffin cells, they are occasionally called chromaffin tumors. Most (90%) are benign tumors so they do not spread to other parts of the body. However, these tumors can cause many problems and if they are not treated and can result in death.

Pheochromocytomas can be found anywhere chromaffin cells are found. They may be found in the heart and in the area around the bladder, but most (90%) are found in the adrenal glands. Every individual has two adrenal glands that are located above the kidneys in the back of the abdomen. Each adrenal gland is made up of two parts: the outer part (called the adrenal cortex) and the inner part (called the adrenal medulla). Pheochromocytomas are found in the adrenal medulla. The adrenal medulla normally secretes two substances, or hormones, called norepinephrine and epinephrine. These two substances, when considered together, are known as adrenaline. Adrenaline is released from the adrenal gland, enters the bloodstream and helps to regulate many things in the body including blood pressure and heart rate. Pheochromocytomas cause the adrenal medulla to secrete too much adrenaline, which in turn causes high blood pressure. The high blood pressure usually causes the other symptoms of the disease.

Pheochromocytomas are rare tumors. They have been reported in babies as young as five days old as well as adults 92 years old. Although they can be found at any time during life, they usually occur in adults between 30 and 40 years of age. Pheochromocytomas are somewhat more common in women than in men.

Causes and symptoms

The cause of most pheochromocytomas is not known. A small minority (about 10-20%) of pheochromocytomas arise because a person has an inherited susceptibility to them. Inherited pheochromocytomas are associated with four separate syndromes: Multiple Endocrine Neoplasia, type 2A (MEN2A), Multiple Endocrine Neoplasia, type 2B (MEN2B), von Hippel-Lindau disease (VHL) and **Neurofibromatosis** type 1 (NF1).

Individuals with pheochromocytomas as part of any of these four syndromes usually have other medical conditions as well. People with MEN2A often have **cancer** (usually **thyroid cancer**) and other hormonal problems. Individuals with MEN2B can also have cancer and hormonal problems, but also have other abnormal physical features. Both MEN2A and MEN2B are due to genetic alterations or mutations in a gene called RET, found at chromosome 10q11.2. Individuals with VHL often have other benign tumors of the central nervous system and pancreas, and can sometimes have renal cell cancer. This syndrome is caused by a mutation in the VHL gene, found at chromosome 3p25-26. Individuals with NF1 often have neurofibromas (benign tumors of the peripheral nervous system). NF1 is caused by mutations in the NF1 gene, found at chromosome 17q11.

All of these disorders are inherited in an autosomal dominant inheritance pattern. With autosomal dominant inheritance, men and women are equally likely to inherit the syndrome. In addition, children of individuals with the disease are at 50% risk of inheriting it. **Genetic testing** is available for these four syndromes (MEN2A, MEN2B, VHL and NF1) but, due to the complexity, **genetic counseling** should be considered before testing.

Most people (90%) with pheochromocytoma have **hypertension**, or high blood pressure. The other symptoms of the disease are extremely variable. These symptoms usually occur in episodes (or attacks) called paroxysms and include:

- headaches
- excess sweating
- racing heart
- rapid breathing
- anxiety/nervousness

- nervous shaking

- pain in the lower chest or upper abdomen

- nausea

- heat intolerance

The episodes can occur as often as 25 times a day or, as infrequently as once every few months. They can last a few minutes, several hours, or days. Usually, the attacks occur several times a week and last for about 15 minutes. After the episode is over, the person feels exhausted and fatigued.

Between the attacks, people with pheochromocytoma can experience the following:

- increased sweating

- cold hands and feet

- weight loss

- constipation

Diagnosis

If a pheochromocytoma is suspected, urine and/or a blood test are usually recommended. A test called "24-hour urinary catacholamines and metanephrines" will be done. This test is designed to look for adrenaline and the break-down products of adrenaline. Since the body gets rid of these hormones in the urine, those testing will need to collect their urine for 24 hours. The laboratory will determine whether or not the levels of hormones are too high. This test is very good at making the diagnosis of pheochromocytoma. Another test called "serum catacholamines" measures the level of adrenaline compounds in the blood. It is not as sensitive as the 24-hour urine test, but can still provide some key information if it shows that the level of adrenaline compounds is too high.

One of the difficulties with these tests is that a person needs to have an attack of symptoms either during the 24-hour urine collection time period or shortly before the blood is drawn for a serum test to ensure the test's accuracy. If a person did not have an episode during that time, the test can be a "false negative". If a doctor suspects the patient has had a "false negative" test, additional tests called "pharmacologic tests" can be ordered. During these tests, a specific drug is given to the patient (usually through an IV) and the levels of hormones are monitored from the patient's blood. These types of tests are only done rarely.

Once a person has been diagnosed with a pheochromocytoma, he or she will undergo tests to identify exactly where in the body the tumor is located. The imaging techniques used are usually computed tomography scan (CT scan) and magnetic resonsance imaging (MRI). A CT scan creates pictures of the interior of the body from computer-analyzed differences in x rays passing through the body. CT scans are performed at a hospital or clinic and take only a few minutes. An MRI is a computerized scanning method that creates pictures of the interior of the body using radio waves and a magnet. An MRI is usually performed at a hospital and takes about 30 minutes.

Treatment

Once a pheochromocytoma is found, more tests will be done to see if the tumor is benign (not cancer) or malignant (cancer). If the tumor is malignant, tests will be done to see how far the cancer has spread. There is no accepted staging system for pheochromocytoma; but an observation of the tumor could provide one of these four indications:

- Localized benign pheochromocytoma means that the tumor is found only in one area, is not cancer, and cannot spread to other tissues of the body.

- Regional pheochromocytoma means that the tumor is malignant and has spread to the lymph nodes around the original cancer. Lymph nodes are small structures found all over the body that make and store infection-fighting cells.

- Metastatic pheochromocytoma means that the tumor is malignant and has spread to other, more distant parts of the body.

- Recurrent pheochromocytoma means that a malignant tumor that was removed has come back.

Treatment in all cases begins with surgical removal of the tumor. Before surgery, medications such as alpha-adrenergic blockers are given to block the effect of the hormones and normalize blood pressure. These medications are usually started seven to 10 days prior to surgery. The surgery of choice is laparoscopic laparotomy, which is a minimally invasive outpatient procedure performed under general or **local anesthesia**. A small incision is made in the abdomen, the laparoscope is inserted, and the tumor is removed. The patient can usually return to normal activities within two weeks. If a laparoscopic laparotomy cannot be done, a traditional laparotomy will be performed. This is a more invasive surgery done under spinal or **general anesthesia** and requires five to seven days in the hospital. Usually patients are able to return to normal activities after four weeks. After surgery, blood and urine tests will be done to make sure hormone levels return to normal. If the hormone levels are

David Gardner. New York: Lange Medical Books/ McGraw-Hill, 2001, pp. 399–421.

Keiser, Harry R. "Pheochromocytoma and Related Tumors.". In *Endocrinology*, edited by Leslie J. DeGroot and J. Larry Jameson, 4th ed. New York: W.B. Saunders Company, 2001, pp. 1862–1883.

PERIODICALS

Barzon, Luisa, and Marco Boscaro. "Diagnosis and Management of Adrenal Incidentalomas." *The Journal of Urology* 163 (February 2000): 398–407.

Young, William F. "Management Approaches to AdrenalIncidentaloma" *Endocrinology and Metabolism Clinics of North America* 29 (March 2000): 159–185.

OTHER

"Pheochromocytoma" *National Cancer Institute CancerWeb* June 29, 2001. < http://www.graylab.ac.uk/cancernet/ 202494.html >.

Lori De Milto
Kristen Mahoney Shannon, M.S. CGC

KEY TERMS

Adrenal medulla—The central core of the adrenal gland.

Laparoscope—An instrument used to examine body cavities during certain types of surgery; for example, surgeries to remove fibroid tumors, or gall bladders, are often removed through the navel rather than cutting into the body.

Paroxysm—A sudden attack of symptoms.

---

still above normal, it may mean that some tumor tissue was not removed. If not all tumor can be removed (as in malignant pheochromocytoma, for example) drugs will be given to control high blood pressure.

If a pheochromocytoma is malignant, radiation therapy and/or **chemotherapy** may be used. **Radiation therapy** uses high-energy x rays to kill cancer cells and shrink tumors. Because there is no evidence that radiation therapy is effective in the treatment of malignant pheochromocytoma, it is not often used for treatment. However, it is useful in the treatment of painful bone metastases if the tumor has spread to the bones. Chemotherapy uses drugs to kill cancer cells. Like radiation therapy, it has not been shown to be effective in the treatment of malignant pheochromocytoma. Chemotherapy, therefore, is only used in rare instances.

Untreated pheochromocytoma can be fatal due to complications of the high blood pressure. In the vast majority of cases, when the tumor is surgically removed, pheochromocytoma is cured. In the minority of cases (10%) where pheochromocytoma is malignant, prognosis depends on how far the cancer has spread, and the patient's age and general health. The overall median five-year survival from the initial time of surgery and diagnosis is approximately 43%.

Prevention

Unfortunately, little is known about environmental and other causes of pheochromocytoma. Some of the tumors are due to inherited predisposition. Because of these factors, pheochromocytoma can not be prevented.

Resources

BOOKS

Goldfien, Alan. "Adrenal Medulla." In *Basic and Clinical Endocrinology*, edited by Francis Greenspan and

---

▌ Phimosis

Definition

A tightening of the foreskin of the penis that may close the opening of the penis.

Description

The foreskin of a newborn boy is always closely contracted around the penis head (glans). Only a small passage allows the urine to pass through. In the first months the foreskin is stuck to the glans and cannot be pulled back and one should not attempt to do so. During the first couple of years, the foreskin will become gradually looser and in many boys it can in time be pulled back without trouble. Half of all three-year-olds can pull back their foreskin. It is not advisable to try pulling the foreskin back using force, since this may cause small cuts in the foreskin with **scars** which could finally cause a regular foreskin contraction.

Foreskin contraction, called phimosis, can last throughout life and not cause any trouble at all. It is a voluntary decision whether to have a **circumcision** operation or not. If any problems do arise, they happen after **puberty**. The contraction may occur for the first time as an adult and usually requires circumcision, the surgical removal of the foreskin.

Causes & symptoms

Phimosis is caused by the inability of the foreskin to retract from around the opening of the penis. In adults, phimosis can lead to chronic inflammation and **cancer**.

Diagnosis

A physician usually diagnoses phimosis when there are persistent problems urinating, when there are recurrent infections under the foreskin, or when the opening to the penis is completely blocked by the foreskin. Phimosis is a tight ring of foreskin often made of scar tissue preventing retraction of the foreskin. It may be primary, or secondary to recurrent infection. It may produce urinary obstruction with ballooning of the foreskin. Phimosis is different than having a non-retractable foreskin, which is normal in many boys.

Treatment

If the foreskin cannot be pulled back into place treatment should be sought. If the blood flow to the penis is restricted then emergency treatment is required and if the foreskin cannot be pulled back a surgical cut to the trapped foreskin may be required. Failure to seek treatment can result in permanent damage to the penis. Once phimosis is diagnosed, the available treatments include topical **corticosteroids**, manual stretching, foreskin surgical repair or **plastic surgery**, and circumcision. Conservative treatments should be tried in the first instance and surgery used as the treatment of last resort.

A number of studies show that phimosis can be safely and effectively treated by the application of topical steroids in 80–90% of cases. Betamethasone cream 0.05% should be applied to the exterior and interior of the tip of the foreskin two or three times a day. The treatment should be discontinued as ineffective after three months if the foreskin has not become retractile during this time.

A number of corrections are available for the adult or adolescent non-retractable foreskin. These include surgery to repair the foreskin, in which an incision is made through the constrictive band of the foreskin. The underlying tissue is spread with forceps to expose the Buck's fascia (the deep, connective tissue of the penis) and the incision is closed with absorbable sutures. This procedure has less risk of disease and infection than circumcision, and allows the foreskin to be retained.

Circumcision is very traumatic to a child. It is essentially irreversible and should be the treatment of last resort. Phimosis due to *balanitis xerotica obliterans* (BXO), a chronic, progressive, hardening skin inflammation of the penis, has been considered the one common absolute indication for circumcision.

Alternative treatment

There are no alternative medicine treatments for phimosis.

Prognosis

In most men, phimosis is not a serious problem and will not require treatment. However, it is not expected to improve on its own. With treatment, phimosis in most males can be managed or corrected.

Prevention

Proper hygiene is the most important preventative measure. The American Academy of Pediatrics recommends that the immature foreskin of boys not be forced back for cleaning. The only person who should clean and retract the foreskin is the boy himself. Bubble bath products and other chemical irritants can cause the foreskin to tighten and it is recommended they should be avoided by males with foreskins.

Resources

BOOKS

Icon Health Publications. *Phimosis: A Medical Dictionary, Bibliography, and Annotated Research Guide to Internet References* San Diego: Icon Health Publications, 2004.

KEY TERMS

Balanitis xerotica obliterans (BXO)—A chronic, progressive, hardening skin inflammation of the penis.

Buck's fascia—The deep connective tissue of the penis.

Circumcision—The removal of all or part of the foreskin from the penis.

Corticosteroids—A synthetic drug similar or identical to a natural corticosteroid, used to reduce inflammation.

Glans—The head of the penis.

Paraphimosis—The entrapment of a retracted foreskin behind the coronal sulcus, a groove that separates the shaft and head of the penis.

PERIODICALS

"GP Registrar: Pictorial-Case Study (Diagnosis of Phimosis)." *GP* (February 11, 2005): 66.

Berk, David R. "Paraphimosis in a Middle-Aged Adult After Intercourse."*American Family Physician* (February 15, 2004): 807.

Choe, Dr. Jong M. "Paraphimosis: Current Treatment Options."*American Family Physician*(December 15, 2000): 2623–2627.

ORGANIZATIONS

American Foundation for Urologic Disease. 1000 Corporate Blvd., Suite 410, Linthicum, MD 21090. (410) 689-3990 or (800) 828-7866. http://www.afud.org.

OTHER

December 19, 2004. Circumcision Information and Resource Pages.*Conservative Treatment of Phimosis: Alternatives to Radical Circumcision* < http://www.cirp.org/library/ treatment/phimosis/ > (Accessed March 31, 2005).

Ken R. Wells

Phlebitis *see* **Thrombophlebitis**

Phlebotomy

Definition

Phlebotomy is the act of drawing or removing blood from the circulatory system through a cut (incision) or puncture in order to obtain a sample for analysis and diagnosis. Phlebotomy is also done as part of the patient's treatment for certain blood disorders.

Purpose

Treatment

Phlebotomy that is part of treatment (therapeutic phlebotomy) is performed to treat polycythemia vera, a condition that causes an elevated red blood cell volume (**hematocrit**). Phlebotomy is also prescribed for patients with disorders that increase the amount of iron in their blood to dangerous levels, such as hemochromatosis, **hepatitis B**, and hepatitis C. Patients with pulmonary edema may undergo phlebotomy procedures to decrease their total blood volume.

Diagnosis

Phlebotomy is also used to remove blood from the body during **blood donation** and for analysis of the substances contained within it.

Precautions

Patients who are anemic or have a history of cardiovascular disease may not be good candidates for phlebotomy.

Description

Phlebotomy, which is also known as venesection, is performed by a nurse or a technician known as a phlebotomist. Blood is usually taken from a vein on the back of the hand or inside of the elbow. Some blood tests, however, may require blood from an artery. The skin over the area is wiped with an antiseptic, and an elastic band is tied around the arm. The band acts as a tourniquet, slowing the blood flow in the arm and making the veins more visible. The patient is asked to make a fist, and the technician feels the veins in order to select an appropriate one. When a vein is selected, the technician inserts a needle into the vein and releases the elastic band. The appropriate amount of blood is drawn and the needle is withdrawn from the vein. The patient's pulse and blood pressure may be monitored during the procedure.

For some tests requiring very small amounts of blood for analysis, the technician uses a finger stick. A lance, or small needle, makes a small cut in the surface of the fingertip, and a small amount of blood is collected in a narrow glass tube. The fingertip may be squeezed to get additional blood to surface.

The amount of blood drawn depends on the purpose of the phlebotomy. Blood donors usually contribute a unit of blood (500 mL) in a session. The volume of blood needed for laboratory analysis varies widely with the type of test being conducted. Therapeutic phlebotomy removes a larger amount of blood than donation and blood analysis require. Phlebotomy for treatment of **hemochromatosis** typically involves removing a unit of blood—or 250 mg of iron—once a week. Phlebotomy sessions are required until iron levels return to a consistently normal level, which may take several months to several years. Phlebotomy for polycythemia vera removes enough blood to keep the patient's hematocrit below 45%. The frequency and duration of sessions depends on the patient's individual needs.

Preparation

Patients having their blood drawn for analysis may be asked to discontinue medications or to avoid food (to fast) for a period of time before the blood test. Patients donating blood will be asked for a brief

KEY TERMS

Finger stick—A technique for collecting a very small amount of blood from the fingertip area.

Hemochromatosis—A genetic disorder known as iron overload disease. Untreated hemochromatosis may cause osteoporosis, arthritis, cirrhosis, heart disease, or diabetes.

Thrombocytosis—A vascular condition characterized by high blood platelet counts.

Tourniquet—Any device that is used to compress a blood vessel to stop bleeding or as part of collecting a blood sample. Phlebotomists usually use an elastic band as a tourniquet.

Venesection—Another name for phlebotomy.

medical history, have their blood pressure taken, and have their hematocrit checked with a finger stick test prior to donation.

Aftercare

After blood is drawn and the needle is removed, pressure is placed on the puncture site with a cotton ball to stop bleeding, and a bandage is applied. It is not uncommon for a patient to feel dizzy or nauseated during or after phlebotomy. The patient may be encouraged to rest for a short period once the procedure is completed. Patients are also instructed to drink plenty of fluids and eat regularly over the next 24 hours to replace lost blood volume. Patients who experience swelling of the puncture site or continued bleeding after phlebotomy should get medical help at once.

Risks

Most patients will have a small bruise or mild soreness at the puncture site for several days. Therapeutic phlebotomy may cause **thrombocytosis** and chronic iron deficiency (anemia) in some patients. As with any invasive procedure, infection is also a risk. This risk can be minimized by the use of prepackaged sterilized equipment and careful attention to proper technique.

Normal results

Normal results include obtaining the needed amount of blood with the minimum of discomfort to the patient.

Resources

PERIODICALS

Wolfe, Yun Lee. "Case of the Ceaseless Fatigue." *Prevention Magazine* July 1997: 88-94.

Paula Anne Ford-Martin

Phobias

Definition

A phobia is an intense but unrealistic fear that can interfere with the ability to socialize, work, or go about everyday life, brought on by an object, event or situation.

Description

Just about everyone is afraid of something—an upcoming job interview or being alone outside after dark. But about 18% of all Americans are tormented by irrational fears that interfere with their daily lives. They are not "crazy"—they know full well their fears are unreasonable–but they can not control the fear. These people have phobias.

Phobias belong to a large group of mental problems known as **anxiety disorders** that include **obsessive-compulsive disorder** (OCD), **panic disorder**, and post-traumatic stress disorder. Phobias themselves can be divided into three specific types:

- specific phobias (formerly called "simple phobias")
- social phobia
- **agoraphobia**

Specific phobias

As its name suggests, a specific phobia is the fear of a particular situation or object, including anything from airplane travel to dentists. Found in one out of every 10 Americans, specific phobias seem to run in families and are roughly twice as likely to appear in women. If the person rarely encounters the feared object, the phobia does not cause much harm. However, if the feared object or situation is common, it can seriously disrupt everyday life. Common examples of specific phobias, which can begin at any age, include fear of snakes, flying, dogs, escalators, elevators, high places, or open spaces.

Social phobia

People with social phobia have deep fears of being watched or judged by others and being embarrassed in public. This may extend to a general fear of social situations—or be more specific or circumscribed, such as a fear of giving speeches or of performing (stage fright). More rarely, people with social phobia may have trouble using a public restroom, eating in a restaurant, or signing their name in front of others.

Social phobia is not the same as **shyness**. Shy people may feel uncomfortable with others, but they don't experience severe **anxiety**, they don't worry excessively about social situations beforehand, and they don't avoid events that make them feel self-conscious. On the other hand, people with social phobia may not be shy–they may feel perfectly comfortable with people except in specific situations. Social phobias may be only mildly irritating, or they may significantly interfere with daily life. It is not unusual for people with social phobia to turn down job offers or avoid relationships because of their fears.

Agoraphobia

Agoraphobia is the intense fear of feeling trapped and having a panic attack in a public place. It usually begins between ages 15 and 35, and affects three times as many women as men—about 3% of the population.

An episode of spontaneous panic is usually the initial trigger for the development of agoraphobia. After an initial panic attack, the person becomes afraid of experiencing a second one. Patients literally "fear the fear," and worry incessantly about when and where the next attack may occur. As they begin to avoid the places or situations in which the panic attack occurred, their fear generalizes. Eventually the person completely avoids public places. In severe cases, people with agoraphobia can no longer leave their homes for fear of experiencing a panic attack.

Causes and symptoms

Experts don't really know why phobias develop, although research suggests the tendency to develop phobias may be a complex interaction between heredity and environment. Some hypersensitive people have unique chemical reactions in the brain that cause them to respond much more strongly to **stress**. These people also may be especially sensitive to **caffeine**, which triggers certain brain chemical responses.

Advances in neuroimaging have also led researchers to identify certain parts of the brain and specific neural pathways that are associated with phobias. One part of the brain that is currently being studied is the amygdala, an almond-shaped body of nerve cells involved in normal fear conditioning. Another area of the brain that appears to be linked to phobias is the posterior cerebellum.

While experts believe the tendency to develop phobias runs in families and may be hereditary, a specific stressful event usually triggers the development of a specific phobia or agoraphobia. For example, someone predisposed to develop phobias who experiences severe turbulence during a flight might go on to develop a phobia about flying. What scientists don't understand is why some people who experience a frightening or stressful event develop a phobia and others do not.

Social phobia typically appears in childhood or adolescence, sometimes following an upsetting or humiliating experience. Certain vulnerable children who have had unpleasant social experiences (such as being rejected) or who have poor social skills may develop social phobias. The condition also may be related to low self-esteem, unassertive personality, and feelings of inferiority.

A person with agoraphobia may have a panic attack at any time, for no apparent reason. While the attack may last only a minute or so, the person remembers the feelings of panic so strongly that the possibility of another attack becomes terrifying. For this reason, people with agoraphobia avoid places where they might not be able to escape if a panic attack occurs. As the fear of an attack escalates, the person's world narrows.

While the specific trigger may differ, the symptoms of different phobias are remarkably similar: e.g., feelings of terror and impending doom, rapid heartbeat and breathing, sweaty palms, and other features of a panic attack. Patients may experience severe anxiety symptoms in anticipating a phobic trigger. For example, someone who is afraid to fly may begin having episodes of pounding heart and sweating palms at the mere thought of getting on a plane in two weeks.

Diagnosis

A mental health professional can diagnose phobias after a detailed interview and discussion of both mental and physical symptoms. Social phobia is often associated with other anxiety disorders, depression, or **substance abuse**.

Treatment

People who have a specific phobia that is easy to avoid (such as snakes) and that doesn't interfere with their lives may not need to get help. When phobias do interfere with a person's daily life, a combination of psychotherapy and medication can be quite effective. While most health insurance covers some form of mental health care, most do not cover outpatient care completely, and most have a yearly or lifetime maximum.

Medication can block the feelings of panic, and when combined with **cognitive-behavioral therapy**, can be quite effective in reducing specific phobias and agoraphobia.

Cognitive-behavioral therapy adds a cognitive approach to more traditional behavioral therapy. It teaches patients how to change their thoughts, behavior, and attitudes, while providing techniques to lessen anxiety, such as deep breathing, muscle relaxation, and refocusing.

One cognitive-behavioral therapy is desensitization (also known as exposure therapy), in which people are gradually exposed to the frightening object or event until they become used to it and their physical symptoms decrease. For example, someone who is afraid of snakes might first be shown a photo of a snake. Once the person can look at a photo without anxiety, he might then be shown a video of a snake. Each step is repeated until the symptoms of fear (such as pounding heart and sweating palms) disappear. Eventually, the person might reach the point where he can actually touch a live snake. Three fourths of patients are significantly improved with this type of treatment.

Another more dramatic cognitive-behavioral approach is called flooding. It exposes the person immediately to the feared object or situation. The person remains in the situation until the anxiety lessens.

Several drugs are used to treat specific phobias by controlling symptoms and helping to prevent panic attacks. These include anti-anxiety drugs (**benzodiazepines**) such as alprazolam (Xanax) or diazepam (Valium). Blood pressure medications called **beta blockers**, such as propranolol (Inderal) and atenolol (Tenormin), appear to work well in the treatment of circumscribed social phobia, when anxiety gets in the way of performance, such as public speaking. These drugs reduce overstimulation, thereby controlling the physical symptoms of anxiety.

In addition, some antidepressants may be effective when used together with cognitive-behavioral therapy. These include the monoamine oxidase inhibitors (MAO inhibitors) phenelzine (Nardil) and tranylcypromine (Parnate), as well as **selective serotonin reuptake inhibitors** (SSRIs) like fluoxetine (Prozac), paroxetine (Paxil), sertraline (Zoloft) and fluvoxamine (Luvox).

A medication that shows promise as a treatment for social phobia is valproic acid (Depakene or Depakote), which is usually prescribed to treat seizures or to prevent migraine headaches. Researchers conducting a twelve-week trial with 17 patients found that about half the patients experienced a significant improvement in their social anxiety symptoms while taking the medication. Further studies are underway.

In all types of phobias, symptoms may be eased by lifestyle changes, such as:

- eliminating caffeine
- cutting down on alcohol
- eating a good diet
- getting plenty of **exercise**
- reducing stress

Treating agoraphobia is more difficult than other phobias because there are often so many fears involved, such as open spaces, traffic, elevators, and escalators. Treatment includes cognitive-behavioral therapy with antidepressants or anti-anxiety drugs. Paxil and Zoloft are used to treat panic disorders with or without agoraphobia.

Prognosis

Phobias are among the most treatable mental health problems; depending on the severity of the condition and the type of phobia, most properly treated patients can go on to lead normal lives. Research suggests that once a person overcomes the phobia, the problem may not return for many years—if at all.

Untreated phobias are another matter. Only about 20% of specific phobias will go away without treatment, and agoraphobia will get worse with time if untreated. Social phobias tend to be chronic, and will not likely go away without treatment. Moreover, untreated phobias can lead to other problems, including depression, **alcoholism**, and feelings of shame and low self-esteem.

A group of researchers in Boston reported in 2003 that phobic anxiety appears to be a risk factor for Parkinson's disease (PD) in males, although it is not yet known whether phobias cause PD or simply share an underlying biological cause.

While most specific phobias appear in childhood and subsequently fade away, those that remain in adulthood often need to be treated. Unfortunately, most people never get the help they need; only about 25% of people with phobias ever seek help to deal with their condition.

KEY TERMS

Agoraphobia—An intense fear of being trapped in a crowded, open, or public space where it may be hard to escape, combined with the dread of having a panic attack.

Benzodiazepine—A class of drugs that have a hypnotic and sedative action, used mainly as tranquilizers to control symptoms of anxiety.

Beta blockers—A group of drugs that are usually prescribed to treat heart conditions, but that also are used to reduce the physical symptoms of anxiety and phobias, such as sweating and palpitations.

Monoamine oxidase inhibitors (MAO inhibitors)—A class of antidepressants used to treat social phobia.

Neuroimaging—The use of x ray studies and magnetic resonance imaging (MRIs) to detect abnormalities or trace pathways of nerve activity in the central nervous system.

Selective serotonin reuptake inhibitors (SSRIs)—A class of antidepressants that work by blocking the reabsorption of serotonin in the brain, raising the levels of serotonin. SSRIs include Prozac, Zoloft, and Paxil.

Serotonin—One of three major types of neurotransmitters found in the brain that is linked to emotions.

Social phobia—Fear of being judged or ridiculed by others; fear of being embarrassed in public.

Prevention

There is no known way to prevent the development of phobias. Medication and cognitive-behavioral therapy may help prevent the recurrence of symptoms once they have been diagnosed.

Resources

BOOKS

American Psychiatric Association.*Diagnostic and Statistical Manual of Mental Disorders.* 4th ed., revised. Washington, DC: American Psychiatric Association, 2000.

Beers, Mark H., MD, and Robert Berkow, MD., editors. "Phobic Disorders." In *The Merck Manual of Diagnosis and Therapy.* Whitehouse Station, NJ: Merck Research Laboratories, 2004.

PERIODICALS

Kinrys, G., M. H. Pollack, N. M. Simon, et al. "Valproic Acid for the Treatment of Social Anxiety Disorder."
International Clinical Psychopharmacology 18 (May 2003): 169–172.

Ploghaus, A., L. Becerra, C. Borras, and D. Borsook. "Neural Circuitry Underlying Pain Modulation: Expectation, Hypnosis, Placebo." *Trends in Cognitive Science* 7 (May 2003): 197–200.

Rauch, S. L., L. M. Shin, and C. I. Wright. "Neuroimaging Studies of Amygdala Function in Anxiety Disorders." *Annals of the New York Academy of Sciences* 985 (April 2003): 389–410.

Weisskopf, M. G., H. Chen, M. A. Schwarzschild, et al. "Prospective Study of Phobic Anxiety and Risk of Parkinson's Disease." *Movement Disorders* 18 (June 2003): 646–651.

ORGANIZATIONS

Agoraphobics Building Independent Lives. 1418 Lorraine Ave., Richmond, VA 23227.

Agoraphobics In Motion. 605 W. 11 Mile Rd., Royal Oak, MI 48067.

American Psychiatric Association (APA). 1400 K Street, NW, Washington, DC 20005. (888) 357-7924. < http://www.psych.org >.

Anxiety Disorders Association of America. 11900 Parklawn Dr., Ste. 100, Rockville, MD 20852. (301) 231-9350.

National Anxiety Foundation. 3135 Custer Dr., Lexington, KY 40517. (606) 272-7166. < http://www.lexington-on-line.com/naf.html >.

National Institute of Mental Health (NIMH) Office of Communications. 6001 Executive Boulevard, Room 8184, MSC 9663, Bethesda, MD 20892-9663. (866) 615-NIMH or (301) 443-4513. < http://www.nimh.nih.gov >.

OTHER

Anxiety Network Homepage. < http://www.anxietynetwork.com >.

National Institute of Mental Health (NIMH). *Anxiety Disorders.* NIH Publication No. 02-3879. Bethesda, MD: NIMH, 2002.

Carol A. Turkington
Rebecca J. Frey, PhD

Phospholipidosis *see* **Pulmonary alveolar proteinosis**

Phosphorus imbalance

Definition

Phosphorus imbalance refers to conditions in which the element phosphorus is present in the body at too high a level (hyperphosphatemia) or too low a level (hypophosphatemia).

Description

Almost all of the phosphorus in the body occurs as phosphate (phosphorus combined with four oxygen atoms), and most of the body's phosphate (85%) is located in the skeletal system, where it combines with calcium to give bones their hardness. The remaining amount (15%) exists in the cells of the body, where it plays an important role in the formation of key nucleic acids, such as DNA, and in the process by which the body turns food into energy (metabolism). The body regulates phosphate levels in the blood through the controlled release of parathyroid hormone (PTH) from the parathyroid gland and calcitonin from the thyroid gland. PTH keeps phosphate levels from becoming too high by stimulating the excretion of phosphate in urine and causing the release of calcium from bones (phosphate blood levels are inversely proportional to calcium blood levels). Calcitonin keeps phosphate blood levels in check by moving phosphates out of the blood and into the bone matrix to form a mineral salt with calcium.

Most phosphorus imbalances develop gradually and are the result of other conditions or disorders, such as **malnutrition**, poor kidney function, or a malfunctioning gland.

Causes and symptoms

Hypophosphatemia

Hypophosphatemia (low blood phosphate) has various causes. **Hyperparathyroidism**, a condition in which the parathyroid gland produces too much PTH, is one primary cause. Poor kidney function, in which the renal tubules do not adequately reabsorb phosphorus, can result in hypophosphatemia, as can overuse of **diuretics**, such as theophylline, and antacids containing aluminum hydroxide. Problems involving the intestinal absorption of phosphate, such as chronic **diarrhea** or a deficiency of vitamin D (needed by the intestines to properly absorb phosphates) can cause the condition. Malnutrition due to chronic alcoholism can result in an inadequate intake of phosphorus. Recovery from conditions such as **diabetic ketoacidosis** or severe burns can provoke hypophosphatemia, since the body must use larger-than-normal amounts of phosphate. Respiratory alkalosis, brought on by hyperventilation, can also result in temporary hypophosphatemia.

Symptoms generally occur only when phosphate levels have decreased profoundly. They include muscle weakness, **tingling** sensations, **tremors**, and bone weakness. Hypophosphatemia may also result in confusion and memory loss, seizures, and coma.

Hyperphosphatemia

Hyperphosphatemia (high blood phosphate) also has various causes. It is most often caused by a decline in the normal excretion of phosphate in urine as a result of kidney failure or impaired function. **Hypoparathyroidism**, a condition in which the parathyroid gland does not produce enough PTH, or pseudoparathyroidism, a condition in which the kidneys lose their ability to respond to PTH, can also contribute to decreased phosphate excretion. Hyperphosphatemia can also result from the overuse of **laxatives** or enemas that contain phosphate. **Hypocalcemia** (abnormally low blood calcium) can cause phosphate blood levels to increase abnormally. A side-effect of hyperphosphatemia is the formation of calcium-phosphate crystals in the blood and soft tissue.

Hyperphosphatemia is generally asymptomatic; however, it can occur in conjunction with hypocalcemia, the symptoms of which are **numbness and tingling** in the extremities, **muscle cramps** and spasms, depression, memory loss, and convulsions. When calcium-phosphate crystals build up in the blood vessels, they can cause arteriosclerosis, which can lead to heart attacks or strokes. When the crystals build up in the skin, they can cause severe itching.

Diagnosis

Disorders of phosphate metabolism are assessed by measuring serum or plasma levels of phosphate and calcium. Hypophosphatemia is diagnosed if the blood phosphate level is less than 2.5 milligrams per deciliter of blood. Hyperphosphatemia is diagnosed if the blood phosphate level is above 4.5 milligrams per deciliter of blood. Appropriate tests are also used to determine if the underlying cause of the imbalance, including assessments of kidney function, dietary intake, and appropriate hormone levels.

Treatment

Treatment of phosphorus imbalances focuses on correcting the underlying cause of the imbalance and restoring equilibrium. Treating the underlying condition may involve surgical removal of the parathyroid gland in the case of hypophosphatemia caused by hyperparathyroidism; initiating hormone therapy in cases of hyperphosphatemia caused by hypoparathyroidism; ceasing intake of drugs or medications that contribute to phosphorus imbalance; or instigating measures to restore proper kidney function.

Restoring phosphorus equilibrium in cases of mild hypophosphatemia may include drinking a prescribed solution that is rich in phosphorus; however, since this solution can cause diarrhea, many doctors recommend that patients drink 1 qt (0.9 L) of skim milk per day instead, since milk and other diary products are significant sources of phosphate. Other phosphate-rich foods include green, leafy vegetables; peas and beans; nuts; chocolate; beef liver; turkey; and some cola drinks. Severe hypophosphatemia may be treated with the administration of an intravenous solution containing phosphate.

Restoring phosphorus equilibrium in cases of mild hyperphosphatemia involves restricting intake of phosphorus-rich foods and taking a calcium-based antacid that binds to the phosphate and blocks its absorption in the intestines. In cases of severe hyperphosphatemia, an intravenous infusion of calcium gluconate may be administered. Dialysis may also be required in severe cases to help remove excess phosphate from the blood.

Prognosis

The prognosis for treating hyperphosphatemia and hypophosphatemia are excellent, though in cases where these problems are due to genetic disease, lifelong hormone treatment may be necessary.

Prevention

Phosphorus imbalances caused by hormonal disorders or other genetically determined conditions cannot be prevented. Hypophosphatemia resulting from poor dietary intake can be prevented by eating foods rich in phosphates, and hypophosphatemia caused by overuse of diuretics or **antacids** can be prevented by strictly following instructions concerning proper dosages, as can hyperphosphatemia due to excessive use of **enemas** or laxative. Finally, patients on dialysis or who are being fed intravenously should be monitored closely to prevent phosphorus imbalances.

Resources

PERIODICALS

Barcia, J. P., C. F. Strife, and C. B. Langman. "Infantile Hypophosphatemia: Treatment Options to Control Hypercalcemia, Hypercalciuria, and ChronicBone Demineralization." *Journal of Pediatrics* 130 (1997): 825-828.

Tom Brody, PhD

Photoallergy *see* **Photosensitivity**

Photokeratitis *see* **Keratitis**

Photorefractive keratectomy and laser-assisted in-situ keratomileusis

Definition

Photorefractive keratectomy (PRK) and laser-assisted in-situ keratomileusis (LASIK) are two similar surgical techniques that use an excimer laser to correct nearsightedness (**myopia**) by reshaping the cornea. The cornea is the clear outer structure of the eye that lies in front of the colored part of the eye (iris). PRK and LASIK are two forms of vision-correcting (refractive) surgery. The two techniques differ in how the surface layer of the cornea is treated. As of mid 1998, two eximer lasers (Summit and Visx) had been approved for laser vision correction (refractive surgery using a laser) in the PRK procedure. Since then, Visx, Summit, and other lasers have received approval by the Food and Drug Administration (FDA) for use in LASIK procedures.

Purpose

The purpose of both LASIK and PRK is to correct nearsightedness in persons who don't want to, or can't, wear eye glasses or contact lenses. Most patients are able to see well enough to pass a driver's license exam without glasses or contact lenses after the operation. After approximately age 40, the lens in the eye stiffens making it harder to focus up close. Because laser vision correction only affects the cornea, the procedures do not eliminate the need for reading glasses. Patients should be wary of any ads that "guarantee" 20/20 vision. Patients should also make sure that the laser being used is approved by the FDA.

Precautions

Patients should be over 18 years of age, have healthy corneas, and have vision that has been stable for the past year. People who may not be good candidates for these procedures are pregnant women or women who are breastfeeding (vision may not be stable); people with scarred corneas or macular disease; people with autoimmune diseases (i.e., systemic lupus erythematosus or **rheumatoid arthritis**); or people with diabetes. Patients with **glaucoma** should not have LASIK because the intraocular pressure (IOP) of the eye is raised during the procedure. A patient with persistent lid infections (i.e., blepharitis) may not be a good candidate because of an increased risk of infection. An ophthalmologist who specializes in laser vision correction can determine who would be likely to benefit from the operation and suggest which of the two operations might be more appropriate for any given patient.

If a patient is thinking of having **cataract surgery**, they should discuss it with the doctor. During cataract surgery an intraocular lens (IOL) will be inserted and that alone may correct distance vision.

Description

PRK and LASIK are both performed with an excimer laser, which uses a cold beam of ultraviolet light to sculpt or reshape the cornea so that light will focus properly on the retina. The cornea is the major focusing structure of the eye. The retina sends the image focused on it to the brain. In myopia, the cornea is either too steep or the eye is too long for a clear image to be focused on the retina. PRK and LASIK flatten out the cornea so that the image will focus more precisely on the retina.

In PRK, the surface of the cornea is removed by the laser. In LASIK, the outer layer of the cornea is sliced, lifted, moved aside while the cornea is reshaped with the laser, then replaced to speed healing. Both procedures cause the cornea to become flatter, which corrects the nearsighted vision.

At least one laser has been approved to treat mild **astigmatism** as of 2000. Correcting farsightedness (**hyperopia**) may be possible in the future.

These laser vision-correcting procedures are rapidly replacing radial keratotomy (RK), an earlier form of refractive surgery that involved cutting the cornea with a scalpel in a pattern of radiating spokes. RK has declined in popularity since the approval of the excimer laser in 1995, falling from a high of 250,000 procedures performed per year in 1994 to 50,000 in 1997.

For both LASIK and PRK, the patient's eye is numbed with anesthetic drops. No injections are necessary. The patient is awake and relaxed during the procedure.

LASIK is sometimes referred to as a "flap and zap" procedure because a thin flap of tissue is temporarily removed from the surface of the cornea and the underlying cornea is then "zapped" with a laser. Prior to the surgery, the surface of the cornea is marked with a dye marker so that the flap of cornea can be precisely aligned when it is replaced. The doctor places a suction ring on the eye to hold it steady. During this part of the operation, which lasts only a few seconds, the patient is not able to see. A surgical instrument called a microkeratome is passed over the cornea to create a very thin flap of tissue. The IOP is increased at this time which is why it is contraindicated in patients with glaucoma. This thin tissue layer is folded back. The cornea is reshaped with the laser beam and the cell layer is replaced. Because the cell layer is not permanently removed, patients have a faster recovery time and experience far less discomfort than with PRK. An antibiotic drop is put in and the eye is patched until the following day's checkup.

In PRK, a small area of the surface layer of the cornea is vaporized. It takes about three days for the surface cells to grow back and vision will be blurred. Some patients describe it as "looking through Vaseline." PRK is generally recommended for patient's with mild to moderate myopia (usually under -5.00 diopters).

With both PRK and LASIK, there is a loud tapping sound from the laser and a burning smell as the cornea is reshaped. The surgery itself is painless and takes only a minute or two. Patients are usually able to return home immediately after surgery. Most patients wait (up to six months) before they have the second one done. This allows the first eye to heal and to see if there were complications from the surgery.

The cost of these procedures can vary with geographic area and the doctor. In general, the procedure costs $1,350–$2,500 per eye for PRK and about $500 more per eye for LASIK. PRK and LASIK are generally not covered by insurance. However, insurance may cover these procedures for people in certain occupations, such as police officers and firefighters.

Preparation

If a patient wears contact lenses, they should not be worn for a few weeks prior to surgery. It also is important to discontinue contact lens wear prior to the visual exams to make sure vision is stable. The doctor should be advised of contact lens wear.

Upon arrival at the doctor's office on the day of surgery, patients are given some eye drops and a sedative, such as Valium, to relax them. Their vision is tested. They rest while waiting for the sedative to take effect. Immediately before the surgery, patients are given local anesthetic eye drops.

Aftercare

After surgery, antibiotic drops are placed in the eye and the eye may be patched. The patient returns for a follow-up visit the next day. The patient is usually given a prescription for eyedrops (usually antibiotic and anti-inflammatory). Patients who have had PRK usually feel mild discomfort for one to three days after the procedure. They may need a bandage contact lens. Patients who have had LASIK generally have less, or even no discomfort after the surgery. After LASIK, antibiotic and anti-inflammatory drops are generally necessary for one week. After PRK, steroidal eye drops may be necessary for months. Because steroids may increase the possibility of glaucoma or **cataracts**, it is a big drawback to the procedure. The patient should speak with the doctor to see how long follow-up medications will be necessary.

Most patients return to work within one to three days after the procedure, although visual recovery from PRK may take as long as four weeks. An eye shield may be used for about one week at night and patients may be sensitive to bright light for a few days. Patients may be asked by their doctor to keep water out of their eye for a week and to avoid mascara or eyeliner during this period.

Risks

There is a risk of under- or over-correction with either of these procedures. If vision is under-corrected, a second procedure can be performed to achieve results that may be closer to 20/20 vision. About 5–10% of PRK patients return for an adjustment, as do 10–25% of LASIK patients. People with higher degrees of myopia have vision that is harder to correct and usually have LASIK surgery rather than PRK. This may account for the higher incidence of adjustments for LASIK patients. Patients with very high myopia (over -15.00 diopters) may experience improvement after LASIK, but they are not likely to achieve 20/40 vision without glasses. However, their glasses will not need to be as thick or heavy after the surgery. However, most patients, especially those with less extreme myopia, do not need glasses after the surgery.

Haze is another possible side effect. Although hazy vision is unlikely, it is more likely to occur after PRK than after LASIK. This haze usually clears up. Corneal scarring, halos, or glare at night, or an irritating bump on the cornea are other possible side effects. As with any eye surgery, infection is possible, but rare. Loss of vision is possible with these procedures, but this complication is extremely rare.

Most complications from LASIK are related to the creation and realignment of the flap. The microkeratome must be in good-working order and sharp. LASIK requires a great deal of skill on the part of the surgeon and the complication rate is related to the experience level of the surgeon. In one study, the rate of LASIK complications declined from 3% for

KEY TERMS

Blepharitits— An inflammation of the eyelid.

Cataract—A condition in which the lens of the eye turns cloudy and interferes with vision.

Cornea—The clear, curved tissue layer in front of the eye. It lies in front of the colored part of the eye (iris) and the black hole in the center of the iris (pupil).

Diopter (D)—A unit of measure of the power or strength of a lens.

Excimer laser—An instrument that is used to vaporize tissue with a cold, coherent beam of light with a single wavelength in the ultraviolet range.

Intraocular lens (IOL) implant—A small, plastic device (IOL) that is usually implanted in the lens capsule of the eye to correct vision after the lens of the eye is removed. This is the implant is used in cataract surgery.

Macular degeneration—A condition usually associated with age in which the area of the retina called the macula is impaired due to hardening of the arteries (arteriosclerosis). This condition interferes with vision.

Microkeratome—A precision surgical instrument that can slice an extremely thin layer of tissue from the surface of the cornea.

Myopia—A vision problem in which distant objects appear blurry. Myopia results when the cornea is too steep or the eye is too long and the light doesn't focus properly on the retina. People who are myopic or nearsighted can usually see near objects clearly, but not far objects.

Refractive surgery—A surgical procedure that corrects visual defects.

Retina—The sensory tissue in the back of the eye that is responsible for collecting visual images and sending them to the brain.

surgeons during their first three months using this technique, to 1% after a year's experience in the technique, to 0% after 18 months experience.

Normal results

Most patients experience improvement in their vision immediately after the operation and about half of LASIK patients are able to see 20/30 within one day of the surgery. Vision tends to become sharper over the next few days and then stabilizes; however, it is possible to have shifts in myopia for the next few months. Vision clears and stabilizes faster after LASIK than after PRK. Final vision is achieved within three to six months with LASIK and six to eight months with PRK. The vast majority of patients (95% for people with low to moderate myopia and 75% for people with high levels of myopia) are able to see 20/40 after either of these procedures and are able to pass a driver's license test without glasses or contact lenses.

LASIK is more complicated than PRK because of the addition of the microkeratome procedure. However, LASIK generally has faster recovery time, less **pain**, and less chance of halos and scarring than PRK. LASIK can treat higher degrees of myopia (-5.00–25.00 diopters). LASIK also requires less use of steroids. Patients need to speak with qualified, experienced eye surgeons to help in choosing the procedure that is right for them.

Resources

ORGANIZATIONS

American Academy of Ophthalmology. 655 Beach Street, P.O. Box 7424, San Francisco, CA 94120-7424. < http://www.eyenet.org >.

American Society of Cataract and Refractive Surgery. 4000 Legato Road, Suite 850, Fairfax, VA 22033-4055. (703) 591-2220. < http://www.ascrs.org >.

Louann W. Murray, PhD

Photosensitivity

Definition

Photosensitivity refers to any increase in the reactivity of the skin to sunlight.

Description

The skin is a carefully designed interface between our bodies and the outside world. It is infection-proof when intact, nearly waterproof, and filled with protective mechanisms. Sunlight threatens the health of the skin. Normal skin is highly variable in its ability to resist sun damage. Natural skin pigmentation is its main protection. The term photosensitivity refers to any increase beyond what is considered normal variation.

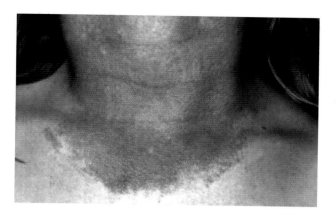

A skin rash on the front of a woman's neck caused by a photosensitive reaction to sunlight. *(Photograph by Dr. P. Marazzi, Photo Researchers, Inc. Reproduced by permission.)*

Causes and symptoms

There are over three dozen diseases, two dozen drugs, a variety of herbal preparations, and several perfume and cosmetic components that can cause photosensitivity. There are also several different types of reaction to sunlight—phototoxicity, photoallergy, and polymorphous light eruption. In addition, prolonged exposure to sunlight, even in normal skin, leads to skin **aging** and **cancer**. These effects are accelerated in patients who have photosensitivity.

- Phototoxicity is a severely exaggerated reaction to sunlight caused by a new chemical in the skin. The primary symptom is **sunburn**, which is rapid and can be severe enough to blister (a second degree burn). The chemicals associated with phototoxicity are usually drugs. The list includes several common antibiotics—quinolones, **sulfonamides**, and **tetracyclines**; **diuretics** (water pills); major tranquilizers; oral diabetes medication; and cancer medicines. There are also some dermatologic drugs, both topical and oral, that can sensitize skin.

- Photoallergy produces an intense **itching** rash on exposure to sunlight. Patients develop chronic skin changes (lichen simplex) as a result of scratching. Some of the agents that cause phototoxicity can also cause photoallergy. Some cosmetic and perfume ingredients, including a compound that was formerly used in sunscreens—para-amino benzoic acid (PABA)—can do this. Most sunscreen preparations in the early 2000s, however, no longer include PABA.

- Polymorphous light eruption (PLE) resembles photoallergy in its production of intensely itching **rashes** in sunlight. However, this condition lessens with continued light exposure, and so is seen mostly in the spring. Also, there does not seem to be an identifiable chemical involved. PLE is most likely to develop in fair-skinned individuals. It is estimated to affect about 10% of the United States population compared to 21% of the Swedish population. The female: male ratio is 2.5: 1, but it is thought that the imbalance may be due to the fact that women are more likely than men to seek treatment for PLE.

- There is a form of inherited PLE that affects Native Americans. The inheritance pattern is autosomal dominant.

Diseases of several kinds increase skin sensitivity:

- A hereditary disease called xeroderma pigmentosum includes a defect in repair mechanisms that greatly accelerates skin damage from sunlight.

- A family of metabolic diseases called **porphyrias** produce chemicals (porphyrins) that absorb sunlight in the skin and thereby cause damage.

- Albinos lack skin pigment through a genetic defect and are thus very sensitive to light.

- Malnutrition, specifically a deficiency of niacin known as **pellagra**, sensitizes the skin.

- Several diseases like **acne**, **systemic lupus erythematosus**, **rosacea**, and herpes simplex (**fever** blisters) decrease the resistance of the skin to sun damage. Rosacea is sometimes described as a photoaggravated skin disorder because its symptoms increase in severity when patients are exposed to sunlight.

- Photosensitivity is increasingly recognized as a common development in HIV-positive patients. Risk factors for photosensitivity in this group include African American ethnicity and treatment with highly active antiretroviral therapy (HAART).

Diagnosis

The pattern of appearance on the skin, a history of drug or chemical exposure, and the timing of the symptoms often suggests a diagnosis. A **skin biopsy** may be needed for further clarification.

Treatment

Removal of the offending drug or chemical is primary. Direct sunlight exposure should be limited. Some people must avoid sunlight altogether, while others can tolerate some direct sunlight with the aid of **sunscreens**.

Prevention

A sunscreen with an SPF of 15 or greater protects most skin from damage. Such protective garments as hats and long-sleeved shirts are highly recommended in addition.

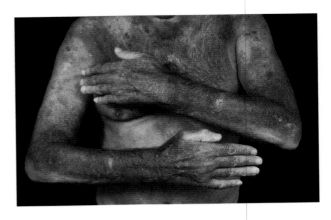

This person had a photoxic reaction after taking an antibiotic drug. *(Photo Researchers, Inc. Reproduced by permission.)*

KEY TERMS

Albino—A person or animal lacking normal coloring in the eyes, hair, and skin due to a hereditary inability to produce the skin pigment melanin. The condition itself is called albinism.

Biopsy—Surgical removal of tissue for examination.

Rosacea—A chronic skin disease characterized by persistent redness of the skin and periodic outbreaks of pustules, usually affecting the middle third of the face.

Resources

BOOKS

Beers, Mark H., MD, and Robert Berkow, MD., editors. "Pigmentation Disorders." Section 10, Chapter 123 In *The Merck Manual of Diagnosis and Therapy*. Whitehouse Station, NJ: Merck Research Laboratories, 2002.

Beers, Mark H., MD, and Robert Berkow, MD., editors. "Reactions to Sunlight." In *The Merck Manual of Diagnosis and Therapy*. Whitehouse Station, NJ: Merck Research Laboratories, 2004.

PERIODICALS

Bilu, D., A. J. Mamelak, R. H. Nguyen, et al. "Clinical and Epidemiologic Characterization of Photosensitivity in HIV-Positive Individuals." *Photodermatology, Photoimmunology and Photomedicine* 20 (August 2004): 175–183.

Ciocon, J. O., D. G. Ciocon, and D. J. Galindo. "Dietary Supplements in Primary Care. Botanicals Can Affect Surgical Outcomes and Follow-Up." *Geriatrics* 59 (September 2004): 20–24.

Levy, Stanley B., MD. "Sunscreens and Photoprotection." *eMedicine* November 25, 2002. < http://www.emedicine.com/derm/topic510.htm >.

Murphy, G. "Ultraviolet Light and Rosacea." *Cutis* 74, Supplement 3 (September 2004): 13–16, 32–34.

Palmer, R. A., C. B. van de Pas, E. Campalani, et al. "A Simple Method to Assess Severity of Polymorphic Light Eruption." *British Journal of Dermatology* 151 (September 2004): 645–652.

Shirin, Sophie, MD, Raul DelRosario, MD, and Ada Winkielman, MD. "Polymorphous Light Eruption." *eMedicine* October 16, 2003. < http://www.emedicine.com/derm/topic342.htm >.

ORGANIZATIONS

American Academy of Dermatology (AAD). P. O. Box 4014, Schaumburg, IL 60168-4014. (847) 330-0230. < http://www.aad.org >.

United States Food and Drug Administration (FDA). 5600 Fishers Lane, Rockville, MD 20857-0001. (888) INFO-FDA. < http://www.fda.gov >.

J. Ricker Polsdorfer, MD
Rebecca J. Frey, PhD

Phototherapy

Definition

Phototherapy, or light therapy, is the administration of doses of bright light in order to normalize the body's internal clock and/or relieve depression.

Purpose

Phototherapy is prescribed primarily to treat seasonal affective disorder (SAD), a mood disorder characterized by depression in the winter months, and is occasionally employed to treat **insomnia and jet lag**. The exact mechanisms by which the treatment works are not known, but the bright light employed in phototherapy may act to readjust the body's circadian (daily) rhythms, or internal clock. Other popular theories are that light triggers the production of serotonin, a neurotransmitter believed to be related to **depressive disorders**, or that it influences the body's production of melatonin, a hormone derived from serotonin that may be related to circadian rhythms.

Precautions

Patients with eye problems should see an ophthalmologist regularly, both before and during phototherapy. Because some ultraviolet rays are emitted by the light boxes used in phototherapy, patients taking photosensitizing medications (medications making the skin more sensitive to light) and those who have sun-sensitive skin should consult with their physician before beginning treatment. Patients with medical conditions that make them sensitive to ultraviolet rays should also be seen by a physician before starting phototherapy. Patients who have a history of mood swings or **mania** should be monitored closely, since phototherapy may cause excessive mood elevation in some individuals.

Description

Phototherapy is generally administered at home. The most commonly used phototherapy equipment is a portable lighting device known as a light box. The box may be mounted upright to a wall, or slanted downwards towards a table. The patient sits in front of the box for a prescribed period of time (anywhere from 15 minutes to several hours). Some patients with SAD undergo phototherapy sessions two or three times a day, others only once. The time of day and number of times treatment is administered depend on the physical needs and lifestyle of the individual patient. If phototherapy has been prescribed for the treatment of SAD, it typically begins in the fall months as the days begin to shorten, and continues throughout the winter and possibly the early spring.

The light from a slanted light box is designed to focus on the table it sits upon, so patients may look down to read or do other sedentary activities during therapy. Patients using an upright light box must face the light source (although they need not look directly into the light). The light sources in these light boxes typically range from 2,500–10,000 lux. (In contrast, average indoor lighting is 300–500 lux; a sunny summer day is about 100,000 lux).

Phototherapy prescribed for the treatment of SAD may be covered by insurance. Individuals requiring phototherapy should check with their insurance company to see if the cost of renting or purchasing a light box is covered.

Aftercare

Patients beginning light therapy for SAD may need to adjust the length, frequency, and timing of their phototherapy sessions to achieve the maximum benefit. These patients should keep their doctor informed of their progress and the status of their depressive symptoms. Occasionally, antidepressants and/or psychotherapy may be recommended as an adjunct to phototherapy.

KEY TERMS

Circadian rhythm—The rhythmic repetition of certain phenomena in living organisms at about the same time each day.

Lux—A standard unit of measure for illumination.

Neurotransmitter—A chemical in the brain that transmits messages between neurons, or nerve cells.

Photosensitivity—An abnormally heightened reaction to light.

Seasonal affective disorder (SAD)—A mood disorder characterized by depression during the winter months. An estimated 11 million Americans experience SAD.

Risks

An abnormally elevated or expansive mood (hypomania) may occur, but it is usually temporary. Some patients undergoing phototherapy treatment report side effects of eyestrain, headaches, insomnia, **fatigue**, **sunburn**, and dry eyes or nose. Most of these effects can be managed by adjusting the timing and duration of the phototherapy sessions. A strong sun block and eye and nose drops can alleviate the other problems. Long-term studies have shown no negative effects to the eye function of individuals undergoing phototherapy treatments.

Normal results

Patients with SAD typically report an alleviation of depressive symptoms within two to 14 days after beginning phototherapy.

Resources

ORGANIZATIONS

National Institute of Mental Health. Mental Health Public Inquiries, 5600 Fishers Lane, Room 15C-05, Rockville, MD 20857. (888) 826-9438. < http://www.nimh.nih.gov >.

Society for Light Treatment and Biological Rhythms. P.O. Box 591687, 174 Cook St., San Francisco, CA 94159-1687. < http://www.websciences.org/sltbr >.

Paula Anne Ford-Martin

Phototoxic reaction *see* **Photosensitivity**

Phycomycosis *see* **Mucormycosis**

Physical allergy

Definition

Physical **allergies** are allergic reactions to cold, sunlight, heat, or minor injury.

Description

The immune system is designed to protect the body from harmful invaders such as germs. Occasionally, it goes awry and attacks harmless or mildly noxious agents, doing more harm than good. This event is termed allergy if the target is from the outside—like pollen or bee venom—and autoimmunity if it is caused by one of the body's own components.

The immune system usually responds only to certain kinds of chemicals, namely proteins. However, non-proteins can trigger the same sort of response, probably by altering a protein to make it look like a target. Physical allergy refers to reactions in which a protein is not the initial inciting agent.

Sometimes it takes a combination of elements to produce an allergic reaction. A classic example is drugs that are capable of sensitizing the skin to sunlight. The result is phototoxicity, which appears as an increased sensitivity to sunlight or as localized skin **rashes** on sun-exposed areas.

Causes and symptoms

- Minor injury, such as scratching, causes itchy welts to develop in about 5% of people. The presence of itchy welts (urticaria) is a condition called dermographism.

- Cold can change certain proteins in the blood so that they induce an immune reaction. This may indicate that there are abnormal proteins in the blood from a disease of the bone marrow. The reaction may also involve the lungs and circulation, producing **wheezing** and **fainting**.

- Heat allergies can be caused by **exercise** or even strong emotions in sensitive people.

- Sunlight, even without drugs, causes immediate urticaria in some people. This may be a symptom of porphyria—a genetic metabolic defect.

- Elements like nickel and chromium, although not proteins, commonly cause skin rashes, and iodine allergy causes skin rashes and sores in the mouth in allergic individuals.

- Pressure or vibration can also cause urticaria.

- Water contact can cause aquagenic urticaria, presumably due to chlorine or some other trace chemical in the water, although distilled water has been known to cause this reaction.

When the inflammatory reaction involves deeper layers of the skin, urticaria becomes angioedema. The skin, especially the lips and eyelids, swells. The tongue, throat, and parts of the digestive tract may also be involved. Angioedema may be due to physical agents. Often the cause remains unknown.

Diagnosis

Visual examination of the symptoms usually diagnoses the reaction. Further skin tests and review of the patient's **photosensitivity** may reveal a cause.

Treatment

Removing the offending agent is the first step to treatment. If sun is involved, shade and sunscreens are necessary. The reaction can usually be controlled with epinephrine, **antihistamines**, or cortisone-like drugs. Urticaria may be treated with antihistamines such as diphenhydramine (Benadryl) or desloratadine (Clarinex). Clarinex is non-sedating, meaning it will not make patients drowsy. Itching can be controlled with cold packs or commercial topical agents that contain menthol, camphor, eucalyptus oil, aloe, antihistamines, or cortisone preparations.

Prognosis

If the causative agent has been diagnosed, avoidance of or protection against the allergen cures the allergy. Usually, allergies can be managed through treatment.

Resources

PERIODICALS

Kirn, F. Timothy. "Desloratadine Improves Urticaria in Clinical Setting." *Skin & Allergy News* September 2004: 41.

J. Ricker Polsdorfer, MD
Teresa G. Odle

Physical examination

Definition

A physical examination is an evaluation of the body and its functions using inspection, palpation (feeling with the hands), percussion (tapping with the fingers), and auscultation (listening). A complete health assessment also includes gathering information about a person's medical history and lifestyle, doing laboratory tests, and screening for disease.

Purpose

The annual physical examination has been replaced by the periodic health examination. How often this is done depends on the patient's age, sex, and risk factors for disease. The United States Preventative Services Task Force (USPSTF) has developed guidelines for preventative health examinations that health care professionals widely follow. Organizations that promote detection and prevention of specific diseases, like the American Cancer Society, generally recommend more intensive or frequent examinations.

A comprehensive physical examination provides an opportunity for the healthcare professional to obtain baseline information about the patient for future use, and to establish a relationship before problems happen. It provides an opportunity to answer questions and teach good health practices. Detecting a problem in its early stages can have good long-term results.

Precautions

The patient should be comfortable and treated with respect throughout the examination. As the examination procedes, the examiner should explain what he or she is doing and share any relevant findings.

Description

A complete physical examination usually starts at the head and proceeds all the way to the toes. However, the exact procedure will vary according to the needs of the patient and the preferences of the examiner. An average examination takes about 30 minutes. The cost of the examination will depend on the charge for the professional's time and any tests that are done. Most health plans cover routine physical examinations including some tests.

The examination

First, the examiner will observe the patient's appearance, general health, and behavior, along with measuring height and weight. The vital signs—including pulse, breathing rate, body temperature, and blood pressure—are recorded.

With the patient sitting up, the following systems are reviewed:

- Skin. The exposed areas of the skin are observed; the size and shape of any lesions are noted.

- Head. The hair, scalp, skull, and face are examined.

- Eyes. The external structures are observed. The internal structures can be observed using an ophthalmoscope (a lighted instrument) in a darkened room.

- Ears. The external structures are inspected. A lighted instrument called an otoscope may be used to inspect internal structures.

- Nose and sinuses. The external nose is examined. The nasal mucosa and internal structures can be observed with the use of a penlight and a nasal speculum.

- Mouth and pharynx. The lips, gums, teeth, roof of the mouth, tongue, and pharynx are inspected.

- Neck. The lymph nodes on both sides of the neck and the thyroid gland are palpated (examined by feeling with the fingers).

- Back. The spine and muscles of the back are palpated and checked for tenderness. The upper back, where the lungs are located, is palpated on the right and left sides and a stethoscope is used to listen for breath sounds.

- Breasts and armpits. A woman's breasts are inspected with the arms relaxed and then raised. In both men and women, the lymph nodes in the armpits are felt with the examiner's hands. While the patient is still sitting, movement of the joints in the hands, arms, shoulders, neck, and jaw can be checked.

Then while the patient is lying down on the examining table, the examination includes:

- Breasts. The breasts are palpated and inspected for lumps.

- Front of chest and lungs. The area is inspected with the fingers, using palpation and percussion. A stethoscope is used to listen to the internal breath sounds.

The head should be slightly raised for:

- Heart. A stethoscope is used to listen to the heart's rate and rhythm. The blood vessels in the neck are observed and palpated.

The patient should lie flat for:

- Abdomen. Light and deep palpation is used on the abdomen to feel the outlines of internal organs including the liver, spleen, kidneys, and aorta, a large blood vessel.

- Rectum and anus. With the patient lying on the left side, the outside areas are observed. An internal digital examination (using a finger), is usually done if the patient is over 40 years old. In men, the prostate gland is also palpated.

- Reproductive organs. The external sex organs are inspected and the area is examined for hernias. In men, the scrotum is palpated. In women, a pelvic examination is done using a speculum and a Papamnicolaou test (**Pap test**) may be taken.

- Legs. With the patient lying flat, the legs are inspected for swelling, and pulses in the knee, thigh, and foot area are found. The groin area is palpated for the presence of lymph nodes. The joints and muscles are observed.

- Musculoskeletel system. With the patient standing, the straightness of the spine and the alignment of the legs and feet is noted.

- Blood vessels. The presence of any abnormally enlarged veins (varicose), usually in the legs, is noted.

In addition to evaluating the patient's alertness and mental ability during the initial conversation, additional inspection of the nervous system may be indicated:

- Neurologic screen. The patient's ability to take a few steps, hop, and do deep knee bends is observed. The strength of the hand grip is felt. With the patient sitting down, the reflexes in the knees and feet can be tested with a small hammer. The sense of touch in the hands and feet can be evaluated by testing reaction to **pain** and vibration.

- Sometimes additional time is spent examining the 12 nerves in the head (cranial) that are connected directly to the brain. They control the sense of smell, strength of muscles in the head, reflexes in the eye, facial movements, gag reflex, and muscles in the jaw. General muscle tone and coordination, and the reaction of the abdominal area to stimulants like pain, temperature, and touch would also be evaluated.

Preparation

Before visiting the health care professional, the patient should write down important facts and dates about his or her own medical history, as well as those

KEY TERMS

Auscultation—The process of listening to sounds that are produced in the body. Direct auscultation uses the ear alone, such as when listening to the grating of a moving joint. Indirect auscultation involves the use of a stethoscope to amplify the sounds from within the body, like a heartbeat.

Hernia—The bulging of an organ, or part of an organ, through the tissues normally containing it; also called a rupture.

Inspection—The visual examination of the body using the eyes and a lighted instrument if needed. The sense of smell may also be used.

Ophthalmoscope—Lighted device for studying the interior of the eyeball.

Otoscope—An instrument with a light for examining the internal ear.

Palpation—The examination of the body using the sense of touch. There are two types: light and deep.

Percussion—An assessment method in which the surface of the body is struck with the fingertips to obtain sounds that can be heard or vibrations that can be felt. It can determine the position, size, and consistency of an internal organ. It is done over the chest to determine the presence of normal air content in the lungs, and over the abdomen to evaluate air in the loops of the intestine.

Reflex—An automatic response to a stimulus.

Speculum—An instrument for enlarging the opening of any canal or cavity in order to facilitate inspection of its interior.

Stethoscope—A Y-shaped instrument that amplifies body sounds such as heartbeat, breathing, and air in the intestine. Used in auscultation.

Varicose veins—The permanent enlargement and twisting of veins, usually in the legs. They are most often seen in people with occupations requiring long periods of standing, and in pregnant women.

The patient usually removes all clothing and puts on a loose-fitting hospital gown. An additional sheet is provided to keep the patient covered and comfortable during the examination.

Aftercare

Once the physical examination has been completed, the patient and the examiner should review what laboratory tests have been ordered and how the results will be shared with the patient. The medical professional should discuss any recommendations for treatment and follow-up visits. Special instructions should be put in writing. This is also an opportunity for the patient to ask any remaining questions about his or her own health concerns.

Normal results

Normal results of a physical examination correspond to the healthy appearance and normal functioning of the body. For example, appropriate reflexes will be present, no suspicious lumps or lesions will be found, and vital signs will be normal.

Abnormal results

Abnormal results of a physical examination include any findings that indicated the presence of a disorder, disease, or underlying condition. For example, the presence of lumps or lesions, fever, muscle weakness or lack of tone, poor reflex response, heart arhythmia, or swelling of lymph nodes will point to a possible health problem.

Resources

BOOKS

Bates, Barbara. *A Guide to Physical Examination and History Taking*. Philadelphia: Lippincott Co., 1995.

Karen Ericson, RN

Physical therapy *see* **Rehabilitation**

of family members. He or she should have a list of all medications with their doses or bring the actual bottles of medicine along. If there are specific concerns about anything, writing them down is a good idea.

Before the physical examination begins, the bladder should be emptied and a urine specimen can be collected in a small container. For some blood tests, the patient may be told ahead of time not to eat or drink after midnight.

Pica

Definition

Pica is the persistent craving and compulsive eating of nonfood substances. The Diagnostic and Statistical Manual of Mental Disorders, fourth edition, classifies it as a feeding and eating disorder of childhood.

Description

The puzzling phenomenon of pica has been recognized and described since ancient times. Pica has been observed in ethnic groups worldwide, in both primitive and modernized cultures, in both sexes, and in all age groups. The word pica comes from the Latin name for magpie, a bird known for its unusual and indiscriminate eating habits. In addition to humans, pica has been observed in other animals, including the chimpanzee.

Pica in humans has many different subgroups, defined by the substance that is ingested. Some of the most commonly described types of pica are eating earth, soil or clay (geophagia), ice (pagophagia) and starch (amylophagia). However, pica involving dozens of other substances, including cigarette butts and ashes, hair, paint chips, and paper have also been reported. In one unusual case, the patient ingested transdermal patches of fentanyl, an opioid medication given for severe **pain**. Eating the skin patch increased the patient's dose of the drug by a factor of 10.

Although pica can occur in individuals of any background, a higher incidence of pica is associated with:

- **pregnancy**
- developmental delay and **mental retardation**
- psychiatric disease and **autism**
- early childhood
- poor **nutrition** or low blood levels of iron and other minerals
- certain cultural or religious traditions

Causes and symptoms

Evidence suggests that there may be several causes of pica. One widely held theory points to iron deficiency as a major cause of pica. Several reports have described pica in individuals with documented iron deficiency, although there has been uncertainty as to whether the iron deficiency was a cause of pica or a result of it. Because some substances, such as clay, are believed to block the absorption of iron into the bloodstream, it was thought that low blood levels of iron could be the direct result of pica. However, some studies have shown that pica cravings in individuals with iron deficiency stop once iron supplements are given to correct the deficiency. Another study looked specifically at the rate of iron absorption during pica conditions and normal dietary behavior, and showed that the iron absorption was not decreased by pica. In addition, low blood levels of iron commonly occur in pregnant women and those with poor nutrition, two populations at higher risk for pica. Such findings offer strong support of iron deficiency as a cause, rather than result, of pica.

Other reports suggest that pica may have a psychological basis and may even fall into the spectrum of **obsessive-compulsive disorder**. Pica has a higher incidence in populations with an underlying diagnosis involving mental functioning. These diagnoses include psychiatric conditions like schizophrenia, developmental disorders including autism, and conditions with mental retardation. These conditions are not characterized by iron deficiency, which supports a psychological component in the cause of pica.

Cultural and religious traditions may also play a role in pica behavior. In some cultures, nonfood substances are believed to have positive health or spiritual effects. Among some African Americans in the south, ingesting a particular kind of white clay is believed to promote health and reduce morning sickness during pregnancy. Other cultures practice pica out of belief that eating a particular substance may promote fertility or bring good luck.

The hallmark feature of pica, consistently consuming nonfood substances, often does not present publicly. People may be embarrassed to admit to these unusual eating habits, and may hide it from their family and physician. In other cases, an individual may not report the pica to a physician simply because of a lack of knowledge of pica's potential medical significance.

Because the eating behaviors of pica are not usually detected or reported, it is the complications of the behavior that bring it to attention. Complications vary, depending on the type of pica. Geophagia has potential side effects that most commonly affect the intestine and bowel. Complications can include **constipation**, cramping, pain, obstruction caused by formation of an indigestible mass, perforation from sharp objects like rocks or gravel, and contamination and infection from soil-dwelling parasites.

Amylophagia usually involves the consumption of cornstarch and, less frequently, laundry starch. The high caloric content of starch can cause excessive weight gain, while at the same time leading to **malnutrition**, as starch contributes "empty" calories lacking **vitamins** and **minerals**. Amylophagia during pregnancy can mimic **gestational diabetes** in its presentation and even in its potential harmful effects on the fetus.

Pica involving the ingestion of substances such as lead-based paint or paper containing mercury can cause symptoms of toxic **poisoning**. Compulsive consumption of even a seemingly harmless substance like ice (pagophagia) can have negative side effects, including decreased absorption of nutrients by the gut.

Diagnosis

In order for the diagnosis of pica to be made, there must be a history of persistent consumption of a nonfood substance continuing for a minimum period of one month. Infants and toddlers are typically excluded from this diagnosis since mouthing objects is a normal developmental behavior at that age. Individuals with mental retardation who function at or below an approximate cognitive level of 18 months may also be exempt form this diagnosis.

Pica is most often diagnosed when a report of such behaviors can be provided by the patient or documented by another individual. In other cases, pica is diagnosed after studies have been performed to assess the presenting symptoms. For example, imaging studies ordered to assess severe gastrointestinal complaints may reveal intestinal blockage with an opaque substance; such a finding is suggestive of pica. Biopsy of intestinal contents can also reveal findings, such as parasitic infection, consistent with pica. Pica may also be suspected if abnormal levels of certain minerals or chemicals are detected in the blood.

Pica in pregnant women is sometimes diagnosed after **childbirth** because of a health problem in the newborn caused by the substance(s) ingested by the mother. In one instance reported in Chicago, a newborn girl was treated for **lead poisoning** caused by her mother's eating fragments of lead-glazed pottery during pregnancy.

Treatment

Treatment of pica will often depend on the cause and type of pica. Conventional medical treatment may be appropriate in certain situations. For example, supplementation with iron-containing vitamins has been shown to cause the unusual cravings to subside in some iron-deficient patients.

Medical complications and health threats, including high lead levels, bowel perforation or intestinal obstruction, will require additional medical management, beyond addressing the underlying issue of pica.

Alternative treatment

Because most cases of pica do not have an obvious medical cause, treatment with counseling, education, and nutritional management is often more successful

---

KEY TERMS

Amylophagia—The compulsive eating of purified starch, typically cornstarch or laundry starch.

Geophagia—The compulsive eating of earthy substances, including sand, soil, and clay.

Pagophagia—The compulsive eating of ice.

---

and more appropriate than treatment with medication. Some therapists specializing in eating disorders may have expertise in treating pica.

Prognosis

The prognosis for individuals with pica varies greatly, according to the type and amount of substance ingested, the extent of presenting side effects, and the success of treatment. Many of the side effects and complications of pica can be reversed once the behavior is stopped, while other complications, including infection and bowel perforation, pose significant health threats and if not successfully treated may result in **death**.

When seen in children, pica behavior tends to lessen with age. However, individuals with a history of pica are more likely to experience it again. Counseling and nutritional education can reduce the risk of recurrence.

Prevention

There are no known methods of preventing pica. However, once pica is known or suspected, measures can be taken to reduce further ingestion of nonfood substances. Removing the particular substance from readily accessible areas can be helpful. Close observation of the individual with pica may limit inappropriate eating behaviors.

Resources

BOOKS

American Psychiatric Association. *Diagnostic and Statistical Manual of Mental Disorders*. 4th ed, revised. Washington, DC: American Psychiatric Association, 2000.

Beers, Mark H., MD, and Robert Berkow, MD., editors. "Anemias." In *The Merck Manual of Diagnosis and Therapy*. Whitehouse Station, NJ: Merck Research Laboratories, 2004.

Beers, Mark H., MD, and Robert Berkow, MD., editors. "Malnutrition." Section 1, Chapter 2 In *The Merck*

Manual of Diagnosis and Therapy. Whitehouse Station, NJ: Merck Research Laboratories, 2002.

PERIODICALS

Jackson, W. Clay. "Amylophagia Presenting as Gestational Diabetes." *Archives of Family Medicine* 9 (July 2000): 649–652.

Kirschner, Jeffrey. "Management of Pica: A Medical Enigma." *American Family Physician* 63, no. 6 (March 15, 2001): 1169. < http://www.aafp.org/afp/20010315/tips/9.html > .

Liappas, I. A., N. P. Dimopoulos, E. Mellos, et al. "Oral Transmucosal Abuse of Transdermal Fentanyl." *Journal of Psychopharmacology* 18 (June 2004): 277–280.

Moya, J., C. F. Bearer, and R. A. Etzel. "Children's Behavior and Physiology and How It Affects Exposure to Environmental Contaminants." *Pediatrics* 113 (April 2004): 996–1006.

Mycyk, M. B., and J. B. Leikin. "Combined Exchange Transfusion and Chelation Therapy for Neonatal Lead Poisoning." *Annals of Pharmacotherapy* 38 (May 2004): 821–824.

ORGANIZATIONS

American Academy of Child and Adolescent Psychiatry. 3615 Wisconsin Avenue, NW, Washington, DC 20016-3007. (202) 966-7300. Fax: (202) 966-2891. < http://www.aacap.org > .

OTHER

"Pica: Dirt Eating or 'Geophagy'." Support, Concern and Resources For Eating Disorders, 2000. < http://www.eating-disorder.org/pica.html >.

"Pica." KidsHealth. The Nemours Foundation, 2001. < http://kidshealth.org/parent/emotions/behavior/pica.html >.

Stefanie B. N. Dugan, M.S.
Rebecca J. Frey, PhD

Pickwickian syndrome

Definition

A group of symptoms that generally accompany massive **obesity**.

Description

Pickwickian syndrome is a complex of symptoms that primarily affect patients with extreme obesity. The syndrome is named after a character in a Charles Dickens novel, *The Pickwick Papers*, who seemed to show some of the traits of this disease.

KEY TERMS

Latency—The period of inactivity between the time a stimulus is provided and the time a response occurs.

Obesity—Exceeding one's normal weight by 20%. A person suffering from extreme obesity would exceed their normal weight by a much higher percentage.

Pulmonary system—Lungs and respiratory system of the body.

The major health problem that occurs in patients with this disease is **sleep apnea**. This is caused in part by the excess amounts of fatty tissue surrounding the chest muscles. This excess fat places a strain on the heart, lungs, and diaphragm of the patient, making it difficult to breathe.

Causes and symptoms

The major cause of Pickwickian syndrome is extreme obesity. This obesity places an excessive load on the pulmonary system. The role of genetics is also being studied. Symptoms of Pickwickian syndrome include excessive daytime sleepiness, shortness of breath due to elevated blood carbon dioxide pressure, disturbed sleep at night, and flushed face. The skin can also have a bluish tint, and the patient may have high blood pressure, an enlarged liver, and an abnormally high red blood cell count.

Diagnosis

Some tests that can be used to diagnose this condition include **echocardiography** to determine heart enlargement or **pulmonary hypertension**. Giving the patient multiple sleep latency tests can help give an objective measurement of daytime sleepiness. Magnetic resonance imaging (MRI), computed tomography (CT) scans, or fiberoptic evaluation of the upper airway may also be used.

Treatment

The primary treatment for Pickwickian syndrome is focused on weight loss and increased physical activity. Also, medroxyprogesterone may help improve the condition.

Prognosis

Pickwickian sydnrome is entirely reversible if it is diagnosed and treated properly. If the problem goes undiagnosed, the outcome can be fatal.

Prevention

Prevention of Pickwickian syndrome can be achieved by maintaining a healthy body weight and getting the proper amount of **exercise**. For prevention of the sleep apnea that generally accompanies Pickwickian syndrome, there are several possible treatments. If the sleep apnea is only present when the patient is flat on their back, a tennis ball can be sewn into the sleep clothes to remind the patient not to sleep on their back. For more severe cases of sleep apnea, a **tonsillectomy** or the use of dental appliances may be recommended.

Resources

BOOKS

Dambro, Mark R. *The 5-Minute Clinical Consult.* Baltimore: Williams & Wilkins, 2001.

Tierney, Lawrence, et. al. *Current Medical Diagnosis and Treatment.* Los Altos: Lange Medical Publications, 2001.

PERIODICALS

"'Apples' and 'Pears': Defining the Shape of the Problem." *FP Report* 6 (November2000).

Kushner, Robert F., and Roland L. Weinsier. "Evlauation of theObese Patient." *Medical Clinics of North America* 84 (March2000).

Kim A. Sharp, M.Ln.

PID *see* Pelvic inflammatory disease

Piercing and tattoos

Definition

Body piercing and tattoos are a popular form of body art that have been practiced throughout history by various cultures.

Description

Various cultures have embraced adorning their bodies with piercings and tattoos throughout history. In 1992, the 4,000-year-old body of a tattooed man was discovered in a glacier on the Austrian border, and historical research has shown that Egyptians identified tattooing with fertility and nobility in the period from 4000–2000 BC Similar to tattooing, body piercing also has a rich history, which includes being used as a symbol of royalty and courage. In some hunting and gathering societies, body piercing and tattoos have long been used in initiation rites and as socialization/enculturation symbols.

In today's industrialized cultures, tattoos and piercing are a popular art form shared by people of all ages. They also are indicative of a psychology of **self-mutilation**, defiance, independence, and belonging, as for example in prison or gang cultures.

Popular piercing sites include the ear, nasal septum, eyebrow, tongue, cheek, navel, labia, and penis. Tattoos permanently mark various areas on the body.

Piercing is performed quickly and without anesthesia by either a spring-loaded ear-piercing gun or piercing needles, with the needle diameter varying from six to 18 gauge. The skin is cleaned, then the needle and jewelry are inserted through the tissue in one swift motion. Piercing is typically completed in tattoo or beauty parlors.

Originating from the Tahitian word tattau, meaning "to mark," tattoos are relatively permanent marks or designs on the skin. An electric needle injects colored pigment into small deep holes made in the skin to form the tattoo. Prison tattoo techniques are usually very crude, in marked contrast to the highly skilled art practiced in Japan and also performed in America and Europe. In recent years, the ancient art of Mehndi, or temporary tattooing of the skin with a paste made of henna has become popular America and around the world. Henna is a stain normally made for hair, and therefore exempt from U.S. Food and Drug Administration (FDA) regulation. Although seemingly safe because it does not pierce the skin, henna tattoos using black henna, a paste that contains parahenylenediamine, can actually be dangerous when absorbed into the skin of some people.

Causes and symptoms

While piercing and tattooing are popular, both present definite health risks. Tattoos can lead to the transmission of infectious diseases, such as hepatitis B and C, and theoretically HIV, when proper sterilization and safety procedures are not followed. Black henna tattoos can cause significant **allergies** and **rashes**, leading to renal (kidney) failure and even **death** in those who are sensitive to their ingredients. These types of tattoos have appeared particularly dangerous to young children. Body piercing also presents the risk of chronic infection, scarring, **hepatitis B** and C, **tetanus**, and skin allergies to the jewelry that is used. A recent Mayo Clinic study reported that 17% of college students with piercings suffered a medical complication such as infection or tearing. Use of piercing guns and preferences for upper ear piercing have led to increased infections in recent years. The force of the gun's delivery further complicates matters around the delicate cartilage of the upper ear and some people require surgical intervention.

Body piercing and tattooing are unregulated in most United States, but illegal in some. The American Dental Association (ADA) opposes oral (tongue, lip or cheek) piercing, and the American Academy of Dermatology is against all forms of body piercing except ear lobe piercing.

Diagnosis

Some of the signs of an infection from either piercing or tattoos are obvious, such as inflammation of the pierced or tattooed area, while the symptoms of hepatitis C, the most common blood-borne infection in the United States, may not be so obvious. Allergic responses to tattoos may occur due to the pigment compounds used, such as oxides of iron, mercury, chromium, cadmium, and cobalt and synthetic organic dyes. Symptoms of an allergic reaction include swelling, redness and severe **itching**. Symptoms of henna tattoo reactions are an eczema-like rash around the tattoo site. The patch should be tested for reaction severity before it proceeds to anaphylactic **shock**, or severe allergic reaction.

Most infections from piercing are due to the use of non-sterile techniques. The skin pathogens streptococcus and staphylococcus are most frequently involved in skin infections from piercing. The fleshy tissue around the pierced area may weaken and tear, leading for example, to a badly disfigured earlobe. Other common complications include contact dermatitis and **scars**. Piercing can result in **endocarditis**, urethral rupture, and a serious infection of the penis foreskin leading to severe disability or even death.

Treatment

Treatment of a local infection from piercing includes warm compresses and antibacterial ointment for local infections, to a five-day course of oral antibiotic therapy. If hepatitis B or C is confirmed, a series of diet and lifestyle changes, such as the elimination of alcohol, is recommended to control the disease.

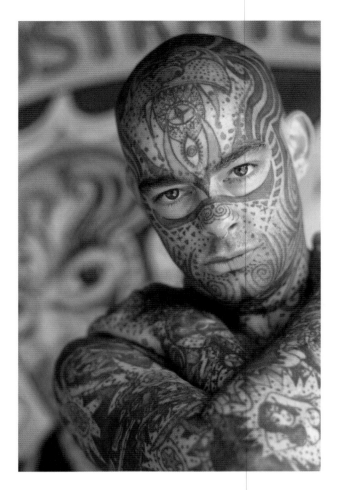

Tattoo artist Michael Wilson displaying his own tattoos and piercings. *(Photograph by Susan Mc Cartney, Photo Researchers. Reproduced by permission.)*

There are four methods to remove tattoos, including: surgical removal that involves cutting the tattoo away; sanding the skin with a wire brush to remove the epidermis and dermis layers in a process called dermabrasion; using a salt solution to soak the tattooed skin (salabrasion); and scarification, removing the tattoo with an acid solution to form a scar in its place. Topical steroids can often treat reactions to henna tattoos, but improvement may take several weeks.

Prognosis

Depending on the type of infection resulting from either piercing or tattoos, the treatment and prognosis vary. Minor infections respond well to antibiotic therapy, while blood borne diseases such as hepatitis B and C cause life-altering results. Disfigurement may or may not be fully correctable by later **plastic surgery**.

"Perichondritis: A Complication of Piercing Auricular Cartridge." *Postgraduate Medical Journal* January 2003: 29–31.

Sullivan, Michele G. "Henna Tattoos Tied to Bad Allergic Reactions." *Family Practice News* May 15, 2003: 16.

Weir, Erica. "Navel Gazing: A Clinical Glimpse at Body Piercing." *Canadian Medical Association Journal* (March 2001): 864.

Beth A. Kapes
Teresa G. Odle

Patients particularly sensitive or allergic to the ingredients in black henna may suffer serious consequences, even death, if their reaction progresses. Others may be left with scarring or altered pigmentation along the tattoo design.

Prevention

The best way to prevent infection from piercing or tattoos is not to get one in the first place. Procedures should be performed in a sterile environment by an experienced professional. The person performing the procedure should remove a new needle from the plastic in front of you and should put on a new pair of sterile gloves. Anyone considering a henna tattoo should require proof from the artists that he or she is using pure, safe brown henna, not the unsafe black henna.

Piercing should be completed with smoothly polished jewelry made of 14 or 18 carat gold, titanium, surgical steel or niobium. An allergic reaction can result with the use of jewelry made of brass plate or containing a nickel alloy. Healing time from a piercing range from six months to two years. A piercing should be completed in a sterile environment that uses every precaution to reduce the risk of infection. Excessive force, such as exerting a strong pull, should never be applied to jewelry inserted into pierced body parts to avoid tearing and injuring the tissues.

Resources

PERIODICALS

Abbasi, Kamran. "Body Piercing." *British Medical Journal* April 14, 2001: 936.

Brown, Kelli McCormack, Paula Perlmutter, and Robert J. McDermott. "Youth and Tattoos: What School Health Personnel Should Know." *Journal of School Health* November 2000: 355.

Califano, Julie. "Piercing Peril: Adorning Your Body can Backfire Big Time." *Cosmopolitan* (April 2003: 112.

Edy, Carolyn. "Body Piercing Woes: One More Reason to Think Twice Before Getting Your Navel Pierced." *Yoga Journal* June 30, 2000: 36.

"Hazards with Henna Tattoos." *Pulse* June 23, 2003: 60.

Pilates

Definition

Pilates or Physical Mind method, is a series of non-impact exercises designed by Joseph Pilates to develop strength, flexibility, balance, and inner awareness.

Purpose

Pilates is a form of strength and flexibility training that can be done by someone at any level of fitness. The exercises can also be adapted for people who have limited movement or who use wheel chairs. It is an engaging **exercise** program that people want to do. Pilates promotes a feeling of physical and mental well-being and also develops inner physical awareness. Since this method strengthens and lengthens the muscles without creating bulk, it is particularly beneficial for dancers and actors. Pilates is also helpful in preventing and rehabilitating from injuries, improving posture, and increasing flexibility, circulation, and balance. Pregnant women who do these exercises can develop body alignment, improve concentration, and develop body shape and tone after **pregnancy**. According to Joseph Pilates, "You will feel better in 10 sessions, look better in 20 sessions and have a completely new body in 30 sessions."

Although Pilates is often associated with dancers, athletes, and younger people in general who are interested in improving their physical strength and flexibility, a simplified version of some Pilates exercises is also being used as of 2003 to lower the risk of hospital-related deconditioning in older adults. A Canadian study of hospitalized patients over the age of 70 found that those who were given a set of Pilates exercises that could be performed in bed recovered more rapidly than a control group given a set of passive range-of-motion exercises.

Description

Origins

Joseph Pilates (pronounced pie-LAH-tes), the founder of the Pilates method (also simply referred to as "the method") was born in Germany in 1880. As a frail child with **rickets**, **asthma**, and **rheumatic fever**, he was determined to become stronger. He dedicated himself to building both his body and his mind through practices which included **yoga**, zen, and ancient Roman and Greek exercises. His conditioning regime worked and he became an accomplished gymnast, skier, boxer, and diver.

While interned in England during World War I for being a German citizen, Pilates became a nurse. During this time, he designed a unique system of hooking springs and straps to a hospital bed in order to help his disabled and immobilized patients regain strength and movement. It was through these experiments that he recognized the importance of training the core abdominal and back muscles to stabilize the torso and allow the entire body to move freely. This experimentation provided the foundation for his style of conditioning and the specialized exercise equipment associated with the Pilates method.

Pilates emigrated to the United States in 1926 after the German government invited him to use his conditioning methods to train the army. That same year he opened the first Pilates studio in New York City. Over the years, dancers, actors, and athletes flocked to his studio to heal, condition, and align their bodies.

Joseph Pilates died at age 87 in a fire at his studio. Although his strength enabled him to escape the flames by hanging from the rafters for over an hour, he died from **smoke inhalation**. He believed that ideal fitness is "the attainment and maintenance of a uniformly developed body with a sound mind fully capable of naturally, easily, and satisfactorily preforming our many and varied daily tasks with spontaneous zest and pleasure."

During the initial meeting, an instructor will analyze the client's posture and movement and design a specific training program. Once the program has been created, the sessions usually follow a basic pattern. A session generally begins with mat work and passive and active stretching. In passive stretching, the instructor moves and presses the client's body to stretch and elongate the muscles. During the active stretching period, the client preforms the stretches while the instructor watches their form and breathing. These exercises warm up the muscles in preparation for the machine work. The machines help the client to maintain the correct positioning required for each exercise.

There are over 500 exercises that were developed by Joseph Pilates. "Classical" exercises, according to the Pilates Studio in New York involve several principles. These include concentration, centering, flowing movement, and breath. Some instructors teach only the classical exercises originally taught by Joseph Pilates. Others design new exercises that are variations upon these classical forms in order to make the exercises more accessible for a specific person.

There are two primary exercise machines used for Pilates, the Universal Reformer and the Cadillac, and several smaller pieces of equipment. The Reformer resembles a single bed frame and is equipped with a carriage that slides back and forth and adjustable springs that are used to regulate tension and resistance. Cables, bars, straps, and pulleys allow the exercises to be done from a variety of positions. Instructors usually work with their clients on the machines for 20–45 minutes. During this time, they are observing and giving feedback about alignment, breathing, and precision of movement. The exercises are done slowly and carefully so that the movements are smooth and flowing. This requires focused concentration and muscle control. The session ends with light stretching and a cool-down period.

Once the basics are learned from an instructor, from either one-on-one lessons or in a class, it is possible to train at home using videos. Exercise equipment for use at home is also available and many exercises can be preformed on a mat.

A private session costs between $45–75 dollars, depending on the part of the country one is in. This method is not specifically covered by insurance although it may be covered when the instructor is a licensed physical therapist.

Precautions

The Pilates method is not a substitute for good physical therapy, although it has been increasingly used and recommended by physical therapists since the mid-1980s. People with chronic injuries are advised to see a physician.

Research and general acceptance

As of early 2004, several physical therapists and gerontologists have done research studies on the Pilates method, although much more work needs to be done in this area. One recent finding is that the method should not be used by patients with lower back **pain**, as it appears to be ineffective in treating this condition.

The appeal of the Pilates method to a wide population, coupled with a new interest in it on the part of **rehabilitation** therapists, suggests that further studies may soon be underway. Dancers and actors originally embraced the Pilates method as a form of strength training that did not create muscle bulk. Professional and amateur athletes also use these exercises to prevent reinjury. Sedentary people find Pilates to be a gentle, non-impact approach to conditioning. Pilates equipment and classes can be found in hospitals, health clubs, spas, and gyms.

Resources

BOOKS

Pilates, Joseph H., et al. *The Complete Writings of Joseph Pilates: Return to Life Through Contrology and Your Health.* New York: Bantam Doubleday, 2000.

Siler, Brooke. *The Pilates Body: The Ultimate At-Home Guide to Strengthening, Lengthening and Toning Your Body-Without Machines.* New York: Bantam Doubleday, 2000.

PERIODICALS

Anderson, Brent D. "Pushing for Pilates." *Rehab Management* 14 (June-July 2001): 23–25.

Blum, C. L. "Chiropractic and Pilates Therapy for the Treatment of Adult Scoliosis." *Journal of Manipulative and Physiological Therapeutics* 25 (May 2002): E3.

Coleman-Brown, L., and V. Haley-Kanigel. "Movement with Meaning." *Rehab Management* 16 (July 2003): 28–32.

Maher, C. G. "Effective Physical Treatment for Chronic Low Back Pain." *Orthopedic Clinics of North America* 35 (January 2004): 57–64.

Mallery, L. H., E. A. MacDonald, C. L. Hubley-Kozey, et al. "The Feasibility of Performing Resistance Exercise with Acutely Ill Hospitalized Older Adults." *BMC Geriatrics* 3 (October 7, 2003): 3.

ORGANIZATIONS

Physical Mind Institute. 1807 Second Street, Suite 15/16, Santa Fe, New Mexico 87505. (505) 988-1990 or (800) 505-1990. Fax: (505) 988-2837. themethod@trail.com.

Pilates Studio. 2121 Broadway, Suite 201, New York, New York, 10023-1786. (800)474-5283 or (888) 474-5283 or (212) 875-0189. Fax: (212) 769-2368. <http:\\www.pilates-studio.com>.

Linda Chrisman
Rebecca J. Frey, PhD

Piles *see* **Hemorrhoids**

Pinguecula and pterygium

Definition

Pinguecula and pterygium are both non-malignant, slow-growing proliferations of conjunctival connective tissue in the eye. Pterygia, but not pingueculae, extend over the cornea.

Description

The outer layer of the eyeball consists of the tough white sclera and the transparent cornea. The cornea lies in front of the colored part of the eye (iris). Overlying the sclera is a transparent mucous membrane called the conjunctiva. The conjunctiva lines the inside of the lids (palpebral conjunctiva) and covers the sclera (bulbar conjunctiva).

Pingueculae and pterygia are common in adults, and their incidence increases with age. Pterygia are less common than pingueculae.

Pingueculae are seen as small, raised, thickenings of the conjunctiva. They may be yellow, gray, white, or colorless. They are almost always to one side of the iris–not above or below–and usually on the side closest to the nose. A pinguecula may develop into a pterygium.

Pterygia are conjunctival thickenings that may have blood vessels associated with them. They often have a triangular-shaped appearance. The pterygia may also grow over the cornea and may therefore affect vision.

Causes and symptoms

Causes

The cause or causes of these disorders are unknown, but they are more frequent in people who live in sunny and windy climates and people whose jobs expose them to ultraviolet (UV) light (for example, farmers and arc welders). Pingueculae and pterygia also occur in older people. It is thought these growths are the result of UV or infrared light and

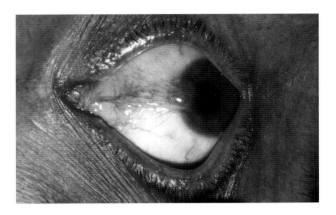

Pterygium, an overgrowth of the cornea, is usually on the inner side of the eye by thickened and degenerative conjunctiva. *(Photo Researchers, Inc. Reproduced by permission.)*

irritation. It is also believed that prolonged exposure to these risk factors (that is, UV light) increases the chances of occurrence.

Symptoms

Although some people with pinguecula constantly feel like they have a foreign body in their eye, most are asymptomatic. Because the lids can no longer spread the tears over a smooth area, dry areas may result. Some people with a pterygium are also asymptomatic; some feel like they have a foreign body in their eye. Because a pterygium can stretch and distort the cornea, some people acquire **astigmatism** from a pterygium.

Diagnosis

An eye doctor (ophthalmologist or optometrist) can usually diagnose pinguecula and pterygia by external observation, generally using an instrument called a slit lamp. A slit lamp is a microscope with a light source and magnifies the structures of the eye for the examiner. However, because pinguecula and pterygia can sometimes look similar to more serious eye growths, it is important for people to have them checked by an eye care professional.

Treatment

Usually, no treatment is needed. Artificial tears can be used to relieve the sensation of a foreign body in the eye and to protect against dryness. Surgery to remove the pinguecula or pterygium is advisable when the effect on the cornea causes visual defects or when the thickening is causing excessive and recurrent discomfort or inflammation. Sometimes surgical

removal is also performed for cosmetic reasons. However, healing from this type of surgery, although usually painless, takes many weeks, and there is a high rate of recurrence (as high as 50–60% in some regions). Accordingly, surgery is avoided unless problems due to the pinguecula or pterygium are significant.

Several methods have been used to attempt to reduce the recurrence of the pinguecula or pterygium after surgery. One method that should be abandoned is beta radiation. Although it is effective at slowing the regrowth of pingueculae and pterygia, it can cause **cataracts**. A preferable method is the topical application of the anticancer drug, mitomycin-C.

Prognosis

Most pingueculae and pterygia grow slowly and almost never cause significant damage, so the prognosis is excellent. Again, a diagnosis must be made to rule out other more serious disorders.

Prevention

There is nothing that has been clearly shown to prevent these disorders, or to prevent a pinguecula from progressing to a pterygium. However, the presence of pingueculae and pterygia have been linked to exposure to UV radiation. For that reason, UV exposure should be reduced. The American Optometric Association (AOA) suggests that sunglasses should block 99–100% of UV-A and UV-B rays. Patients should speak to their eye care professionals about protective coatings on sunglasses or regular spectacles. Protecting the eyes from sunlight, dust, and other environmental irritants is a good idea.

Resources

ORGANIZATIONS

New York University (NYU), Department of Ophthalmology. 550 First Ave., New York, NY 10016. (212) 263-6433. < http://ophth-www.med.nyu.edu/Ophth >.

Lorraine Lica, PhD

Pinkeye *see* **Conjunctivitis**

Pinta

Definition

A bacterial infection of the skin which causes red to bluish-black colored spots.

Description

Pinta is a skin infection caused by the bacterium *Treponema carateum*, a relative of the bacterium which causes **syphilis**. The word "pinta" comes from the Spanish and means "painted." Pinta is also known as "azula" (blue), and "mal de pinto" (pinto sickness). It is one of several infections caused by different *Treponema* bacteria, which are called "endemic" or "non-venereal" treponematoses.

Pinta is primarily found in rural, poverty-stricken areas of northern South America, Mexico, and the Caribbean. The disease is usually acquired during childhood and is spread from one person to another by direct skin-to-skin contact. The bacteria enter the skin through a small cut, scratch, or other skin damage. Once inside the skin, the warmth and moisture allow the bacteria to multiply. The bacterial infection causes red, scaly lesions on the skin.

Causes and symptoms

Pinta is caused by an infection with the bacterium *Treponema carateum*. Persons at risk for pinta are those who live in rural, poverty-stricken, overcrowded regions of South America, Mexico, and the Caribbean. Symptoms of pinta occur within two to four weeks after exposure to the bacteria. The first sign of infection is a red, scaly, slowly enlarging bump on the skin. This is called the "primary lesion." The primary lesion usually appears at the site where the bacteria entered the skin. This is often on the arms, legs, or face. The smaller lesions which form around the primary lesion are called "satellite lesions." Lymph nodes located near the infected area will become enlarged, but are painless.

The second stage of pinta occurs between one and 12 months after the primary lesion stage. Many flat, red, scaly, itchy lesions called "pintids" occur either near the primary lesion, or scattered around the body. Pintid lesions progress through a range of color changes, from red to bluish-black. The skin of older lesions will become depigmented (loss of normal color).

Diagnosis

Pinta can be diagnosed by dermatologists (doctors who specialize in skin diseases) and infectious disease specialists. The appearance of the lesions helps in the diagnosis. A blood sample will be taken from the patient's arm to test for antibodies to *Treponema carateum*. A scraping of a lesion will be examined under the microscope to look for *Treponema* bacteria. The results of these tests should be available within one to two days.

Treatment

Pinta is treated with benzathine penicillin G (Bicillin), given as a single injection.

Prognosis

Treatment will result in a complete cure but will not undo any skin damage caused by the late stages of disease. Spread of pinta to the eyes can cause eyelid deformities.

Prevention

Good personal hygiene and general health may help prevent infections. In general, avoid physical contact with persons who have **skin lesions**.

Resources

OTHER

Mayo Clinic Online. March 5, 1998. < http://www.mayohealth.org >.

Belinda Rowland, PhD

> ## KEY TERMS
>
> **Lesion**—An abnormal change in skin due to disease.

Pinworm infection *see* **Enterobiasis**

Pituitary adenoma *see* **Pituitary tumors**

Pituitary dwarfism

Definition

Dwarfism is a condition in which the growth of the individual is very slow or delayed. There are many forms of dwarfism. The word pituitary is in reference to the pituitary gland in the body. This gland regulates certain chemicals (hormones) in the body. Therefore, pituitary dwarfism is decreased bodily growth due to hormonal problems. The end result is a proportionate little person, because the height as well as the growth of all other structures of the individual are decreased.

Description

Pituitary dwarfism is caused by problems arising in the pituitary gland. The pituitary gland is also called the hypophysis. The pituitary gland is divided into two halves: the anterior (front) and posterior (back) halves. The anterior half produces six hormones: growth hormone, adrenocorticotropin (corticotropin), thyroid stimulating homone (thyrotropin), prolactin, follicle stimulating hormone, and lutenizing hormone. The posterior pituitary gland only produces two hormones. It produces antidiuretic hormone (vasopressin) and oxytocin.

Most forms of dwarfism are a result of decreased production of hormones from the anterior half of the pituitary gland. The most common form is due to decreases of growth hormone which will be discussed here. These decreases during childhood cause the individual's arms, legs, and other structures to develop normal proportions for their bodies, but at a decreased rate.

When all of the hormones of the anterior pituitary gland are not produced, this is called panhypopituitarism. Another type of dwarfism occurs when only the growth hormone is decreased. Dwarfism can also result from a lack of somatomedin C (also called insulin like growth factor, IGF-1) production. Somatomedin C is a hormone produced in the liver that increases bone growth when growth hormone is present. The African pygmy and the Levi-Lorain dwarfs lack the ability to produce somatomedin C in response to growth hormone. All causes of dwarfism lead to a proportionate little person.

Growth is the body's response to different hormones. The forebrain contains a small organ called the hypothalamus, which is responsible for releasing hormones in response to the body's needs for purposes of regulation. Growth hormone is produced in the anterior pituitary gland when growth hormone-releasing hormone (GHRH), is released by the hypothalamus. Growth hormone is then released and stimulates the liver to produce IGF-1. In return, IGF-1 stimulates the long bones to grow in length. Thus, growth can be slowed down or stopped if there is a problem making any of these hormones or if there is a problem with the cells receiving these hormones.

Some estimates show that there are between 10,000 and 15,000 children in the United States who have growth problems due to a deficiency of growth hormone.

Causes and symptoms

Pituitary dwarfism has been shown to run in families. New investigations are underway to determine the specific cause and location of the gene responsible for dwarfism. The human cell contains 46 chromosomes arranged in 23 pairs. Most of the genes in the two chromosomes of each pair are identical or almost identical with each other. However, with dwarfism, there appears to be disruption on different areas of chromosome 3 and 7. Some studies have isolated defects for the production of pituitary hormones to the short arm (the "p" end) of chromosome 3 at a specific location of 3p11. Other studies have found changes on the short arm of chromosome 7.

A child with a growth hormone deficiency is often small with an immature face and chubby body build. The child's growth will slow down and not follow the normal growth curve patterns. In cases of tumor, most commonly craniopharyngioma (a tumor near the pituitary gland), children and adolescents may present with neurological symptoms such as headaches, **vomiting**, and problems with vision. The patient may also have symptoms of double vision. Symptoms such as truly bizarre and excessive drinking behaviors (polydipsia) and sleep disturbances may be common.

Diagnosis

The primary symptom of pituitary dwarfism is lack of height. Therefore, a change in the individual's growth habits will help lead to a diagnosis. Another diagnostic technique uses an x ray of the child's hand to determine the child's bone age by comparing this to the child's actual chronological age. The bone age in

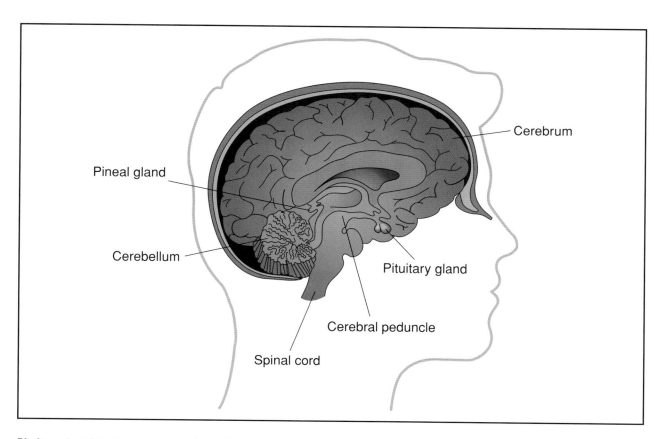

Cerebrum

Pineal gland

Cerebellum

Pituitary gland

Cerebral peduncle

Spinal cord

Pituitary dwarfism is a condition of growth retardation characterized by patients who are very short but have normal body proportions. It is caused by a dysfunction of the pituitary gland, the pea-sized mass of tissue located at the base of the brain. (Illustration by Electronic Illustrators Group.)

affected children is usually two years or more behind the chronological age. This means that if a child is ten years old, his or her bones will look like they are those of an eight-year-old child. The levels of growth hormone and somatomedin C must also be measured with blood tests.

Hypopituitarism may be gained or acquired following birth for several reasons. It could be due to trauma to the pituitary gland such as a fall or following surgery to the brain for removal of a tumor. It may also be due to the child's environment (deprivational dwarfism).

On examination by the doctor there may be optic nerve atrophy, if the dwarfism is due to a type of tumor. X rays of the area where the pituitary gland is located (sella turcica) or more advanced imaging such as **magnetic resonance imaging** (MRI) or computed tomography CT may show changes of the pituitary gland itself. Computed tomography, is an advanced form of x ray that will help determine the integrity of the bone and how much calcification the tumor is producing. Magnetic resonance imaging, will also

help in the diagnosis. MRI is a type of imaging device that can visualize soft tissues such as muscle and fat.

If the dwarfism is due to environmental and emotional problems, the individual may be hospitalization to monitor hormone levels. Following a few days of hospitalized, hormone levels may become normal due to avoidance of the original environment.

Treatment

The main course of therapy is growth **hormone replacement therapy** when there is lack of growth hormone in the body. A pediatric endocrinologist, a doctor specializing in the hormones of children, usually administers this type of therapy before a child's growth plates have fused or joined together. Once the growth plates have fused, GH replacement therapy is rarely effective.

Growth hormone used to be collected from recently deceased humans. However, frequent disease complications resulting from human growth hormone collected from deceased bodies, lead to the banning of

KEY TERMS

Adrenocorticotropin (corticotrophin)—A hormone that acts on cells of the adrenal cortex, causing them to produce male sex hormones and hormones that control water and mineral balance in the body.

Antidiuretic hormone (vasopressin)—A hormone that acts on the kidneys to regulate water balance.

Craniopharyngioma—A tumor near the pituitary gland in the craniopharyngeal canal that often results in intracranial pressure.

Deprivational dwarfism—A condition where emotional disturbances are associated with growth failure and abnormalities of pituitary function.

Follicle-stimulating hormone (FSH)—A hormone that in females stimulates estrogen and in males stimulates sperm production.

Growth hormone—A hormone that eventually stimulates growth. Also called somatotropin.

Hormone—A chemical messenger produced by the body that is involved in regulating specific bodily functions such as growth, development, and reproduction.

Luteinizing hormone—A hormone secreted by the pituitary gland that regulates the menstrual cycle and triggers ovulation in females. In males it stimulates the testes to produce testosterone.

Oxytocin—A hormone that stimulates the uterus to contract during child birth and the breasts to release milk.

Panhypopituitarism—Generalized decrease of all of the anterior pituitary hormones.

Prolactin—A hormone that helps the breast prepare for milk production during pregnancy.

Puberty—Point in development when the gonads begin to function and secondary sexual characteristics begin to appear.

Thyroid stimulating hormone (thyrotropin)—A hormone that stimulates the thyroid gland to produce hormones that regulate metabolism.

this method. In the mid-1980s, techniques were discovered that could produce growth hormones in the lab. Now, the only growth hormone used for treatment is that made in a laboratory.

A careful balancing of all of the hormones produced by the pituitary gland is necessary for patients with panhypopituitarism. This form of dwarfism is very difficult to manage.

Prognosis

The prognosis for each type of dwarfism varies. A panhypopituitarism dwarf does not pass through the initial onset of adult sexual development (**puberty**) and never produces enough gonadotropic hormones to develop adult sexual function. These individuals also have several other medical conditions. Dwarfism due to only growth hormone deficiency has a different prognosis. These individuals do pass through puberty and mature sexually, however, they remain proportionately small in stature.

If the individual is lacking only growth hormone then growth hormone replacement therapy can be administered. The success of treatment with growth hormone varies however. An increase in height of 4–6 in (10–15 cm) can occur in the first year of treatment. Following this first year, the response to the hormone is not as successful. Therefore the amount of growth hormone administered must be tripled to maintain this rate. Long-term use is considered successful if the individual grows at least 0.75 in (2 cm) per year more than they would without the hormone. However, if the growth hormone treatment is not administered before the long bones—such as the legs and arms—fuse, then the individual will never grow. This fusion is completed by adult age.

Improvement for individuals with dwarfism due to other causes such as a tumor, varies greatly. If the dwarfism is due to deprevational causes, then removing a child from that environment should help to alleviate the problem.

Resources

BOOKS

Beers, Mark H., Robert Berkow, and Mark Burs. "Pituitary Dwarfism." In *Merck Manual*. Rahway, NJ: Merck & Co., Inc., 2004.

ORGANIZATIONS

Human Growth Foundation. 997 Glen Cove Ave., Glen Head, NY 11545. (800) 451-6434. Fax: (516) 671-4055. < http://www.hgfound.org >.

Little People of America, Inc. National Headquarters, PO Box 745, Lubbock, TX 79408. (806) 737-8186 or (888) LPA-2001. lpadatabase@juno.com. < http://www.lpaonline.org >.

OTHER

"Clinical Growth Charts by the National Center for Health Statistics." *Center for Disease Control.* < http://

www.cdc.gov/nchs/about/major/nhanes/growthcharts/
clinical_charts.htm >.

"Entry 312000: Panhypopituitarism; PHP." *OMIM—
Online Mendelian Inherichance in Man..* National
Institutes of Health. <http://www.ncbi.nlm.nih.gov/
htbin-post/Omim/dispmim?312000>.

Hill, Mark. "Development of the Endocrine System—
Pituitary." *The University of New South Wales, Sydney,
Australia—Department of Embryology.* <http://anato-
my.med.unsw.edu.au/CBL/Embryo/OMIMfind/
endocrine/pitlist.htm >.

Jason S. Schliesser, DC

Pituitary gland removal *see*
Hypophysectomy

Pituitary tumors

Definition

Pituitary tumors are abnormal growths on the
pituitary gland. Some tumors secrete hormones normally made by the pituitary gland.

Description

Located in the center of the brain, the pituitary
gland manufactures and secretes hormones that
regulate growth, sexual development and functioning, and the fluid balance of the body. About 10%
of all cancers in the skull are pituitary tumors.
Pituitary adenomas (adenomas are tumors that
grow from gland tissues) and pituitary tumors in
children and adolescencents (craniopharyngiomas)
are the most common types of pituitary tumors.
They are usually benign and grow slowly. Even
malignant pituitary tumors rarely spread to other
parts of the body.

Pituitary adenomas do not secrete hormones but
are likely to be larger and more invasive than tumors
that do. Craniopharyngiomas are benign tumors that
are extremely difficult to remove. Radiation does not
stop them from spreading throughout the pituitary
gland. Craniopharyngiomas account for less than
5% of all brain tumors. Pituitary tumors usually
develop between the ages of 30 and 40, but half of all
craniopharyngiomas occur in children, with symptoms most often appearing between the ages of five
and ten.

Causes and symptoms

The cause of pituitary tumors is not known, but
may be genetic. Symptoms related to tumor location,
size, and pressure on neighboring structures include:

- persistent **headache** on one or both sides, or in the
center of the forehead

- blurred or double vision; loss of peripheral vision

- drooping eyelid caused by pressure on nerves leading
to the eye

- seizures

Symptoms related to hormonal imbalance
include:

- excessive sweating

- loss of appetite

- loss of interest in sex

- inability to tolerate cold temperatures

- nausea

- high levels of sodium in the blood

- menstrual problems

- excessive thirst

- frequent urination

- dry skin

- constipation

- premature or delayed **puberty**

- delayed growth in children

- galactorrea (milk secretion in the absence of **pregnancy** or breast feeding)

- low blood pressure

- low blood sugar

Diagnosis

As many as 40% of all pituitary tumors do not
release excessive quantities of hormones into the
blood. Known as clinically nonfunctioning, these
tumors are difficult to distinguish from tumors that
produce similar symptoms. They may grow to be quite
large before they are diagnosed.

Endocrinologists and neuroendocrinologists base
the diagnosis of pituitary tumors on:

- the patient's own observations and medical history

- physical examination

- laboratory studies of the patient's blood and cerebrospinal fluid

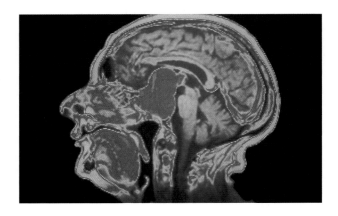

Colorized MRI showing large pituitary tumor at center in pink.
(Mehau Kulyk, Photo Researchers. Reproduced by permission.)

- x rays of the skull and other studies that provide images of the inside of the brain (CT, MRI)
- vision tests
- urinalysis

Treatment

Some pituitary tumors stabilize without treatment, but a neurosurgeon will operate at once to remove the tumor (adenectomy) or pituitary gland (**hypophysectomy**) of a patient whose vision is deteriorating rapidly. Patients who have pituitary apoplexy may experience very severe headaches, have symptoms of stiff neck, and sensitivity to light. This condition is considered an emergency. Magnetic resonance imaging (MRI) is the best imaging technique for patients with these symptoms. If the tumor is small, surgery may be done through the nose. If the tumor is large, it may require opening the skull for **tumor removal**. Selected patients do well with proton beam radiosurgery (the use of high energy particles in the form of a high energy beam to destroy an overactive gland).

Treatment is determined by the type of tumor and by whether it has invaded tissues adjacent to the pituitary gland. Hormone-secreting tumors can be successfully treated with surgery, radiation, bromocriptine (Parlodel), Sandostatin (Octreotide), or other somatostatin analogues (drugs similar to somatostatin). Surgery is usually used to remove all or part of a tumor within the gland or the area surrounding it, and may be combined with radiation therapy to treat tumors that extend beyond the pituitary gland. Removal of the pituitary gland requires life-long **hormone replacement therapy**.

Radiation therapy can provide long-term control of the disease if it recurs after surgery, and radioactive pellets can be implanted in the brain to treat craniopharyngiomas. CV205-502, a new dopamine agonist (a drug that increases the effect of another, in this instance dopamine) can control symptoms of patients who do not respond to bromocriptine.

Prognosis

Pituitary tumors are usually curable. Following surgery, adults may gradually resume their normal activities, and children may return to school when the effects of the operation have diminished, and appetite and sense of well-being have returned. Patients should wear medical identification tags identifying their condition and the hormonal replacement medicines they take.

Resources

ORGANIZATIONS

American Brain Tumor Association. 2770 River Road, Des Plaines, IL 60018. (800) 886-2289. < http://www.abta.org >.

Brain Tumor Information Services. Box 405, Room J341, University of Chicago Hospitals, 5841 S. Maryland Ave., Chicago, IL 60637. (312) 684-1400.

Maureen Haggerty

Pityriasis rosea

Definition

Pityriasis rosea is a mild, noncontagious skin disorder common among children and young adults, and characterized by a single round spot on the body, followed later by a rash of colored spots on the body and upper arms.

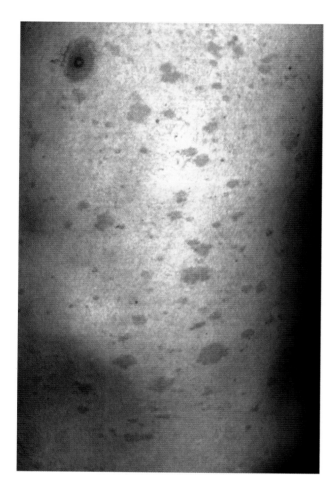

The torso of a man covered with pityriasis rosea. The cause of this disorder is thought to be due to a viral infection. It often appears on the torso and upper parts of the limbs of young people and may be contagious. *(Photograph by Dr. P. Marazzi, Photo Researchers, Inc. Reproduced by permission.)*

Description

Pityriasis rosea is most common in young adults, and appears up to 50% more often in women. Its cause is unknown; however, some scientists believe that the rash is an immune response to some type of infection in the body.

Causes and symptoms

Doctors do not think that pityriasis rosea is contagious, but the cause is unknown. Some experts suspect the rash, which is most common in spring and fall, may be triggered by a virus, but no infectious agent has ever been found.

It is not sexually transmitted, and does not appear to be contagious from one person to the next.

Sometimes, before the symptoms appear, people experience preliminary sensations including **fever**, malaise, sore throat, or **headache**. Symptoms begin with a single, large round spot called a "herald patch" on the body, followed days or weeks later by slightly raised, scaly-edged round or oval pink-copper colored spots on the trunk and upper arms. The spots, which have a wrinkled center and a sharp border, sometimes resemble a Christmas tree. They may be mild to severely itchy, and they can spread to other parts of the body.

Diagnosis

A physician can diagnose the condition with blood tests, skin scrapings, or a biopsy of the lesion.

Treatment

The rash usually clears up on its own, although a physician should rule out other conditions that may cause a similar rash (such as **syphilis**).

Treatment includes external and internal medications for **itching** and inflammation. Mild inflammation and itching can be relieved with antihistamine drugs or calamine lotion, zinc oxide, or other mild lubricants or anti-itching creams. Gentle, soothing strokes should be used to apply the ointments, since vigorous rubbing may cause the lesions to spread. More severe itching and inflammation is treated with topical steroids. Moderate exposure to sun or ultraviolet light may help heal the lesions, but patients should avoid being sunburned.

Soap makes the rash more uncomfortable; patients should bathe or shower with plain lukewarm water, and apply a thin coating of bath oil to freshly-dried skin afterwards.

Prognosis

These spots, which may be itchy, last for 3–12 weeks. Symptoms rarely recur.

Resources

ORGANIZATIONS

American Academy of Dermatology. 930 N. Meacham Road, P.O. Box 4014, Schaumburg, IL 60168-4014. (847) 330-0230. Fax: (847) 330-0050. < http://www.aad.org >.

Carol A. Turkington

PKU *see* **Phenylketonuria**

Placenta previa

Definition

Placenta previa is a condition that occurs during **pregnancy** when the placenta is abnormally placed, and partially or totally covers the cervix.

Description

The uterus is the muscular organ that contains the developing baby during pregnancy. The lowest segment of the uterus is a narrowed portion called the cervix. This cervix has an opening (the os) that leads into the vagina, or birth canal. The placenta is the organ that attaches to the wall of the uterus during pregnancy. The placenta allows nutrients and oxygen from the mother's blood circulation to pass into the developing baby (the fetus) via the umbilical cord.

During labor, the muscles of the uterus contract repeatedly. This allows the cervix to begin to grow thinner (called effacement) and more open (dilatation). Eventually, the cervix will become completely effaced and dilated, and the baby can leave the uterus and enter the birth canal. Under normal circumstances, the baby will emerge through the mother's vagina during birth.

In placenta previa, the placenta develops in an abnormal location. Normally, the placenta should develop relatively high up in the uterus, on the front or back wall. In about one in 200 births, the placenta will be located low in the uterus, partially or totally covering the os. This causes particular problems in late pregnancy, when the lower part of the uterus begins to take on a new formation in preparation for delivery. As the cervix begins to efface and dilate, the attachments of the placenta to the uterus are damaged, resulting in bleeding.

Causes and symptoms

While the actual cause of placenta previa is unknown, certain factors increase the risk of a woman developing the condition. These factors include:

- having abnormalities of the uterus
- being older in age
- having had other babies
- having a prior delivery by **cesarean section**
- smoking cigarettes

When a pregnancy involves more than one baby (twins, triplets, etc.), the placenta will be considerably larger than for a single pregnancy. This also increases the chance of placenta previa.

Placenta previa may cause a number of problems. It is thought to be responsible for about 5% of all miscarriages. It frequently causes very light bleeding (spotting) early in pregnancy. Sometime after 28 weeks of pregnancy (most pregnancies last about 40 weeks), placenta previa can cause episodes of significant bleeding. Usually, the bleeding occurs suddenly and is bright red. The woman rarely experiences any accompanying **pain**, although about 10% of the time the placenta may begin separating from the uterine wall (called abruptio placentae), resulting in pain. The bleeding usually stops on its own. About 25% of such patients will go into labor within the next several days. Sometimes, placenta previa does not cause bleeding until labor has already begun.

Placenta previa puts both the mother and the fetus at high risk. The mother is at risk of severe and uncontrollable bleeding (hemorrhage), with dangerous blood loss. If the mother's bleeding is quite severe, this puts the fetus at risk of becoming oxygen deprived. The fetus' only source of oxygen is the mother's blood. The mother's blood loss, coupled with certain changes that take place in response to that blood loss, decreases the amount of blood going to the placenta, and ultimately to the fetus. Furthermore, placenta previa increases the risk of preterm labor, and the possibility that the baby will be delivered prematurely.

Diagnosis

Diagnosis of placenta previa is suspected whenever bright red, painless vaginal bleeding occurs during the course of a pregnancy. The diagnosis can be confirmed by performing an ultrasound examination. This will allow the location of the placenta to be evaluated.

KEY TERMS

Cesarean section—Delivery of a baby through an incision in the mother's abdomen instead of through the vagina.

Labor—The process during which the uterus contracts, and the cervix opens to allow the passage of a baby into the vagina.

Placenta—The organ that provides oxygen and nutrition from the mother to the baby during pregnancy. The placenta is attached to the wall of the uterus and leads to the baby via the umbilical cord.

Umbilical cord—The blood vessels that allow the developing baby to receive nutrition and oxygen from its mother; the blood vessels also eliminate the baby's waste products. One end of the umbilical cord is attached to the placenta and the other end is attached to the baby's belly button (umbilicus).

Vagina—The birth canal; the passage from the cervix of the uterus to the opening leading outside of a woman's body.

While many conditions during pregnancy require a pelvic examination, in which the health care provider's fingers are inserted into the patient's vagina, such an examination should never be performed if there is any suspicion of placenta previa. Such an examination can disturb the already susceptible placenta, resulting in hemorrhage.

Sometimes placenta previa is found early in a pregnancy, during an ultrasound examination performed for another reason. In these cases, it is wise to have a repeat ultrasound performed later in pregnancy (during the last third of the pregnancy, called the third trimester). A large percentage of these women will have a low-lying placenta, but not a true placenta previa where some or all of the os is covered.

Treatment

Treatment depends on how far along in the pregnancy the bleeding occurs. When the pregnancy is less than 36 weeks along, the fetus is not sufficiently developed to allow delivery without a high risk of complications. Therefore, a woman with placenta previa is treated with bed rest, blood transfusions as necessary, and medications to prevent labor. After 36 weeks, the baby can be delivered via cesarean section. This is

almost always the preferred method of delivery in order to avoid further bleeding from the low-lying placenta.

Prognosis

In cases of placenta previa, the prognosis for the mother is very good. However, there is a 15–20% chance the infant will not survive. This is 10 times the **death** rate associated with normal pregnancies. About 60% of these deaths occur because the baby delivered was too premature to survive.

Prevention

There are no known ways to insure the appropriate placement of the placenta in the uterus. However, careful treatment of the problem can result in the best chance for a good outcome for both mother and baby.

Resources

ORGANIZATIONS

American College of Obstetricians and Gynecologists. 409 12th Street, S.W., P.O. Box 96920, Wasington, DC 20090-6920. .

Rosalyn Carson-DeWitt, MD

Placental abruption

Definition

Placental abruption occurs when the placenta separates from the wall of the uterus prior to the birth of the baby. This can result in severe, uncontrollable bleeding (hemorrhage).

Description

The uterus is the muscular organ that contains the developing baby during **pregnancy**. The lowest segment of the uterus is a narrowed portion called the cervix. This cervix has an opening (the os) that leads into the vagina, or birth canal. The placenta is the organ that attaches to the wall of the uterus during pregnancy. The placenta allows nutrients and oxygen from the mother's blood circulation to pass into the developing baby (the fetus) via the umbilical cord.

During labor, the muscles of the uterus contract repeatedly. This allows the cervix to begin to grow thinner (called effacement) and more open (dilatation). Eventually, the cervix will become completely effaced and dilated, and the baby can leave the uterus and enter the birth canal. Under normal circumstances, the baby will go through the mother's vagina during birth.

During a normal labor and delivery, the baby is born first. Several minutes to 30 minutes later, the placenta separates from the wall of the uterus and is delivered. This sequence is necessary because the baby relies on the placenta to provide oxygen until he or she begins to breathe independently.

Placental abruption occurs when the placenta separates from the uterus before the birth of the baby. Placental abruption occurs in about one out of every 200 deliveries. African-American and Latin-American women have a greater risk of this complication than do Caucasian women. It was once believed that the risk of placental abruption increased in women who gave birth to many children, but this association is still being researched.

Causes and symptoms

The cause of placental abruption is unknown. However, a number of risk factors have been identified. These factors include:

- older age of the mother
- history of placental abruption during a previous pregnancy
- high blood pressure
- certain disease states (diabetes, collagen vascular diseases)
- the presence of a type of uterine tumor called a leiomyoma
- twins, triplets, or other multiple pregnancies
- cigarette **smoking**
- heavy alcohol use
- **cocaine** use
- malformations of the uterus
- malformations of the placenta
- injury to the abdomen (as might occur in a car accident)

Symptoms of placental abruption include bleeding from the vagina, severe **pain** in the abdomen or back, and tenderness of the uterus. Depending on the severity of the bleeding, the mother may experience a drop in blood pressure, followed by symptoms of organ failure as her organs are deprived of oxygen. Sometimes, there is no visible vaginal bleeding.

Instead, the bleeding is said to be "concealed." In this case, the bleeding is trapped behind the placenta, or there may be bleeding into the muscle of the uterus. Many patients will have abnormal contractions of the uterus, particularly extremely hard, prolonged contractions. Placental abruption can be total (in which case the fetus will almost always die in the uterus), or partial.

Placental abruption can also cause a very serious complication called consumptive coagulopathy. A series of reactions begin that involve the elements of the blood responsible for clotting. These clotting elements are bound together and used up by these reactions. This increases the risk of uncontrollable bleeding and may contribute to severe bleeding from the uterus, as well as causing bleeding from other locations (nose, urinary tract, etc.).

Placental abruption is risky for both the mother and the fetus. It is dangerous for the mother because of blood loss, loss of clotting ability, and oxygen deprivation to her organs (especially the kidneys and heart). This condition is dangerous for the fetus because of oxygen deprivation, too, since the mother's blood is the fetus' only source of oxygen. Because the abrupting placenta is attached to the umbilical cord, and the umbilical cord is an extension of the fetus' circulatory system, the fetus is also at risk of hemorrhaging. The fetus may die from these stresses, or may be born with damage due to oxygen deprivation. If the abruption occurs well before the baby was due to be delivered, early delivery may cause the baby to suffer complications of premature birth.

Diagnosis

Diagnosis of placental abruption relies heavily on the patient's report of her symptoms and a **physical examination** performed by a health care provider. Ultrasound can sometimes be used to diagnose an abruption, but there is a high rate of missed or incorrect diagnoses associated with this tool when used for this purpose. Blood will be taken from the mother and tested to evaluate the possibility of life-threatening problems with the mother's clotting system.

Treatment

The first line of treatment for placental abruption involves replacing the mother's lost blood with blood transfusions and fluids given through a needle in a vein. Oxygen will be administered, usually by a mask or through tubes leading to the nose. When the placental separation is severe, treatment may require

KEY TERMS

Cesarean section—Delivery of a baby through an incision in the mother's abdomen, instead of through the vagina.

Labor—The process during which the uterus contracts, and the cervix opens to allow the passage of a baby into the vagina.

Placenta—The organ that provides oxygen and nutrition from the mother to the baby during pregnancy. The placenta is attached to the wall of the uterus and leads to the baby via the umbilical cord.

Umbilical cord—The blood vessels that allow the developing baby to receive nutrition and oxygen from its mother; the blood vessels also eliminate the baby's waste products. One end of the umbilical cord is attached to the placenta and the other end is attached to the baby's belly button (umbilicus).

Uterus—The muscular organ that contains the developing baby during pregnancy.

Vagina—The birth canal; the passage from the cervix of the uterus to the opening leading outside of a woman's body.

---

prompt delivery of the baby. However, delivery may be delayed when the placental separation is not as severe, and when the fetus is too immature to insure a healthy baby if delivered. The baby is delivered vaginally when possible. However, a **cesarean section** may be performed to deliver the baby more quickly if the abruption is quite severe or if the baby is in distress.

Prognosis

The prognosis for cases of placental abruption varies, depending on the severity of the abruption. The risk of **death** for the mother ranges up to 5%, usually due to severe blood loss, **heart failure**, and kidney failure. In cases of severe abruption, 50–80% of all fetuses die. Among those who survive, nearly half will have lifelong problems due to oxygen deprivation in the uterus and premature birth.

Prevention

Some of the causes of placental abruption are preventable. These include cigarette smoking, alcohol **abuse**, and cocaine use. Other causes of abruption may

not be avoidable, like diabetes or high blood pressure. These diseases should be carefully treated. Patients with conditions known to increase the risk of placental abruption should be carefully monitored for signs and symptoms of this complication.

Resources

ORGANIZATIONS

American College of Obstetricians and Gynecologists. 409 12th Street, S.W., P.O. Box 96920, Washington, DC 20090-6920.

Rosalyn Carson-DeWitt, MD

Plague

Definition

Plague is a serious, potentially life-threatening infectious disease that is usually transmitted to humans by the bites of rodent fleas. It was one of the scourges of early human history. There are three major forms of the disease: bubonic, septicemic, and pneumonic.

Description

Plague has been responsible for three great world pandemics, which caused millions of deaths and significantly altered the course of history. A pandemic is a disease occurring in epidemic form throughout the entire population of a country, a people, or the world. Although the cause of the plague was not identified until the third pandemic in 1894, scientists are virtually certain that the first two pandemics were plague because a number of the survivors wrote about their experiences and described the symptoms.

The first great pandemic appeared in AD 542 and lasted for 60 years. It killed millions of citizens, particularly people living along the Mediterranean Sea. This sea was the busiest, coastal trade route at that time and connected what is now southern Europe, northern Africa, and parts of coastal Asia. This pandemic is sometimes referred to as the Plague of Justinian, named for the great emperor of Byzantium who was ruling at the beginning of the outbreak. According to the historian Procopius, this outbreak of plague killed 10,000 people per day at its height just within the city of Constantinople.

The second pandemic occurred during the fourteenth century, and was called the Black Death because its main symptom was the appearance of black patches (caused by bleeding) on the skin. It was also a subject found in many European paintings, drawings, plays, and writings of that time. The connections between large active trading ports, rats coming off the ships, and the severe outbreaks of the plague were understood by people at the time. This was the most severe of the three, beginning in the mid-1300s with an origin in central Asia and lasting for 400 years. Between a fourth and a third of the entire European population died within a few years after plague was first introduced. Some smaller villages and towns were completely wiped out.

The final pandemic began in northern China, reaching Canton and Hong Kong by 1894. From there, it spread to all continents, killing millions.

The great pandemics of the past occurred when wild rodents spread the disease to rats in cities, and then to humans when the rats died. Another route for infection came from rats coming off ships that had traveled from heavily infected areas. Generally, these were busy coastal or inland trade routes. Plague was introduced into the United States during this pandemic and it spread from the West towards the Midwest and became endemic in the Southwest of the United States.

About 10–15 Americans living in the southwestern United States contract plague each year during the spring and summer. The last rat-borne epidemic in the United States occurred in Los Angeles in 1924–25. Since then, all plague cases in this country have been sporadic, acquired from wild rodents or their fleas. Plague can also be acquired from ground squirrels and prairie dogs in parts of Arizona, New Mexico, California, Colorado, and Nevada. Around the world, there are between 1,000 and 2,000 cases of plague each year. Recent outbreaks in humans occurred in Africa, South America, and Southeast Asia.

Some people and/or animals with bubonic plague go on to develop **pneumonia** (pneumonic plague). This can spread to others via infected droplets during coughing or sneezing.

Plague is one of three diseases still subject to international health regulations. These rules require that all confirmed cases be reported to the World Health Organization (WHO) within 24 hours of diagnosis. According to the regulations, passengers on an international voyage who have been to an area where there is an epidemic of pneumonic plague must be placed in isolation for six days before being allowed to leave.

While plague is found in several countries, there is little risk to United States travelers within endemic areas (limited locales where a disease is known to be present) if they restrict their travel to urban areas with modern hotel accommodations.

Over the past few years, this infection primarily of antiquity has become a modern issue. This change has occurred because of the concerns about the use of plague as a weapon of biological warfare or terrorism (bioterrorism). Along with **anthrax** and **smallpox**, plague is considered to be a significant risk. In this scenario, the primary manifestation is likely to be pneumonic plague transmitted by clandestine aerosols. It has been reported that during World War II the Japanese dropped "bombs" containing plague-infected fleas in China as a form of biowarfare.

Causes and symptoms

Fleas carry the bacterium *Yersinia pestis*, formerly known as *Pasteurella pestis*. The plague bacillus can be stained with Giemsa stain and typically looks like a safety pin under the microscope. When a flea bites an infected rodent, it swallows the plague bacteria. The bacteria are passed on when the fleas, in turn, bite a human. Interestingly, the plague bacterium grows in the gullet of the flea, obstructing it and not allowing the flea to eat. Transmission occurs during abortive feeding with regurgitation of bacteria into the feeding site. Humans also may become infected if they have a break or cut in the skin and come in direct contact with body fluids or tissues of infected animals.

More than 100 species of fleas have been reported to be naturally infected with plague; in the western United States, the most common source of plague is the golden-manteled ground squirrel flea. Chipmunks and prairie dogs have also been identified as hosts of infected fleas.

Since 1924, there have been no documented cases in the United States of human-to-human spread of plague from droplets. All but one of the few pneumonic cases have been associated with handling infected cats. While dogs and cats can become infected, dogs rarely show signs of illness and are not believed to spread disease to humans. However, plague has been spread from infected coyotes (wild dogs) to humans. In parts of central Asia, gerbils have been identified as the source of cases of bubonic plague in humans.

Bubonic plague

Two to five days after infection, patients experience a sudden **fever**, chills, seizures, and severe

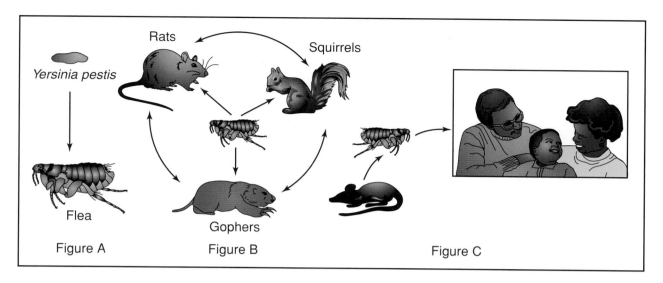

Yersinia pestis

Rats

Squirrels

Flea

Gophers

Figure A

Figure B

Figure C

Plague is a serious infectious disease transmitted by the bites of rat fleas. There are three major forms of plague: bubonic, pneumonic, and septicemic. As illustrated above, fleas carry the bacterium *Yersinia pestis*. When a flea bites an infected rodent, it becomes a vector and then passes the plague bacteria when it bites a human. *(Illustration by Electronic Illustrators Group.)*

headaches, followed by the appearance of swellings or "buboes" in armpits, groin, and neck. The most commonly affected sites are the lymph glands near the site of the first infection. As the bacteria multiply in the glands, the lymph node becomes swollen. As the nodes collect fluid, they become extremely tender. Occasionally, the bacteria will cause an ulcer at the point of the first infection.

Septicemic plague

Bacteria that invade the bloodstream directly (without involving the lymph nodes) cause septicemic plague. (Bubonic plague also can progress to septicemic plague if not treated appropriately.) Septicemic plague that does not involve the lymph glands is particularly dangerous because it can be hard to diagnose the disease. The bacteria usually spread to other sites, including the liver, kidneys, spleen, lungs, and sometimes the eyes, or the lining of the brain. Symptoms include fever, chills, prostration, abdominal **pain**, **shock**, and bleeding into the skin and organs.

Pneumonic plague

Pneumonic plague may occur as a direct infection (primary) or as a result of untreated bubonic or septicemic plague (secondary). Primary pneumonic plague is caused by inhaling infective drops from another person or animal with pneumonic plague. Symptoms, which appear within one to three days after infection, include a severe, overwhelming pneumonia, with shortness of breath, high fever, and blood

in the phlegm. If untreated, half the patients will die; if blood **poisoning** occurs as an early complication, patients may die even before the buboes appear.

Life-threatening complications of plague include shock, high fever, problems with blood clotting, and convulsions.

Diagnosis

Plague should be suspected if there are painful buboes, fever, exhaustion, and a history of possible exposure to rodents, rabbits, or fleas in the West or Southwest. The patient should be isolated. Chest x rays are taken, as well as blood cultures, antigen testing, and examination of lymph node specimens. Blood cultures should be taken 30 minutes apart, before treatment.

A group of German researchers reported in 2004 on a standardized enzyme-linked immunosorbent assay (ELISA) kit for the rapid diagnosis of plague. The test kit was developed by the German military and has a high degree of accuracy as well as speed in identifying the plague bacillus. The kit could be useful in the event of a bioterrorist attack as well as in countries without advanced microbiology laboratories.

Treatment

As soon as plague is suspected, the patient should be isolated, and local and state departments notified. Drug treatment reduces the risk of **death** to less

KEY TERMS

Bioterrorism—The use of disease agents to terrorize or intimidate a civilian population.

Buboes—Smooth, oval, reddened, and very painful swellings in the armpits, groin, or neck that occur as a result of infection with the plague.

Endemic—A disease that occurs naturally in a geographic area or population group.

Epidemic—A disease that occurs throughout part of the population of a country.

Pandemic—A disease that occurs throughout a regional group, the population of a country, or the world.

Septicemia—The medical term for blood poisoning, in which bacteria have invaded the bloodstream and circulates throughout the body.

than 5%. The preferred treatment is streptomycin administered as soon as possible. Alternatives include gentamicin, chloramphenicol, tetracycline, or trimethoprim/sulfamethoxazole.

Prognosis

Plague can be treated successfully if it is caught early; the mortality rate for treated disease is 1–15% but 40–60% in untreated cases. Untreated pneumonic plague is almost always fatal, however, and the chances of survival are very low unless specific antibiotic treatment is started within 15–18 hours after symptoms appear. The presence of plague bacteria in a blood smear is a grave sign and indicates septicemic plague. Septicemic plague has a mortality rate of 40% in treated cases and 100% in untreated cases.

Prevention

Anyone who has come in contact with a plague pneumonia victim should be given antibiotics, since untreated pneumonic plague patients can pass on their illness to close contacts throughout the course of the illness. All plague patients should be isolated for 48 hours after antibiotic treatment begins. Pneumonic plague patients should be completely isolated until sputum cultures show no sign of infection.

Residents of areas where plague is found should keep rodents out of their homes. Anyone working in a rodent-infested area should wear insect repellent on skin and clothing. Pets can be treated with insecticidal dust and kept indoors. Handling sick or dead animals (especially rodents and cats) should be avoided.

Plague vaccines have been used with varying effectiveness since the late nineteenth century. Experts believe that **vaccination** lowers the chance of infection and the severity of the disease. However, the effectiveness of the vaccine against pneumonic plague is not clearly known.

Vaccinations against plague are not required to enter any country. Because immunization requires multiple doses over a 6–10 month period, plague vaccine is not recommended for quick protection during outbreaks. Moreover, its unpleasant side effects make it a poor choice unless there is a substantial long-term risk of infection. The safety of the vaccine for those under age 18 has not been established. Pregnant women should not be vaccinated unless the need for protection is greater than the risk to the unborn child. Even those who receive the vaccine may not be completely protected. The inadequacy of the vaccines available as of the early 2000s explains why it is important to protect against rodents, fleas, and people with plague. A team of researchers in the United Kingdom reported in the summer of 2004 that an injected subunit vaccine is likely to offer the best protection against both bubonic and pneumonic forms of plague.

Resources

BOOKS

Beers, Mark H., MD, and Robert Berkow, MD., editors. "Plague (Bubonic Plague; Pestis; Black Death)." In *The Merck Manual of Diagnosis and Therapy.* Whitehouse Station, NJ: Merck Research Laboratories, 2004.

PERIODICALS

Davis, S., M. Begon, L. DeBruyn, et al. "Predictive Thresholds for Plague in Kazakhstan." *Science* 304 (April 30, 2004): 736–738.

Gani, R., and S. Leach. "Epidemiologic Determinants for Modeling Pneumonic Plague Outbreaks." *Emerging Infectious Diseases* 10 (April 2004): 608–614.

Splettstoesser, W. D., L. Rahalison, R. Grunow, et al. "Evaluation of a Standardized F1 Capsular Antigen Capture ELISA Test Kit for the Rapid Diagnosis of Plague." *FEMS Immunology and Medical Microbiology* 41 (June 1, 2004): 149–155.

Titball, R. W., and E. D. Williamson. "*Yersinia pestis* (Plague) Vaccines." *Expert Opinion on Biological Therapy* 4 (June 2004): 965–973.

Velendzas, Demetres, MD, and Susan Dufel, MD. "Plague." *eMedicine* December 2, 2004. < http:// www.emedicine.com/EMERG/topic428.htm >.

ORGANIZATIONS

Centers for Disease Control. 1600 Clifton Rd., NE, Atlanta, GA 30333. (800) 311-3435, (404) 639-3311. < http://www.cdc.gov >.

National Institute of Allergies and Infectious Diseases, Division of Microbiology and Infectious Diseases. Bldg. 31, Rm. 7A-50, 31 Center Drive MSC 2520, Bethesda, MD 20892.

World Health Organization. Division of Emerging and Other Communicable Diseases Surveillance and Control. 1211 Geneva 27, Switzerland.

OTHER

Bacterial Diseases (Healthtouch). < http://www.health-touch.com/level1/leaflets/105825/105826.htm >.

Bug Bytes. < http://www.isumc.edu/bugbytes/ >.

Centers for Disease Control. < http://www.cdc.gov/travel/travel.html >.

Infectious Diseases Weblink. < http://pages.prodigy.net/pdeziel/ >.

International Society of Travel Medicine. < http://www.istm.org >.

World Health Organization. < http://www.who.ch/ >.

Arnold Cua, MD
Rebecca J. Frey, PhD

Plaque *see* **Skin lesions**

Plasma cell myeloma *see* **Multiple myeloma**

Plasma renin activity

Definition

Renin is an enzyme released by the kidney to help control the body's sodium-potassium balance, fluid volume, and blood pressure.

Purpose

Plasma renin activity (PRA), also called plasma renin assay, may be used to screen for high blood pressure (**hypertension**) of kidney origin, and may help plan treatment of essential hypertension, a genetic disease often aggravated by excess sodium intake. PRA is also used to further evaluate a diagnosis of excess aldosterone, a hormone secreted by the adrenal cortex, in a condition called Conn's syndrome.

Precautions

Patients taking **diuretics**, antihypertensives, **vasodilators**, **oral contraceptives**, and licorice should discontinue use of these substances for two to four weeks before the test. It should be noted that renin is increased in **pregnancy** and in **diets** with reduced salt intake. Also, since renin is affected by body position, as well as by diurnal (daily) variation, blood samples should be drawn in the morning, and the position of the patient (sitting or lying down) should be noted.

Description

When the kidneys release the enzyme renin in response to certain conditions (high blood potassium, low blood sodium, decreased blood volume), it is the first step in what is called the renin-angiotensin-aldosterone cycle. This cycle includes the conversion of angiotensinogen to angiotensin I, which in turn is converted to angiotensin II, in the lung. Angiotensin II is a powerful blood vessel constrictor, and its action stimulates the release of aldosterone from an area of the adrenal glands called the adrenal cortex. Together, angiotensin and aldosterone increase the blood volume, the blood pressure, and the blood sodium to re-establish the body's sodium-potassium and fluid volume balance. Primary aldosteronism, the symptoms of which include hypertension and low blood potassium (**hypokalemia**), is considered "low-renin aldosteronism."

Renin itself is not actually measured in the PRA test, because renin can be measured only with great difficulty even in research laboratories. In the most commonly used renin assay, the test actually determines, by a procedure called radioimmunoassay, the rate of angiotensin I generation per unit time, while the PRC (plasma renin concentration) measures the maximum renin effect.

Both the PRA and the PRC are extremely difficult to perform. Not only is renin itself unstable, but the patient's body position and the time of day affect the results. Also, the sample must be collected properly: drawn into a chilled syringe and collection tube, placed on ice, and sent to the performing laboratory immediately. Even if all these procedures are followed, results can vary significantly.

A determination of the PRA and a measurement of the plasma aldosterone level are used in the differential diagnosis of primary and secondary **hyperaldosteronism**. Patients with primary hyperaldosteronism (caused by an adrenal tumor that overproduces aldosterone) will have an increased aldosterone level with decreased renin activity. Conversely, patients with secondary hyperaldosteronism (caused by certain types of **kidney disease**) will have increased levels of renin.

KEY TERMS

Aldosteronism—A disorder caused by excessive production of the hormone aldosterone, which is produced by a part of the adrenal glands called the adrenal cortex. Causes include a tumor of the adrenal gland (Conn's syndrome), or a disorder reducing the blood flow through the kidney. This leads to overproduction of renin and angiotensin, and in turn causes excessive aldosterone production. Symptoms include hypertension, impaired kidney function, thirst and muscle weakness.

Conn's syndrome—A disorder caused by excessive aldosterone secretion by a benign tumor of one of the adrenal glands. This results in malfunction of the body's salt and water balance and subsequently causes hypertension. Symptoms include thirst, muscle weakness, and excessive urination.

Renin stimulation test

The renin stimulation test is performed to help diagnose and distinguish the two forms of hyperaldosteronism. With the patient having been on a low-salt diet and lying down for the test, a blood sample for PRA is obtained. The PRA is repeated with the patient still on the low salt diet but now standing upright. In cases of primary hyperaldosteronism, the blood volume is greatly expanded, and a change in position or reduced salt intake does not result in decreased kidney blood flow or decreased blood sodium. As a result, renin levels do not increase. However, in secondary hyperaldosteronism, blood sodium levels decrease with a lowered salt intake, and when the patient is standing upright, the kidney blood flow decreases as well. Consequently, renin levels do increase.

Captopril test

The captopril test is a screening test for hypertension of kidney origin (**renovascular hypertension**). For this test, a baseline PRA test is done first, then the patient receives an oral dose of captopril, which is an angiotensin-converting enzyme (ACE) inhibitor. Blood pressure measurements are taken at this time and again at 60 minutes when another PRA test is done. Patients with kidney-based hypertension demonstrate greater falls in blood pressure and increases in PRA after captopril administration than do those with essential hypertension. Consequently, the captopril test is an excellent screening procedure to determine the need for a more invasive radiographic evaluation such as renal arteriography.

Preparation

This test requires a blood sample. For the PRA, the patient should maintain a normal diet with a restricted amount of sodium (approximately 3 g per day) for three days before the test. It is recommended that the patient be **fasting** (nothing to eat or drink) from midnight the day of the test.

Risks

Risks for this test are minimal, but may include slight bleeding from the puncture site, fainting or feeling lightheaded after venipuncture, or hematoma (blood accumulating under the puncture site).

Normal results

Reference values for the PRA test are laboratory-specific and depend upon the kind of diet (sodium restricted or normal), the age of the patient, and the patient's posture at the time of the test. Values are also affected if renin has been stimulated or if the patient has received an ACE inhibitor, like captopril.

Abnormal results

Increased PRA levels are seen in essential hypertension (uncommon), malignant hypertension, and kidney-based (renovascular) hypertension. Renin-producing renal tumors, while rare, can also cause elevated levels, as can **cirrhosis**, low blood volume due to hemorrhage, and diminished adrenal function (Addison's disease). Decreased renin levels may indicate increased blood volume due to a high-sodium diet, salt-retaining steroids, primary aldosteronism, licorice ingestion syndrome, or essential hypertension with low renin levels.

Resources

BOOKS

Pagana, Kathleen Deska. *Mosby's Manual of Diagnosticand Laboratory Tests.* St. Louis: Mosby, Inc., 1998.

Janis O. Flores

Plasmapheresis

Definition

Plasmapheresis is a blood purification procedure used to treat several autoimmune diseases. It is also known as therapeutic plasma exchange.

Purpose

In an autoimmune disease, the immune system attacks the body's own tissues. In many autoimmune diseases, the chief weapons of attack are antibodies, proteins that circulate in the bloodstream until they meet and bind with the target tissue. Once bound, they impair the functions of the target, and signal other immune components to respond as well.

Plasmapheresis is used to remove antibodies from the bloodstream, thereby preventing them from attacking their targets. It does not directly affect the immune system's ability to make more antibodies, and therefore may only offer temporary benefit. This procedure is most useful in acute, self-limited disorders such as **Guillain-Barré syndrome,** or when chronic disorders, such as **myasthenia gravis**, become more severe in symptoms. In these instances, a rapid improvement could save the patient's life. Neurologic diseases comprise 90% of the diseases that could profit from plasmapheresis.

Precautions

Patients with clotting disorders may not be suitable candidates for plasmapheresis.

Description

The basic procedure consists of removal of blood, separation of blood cells from plasma, and return of these blood cells to the body's circulation, diluted with fresh plasma or a substitute. Because of concerns over viral infection and allergic reaction, fresh plasma is not routinely used. Instead, the most common substitute is saline solution with sterilized human albumin protein. During the course of a single session, two to three liters of plasma is removed and replaced.

Plasmapheresis requires insertion of a venous catheter, either in a limb or central vein. Central veins allow higher flow rates and are more convenient for repeat procedures, but are more often the site of complications, especially bacterial infection.

When blood is outside the body, it must be treated to prevent it from clotting. While most of the anticlotting agent is removed from the blood during treatment, some is returned to the patient.

Three procedures are available:

- "Discontinuous flow centrifugation." Only one venous catheter line is required. Approximately 300 ml of blood is removed at a time and centrifuged to separate plasma from blood cells.
- "Continuous flow centrifugation." Two venous lines are used. This method requires slightly less blood volume to be out of the body at any one time.
- "Plasma filtration." Two venous lines are used. The pasma is filtered using standard hemodialysis equipment. It requires less than 100 ml of blood to be outside the body at one time.

A single plasmapheresis session may be effective, although it is more common to have several sessions per week over the course of two weeks or more.

Preparation

Good **nutrition** and plenty of rest make the procedure less stressful. The treating physician determines which of the patient's medications should be discontinued before the plasmapheresis session.

Aftercare

The patient may experience **dizziness**, **nausea**, numbness, tingling, or lightheadedness during or after the procedure. These effects usually pass quickly, allowing the patient to return to normal activities the same day.

Risks

Reinfusion (replacement) with human plasma may cause **anaphylaxis**, a life threatening allergic reaction. All procedures may cause a mild allergic reaction, leading to **fever**, chills, and rash. Bacterial infection is a risk, especially when a central venous catheter is used. Reaction to the citrate anticoagulant used may cause cramps and **numbness**, though these usually resolve on their own. Patients with impaired kidney function may require drug treatment for the effects of citrate metabolism.

Plasma contains clotting agents, chemicals that allow the blood to coagulate into a solid clot. Plasma exchange removes these. Bleeding complications are rare following plasmapheresis, but may require replacement of clotting factors.

Normal results

Plasmapheresis is an effective temporary treatment for:

- Guillain-Barré syndrome (an acute neurological disorder following a viral infection that produces progressive muscle weakness and **paralysis**)
- Myasthenia gravis (an autoimmune disease that causes muscle weakness)
- chronic inflammatory demyelinating polyneuropathy (a chronic neurological disorder caused by destruction of the myelin sheath of peripheral nerves, which produces symptoms similar to Guillain-Barré syndrome)
- thrombotic thrombocytopenic purpura (a rare blood disorder)
- Paraproteinemic peripheral neuropathies (a neurological disorder affecting the peripheral nerves)
- blood that is too thick (hyperviscosity)

Other conditions may respond to plasmapheresis as well. Beneficial effects are usually seen within several days. Effects commonly last up to several months, although longer-lasting changes are possible, presumably by inducing shifts in immune response.

Resources

BOOKS

Samuels, Martin, and Steven Feske, editors. *Office Practice of Neurology.* New York: Churchill Livingstone, 1996.

Richard Robinson

Plasmodium infection *see* **Malaria**

Plastic, cosmetic, and reconstructive surgery

Definition

Plastic, cosmetic, and reconstructive surgery refers to a variety of operations performed in order to repair or restore body parts to look normal, or to change a body part to look better. These types of surgery are highly specialized. They are characterized by careful preparation of the patient's skin and tissues, by precise cutting and suturing techniques, and by care taken to minimize scarring. Recent advances in the development of miniaturized instruments, new materials for artificial limbs and body parts, and improved surgical techniques have expanded the range of plastic surgery operations that can be performed.

Purpose

Although these three types of surgery share some common techniques and approaches, they have somewhat different emphases. Plastic surgery is usually performed to treat **birth defects** and to remove skin blemishes such as **warts**, **acne scars**, or **birthmarks**. Cosmetic surgery procedures are performed to make the patient look younger or enhance his or her appearance in other ways. Reconstructive surgery is used to reattach body parts severed in combat or accidents, to perform skin grafts after severe **burns**, or to reconstruct parts of the patient's body that were missing at birth or removed by surgery. Reconstructive surgery is the oldest form of plastic surgery, having developed out of the need to treat wounded soldiers in wartime.

Precautions

Medical

Some patients should not have plastic surgery because of certain medical risks. These groups include:

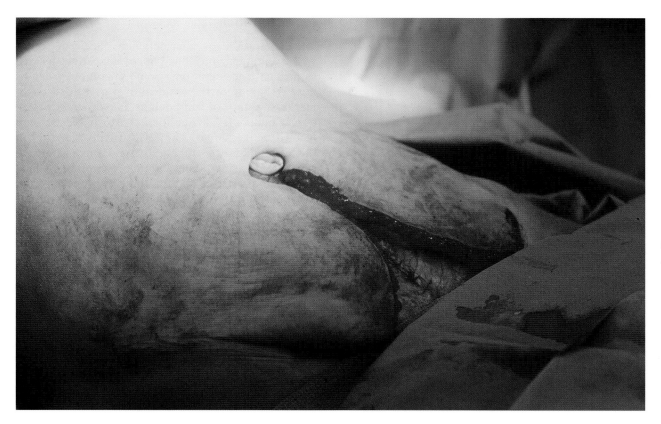

A patient undergoing abdominoplasty. *(Photo Researchers, Inc. Reproduced by permission)*

- patients recovering from a **heart attack**, severe infection (for example, **pneumonia**), or other serious illness

- patients with infectious hepatitis or HIV infection

- **cancer** patients whose cancer might spread (metastasize)

- patients who are extremely overweight. Patients who are more than 30% overweight should not have **liposuction**

- patients with blood clotting disorders

Psychological

Plastic, cosmetic, and reconstructive surgeries have an important psychological dimension because of the high value placed on outward appearance in Western society. Many people who are born with visible deformities or disfigured by accidents later in life develop emotional problems related to social rejection. Other people work in fields such as acting, modeling, media journalism, and even politics, where their employment depends on how they look. Some people have unrealistic expectations of cosmetic surgery and think that it will solve all their life problems. It is important for anyone considering nonemergency plastic or cosmetic surgery to be realistic about its results. One type of psychiatric disorder, called **body dysmorphic disorder**, is characterized by an excessive preoccupation with imaginary or minor flaws in appearance. Patients with this disorder frequently seek unnecessary plastic surgery.

Description

Plastic surgery

Plastic surgery includes a number of different procedures that usually involve skin. Operations to remove excess fat from the abdomen ("tummy tucks"), dermabrasion to remove acne scars or **tattoos**, and reshaping the cartilage in children's ears (otoplasty) are common applications of plastic surgery.

Cosmetic surgery

Most cosmetic surgery is done on the face. It is intended either to correct disfigurement or to enhance the patient's features. The most common cosmetic

The Top 10 Elective Cosmetic Surgeries In The U.S. (1999)			
Procedure	Female Patients	Male Patients	Total
Liposuction	201,083	29,782	230,865
Breast augmentation	167,318	0	167,318
Eyelid surgery	120,160	21,859	142,033
Face lift	66,096	6,697	72,793
Tummy tuck	52,888	2,089	54,977
Collagen injections	48,989	4,208	53,197
Chemical peel	47,359	4,215	51,589
Laser skin resurfacing	46,162	4,343	50,505
Rhinoplasty	34,761	11,831	46,596
Forehead lift	36,995	3,962	40,969

procedure for children is correction of a **cleft lip** or palate. In adults, the most common procedures are remodeling of the nose (rhinoplasty), removal of baggy skin around the eyelids (**blepharoplasty**), facelifts (rhytidectomy), or changing the size of the breasts (mammoplasty). Although many people still think of cosmetic surgery as only for women, growing numbers of men are choosing to have facelifts and eyelid surgery, as well as hair transplants and "tummy tucks."

Reconstructive surgery

Reconstructive surgery is often performed on cancer patients as well as on burn and accident victims. It may involve the rebuilding of severely fractured bones, as well as skin grafting. Reconstructive surgery includes such procedures as the reattachment of an amputated finger or toe, or implanting a prosthesis. Prostheses are artificial structures and materials that are used to replace missing limbs or teeth, or arthritic hip and knee joints.

In cancer patients, reconstructive surgery is done to restore the function as well as the appearance of the face and other parts of the body. The most commonly performed reconstructive surgeries of cancer patients are **breast reconstruction**, **laceration repair**, scar revision, and **tumor removal**.

The most challenging area of reconstructive surgery involves the structures of the face, neck, and jaw because trauma or cancer treatments often affect the patient's ability to see, eat, taste, swallow, speak, and hear as well as his or her external appearance. The surgeon must try to retain as much sensation as possible when performing skin or bone grafts in the head and neck as well as recreate a reasonably normal appearance.

Preparation

Preparation for nonemergency plastic or reconstructive surgery includes patient education, as well as medical considerations. Some operations, such as nose reshaping or the removal of warts, small birthmarks, and tattoos can be done as outpatient procedures under local anesthesia. Most plastic and reconstructive surgery, however, involves a stay in the hospital and general anesthesia. Patients are typically asked to stop taking certain prescription medications that affect bleeding for about two weeks before the procedure and to stop **smoking** for at least a week before the operation.

Preparation for reconstructive surgery following cancer treatment may require much more extensive counseling and discussion of possible alternatives to the surgery.

Medical preparation

Preparation for plastic surgery includes the surgeon's detailed assessment of the parts of the patient's body that will be involved. Skin grafts require evaluating suitable areas of the patient's skin for the right color and texture to match the skin at the graft site. Facelifts and cosmetic surgery in the eye area require very close attention to the texture of the skin and the placement of surgical cuts (incisions).

Patients scheduled for plastic surgery under **general anesthesia** will be given a **physical examination**, blood and urine tests, and other tests to make sure that they do not have any previously undetected health problems or blood clotting disorders. The doctor will check the list of prescription medications that the patient may be taking to make sure that none of them will interfere with normal blood clotting or interact with the anesthetic.

Patients are asked to avoid using **aspirin** or medications containing aspirin for a week to two weeks before surgery, because these drugs lengthen the time of blood clotting. Smokers are asked to stop smoking two weeks before surgery because smoking interferes with the healing process. For some types of plastic surgery, the patient may be asked to donate several units of his or her own blood before the procedure, in case a **transfusion** is needed during the operation. The patient will be asked to sign a consent form before the operation.

Patient education

The doctor will meet with the patient before the operation is scheduled, in order to explain the procedure and to be sure that the patient is realistic about the expected results. This consideration is particularly important if the patient is having cosmetic surgery.

Aftercare

Medical

Medical aftercare following plastic surgery under general anesthesia includes bringing the patient to a recovery room, monitoring his or her vital signs, and giving medications to relieve pain as necessary. Patients who have had fat removed from the abdomen may be kept in bed for as long as two weeks. Patients who have had mammoplasties, breast reconstruction, and some types of facial surgery typically remain in the hospital for a week after the operation. Patients who have had liposuction or eyelid surgery are usually sent home in a day or two.

Patients who have had outpatient procedures are usually given **antibiotics** to prevent infection and are sent home as soon as their vital signs are normal.

Psychological

Some patients may need follow-up psychotherapy or counseling after plastic or reconstructive surgery. These patients typically include children whose schooling and social relationships have been affected by birth defects, as well as patients of any age whose deformities or disfigurements were caused by trauma from accidents, war injuries, or violent crime.

Risks

The risks associated with plastic, cosmetic, and reconstructive surgery include the postoperative complications that can occur with any surgical operation under anesthesia. These complications include wound infection, internal bleeding, pneumonia, and reactions to the anesthesia.

In addition to these general risks, plastic, cosmetic, and reconstructive surgery carry specific risks:

- formation of undesirable scar tissue
- persistent **pain**, redness, or swelling in the area of the surgery
- infection inside the body related to inserting a prosthesis. These infections can result from contamination at the time of surgery or from bacteria migrating into the area around the prosthesis at a later time
- anemia or fat embolisms from liposuction
- rejection of skin grafts or tissue transplants

- loss of normal feeling or function in the area of the operation (for example, it is not unusual for women who have had mammoplasties to lose sensation in their nipples)
- complications resulting from unforeseen technological problems (the best-known example of this problem was the discovery in the mid-1990s that breast implants made with silicone gel could leak into the patient's body).

Normal results

Normal results include the patient's recovery from the surgery with satisfactory results and without complications.

Resources

PERIODICALS

Cordeiro, P. G., A. L. Pusic, J. J. Disa, et al. "Irradiation after Immediate Tissue Expander/Implant Breast Reconstruction: Outcomes, Complications, Aesthetic Results, and Satisfaction among 156 Patients." *Plastic and Reconstructive Surgery* 113 (March 2004): 877–881.

Dupin, C., S. Metzinger, and R. Rizzuto. "Lip Reconstruction after Ablation for Skin Malignancies." *Clinics in Plastic Surgery* 31 (January 2004): 69–85.

Guerra, A. B., S. E. Metzinger, R. S. Bidros, et al. "Bilateral Breast Reconstruction with the Deep Inferior Epigastric Perforator (DIEP) Flap: An Experience with 280 Flaps." *Annals of Plastic Surgery* 52 (March 2004): 246–252.

Hofstra, E. I., S. O. Hofer, J. M. Nauta et al. "Oral Functional Outcome after Intraoral Reconstruction with Nasolabial Flaps." *British Journal of Plastic Surgery* 57 (March 2004): 150–155.

Losken, A., G. W. Carlson, M. B. Schoemann, et al. "Factors That Influence the Completion of Breast Reconstruction." *Annals of Plastic Surgery* 52 (March 2004): 258–261.

Patrick, C. W. "Breast Tissue Engineering." *Annual Review of Biomedical Engineering* 6 (2004): 109–130.

ORGANIZATIONS

American Academy of Facial Plastic and Reconstructive Surgery (AAFPRS). 310 South Henry Street, Alexandria, VA 22314. (703) 299-9291. < http://www.facemd.org >.

American Medical Association. 515 N. State St., Chicago, IL 60612. (312) 464-5000. < http://www.ama-assn.org >.

American Society of Plastic Surgeons (ASPS). 444 East Algonquin Road, Arlington Heights, IL 60005. (847) 228-9900. < www.plasticsurgery.org >.

Rebecca J. Frey, PhD

Platelet aggregation test

Definition

Platelets are disk-shaped blood cells that are also called thrombocytes. They play a major role in the blood-clotting process. The platelet aggregation test is a measure of platelet function.

Purpose

The platelet aggregation test aids in the evaluation of bleeding disorders by measuring the rate and degree to which platelets form a clump (aggregate) after the addition of a chemical that stimulates clumping (aggregation).

Precautions

There are many medications that can affect the results of the platelet aggregation test. The patient should discontinue as many as possible beforehand. Some of the drugs that can decrease platelet aggregation include **aspirin**, some **antibiotics**, **beta blockers**, dextran (Macrodex), alcohol, heparin (Lipo-Hepin), nonsteroidal anti-inflammatory drugs (NSAIDs), **tricyclic antidepressants**, and warfarin (Coumadin).

Description

There are many factors involved in blood clotting (coagulation). One of the first steps in the process involves small cells in the bloodstream called platelets, which are produced in the bone marrow. Platelets gather at the site of an injury and clump together to form a plug, or aggregate, that helps to limit the loss of blood and promote healing.

Inherited bleeding disorders (e.g., **hemophilia** or von Willebrand's disease) and acquired bleeding problems that occur because of another disorder or a medication can affect the number of platelets and their level of function. When these problems are present, the result is a drop in platelet aggregation and a lengthened bleeding time.

The platelet aggregation test uses a machine called an aggregometer to measure the cloudiness (turbidity) of blood plasma. Several different substances called agonists are used in the test. These agonists include adenosine diphosphate, epinephrine, thrombin, collagen, and ristocetin. The addition of an agonist to a plasma sample causes the platelets to clump together, making the fluid more transparent. The aggregometer then measures the increased light transmission through the specimen.

Preparation

The test requires a blood sample. The patient should either avoid food and drink altogether for eight hours before the test, or eat only nonfat foods. High levels of fatty substances in the blood can affect test results.

Because the use of aspirin and/or aspirin compounds can directly affect test results, the patient should avoid these medications for two weeks before the test. If the patient must take aspirin and the test cannot be postponed, the laboratory should be notified and asked to verify the presence of aspirin in the blood plasma. If the results are abnormal, aspirin use must be discontinued and the test repeated in two weeks.

Aftercare

Because the platelet aggregation test is ordered when some type of bleeding problem is suspected, the patient should be cautioned to watch the puncture site for signs of additional bleeding.

Risks

Risks for this test are minimal in normal individuals. Patients with bleeding disorders, however, may have prolonged bleeding from the puncture wound or the formation of a bruise (hematoma) under the skin where the blood was withdrawn.

KEY TERMS

Aggregation—The blood cell clumping process that is measured in the platelet aggregation test.

Agonist—A chemical that is added to the blood sample in the platelet aggregation test to stimulate the clumping process.

Hemophilia—An inherited bleeding disorder caused by a deficiency of factor VIII, one of a series of blood proteins essential for blood clotting.

Platelets—Small, round, disk-shaped blood cells that are involved in clot formation. The platelet aggregation test measures the clumping ability of platelets.

Turbidity—The cloudiness or lack of transparency of a solution.

von Willebrand's disease—An inherited lifelong bleeding disorder caused by an abnormal gene, similar to hemophilia. The gene defect results in a decreased blood concentration of a substance called von Willebrand's factor (vWF).

Normal results

The normal time for platelet aggregation varies somewhat depending on the laboratory, the temperature, the shape of the vial in which the test is performed, and the patient's response to different agonists. For example, the difference between the response to ristocetin and other products should be noted because ristocetin triggers aggregation through a different mechanism than other agonists.

Abnormal results

Prolonged platelet aggregation time can be found in such congenital disorders as hemophilia and von Willebrand's disease, as well as in some connective tissue disorders. Prolonged aggregation times can also occur in leukemia or myeloma; after recent heart/lung bypass or **kidney dialysis**; and after taking certain drugs.

Resources

BOOKS

Pagana, Kathleen Deska. *Mosby's Manual of Diagnosticand Laboratory Tests*. St. Louis: Mosby, Inc., 1998.

Janis O. Flores

Platelet count

Definition

A platelet count is a diagnostic test that determines the number of platelets in the patient's blood. Platelets, which are also called thrombocytes, are small disk-shaped blood cells produced in the bone marrow and involved in the process of blood clotting. There are normally between 150,000-450,000 platelets in each microliter of blood. Low platelet counts or abnormally shaped platelets are associated with bleeding disorders. High platelet counts sometimes indicate disorders of the bone marrow.

Purpose

The primary functions of a platelet count are to assist in the diagnosis of bleeding disorders and to monitor patients who are being treated for any disease involving bone marrow failure. Patients who have leukemia, **polycythemia vera**, or **aplastic anemia** are given periodic platelet count tests to monitor their health.

Description

Blood collection and storage

Platelet counts use a freshly-collected blood specimen to which a chemical called EDTA has been added to prevent clotting before the test begins. About 5 mL of blood are drawn from a vein in the patient's inner elbow region. Blood drawn from a vein helps to produce a more accurate count than blood drawn from a fingertip. Collection of the sample takes only a few minutes.

After collection, the mean platelet volume of EDTA-blood will increase over time. This increase is caused by a change in the shape of the platelets after removal from the body. The changing volume is relatively stable for a period of one to three hours after collection. This period is the best time to count the sample when using electronic instruments, because the platelets will be within a standard size range.

Counting methods

Platelets can be observed in a direct blood smear for approximate quantity and shape. A direct smear is made by placing a drop of blood onto a microscope slide and spreading it into a thin layer. After staining to make the various blood cells easier to see and distinguish, a laboratory technician views the smear through a light microscope. Accurate assessment of the number of platelets requires other methods of counting. There are three methods used to count platelets; hemacytometer, voltage-pulse counting, and electro-optical counting.

HEMACYTOMETER COUNTING. The microscopic method uses a phase contrast microscope to view blood on a hemacytometer slide. A sample of the diluted blood mixture is placed in a hemacytometer, which is an instrument with a grid etched into its surface to guide the counting. For a proper count, the platelets should be evenly distributed in the hemacytometer. Counts made from samples with platelet clumping are considered unreliable. Clumping can be caused by several factors, such as clotting before addition of the anticoagulant and allowing the blood to remain in contact with a capillary blood vessel during collection. Errors in platelet counting are more common when blood is collected from capillaries than from veins.

ELECTRONIC COUNTING. Electronic counting of platelets is the most common method. There are two types of electronic counting, voltage-pulse and electro-optical counting systems. In both systems, the collected blood is diluted and counted by passing the blood through an electronic counter. The instruments are set to count only particles within the proper size range for platelets. The upper and lower levels of the size range are called size exclusion limits. Any cells or material larger or smaller than the size exclusion limits will not be counted. Any object in the proper size range is counted, however, even if it isn't a platelet. For these instruments to work properly, the sample must not contain other material that might mistakenly be counted as platelets. Electronic counting instruments sometimes produce artificially low platelet counts. If a platelet and another blood cell pass through the counter at the same time, the instrument will not count the larger cell because of the size exclusion limits, which will cause the instrument to accidentally miss the platelet. Clumps of platelets will not be counted because clumps exceed the upper size exclusion limit for platelets. In addition, if the patient has a high white blood cell count, electronic counting may yield an unusually low platelet count because white blood cells may filter out some of the platelets before the sample is counted. On the other hand, if the red blood cells in the sample have burst, their fragments will be falsely counted as platelets.

Aftercare

Because platelet counts are sometimes ordered to diagnose or monitor bleeding disorders, patients with

---

KEY TERMS

Capillaries—The smallest of the blood vessels that bring oxygenated blood to tissues.

EDTA—A colorless compound used to keep blood samples from clotting before tests are run. Its chemical name is ethylene-diamine-tetra-acetic acid.

Hemocytometer—An instrument used to count platelets or other blood cells.

Phase contrast microscope—A light microscope in which light is focused on the sample at an angle to produce a clearer image.

Thrombocyte—Another name for platelet.

Thrombocytopenia—An abnormally low platelet count.

Thrombocytosis—An abnormally high platelet count. It occurs in polycythemia vera and other disorders in which the bone marrow produces too many platelets.

---

these disorders should be cautioned to watch the puncture site for signs of additional bleeding.

Risks

Risks for a platelet count test are minimal in normal individuals. Patients with bleeding disorders, however, may have prolonged bleeding from the puncture wound or the formation of a bruise (hematoma) under the skin where the blood was withdrawn.

Normal results

The normal range for a platelet count is 150,000-450,000 platelets per microliter of blood.

Abnormal results

An abnormally low platelet level (**thrombocytopenia**) is a condition that may result from increased destruction of platelets, decreased production, or increased usage of platelets. In **idiopathic thrombocytopenic purpura** (ITP), platelets are destroyed at abnormally high rates. **Hypersplenism** is characterized by the collection (sequestration) of platelets in the spleen. Disseminated intravascular coagulation (DIC) is a condition in which **blood clots** occur within blood vessels in a number of tissues. All of these diseases produce reduced platelet counts.

Abnormally high platelet levels (**thrombocytosis**) may indicate either a benign reaction to an infection, surgery, or certain medications; or a disease like polycythemia vera, in which the bone marrow produces too many platelets too quickly.

Resources

BOOKS

Berktow, Robert, et al., editors. *Merck Manual of Medical Information*. Whitehouse Station, NJ: Merck Research Laboratories, 2004.

John T. Lohr, PhD

Platelet function disorders

Definition

Platelets are elements within the bloodstream that recognize and cling to damaged areas inside blood vessels. When they do this, the platelets trigger a series of chemical changes that result in the formation of a blood clot. There are certain hereditary disorders that affect platelet function and impair their ability to start the process of blood clot formation. One result is the possibility of excessive bleeding from minor injuries or menstrual flow.

Description

Platelets are formed in the bone marrow–a spongy tissue located inside the long bones of the body–as fragments of a large precursor cell (a megakaryocyte). These fragments circulate in the bloodstream and form the first line of defense against blood escaping from injured blood vessels.

Damaged blood vessels release a chemical signal that increases the stickiness of platelets in the area of the injury. The sticky platelets adhere to the damaged area and gradually form a platelet plug. At the same time, the platelets release a series of chemical signals that prompt other factors in the blood to reinforce the platelet plug. Between the platelet and its reinforcements, a sturdy clot is created that acts as a patch while the damaged area heals.

There are several hereditary disorders characterized by some impairment of the platelet's action. Examples include von Willebrand's disease, Glanzmann's thrombasthenia, and **Wiskott-Aldrich syndrome**. Vulnerable aspects of platelet function include errors in the production of the platelets themselves or errors in the formation, storage, or release of their chemical signals. These defects can prevent platelets from responding to injuries or from prompting the action of other factors involved in clot formation.

Causes and symptoms

Platelet function disorders can be inherited, but they may also occur as a symptom of acquired diseases or as a side effect of certain drugs, including **aspirin**. Common symptoms of platelet function disorders include bleeding from the nose, mouth, vagina, or anus; pinpoint **bruises** and purplish patches on the skin; and abnormally heavy menstrual bleeding.

Diagnosis

In diagnosing platelet function disorders, specific tests are needed to determine whether the problem is caused by low numbers of platelets or impaired platelet function. A blood **platelet count** and **bleeding time** are common screening tests. If these tests confirm that the symptoms are due to impaired platelet function, further tests are done–such as platelet aggregation or an analysis of the platelet proteins–that pinpoint the exact nature of the defect.

Treatment

Treatment is intended to prevent bleeding and stop it quickly when it occurs. For example, patients are advised to be careful when they brush their teeth to reduce damage to the gums. They are also warned against taking medications that interfere with platelet function. Some patients may require iron and folate supplements to counteract potential anemia. Platelet transfusions may be necessary to prevent life-threatening hemorrhaging in some cases. Bone marrow transplantation can cure certain disorders but also carries some serious risks. Hormone therapy is useful in treating heavy menstrual bleeding. Von Willebrand's disease can be treated with desmopressin (DDAVP, Stimate).

Prognosis

The outcome depends on the specific disorder and the severity of its symptoms. Platelet function disorders range from life-threatening conditions to easily treated or little-noticed problems.

Prevention

Inherited platelet function disorders cannot be prevented except by **genetic counseling**; however,

KEY TERMS

Anemia—A condition in which inadequate quantities of hemoglobin and red blood cells are produced.

Bone marrow—A spongy tissue located within the body's flat bones–including the hip and breast bones and the skull. Marrow contains stem cells, the precursors to platelets and red and white blood cells.

Hemoglobin—The substance inside red blood cells that enables them to carry oxygen.

Megakaryocyte—A large bone marrow cell with a lobed nucleus that is the precursor cell of blood platelets.

Platelets—Fragments of a large precursor cell (a megakaryocyte) found in the bone marrow. These fragments adhere to areas of blood vessel damage and release chemical signals that direct the formation of a blood clot.

some acquired function disorders may be guarded against by avoiding substances that trigger the disorder.

Resources

PERIODICALS

Liesner, R. J., and S. J. Machin. "Platelet Disorders."*British Medical Journal* 314, no. 7083 (1997): 809.

Julia Barrett

Pleural biopsy

Definition

The pleura is the membrane that lines the lungs and chest cavity. A pleural biopsy is the removal of pleural tissue for examination.

Purpose

Pleural biopsy is done to differentiate between benign and malignant disease, to diagnose viral, fungal, or parasitic diseases, and to identify a condition called collagen vascular disease of the pleura. It is also ordered when a **chest x ray** indicates a pleural-based tumor, reaction, or thickening of the lining.

Precautions

Because pleural biopsy is an invasive procedure, it is not recommended for patients with severe bleeding disorders.

Description

Pleural biopsy is usually ordered when pleural fluid obtained by another procedure called thoracentesis (aspiration of pleural fluid) suggests infection, signs of **cancer**, or **tuberculosis**. Pleural biopsies are 85–90% accurate in diagnosing these diseases.

The procedure most often performed for pleural biopsy is called a percutaneous (passage through the skin by needle puncture) needle biopsy. The procedure takes 30–45 minutes, although the biopsy needle itself remains in the pleura for less than one minute. This type of biopsy is usually performed by a physician at bedside, if the patient is hospitalized, or in the doctor's office under local anesthetic.

The actual procedure begins with the patient in a sitting position, shoulders and arms elevated and supported. The skin overlying the biopsy site is anesthetized and a small incision is made to allow insertion of the biopsy needle. This needle is inserted with a cannula (a plastic or metal tube) until fluid is removed. Then the inner needle is removed and a trocar (an instrument for withdrawing fluid from a cavity) is inserted to obtain the actual biopsy specimen. As many as three separate specimens are taken from different sites during the procedure. These specimens are then placed into a fixative solution and sent to the laboratory for tissue (histologic) examination.

Preparation

Preparations for this procedure vary, depending on the type of procedure requested. Pleural biopsy can be performed in several ways: percutaneous needle biopsy (described above), by thoracoscopy (insertion of a visual device called a laparoscope into the pleural space for inspection), or by open pleural biopsy, which requires general anesthesia.

Aftercare

Potential complications of this procedure include bleeding or injury to the lung, or a condition called **pneumothorax**, in which air enters the pleural cavity (the space between the two layers of pleura lining the lungs and the chest wall). Because of these possibilities, the patient is to report any shortness of breath, and to note any signs of bleeding, decreased blood pressure, or increased pulse rate.

Risks

Risks for this procedure include respiratory distress on the side of the biopsy, as well as bleeding, possible shoulder **pain**, pneumothorax (immediate) or pneumonia (delayed).

Normal results

Normal findings indicate no evidence of any pathologic or disease conditions.

Abnormal results

Abnormal findings include tumors called neoplasms (any new or abnormal growth) that can be either benign or malignant. Pleural tumors are divided into two classifications: primary (mesothelioma), or metastatic (arising from cancer sites elsewhere in the body). These tumors are often associated with an accumulation of fluid between the pleural layers called a **pleural effusion**, which itself may be caused by **pneumonia**, **heart failure**, cancer, or blood clot in the lungs (pulmonary embolism).

Other causes of abnormal findings include viral, fungal, or parasitic infections, and tuberculosis.

Resources

BOOKS

Pagana, Kathleen Deska. *Mosby's Manual of Diagnostic and Laboratory Tests*. St. Louis: Mosby, Inc., 1998.

Janis O. Flores

Pleural effusion

Definition

Pleural effusion occurs when too much fluid collects in the pleural space (the space between the two layers of the pleura). It is commonly known as "water on the lungs." It is characterized by **shortness of breath**, chest **pain**, gastric discomfort (**dyspepsia**), and cough.

Description

There are two thin membranes in the chest, one (the visceral pleura) lining the lungs, and the other (the parietal pleura) covering the inside of the chest wall. Normally, small blood vessels in the pleural linings produce a small amount of fluid that lubricates the opposed pleural membranes so that they can glide smoothly against one another during breathing movements. Any extra fluid is taken up by blood and lymph vessels, maintaining a balance. When either too much fluid forms or something prevents its removal, the result is an excess of pleural fluid–an effusion. The most common causes are disease of the heart or lungs, and inflammation or infection of the pleura.

Pleural effusion itself is not a disease as much as a result of many different diseases. For this reason, there is no "typical" patient in terms of age, sex, or other characteristics. Instead, anyone who develops one of the many conditions that can produce an effusion may be affected.

There are two types of pleural effusion: the transudate and the exudate. This is a very important point because the two types of fluid are very different, and which type is present points to what sort of disease is likely to have produced the effusion. It also can suggest the best approach to treatment.

Transudates

A transudate is a clear fluid, similar to blood serum, that forms not because the pleural surfaces themselves are diseased, but because the forces that normally produce and remove pleural fluid at the same rate are out of balance. When the heart fails, pressure in the small blood vessels that remove pleural fluid is increased and fluid "backs up" in the pleural space, forming an effusion. Or, if too little protein is present in the blood, the vessels are less able to hold the fluid part of blood within them and it leaks out into the pleural space. This can result from disease of the liver or kidneys, or from **malnutrition**.

Exudates

An exudate–which often is a cloudy fluid, containing cells and much protein–results from disease of the pleura itself. The causes are many and varied. Among the most common are infections such as bacterial **pneumonia** and **tuberculosis**; **blood clots** in the lungs; and connective tissue diseases, such as rheumatoid arthritis. **Cancer** and disease in organs such as the pancreas also may give rise to an exudative pleural effusion.

Special types of pleural effusion

Some of the pleural disorders that produce an exudate also cause bleeding into the pleural space. If the effusion contains half or more of the number of red blood cells present in the blood itself, it is called hemothorax. When a pleural effusion has a milky appearance and contains a large amount of fat, it is called chylothorax. Lymph fluid that drains from tissues throughout the body into small lymph vessels finally collects in a large duct (the thoracic duct) running through the chest to empty into a major vein. When this fluid, or chyle, leaks out of the duct into the pleural space, chylothorax is the result. Cancer in the chest is a common cause.

Causes and symptoms

Causes of transudative pleural effusion

Among the most important specific causes of a transudative pleural effusion are:

- Congestive **heart failure**. This causes pleural effusions in about 40% of patients and is often present on both sides of the chest. Heart failure is the most common cause of bilateral (two-sided) effusion. When only one side is affected it usually is the right (because patients usually lie on their right side).

- Pericarditis. This is an inflammation of the pericardium, the membrane covering the heart.

- Too much fluid in the body tissues, which spills over into the pleural space. This is seen in some forms of **kidney disease**; when patients have bowel disease and absorb too little of what they eat; and when an excessive amount of fluid is given intravenously.

- Liver disease. About 5% of patients with a chronic scarring disease of the liver called cirrhosis develop pleural effusion.

Causes of exudative pleural effusions

A wide range of conditions may be the cause of an exudative pleural effusion:

- Pleural tumors account for up to 40% of one-sided pleural effusions. They may arise in the pleura itself (**mesothelioma**), or from other sites, notably the lung.

- Tuberculosis in the lungs may produce a long-lasting exudative pleural effusion.

- Pneumonia affects about three million persons each year, and four of every ten patients will develop pleural effusion. If effective treatment is not provided, an extensive effusion can form that is very difficult to treat.

- Patients with any of a wide range of infections by a virus, fungus, or parasite that involve the lungs may have pleural effusion.

- Up to half of all patients who develop blood clots in their lungs (**pulmonary embolism**) will have pleural effusion, and this sometimes is the only sign of **embolism**.

- Connective tissue diseases, including **rheumatoid arthritis**, lupus, and **Sjögren's syndrome** may be complicated by pleural effusion.

- Patients with disease of the liver or pancreas may have an exudative effusion, and the same is true for any patient who undergoes extensive abdominal surgery. About 30% of patients who undergo heart surgery will develop an effusion.

- Injury to the chest may produce pleural effusion in the form of either hemothorax or chylothorax.

Symptoms

The key symptom of a pleural effusion is shortness of breath. Fluid filling the pleural space makes it hard for the lungs to fully expand, causing the patient to take many breaths so as to get enough oxygen. When the parietal pleura is irritated, the patient may have mild pain that quickly passes or, sometimes, a sharp, stabbing pleuritic type of pain. Some patients will have a dry cough. Occasionally a patient will have no symptoms at all. This is more likely when the effusion results from recent abdominal surgery, cancer, or tuberculosis. Tapping on the chest will show that the usual crisp sounds have become dull, and on listening with a stethoscope the normal breath sounds are muted. If the pleura is inflamed, there may be a scratchy sound called a "pleural friction rub."

Diagnosis

When pleural effusion is suspected, the best way to confirm it is to take chest x rays, both straight-on and from the side. The fluid itself can be seen at the bottom of the lung or lungs, hiding the normal lung structure. If heart failure is present, the x-ray shadow of the heart will be enlarged. An ultrasound scan may disclose a small effusion that caused no abnormal findings during chest examination. A computed tomography scan is very helpful if the lungs themselves are diseased.

In order to learn what has caused the effusion, a needle or catheter is often used to obtain a fluid sample, which is examined for cells and its chemical makeup. This procedure, called a thoracentesis, is the way to determine whether an effusion is a transudate or exudate, giving a clue as to the underlying cause. In some cases–for instance when cancer or bacterial infection is present–the specific cause can be determined and the correct treatment planned. Culturing a fluid sample can identify the bacteria that cause tuberculosis or other forms of pleural infection. The next diagnostic step is to take a tissue sample, or **pleural biopsy**, and examine it under a microscope. If the effusion is caused by lung disease, placing a viewing tube (bronchoscope) through the large air passages will allow the examiner to see the abnormal appearance of the lungs.

Treatment

The best way to clear up a pleural effusion is to direct treatment at what is causing it, rather than treating the effusion itself. If heart failure is reversed or a lung infection is cured by antibiotics, the effusion will usually resolve. However, if the cause is not known, even after extensive tests, or no effective treatment is at hand, the fluid can be drained away by placing a large-bore needle or catheter into the pleural space, just as in diagnostic **thoracentesis**. If necessary, this can be repeated as often as is needed to control the amount of fluid in the pleural space. If large effusions continue to recur, a drug or material that irritates the pleural membranes can be injected to deliberately inflame them and cause them to adhere close together–a process called sclerosis. This will prevent further effusion by eliminating the pleural space. In the most severe cases, open surgery with removal of a rib may be necessary to drain all the fluid and close the pleural space.

Prognosis

When the cause of pleural effusion can be determined and effectively treated, the effusion itself will reliably clear up and should not recur. In many other cases, sclerosis will prevent sizable effusions from recurring. Whenever a large effusion causes a patient to be short of breath, thoracentesis will make breathing easier, and it may be repeated if necessary. To a great extent, the outlook for patients with pleural effusion depends on the primary cause of effusion and whether it can be eliminated. Some forms of pleural effusion, such as that seen after abdominal surgery, are only temporary and will clear without specific treatment. If heart failure can be controlled, the patient will remain free of pleural effusion. If, on the other hand, effusion is caused by cancer that cannot be controlled, other effects of the disease probably will become more important.

Prevention

Because pleural effusion is a secondary effect of many different conditions, the key to preventing it is to promptly diagnose the primary disease and provide effective treatment. Timely treatment of infections such as tuberculosis and pneumonia will prevent many effusions. When effusion occurs as a drug side-effect, withdrawing the drug or using a different one may solve the problem. On rare occasions, an effusion occurs because fluid meant for a vein is mistakenly injected into the pleural space. This can be prevented by making sure that proper technique is used.

Resources

ORGANIZATIONS

American Lung Association. 1740 Broadway, New York, NY 10019. (800) 586-4872. <http://www.lungusa.org>.

National Heart, Lung and Blood Institute. P.O. Box 30105, Bethesda, MD 20824-0105. (301) 251-1222. <http://www.nhlbi.nih.gov>.

David A. Cramer, MD

Pleural fluid analysis *see* **Thoracentesis**

Pleurisy

Definition

Pleurisy is an inflammation of the membrane that surrounds and protects the lungs (the pleura). Inflammation occurs when an infection or damaging agent irritates the pleural surface. As a consequence, sharp chest pains are the primary symptom of pleurisy.

Description

Pleurisy, also called pleuritis, is a condition that generally stems from an existing respiratory infection, disease, or injury. In people who have otherwise good health, respiratory infections or **pneumonia** are the main causes of pleurisy. This condition used to be more common, but with the advent of **antibiotics** and modern disease therapies, pleurisy has become less prevalent.

The pleura is a double-layered structure made up of an inner membrane, which surrounds the lungs, and an outer membrane, which lines the chest cavity. The pleural membranes are very thin, close together, and have a fluid coating in the narrow space between them. This liquid acts as a lubricant, so that when the lungs inflate and deflate during breathing, the pleural surfaces can easily glide over one another.

Pleurisy occurs when the pleural surfaces rub against one another, due to irritation and inflammation. Infection within the pleural space is the most common irritant, although the abnormal presence of air, blood, or cells can also initiate pleurisy. These disturbances all act to displace the normal pleural fluid, which forces the membranes to rub, rather than glide, against one another. This rubbing irritates nerve endings in the outer membrane and causes **pain**. Pleurisy

also causes a chest noise that ranges from a faint squeak to a loud creak. This characteristic sound is called a "friction rub."

Pleurisy cases are classified either as having pleural effusion or as being "dry." **Pleural effusion** is more common and refers to an accumulation of fluid within the pleural space; dry pleurisy is inflammation without fluid build-up. Less pain occurs with pleural effusion because the fluid forces the membrane surfaces apart. However, pleural effusion causes additional complications because it places pressure on the lungs. This leads to respiratory distress and possible lung collapse.

Causes and symptoms

A variety of conditions can give rise to pleurisy. The following list represents the most common sources of pleural inflammation.

- infections, including pneumonia, **tuberculosis**, and other bacterial or viral respiratory infections
- immune disorders, including systemic lupus erythematosus, rheumatoid arthritis, and **sarcoidosis**
- diseases, including **cancer**, **pancreatitis**, liver **cirrhosis**, and heart or kidney failure
- injury, from a rib fracture, collapsed lung, esophagus rupture, blood clot, or material such as asbestos
- drug reactions, from certain drugs used to treat tuberculosis (isoniazid), cancer (methotrexate, procarbazine), or the immune disorders mentioned above (hydralazine, procainamide, phenytoin, quinidine)

Symptomatic pain

The hallmark symptom of pleurisy is sudden, intense chest pain that is usually located over the area of inflammation. Although the pain can be constant, it is usually most severe when the lungs move during breathing, coughing, sneezing, or even talking. The pain is usually described as shooting or stabbing, but in minor cases it resembles a mild cramp. When pleurisy occurs in certain locations, such as near the diaphragm, the pain may be felt in other areas such as the neck, shoulder, or abdomen (referred pain). Another indication of pleurisy is that holding one's breath or exerting pressure against the chest causes pain relief.

Breathing difficulties

Pleurisy is also characterized by certain respiratory symptoms. In response to the pain, pleurisy patients commonly have a rapid, shallow breathing pattern. Pleural effusion can also cause **shortness of breath**, as excess fluid makes expanding the lungs difficult. If severe breathing difficulties persist, patients may experience a blue colored complexion (**cyanosis**).

Additional symptoms of pleurisy are specific to the illness that triggers the condition. Thus, if infection is the cause, then chills, **fever**, and **fatigue** will be likely pleurisy symptoms.

Diagnosis

The distinctive pain of pleurisy is normally the first clue physicians use for diagnosis. Doctors usually feel the chest to find the most painful area, which is the likely site of inflammation. A stethoscope is also used to listen for abnormal chest sounds as the patient breathes. If the doctor hears the characteristic friction rub, the diagnosis of pleurisy can be confirmed. Sometimes, a friction rub is masked by the presence of pleural effusion and further examination is needed for an accurate diagnosis.

Identifying the actual illness that causes pleurisy is more difficult. To make this diagnosis, doctors must evaluate the patient's history, additional symptoms, and laboratory test results. A chest x ray may also be taken to look for signs of accumulated fluid and other abnormalities. Possible causes, such as pneumonia, fractured ribs, esophagus rupture, and lung tumors may be detected on an x ray. Computed tomography scan (CT scan) and ultrasound scans are more powerful diagnostic tools used to visualize the chest cavity. Images from these techniques more clearly pinpoint the location of excess fluid or other suspected problems.

The most helpful information in diagnosing the cause of pleurisy is a fluid analysis. Once the doctor knows the precise location of fluid accumulation, a sample is removed using a procedure called **thoracentesis**. In this technique, a fine needle is inserted into the chest to reach the pleural space and extract fluid. The fluid's appearance and composition is thoroughly examined to help doctors understand how the fluid was produced. Several laboratory tests are performed to analyze the chemical components of the fluid. These tests also determine whether infection-causing bacteria or viruses are present. In addition, cells within the fluid are identified and counted. Cancerous cells can also be detected to learn whether the pleurisy is caused by a malignancy.

In certain instances, such as dry pleurisy, or when a fluid analysis is not informative, a biopsy of the pleura may be needed for microscopic analysis. A sample of pleural tissue can be obtained several ways: with a biopsy needle, by making a small incision in the chest wall, or by using a thoracoscope (a video-assisted instrument for viewing the pleural space and collecting samples).

Treatment

Pain management

The pain of pleurisy is usually treated with analgesic and anti-inflammatory drugs, such as acetaminophen, ibuprofen, and indomethacin. People with pleurisy may also receive relief from lying on the painful side. Sometimes, a painful **cough** will be controlled with codeine-based cough syrups. However, as the pain eases, a person with pleurisy should try to breathe deeply and cough to clear any congestion, otherwise pneumonia may occur. Rest is also important to aid in the recovery process.

Treating the source

The treatment used to cure pleurisy is ultimately defined by the underlying cause. Thus, pleurisy from a bacterial infection can be successfully treated with antibiotics, while no treatment is given for viral infections that must run their course. Specific therapies designed for more chronic illnesses can often cause pleurisy to subside. For example, tuberculosis pleurisy is treated with standard anti-tuberculosis drugs. With some illnesses, excess fluid continues to accumulate and causes severe respiratory distress. In these individuals, the fluid may be removed by thoracentesis, or the doctor may insert a chest tube to drain large amounts. If left untreated, a more serious infection may develop within the fluid, called **empyema**.

Alternative treatment

Alternative treatments can be used in conjunction with conventional treatment to help heal pleurisy. **Acupuncture** and botanical medicines are alternative approaches for alleviating pleural pain and breathing problems. An herbal remedy commonly recommended is pleurisy root (*Asclepias tuberosa*), so named because of its use by early American settlers who learned of this medicinal plant from Native Americans. Pleurisy root helps to ease pain, inflammation, and breathing difficulties brought on by pleurisy. This herb is often used in conjunction with mullein (*Verbascum thapsus*) or elecampane (*Inula helenium*), which serve as **expectorants** to clear excess mucus from the lungs. In addition, there are many

KEY TERMS

Effusion—The accumulation of fluid within a cavity, such as the pleural space.

Empyema—An infection that causes pus to accumulate in the pleural space. The pus may cause a tear in the pleural membrane, which allows the infection to spread to other areas in the body. Intravenous antibiotics are often given to control the infection.

Inflammation—An accumulation of fluid and cells within tissue that is often caused by infection and the immune response that occurs as a result.

Pneumonia—A condition caused by bacterial or viral infection that is characterized by inflammation of the lungs and fluid within the air passages. Pneumonia is often an underlying cause of pleurisy.

Referred pain—The presence of pain in an area other than where it originates. In some pleurisy cases, referred pain occurs in the neck, shoulder, or abdomen.

other respiratory herbs that are used as expectorants or for other actions on the respiratory system. Herbs thought to combat infection, such as **echinacea** (*Echinacea* spp.) are also included in herbal pleurisy remedies. Anitviral herbs, such as *Lomatium dissectum* and *Ligusticum porteri*, can be used if the pleurisy is of viral origin. **Traditional Chinese medicine** uses the herb ephedra (*Ephedra sinica*), which acts to open air passages and alleviate respiratory difficulties in pleurisy patients. Dietary recommendations include eating fresh fruits and vegetables, adequate protein, and good quality fats (omega–3 fatty acids are anti-inflammatory and are found in fish and flax oil). Taking certain nutritional supplements, especially large doeses of vitamin C, may also provide health benefits to people with pleurisy. Contrast **hydrotherapy** applied to the chest and back, along with compresses (cloths soaked in an herbal solution) or poultices (crushed herbs applied directly to the skin) of respiratory herbs, can assist in the healing process. Homeopathic treatment, guided by a trained practitioner, can be effective in resolving pleurisy.

Prognosis

Prompt diagnosis, followed by appropriate treatment, ensures a good recovery for most pleurisy patients. Generally speaking, the prognosis for pleurisy is linked to the seriousness of its cause. Therefore, the outcome of pleurisy caused by a disease such as cancer will vary depending on the type and location of the tumor.

Prevention

Preventing pleurisy is often a matter of providing early medical attention to conditions that can cause pleural inflammation. Along this line, appropriate antibiotic treatment of bacterial respiratory infections may successfully prevent some cases of pleurisy. Maintaining a healthy lifestyle and avoiding exposure to harmful substances (for example, asbestos) are more general preventative measures.

Resources

ORGANIZATIONS

American Lung Association. 1740 Broadway, New York, NY 10019. (800) 586-4872. < http:// www.lungusa.org >.

National Heart, Lung and Blood Institute. P.O. Box 30105, Bethesda, MD 20824-0105. (301) 251-1222. < http:// www.nhlbi.nih.gov >.

Julie A. Gelderloos

Pleuritis *see* **Pleurisy**

Plumbism *see* **Lead poisoning**

PMS *see* **Premenstrual syndrome**

Pneumococcal pneumonia

Definition

Pneumococcal **pneumonia** is a common but serious infection and inflammation of the lungs. It is caused by the bacterium *Streptococcus pneumoniae*.

Description

The gram-positive, spherical bacteria, *Streptococcus pneumoniae*, is the cause of many human diseases, including pneumonia. Although the bacteria can normally be found in the nose and throat of healthy individuals, it can grow and cause infection when the immune system is weakened. Infection usually begins with the upper respiratory tract and then travels into the lungs. Pneumonia occurs when the bacteria find their way deep into the lungs, to the area called the alveoli, or air sacs. This is the functional part of the lungs where oxygen is absorbed into the blood. Once in the alveoli, *Streptococcus pneumoniae* begin to grow and multiply. White blood cells and immune proteins from the blood also accumulate at the site of infection in the alveoli. As the alveoli fill with these substances and fluid, they can no longer function in the exchange of oxygen. This fluid filling of the lungs is how pneumonia is defined.

Those people most at risk of developing pneumococcal pneumonia have a weakened immune system. This includes the elderly, infants, **cancer** patients, AIDS patients, post-operative patients, alcoholics, and those with diabetes. Pneumococcal pneumonia is a disease that has a high rate of hospital transmission, putting hospital patients at greater risk. Prior lung infections also makes someone more likely to develop pneumococcal pneumonia. The disease can be most severe in patients who have had their spleen removed. It is the spleen that is responsible for removing the bacteria from the blood. Cases of pneumonia, which is spread by close contact, seem to occur most often between November through April. If not treated, the disease can spread, causing continually decreasing lung function, heart problems, and arthritis.

Causes and symptoms

Symptoms of bacterial pneumonia include a **cough**, sputum (mucus) production that may be pus-like or bloody, shaking and chills, **fever**, and chest **pain**. Symptoms often have an abrupt beginning and occur after an upper respiratory infection such as a cold. Symptoms may differ somewhat in the elderly, with minimal cough, no sputum and no fever, but rather tiredness and confusion leading to **hypothermia** and **shock**.

Diagnosis

The presence of symptoms and a physical exam that reveals abnormal lung sounds usually suggest the presence of pneumonia. Diagnosis is typically made from an x ray of the lungs, which indicates the accumulation of fluid. Additional tests that may be done include a complete blood count, a sputum sample for microscopic examination and culture for *Streptococcus pneumoniae*, and possibly blood cultures.

Treatment

Depending on the severity of the disease, **antibiotics** are given either at home or in the hospital. Historically, the treatment for pneumococcal pneumonia has been penicillin. An increasing number of cases of pneumococcal pneumonia have become partially or completely resistant to penicillin, making it less effective in treating this disease. Other effective antibiotics include amoxicillin and erythromycin. If these antibiotics are not effective, vancomycin or cephalosporin may alternatively be used.

Symptoms associated with pneumococcal pneumonia can also be treated. For instance, fever can be treated with **aspirin** or **acetaminophen**. Supplemental oxygen and intravenous fluids may help. Patients are advised to get plenty of rest and take increased amounts of fluids. Coughing should be promoted because it helps to clear the lungs of fluid.

Alternative treatment

Being a serious, sometimes fatal disease, pneumococcal pneumonia is best treated as soon as possible with antibiotics. However, there are alternative treatments that both support this conventional treatment and prevent recurrences. Maintaining a healthy immune system is important. One way to do this is by taking the herb, **echinacea** (*Echinacea* spp.). Getting plenty of rest and reducing **stress** can help the body heal. Some practitioners feel that mucus-producing foods (including dairy products, eggs, gluten-rich grains such as wheat, oats, rye, as well as sugar) can contribute to the lung congestion that accompanies pneumonia. Decreasing these foods and increasing the amount of fresh fruits and vegetables may help to decrease lung congestion. Adequate protein in the diet is also essential for the body to produce antibodies. Contrast and constitutional **hydrotherapy** can be very helpful in treating cases of pneumonia. Other alternative therapies, including acupuncture, Chinese herbal medicine, and homeopathy, can be very useful during the recovery phase, helping the body to rebuild after the illness and contributing to the prevention of recurrences.

Prognosis

Simple, uncomplicated cases of pneumococcal pneumonia will begin to respond to antibiotics in 48 to72 hours. Full recovery from pneumonia, however, is greatly dependent on the age and overall health of the individual. Normally, healthy and younger patients can recover in only a few days, while the elderly or otherwise weakened individuals may not recover for several weeks. Complications may develop which give a poorer prognosis. Even when promptly and properly diagnosed, such weakened patients may die of their pneumonia.

KEY TERMS

Acetaminophen—A drug used for pain relief as well as to decrease fever. A common trade name for the drug is Tylenol.

Aspirin—A commonly used drug for pain relief and to decrease fever.

Bronchi—Two main branches of the trachea that go into the lungs. This then further divides into the bronchioles and alveoli.

Sputum—A substance that comes up from the throat when coughing or clearing the throat. It is important since it contains materials from the lungs.

Prevention

Vaccination

Recently, a **vaccination** has become available for the prevention of pneumococcal pneumonia. This vaccination is generally recommended for people with a high likelihood of developing pneumococcal infection or for those in whom a serious complication of infection is likely to develop. This would include persons over the age of 65, as well as those with:

- chronic pulmonary disease
- advanced cardiovascular disease
- diabetes mellitus
- alcoholism
- cirrhosis
- chronic kidney disease
- spleen dysfunction, or removal of spleen
- immunosuppression (cancer, organ transplant or AIDS)
- sickle cell anemia

Unfortunately, those people for whom the vaccination is most recommended are also those who are least likely to respond favorably to a vaccination. Therefore, the overall effectiveness of this vaccine remains questionable.

Antibiotics

The use of oral penicillin to prevent infection may be recommended for some patients at high risk, such as children with **sickle cell disease** and those with a spleen removed. This treatment, however, must be weighed with the increased likelihood of developing penicillin-resistant infections.

Resources

ORGANIZATIONS

American Lung Association. 1740 Broadway, New York, NY 10019. (800) 586-4872. < http://www.lungusa.org >.

Centers for Disease Control and Prevention. 1600 Clifton Rd., NE, Atlanta, GA 30333. (800) 311-3435, (404) 639-3311. < http://www.cdc.gov >.

Cindy L. A. Jones, PhD

Pneumocystis pneumonia

Definition

Pneumocystis **pneumonia** is a lung infection that occurs primarily in people with weakened immune systems–especially people who are HIV-positive. The disease agent is an organism whose biological classification is still uncertain. *Pneumocystis carinii* was originally thought to be a one-celled organism (a protozoan), but more recent research suggests that it is a fungus. Although its life cycle is known to have three stages, its method of reproduction is not yet completely understood. The complete name of the disease is *Pneumocystis carinii* pneumonia, often shortened to PCP. PCP is also sometimes called pneumocystosis.

Description

Pneumonia as a general term refers to a severe lung inflammation. In pneumocystis pneumonia, this inflammation is caused by the growth of *Pneumocystis carinii*, a fungus-like organism that is widespread in the environment. PCP is ordinarily a rare disease, affecting only people with weakened immune systems. Many of these people are patients receiving drugs for organ transplants or **cancer** treatment. With the rising incidence of **AIDS**, however, PCP has become primarily associated with AIDS patients. In fact, as many as 75% of AIDS patients have developed PCP. It has also been the leading cause of **death** in AIDS patients.

Transmission

The organism that causes PCP is widely distributed in nature and is transmitted through the air. When the organism is inhaled, it enters the upper respiratory tract and infects the tiny air sacs at the ends of the smaller air tubes (bronchioles) in the lungs. These tiny air sacs are called alveoli. Under a microscope, alveoli look like groups of hollow spheres resembling grape clusters. The exchange of oxygen with the blood takes place in the alveoli. It appears that *P. carinii* lives in the fluid in the lining of the alveoli.

Person-to-person infection does not appear to be very common; however, clusters of PCP outbreaks in hospitals and groups of immunocompromised people indicate that patients with active PCP should not be exposed to others with weakened immune systems. It is thought that many people actually acquire mild *Pneumocystis carinii* infections from time to time, but are protected by their immune systems from developing a full-blown case of the disease.

Causes and symptoms

Causes

P. carinii is an opportunistic organism. This means that it causes disease only under certain conditions, as when a person is immunocompromised. Under these circumstances, *P. carinii* can multiply and cause pneumonia. The mechanisms of the organism's growth within the alveoli are not fully understood. As the pneumocystis organism continues to replicate, it gradually fills the alveoli. As the pneumonia becomes more severe, fluid accumulates and tissue scarring occurs. These changes result in decreased respiratory function and lower levels of oxygen in the blood.

High-risk groups

Some patients are at greater risk of developing PCP. These high-risk groups include:

- premature infants
- patients with **immunodeficiency** diseases, including **severe combined immunodeficiency** disease (SCID) and acquired immunodeficiency syndrome (AIDS),
- patients receiving immunosuppressive drugs, especially cortisone-like drugs (**corticosteroids**)
- Patients with protein malnutrition.

AIDS is currently the most common risk factor for PCP in the United States. PCP is, however, also found in countries with widespread hunger and poor hygiene.

Symptoms

The incubation period of PCP is not definitely known, but is thought to be between four and eight weeks. The major symptoms include **shortness of breath**, **fever**, and a nonproductive **cough**. Less common symptoms include production of sputum, blood in the sputum, difficulty breathing, and chest **pain**. Most patients will have symptoms for one to two weeks before seeing a physician. Occasionally, the disease will spread outside of the lung to other organs, including the lymph nodes, spleen, liver, or bone marrow.

Diagnosis

The diagnosis of PCP begins with a thorough **physical examination** and blood tests. Although imaging studies are helpful in identifying abnormal areas in the lungs, the diagnosis of PCP must be confirmed by microscopic identification of the organism in the lung. Samples may be taken from the patient's sputum, or may be obtained via **bronchoscopy** or **lung biopsy**. Because of the severity of the disease, many physicians will proceed to treat patients with symptoms of pneumocystis pneumonia if they belong to a high-risk group, without the formality of an actual diagnosis. The severity of PCP can be measured by x-ray studies and by determining the amount of oxygen and carbon dioxide present in the patient's blood.

Treatment

Treatment for PCP involves the use of **antibiotics**. These include trimethoprim-sulfamethoxazole (TMP-SMX, Bactrim, Septra) and pentamidine isoethionate (Nebupent, Pentam 300). Both of these anti-microbial drugs are equally effective. AIDS patients are typically treated for 21 days, whereas non-AIDS patients are treated for 14 days. TMP-SMX may be highly toxic in AIDS patients, causing severe side effects that include fever, rash, decreased numbers of white blood cells and platelets, and hepatitis. Pentamidine also causes side effects in immunocompromised patients. These side effects include decreased blood pressure, irregular heart beats, the accumulation of nitrogenous waste products in the blood (azotemia), and electrolyte imbalances. Pentamidine can be given in aerosol form to minimize side effects. Alternative drugs can be used for patients experiencing these side effects.

P. carinii appears to be developing resistance to TMP-SMX. In addition, some patients are allergic to the standard antibiotics given for PCP. As a result, other antibiotics for the treatment of PCP are continually under investigation. Some drugs proven to be effective against *P. carinii* include

KEY TERMS

Alveoli—Small, hollow air sacs found in the lungs at the end of the smaller airways (bronchioles). Air exchange occurs in the alveoli.

Azotemia—The presence of excess nitrogenous wastes in the blood.

Biopsy—A procedure in which a piece of tissue is obtained for microscopic study.

Bronchoscopy—A procedure that uses a fiber-optic scope to view the airways in the lung.

Fungus—A member of a group of simple organisms related to yeasts and molds.

Pentamidine isoethionate—An antibiotic used to treat and prevent PCP.

Pneumocystosis—Another name for active PCP infection.

Protozoan—A microorganism belonging to the Protista, which includes the simplest one-celled organisms.

Sputum—A substance obtained from the lungs and bronchial tubes by clearing the throat or coughing. Sputum can be tested for evidence of PCP infection.

Trimethoprim-sulfamethoxazole (TMP-SMX)—An antibiotic used to treat and prevent PCP.

dapsone (DDS) with trimethoprim (Trimpex), clindamycin (Cleocin) with primaquine, as well as atovaquone (Mepron). Paradoxically, corticosteroids have been found to improve the ability of TMP-SMX or pentamidine to treat PCP. As a treatment of last resort, trimetrexate with leucovorin (Wellcovorin) can also be used.

Prognosis

If left untreated, PCP will cause breathing difficulties that will eventually cause death. The prognosis for this disease depends on the amount of damage to the patient's lungs prior to treatment. Prognosis is usually better at a facility that specializes in caring for AIDS patients. Antibiotic treatment of PCP is about 80% effective.

Prevention

Medications

For patients at serious risk for PCP infection, low doses of TMP-SMX, given daily or three times a week,

are effective in preventing PCP. The drug is, however, highly toxic. Researchers are currently evaluating the effectiveness and toxicity of aerosol pentamidine and dapsone in preventing PCP.

Lifestyle modifications

Patients who have previously had PCP often experience a recurrence. Healthy lifestyle choices, including exercising, eating well, and giving up **smoking** may keep the disease at bay.

Resources

ORGANIZATIONS

American Lung Association. 1740 Broadway, New York, NY 10019. (800) 586-4872. < http://www.lungusa.org >.

Centers for Disease Control and Prevention. 1600 Clifton Rd., NE, Atlanta, GA 30333. (800) 311-3435, (404) 639-3311. < http://www.cdc.gov >.

Cindy L. A. Jones, PhD

Pneumonectomy *see* **Lung surgery**

Pneumonia

Definition

Pneumonia is an infection of the lung that can be caused by nearly any class of organism known to cause human infections. These include bacteria, amoebae, viruses, fungi, and parasites. In the United States, pneumonia is the sixth most common disease leading to **death**; 2 million Americans develop pneumonia each year, and 40,000–70,000 die from it. Pneumonia is also the most common fatal infection acquired by already hospitalized patients. In developing countries, pneumonia ties with **diarrhea** as the most common cause of death. Even in nonfatal cases, pneumonia is a significant economic burden on the health care system. One study estimates that people in the American workforce who develop pneumonia cost employers five times as much in health care as the average worker.

According to the Centers for Disease Control and Prevention (CDC), however, the number of deaths from pneumonia in the United States has declined slightly since 2001.

Description

Anatomy of the lung

To better understand pneumonia, it is important to understand the basic anatomic features of the respiratory system. The human respiratory system begins at the nose and mouth, where air is breathed in (inspired) and out (expired). The air tube extending from the nose is called the nasopharynx. The tube carrying air breathed in through the mouth is called the oropharynx. The nasopharynx and the oropharynx merge into the larynx. The oropharynx also carries swallowed substances, including food, water, and salivary secretion, which must pass into the esophagus and then the stomach. The larynx is protected by a trap door called the epiglottis. The epiglottis prevents substances that have been swallowed, as well as substances that have been regurgitated (thrown up), from heading down into the larynx and toward the lungs.

A useful method of picturing the respiratory system is to imagine an upside-down tree. The larynx flows into the trachea, which is the tree trunk, and thus the broadest part of the respiratory tree. The trachea divides into two tree limbs, the right and left bronchi. Each one of these branches off into multiple smaller bronchi, which course through the tissue of the lung. Each bronchus divides into tubes of smaller and smaller diameter, finally ending in the terminal bronchioles. The air sacs of the lung, in which oxygen-carbon dioxide exchange actually takes place, are clustered at the ends of the bronchioles like the leaves of a tree. They are called alveoli.

The tissue of the lung which serves only a supportive role for the bronchi, bronchioles, and alveoli is called the lung stroma.

Function of the respiratory system

The main function of the respiratory system is to provide oxygen, the most important energy source for the body's cells. Inspired air (the air you breath in) contains the oxygen, and travels down the respiratory tree to the alveoli. The oxygen moves out of the alveoli and is sent into circulation throughout the body as part of the red blood cells. The oxygen in the inspired air is exchanged within the alveoli for the waste product of human metabolism, carbon dioxide. The air you breathe out contains the gas called carbon dioxide. This gas leaves the alveoli during expiration. To restate this exchange of gases simply, you breathe in oxygen, you breathe out carbon dioxide

Respiratory system defenses

The healthy human lung is sterile. There are no normally resident bacteria or viruses (unlike the upper respiratory system and parts of the gastrointestinal system, where bacteria dwell even in a healthy state). There are multiple safeguards along the path of the respiratory system. These are designed to keep invading organisms from leading to infection.

The first line of defense includes the hair in the nostrils, which serves as a filter for large particles. The epiglottis is a trap door of sorts, designed to prevent food and other swallowed substances from entering the larynx and then trachea. Sneezing and coughing, both provoked by the presence of irritants within the respiratory system, help to clear such irritants from the respiratory tract.

Mucus, produced through the respiratory system, also serves to trap dust and infectious organisms. Tiny hair like projections (cilia) from cells lining the respiratory tract beat constantly. They move debris trapped by mucus upwards and out of the respiratory tract. This mechanism of protection is referred to as the mucociliary escalator.

Cells lining the respiratory tract produce several types of immune substances which protect against various organisms. Other cells (called macrophages) along the respiratory tract actually ingest and kill invading organisms.

The organisms that cause pneumonia, then, are usually carefully kept from entering the lungs by virtue of these host defenses. However, when an individual encounters a large number of organisms at once, the usual defenses may be overwhelmed, and infection may occur. This can happen either by inhaling contaminated air droplets, or by aspiration of organisms inhabiting the upper airways.

Conditions predisposing to pneumonia

In addition to exposure to sufficient quantities of causative organisms, certain conditions may make an individual more likely to become ill with pneumonia. Certainly, the lack of normal anatomical structure could result in an increased risk of pneumonia. For example, there are certain inherited defects of cilia which result in less effective protection. Cigarette smoke, inhaled directly by a smoker or second-hand by a innocent bystander, interferes significantly with ciliary function, as well as inhibiting macrophage function.

Stroke, seizures, alcohol, and various drugs interfere with the function of the epiglottis. This leads to a

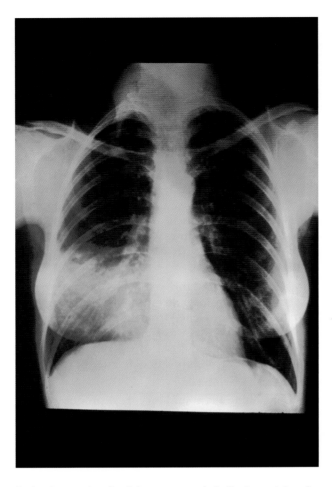

A chest x ray showing lobar pneumonia in the lower lobe of a patient's right lung. The alveoli (air sacs) of the lung become blocked with pus, which forces air out and causes the lung to become solidified. *(Photo Researchers, Inc. Reproduced by permission.)*

leaky seal on the trap door, with possible contamination by swallowed substances and/or regurgitated stomach contents. Alcohol and drugs also interfere with the normal **cough** reflex. This further decreases the chance of clearing unwanted debris from the respiratory tract.

Viruses may interfere with ciliary function, allowing themselves or other microorganism invaders (such as bacteria) access to the lower respiratory tract. One of the most important viruses is HIV (Human **Immunodeficiency** virus), the causative virus in **AIDS** (acquired immunodeficiency syndrome). In recent years this virus has resulted in a huge increase in the incidence of pneumonia. Because AIDS results in a general decreased effectiveness of many aspects of the host's immune system, a patient with AIDS is susceptible to all kinds of pneumonia. This includes some

previously rare parasitic types which would be unable to cause illness in an individual possessing a normal immune system.

The elderly have a less effective mucociliary escalator, as well as changes in their immune system. This causes this age group to be more at risk for the development of pneumonia.

Various chronic conditions predispose a person to infection with pneumonia. These include **asthma, cystic fibrosis**, and neuromuscular diseases which may interfere with the seal of the epiglottis. **Esophageal disorders** may result in stomach contents passing upwards into the esophagus. This increases the risk of aspiration into the lungs of those stomach contents with their resident bacteria. Diabetes, sickle cell anemia, lymphoma, leukemia, and **emphysema** also predispose a person to pneumonia.

Genetic factors also appear to be involved in susceptibility to pneumonia. Certain changes in DNA appear to affect some patients' risk of developing such complications of pneumonia as **septic shock**.

Pneumonia is also one of the most frequent infectious complications of all types of surgery. Many drugs used during and after surgery may increase the risk of aspiration, impair the cough reflex, and cause a patient to underfill their lungs with air. **Pain** after surgery also discourages a patient from breathing deeply enough, and from coughing effectively.

Radiation treatment for **breast cancer** increases the risk of pneumonia in some patients by weakening lung tissue.

Causes and symptoms

The list of organisms which can cause pneumonia is very large, and includes nearly every class of infecting organism: viruses, bacteria, bacteria-like organisms, fungi, and parasites (including certain worms). Different organisms are more frequently encountered by different age groups. Further, other characteristics of an individual may place him or her at greater risk for infection by particular types of organisms:

- Viruses cause the majority of pneumonias in young children (especially respiratory syncytial virus, parainfluenza and **influenza** viruses, and adenovirus).

- Adults are more frequently infected with bacteria (such as *Streptococcus pneumoniae, Haemophilus influenzae,* and *Staphylococcus aureus*).

- Pneumonia in older children and young adults is often caused by the bacteria-like *Mycoplasma pneumoniae* (the cause of what is often referred to as "walking" pneumonia).

- *Pneumocystis carinii* is an extremely important cause of pneumonia in patients with immune problems (such as patients being treated for **cancer** with **chemotherapy**, or patients with AIDS. Classically considered a parasite, it appears to be more related to fungi.

- People who have reason to come into contact with bird droppings, such as poultry workers, are at risk for pneumonia caused by the organism *Chlamydia psittaci.*

- A very large, serious outbreak of pneumonia occurred in 1976, when many people attending an American Legion convention were infected by a previously unknown organism. Subsequently named *Legionella pneumophila,* it causes what is now called "Legionnaire's disease." The organism was traced to air conditioning units in the convention's hotel.

Pneumonia is suspected in any patient who has **fever**, cough, chest pain, **shortness of breath**, and increased respirations (number of breaths per minute). Fever with a shaking chill is even more suspicious. Many patients cough up clumps of sputum, commonly known as spit. These secretions are produced in the alveoli during an infection or other inflammatory condition. They may appear streaked with pus or blood. Severe pneumonia results in the signs of oxygen deprivation. This includes blue appearance of the nail beds or lips (**cyanosis**).

The invading organism causes symptoms, in part, by provoking an overly-strong immune response in the lungs. In other words, the immune system, which should help fight off infections, kicks into such high gear, that it damages the lung tissue and makes it more susceptible to infection. The small blood vessels in the lungs (capillaries) become leaky, and protein-rich fluid seeps into the alveoli. This results in less functional area for oxygen-carbon dioxide exchange. The patient becomes relatively oxygen deprived, while retaining potentially damaging carbon dioxide. The patient breathes faster and faster, in an effort to bring in more oxygen and blow off more carbon dioxide.

Mucus production is increased, and the leaky capillaries may tinge the mucus with blood. Mucus plugs actually further decrease the efficiency of gas exchange in the lung. The alveoli fill further with fluid and debris from the large number of white blood cells being produced to fight the infection.

Consolidation, a feature of bacterial pneumonias, occurs when the alveoli, which are normally hollow air spaces within the lung, instead become solid, due to quantities of fluid and debris.

Viral pneumonias and mycoplasma pneumonias do not result in consolidation. These types of pneumonia primarily infect the walls of the alveoli and the stroma of the lung.

Severe acute respiratory syndrome (SARS)

Severe acute respiratory syndrome, or **SARS**, is a contagious and potentially fatal disease that first appeared in the form of a multi-country outbreak in early February 2003. Later that month, the CDC began to work with the World Health Organization (WHO) to investigate the cause(s) of SARS and to develop guidelines for **infection control**. SARS has been described as an "atypical pneumonia of unknown etiology;" by the end of March 2003, the disease agent was identified as a previously unknown coronavirus.

The early symptoms of SARS include a high fever with chills, **headache**, **muscle cramps**, and weakness. This early phase is followed by respiratory symptoms, usually a dry cough and painful or difficult breathing. Some patients require mechanical ventilation. The mortality rate of SARS is thought to be about 3%.

As of the end of March 2003, the CDC did not have clearly defined recommendations for treating SARS. Treatments that have been used include **antibiotics** known to be effective against bacterial pneumonia; ribavirin and other **antiviral drugs**; and steroids.

Diagnosis

For the most part, diagnosis is based on the patient's report of symptoms, combined with examination of the chest. Listening with a stethoscope will reveal abnormal sounds, and tapping on the patient's back (which should yield a resonant sound due to air filling the alveoli) may instead yield a dull thump if the alveoli are filled with fluid and debris.

Laboratory diagnosis can be made of some bacterial pneumonias by staining sputum with special chemicals and looking at it under a microscope. Identification of the specific type of bacteria may require culturing the sputum (using the sputum sample to grow greater numbers of the bacteria in a lab dish.).

X-ray examination of the chest may reveal certain abnormal changes associated with pneumonia. Localized shadows obscuring areas of the lung may indicate a bacterial pneumonia, while streaky or patchy appearing changes in the x-ray picture may indicate viral or mycoplasma pneumonia. These changes on x ray, however, are known to lag in time behind the patient's actual symptoms.

Treatment

Prior to the discovery of penicillin antibiotics, bacterial pneumonia was almost always fatal. Today, antibiotics, especially given early in the course of the disease, are very effective against bacterial causes of pneumonia. Erythromycin and tetracycline improve recovery time for symptoms of mycoplasma pneumonia. They, do not, however, eradicate the organisms. Amantadine and acyclovir may be helpful against certain viral pneumonias.

A newer antibiotic named linezolid (Zyvox) is being used to treat penicillin-resistant organisms that cause pneumonia. Linezolid is the first of a new line of antibiotics known as oxazolidinones. Another new drug known as ertapenem (Invanz) is reported to be effective in treating bacterial pneumonia.

Prognosis

Prognosis varies according to the type of organism causing the infection. Recovery following pneumonia with *Mycoplasma pneumoniae* is nearly 100%. *Staphylococcus pneumoniae* has a death rate of 30–40%. Similarly, infections with a number of gram negative bacteria (such as those in the gastrointestinal tract which can cause infection following aspiration) have a death rate of 25–50%. *Streptococcus pneumoniae*, the most common organism causing pneumonia, produces a death rate of about 5%. More complications occur in the very young or very old individuals who have multiple areas of the lung infected simultaneously. Individuals with other chronic illnesses (including **cirrhosis** of the liver, congestive **heart failure**, individuals without a functioning spleen, and individuals who have other diseases that result in a weakened immune system, experience complications. Patients with immune disorders, various types of cancer, transplant patients, and AIDS patients also experience complications.

Prevention

Because many bacterial pneumonias occur in patients who are first infected with the influenza virus (the flu), yearly **vaccination** against influenza can decrease the risk of pneumonia for certain patients. This is particularly true of the elderly and people with chronic diseases (such as asthma, cystic

KEY TERMS

Alveoli—The little air sacs clustered at the ends of the bronchioles, in which oxygen-carbon dioxide exchange takes place.

Aspiration—A situation in which solids or liquids which should be swallowed into the stomach are instead breathed into the respiratory system.

Cilia—Hair-like projections from certain types of cells.

Consolidation—A condition in which lung tissue becomes firm and solid rather than elastic and air-filled because it has accumulated fluids and tissue debris.

Coronavirus—One of a family of RNA-containing viruses known to cause severe respiratory illnesses. In March 2003, a previously unknown coronavirus was identified as the causative agent of severe acute respiratory syndrome, or SARS.

Cyanosis—A bluish tinge to the skin that can occur when the blood oxygen level drops too low.

Sputum—Material produced within the alveoli in response to an infectious or inflammatory process.

Stroma—A term used to describe the supportive tissue surrounding a particular structure. An example is that tissue which surrounds and supports the actually functional lung tissue.

fibrosis, other lung or heart diseases, **sickle cell disease**, diabetes, **kidney disease**, and forms of cancer).

A specific vaccine against *Streptococcus pneumoniae* is very protective, and should also be administered to patients with chronic illnesses.

Patients who have decreased immune resistance are at higher risk for infection with *Pneumocystis carinii*. They are frequently put on a regular drug regimen of trimethoprim sulfa and/or inhaled pentamidine to avoid **pneumocystis pneumonia**.

Resources

BOOKS

Beers, Mark H., MD, and Robert Berkow, MD., editors. "Pneumonia." In *The Merck Manual of Diagnosis and Therapy*. Whitehouse Station, NJ: Merck Research Laboratories, 2004.

PERIODICALS

Arias, E., and B. L. Smith. "Deaths: Preliminary Data for 2001." *National Vital Statistics Reports* 51 (March 14, 2003): 1–44.

Birnbaum, Howard G., Melissa Morley, Paul E. Greenberg, et al. "Economic Burden of Pneumonia in an Employed Population." *Archives of Internal Medicine* 161 (December 10, 2001): 2725-2732.

Curran, M., D. Simpson, and C. Perry. "Ertapenem: A Review of Its Use in the Management of Bacterial Infections." *Drugs* 63 (2003): 1855–1878.

Lyseng-Williamson, K. A., and K. L. Goa. "Linezolid: In Infants and Children with Severe Gram-Positive Infections." *Paediatric Drugs* 5 (2003): 419–429.

"New Research Shows That Pneumonia, Septic Shock Run in Families." *Genomics & Genetics Weekly* November 16, 2001: 13.

"Outbreak of Severe Acute Respiratory Syndrome—Worldwide, 2003." *Morbidity and Mortality Weekly Report* 52 (March 21, 2003): 226–228.

"Update: Outbreak of Severe Acute Respiratory Syndrome—Worldwide, 2003." *Morbidity and Mortality Weekly Report* 52 (March 28, 2003): 241–246, 248.

Worcester, Sharon. "Ventilator-Linked Pneumonia." *Internal Medicine News* 34 (October 15, 2001): 32.

Wunderink, R. G., S. K. Cammarata, T. H. Oliphant, et al. "Continuation of a Randomized, Double-Blind, Multicenter Study of Linezolid Versus Vancomycin in the Treatment of Patients with Nosocomial Pneumonia." *Clinical Therapeutics* 25 (March 2003): 980–992.

ORGANIZATIONS

American Lung Association. 1740 Broadway, New York, NY 10019. (800) 586-4872. < http://www.lungusa.org >.

Centers for Disease Control and Prevention. 1600 Clifton Rd., NE, Atlanta, GA 30333. (800) 311-3435, (404) 639-3311. < http://www.cdc.gov >.

Rosalyn Carson-DeWitt, MD
Rebecca J. Frey, PhD

Pneumonitis *see* **Pneumonia**

Pneumothorax

Definition

Pneumothorax is a collection of air or gas in the chest or pleural space that causes part or all of a lung to collapse.

Description

Normally, the pressure in the lungs is greater than the pressure in the pleural space surrounding the lungs. However, if air enters the pleural space, the pressure in the pleura then becomes greater than the pressure in the lungs, causing the lung to collapse partially or completely. Pneumothorax can be either spontaneous or due to trauma.

If a pneumothorax occurs suddenly or for no known reason, it is called a spontaneous pneumothorax. This condition most often strikes tall, thin men between the ages of 20 to 40. In addition, people with lung disorders, such as emphysema, cystic fibrosis, and **tuberculosis**, are at higher risk for spontaneous pneumothorax. Traumatic pneumothorax is the result of accident or injury due to medical procedures performed to the chest cavity, such as **thoracentesis** or mechanical ventilation. Tension pneumothorax is a serious and potentially life-threatening condition that may be caused by traumatic injury, chronic lung disease, or as a complication of a medical procedure. In this type of pneumothorax, air enters the chest cavity, but cannot escape. This greatly increased pressure in the pleural space causes the lung to collapse completely, compresses the heart, and pushes the heart and associated blood vessels toward the unaffected side.

Causes and symptoms

The symptoms of pneumothrax depend on how much air enters the chest, how much the lung collapses, and the extent of lung disease. Symptoms include the following, according to the cause of the pneumothorax:

- Spontaneous pneumothorax. Simple spontaneous pneumothorax is caused by a rupture of a small air sac or fluid-filled sac in the lung. It may be related to activity in otherwise healthy people or may occur during scuba diving or flying at high altitudes. Complicated spontaneous pneumothorax, also generally caused by rupture of a small sac in the lung, occurs in people with lung diseases. The symptoms of complicated spontaneous pneumothorax tend to be worse than those of simple pneumothorax, due to the underlying lung disease. Spontaneous pneumothorax is characterized by dull, sharp, or stabbing chest **pain** that begins suddenly and becomes worse with deep breathing or coughing. Other symptoms are **shortness of breath**, rapid breathing, abnormal breathing movement (that is, little chest wall movement when breathing), and cough.

- Tension pneumothorax. Following trauma, air may enter the chest cavity. A penetrating chest wound allows outside air to enter the chest, causing the lung to collapse. Certain medical procedures performed in the chest cavity, such as thoracentesis,

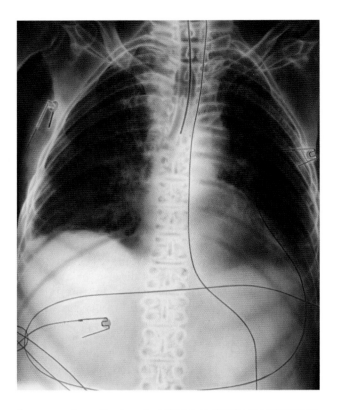

An x ray of a patient undergoing pneumothorax treatment. ECG electrodes attached to chest monitor heartbeat while endotracheal tube is inserted in windpipe. *(Photo Researchers. Reproduced by permission.)*

also may cause a lung to collapse. Tension pneumothorax may be the immediate result of an injury; the delayed complication of a hidden injury, such as a fractured rib, that punctures the lung; or the result of lung damage from asthma, chronic **bronchitis**, or emphysema. Symptoms of tension pneumothorax tend to be severe with sudden onset. There is marked **anxiety**, distended neck veins, weak pulse, decreased breath sounds on the affected side, and a shift of the mediastinum to the opposite side.

Diagnosis

To diagnose pneumothorax, it is necessary for the health care provider to listen to the chest (auscultation) during a **physical examination**. By using a stethoscope, the physician may note that one part of the chest does not transmit the normal sounds of breathing. A **chest x ray** will show the air pocket and the collapsed lung. An electrocardiogram (ECG) will be performed to record the electrical impulses that control the heart's activity. Blood samples may be taken to check for the level of arterial blood gases.

Treatment

A small pneumothorax may resolve on its own, but most require medical treatment. The object of treatment is to remove air from the chest and allow the lung to re-expand. This is done by inserting a needle and syringe (if the pneumothorax is small) or chest tube through the chest wall. This allows the air to escape without allowing any air back in. The lung will then re-expand itself within a few days. Surgery may be needed for repeat occurrences.

Prognosis

Most people recover fully from spontaneous pneumothorax. Up to half of patients with spontaneous pneumothorax experience recurrence. Recovery from a collapsed lung generally takes one to two weeks. Tension pneumothorax can cause **death** rapidly due to inadequate heart output or insufficient blood oxygen (hypoxemia), and must be treated as a medical emergency.

Prevention

Preventive measures for a non-injury related pneumothorax include stopping **smoking** and seeking medical attention for respiratory problems. If the pneumothorax occurs in both lungs or more than once in the same lung, surgery may be needed to prevent it from occurring again.

Resources

ORGANIZATIONS

American Association for Respiratory Care. 11030 Ables Lane, Dallas, Texas 75229. (972) 243-2272. < http://www.aarc.org >.

American Lung Association. 1740 Broadway, New York, NY 10019. (800) 586-4872. < http://www.lungusa.org >.

OTHER

"Spontaneous Pneumothorax." *HealthAnswers.com.*
< http://www.healthanswers.com >.

Lorraine Steefel, RN

Podiatry *see* **Foot care**

Poison ivy and poison oak

Definition

Poison ivy and poison oak are plants that cause an allergic skin reaction in most people who are exposed to them.

Description

Poison ivy, which is generally thought of as a climbing vine, can also grow as a shrub or bush. It has leaves that are elliptical in shape and grow in groups of three on a stem. Poison ivy is common in the United States, except in the southwest, Alaska, and Hawaii. Poison oak, which grows as a shrub, has leaves that are shaped like oak leaves and also grow in groups of three to a stem. Poison oak is common in the United States, especially on the west coast from Mexico to Canada.

Not everyone is sensitive to poison ivy and poison oak; however, nine out of ten people who come in contact with either of the plants will have an allergic reaction to some degree. All parts of the plants are poisonous and the amount of time it takes for an allergic reaction to develop varies from person to person. The extent and severity of the reaction depends on the length of exposure, type of contact, and how sensitive the person is to the plants. If a person is going to have an allergic reaction, it will usually occur within one or two days of exposure. However, some people have a reaction within an hour, whereas others don't experience a reaction until five days after the exposure.

Causes and symptoms

The substance that causes the allergic reaction is the same for both plants. It is an oily resin called urushiol. It only takes a small amount of the resin to cause a reaction. The resin can be transferred to the skin by directly touching the plant or indirectly by coming in contact with something that has touched the plant, such as tools, animals, or clothing. Although animals are rarely affected, they can carry the resin on their fur and transfer it to humans. According to the experts at the University of Maryland Medical Center, the "chemical [resin] can remain active for more than a year."

The symptoms for poison ivy and poison oak are the same. Usually the first symptoms to appear are itchiness and swelling in the areas of contact. The itchy rash that follows is made up of small pimple-like bumps (sometimes referred to as papules), as well as blisters that later break open, ooze, and crust over.

Diagnosis

A diagnosis is made based on the symptoms and a **physical examination** of the patient.

In some cases, people have jobs that make it difficult for them to avoid poison ivy and poison oak, such as people who work in wooded areas or on construction sites, for example. Employees without health insurance may be covered by workers compensation.

Treatment

Anyone who comes in contact with either plant should wash the exposed area with soap and water immediately. Taking a bath immediately after contact is not recommended, because that could spread the resin to other areas of the body. All clothing, including shoes and shoelaces, should be removed carefully and either washed separately or discarded.

For minor cases, hydrocortisone cream and Calamine lotion can provide relief until the symptoms disappear. Over-the-counter Benadryl capsules help with the **itching**. Some people find oatmeal or baking soda baths to be soothing as well. Oral steroids, such as prednisone, are available for more serious cases, especially those affecting the face, eyes, mouth, or genitals. If signs of infection develop, such as pus and a **fever**, patients should contact their doctors.

Patients should consult their physicians before they use any ointments that contain benzocaine or zirconium, because they can cause an allergic reaction that worsens the condition. Antihistamine ointments are not recommended for the same reason. The experts at the Alabama Cooperative Extension System caution that "some people have severe allergic reactions to these plants and can have swelling in the throat, breathing problems, weakness, **dizziness**, and bluish lips." Emergency medical care should be sought if any serious reactions occur.

Prognosis

In most cases, the condition goes away in two weeks.

Prevention

The best prevention is know what the plants look like and to avoid them. A common saying should be kept in mind: Leaves of three, let them be.

People who plan to be in an area where poison ivy and poison oak might be found should wear protective clothing, such as long-sleeved shirts and long pants.

Eradication of the plants should be handled with care. As stated by the experts at the Alabama Cooperative Extension System, "burning can be dangerous and is not recommended for disposal or as a control measure, because the toxic oil from the plant can be carried in the smoke." Instead they recommend spraying the plants with glyphosate, which is commonly known as the brands Roundup or Kleenup.

Resources

OTHER

Common Pesky Plants: Poison Ivy & Poison Oak Alabama Cooperative Extension. [cited march 19, 2005]. <http://www.aces.edu/Tallapoosa/weed-control/poison-ivy.htm>.
Poison Ivy University of Maryland Medical Center. [cited march 19, 2005]. <http://www.umm.edu/>.

Lee Ann Paradise

Poisoning

Definition

Poisoning occurs when any substance interferes with normal body functions after it is swallowed, inhaled, injected, or absorbed. The branch of medicine that deals with the detection and treatment of poisons is known as toxicology.

Description

Poisonings are a common occurrence. About 10 million cases of poisoning occur in the United States each year. In 80% of the cases, the victim is a child under the age of five. About 50 children die each year from poisonings. Curiosity, inability to read warning labels, a desire to imitate adults, and inadequate supervision lead to childhood poisonings.

The elderly are the second most likely group to be poisoned. Mental confusion, poor eyesight, and the use of multiple drugs are the leading reasons why this group has a high rate of accidental poisoning. A substantial number of poisonings also occur as **suicide** attempts or drug overdoses.

Poisons are common in the home and workplace, yet there are basically two major types. One group consists of products that were never meant to be ingested or inhaled, such as shampoo, paint thinner, pesticides, houseplant leaves, and carbon monoxide. The other group contains products that can be ingested in small quantities, but which are harmful if taken in large amounts, such as pharmaceuticals, medicinal herbs, or alcohol. Other types of poisons include the bacterial toxins that cause **food poisoning**, such as *Escherichia coli*; heavy metals, such as the lead found in the paint on older houses; and the venom found in the bites and stings of some animals and insects. The staff at a poison control center and emergency room doctors have the most experience diagnosing and treating poisoning cases.

Causes and symptoms

The effects of poisons are as varied as the poisons themselves; however, the exact mechanisms of only a few are understood. Some poisons interfere with the metabolism. Others destroy the liver or kidneys, such as heavy metals and some pain relief medications, including **acetaminophen** (Tylenol) and nonsteroidal anti-inflammatory drugs (Advil, Ibuprofen). A poison may severely depress the central nervous system, leading to coma and eventual respiratory and circulatory failure. Potential poisons in this category include anesthetics (e.g. ether and chloroform), opiates (e.g., morphine and codeine), and **barbiturates**. Some poisons directly affect the respiratory and circulatory system. Carbon monoxide causes **death** by binding with hemoglobin that would normally transport oxygen throughout the body. Certain corrosive vapors trigger the body to flood the lungs with fluids, effectively drowning the person. Cyanide interferes with respiration at the cellular level. Another group of poisons interferes with the electrochemical impulses that travel between neurons in the nervous system. Yet another group, including cocaine, ergot, strychnine, and some snake venoms, causes potentially fatal seizures.

Severity of symptoms can range from **headache** and nausea to convulsions and death. The type of poison, the amount and time of exposure, and the

Common Household, Industrial, And Agricultural Products Containing Toxic Sustances

Alcohol (rubbing)	FuelAntifreeze	Floor/furniture polish
Arsenic	Gasoline	Art and craft supplies
Glues/adhesives	Automotive fluids	Hemlock
Batteries, automotive	Kerosene	Batteries, household
Mercury	Building products	Metal primers
Cleaning products	Metalworking materials	Cosmetics/personal care items
Mothballs	Cyanide	Oven cleaners
Daffodil bulbs	Paint strppers/thinners	Dieffenbachia
Paints, oil-based or alkyds	Disinfectants/air fresheners	Paints, water-based or latex
Drain openers	Pesticides	Flea collars/insect repellent
English nightshade	Stains/finishes	Ethanol
Strychnine	Foxglove	Wood preservatives

age, size, and health of the victim are all factors which determine the severity of symptoms and the chances for recovery.

Plant poisoning

There are more than 700 species of poisonous plants in the United States. Plants are second only to medicines in causing serious poisoning in children under age five. There is no way to tell by looking at a plant if it is poisonous. Some plants, such as the yew shrub, are almost entirely toxic: needles, bark, seeds, and berries. In other plants, only certain parts are poisonous. The bulb of the hyacinth and daffodil are toxic, but the flowers are not; while the flowers of the jasmine plant are the poisonous part. Moreover, some plants are confusing because portions of them are eaten as food while other parts are poisonous. For example, the fleshy stem (tuber) of the potato plant is nutritious; however, its roots, sprouts, and vines are poisonous. The leaves of tomatoes are poisonous, while the fruit is not. Rhubarb stalks are good to eat, but the leaves are poisonous. Apricots, cherries, peaches, and apples all produce healthful fruit, but their seeds contain a form of cyanide that can kill a child if chewed in sufficient quantities. One hundred milligrams (mg) of moist, crushed apricot seeds can produce 217 mg of cyanide.

Common houseplants that contain some poisonous parts include:

- Aloe
- Amaryllis
- Cyclamen
- Dumb cane (also called Dieffenbachia)
- Philodendron

Common outdoor plants that contain some poisonous part include:

- Bird of paradise flower
- Buttercup
- Castor bean
- Chinaberry tree
- Daffodil
- English ivy
- Eucalyptus
- Foxglove
- Holly
- Horse chestnut
- Iris
- Jack-in-the-pulpit
- Jimsonweed (also called thornapple)
- Larkspur
- Lily-of-the-valley
- Morning glory
- Nightshade (several varieties)
- Oleander
- Potato
- Rhododendron
- Rhubarb
- Sweet pea
- Tomato
- Wisteria
- Yew

Symptoms of plant poisoning range from irritation of the skin or mucous membranes of the mouth and throat to **nausea**, **vomiting**, convulsions, irregular heartbeat, and even death. It is often difficult to tell if a person has eaten a poisonous plant because there are no tell-tale empty containers and no unusual lesions or odors around the mouth.

Many cases of plant poisoning involve plants that contain hallucinogens, such as peyote cactus buttons, certain types of mushrooms, and **marijuana**. A recent case of plant poisoning in France concerned *Datura*, or moonflower, a plant that has become popular with young people trying to imitate Native American **puberty** rites.

Other cases of plant poisoning result from the use of herbal dietary supplements that have been contaminated by toxic substances. The Food and Drug Administration (FDA) has the authority to monitor herbal products on the market and issue warnings about accidental poisoning or other adverse affects associated with these products. For example, in 2002 a manufacturer of nettle capsules found to contain lead recalled the product following a warning from the FDA. Other dietary supplements have been found to contain small quantities of prescription medications or even toxic plants.

Household chemicals

Many products used daily in the home are poisonous if swallowed. These products often contain strong acids or strong bases (alkalis). Toxic household cleaning products include:

- ammonia
- bleach
- dishwashing liquids
- drain openers
- floor waxes and furniture polishes
- laundry detergents, spot cleaners, and fabric softeners
- mildew removers
- oven cleaners
- toilet bowl cleaners

Personal care products found in the home can also be poisonous. These include:

- deodorant
- hairspray
- hair straighteners
- nail polish and polish remover
- perfume
- shampoo

Signs that a person has swallowed one of these substances include evidence of an empty container nearby, nausea or vomiting, and **burns** on the lips and skin around the mouth if the substance was a strong acid or alkali. The chemicals in some of these products may leave a distinctive odor on the breath.

Pharmaceuticals

Both over-the-counter and prescription medicines can help the body heal if taken as directed. However, when taken in large quantities, or with other drugs where there may be an adverse interaction, they can act as poisons. Drug overdoses, both accidental and intentional, are the leading cause of poisoning in adults. Medicinal herbs should be treated like pharmaceuticals and taken only in designated quantities under the supervision of a knowledgeable person. Herbs that have healing qualities when taken in small doses can be toxic in larger doses, or may interact with prescription medications in unpredictable ways.

Drug overdoses cause a range of symptoms, including excitability, sleepiness, confusion, unconsciousness, rapid heartbeat, convulsions, nausea, and changes in blood pressure. The best initial evidence of a **drug overdose** is the presence of an empty container near the victim.

Other causes of poisonings

People can be poisoned by fumes they inhale. Carbon monoxide is the most common form of inhaled poison. Other toxic substances that can be inhaled include:

- farm and garden insecticides and herbicides
- gasoline fumes
- insect repellent
- paint thinner fumes

Diagnosis

Initially, poisoning is suspected if the victim shows changes in behavior and signs or symptoms previously described. **Hallucinations** or other psychiatric symptoms may indicate poisoning by a hallucinogenic plant. Evidence of an empty container or information from the victim are helpful in determining exactly what substance has caused the poisoning. Some acids and alkalis leave burns on the mouth. Petroleum products, such as lighter fluid or kerosene, leave a distinctive odor on the breath. The vomit may be tested to determine the exact composition of the poison. Once hospitalized, the patient may be given blood and urine tests to determine his or her metabolic condition.

Treatment

Treatment for poisoning depends on the poison swallowed or inhaled. Contacting the poison control center or hospital emergency room is the first step in getting proper treatment. The poison control center's telephone number is often listed with emergency numbers on the inside cover of the telephone book, or it can be reached by dialing the operator. The poison control center will ask for specific information about the victim and the poison, then give appropriate first aid instructions. If the patient is to be taken to a hospital, a sample of vomit and the poison container should be taken along, if they are available.

Most cases of plant poisoning are treated by inducing vomiting, if the patient is fully conscious. Vomiting can be induced by taking syrup of **ipecac**, an over-the-counter emetic available at any pharmacy.

For acid, alkali, or petroleum product poisonings, the patient should not vomit. Acids and alkalis can burn the esophagus if they are vomited, and petroleum products can be inhaled into the lungs during vomiting, resulting in **pneumonia**.

Once under medical care, doctors have the option of treating the patient with a specific remedy to counteract the poison (antidote) or with **activated charcoal** to absorb the substance inside the patient's digestive system. In some instances, pumping the stomach may be required. This technique, which is known as gastric lavage, involves introducing 20–30 mL of tap water or 9% saline solution into the patient's digestive tract and removing the stomach contents with a siphon or syringe. The process is repeated until the washings are free of poison. Medical personnel will also provide supportive care as needed, such as intravenous fluids or mechanical ventilation.

If the doctor suspects that the poisoning was not accidental, he or she is required to notify law enforcement authorities. Most cases of malicious poisoning concern family members or acquaintances of the victim, but the number of intentional random poisonings of the general public has increased in recent years. A case reported in 2003 involved the use of nicotine to poison 1700 pounds of ground beef in a Michigan supermarket. Over a hundred persons fell ill after eating the poisoned beef.

Prognosis

The outcome of poisoning varies from complete recovery to death, and depends on the type and amount of the poison, the health of the victim, and the speed with which medical care is obtained.

KEY TERMS

Antidote—A medication or remedy for counteracting the effects of a poison.

Emetic—A medication or substance given to induce vomiting.

Gastric lavage—A technique for washing poison out of the stomach by instilling water or saline solution through a tube, removing the stomach contents by suction, and repeating the process until the washings are free of poison. It is also called stomach pumping.

Toxicology—The branch of medicine that deals with the effects, detection, and treatment of poisons.

Prevention

Most accidental poisonings are preventable. The number of deaths of children from poisoning has declined from about 450 per year in the 1960s to about 50 each year in the 1990s. This decline has occurred mainly because of better packaging of toxic materials and better public education.

Actions to prevent poisonings include:

- removing plants that are poisonous
- keeping medicines and household chemicals locked and in a place inaccessible to children
- keeping medications in child-resistant containers
- never referring to medicine as "candy"
- keeping cleaners and other poisons in their original containers
- disposing of outdated prescription medicines
- not purchasing over-the-counter medications with damaged protective seals or packaging
- avoiding the use of herbal preparations not made by a reputable manufacturer

Resources

BOOKS

Beers, Mark H., MD, and Robert Berkow, MD., editors. "Poisoning." In *The Merck Manual of Diagnosis and Therapy*. Whitehouse Station, NJ: Merck Research Laboratories, 2004.

PERIODICALS

Arouko, H., M. D. Matray, C. Braganca, et al. "Voluntary Poisoning by Ingestion of *Datura stramonium*. Another Cause of Hospitalization in Youth Seeking Strong

---

Sensations." [in French] *Annales de médecine interne* 154, Spec no. 1 (June 2003): S46–S50.

Centers for Disease Control and Prevention. "Nicotine Poisoning After Ingestion of Contaminated Ground Beef—Michigan, 2003. " *Morbidity and Mortality Weekly Report* 52 (May 9, 2003): 413–416.

Hirshon, Jon Mark, MD, MPH. "Plant Poisoning, Herbs." *eMedicine* January 18, 2002. < http://www.emedicine.com/EMERG/topic449.htm >.

Salomone, Joseph A., III, MD. "Toxicity, Hallucinogen." *eMedicine* November 27, 2001. < http:///www.emedicine.com/emerg/topic223.htm >.

ORGANIZATIONS

American Association of Poison Control Centers (AAPCC). 3201 New Mexico Avenue, Suite 330, Washington, DC 20016. (202) 362-7217. POISONING EMERGENCIES: (800) 222-1222. < http://www.aapcc.org >.

National Toxicology Program (NTP) of the National Institute of Environmental Health Sciences (NIEHS). P. O. Box 12233, Research Triangle Park, NC 27709. (919) 541-3419. < http://www.ntp-server.niehs.nih.gov >.

U. S. Food and Drug Administration (FDA). 5600 Fishers Lane, Rockville, MD 20857. (888) 463-6332. < http://www.fda.gov >.

OTHER

Arizona Poison and Drug Information Center Page. < http://www.pharmacy.arizona.edu/centers/poisoncenter >.

"Homeowner Chemical Safety." *Centers for DiseaseControl.* < http://www.cdc.gov/niosh/nasd/docs2/pdfs/as23900.pdf >.

"Poisonous Plant Databases." University of Maryland. < http://www.inform.umd.edu >.

Tish Davidson, A.M.
Rebecca J. Frey, PhD

Polarity therapy

Definition

Polarity therapy is a holistic, energy-based system that includes bodywork, diet, **exercise**, and lifestyle counseling for the purpose of restoring and maintaining proper energy flows throughout the body. The underlying concept of polarity therapy is that all energy within the human body is based in electromagnetic force and that disease results from improperly dissipated energy.

Purpose

Polarity therapy unblocks and recharges the flow of life energy and realigns unbalanced energy as a means of eliminating disease. Patients learn to release tension by addressing the source of the **stress** and by maintaining a healthy demeanor accordingly.

This treatment may be effective to promote health and healing to anyone willing to embrace the appropriate lifestyle. Polarity therapy is reportedly effective for anyone who has been exposed to toxic poisons. Likewise, HIV-positive individuals may find comfort in polarity therapy. Additionally this is an appropriate therapy for relieving general stress, back **pain**, stomach cramps, and other recurring maladies and conditions.

Description

Origins

Austrian-American chiropractor, osteopath, and naturopath Randolph Stone (1888–1981) developed polarity therapy as an integration of Eastern and Western principles and techniques of healing. Stone discovered the ancient principles of the Ayurvedic philosophy in the course of his travels during a sojourn in India. On a life-long quest to learn the fundamentals of human vitality, he also studied **reflexology** and traditional Chinese medicine.

Stone became committed to the principles of Ayurvedic medicine, which he interpreted in conjunction with his scientific and medical knowledge to define polarity therapy. According to the philosophy of Ayurved, which is based in a set of principles called the tridosha—the energy of the human body is centered in five organs or regions (the brain; the cardiopulmonary [heart and lungs] region, the diaphragm, the smaller intestine, and the larger intestine). One of five airs or energy forms controls each respective region: prana in the brain, vyana in the heart and lungs, udana in the diaphragm, samana in the smaller intestine, and apana in the larger intestine. The five airs control all directional motion in the body, with each air in command of a different type of movement. Stone established further that the prana, centered in the brain, ultimately controlled the combined forces of the body. Any impediment or restriction to the flow of prana in turn affects the health of the entire body. The prana force is nurtured through the flow of food and air into the body as well as through our interactions with other living beings and through the intake of the five sensory organs.

Stone devoted much of his life to defining an elaborately detailed cause and effect relationship between the human anatomy and illness, based on the energy flow of the prana. He further attributed electromagnetic energy as the basis of the energy forces. He used the medical symbol of the Caduceus to define the patterns of the flow and described the energy movement in detail in charts of the human body. Polarity therapy is based in charted energy flows. The primary energy pattern is defined in a spiral motion that radiates from the umbilicus and defines the original energy flow of the fetus in the womb.

After determining the exact source of a patient's energy imbalance, the therapist begins the first of a series of bodywork sessions designed to rechannel and release the patient's misdirected prana. This therapy, akin to massage, is based in energetic pressure and involves circulating motions. In performing the regimen, the therapist pays strict attention to the pressure exerted at each location—even to which finger is used to apply pressure at any given point of the patient's anatomy. This technique, which comprises the central regimen or focal point of polarity therapy is very gentle and is unique to polarity therapy. It typically involves subtle rocking movements and cranial holds to stimulate body energy. Although firm, deep pushing touches are employed in conjunction with the massage technique, the polarity therapist never exerts a particularly forceful contact.

To support the bodywork, the therapist often prescribes a diet for the patient, to encourage cleansing and eliminate waste. The precepts of polarity therapy take into consideration specific interactions between different foods and the human energy fields.

Likewise, a series of exercises is frequently prescribed. These exercises, called polarity yoga include squats, stretches, rhythmic movements, deep breathing, and expression of sounds. They can be both energizing and relaxing. Counseling may be included whenever appropriate as a part of a patient's highly individual therapy regimen to promote balance.

Preparations

Therapists take a comprehensive case history from every patient prior to beginning treatment. This preliminary verbal examination often monopolizes the first therapy session. Depending upon circumstances, a therapist might have a need to assess the patient's physical structural balance through observation and physical examination.

Precautions

Polarity therapy is safe for virtually anyone, even the elderly and the most frail patients, because of the intrinsic gentleness of the **massage therapy**.

KEY TERMS

Apana—Life sustaining energy centered in the larger intestine; the fifth of the five airs of Ayurvedic philosophy; the life force governing expulsion activity.

Ayurveda—(Sanskrit, *Ayur,* life, and *veda,* knowledge) Translated as "knowledge of life" or "science of longevity." It became established as the traditional Hindu system of medicine.

Caduceus—The ancient and universal symbol of medicine consisting of the winged staff of Mercury and two intertwining serpents.

Primary energy pattern—A spiral motion that radiates from the umbilicus; the energy pattern associated with a child in the womb.

Prana—Life sustaining energy centered in the human brain; the first of the five airs of Ayurvedic philosophy; the life force governing inspiration and the conscious intellect.

QV—Quantum vacuum, a theory coined by physicists, which defines the interactions of energy that combine to form reality.

Reflexology—Belief that reflex areas in the feet correspond to every part of the body, including organs and glands, and that stimulating the correct reflex area can affect the body part.

Samana—Life sustaining energy of the smaller intestine; the fourth of the five airs of Ayurvedic philosophy; the life force governing side-to-side motion.

Tridosha—The combination of three basic principles of energy, or biological humor, that comprise life, according to Ayurvedic philosophy.

Udana—Life sustaining energy of the diaphragm, the third of the five airs of Ayurvedic philosophy, the life force governing upward motion.

Vyana—Life sustaining energy of the heart and lungs; the second of the five airs of Ayurvedic philosophy; the life force governing circular motion.

Side effects

Highly emotional releases of energy (laughter, tears, or a combination of both) are associated with this therapy.

Research and general acceptance

This is a complementary therapy of holistic, spiritually based treatment, which may be used in conjunction with a medical approach. Polarity therapy is practiced worldwide, but the majority of practitioners are based in the United States. Modern physicists employ concepts similar to Stone's basic theories of polarity in defining the quantum vacuum (QV) as a foundation of all reality. Still, by 2000, this holistic regimen had not achieved the widespread acceptance anticipated by Stone before his death in 1981.

When St. Paul Fire and Marine insurers offered a liability insurance package to therapy providers, the company recognized polarity therapy as an alternative medical treatment along with acupuncture, biofeedback, homeopathy, reflexology, and others.

Resources

PERIODICALS

Modern Medicine August 1, 1999: 15.

ORGANIZATIONS

American Polarity Therapy Association. P.O. Box 19858, Boulder Colorado 80308. (303) 545-2080. Fax: (303) 545-2161.
Trans-Hyperboreau Institute of Science. P.O. Box 2344 Sausalito, California 94966. (415) 331-0230. (800) 485-8095. Fax: (415) 331-0231.

OTHER

Young, Phil. "Prana." June 16, 2000. < http://www.eclipse.co.uk/masterworks/Polarity/PolarityArticles.htm >.

Gloria Cooksey

Polio

Definition

Poliomyelitis, also called polio or infantile **paralysis**, is a highly infectious viral disease that may attack the central nervous system and is characterized by symptoms that range from a mild nonparalytic infection to total paralysis in a matter of hours.

Description

There are three known types of polioviruses (called 1,2, and 3), each causing a different strain of the disease and all are members of the viral family of enteroviruses (viruses that infect the gastrointestinal tract). Type 1 is the cause of epidemics and many cases of paralysis, which is the most severe manifestation of the infection. The virus is usually a harmless parasite of human beings.

Some statistics quote one in 200 infections as leading to paralysis while others state that one in 1,000 cases reach the central nervous system (CNS). When it does reach the CNS, inflammation and destruction of the spinal cord motor cells (anterior horn cells) occurs, which prevents them from sending out impulses to muscles. This causes the muscles to become limp or soft and they cannot contract. This is referred to as flaccid paralysis and is the type found in polio. The extent of the paralysis depends on where the virus strikes and the number of cells that it destroys. Usually, some of the limb muscles are paralyzed; the abdominal muscles or muscles of the back may be paralyzed, affecting posture. The neck muscles may become too weak for the head to be lifted. Paralysis of the face muscles may cause the mouth to twist or the eyelids to droop. Life may be threatened if paralysis of the throat or of the breathing muscles occurs.

Man is the only natural host for polioviruses and it most commonly infects younger children, although older children and adults can be infected. Crowded living conditions and poor hygiene encourage the spread of poliovirus. Risk factors for this paralytic illness include older age, **pregnancy**, abnormalities of the immune system, recent tonsillectomy, and a recent episode of excessively strenuous **exercise** concurrent with the onset of the CNS phase.

Causes and symptoms

Poliovirus can be spread by direct exposure to an infected individual, and more rarely, by eating foods contaminated with waste products from the intestines (feces) and/or droplets of moisture (saliva) from an infected person. Thus, the major route of transmission is fecal-oral, which occurs primarily with poor sanitary conditions. The virus is believed to enter the body through the mouth with primary multiplication occurring in the lymphoid tissues in the throat, where it can persist for about one week. During this time, it is absorbed into the blood and lymphatics from the gastrointestinal tract where it can reside and multiply, sometimes for as long as 17 weeks. Once absorbed, it is widely distributed throughout the body until it ultimately reaches the CNS (the brain and spinal cord). The infection is passed on to others when poor handwashing allows the virus to remain on the hands after eating or using the bathroom. Transmission remains possible while the virus is being excreted and it can be transmitted for as long as the virus remains in the throat or feces. The incubation period ranges from three to 21 days, but cases are most infectious from seven to 10 days before and after the onset of symptoms.

DR. JONAS E. SALK (1914–1995)

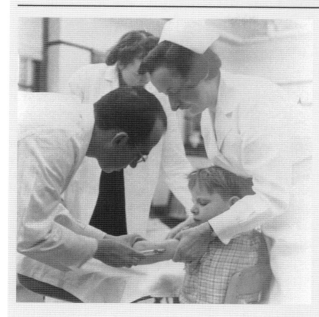

(Library of Congress.)

Jonas Salk was born in New York, New York, on October 28, 1914. He received his medical degree from New York University in 1939. In 1942, Salk began working for a former teacher, Thomas Francis, Jr., to produce influenza vaccines, a project that continued until 1949. That year, as a research professor, Salk began a three-year project sponsored by the National Foundation for Infantile Paralysis, also known as the March of Dimes. Caused by the poliomyelitis virus, polio was also known as infantile paralysis. Periodic outbreaks of the disease, which attacks the nervous system, caused death or a lifetime of paralysis, especially in children. It was a difficult disease to study because sufficient viruses could not be obtained. Unlike bacteria, which can be grown in cultures, viruses need living tissue on which to grow. Once a method for preparing viruses was discovered and improved, sufficient viruses became available for research.

Salk first set out to confirm that there were three virus types responsible for polio and then began to experiment with ways to kill the virus and yet retain its ability to produce an immune response. By 1952, he had produced a dead virus vaccine that worked against the three virus types. He began testing. First the vaccine was tested on monkeys, then on children who had recovered from the disease, and finally on Salk's own family and children, none of whom had ever had the disease. Following large-scale trials in 1954, the vaccine was finally released for public use in 1955. The Salk vaccine was not the first vaccine against polio, but it was the first to be found safe and effective. By 1961, there was a 96 percent reduction in polio cases in the United States.

There are two basic patterns to the virus: the minor illness (abortive type) and the major illness (which may be paralytic or nonparalytic). The minor illness accounts for 80–90% of clinical infections and is found mostly in young children. It is mild and does not involve the CNS. Symptoms include a slight **fever**, **fatigue**, **headache**, sore throat, and **vomiting**, which generally develop three to five days after exposure. Recovery from the minor illness occurs within 24–72 hours. Symptoms of the major illness usually appear without a previous minor illness and generally affect older children and adults.

About 10% of people infected with poliovirus develop severe headache and **pain** and stiffness of the neck and back. This is due to an inflammation of the meninges (tissues which cover the spinal cord and brain). This syndrome is called "aseptic meningitis." The term "aseptic" is used to differentiate this type of **meningitis** from those caused by bacteria. The patient usually recovers completely from this illness within several days.

About 1% of people infected with poliovirus develop the most severe form. Some of these patients may have two to three symptom-free days between the minor illness and the major illness but the symptoms often appear without any previous minor illness. Symptoms again include headache and back and neck pain. The major symptoms, however, are due to invasion of the motor nerves, which are responsible for movement of the muscles. This viral invasion causes inflammation, and then destruction of these nerves. The muscles, therefore, no longer receive any messages from the brain or spinal cord. The muscles become weak, floppy, and then totally paralyzed. All muscle tone is lost in the affected limb and the muscle becomes soft (flaccid). Within a few days, the muscle will begin to decrease in size (atrophy). The affected muscles may be on both sides of the body (symmetric paralysis), but are often on unbalanced parts of the body (asymmetric paralysis). Sensation or the ability to feel is not affected in these paralyzed limbs.

When poliovirus invades the brainstem (the stalk of brain which connects the two cerebral hemispheres with the spinal cord, called bulbar polio), a person may begin to have trouble breathing and swallowing.

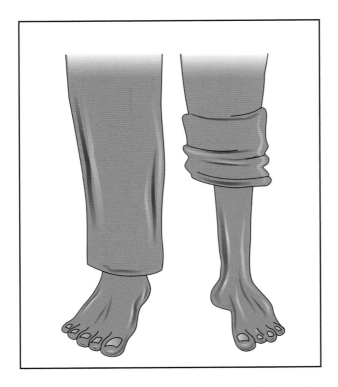

In its most severe form, polio causes paralysis of the muscles of the legs, arms, and respiratory system. All muscle tone is lost in the affected limb, and the muscle becomes flaccid and begins to atrophy, as shown in the illustration above. *(Illustration by Electronic Illustrators Group.)*

If the brainstem is severely affected, the brain's control of such vital functions as heart rate and blood pressure may be disturbed. This can lead to **death**.

The maximum state of paralysis is usually reached within just a few days. The remaining, unaffected nerves then begin the process of attempting to grow branches which can compensate for the destroyed nerves. Fortunately, the nerve cells are not always completely destroyed. By the end of a month, the nerve impulses start to return to the apparently paralyzed muscle and by the end of six months, recovery is almost complete. If the nerve cells are completely destroyed, however, paralysis is permanent.

Diagnosis

Fever and asymmetric flaccid paralysis without sensory loss in a child or young adult almost always indicate poliomyelitis. Using a long, thin needle inserted into the lower back to withdraw spinal fluid (lumbar puncture) will reveal increased white blood cells and no bacteria (aseptic meningitis). Nonparalytic poliomyelitis cannot be distinguished clinically from aseptic meningitis due to other agents. Virus isolated from a throat swab and/or feces or blood tests demonstrating the rise in a specific antibody is required to confirm the diagnosis.

Treatment

There is no specific treatment for polio except symptomatic. Therapy is designed to make the patient more comfortable (pain medications and hot packs to soothe the muscles), and intervention if the muscles responsible for breathing fail (for instance, a ventilator to take over the work of breathing). During active infection, rest on a firm bed is indicated. Physical therapy is the most important part of management of paralytic polio during recovery.

Prognosis

When poliovirus causes only the minor illness or simple aseptic meningitis, the patient can be expected to recover completely. When the patient is diagnosed with the major illness, about 50% will recover completely. About 25% of such patients will have slight disability, and about 25% will have permanent and serious disability. Approximately 1% of all patients with major illness die. The greatest return of muscle function occurs in the first six months, but improvements may continue for two years.

A recently described phenomenon called postpolio syndrome may begin many years after the initial illness. This syndrome is characterized by a very slow, gradual decrease in muscle strength.

Prevention

There are two types of polio immunizations available in the United States. Both of these vaccines take advantage of the fact that infection with polio leads to an immune reaction, which will give the person permanent, lifelong immunity from re-infection with the form of poliovirus for which the person was vaccinated.

The Sabin vaccine (also called the oral polio vaccine or OPV) is given to infants by mouth at the same intervals as the DPT (three doses). It contains the live, but weakened, poliovirus, which make the recipient immune to future infections with poliovirus. Because OPV uses live virus, it has the potential to cause infection in individuals with weak immune defenses (both in the person who receives the vaccine and in close contacts). This is a rare complication, however, occurring in only one in 6.8 million doses administered and

KEY TERMS

Aseptic—Sterile; containing no microorganisms, especially no bacteria.

Asymmetric—Not occurring evenly on both sides of the body.

Atrophy—Shrinking; growing smaller in size.

Brainstem—The stalk of the brain which connects the two cerebral hemispheres with the spinal cord.

DPT—Diphtheria, Pertussis and Tetanus injections.

Epidemic—Refers to a situation in which a particular disease rapidly spreads among many people in the same geographical region over a small time period.

Flaccid—Weak, soft, floppy.

Gastrointestinal—Pertaining to the stomach and intestines.

Lymph/lymphatic—One of the three body fluids that is transparent and a slightly yellow liquid that is collected from the capillary walls into the tissues and circulates back to the blood supply.

Paralysis—The inability to voluntarily move.

Symmetric—Occurring on both sides of the body, in a mirror-image fashion.

Resources

BOOKS

Braunwald MD, E., A. Fauci MD, D. Kasper MD, S. Hauser MD,D. Longo MD, and J. Jameson MD. *Harrison's Principles of Internal Medicine.* NewYork: McGraw-Hill, 2001.

Cecil, R., and L. Goldman. *Cecil Textbook ofMedicine.* Philadelphia: W.B. Saunders, 1999.

PERIODICALS

Centers for Disease Control and Prevention. "Poliomyelitis prevention in the United States: Updated recommendations of the AdvisoryCommittee on Immunization Practices (ACIP)." *MMWR* 2000. < http://www.cdc.gov/ >.

OTHER

World Health Organization. "Global Polio EradicationProgress 2000." < http://www.polioeradication.org/ >.

Linda K. Bennington, CNS

Poliomyelitis *see* **Polio**

Polyangiitis overlap syndrome *see* **Vasculitis**

Polyarteritis nodosa *see* **Vasculitis**

one in every 6.4 million doses from having close contact with someone who received the vaccine.

The Salk vaccine (also called the killed polio vaccine or inactivated polio vaccine) consists of a series of three shots that are given just under the skin. This immunization contains no live virus, just the components of the virus that provoke the recipient's immune system to react as if the recipient were actually infected with the poliovirus. The recipient thus becomes immune to infection with the poliovirus in the future.

In the 13 years following the launching of the Global Polio Eradication Initiative, the number of cases has fallen 99% from an estimated 350,000 cases to less than 3,500 cases worldwide in 2000. At the end of 2000, the number of polio-infected countries was approximately 20, down from 125. The goal of the World Health Organization (WHO) is to have polio eliminated from the planet by the year 2005. The virus has still been identified in Africa and parts of Asia, so travelers to those areas may want to check with their physicians concerning booster vaccinations.

Polycystic kidney disease

Definition

Polycystic **kidney disease** (PKD) is one of the most common of all life-threatening human genetic disorders. It is an incurable genetic disorder characterized by the formation of fluid-filled cysts in the kidneys of affected individuals. These cysts multiply over time. It was originally believed that the cysts eventually caused kidney failure by crowding out the healthy kidney tissue. It is now thought that the kidney damage seen in PKD is actually the result of the body's immune system. The immune system, in its attempts to rid the kidney of the cysts, instead progressively destroys the formerly healthy kidney tissue.

Description

A healthy kidney is about the same size as a human fist. PKD cysts, which can be as small as the head of a pin or as large as a grapefruit, can expand the kidneys until each one is bigger than a football and weighs as much as 38lb (17 kg).

There are two types of PKD: infantile PKD, which generally shows symptoms prior to birth; and adult onset PKD. Individuals affected with infantile PKD are often stillborn. Among the liveborn individuals affected with infantile PKD, very few of these children survive to the age of two. The adult onset form of PKD is much more common. The time and degree of symptom onset in the adult form of PKD can vary widely, even within a single family with two or more affected individuals. Symptoms of this form of PKD usually start to appear between the ages of 20 and 50. Organ deterioration progresses more slowly in adult onset PKD than it does in the infantile form; but, if left untreated, adult onset PKD also eventually leads to kidney failure.

One of the most common of all life-threatening genetic diseases, PKD affects more than 60,000 Americans. Over 12.5 million people worldwide are affected with PKD. Approximately one in every 400 to 1,000 people is affected with ADPKD. Another one in 10,000 affected with ARPKD. PKD is observed in equal numbers in both males and females. PKD is also observed with equal frequency among ethnic groups.

Causes and symptoms

Polycystic kidney disease is expressed as both a recessive and a dominant trait. A recessive genetic trait will not cause disease in a child unless it it inheritied from both parents. A dominant genetic trait can be inherited from just one parent. Those people affected with autosomal dominant PKD (ADPKD) have the much more common adult onset form. Those with autosomal recessive PKD (ARPKD) have the infantile form.

There are mutations on at least three genes that cause adult onset PKD. Approximately 85% of these cases are known to arise from mutations in the PKD1 gene that has been mapped to a region on the short arm of chromosome 16 (16p13.3-p13.12). Another 10–15% of cases of adult onset PKD are thought to be caused by mutations in the PKD2 gene that has been mapped to a region on the long arm of chromosome 4 (4q21-q23). As of early 2001, it is thought that the remainder of the cases of PKD are caused by mutations in the PKD3 gene, which has not yet been mapped. This unidentified "PKD3 gene" may, in fact, be more than one gene.

Adult onset PKD is transmitted from parents to their offspring as a non-sex linked (autosomal) dominant trait. This means that if either parent carries this genetic mutation, there is a 50% chance that their child will inherit this disease. In the case of two affected parents, there is a 75% probability that their children will be affected with adult onset PKD.

Infantile PKD is caused by a non-sex linked (autosomal) recessive genetic mutation that has been mapped to a region on the short arm of chromosome 6 (6p21). Both parents must be carriers of this mutation for their children to be affected with infantile PKD. In the case of two carrier parents, the probability is 25% that their child will be affected by infantile PKD.

A baby born with infantile PKD has floppy, low-set ears, a pointed nose, a small chin, and folds of skin surrounding the eyes (epicanthal folds). Large, rigid masses can be felt on the back of both thighs (flanks), and the baby usually has trouble breathing.

In the early stages of adult onset PKD, many people show no symptoms. Generally, the first symptoms to develop are: high blood pressure (**hypertension**); general **fatigue**; **pain** in the lower back or the backs of the thighs; headaches; and/or urinary tract infections accompanied by frequent urination.

As PKD becomes more advanced, the kidneys' inability to function properly becomes more pronounced. The cysts on the kidney may begin to rupture and the kidneys tend to be much larger than normal. Individuals affected with PKD have a much higher rate of **kidney stones** than the rest of the population at this, and later stages, of the disease. Approximately 60% of those individuals affected with PKD develop cysts in the liver, while 10% develop cysts in the pancreas.

Because the kidneys are primarily responsible for cleaning the blood, individuals affected with PKD often have problems involving the circulatory system. These include: an underproduction of red blood cells which results in an insufficient supply of oxygen to the tissues and organs (anemia); an enlarged heart (cardiac hypertrophy) probably caused by long term hypertension; and, a leakage of the valve between the left chambers (auricle and ventricle) of the heart (**mitral valve prolapse**). Less common (affecting approximately 5% of PKD patients) are brain aneurysms. An aneurysm is an abnormal and localized bulging of the wall of a blood vessel. If an aneurysm within the brain leaks or bursts, it may cause a **stroke** or even **death**.

Other health problems associated with adult onset PKD include: chronic leg or back pain; frequent infections; and herniations of the groin and abdomen, including herniation of the colon (diverticular disease). A herniation, or **hernia**, is caused when a tissue, designed to hold the shape of an underlying tissue,

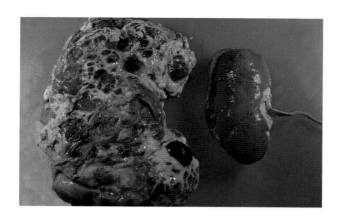

A pair of human kidneys. Tthe left a polycystic kidney, the right a normal kidney. (Photograph by A. Glauberman, Photo Researchers, Inc. Reproduced by permission.)

becomes weakened at a particular spot. The underlying tissue pushes against this weakened area until the area is no longer able to hold back the underlying tissue and the area forms an abnormal bulge through which the underlying tissue projects. Diverticular disease is caused by a weakening of the muscles that hold the shape of the organs of the digestive tract. These muscles weaken allowing these organs, particularly one section of the colon, to form sac-like projections that can trap feces and become infected, or rupture.

In the final stages of PKD, the major symptom is kidney (renal) failure. Renal failure is indicated by an increase of nitrogen (in the form of urea) in the blood (uremia, or uremic **poisoning**). Uremia is a rapidly fatal condition without treatment.

Diagnosis

Many patients who have PKD do not have any symptoms. Their condition may not be discovered unless tests that detect it are performed for other reasons.

When symptoms of PKD are present, the diagnostic procedure begins with a family medical history and **physical examination** of the patient. If several family members have PKD, there is a strong likelihood that the patient has it too. If the disease is advanced, the doctor will be able to feel the patient's enlarged kidneys. Heart murmur, high blood pressure, and other signs of cardiac impairment can also be detected.

Urinalysis and a blood test called creatine clearance can indicate how effectively the kidneys are functioning. Scanning procedures using intravenous dye reveal kidney enlargement or deformity and scarring

caused by cysts. Ultrasound and **computed tomography scans** (CT scans) can reveal kidney enlargement and the cysts that caused it. CT scans can highlight cyst-damaged areas of the kidneys. A sampling of the kidney cells (biopsy) may be performed to verify the diagnosis.

Treatment

There is no way to prevent cysts from forming or becoming enlarged, or to prevent PKD from progressing to kidney failure. Treatment goals include preserving healthy kidney tissue; controlling symptoms and, preventing infection and other complications.

If adult PKD is diagnosed before symptoms become evident, urinalysis and other diagnostic tests are performed at six-week intervals to monitor the patient's health status. If results indicate the presence of infection or another PKD-related health problem, aggressive antibiotic therapy is initiated to prevent inflammation that can accelerate disease progression; iron supplements or infusion of red blood cells are used to treat anemia; and surgery may be needed to drain cysts that bleed, cause pain, have become infected, or interfere with normal kidney function.

Lowering high blood pressure can slow loss of kidney function. Blood-pressure control, which is the cornerstone of PKD treatment, is difficult to achieve. Therapy may include antihypertensive medications, diuretic medications, and/or a low-salt diet. As kidney function declines, some patients need dialysis and/or a kidney transplant.

There is no known way to prevent PKD, but certain lifestyle modifications can help control symptoms. People who have PKD should not drink heavily or smoke. They should not use **aspirin**, non-steroidal anti-inflammatory drugs (NSAIDs), or other prescription or over-the-counter medications that can impair kidney function. Individuals affected with PKD should eat a balanced diet, **exercise** regularly, and maintain a weight appropriate for their height, age, and body type. Regular medical monitoring is also recommended.

Prognosis

There is no known cure for PKD. Those affected with infantile PKD generally die before the age of two. In adults, untreated disease can be rapidly fatal or continue to progress slowly, even after symptoms of kidney failure appear. About half of all adults with PKD also develop kidney failure. Unless the patient undergoes dialysis or has a kidney transplant, this

KEY TERMS

Biopsy—The surgical removal and microscopic examination of living tissue for diagnostic purposes.

Cancer—A disease caused by uncontrolled growth of the body's cells.

Computed tomography (CT) scan—An imaging procedure that produces a three-dimensional picture of organs or structures inside the body, such as the brain.

Cyst—An abnormal sac or closed cavity filled with liquid or semisolid matter.

Diuretics—Medications that increase the excretion of urine.

Kidney—Either of two organs in the lumbar region that filter the blood, excreting the end products of the body's metabolism in the form of urine and regulating the concentrations of hydrogen, sodium, potassium, phosphate and other ions in the body.

Magnetic resonance imaging (MRI)—A technique that employs magnetic fields and radio waves to create detailed images of internal body structures and organs, including the brain.

Ultrasonogram—A procedure where high-frequency sound waves that cannot be heard by human ears are bounced off internal organs and tissues. These sound waves produce a pattern of echoes, which are then used by the computer to create sonograms or pictures of areas inside the body.

Uremic poisoning—Accumulation of waste products in the body.

condition usually leads to death within four years of diagnosis.

Although medical treatment can temporarily alleviate symptoms of PKD, the expanding cysts continue to increase pressure on the kidneys. Kidney failure and uremic poisoning (accumulation of waste products the body is unable to eliminate) generally cause death about 10 years after symptoms first appear.

Medications used to fight **cancer** and reduce elevated cholesterol levels have slowed the advance of PKD in laboratory animals. They may soon be used to treat adults and children who have the disease. Researchers are also evaluating the potential benefits of anti-inflammatory drugs, which may prevent the scarring that destroys kidney function.

Resources

PERIODICALS

Koptides, M., and C. Deltas. "Autosomal dominant polycystic kidney disease: Molecular genetics and molecular pathogenesis." *Human Genetics* August 2000: 115–26.

Pei, Y., A. Paterson, K. Wang, N. He, et al. "Bilineal disease and trans-heterozygotes in autosmal dominant polycystic kidney disease." *American Journal of Human Genetics* February 2001: 355–63.

ORGANIZATIONS

Polycystic Kidney Disease Foundation. 4901 Main Street, Kansas City, MO 64112-2634. (800) PKD-CURE. < http://www.pkdcure.org/home.htm >.

OTHER

Brochert, Adam, MD. "Polycystic Kidney Disease." September 4, 2000. *HealthAnswers.* < http://www.healthanswers.com/library/library_fset.asp >.

Cooper, Joel R. "Treating Polycystic Kidney Disease. What Does the Future Hold?" *Coolware, Inc.* < http://www.coolware.com/health/medical_reporter/kidney1.html >.

Online Mendelian Inheritance in Man (OMIM). February 15, 2001. < http://www.ncbi.nlm.nih.gov/htbin-post/Omim/dispmim?600595 >.

Polycystic Kidney Disease Access Center. < http://www.nhpress.com/pkd/ >.

Paul A. Johnson, Ed.M.

Polycystic ovary syndrome

Definition

Polycystic ovary syndrome (PCOS) is a condition characterized by the accumulation of numerous cysts (fluid-filled sacs) on the ovaries associated with high male hormone levels, chronic anovulation (absent ovulation), and other metabolic disturbances. Classic symptoms include excess facial and body hair, **acne**, **obesity**, irregular menstrual cycles, and **infertility**.

Description

PCOS, also called Stein-Leventhal syndrome, is a group of symptoms caused by underlying hormonal and metabolic disturbances that affect about 6% of premenopausal women. PCOS symptoms appear as early as adolescence in the form of **amenorrhea** (missed periods), obesity, and **hirsutism**, the abnormal growth of body hair.

A disturbance in normal hormonal signals prevents ovulation in women with PCOS. Throughout the cycle, estrogen levels remain steady, luteinizing hormone (LH) levels are high, and follide stimulating hormone (FSH) and progesterone levels are low. Since eggs are rarely or never released from their follicles, multiple **ovarian cysts** develop over time.

One of the most important characteristics of PCOS is hyperandrogenism, the excessive production of male hormones (androgens), particularly testosterone, by the ovaries. This accounts for the male hair-growth patterns and acne in women with PCOS. Hyperandrogenism has been linked with **insulin resistance** (the inability of the body to respond to insulin) and hyperinsulinemia (high blood insulin levels), both of which are common in PCOS.

Causes and symptoms

While the exact cause of PCOS is unknown, it runs in families, so the tendency to develop the syndrome may be inherited. The interaction of hyperinsulinemia and hyperandrogenism is believed to play a role in chronic anovulation in susceptible women.

The numbers and types of PCOS symptoms that appear vary among women. These include:

- Hirsutism. Related to hyperandrogenism, this occurs in 70% of women.

- Obesity. Approximately 40–70% of persons with PCOS are overweight.

- Anovulation and menstrual disturbances. Anovulation appears as amenorrhea in 50% of women, and as heavy uterine bleeding in 30% of women. However, 20% of women with PCOS have normal menstruation.

- Male-pattern hair loss. Some women with PCOS develop bald spots.

- Infertility. Achieving **pregnancy** is difficult for many women with PCOS.

- Polycystic ovaries. Most, but not all, women with PCOS have multiple cysts on their ovaries.

- Skin discoloration. Some women with PCOS have dark patches on their skin.

- Abnormal blood chemistry. Women with PCOS have high levels of low-density lipoprotein (LDL or "bad") cholesterol and triglycerides, and low levels of high-density lipoprotein (HDL or "good") cholesterol.

- Hyperinsulinemia. Some women with PCOS have high blood insulin levels, particularly if they are overweight.

Diagnosis

PCOS is diagnosed when a woman visits her doctor for treatment of symptoms such as hirsutism, obesity, menstrual irregularities, or infertility. Women with PCOS are treated by a gynecologist, a doctor who treats diseases of the female reproductive organs, or a reproductive endocrinologist, a specialist who treats diseases of the body's endocrine (hormones and glands) system and infertility.

PCOS can be difficult to diagnose because its symptoms are similar to those of many other diseases or conditions, and because all of its symptoms may not occur. A doctor takes a complete medical history, including questions about menstruation and reproduction, and weight gain. **Physical examination** includes a pelvic examination to determine the size of the ovaries, and visual inspection of the skin for hirsutism, acne, or other changes. Blood tests are performed to measure levels of luteinizing hormone, follicle stimulating hormone, estrogens, androgens, glucose, and insulin. A glucose-tolerance test may be administered. An ultrasound examination of the ovaries is performed to evaluate their size and shape. Most insurance plans cover the costs of diagnosing and treating PCOS and its related problems.

Treatment

PCOS treatment is aimed at correcting anovulation, restoring normal menstrual periods, improving fertility, eliminating hirsutism and acne, and preventing future complications related to high insulin and blood lipid (fat) levels. Treatment consists of weight loss, drugs or surgery, and hair removal, depending upon which symptoms are most bothersome, and whether a woman desires pregnancy.

Weight loss

In overweight women, weight loss (as little as 5%) through diet and **exercise** may correct hyperandrogenism, and restore normal ovulation and fertility. This is often tried first.

Drugs

HORMONAL DRUGS. Women who do not want to become pregnant and require **contraception** (spontaneous ovulation occurs occasionally among women with PCOS) are treated with low-dose oral contraceptive pills (OCPs). OCPs bring on regular menstrual periods and correct heavy uterine bleeding, as well as hirsutism, although improvement may not be seen for up to a year.

If an infertile woman desires to become pregnant, the first drug usually given to help induce ovulation is clomiphene citrate (Clomid), which results in pregnancy in about 70% of women but can cause multiple births. In the 20–25% of women who do not respond to clomiphene, other drugs that stimulate follicle development and induce ovulation, such as human menstrual gonadotropin (Pergonal) and human chorionic gonadotropin (HCG), are given. However, these drugs have a lower pregnancy rate (less than 30%), a higher rate of **multiple pregnancy** (from 5–30%, depending on the dose of the drug), and a higher risk of medical problems. Women with PCOS have a high rate of **miscarriage** (30%), and may be treated with the gonadotropin-releasing hormone agonist leuprolide (Lupron) to reduce this risk.

Since women with PCOS do not have regular endometrial shedding due to high estrogen levels, they are at increased risk for overgrowth of this tissue and **endometrial cancer**. The drug medroxyprogesterone acetate, when taken for the first 10 days of each month, causes regular shedding of the endometrium, and reduces the risk of **cancer**. However, in most cases, oral contraceptive pills are used instead to bring about regular menstruation.

OTHER DRUGS. Another drug that helps to trigger ovulation is the steroid hormone dexamethasone. This drug acts by reducing the production of androgens by the adrenal glands.

The antiandrogen spironolactone (Aldactazide), which is usually given with an oral contraceptive, improves hirsutism and male-pattern baldness by reducing androgen production, but has no effect on fertility. The drug causes abnormal uterine bleeding and is linked with **birth defects** if taken during pregnancy. Another antiandrogen used to treat hirsutism, flutamide (Eulexin), can cause liver abnormalities, **fatigue**, mood swings, and loss of sexual desire. A drug used to reduce insulin levels, metformin (Glucophage), has shown promising results in women with PCOS hirsutism, but its effects on infertility and other PCOS symptoms are unknown. Drug treatment of hirsutism is long-term, and improvement may not be seen for up to a year or longer.

Acne is treated with **antibiotics**, antiandrogens, and other drugs such as retinoic acids (vitamin A compounds).

Surgical treatment

Surgical treatment of PCOS may be performed if drug treatment fails, but it is not common. A wedge resection, the surgical removal of part of the ovary and cysts through a laparoscope (an instrument inserted into the pelvis through a small incision), or an abdominal incision, reduces androgen production and restores ovulation. Although laparoscopic surgery is less likely to cause scar tissue formation than abdominal surgery, both are associated with the potential for scarring that may require additional surgery. Laparoscopic ovarian drilling is another type of laparoscopic surgery used to treat PCOS. The ovarian cysts are penetrated with a laser beam and some of the fluid is drained off. Between 50–65% of women may become pregnant after either type of surgery.

Some cases of severe hirsutism are treated by removal of the uterus (**hysterectomy**) and the ovaries (oopherectomy), followed by estrogen replacement therapy.

Other treatment

Hirsutism may be treated by hair removal techniques such as shaving, depilatories (chemicals that break down the structure of the hair), tweezing, waxing, electrolysis (destruction of the hair root by an electrical current), or the destruction of hair follicles by laser therapy. However, the treatments may have to be repeated.

Alternative treatment

PCOS can be addressed using many types of alternative treatment. The rebalancing of hormones is a primary focus of all these therapies. **Acupuncture** works on the body's energy flow according to the meridian system. Chinese herbs, such as *gui zhi fu ling wan*, can be effective. In **naturopathic medicine**, treatment focuses on helping the liver function more optimally in the horomonal balancing process. Dietary changes, including reducing animal products and fats, while increasing foods that nourish the liver such as carrots, dark green vegetables, lemons, and beets, can be beneficial. Essential fatty acids, including flax oil, evening primrose oil (*Oenothera biennis*), and black currant oil, act as anti-inflammatories and hormonal regulators. Western herbal medicine uses phytoestrogen and phytoprogesteronic herbs, such as blue cohosh (*Caulophyllum thalictroides*) and false unicorn root (*Chamaelirium luteum*), as well as liver herbs, like dandelion (*Taraxacum mongolicum*), to work toward hormonal balance. Supplementation with antioxidants, including zinc, and **vitamins** A, E, and C, is also recommended. Constitutional homeopathy can bring about a deep level of healing with the correct remedies.

KEY TERMS

Androgens—Male sex hormones produced by the adrenal glands and testes, the male sex glands.

Anovulation—The absence of ovulation.

Antiandrogens—Drugs that inhibit androgen production.

Estrogens—Hormones produced by the ovaries, the female sex glands.

Follicle stimulating hormone—A hormone that stimulates the growth and maturation of mature eggs in the ovary.

Gynecologist—A physician with specialized training in diseases and conditions of the female reproductive system.

Hirsutism—An abnormal growth of hair on the face and other parts of the body caused by an excess of androgens.

Hyperandrogenism—The excessive secretion of androgens.

Hyperinsulinemia—High blood insulin levels.

Insulin resistance—An inability to respond to insulin, a hormone produced by the pancreas that helps the body to use glucose.

Laparoscope—An instrument inserted into the pelvis through a small incision.

Luteinizing hormone—A hormone that stimulates the secretion of sex hormones by the ovary.

Ovarian follicles—Structures found within the ovary that produce eggs.

Prognosis

With proper diagnosis and treatment, most PCOS symptoms can be adequately controlled or eliminated. Infertility can be corrected and pregnancy achieved in most women although, in some, hormonal disturbances and anovulation may recur. Women should be monitored for endometrial cancer. Because of the high rate of hyperinsulinemia seen in PCOS, women with the disorder should have their glucose levels checked regularly to watch for the development of diabetes. Blood pressure and cholesterol screening are also needed because these women also tend to have high levels of LDL cholesterol and triglycerides, which put them at risk for developing heart disease.

Prevention

There is no known way to prevent PCOS, but if diagnosed and treated early, risks for complications such as and heart disease and diabetes may be minimized. Weight control through diet and exercise stabilizes hormones and lowers insulin levels.

Resources

BOOKS

DeGroot, Leslie J., and J. Larry Jameson. *Endocribnology.* 4th ed. Philadelphia: W B Saunders, 2001.

Genazzani, A. R., and F. Petraglia. *Advances in Gynecological Endocrinology.* London: Parthenon Press, 2001.

Nader, Shala. *Case Studies in Reproductive Endocrinology.* London: Edward Arnold, 2000.

Speroff, Leon. *Handbook for Clinical Gynecologic Endocrinology and Infertility* Philadelphia: Lippincott Williams & Wilkins, 2001.

Spratt, Daniel, and Nanette Santoro. *Endocrinology and Management of Reproduction and Fertility: Practical Diagnosis and Treatment.* Totowa, NJ: Humana Press, 2001.

PERIODICALS

Bracero, N., H. A. Zacur. "Polycystic ovary syndrome and hyperprolactinemia." *Obstetrics and Gynecology Clinics of North America* 28, no. 1 (2001): 77-84.

Calvo, R.M., et al. "Role of the follistatin gene in women with polycystic ovary syndrome." *Fertility and Sterility* 75, no. 5 (2001): 1020-102.

Dejager, S., et al. "Smaller LDL particle size in women with polycystic ovary syndrome compared to controls." *Clinical Endocrinology* (Oxford) 54, no. 4 (2001): 455–462.

Heinonen, S., et al. "Apolipoprotein E alleles in women with polycystic ovary syndrome." *Fertility and Sterility* 75, no. 5 (2001): 878-880.

Hoeger, K. "Obesity and weight loss in polycystic ovary syndrome." *Obstetrics and Gynecology Clinics of North America* 28, no. 1 (2001): 85-97.

Iuorno, M. J., and J. E. Nestler. "Insulin-lowering drugs in polycystic ovary syndrome." *Obstetrics and Gynecology Clinics of North America* 28, no. 1 (2001): 153-164.

Kalro, B. N., T. L. Loucks, and S. L. Berga. "Neuromodulation in polycystic ovary syndrome." *Obstetrics and Gynecology Clinics of North America* 28, no. 1 (2001): 35-62.

Legro, R. S. "Diabetes prevalence and risk factors in polycystic ovary syndrome." *Obstetrics and Gynecology Clinics of North America* 28, no. 1 (2001): 99-109.

Lewis, V. "Polycystic ovary syndrome. A diagnostic challenge." *Obstetrics and Gynecology Clinics of North America* 28, no. 1: 1-20.

Moran, C., and R. Azziz. "The role of the adrenal cortex in polycystic ovary syndrome." *Obstetrics and Gynecology Clinics of North America* 28, no. 1 (2001): 63-75.

Padmanabhan, V., et al. "Dynamics of bioactive follicle-stimulating hormone secretion in women with polycystic ovary syndrome: effects of estradiol and progesterone." *Fertility and Sterility* 75, no. 5 (2001): 881-888.

Phipps, W. R. "Polycystic ovary syndrome and ovulation induction." *Obstetrics and Gynecology Clinics of North America* 28, no. 1 (2001): 165-182.

Talbott, E. O., et al. "Cardiovascular risk in women with polycystic ovary syndrome." *Obstetrics and Gynecology Clinics of North America* 28, no. 1 (2001): 111-133.

Zacur, H. A. "Polycystic ovary syndrome, hyperandrogenism, and insulin resistance." *Obstetrics and Gynecology Clinics of North America* 28, no. 1 (2001): 21-33.

Zborowski, J. V., et al. "Polycystic ovary syndrome, androgen excess, and the impact on bone." *Obstetrics and Gynecology Clinics of North America* 28, no. 1 (2001): 135–151.

ORGANIZATIONS

American Academy of Family Physicians. 11400 Tomahawk Creek Parkway, Leawood, KS 66211-2672. (913) 906-6000. < http://www.aafp.org/ >. fp@aafp.org.

American Medical Association. 515 N. State Street, Chicago, IL 60610. (312) 464-5000. < http://www.ama-assn.org/ >.

Polycystic Ovarian Syndrome Association. PO Box 80517, Portlabd, OR 97280. (877) 775-7267. < http://www.pcosupport.org/ >. info@pcossupport.org.

OTHER

American Academy of Family Physicians. < http://www.aafp.org/afp/20000901/1079.html >.

Jewish Hospital of Cincinnati. < http://uc.edu/~gartsips/polycyst.htm >.

Merck Manual. < http://www.merck.com/pubs/mmanual/section18/chapter235/235d.htm >.

Vanderbilt University School of Medicine. < http://www.mc.vanderbilt.edu/peds/pidl/adolesc/polcysov.htm >.

Women's Health-UK. < http://www.womens-health.co.uk/pcos.htm >.

L. Fleming Fallon, Jr., MD, DrPH

Polycythemia *see* **Secondary polycythemia**

Polycythemia rubra vera *see* **Polycythemia vera**

Polycythemia vera

Definition

Polycythemia vera (PV) is a chronic blood disorder marked by an abnormal increase in three types of blood cells produced by bone marrow: red blood cells (RBCs), white blood cells (WBCs), and platelets. PV is called a myeloproliferative disorder, which means that the bone marrow is producing too many cells too quickly. Most of the symptoms of PV are related to the increased volume of the patient's blood and its greater thickness (high viscosity). PV sometimes evolves into a different myeloproliferative disorder or into acute leukemia.

Description

Polycythemia vera is a relatively common progressive disorder that develops over a course of 10–20 years. In the United States, PV affects about one person in every 200,000. PV has several other names, including splenomegalic polycythemia, Vaquez-Osler syndrome, erythremia, and primary polycythemia. Primary polycythemia means that the disorder is not caused or triggered by other illnesses. PV most commonly affects middle-aged adults. It is rarely seen in children or young adults and does not appear to run in families. The male/female ratio is 2:1.

Risk factors for polycythemia vera include:

- Caucasian race
- male sex
- age between 40 and 60

Causes and symptoms

The cause of PV remains uncertain. In general, the increased mass of red blood cells in the patient's blood causes both hemorrhage and abnormal formation of **blood clots** in the circulatory system (thrombosis). The reasons for these changes in clotting patterns are not yet fully understood.

Early symptoms

The symptoms of early PV may be minimal–it is not unusual for the disorder to be discovered during a routine blood test. More often, however, patients have symptoms that include headaches, ringing in the ears, tiring easily, memory problems, difficulty breathing, giddiness or lightheadedness, **hypertension**, visual problems, or **tingling** or burning sensations in their hands or feet. Another common symptom is **itching** (pruritus). Pruritus related to PV is often worse after the patient takes a warm bath or shower.

Some patients' early symptoms include unusually heavy bleeding from minor cuts, nosebleeds, stomach ulcers, or bone **pain**. In a few cases, the first symptom is the development of blood clots in an unusual part of the circulatory system (e.g., the liver).

Later symptoms and complications

As the disease progresses, patients with PV may have episodes of hemorrhage or thrombosis. Thrombosis is the most frequent cause of **death** from PV. Other complications include a high level of uric acid in the blood and an increased risk of peptic ulcer disease. About 10% of PV patients eventually develop **gout**; another 10% develop peptic ulcers.

Spent phase

The spent phase is a development in late PV that affects about 30% of patients. The bone marrow eventually fails and the patient becomes severely anemic, requiring repeated blood transfusions. The spleen and liver become greatly enlarged–in the later stages of PV, the patient's spleen may fill the entire left side of the abdomen.

Diagnosis

Physical examination

PV is often a diagnosis of exclusion, which means that the doctor will first rule out other possible causes of the patient's symptoms. The doctor can detect some signs of the disorder during a **physical examination**. Patients with PV will have an enlarged spleen (splenomegaly) in 75% of cases. About 50% will have a slightly enlarged liver. The doctor can feel these changes when he or she presses on (palpates) the patient's abdomen while the patient is lying flat. An **eye examination** will usually reveal swollen veins at the back of the eye. Patients with PV often have unusually red complexions; mottled red patches on their legs, feet, or hands; or swelling at the ends of the fingers.

Diagnostic criteria for PV

Accurate diagnosis of PV is critical because its treatment may require the use of drugs with the potential to cause leukemia. The results of the patient's blood tests are evaluated according to criteria worked out around 1970 by the Polycythemia Vera Study Group. The patient is considered to have PV if all three major criteria are met; or if the first two major criteria and any two minor criteria are met.

Major criteria:

- red blood cell mass greater than 36 mL/kg in males, greater than 32 mL/kg in females
- arterial oxygen level greater than 92%
- splenomegaly

Minor criteria:

- platelet count greater than 400,000/mm^3
- WBC greater than 12,000/mm^3 without **fever** or infection
- leukocyte alkaline phosphatase (LAP) score greater than 100 with increased blood serum levels of vitamin B$_{12}$

Laboratory testing

BLOOD TESTS. The diagnosis of PV depends on a set of findings from blood tests. The most important single measurement is the patient's red blood cell mass as a proportion of the total blood volume. This measurement is made by tagging RBCs with radioactive chromium (^{51}Cr) in order to determine the patient's RBC volume. While a few patients with PV may have a red cell mass level within the normal range if they have had recent heavy bleeding, a high score may eliminate the need for some other tests. A score higher than 36 mL/kg for males and 32 mL/kg for females on the ^{51}Cr test suggests PV. Measurements of the oxygen level in the patient's arterial blood, of the concentration of vitamin B$_{12}$ in the blood serum, and of leukocyte alkaline phosphatase (LAP) staining can be used to distinguish PV from certain types of leukemia or from other types of polycythemia. LAP staining measures the intensity of enzyme activity in a type of white blood cell called a neutrophil. In PV, the LAP score is higher than normal whereas in leukemia it is below normal.

BONE MARROW TESTS. Bone marrow testing can be used as part of the diagnostic process. A sample of marrow can be cultured to see if red blood cell colonies develop without the addition of a hormone that stimulates RBC production. The growth of a cell colony without added hormone indicates PV. Bone marrow testing is also important in monitoring the progress of the disease, particularly during the spent phase.

GENETIC TESTING. Genetic testing can be used to rule out the possibility of chronic myeloid leukemia. Patients with this disease have a characteristic chromosomal abnormality called the Philadelphia chromosome. The Philadelphia chromosome does *not* occur in patients with PV.

Imaging studies

Imaging studies are not necessary to make the diagnosis of PV. In some cases, however, imaging studies can detect enlargement of the spleen that the doctor may not be able to feel during the physical examination.

Treatment

Treatment of PV is tailored to the individual patient according to his or her age, the severity of the symptoms and complications, and the stage of the disease.

Phlebotomy

Phlebotomy is the withdrawal of blood from a vein. It is the first line of treatment for patients with PV. Phlebotomy is used to bring down the ratio of red blood cells to fluid volume (the **hematocrit**) in the patient's blood to a level below 45%. In most cases the doctor will withdraw about 500 mL of blood (about 15 fluid ounces) once or twice a week until the hematocrit is low enough. Phlebotomy is considered the best course of treatment for patients younger than 60 and for women of childbearing age. Its drawback is that patients remain at some risk for either thrombosis or hemorrhage.

Myelosuppression

Myelosuppressive therapies are used to slow down the body's production of blood cells. They are given to patients who are older than 60 and at high risk for thrombosis. These therapies, however, increase the patient's risk of developing leukemia. The substances most frequently used as of 1998 include hydroxyurea (Hydrea), interferon alfa (Intron), or radioactive phosphorus (^{32}P). ^{32}P is used only in elderly patients with life expectancies of less than five years because it causes leukemia in about 10% of patients. Interferon alfa is expensive and causes side effects resembling the symptoms of influenza but is an option for some younger PV patients.

Investigational treatment

The Food and Drug Administration (FDA) has approved the use of anagrelide, an orphan drug, for investigational use in the treatment of PV. Anagrelide has moderate side effects and controls the platelet level in over 90% of patients.

Treatment of complications

The itching caused by PV is often difficult to control. Patients with pruritus are given diphenhydramine (Benadryl) or another antihistamine. Patients with high levels of uric acid are usually given allopurinol (Lopurin, Zyloprim) by mouth. Supportive care includes advice about diet–splenomegaly often makes patients feel full after eating only a little food. This

---

KEY TERMS

Anagrelide—An orphan drug that is approved for treating PV patients on an investigational basis. Anagrelide works by controlling the level of platelets in the blood.

Leukocyte alkaline phosphatase (LAP) test—A blood test that measures the level of enzyme activity in a type of white blood cell called neutrophils.

Myeloproliferative disorder—A disorder in which the bone marrow produces too many cells too rapidly.

Myelosuppressive therapy—Any form of treatment that is aimed at slowing down the rate of blood cell production.

Orphan drug—A drug that is known to be useful in treatment but lacks sufficient funding for further research and development.

Philadelphia chromosome—An abnormal chromosome that is found in patients with a chronic form of leukemia but not in PV patients.

Phlebotomy—Drawing blood from a patient's vein as part of diagnosis or therapy. Phlebotomy is sometimes called venesection. It is an important part of the treatment of PV.

Pruritus—An itching sensation or feeling. In PV the itching is not confined to a specific part of the body and is usually worse after a warm bath or shower.

Spent phase—A late development in PV leading to failure of the bone marrow and severe anemia.

Splenomegaly—Abnormal enlargement of the spleen. Splenomegaly is a major diagnostic criterion of PV.

---

problem can be minimized by advising patients to eat small meals followed by rest periods.

Because of the clotting problems related to PV, patients should not undergo surgery until their blood counts are close to normal levels. Female patients of childbearing age should be warned about the dangers of **pregnancy** related to their clotting abnormalities.

Prognosis

The prognosis for untreated polycythemia vera is poor; 50% of patients die within 18 months after diagnosis. Death usually results from heart failure, leukemia, or hemorrhage. Patients being treated for

PV can expect to live between 11 and 15 years on average after diagnosis.

Resources

ORGANIZATIONS

National Heart, Lung and Blood Institute. P.O. Box 30105, Bethesda, MD 20824-0105. (301) 251-1222. < http://www.nhlbi.nih.gov >.

National Organization for Rare Disorders. P.O. Box 8923, New Fairfield, CT 06812-8923. (800) 999-6673. < http://www.rarediseases.org >.

Rebecca J. Frey, PhD

Polydactyly and syndactyly

Definition

Polydactyly and syndactyly are congenital irregularities of the hands and feet. Polydactyly is the occurrence of extra fingers or toes, and syndactyly is the webbing or fusing together of two or more fingers or toes.

Description

Polydactyly can vary from an unnoticeable rudimentary finger or toe to fully developed extra digits.

Syndactyly also exhibits a large degree of variation. Digits can be partially fused or fused along their entire length. The fusion can be simple with the digits connected only by skin, or it can be complicated with shared bones, nerves, vessels, or nails.

Polydactyly and syndactyly can occur simultaneously when extra digits are fused. This condition is known as polysyndactyly.

Causes and symptoms

Polydactyly and syndactyly are due to errors in the process of fetal development. For example, syndactyly results from the failure of the programmed cell death that normally occurs between digits. Most often these errors are due to genetic defects.

Polydactyly and syndactyly can both occur by themselves as isolated conditions or in conjunction with other symptoms as one aspect of a multi-symptom disease. There are several forms of isolated syndactyly and several forms of isolated polydactyly; each of these, where the genetics is understood, is caused by an autosomal dominant gene. This means that since

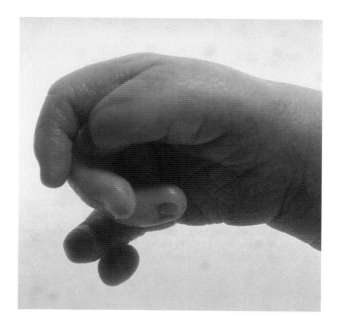

Polydactyly is the occurrence of extra or partial fingers or toes. *(Custom Medical Stock Photo. Reproduced by permission.)*

the gene is autosomal (not sex-linked), males and females are equally likely to inherit the trait. This also means that since the gene is dominant, children who have only one parent with the trait have a 50% chance of inheriting it. However, people in the same family carrying the same gene can have different degrees of polydactyly or syndactyly.

Polydactyly and syndactyly are also possible outcomes of a large number of rare inherited and developmental disorders. One or both of them can be present in over 100 different disorders where they are minor features compared to other characteristics of these diseases.

For example, polydactyly is a characteristic of Meckel syndrome and Laurence-Moon-Biedl syndrome. Polydactyly may also be present in Patau's syndrome, asphyxiating thoracic dystrophy, hereditary spherocytic hemolytic anemia, Moebius syndrome, VACTERL association, and Klippel-Trenaunay syndrome.

Syndactyly is a characteristic of Apert syndrome, Poland syndrome, Jarcho-Levin syndrome, oral-facial-digital syndrome, Pfeiffer syndrome, and Edwards syndrome. Syndactyly may also occur with Gordon syndrome, Fraser syndrome, Greig cephalopolysyndactyly, phenylketonuria, Saethre-Chotzen syndrome, Russell-Silver syndrome, and triploidy.

In some isolated cases of polydactyly or syndactyly, it is not possible to determine the cause. Some of these cases might nevertheless be due to genetic defects; sometimes there is too little information to demonstrate

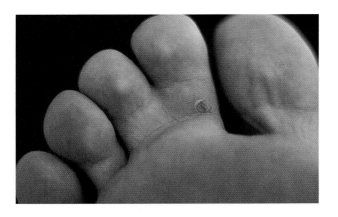

Syndactyly is the webbing or fusing together of two or more fingers or toes. *(Photograph by Keith, Custom Medical Stock Photo. Reproduced by permission.)*

a genetic cause. Some cases might be due to external factors like exposure to toxins or womb anomalies.

Diagnosis

Polydactyly and syndactyly can be diagnosed by external observation, x ray, and fetal sonogram.

Treatment

Polydactyly can be corrected by surgical removal of the extra digit or partial digit. Syndactyly can also be corrected surgically, usually with the addition of a skin graft from the groin.

Prognosis

The prognosis for isolated polydactyly and syndactyly is excellent. When polydactyly or syndactyly are part of a larger condition, the prognosis depends on the condition. Many of these conditions are quite serious, and early death may be the probable outcome.

Prevention

There is no known prevention for these conditions.

Resources

ORGANIZATIONS

March of Dimes Birth Defects Foundation. 1275 Mamaroneck Ave., White Plains, NY 10605. (914) 428-7100. resourcecenter@modimes.org. < http://www.modimes.org >.

National Institute of Child Health and Human Development. Bldg 31, Room 2A32, MSC 2425, 31 Center Drive, Bethesda, MD 20892-2425. (800) 505-2742. < http://www.nichd.nih.gov/sids/sids.htm >.

> **KEY TERMS**
>
> **Autosomal chromosome**—One of the non-X or non-Y chromosomes.
>
> **Congenital**—A condition present at birth.
>
> **Digit**—A finger or a toe.
>
> **Dominant trait**—A genetic trait that will always express itself when present as one of a pair of genes (as opposed to a recessive trait where two copies of the gene are necessary to give the individual the trait).
>
> **Gene**—A portion of a DNA molecule that either codes for a protein or RNA molecule or has a regulatory function.
>
> **Triploidy**—The condition where an individual has three entire sets of chromosomes instead of the usual two.
>
> **Trisomy**—An abnormal condition where three copies of one chromosome are present in the cells of an individual's body instead of two, the normal number.

OTHER

OMIM Home Page, Online Mendelian Inheritance in Man. < http://www.ncbi.nlm.nih.gov/Omim >.

Lorraine Lica, PhD

Polyendocrine deficiency syndromes *see* **Polyglandular deficiency syndromes**

Polyglandular deficiency syndromes

Definition

Polyglandular deficiency syndromes are disorders characterized by the failure of more than one endocrine gland to make hormones in sufficient quantities for the body to function normally.

Description

the endocrine system is a diverse group of glands located all over the body that work together to regulate the body's metabolic activities. It includes:

- the pituitary gland, located deep in the brain, is considered the "master gland" that regulates many of the others

- the thyroid gland is located in the neck and sets the metabolic speed of many processes,

- the parathyroid glands, attached to the back of the thyroid, regulate calcium balance,

- the adrenal glands are located on top of the kidneys and make four separate kinds of hormones,

- the gonads (sex organs) produce sex hormones,

- the pancreas is responsible for the production of digestive juices, insulin, and glucagon.

There are over a dozen different syndromes that involve failure of more than one endocrine gland.

Causes and symptoms

The cause of polyglandular deficiency syndromes is usually an autoimmune response—a condition in which the body generates antibodies to its own tissues. The immune system may attack one or more glands; however, because of their inter dependence, the destruction of one gland can often lead to the impairment of another. Other causes may include infectious disease; insufficient blood flow to the glands due to an obstruction such as a blood clot; or the presence of a tumor.

Doctors usually group polyglandular deficiency syndromes into three types:

- Type I occurs during childhood and is characterized by failure of the adrenals, parathyroids, thyroid, and gonads combined with hepatitis, hair loss, skin pigment changes, and inability of the bowel to absorb adequate **nutrition**. These children also get a persistent skin fungus infection called candidiasis.

- Type II occurs during adulthood and is characterized by failure of the adrenals, thyroid (Schmidt's syndrome), and gonads combined with similar nutritional failures and hair and skin changes. These patients also have **myasthenia gravis**. This type of polyglandular deficiency syndrome often produces insulin-dependent diabetes mellitus (IDDM).

- Type III disease may produce diabetes or adrenal failure combined with thyroid problems. It may also include baldness (**alopecia**), anemia, and **vitiligo** (condition characterized by white patches on normally pigmented skin).

Not all symptoms of any syndrome appear at once or in the same patient.

KEY TERMS

Antibody—A weapon in the body's immune defense arsenal that attacks a specific antigen.

Congenital—Present at birth.

Myasthenia gravis—A disease that causes muscle weakness.

Rubella—German measles.

Syndrome—A collection of abnormalities that occur often enough to suggest they have a common cause.

Diagnosis

Because these diseases evolve over time, the final diagnosis may not appear for years. A family history is very helpful in knowing what to expect. Any single endocrine abnormality should heighten suspicion that there are others, since they so often occur together, both as underproduction and overproduction of hormones. Most hormone levels can be monitored through blood tests. Many of the antibodies that characterize these conditions can also be found by blood testing.

Treatment

Fortunately there are replacements available for all the missing hormones. Careful balancing of them all can provide a reasonably comfortable quality of life for these patients.

Resources

BOOKS

Sherman, Steven I., and Robert F. Gagel. "Disorders Affecting Multiple Endocrine Systems." In *Harrison's Principles of Internal Medicine*, edited by Anthony S. Fauci, et al. New York: McGraw-Hill, 1997.

J. Ricker Polsdorfer, MD

Polyhydramnios and oligohydramnios

Definition

Polyhydramnios is a high level and oligohydramnios is low level of amniotic fluid.

Description

Amniotic fluid is the liquid that surrounds the developing fetus during **pregnancy**. It is contained within the amniotic membrane that forms the amniotic sac (bag of waters). During the first three months after conception (first trimester), amniotic fluid is mainly derived from the blood plasma that diffuses through the thin tissues of the fetus into the surrounding space. After the fetal kidneys form and become functional at about 10–11 weeks, fetal urine becomes the main source of amniotic fluid and remains so for the rest of the pregnancy. In addition, the lungs also produce liquid that becomes part of the amniotic fluid. Other contributions come from fetal oral and nasal secretions and from the fetal surface of the placenta. Amniotic fluid removal is largely due to fetal swallowing and absorption into the fetal blood. Uptake also occurs across the placental surface. The volume of amniotic fluid normally increases throughout pregnancy, reaching a peak at about 32–33 weeks and remaining fairly constant or decreasing slightly thereafter. There is a wide range of normal fluid volumes with an average of 700–800 ml at 32–33 weeks. Through the processes of swallowing and urination, a fetus can recycle the entire volume in less than 24 hours. Because the normal values for amniotic fluid volume increase during pregnancy, the actual volume that constitutes polyhydramnios is dependent on the gestational age of the fetus. During the last two months of pregnancy, polyhydramnios usually refers to amniotic fluid volumes greater than 1,700–1,900 ml. Severe cases are associated with much greater fluid volume excesses. The range of fluid values diagnostic of oligohydramnios is not as wide as that for polyhydramnios. Less than 300 ml, or lower than the 5% percentile for gestational age, is usually considered the upper threshold.

Causes and symptoms

Polyhydramnios, also referred to as hydramnios, can have any one of a number of causes related either to an underlying maternal or fetal condition. Maternal diabetes, which is associated with a macrosomic (enlarged) fetus, is a common cause. The medication lithium, used to treat depression, can also increase amniotic fluid levels. Twin gestations are prone to polyhydramnios. Infections passed from mother to fetus such as **rubella**, cytomegalovirus, and **toxoplasmosis**, can also result in damage to the fetus and elevated amniotic fluid levels. Fetal abnormalities, including many that are life-threatening or lead to a significant impairment in the quality of life, are found in up to a quarter of all patients. For this reason, the initial finding of excess amniotic fluid should be followed by thorough diagnostic studies to determine the cause and the prognosis.

Because fetal swallowing is a major factor in amniotic fluid removal, fetal abnormalities that prevent fluid uptake should be investigated. These include gastrointestinal obstructions such as **esophageal atresia** and duodenal atresia, as well as neurological conditions that affect swallowing including anencephaly. Certain cardiac abnormalities, kidney disorders, and genetic conditions such as **myotonic dystrophy** and alpha-thalassemia can also cause polyhydramnios. Fetal chromosome abnormalities are frequently associated with elevated amniotic fluid levels. The more severe the polyhydramnios the more likely it is that fetal abnormalities will be present. In addition, there are other, infrequent causes, and in a number of cases, no cause can be found. Polyhydramnios can lead to maternal abdominal discomfort and respiratory difficulties as well as preterm labor. When polyhydramnios is associated with fetal abnormalities, perinatal mortality is significantly increased.

Oligohydramnios is most commonly associated with abnormalities of the fetal kidneys. Since fetal urine is the main source of amniotic fluid in the latter two-thirds of pregnancy, any condition that interferes with fetal urine production can lead to oligohydramnios. Renal agenesis, cystic kidneys, and bladder outlet obstructions are common. Meckel-Gruber syndrome, a lethal autosomal recessive genetic disorder featuring brain and kidney abnormalities and extra digits is one specific cause. Placental insufficiency and fetal growh retardation can also result in oligohydramnios. **Premature rupture of membranes**, especially between 16 and 24 weeks is another cause and, because amniotic fluid is important in lung growth, it can lead to underdevelopment of the lungs (pulmonary hypoplasia). In general, regardless of the cause, oligohydramnios that arises early in a pregnancy, can cause hypoplastic lungs. It can also result in space limitations within the amniotic sac that cause fetal compression and orthopedic abnormalities such as clubbed feet in the newborn. In general, oligohydramnios that begins near the time of delivery is associated with a better outcome than cases than have an onset earlier in pregnancy.

Diagnosis

In current obstetrical practice, polyhydramnios and oligohydramnios are usually detected during a routine prenatal ultrasound. If the ultrasonographer suspects that excess or reduced fluid is present, it is customary to take measurements of pockets of fluid visualized around the fetus, calculate the amniotic fluid index (AFI), and compare it to AFI values found in standard tables. Subsequent ultrasound measurements can then be used to track the increase or decrease in fluid.

It is extremely important that the cause of an abnormal AFI be sought. Because of the high risk of fetal abnormalities, detailed ultrasound exams (targeted exams) should then be performed. The mother should be counseled about the possible complications and offered additional testing as necessary. For example, an **amniocentesis** for prenatal chromosome analysis may be important because of the high risk of fetal chromosome abnormalities. This test is usually indicated if fetal abnormalities are suspected on the basis of the ultrasound exam. An amniocentesis can also be used to check for fetal infections and some rare single gene defects.

Treatment

Effective treatments for polyhydramnios and oligohydramnios are limited. To relieve maternal discomfort, an excess fluid level can be reduced by inserting a needle into the amniotic sac and using a syringe to withdraw excess fluid. This can be done repeatedly, if necessary. In oligohydramnios, the opposite approach of adding fluid either by increasing oral intake in the mother or by directly infusing saline into the amniotic sac has been tried in select cases. If the cause of oligohydramnios is a fetal bladder obstruction, it may be possible to place a small tube in the bladder to shunt the fluid into the amniotic sac.

Alternative treatment

In select cases where polyhydramnios is thought to be due to an increased output of fetal urine, the drug indomethicin has been used with some success, but there is concern about side effects, particularly on the fetus. Another similar drug, sulindac, is currently being investigated. If oligohydramnios is due to premature rupture of the membranes, a protocol to manage complications should be instituted.

Prognosis

The prognosis for both polyhydramnios and oligohydramnios depends on the cause. If excess or reduced amniotic fluid is the result of an underlying

fetal abnormality, the nature of that abnormality will determine the prognosis. This is one reason why it is important to perform the necessary follow-up studies. A woman who has been diagnosed with polyhydramnios or oligohydramnios needs to be made fully aware of the types of testing available and carefully counseled about the diagnosis and its impact on the chance for a successful pregnancy outcome and a healthy infant.

Prevention

In order to prevent polyhydramnios or oligohydramnios, it would be necessary to prevent the underlying cause. Good control of maternal diabetes and the prevention of infections transmittable from mother to fetus are two approaches for a subset of cases, but, in general, prevention is not possible.

Resources

BOOKS

Cunningham, F. Gary. *Williams Obstetrics.* New York; McGraw-Hill, 2001

Rodeck, Charles H., and Martin J. Whittle. *Fetal Medicine, Basic Science and Clinical Practice.* New York, Churchill Livingstone, 1999.

PERIODICALS

Kilpactrick, Sarah J. "Therapeutic Interventions for Oligohydramnios: Amnioinfusion and Maternal Hydration" *Clinical Obstetric and GYN* 40, no. 2 (June 1996): 266-279.

Sallie Boineau Freeman, PhD

Polymyalgia rheumatica

Definition

Polymyalgia rheumatica is a syndrome that causes **pain** and stiffness in the hips and shoulders of people over the age of 50.

Description

Although the major characteristics of this condition are just pain and stiffness, there are reasons to believe it is more than just old-fashioned rheumatism. Patients are commonly so afflicted that their muscles atrophy from disuse. A similar complaint of such weakness is also seen in serious muscle diseases. Moreover, some patients develop arthritis or a disease called giant cell arteritis or **temporal arteritis.**

Causes and symptoms

This condition may arise as often as once in every 2,000 people. Rarely does it affect people under 50 years old. The average age is 70; women are afflicted twice as often as men. Along with the pain and stiffness of larger muscles, **headache** may add to the discomfort. The scalp is often tender. Pain is usually worse at night. There may be fever and weight loss before the full disease appears. Patients complain that stiffness is worse in the morning and returns if they have been inactive for any period of time, a condition called gelling. Sometimes the stiffness is severe enough that it causes frozen shoulder.

KEY TERMS

Anemia—A condition in which the blood lacks enough red blood cells (hemoglobin).

Atrophy—Wasting away of a body part.

Frozen shoulder—A shoulder that becomes scarred and cannot move.

Giant cell arteritis—Also called temporal arteritis. A condition which causes the inflammation of temporal arteries. It can cause blindness when the inflammation effects the ophthalmic artery.

NSAIDs—Non-steroidal anti-inflammatory drugs like aspirin, ibuprofen, and naproxen.

Syndrome—A collection of abnormalities that occur often enough to suggest they have a common cause.

Diagnosis

Symptoms are usually present for over a month by the time patients seek medical attention. A mild anemia is often is often present. One blood test, called an erythrocyte sedimentation rate, is very high, much more so than in most other diseases. The most important issue in evaluating polymyalgia rheumatica is to check for giant cell arteritis. Giant cell arteritis can lead to blindness if lift untreated.

Treatment

Polymyalgia rheumatica responds dramatically to cortisone-like drugs in modest doses. In fact, one part of confirming the diagnosis is to observe the response to this treatment. It may also respond to **nonsteroidal anti-inflammatory drugs** (NSAIDs). Temporal arteritis is also treated with cortisone, but in higher doses.

Prognosis

The disease often remits after a while, with no further treatment required.

Resources

BOOKS

Griggs, Robert C. "Episodic Muscle Spasms, Cramps, andWeakness." In *Harrison's Principles of Internal Medicine*, edited by Anthony S. Fauci, et al. New York: McGraw-Hill, 1997.

J. Ricker Polsdorfer, MD

Polymyositis

Definition

Polymyositis is an inflammatory muscle disease causing weakness and **pain**. **Dermatomyositis** is identical to polymyositis with the addition of a characteristic skin rash.

Description

Polymyositis (PM) is an inflammatory disorder in which muscle tissue becomes inflamed and deteriorates, causing weakness and pain. It is one of several types of inflammatory muscle disease, or myopathy. Others include dermatomyositis (DM) and inclusion body **myositis**. All three types are progressive conditions, usually beginning in adulthood. A fourth type, juvenile dermatomyositis, occurs in children. Although PM and DM can occur at any age, 60% of cases appear between the ages of 30 and 60. Females are affected twice as often as males.

Causes and symptoms

Causes

The cause of PM and DM is not known, but it is suspected that a variety of factors may play a role in the development of these diseases. PM and DM may be autoimmune diseases, caused by the immune system's attack on the body's own tissue. The reason for this attack is unknown, although some researchers believe that a combination of immune system susceptibility and an environmental trigger may explain at least some cases. Known environmental agents associated with PM and DM include infectious agents such as *Toxoplasma*, *Borrella* (**Lyme disease** bacterium), and coxsackievirus. Most cases, however, have no obvious triggers (direct causative agents). There may also be a genetic component in the development of PM and DM.

Symptoms

The early symptoms of PM and DM are slowly progressing muscle weakness, usually symmetrical between the two sides of the body. PM and DM affect primarily the muscles of the trunk and those closest to the trunk, while the hands, feet, and face usually are not involved. Weakness may cause difficulty walking, standing, and lifting objects. Rarely, the muscles of breathing may be affected. Weakness of themuscles used for swallowing can cause difficulty with swallowing (dysphagia). Joint pain and/or swelling also may be present. Later in the course of these diseases, muscle wasting or shortening (contracture) may develop in the arms or legs. Heart abnormalities, including electrocardiogram (ECG) changes and **arrhythmias**, develop at some time during the coursed of these diseases in about 30% of patients.

Dermatomyositis is marked by a skin rash. The rash is dusky, reddish, or lilac in color, and is most often seen on the eyelids, cheeks, bridge of the nose, and knuckles, as well as on the back, upper chest, knees, and elbows. The rash often appears before the muscle weakness.

Diagnosis

PM and DM are often difficult diseases to diagnose, because they are rare, because symptoms come on slowly, and because they can be mistaken for other diseases that cause muscle weakness, especially limb girdle **muscular dystrophy**.

Accurate diagnosis involves:

- A neurological exam.

- Blood tests to determine the level of the muscle enzyme creatine kinase, whose presence in the circulation indicates muscle damage.

- Electromyography, an electrical test of muscle function.

- Muscle biopsy, in which a small sample of affected muscle is surgically removed for microscopic analysis. A biopsy revealing muscle cells surrounded by immune system cells is a strong indicator of myositis.

Treatment

PM and DM respond to high doses of immunosuppressant drugs in most cases. The most common medication used is the corticosteroid prednisone. Prednisone therapy usually leads to improvement within two or three months, at which point the dose can be tapered to a lower level to avoid the significant side effects associated with high doses of prednisone. Unresponsive patients are often given a replacement or supplementary immunosuppressant, such as azathioprine, cyclosporine, or methotrexate. Intravenous immunoglobulin treatments may help some people who are unresponsive to other immunosuppressants.

Pain can usually be controlled with an over-the-counter analgesic, such as **aspirin**, ibuprofen, or naproxen. A speech-language therapist can help suggest exercises and tips to improve difficulty in swallowing. Avoiding weight gain helps prevent overtaxing weakened muscles.

Alternative treatment

As with all autoimmune conditions, food allergies/intolerances and environmental triggers may be contributing factors. For **food allergies** and intolerances, an elimination challenge diet can be used under the supervision of a trained practitioner, naturopath, or nutritionist, to identify trigger foods. These foods can then be eliminated from the person's diet. For environmental triggers, it is helpful to identify the source so that it can be avoided or eliminated. A thorough **detoxification** program can help alleviate symptoms and change the course of the disease. Dietary changes from processed foods to whole foods that do not include allergen triggers can have significant results. Nutrient supplements, especially the antioxidants zinc, selenium, and **vitamins** A, C, and E, can be beneficial. Constitutional homeopathic treatment can work at a deep level to rebalance the whole person. **Acupuncture** and Chinese herbs can be effective in symptom alleviation and deep healing. Visualization, guided imagery, and hypnosis for **pain management** are also useful.

Prognosis

The progression of PM and DM varies considerably from person to person. Immunosuppressants can improve strength, although not all patients respond, and relapses may occur. PM and DM can lead to increasing weakness and disability, although the life span usually is not significantly affected. About half of the patients recover and can discontinue treatment within five years of the onset of their symptoms. About 20% still have active disease requiring ongoing treatment after five years, and about 30% have inactive disease but some remaining muscle weakness.

Prevention

There is no known way to prevent myositis, except to avoid exposure to those environmental agents that may be associated with some cases.

Resources

ORGANIZATIONS

Dermatomyositis and Polymyositis Support Group. 146 Newtown Road, Southampton, SO2 9HR, U.K.

Muscular Dystrophy Association. 3300 East Sunrise Drive, Tucson, AZ 85718. (800) 572-1717. <http://www.mdausa.org>.

Myositis Association of America. 600-D University Boulevard, Harrisonburg, VA 22801. (540) 433-7686. <http://www.myositis.org>.

National Institutes of Health. National Institute of Arthritis and Musculoskeletal and Skin Diseases. 900 Rockville Pike, Bethesda, MD 20892. (301) 496-8188. <http://www.hih.gov.niams>.

Richard Robinson

Polyneuritis *see* **Peripheral neuropathy**

Polysomnography

Definition

The word polysomnography, derived from the Greek roots "poly," meaning many, "somno," meaning sleep, and "graphy" meaning to write, refers to multiple tests performed on patients while they sleep. Polysomnography is an overnight test to evaluate **sleep disorders**. Polysomnography generally includes monitoring of the patient's airflow through the nose and mouth, blood pressure, electrocardiographic activity, blood oxygen level, brain wave pattern, eye movement, and the movement of respiratory muscle and limbs.

Purpose

Polysomnography is used to help diagnose and evaluate a number of sleep disorders. For instance, it can help diagnose **sleep apnea**, a common disorder in middle-aged and elderly obese men, in which the muscles of the soft palate in the back of the throat relax and close off the airway during sleep. This may cause the person to snore loudly and gasp for air at night, and to be excessively sleepy and doze off during the day. Another syndrome often evaluated by polysomnography is **narcolepsy**. In narcolepsy, people have sudden attacks of sleep and/or cataplexy (temporary loss of muscle tone caused by moments of emotion, such as fear, anger, or surprise, which causes people to slump or fall over), sleep **paralysis** or **hallucinations** at the onset of sleep. Polysomnography is often used to evaluate parasomnias (abnormal behaviors or movements during sleep), such as sleep walking, talking in one's sleep, nightmares, and bedwetting. It can also be used to detect or evaluate seizures that occur in the middle of the night, when the patient and his or her family are unlikely to be aware of them.

Precautions

Polysomnography is extremely safe and no special precautions need to be taken.

Description

Polysomnography requires an overnight stay in a sleep laboratory. During this stay, while the patient sleeps, he or she is monitored in a number of ways that can provide very useful information.

One form of monitoring is **electroencephalography** (EEG), in which electrodes are attached to the patient's scalp in order to record his or her brain wave activity. The electroencephalograph records brain wave activity from different parts of the brain and charts them on a graph. The EEG not only helps doctors establish what stage of sleep the patient is in, but may also detect seizures.

Another form of monitoring is continuous electro-oculography (EOG), which records eye movement and is used to determine when the patient is going through a stage of sleep called rapid-eye-movement (REM) sleep. Both EEG and EOG can be helpful in determining sleep latency (the time that transpires between lights out and the onset of sleep), total sleep time, the time spent in each sleep stage, and the number of arousals from sleep.

The air flow through the patient's nose and mouth are measured by heat-sensitive devices called thermistors. This can help detect episodes of apnea (stopped breathing), or hypnopea (inadequate breathing). Another test called pulse oximetry measures the amount of oxygen in the blood, and can be used to assess the degree of oxygen **starvation** during episodes of hypnopea or apnea.

The electrical activity of the patient's heart is also measured on an electrocardiogram, or ECG. Electrodes are affixed to the patient's chest and they pick up electrical activity from various areas of the heart. They help detect cardiac arrythmias (abnormal heart rhythms), which may occur during periods of sleep apnea. Blood pressure is also measured: sometimes episodes of sleep apnea can dangerously elevate blood pressure.

In some cases, sleep laboratories monitor the movement of limbs during sleep. This can be helpful in detecting such sleep disorders as periodic limb movements.

Preparation

The patient may be asked to discontinue taking any medications used to help him/her sleep. Before the patient goes to sleep, the technician hooks him or her up to all of the monitors being used.

Aftercare

Once the test is over, the monitors are detached from the patient. No special measures need to be taken after polysomnography.

Normal results

A normal result in polysomnography shows normal results for all parameters (EEG, ECG, blood pressure, eye movement, air flow, pulse oximetry, etc.) monitored throughout all stages of sleep.

Abnormal results

Polysomnography may yield a number of abnormal results, indicating a number of potential disorders. For instance, abnormal transitions in and out of various stages of sleep, as documented by the EEG and the EOG, may be a sign of narcolepsy. Reduced air flow through the nose and mouth, along with a fall in oxygenation of the blood, may indicate apnea or hypopnea. If apnea is accompanied by abnormalities in ECG or elevations in blood pressure, this can indicate that sleep apnea may be particularly harmful. Frequent movement of limbs may indicate a sleep disorder called periodic limb movement.

Resources

ORGANIZATIONS

National Heart, Lung and Blood Institute. P.O. Box 30105, Bethesda, MD 20824-0105. (301) 251-1222. < http://www.nhlbi.nih.gov >.

Robert Scott Dinsmoor

Pompe's disease *see* **Glycogen storage diseases**

Porphyrias

Definition

The porphyrias are disorders in which the body produces too much porphyrin and insufficient heme (an iron-containing nonprotein portion of the hemoglobin molecule). Porphyrin is a foundation structure for heme and certain enzymes. Excess porphyrins are excreted as waste in the urine and stool. Overproduction and overexcretion of porphyrins causes low, unhealthy levels of heme and certain important enzymes, creating various physical symptoms.

Description

Biosynthesis of heme is a multistep process that begins with simple molecules and ends with a large, complex heme molecule. Each step of the chemical pathway is directed by its own task-specific protein, called an enzyme. As a heme precursor molecule moves through each step, an enzyme modifies the precursor in some way. If a precursor molecule is not modified, it cannot proceed to the next step, causing a buildup of that specific precursor.

This situation is the main characteristic of the porphyrias. Owing to a defect in one of the enzymes of the heme biosynthesis pathway, protoporphyrins or porphyrins (heme precursors) are prevented from proceeding further along the pathway. These precursors accumulate at the stage of the enzyme defect causing an array of physical symptoms in an affected person. Specific symptoms depend on the point at which heme biosynthesis is blocked and which precursors accumulate. In general, the porphyrias primarily affect the skin and the nervous system. Symptoms can be debilitating or life threatening in some cases. Porphyria is most commonly an inherited condition. It can also, however, be acquired after exposure to poisonous substances.

Heme

Heme is produced in several tissues in the body, but its primary biosynthesis sites are the liver and the bone marrow. Heme synthesis for immature red blood cells, namely the erythroblasts and the reticulocytes, occurs in the bone marrow.

Although production is concentrated in the liver and bone marrow, heme is utilized in various capacities in virtually every tissue in the body. In most cells, heme is a key building block in the construction of factors that oversee metabolism and transport of oxygen and energy. In the liver, heme is a component of several vital enzymes, particularly cytochrome P450. Cytochrome P450 is involved in the metabolism of chemicals, **vitamins**, fatty acids, and hormones; it is very important in transforming toxic substances into easily excretable materials. In immature red blood cells, heme is the featured component of hemoglobin. Hemoglobin is the red pigment that gives red blood cells their characteristic color and their essential ability to transport oxygen.

Heme biosynthesis

The heme molecule is composed of porphyrin and an iron atom. Much of the heme biosynthesis pathway is dedicated to constructing the porphyrin molecule. Porphyrin is a large molecule shaped like a four-leaf clover. An iron atom is placed at its center point in the last step of heme biosynthesis.

The production of heme may be compared to a factory assembly line. At the start of the line, raw materials are fed into the process. At specific points along the line, an addition or adjustment is made to further development. Once additions and adjustments are complete, the final product rolls off the end of the line.

The heme "assembly line" is an eight-step process, requiring eight different and properly functioning enzymes:

1. delta-aminolevulinic acid synthase
2. delta-aminolevulinic acid dehydratase
3. porphobilogen deaminase
4. uroporphyrinogen III cosynthase
5. uroporphyrinogen decarboxylase
6. coproporphyrinogen oxidase
7. protoporphyrinogen oxidase
8. ferrochelatase

The control of heme biosynthesis is complex. Various chemical signals can trigger increased or decreased production. These signals can affect the enzymes themselves or the production of these enzymes, starting at the genetic level. For example, one point at which heme biosynthesis may be controlled is at the first step. When heme levels are low, greater quantities of delta-aminolevulinic acid (ALA) synthase are produced. As a result, larger quantities of heme precursors are fed into the biosynthesis pathway to step up heme production.

Porphyrias

Under normal circumstances, when heme concentrations are at an appropriate level, precursor production decreases. However, a glitch in the biosynthesis pathway—represented by a defective enzyme—means that heme biosynthesis does not reach completion. Because heme levels remain low, the synthesis pathway continues to churn out precursor molecules in an attempt to correct the heme deficit.

The net effect of this continued production is an abnormal accumulation of precursor molecules and development of some type of porphyria. Each type of porphyria corresponds with a specific enzyme defect and an accumulation of the associated precursor. Although there are eight steps in heme biosynthesis, there are only seven types of porphyrias; a defect in ALA synthase activity does not have a corresponding porphyria.

Enzymes involved in heme biosynthesis display subtle, tissue-specific variations; therefore, heme biosynthesis may be impeded in the liver, but normal in the immature red blood cells, or vice versa. Incidence of porphyria varies widely between types and occasionally by geographic location. Although certain porphyrias are more common than others, their greater frequency is only relative to other types. All porphyrias are considered to be rare disorders.

In the past, the porphyrias were divided into two general categories based on the location of the porphyrin production. Porphyrias affecting heme biosynthesis in the liver were referred to as hepatic porphyrias. Porphyrias that affect heme biosynthesis in immature red blood cells were referred to as erythropoietic porphyrias (erythropoiesis is the process through which red blood cells are produced). As of 2001, porphyrias were usually grouped into acute and non-acute types. Acute porphyrias produce severe attacks of **pain** and neurological effects. Non-acute porphyrias present as chronic diseases.

The acute porphyrias, and the heme biosynthesis steps at which enzyme defects occur, are:

- ALA dehydratase deficiency porphyria (step 2). This porphyria type is very rare. The inheritance pattern appears to be autosomal recessive. In autosomal recessively inherited disorders, a person must inherit two defective genes, one from each parent. A parent with only one gene for an autosomal recessive disorder does not display symptoms of the disease.

- Acute intermittent porphyria (step 3). Acute intermittent porphyria (AIP) is also known as Swedish porphyria, pyrroloporphyria, and intermittent acute porphyria. AIP is inherited as an autosomal dominant trait, which means that only one copy of the defective gene needs to be present for the disorder to occur. Simply inheriting this gene, however, does not necessarily mean that a person will develop the disease. Approximately five to 10 per 100,000 people in the United States carry a gene for AIP, but only 10% of these people ever develop symptoms of the disease.

- Hereditary coproporphyria (step 6). Hereditary coproporphyria (HCP) is inherited in an autosomal dominant manner. As with all porphyrias, it is an uncommon ailment. By 1977, only 111 cases of HCP were recorded; in Denmark, the estimated incidence is two in one million people.

- Variegate porphyria (step 7). Variegate porphyria (VP) is also known as porphyria variegata, protocoproporphyria, South African genetic porphyria, and Royal malady (supposedly King George III of England and Mary, Queen of Scots, suffered from VP). VP is inherited in an autosomal dominant manner and is especially prominent in South Africans of Dutch descent. Among that population, the incidence is approximately three in 1,000 persons. It is estimated that there are 10,000 cases of VP in South Africa. Interestingly, it appears that the affected South Africans are descendants of two Dutch settlers who came to South Africa in 1680. Among other populations, the incidence of VP is estimated to be one to two cases per 100,000 persons.

The non-acute porphyrias, and the steps of heme biosynthesis at which they occur, are:

- Congenital erythropoietic porphyria (step 4). Congenital erythropoietic porphyria (CEP) is also called Gunther's disease, erythropoietic porphyria, congenital porphyria, congenital hematoporphyria, and erythropoietic uroporphyria. CEP is inherited in an autosomal recessive manner. It is a rare disease, estimated to affect fewer than one in one million people. Onset of dramatic symptoms usually occurs in infancy, but may hold off until adulthood.

- Porphyria cutanea tarda (step 5). Porphyria cutanea tarda (PCT) is also called symptomatic porphyria, porphyria cutanea symptomatica, and idiosyncratic porphyria. PCT may be acquired, typically as a result of disease (especially **hepatitis C**), drug or alcohol use, or exposure to certain poisons. PCT may also be inherited as an autosomal dominant disorder, however most people remain latent—that is, symptoms never develop. PCT is the most common of the porphyrias, but the incidence of PCT is not well defined.

- Hepatoerythopoietic porphyria (step 5). Hepatoerythopoietic porphyria (HEP) affects heme biosynthesis in both the liver and the bone marrow. HEP results from a defect in uroporphyrinogen decarboxylase activity (step 5), and is caused by defects in the same gene as PCT. Disease symptoms, however, strongly resemble congenital erythropoietic porphyria. HEP seems to be inherited in an autosomal recessive manner.

- Erythropoietic protoporphyria (step 8). Also known as protoporphyria and erythrohepatic protoporphyria, erythropoietic protoporphyria (EPP) is more common than CEP; more than 300 cases have been reported. In these cases, onset of symptoms typically occurred in childhood.

Causes and symptoms

General characteristics

The underlying cause of all porphyrias is a defective enzyme important to the heme biosynthesis pathway. Porphyrias are inheritable conditions. In virtually all cases of porphyria an inherited factor causes the enzyme's defect. An environmental trigger—such as diet, drugs, or sun exposure—may be necessary before any symptoms develop. In many cases, symptoms do not develop. These asymptomatic individuals may be completely unaware that they have a gene for porphyria.

All of the hepatic porphyrias—except porphyria cutanea tarda—follow a pattern of acute attacks separated by periods during which no symptoms are present. For this reason, this group is often referred to as the acute porphyrias. The erythropoietic porphyrias and porphyria cutanea tarda do not follow this pattern and are considered to be chronic conditions.

The specific symptoms of each porphyria vary based on which enzyme is affected and whether that enzyme occurs in the liver or in the bone marrow. The severity of symptoms can vary widely, even within the same type of porphyria. If the porphyria becomes symptomatic, the common factor between all types is an abnormal accumulation of protoporphyrins or porphyrin.

ALA dehydratase porphyria (ADP)

ADP is characterized by a deficiency of ALA dehydratase. ADP is caused by mutations in the delta-aminolevulinate dehydratase gene (ALAD) at 9q34. Of the few cases on record, the prominent symptoms are **vomiting**, pain in the abdomen, arms, and legs, and neuropathy. (Neuropathy refers to nerve damage that can cause pain, **numbness**, or paralysis.) The nerve damage associated with ADP could cause breathing impairment or lead to weakness or **paralysis** of the arms and legs.

Acute intermittent porphyria (AIP)

AIP is caused by a deficiency of porphobilogen deaminase, which occurs due to mutations in the hydroxymethylbilane synthase gene (HMBS) located at 11q23.3. Symptoms of AIP usually do not occur unless a person with the deficiency encounters a trigger substance. Trigger substances can include hormones (for example oral contraceptives, menstruation, **pregnancy**), drugs, and dietary factors. Most people with this deficiency never develop symptoms.

Attacks occur after **puberty** and commonly feature severe abdominal pain, **nausea**, vomiting, and **constipation**. Muscle weakness and pain in the back, arms, and legs are also typical symptoms. During an attack, the urine is a deep reddish color. The central nervous system may also be involved. Possible psychological symptoms include **hallucinations**, confusion, seizures, and mood changes.

Congenital erythropoietic porphyria (CEP)

CEP is caused by a deficiency of uroporphyrinogen III cosynthase due to mutations in the uroporphyrinogen III cosynthase gene (UROS) located at 10q25.2-q26.3. Symptoms are often apparent in infancy and include reddish urine and possibly an enlarged spleen. The skin is unusually sensitive to light and blisters easily if exposed to sunlight. (Sunlight induces protoporphyrin changes in the plasma and skin. These altered protoporphyrin molecules can cause skin damage.) Increased hair growth is common. Damage from recurrent blistering and associated skin infections can be severe. In some cases facial features and fingers may be lost to recurrent damage and infection. Deposits of protoporphyrins can sometimes lead to red staining of the teeth and bones.

Porphyria cutanea tarda (PCT)

PCT is caused by deficient uroporphyrinogen decarboxylase. PCT is caused by mutations in the uroporphyrinogen decarboxylase gene (UROD) located at 1p34. PCT may occur as an acquired or an inherited condition. The acquired form usually does not appear until adulthood. The inherited form may appear in childhood, but often demonstrates no symptoms. Early symptoms include blistering on the hands, face, and arms following minor injuries or exposure to sunlight. Lightening or darkening of the skin may occur along with increased hair growth or loss of hair. Liver function is abnormal but the signs are mild.

Hepatoerythopoietic porphyria (HEP)

HEP is linked to a deficiency of uroporphyrinogen decarboxylase in both the liver and the bone marrow. HEP is an autosomal recessive disease caused by mutations in the gene responsible for PCT, the uroporphyrinogen decarboxylase gene (UROD), located at 1p34. The gene is shared, but the mutations, inheritance, and specific symptoms of these two diseases are different. The symptoms of HEP resemble those of CEP.

Hereditary coproporphyria (HCP)

HCP is similar to AIP, but the symptoms are typically milder. HCP is caused by a deficiency of coproporphyrinogen oxidase due to mutations in a gene by the same name at 3q12. The greatest difference between HCP and AIP is that people with HCP may have some skin sensitivity to sunlight. However, extensive damage to the skin is rarely seen.

Variegate porphyria (VP)

VP is caused by a deficiency of protoporphyrinogen oxidase. There is scientific evidence that VP is caused by mutation in the gene for protoporphyrinogen oxidase located at 1q22. Like AIP, symptoms of VP occur only during attacks. Major symptoms of this type of porphyria include neurological problems and sensitivity to light. Areas of the skin that are exposed to sunlight are susceptible to burning, blistering, and scarring.

Erythropoietic protoporphyria (EPP)

Owing to deficient ferrochelatase, the last step in the heme biosynthesis pathway—the insertion of an iron atom into a porphyrin molecule—cannot be completed. This enzyme deficiency is caused by mutations in the ferrochelatase gene (FECH) located at 18q21.3. The major symptoms of this disorder are related to sensitivity to light—including both artificial and natural light sources. Following exposure to light, a person with EPP experiences burning, **itching**, swelling, and reddening of the skin. Blistering and scarring may occur but are neither common nor severe. EPP is associated with increased risks for **gallstones** and liver complications. Symptoms can appear in childhood and tend to be more severe during the summer when exposure to sunlight is more likely.

Diagnosis

Depending on the array of symptoms an individual may exhibit, the possibility of porphyria may not immediately come to a physician's mind. In the absence of a family history of porphyria, non-specific symptoms, such as abdominal pain and vomiting, may be attributed to other disorders. Neurological symptoms, including confusion and hallucinations, can lead to an initial suspicion of psychiatric disease. Diagnosis is more easily accomplished in cases in which non-specific symptoms appear in combination with symptoms more specific to porphyria, like neuropathy, sensitivity to sunlight, or certain other manifestations. Certain symptoms, such as urine the color of port wine, are hallmark signs very specific to porphyria. DNA analysis is not yet of routine diagnostic value.

A common initial test measures protoporphyrins in the urine. However, if skin sensitivity to light is a symptom, a blood plasma test is indicated. If these tests reveal abnormal levels of protoporphyrins, further tests are done to measure heme precursor levels in red blood cells and the stool. The presence and estimated quantity of porphyrin and protoporphyrins in biological samples are easily detected using spectrofluorometric testing. Spectrofluorometric testing uses a spectrofluorometer that directs light of a specific strength at a fluid sample. The porphyrins and protoporphyrins in the sample absorb the light energy and fluoresce, or glow. The spectrofluorometer detects and measures fluorescence, which indicates the amount of porphyrins and protoporphyrins in the sample.

Whether heme precursors occur in the blood, urine, or stool gives some indication of the type of porphyria, but more detailed biochemical testing is required to determine their exact identity. Making this determination yields a strong indicator of which enzyme in the heme biosynthesis pathway is defective; which, in turn, allows a diagnosis of the particular type of porphyria.

Biochemical tests rely on the color, chemical properties, and other unique features of each heme precursor. For example, a screening test for acute intermittent porphyria (AIP) is the Watson-Schwartz test. In this test, a special dye is added to a urine sample. If one of two heme precursors—porphobilinogen or urobilinogen—is present, the sample turns pink or red. Further testing is necessary to determine whether the precursor present is porphobilinogen or urobilinogen—only porphobilinogen is indicative of AIP.

Other biochemical tests rely on the fact that heme precursors become less soluble in water (able to be dissolved in water) as they progress further through the heme biosynthesis pathway. For example, to determine whether the Watson-Schwartz urine test is positive for porphobilinogen or urobilinogen, chloroform is added to the test tube. Chloroform is a water-insoluble substance. Even after vigorous mixing, the water and chloroform separate into two distinct layers.

Urobilinogen is slightly insoluble in water, while porphobilinogen tends to be water soluble. The porphobilinogen mixes more readily in water than chloroform, so if the water layer is pink (from the dye added to the urine sample), that indicates the presence of porphobilinogen, and a diagnosis of AIP is probable.

As a final test, measuring specific enzymes and their activities may be done for some types of porphyrias; however, such tests are not done as a screening method. Certain enzymes, such as porphobilinogen deaminase (the defective enzyme in AIP), can be easily extracted from red blood cells; other enzymes, however, are less readily collected or tested. Basically, an enzyme test involves adding a certain amount of the enzyme to a test tube that contains the precursor it is supposed to modify. Both the production of modified precursor and the rate at which it appears can be measured using laboratory equipment. If a modified precursor is produced, the test indicates that the enzyme is doing its job. The rate at which the modified precursor is produced can be compared to a standard to measure the efficiency of the enzyme.

Treatment

Treatment for porphyria revolves around avoiding acute attacks, limiting potential effects, and treating symptoms. Treatment options vary depending on the specific type of porphyria diagnosed. **Gene therapy** has been successful for both CEP and EPP. In the future, scientists expect development of gene therapy for the remaining porphyrias. Given the rarity of ALA dehydratase porphyria, definitive treatment guidelines for this rare type have not been developed.

Acute intermittent porphyria, hereditary coproporphyria, and variegate porphyria

Treatment for acute intermittent porphyria, hereditary coproporphyria, and variegate porphyria follows the same basic regime. A person who has been diagnosed with one of these porphyrias can prevent most attacks by avoiding precipitating factors, such as certain drugs that have been identified as triggers for acute porphyria attacks. Individuals must maintain adequate nutrition, particularly with respect to carbohydrates. In some cases, an attack can be stopped by increasing carbohydrate consumption or by receiving carbohydrates intravenously. In 2004, a report from Turkey revealed successful treatment of an acute intermittent porphyria attack with a drug called fluoxetine.

When attacks occur prompt medical attention is necessary. Pain is usually severe, and narcotic **analgesics** are the best option for relief. Phenothiazines can be used to counter nausea, vomiting, and **anxiety**, and chloral hydrate or diazepam is useful for **sedation** or to induce sleep. Hematin, a drug administered intravenously, may be used to halt an attack. Hematin seems to work by signaling the pathway of heme biosynthesis to slow production of precursors. Women, who tend to develop symptoms more frequently than men owing to hormonal fluctuations, may find ovulation-inhibiting hormone therapy to be helpful.

Gene therapy is a possible future treatment for these porphyrias. An experimental animal model of AIP has been developed and research is in progress.

Congenital erythropoietic porphyria

The key points of congenital erythropoietic porphyria treatment are avoiding exposure to sunlight and prevention of skin trauma or skin infection. Liberal use of **sunscreens** and consumption of beta-carotene supplements can provide some protection from sun-induced damage. Medical treatments such as removing the spleen or administering transfusions of red blood cells can create short-term benefits, but these treatments do not offer a cure. Remission can sometimes be achieved after treatment with oral doses of activated charcoal. Severely affected patients may be offered bone marrow transplantation which appears to confer long-term benefit.

Porphyria cutanea tarda

As with other porphyrias, the first line of defense is avoidance of factors, especially alcohol, that could bring about symptoms. Regular blood withdrawal is a proven therapy for pushing symptoms into remission. If an individual is anemic or cannot have blood drawn for other reasons, chloroquine therapy may be used.

Erythropoietic protoporphyria

Avoiding sunlight, using sunscreens, and taking beta-carotene supplements are typical treatment options for erythropoietic protoporphyria. The drug cholestyramine may reduce the skin's sensitivity to sunlight as well as the accumulated heme precursors in the liver. **Liver transplantation** has been used in cases of liver failure. In 2004, a report in a medical journal told of one case of successful treatment of a 19-year-old patient with acute intermittent porphyria with liver transplantation. While she had only been studied for 1.5 years, the authors said her quality of life was good and they hoped that the procedure would offer cure for select patients with severe forms of the disease.

Alternative treatment

Acute porphyria attacks can be life-threatening events, so attempts at self-treatment can be dangerous. Alternative treatments can be useful adjuncts to conventional therapy. For example, some people may find relief for the pain associated with acute intermittent porphyria, hereditary coproporphyria, or variegate porphyria through **acupuncture** or hypnosis. Relaxation techniques, such as **yoga** or **meditation**, may also prove helpful in pain management.

Prognosis

Even when porphyria is inherited, symptom development depends on a variety of factors. In the majority of cases, a person remains asymptomatic throughout life. About one percent of acute attacks can be fatal. Other symptoms may be associated with temporarily debilitating or permanently disfiguring consequences. Measures to avoid these consequences are not always successful, regardless of how diligently they are pursued. Although pregnancy has been known to trigger porphyria attacks, dangers associated with pregnancy as not as great as was once thought.

Prevention

For the most part, the porphyrias are attributable to inherited genes; such inheritance cannot be prevented. However, symptoms can be limited or prevented by avoiding factors that trigger symptom development.

People with a family history of an acute porphyria should be screened for the disease. Even if symptoms are absent, it is useful to know about the presence of the gene to assess the risks of developing the associated porphyria. This knowledge also reveals whether a person's offspring may be at risk. Prenatal testing for certain porphyrias is possible. Prenatal diagnosis of congenital erythropoietic porphyria has been successfully accomplished. Any prenatal tests, however, would not indicate whether a child would develop porphyria symptoms; only that the potential is there.

Resources

BOOKS

Deats-O'Reilly, Diana. *Porphyria: The UnknownDisease.* Grand Forks, N.D.: Porphyrin Publications Press/ Educational Services,1999.

PERIODICALS

"Fluoxetine Treats Acute Intermittent Porphyria Safely and Effectively." *Drug Week* January 16, 2004: 292.
Gordon, Neal. "The Acute Porphyrias." *Brain & Development* 21 (September 1999): 373–77.

Thadani, Helen, et al. "Diagnosis and Management of Porphyria."*British Medical Journal* 320 (June 2000): 1647–51.

KEY TERMS

Autosomal dominant—A pattern of genetic inheritance in which only one abnormal gene is needed to display the trait or disease.

Autosomal recessive—A pattern of genetic inheritance in which two abnormal genes are needed to display the trait or disease.

Biosynthesis—The manufacture of materials in a biological system.

Bone marrow—A spongy tissue located in the hollow centers of certain bones, such as the skull and hip bones. Bone marrow is the site of blood cell generation.

Enzyme—A protein that catalyzes a biochemical reaction or change without changing its own structure or function.

Erythropoiesis—The process through which new red blood cells are created; it begins in the bone marrow.

Erythropoietic—Referring to the creation of new red blood cells.

Gene—A building block of inheritance, which contains the instructions for the production of a particular protein, and is made up of a molecular sequence found at a section of DNA. Each gene is found on a precise location on a chromosome.

Hematin—A drug administered intravenously to halt an acute porphyria attack. It causes heme biosynthesis to decrease, preventing the further accumulation of heme precursors.

Heme—The iron-containing molecule in hemoglobin that serves as the site for oxygen binding.

Hemoglobin—Protein-iron compound in the blood that carries oxygen to the cells and carries carbon dioxide away from the cells.

Hepatic—Referring to the liver.

Neuropathy—A condition caused by nerve damage. Major symptoms include weakness, numbness, paralysis, or pain in the affected area.

Porphyrin—A large molecule shaped like a four-leaf clover. Combined with an iron atom, it forms a heme molecule.

Protoporphyrin—A precursor molecule to the porphyrin molecule.

Zahir, Soonawalla F., et al. "Liver Transplantation as a Cure for Acute Intermittent Porphyria." *The Lancet* February 28, 2004: 705.

ORGANIZATIONS

American Porphyria Foundation. PO Box 22712, Houston, TX 77227. (713) 266-9617. < http://www.enterprise.net/apf/ >.

OTHER

Gene Clinics. < http://www.geneclinics.org >.
National Institute of Diabetes & Digestive & KidneyDiseases. < http://www.niddk.nih.gov >.
Online Mendelian Inheritance in Man (OMIM). < http://www3.ncbi.nlm.nih.gov/Omim >.

Julia Barrett
Judy C. Hawkins, MS
Teresa G. Odle

Port-wine stain *see* **Birthmarks**

Portacaval shunting *see* **Portal vein bypass**

Portal-systemic encephalopathy *see* **Liver encephalopathy**

Portal vein bypass

Definition

Portal vein bypass surgery diverts blood from the portal vein into another vein. It is performed when pressure in the portal vein is so high that it causes internal bleeding from blood vessels in the esophagus.

Purpose

The portal vein carries blood from the stomach and abdominal organs to the liver. It is a major vein that splits into many branches. High pressure in the portal vein causes swelling and bleeding from blood vessels in the esophagus. This situation occurs when the liver is damaged from **cirrhosis** of the liver, a condition usually caused by prolonged, excessive alcohol consumption.

Massive internal bleeding caused by high pressure in the portal vein occurs in about 40% of patients with cirrhosis. It is initially fatal in at least half of these patients. Patients who survive are likely to experience bleeding recurrence. Portal vein bypass, also called portacaval shunting, is performed on these surviving patients to control bleeding.

Precautions

Most patients who need portal vein bypass surgery not only have **liver disease** and poor liver function, but also suffer from an enlarged spleen, jaundice, and damage to the vascular system brought on by years of **alcoholism**. They are likely to experience serious complications during surgery. Some patients are aggressively uncooperative with medical personnel. Under these conditions, half the patients may not survive the operation.

Description

A choice of portal vein bypasses is available. Portal vein bypass is usually performed as an emergency operation in a hospital under **general anesthesia**. The surgeon makes an abdominal incision and finds the portal vein. In portacaval shunting, blood from the portal vein is diverted into the inferior vena cava. This is the most common bypass. In splenorenal shunting, the splenic vein (a part of the portal vein), is connected to the renal vein. A mesocaval shunt connects the superior mesenteric vein (another part of the portal vein) to the inferior vena cava.

Portal pressure can also be reduced in a procedure called transvenous intrahepatic portosystemic shunt (TIPS). A catheter is threaded into the portal vein, and an expandable balloon or wire mesh is inserted to divert blood from the portal vein to the hepatic vein. The rate of serious complications in TIPS is only 1–2%. The operation cannot be performed at all hospitals, but is becoming the preferred treatment for reducing portal pressure.

Preparation

Standard preoperative blood and urine tests are performed, and liver function is evaluated. The heart and arterial blood pressure are monitored both during and after the operation.

Aftercare

The patient will be connected to a heart monitor and fed through a nasogastric tube. Vital functions are monitored through blood and urine tests. Patients receive **pain** medication and **antibiotics**. Once released from the hospital, patients are expected to abstain from alcohol and follow a diet and medication schedule designed to reduce the risks of re-bleeding.

Risks

Portal vein bypass surgery is high risk because it is performed on patients who are generally in poor health. Only half the patients survive, although the chances of survival are greater with TIPS surgery. Those patients who survive the operation still face the risk of **heart failure**, brain disease due to a decrease in the liver's conversion of waste products (**liver encephalopathy**), hemorrhage, lung complications, infection, **coma**, and **death**.

Normal results

The survival rate is directly related to the amount of liver damage patients have. The less damage, the more likely the patient is to recover. Cooperation with restrictions on alcohol and diet affect long-term survival.

Resources

BOOKS

McPhee, Stephen, et al., editors. *Current Medical Diagnosis and Treatment, 1998.* 37th ed. Stamford: Appleton & Lange, 1997.

Tish Davidson, A.M.

Positron emission tomography (PET)

Definition

Positron emission tomography (PET) is a scanning technique used in conjunction with small amounts of radiolabeled compounds to visualize brain anatomy and function.

Purpose

PET was the first scanning method to provide information on brain function as well as anatomy. This information includes data on blood flow, oxygen

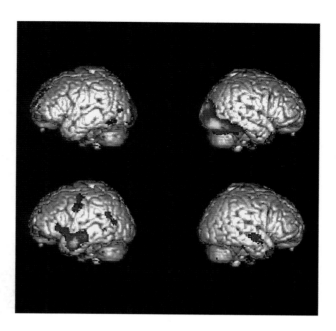

A PET scan showing brain activity while patient recognizes faces—left sides at left/right sides at right. Activity is prevalent in temporal lobe (bottom scans). *(Photo Researchers. Reproduced by permission.)*

consumption, glucose metabolism, and concentrations of various molecules in brain tissue.

PET has been used to study brain activity in various neurological diseases and disorders, including **stroke**; epilepsy; Alzheimer's disease, Parkinson's disease, and Huntington's disease; and in some psychiatric disorders, such as schizophrenia, depression, **obsessive-compulsive disorder**, **attention-deficit/hyperactivity disorder**, and Tourette syndrome. PET studies have helped to identify the brain mechanisms that operate in drug **addiction**, and to shed light on the mechanisms by which individual drugs work. PET is also proving to be more accurate than other methods in the diagnosis of many types of **cancer**. In the treatment of cancer, PET can be used to determine more quickly than conventional tests whether a given therapy is working. PET scans also give accurate and detailed information on heart disease, particularly in women, in whom breast tissue can interfere with other types of tests.

Description

A very small amount of a radiolabeled compound is inhaled by or injected into the patient. The injected or inhaled compound accumulates in the tissue to be studied. As the radioactive atoms in the compound decay, they release smaller particles called positrons, which are positively charged. When

KEY TERMS

Electron—One of the small particles that make up an atom. An electron has the same mass and amount of charge as a positron, but the electron has a negative charge.

Gamma ray—A high-energy photon, emitted by radioactive substances.

Half-life—The time required for half of the atoms in a radioactive substance to disintegrate.

Photon—A light particle.

Positron—One of the small particles that make up an atom. A positron has the same mass and amount of charge as an electron, but the positron has a positive charge.

a positron collides with an electron (negatively charged), they are both annihilated, and two photons (light particles) are emitted. The photons move in opposite directions and are picked up by the detector ring of the PET scanner. A computer uses this information to generate three-dimensional, cross-sectional images that represent the biological activity where the radiolabeled compound has accumulated.

A related technique is called single photon emission computed tomography (CT) scan (SPECT). SPECT is similar to PET, but the compounds used contain heavier, longer-lived radioactive atoms that emit high-energy photons, called gamma rays, instead of positrons. SPECT is used for many of the same applications as PET, and is less expensive than PET, but the resulting picture is usually less sharp than a PET image and reveals less information about the brain.

Risks

Some of radioactive compounds used for PET or SPECT scanning can persist for a long time in the body. Even though only a small amount is injected each time, the long half-lives of these compounds can limit the number of times a patient can be scanned.

Resources

PERIODICALS

"Studies Argue for Wider Use of PET for Cancer Patients." *Cancer Weekly Plus* December 15, 1997: 9.

Lisa Christenson, PhD

▌Post-concussion syndrome

Definition

Post-concussion syndrome (PCS) is a common but controversial disorder that presents with variety of symptoms including—but not limited to—headache, **dizziness**, **fatigue**, and personality changes.

Description

PCS occurs in approximately 23–93% of persons with mild to severe head injuries. It is estimated that a neurologist (a physician who specializes in nerve and brain disorders) sees five patients with PCS per month. There is no accurate correlation between the severity of injury and the development of PCS symptoms, since signs of the disorder can occur in someone who was just dazed by an injury. Some studies suggest that PCS symptoms occur at a higher rate in patients who were unconscious after trauma.

Causes and symptoms

PCS is most commonly caused by minor **head injury** called a **concussion**. The majority of patients with minor head injury characteristically develop PCS with distinct symptoms. Patients may report problems with concentration, recent memory, and abstract thinking. Additionally, patients may develop dizziness, irritability, fatigue, and personality changes. Elderly patients are particularly affected by disequilibrium and chronic dizziness even after minor trauma.

Diagnosis

There are no specific or reliable tests to diagnose PCS. A neuropsychologist can perform an in-depth neuropsychologic assessment that can determine presence or absence and extent of impairment. These tests may be performed for medical purposes.

Treatment

Treatment for PCS can be extensive. Medications for **headache** and **pain** may be indicated (analgesics and muscle relaxants). Antidepressants may be given to improve **insomnia**, irritability, or anxiety. Pain control could be achieved with **acupuncture**, nerve blocks, or transcutaneous electrical nerve stimulation (TENS, electrical stimulation of muscle groups). It is important for clinicians to educate caretakers and to provide

KEY TERMS

Disequilibrium—Difficulty with equilibrium that can mean a deficiency in balance and/or orientation.

Neuropsychologist—A clinical psychologist who specializes in assessing psychological status caused by a brain disorder.

referrals for family therapy and cognitive **rehabilitation** for the affected person.

Prognosis

The overall outcome is difficult to assess. Limited interpretation in literature is primarily due to the subjective nature of symptoms. Patient recovery is directed and evaluated by cognitive function changes, subjective symptoms, and return to work. Most cases of PCS can be a financial strain and threaten family stability. There may be compensation and litigation claims, which is often stressful and aggravates symptoms.

Resources

BOOKS

Coper, Paul R., and John G. Golfinos, et al, editors. *Head Injury*. 4th ed. New York: McGraw-Hill, 2000.
Goetz, Christopher G., et al., editors. *Textbook of Clinical Neurology*. 1st ed. Philadelphia: W. B. Saunders Company, 1999.
Goldman, Lee, et al. *Cecil's Textbook of Medicine*. 21st ed. Philadelphia: W. B. Saunders Company, 2000.

Laith Farid Gulli, M.D.

Post-herpetic neuralgia *see* **Neuralgia**

Post-traumatic stress disorder

Definition

Post-traumatic **stress** disorder (PTSD) is a debilitating psychological condition triggered by a major traumatic event, such as **rape**, war, a terrorist act, **death** of a loved one, a natural disaster, or a catastrophic accident. It is marked by upsetting memories or thoughts of the ordeal, "blunting" of emotions, increased arousal, and sometimes severe personality changes.

Description

Officially termed post-traumatic stress disorder since 1980, PTSD was once known as shell shock or battle **fatigue** because of its more common manifestation in war veterans. However in the past 20 years, PTSD has been diagnosed in rape victims and victims of violent crime; survivors of natural disasters; the families of loved ones lost in the downing of Flight 103 over Lockerbie, Scotland; and survivors of the 1993 World Trade Center bombing, the 1995 Oklahoma City bombing, the random school and workplace shootings, and the release of poisonous gas in a Japanese subway; and, most recently, in the September 11, 2001, World Trade Center and Pentagon terrorist attacks. PTSD can affect adults of all ages. Statistics gathered from past events indicate that the risk of PTSD increases in order of the following factors.

- female gender
- middle-aged (40 to 60 years old)
- little or no experience coping with traumatic events
- ethnic minority
- lower socioeconomic status (SES)
- children in the home
- women with spouses exhibiting PTSD symptoms
- pre-existing psychiatric conditions
- primary exposure to the event including injury, life-threatening situation, and loss
- living in traumatized community

For example, over a third of the Oklahoma City bombing survivors developed PTSD and over half showed signs of **anxiety**, depression, and alcohol **abuse**. Over one year later, Oklahomans in general had a increased use of alcohol and tobacco products, as well as PTSD symptoms.

Children are also susceptible to PTSD and their risk is increased exponentially as their exposure to the event increases. Children experiencing abuse, the death of a parent, or those located in a community suffering a traumatic event can develop PTSD. Two years after the Oklahoma City bombing, 16% of children in a 100 mile radius of Oklahoma City with no direct exposure to the bombing had increased symptoms of PTSD. Weak parental response to the event, having a parent suffering from PTSD symptoms, and increased exposure to the event via the media all increase the possibility of the child developing PTSD symptoms.

Causes and symptoms

Specific causes for the onset of PTSD following a trauma aren't clearly defined, although experts suspect it may be influenced both by the severity of the event, by the person's personality and genetic make-up, and by whether or not the trauma was expected. First response emergency personnel and individuals directly involved in the event or those children and families who have lost loved ones are more likely to experience PTSD. Natural disasters account for about a 5% rate of PTSD, while there is a 50% rate of PTSD among rape and Holocaust survivors.

Media coverage plays a new role in both adult and pediatric onset of PTSD symptoms. The heightened level of news footage of actual traumatic events, such as the Oklahoma City bombing and the terrorist attack on the World Trade Center and the Pentagon, increases the exposure to the violence, injury, and death associated with the event and may reinforce PTSD symptoms in individuals, especially young children who cannot distinguish between the actual event and the repeated viewing of the event in the media.

PTSD symptoms are distinct and prolonged stress reactions that naturally occur during a highly stressful event. Common symptoms are:

- hyperalertness
- fear and anxiety
- nightmares and flashbacks
- sight, sound, and smell recollection
- avoidance of recall situations
- anger and irritability
- guilt
- depression
- increased substance abuse
- negative world view
- decreased sexual activity

Symptoms usually begin within three months of the trauma, although sometimes PTSD doesn't develop until years after the initial trauma occurred. Once the symptoms begin, they may fade away again within six months. Others suffer with the symptoms for far longer and in some cases, the problem may become chronic.

Among the most troubling symptoms of PTSD are flashbacks, which can be triggered by sounds, smells, feelings, or images. During a flashback, the person relives the traumatic event and may completely lose touch with reality, suffering through the trauma for minutes or hours at a time, believing that the traumatizing event is actually happening all over again.

For a diagnosis of PTSD, symptoms must include at least one of the following so-called "intrusive" symptoms:

- flashbacks
- sleep disorders: nightmares or night terrors
- intense distress when exposed to events that are associated with the trauma

In addition, the person must have at least three of the following "avoidance" symptoms that affect interactions with others:

- trying to avoid thinking or feeling about the trauma
- inability to remember the event
- inability to experience emotion, as well as a loss of interest in former pleasures (psychic numbing or blunting)
- a sense of a shortened future

Finally, there must be evidence of increased arousal, including at least two of the following:

- problems falling asleep
- startle reactions: hyperalertness and strong reactions to unexpected noises
- memory problems
- concentration problems
- moodiness
- violence

In addition to the above symptoms, children with PTSD may experience learning disabilities and memory or attention problems. They may become more dependent, anxious, or even self-abusing.

Recovery may be slowed by injuries, damage to property, loss of employment, or other major problems in the community due to disaster.

Diagnosis

Not every person who experiences a traumatic event will experience PTSD. A mental health professional will diagnose the condition if the symptoms of stress last for more than a month after a traumatic event. While a formal diagnosis of PTSD is made only in the wake of a severe trauma, it is possible to have a mild PTSD-like reaction following less severe stress.

Treatment

Several factors have shown to be important in the treatment of post-traumatic stress. These include proximity of the treatment to the site of the event, immediate intervention of therapy as soon as possible, and the expectation that the individual will eventually return to more normal functions. The most helpful treatment of prolonged PTSD appears to be a combination of medication along with supportive and cognitive-behavioral therapies.

Emergency care

Immediate intervention is important for individuals directly affected by the traumatic event. Emergency care workers focus on achieving the following during the hours and days following the trauma.

- protect survivors from further danger
- treat immediate injuries
- provide food, shelter, fluids, and clothing
- provide safe zone
- locate separated loved ones
- reconnect loved ones
- provide normal social contact
- help reestablish routines
- help resolve transportation, housing, or other issues caused by disaster
- provide grief counseling, **stress reduction**, and other consultation to enable survivors and families to return to normal life

As well as providing care to others, emergency personnel often need the same support as the survivors. Operational debriefing is used to organize the emergency response and to disseminate information and sense of purpose to the first responders. Critical Incident Stress Debriefing (CISD) is a formal group invention designed to include various crisis intervention, such as information disbursement, one-on-one counseling, consultation, family crisis intervention, and referrals. CISD is not useful for survivors and is an interim support for first responders until they are able to receive therapy.

Medications

Medications used to reduce the symptoms of PTSD include anxiety-reducing medications and antidepressants, especially the **selective serotonin reuptake inhibitors** (SSRIs) such as fluoxetine (Prozac) and sertraline HCl (Zoloft). In 2001, the U.S. Food and Drug Administration (FDA) approved Zoloft as a long-term treatment for PTSD. In a controlled study, Zoloft was effective in safely improving symptoms of PTSD over a period of 28 weeks and reducing the risk of relapse.

Sleep problems can be lessened with brief treatment with an anti-anxiety drug, such as a benzodiazepine like alprazolam (Xanax), but long-term usage can lead to disturbing side effects, such as increased anger, drug tolerance, dependency, and abuse.

Therapy

Several types of therapy may be useful and they are often combined in a multi-faceted approach to understand and treat this condition.

- Cognitive-behavioral therapy focuses on changing specific actions and thoughts through repetitive review of traumatic events, identification of negative behaviors and thoughts, and stress management.

- Group therapy has been useful in decreasing psychological distress, depression, and anxiety in some PTSD sufferers such as sexually abused women and war veterans.

- Psychological debriefing has been widely used to treat victims of natural disasters and other traumatic events such as bombings and workplace shootings, however, recent research shows that psychological debriefing may increase the stress response. Since this type of debriefing focuses on the emotional response of the survivor, it is not recommended for individuals experiencing an extreme level of grief.

Alternative treatment

Several means of alternative treatment may be helpful in combination with conventional therapy for reduction of the symptoms of post-traumatic stress disorder. These include relaxation training, breathing techniques, spiritual treatment, and drama therapy where the event is re-enacted.

Prognosis

The severity of the illness depends in part on whether the trauma was unexpected, the severity of the trauma, how chronic the trauma was (such as for victims of sexual abuse), and the person's readiness to embrace the recovery process. With appropriate medication, emotional support, counseling, and follow-up care, most people show significant improvement. However, prolonged exposure to severe trauma, such as experienced by victims of prolonged physical or sexual abuse and survivors of the Holocaust, may cause permanent psychological **scars**.

Prevention

More studies are needed to determine if PTSD can actually be prevented. Some measures that have been explored include controlling exposure to traumatic events through safety and security measures, psychological preparation for individuals who will be exposed to traumatic events (i.e. policemen, paramedics, soldiers), and stress inoculation training (rehearsal of the event with small doses of the stressful situation).

Resources

PERIODICALS

DiGiovanni, C. "Domestic Terrorism with Chemical or Biological Agents: Psychiatric Aspects." *American Journal of Psychiatry* 156 (1999): 1500-1505.

North, C., S. Nixon, S. Hariat, S. Mallonee, et al. "Psychiatric Disorders Among Survivors of the Oklahoma City Bombing." *Journal of the American Medical Association* 282 (1999): 755-762.

Pfefferbaum, B., R. Gurwitch, N. McDonald, et al. "Posttraumatic Stress Among Children After the Death of a Friend or Acquaintance in a Terrorist Bombing." *Psychiatric Services* 51 (2000): 386-388.

"Sertraline HCl Approved for Long-Term Use." *Women's Health Weekly* September 20, 2001.

Sloan, M. "Response to Media Coverage of Terrorism" *Journal of Conflict Resolution* 44 (2000): 508-522.

Smith, D, E. Christiansen, R. Vincent, and N. Hann. "Population Effects of the Bombing of Oklahoma City." *Journal of Oklahoma State Medical Association* 92 (1999): 193-198.

ORGANIZATIONS

American Psychiatric Association. 1400 K St., NW, Washington, DC 20005.

Anxiety Disorders Association of America. 11900 Parklawn Dr., Ste. 100, Rockville, MD 20852. (301) 231-9350.

Freedom From Fear. 308 Seaview Ave., Staten Island, NY 10305. (718) 351-1717.

National Anxiety Foundation. 3135 Custer Dr., Lexington, KY 40517. (606) 272-7166.

National Center for Post-Traumatic Stress Disorder. < http://www.dartmouth.edu/dms/ptsd >.

National Institute of Mental Health. Rm 15C-05, 5600 Fishers Lane, Rockville, MD 20857.

Society for Traumatic Stress Studies, 60 Revere Dr., Ste. 500, Northbrook, IL 60062. (708) 480-9080.

Jacqueline L. Longe
Jill Granger, MS

Postmenopausal bleeding

Definition

Postmenopausal bleeding is bleeding from the reproductive system that occurs six months or more after menstrual periods have stopped due to **menopause**.

Description

Menopause, the end of ovulation and menstrual periods, naturally occurs for most women age 40–55 years. The process of ending ovulation and menstruation is gradual, spanning one to two years.

Postmenopausal bleeding is bleeding that occurs after menopause has been established for at least six months. It is different from infrequent, irregular periods (**oligomenorrhea**) that occur around the time of menopause.

Many women experience some postmenopausal bleeding. However, postmenopausal bleeding is not normal. Because it can be a symptom of a serious medical condition, any episodes of postmenopausal bleeding should be brought to the attention of a woman's doctor.

Women taking estrogen (called hormone replacement therapy or HRT) are more likely to experience postmenopausal bleeding. So are obese women, because fat cells transform male hormones (androgens) secreted by the adrenal gland into estrogen.

Causes and symptoms

Postmenopausal bleeding can originate in different parts of the reproductive system. Bleeding from the vagina may occur because when estrogen secretion stops, the vagina dries out and can diminish (atrophy). This is the most common cause of bleeding from the lower reproductive tract.

Lesions and cracks on the vulva may also bleed. Sometimes bleeding occurs after intercourse. Bleeding can occur with or without an associated infection.

Bleeding from the upper reproductive system can be caused by:

- hormone replacements
- **endometrial cancer**
- endometrial polyps
- cervical **cancer**
- cervical lesions
- uterine tumors
- ovarian cancer
- estrogen-secreting tumors in other parts of the body

The most common cause of postmenopausal bleeding is HRT. The estrogen in the replacement therapy eases the symptoms of menopause (like hot flashes), and decreases the risk of osteoporosis. Sometimes this supplemental estrogen stimulates the uterine lining to grow. When the lining is shed, post-menopausal bleeding occurs. Most women on HRT usually take the hormone progesterone with the estrogen, and may have monthly withdrawal bleeding. This is a normal side effect.

About 5–10% of postmenopausal bleeding is due to endometrial cancer or its precursors. Uterine hyperplasia, the abnormal growth of uterine cells, can be a precursor to cancer.

Diagnosis

Diagnosis of postmenopausal bleeding begins with the patient. The doctor will ask for a detailed history of how long postmenopausal bleeding has occurred. A woman can assist the doctor by keeping a record of the time, frequency, length, and quantity of bleeding. She should also tell the doctor about any medications she is taking, especially any estrogens or steroids.

After taking the woman's history, the doctor does a pelvic examination and **Pap test**. The doctor will examine the vulva and vagina for signs of atrophy, and will feel for any sign of uterine polyps. Depending on the results of this examination, the doctor may want to do more extensive testing.

Invasive diagnostic procedures

Endometrial biopsy allows the doctor to sample small areas of the uterine lining, while cervical biopsy allows the cervix to be sampled. Tissues are then examined for any abnormalities. This is a simple office procedure.

Dilatation and curettage (D & C) is often necessary for definitive diagnosis. This is done under either general or **local anesthesia**. After examining the tissues collected by an endometrial biopsy or D & C, the doctor may order additional tests to determine if an estrogen-secreting tumor is present on the ovaries or in another part of the body.

Non-invasive diagnostic procedures

With concerns about the rising cost of health care, vaginal probe ultrasound is increasingly being used more than endometrial biopsy to evaluate women with postmenopausal bleeding. Vaginal ultrasound measures the thickness of the endometrium. When the endometrial stripe is less than 0.2 in (5 mm) thick, the chance of cancer is less than 1%. The disadvantage of vaginal ultrasound is that it often does not show polyps and fibroids in the uterus.

A refinement of vaginal probe ultrasound is saline infusion sonography (SIS). A salt water (saline) solution is injected into the uterus with a small tube (catheter) before the vaginal probe is inserted. The presence of liquid in the uterus helps make any structural abnormalities more distinct. These two non-invasive procedures cause less discomfort than endometrial biopsies and D & Cs, but D & C still remains the definitive test for diagnosing uterine cancer.

Treatment

It is common for women just beginning HRT to experience some bleeding. Most women who are on HRT also take progesterone with the estrogen and may have monthly withdrawal bleeding. Again, this is a normal side effect that usually does not require treatment.

Postmenopausal bleeding due to bleeding of the vagina or vulva can be treated with local application of estrogen or HRT.

When diagnosis indicates cancer, some form of surgery is required. The uterus, cervix, ovaries, and fallopian tubes may all be removed depending on the type and location of the cancer. If the problem is estrogen- or androgen-producing tumors elsewhere in the body, these must also be surgically removed.

KEY TERMS

Dilation and curettage (D & C)—A procedure performed under anesthesia during which the cervix is opened more (or dilated) and tissue lining the uterus is scraped out with a metal, spoon-shaped instrument or a suction tube. The procedure can be used to diagnose a problem or to remove growths (polyps).

Endometrial biopsy—The removal of uterine tissue samples either by suction or scraping; the cervix is not dilated. The procedure has a lower rate of diagnostic accuracy than D & C, but can be done as an office procedure under local anesthesia.

Endometrium—The tissue lining the inside of the uterus.

Fibroid tumors—Non-cancerous (benign) growths in the uterus. These growths occur in 30–40% of women over age 40, and do not need to be removed unless they are causing symptoms that interfere with a woman's normal activities.

Osteoporosis—The excessive loss of calcium from the bones, causing the bones to become fragile and break easily. Postmenopausal women are especially vulnerable to this condition because estrogen, a hormone that protects bones against calcium loss, decreases drastically after menopause.

Postmenopausal bleeding that is not due to cancer and cannot be controlled by any other treatment usually requires a **hysterectomy**.

Prognosis

Response to treatment for postmenopausal bleeding is highly individual and is not easy to predict. The outcome depends largely on the reason for the bleeding. Many women are successfully treated with hormones. As a last resort, hysterectomy removes the source of the problem by removing the uterus. However, this operation is not without risk and the possibility of complications. The prognosis for women who have various kinds of reproductive cancer varies with the type of cancer and the stage at which the cancer is diagnosed.

Prevention

Postmenopausal bleeding is not a preventable disorder. However, maintaining a healthy weight will decrease the chances of it occurring.

Resources

ORGANIZATIONS

American Cancer Society. 1599 Clifton Rd., NE, Atlanta, GA 30329-4251. (800) 227-2345. <http://www.cancer.org>.

National Cancer Institute. Building 31, Room 10A31, 31 Center Drive, MSC 2580, Bethesda, MD 20892-2580. (800) 422-6237. <http://www.nci.nih.gov>.

Tish Davidson, A.M.

Postpartum blues *see* **Postpartum depression**

Postpartum depression

Definition

Postpartum depression is a mood disorder that begins after **childbirth** and usually lasts beyond six weeks.

Description

The onset of postpartum depression tends to be gradual and may persist for many months, or develop into a second bout following a subsequent pregnancy. Postpartum depression affects approximately 15% of all childbearing women. Mild to moderate cases are sometimes unrecognized by women themselves. Many women feel ashamed if they are not coping and so may conceal their difficulties. This is a serious problem that disrupts women's lives and can have effects on the baby, other children, her partner, and other relationships. Levels of depression for fathers also increase significantly.

Postpartum depression is often divided into two types: early onset and late onset. An early onset most often seems like the "blues," a mild brief experience during the first days or weeks after birth. During the first week after the birth up to 80% of mothers will experience the "baby blues." This is usually a time of extra sensitivity and symptoms include tearfulness, irritability, **anxiety**, and mood changes, which tend to peak between three to five days after childbirth. The symptoms normally disappear within two weeks without requiring specific treatment apart from understanding, support, skill, and practice. In short, some depression, tiredness, and anxiety may fall within the "normal" range of reactions to giving birth.

Late onset appears several weeks after the birth. This involves a slowly growing feeling of sadness, depression, lack of energy, chronic tiredness, inability to sleep, change in appetite, significant weight loss or gain, and difficulty caring for the baby.

Causes and symptoms

As of 2006, experts cannot say what causes postpartum depression. Most likely, it is caused by many factors that vary from individual to individual. Mothers commonly experience some degree of depression during the first weeks after birth. **Pregnancy** and birth are accompanied by sudden hormonal changes that affect emotions. Additionally, the 24-hour responsibility for a newborn infant represents a major psychological and lifestyle adjustment for most mothers, even after the first child. These physical and emotional stresses are usually accompanied by inadequate rest until the baby's routine stabilizes, so **fatigue** and depression are not unusual.

Experiences vary considerably but usually include several symptoms.

Feelings:

- persistent low mood
- inadequacy, failure, hopelessness, helplessness
- exhaustion, emptiness, sadness, tearfulness
- guilt, shame, worthlessness
- confusion, anxiety, and panic
- fear for the baby and of the baby
- fear of being alone or going out

Behaviors:

- lack of interest or pleasure in usual activities
- insomnia or excessive sleep, nightmares
- not eating or overeating
- decreased energy and motivation
- withdrawal from social contact
- poor self-care
- inability to cope with routine tasks

Thoughts:

- inability to think clearly and make decisions
- lack of concentration and poor memory
- running away from everything
- fear of being rejected by partner
- worry about harm or **death** to partner or baby
- ideas about suicide

Some symptoms may not indicate a severe problem. However, persistent low mood or loss of interest or pleasure in activities, along with four other symptoms occurring together for a period of at least two weeks, indicate clinical depression, and require adequate treatment.

There are several important risk factors for postpartum depression, including:

- **stress**
- lack of sleep
- poor **nutrition**
- lack of support from one's partner, family or friends
- family history of depression
- labor/delivery complications for mother or baby
- premature or postmature delivery
- problems with the baby's health
- separation of mother and baby
- A difficult baby (temperament, feeding, sleeping, settling problems)
- preexisting neurosis or **psychosis**

Diagnosis

There is no diagnostic test for postpartum depression. However, it is important to understand that it is, nonetheless, a real illness, and like a physical ailment, it has specific symptoms.

Treatment

Several treatment options exist, including medication, psychotherapy, counseling, and group treatment and support strategies, depending on the woman's needs. One effective treatment combines antidepressant medication and psychotherapy. These types of medication are often effective when used for 3 to 4 weeks. Any medication use must be carefully considered if the woman are breast-feeding, but with some medications, continuing breast-feeding is safe. Nevertheless, medication alone is never sufficient and should always be accompanied by counseling or other support services.

Alternative treatment

Postpartum depression can be effectively alleviated through counseling and support groups, so that the mother doesn't feel she is alone in her feelings. Constitutional homeopathy can be the most effective treatment of the alternative therapies because it acts on the emotional level where postpartum depression is felt. **Acupuncture**, Chinese herbs, and Western herbs can all help the mother suffering from postpartum depression come back to a state of balance. Seeking help from a practitioner allows the new mother to feel supported and cared for and allows for more effective treatment.

A new mother also should remember that this time of stress does not last forever. In addition, there are useful things she can do for herself, including:

- valuing her role as a mother and trusting her own judgment

- making each day as simple as possible

- avoiding extra pressures or unnecessary tasks

- trying to involve her partner more in the care of the baby from the beginning

- discussing with her partner how both can share the household chores and responsibilities

- scheduling frequent outings, such as walks and short visits with friends

- having the baby sleep in a separate room so she sleeps more restfully

- sharing her feelings with her partner or a friend who is a good listener

- talking with other mothers to help keep problems in perspective

- trying to sleep or rest when the baby is sleeping

- taking care of her health and well-being.

- not losing her sense of humor

Prognosis

With support from friends and family, mild postpartum depression usually disappears quickly. If depression becomes severe, a mother cannot care for herself and the baby, and in rare cases, hospitalization may be necessary. Yet, medication, counseling, and support from others usually cures even severe depression in 3–6 months.

Prevention

Exercise can help enhance a new mother's emotional well-being. New mothers should also try to cultivate good sleeping habits and learn to rest when they feel physically or emotionally tired. It's important for a woman to learn to recognize her own warning signs of fatigue, respond to them by taking a break.

Resources

ORGANIZATIONS

Depression After Delivery (D.A.D.). P.O. Box 1282, Morrisville, PA 19067. (800) 944-4773.
Postpartum Support International. 927 North Kellog Ave., Santa Barbara, CA 93111. (805) 967-7636.

David James Doermann

Postpartum psychosis *see* **Postpartum depression**

Postpolio syndrome

Definition

Postpolio syndrome (PPS) is a condition that strikes survivors of the disease **polio**. PPS occurs about 20–30 years after the original bout with polio, and causes slow but progressive weakening of muscles.

Description

Polio is a disease caused by the poliovirus. It most commonly infects younger children, although it can also infect older children and adults. About 90% of people infected by poliovirus develop only a mild case or no illness at all. However, infected people can continue to spread the virus to others. In its most severe form polio causes **paralysis** of the muscles of the legs, arms, and respiratory system.

About 1% of all people infected with poliovirus develop the actual disease known as polio. In these cases, the virus (which enters the person's body through the mouth) multiplies rapidly within the intestine. The viruses then invade the nearby lymphatic system. Eventually, poliovirus enters the bloodstream, which allows it to gain access to the central nervous system or CNS (the brain and spinal cord). The virus may actually infect a nerve elsewhere in the body, and then spread along that nerve to enter the brain.

The major illness associated with poliovirus often follows a mild illness, which has symptoms of **fever**, **nausea**, and **vomiting**. However, after a symptom-free interval of several days, the patient who is on the way to a major illness develops new symptoms such as **headache** and back and neck **pain**. These symptoms are due to invasion of the nervous system. The motor nerves (those nerves responsible for movement of the muscles) become inflamed, injured, and destroyed. The muscles, therefore, no longer receive any messages from the brain or spinal cord. The muscles become weak, floppy, and then totally paralyzed (unable to move). All muscle tone is lost in the affected limb, and the muscle begins to decrease in size (atrophy). The affected muscles are often only on one side (asymmetric paralysis) of the body. Sensation (the person's ability to feel) is not affected in these paralyzed limbs.

The maximum state of paralysis is usually reached within just a few days. The remaining, unaffected nerves then begin the process of attempting to grow branches to compensate (make up for) the destroyed nerves. This process continues for about six months. Whatever function has not been regained in this amount of time will usually be permanently lost.

Causes and symptoms

PPS occurs in about 25% of patients, several decades after their original infection with polio. However, long-term follow-up indicates that two thirds of polio survivors may experience new weakness. Several theories exist as to the cause of this syndrome.

One such theory has looked at the way function is regained by polio survivors. Three mechanisms seem to be at work:

• injured nerves recuperate and begin functioning again

• muscles that still have working nerve connections grow in size and strength, in order to take over for other paralyzed muscles

• working nerves begin to send small branches out to muscles whose original nerves were destroyed by polio

As a person ages, injured nerves that were able to regain function may fail again, as may muscles that have been over-worked for years in order to compensate for other paralyzed muscles. Even the uninjured nerves that provided new nerve twigs to the muscles may begin to falter after years of relative over-activity. This theory, then, suggests that the body's ability to compensate for destroyed nerves may eventually begin to fail. The compensating nerves and muscles grow older, and because they've been working so much harder over the years, they wear out relatively sooner than would be expected of normal nerves and muscles. Some researchers look at this situation as a form of premature **aging**, brought on by overuse.

Other researchers note that normal aging includes the loss of a fair number of motor nerves. When a patient has already lost motor nerves through polio, normal loss of motor nerves through aging may cause

the number of remaining working nerves to drop low enough to cause symptoms of weakness.

Other theories of PPS include the possibility that particles of the original polioviruses remain in the body. These particles may exert a negative effect, decades later, or they may cause the body's immune system to produce substances originally intended to fight the invading virus, but which may accidentally set off a variety of reactions within the body that actually serve to interfere with the normal functioning of the nerves and muscles.

Still other researchers are looking at the possibility that polio patients have important spinal cord changes which, over time, affect the nerves responsible for movement.

The symptoms of PPS include generalized **fatigue**, low energy, progressively increasing muscle weakness, shrinking muscle size (atrophy), involuntary twitching of the muscle fibers (fasciculations), painful muscles and joints, difficulties with breathing and swallowing, and sleep problems.

Survivors of polio may also develop arthritis of the spine, shoulders, or arms, related to the long-term use of crutches or overcompensation for weak leg muscles.

Diagnosis

Diagnosis is primarily through history. When a patient who has recovered from polio some decades previously begins to experience muscle weakness, PPS must be strongly suspected.

Treatment

Just as there are no treatments available to reverse the original damage of polio, there are also no treatments available to reverse the damaging effects of post polio syndrome. Attempts can be made to relieve some of the symptoms, however.

Pain and inflammation of the muscles and joints can be treated with anti-inflammatory medications, application of hot packs, stretching exercises, and physical therapy. Exercises to maintain/increase flexibility are particularly important. However, an **exercise** regimen must be carefully designed, so as not to strain already fatigued muscles and nerves.

Some patients will require new types of braces to provide support for weakening muscles. Others will need to use wheelchairs or motorized scooters to maintain mobility.

Sleep problems and respiratory difficulties may be related to each other. If breathing is labored during

Asymmetric—Not occurring equally on both sides of the body.

Atrophy—Shrinking, growing smaller in size.

Flaccid—Weak, soft, floppy.

Paralysis—The inability to voluntarily move.

sleep, the blood's oxygen content may drop low enough to interfere with the quality of sleep. This may require oxygen supplementation, or even the use of a machine to aid in breathing.

Prognosis

Prognosis for patients with post polio syndrome is relatively good. It is a very slow, gradually progressing syndrome. Only about 20% of all patients with PPS will need to rely on new aids for mobility or breathing. It appears that the PPS symptoms reach their most severe about 30–34 years after original diagnosis of polio.

Prevention

There is no way to prevent PPS. However, paying attention to what types of exertion worsen symptoms may slow the progression of the syndrome.

Resources

ORGANIZATIONS

International Polio Network. 4207 Lindell Blvd., Suite 110, St. Louis, MO 63108-2915. (314) 534-0475.

March of Dimes Birth Defects Foundation. 1275 Mamaroneck Ave., White Plains, NY 10605. (914) 428-7100. resourcecenter@modimes.org. <http://www.modimes.org>.

Polio Survivors Association. 12720 Lareina Ave., Downey, CA 90242. (310) 862-4508.

Rosalyn Carson-DeWitt, MD

Postpoliomyelitis muscular atrophy *see*
Postpolio syndrome

Postpoliomyelitis syndrome *see* **Postpolio syndrome**

Poststreptococcal glomerulonephritis *see*
Acute poststreptococcal glomerulonephritis

Postural drainage *see* **Chest physical therapy**

Postural hypotension *see* **Orthostatic hypotension**

Postviral thrombocytopenia *see* **Idiopathic thrombocytopenic purpura**

Potassium hydroxide test *see* **KOH test**

Potassium imbalance *see* **Hyperkalemia; Hypokalemia**

PPD skin test *see* **Tuberculin skin test**

Prader-Willi syndrome

Definition

Prader-Willi syndrome (PWS) is a genetic condition caused by the absence of chromosomal material from chromosome 15. The genetic basis of PWS is complex. Characteristics of the syndrome include developmental delay, poor muscle tone, short stature, small hands and feet, incomplete sexual development, and unique facial features. Insatiable appetite is a classic feature of PWS. This uncontrollable appetite can lead to health problems and behavior disturbances.

Description

The first patients with features of PWS were described by Dr. Prader, Dr. Willi, and Dr. Lambert in 1956. Since that time, the complex genetic basis of PWS has begun to be understood. Initially, scientists found that individuals with PWS have a portion of genetic material deleted (erased) from chromosome 15. In order to have PWS, the genetic material must be deleted from the chromosome 15 received from one's father. If the deletion is on the chromosome 15 inherited from one's mother a different syndrome develops. This was an important discovery. It demonstrated for the first time that the genes inherited from one's mother can be expressed differently than the genes inherited from one's father.

Over time, scientists realized that some individuals with PWS do not have genetic material deleted from chromosome 15. Further studies found that these patients inherit both copies of chromosome 15 from their mother. This is not typical. Normally, an individual receives one chromosome 15 from their father and one chromosome 15 from their mother.

When a person receives both chromosomes from the same parent it is called "uniparental disomy". "When a person receives both chromosomes from his or her mother it is called "maternal uniparental disomy."

Scientists are still discovering other causes of PWS. A small number of patients with PWS have a change (mutation) in the genetic material on the chromosome 15 inherited from their father. This mutation prevents certain genes on chromosome 15 from working properly. PWS develops when these genes do not work normally.

Newborns with PWS generally have poor muscle tone, (hypotonia) and do not feed well. This can lead to poor weight gain and **failure to thrive**. Genitalia can be smaller than normal. Hands and feet are also typically smaller than normal. Some patients with PWS have unique facial characteristics. These unique facial features are typically subtle and detectable only by physicians.

As children with PWS age, development is typically slower than normal. Developmental milestones, such as crawling, walking and talking occur later than usual. Developmental delay continues into adulthood for approximately 50% of individuals with PWS. At about one to two years of age, children with PWS develop an uncontrollable, insatiable appetite. Left to their own devices, individuals with PWS will eat until they suffer from life-threatening **obesity**. The desire to eat can lead to significant behavior problems.

The symptoms and features of PWS require life long support and care. If food intake is strictly monitored and various therapies provided, individuals with PWS have a normal life expectancy.

PWS affects approximately 1 in 10,000 to 25,000 live births. It is the most common genetic cause of life-threatening obesity. It affects both males and females. PWS can be seen in all races and ethnic groups.

Causes and symptoms

In order to comprehend the various causes of PWS, the nature of chromosomes and genes must be well understood. Human beings have 46 chromosomes in the cells of their body. Chromosomes contain genes, which regulate the function and development of the body. An individual's chromosomes are inherited from his/her parents. Each parent normally gives a child 23 chromosomes. A child receives 23 chromosomes from the egg and 23 chromosomes from the sperm.

The 46 chromosomes in the human body are divided into pairs based on their physical characteristics. Each pair is assigned a number or a letter. When viewed under a microscope, chromosomes within the same pair appear identical because they contain the same genes.

Most chromosomes have a constriction near the center called the centromere. The centromere separates the chromosome into long and short arms. The short arm of a chromosome is called the "p arm." the long arm and is called the "q arm,"

Chromosomes in the same pair contain the same genes. However, some genes work differently depending on if they were inherited from the egg or the sperm. Sometimes, genes are silenced when inherited from the mother. Other times, genes are silenced when inherited from the father. When genes in a certain region on a chromosome are silenced, they are said to be "imprinted." Imprinting is a normal process that does not typically cause disease. If normal imprinting is disrupted a genetic disease can develop.

Individuals have two complete copies of chromosome 15. One chromosome 15 is inherited from the mother, or "maternal" in origin. The other chromosome 15 is inherited from the father, or is "paternal" in origin.

Chromosome 15 contains many different genes. There are several genes found on the q arm of chromosome 15 that are imprinted. A gene called "SNPRN" is an example of one of these genes. It is normally imprinted, or silenced, if inherited from the mother. The imprinting of this group of maternal genes does not typically cause disease. The genes in this region should not be imprinted if paternal in origin. Normal development depends on these paternal genes being present and active. If these genes are deleted, not inherited, or incorrectly imprinted PWS develops.

Seventy percent of the cases of PWS are caused when a piece of material is deleted, or erased, from the paternal chromosome 15. This deletion occurs in a specific region on the q arm of chromosome 15. The piece of chromosomal material that is deleted contains genes that must be present for normal development. These paternal genes must be working normally, because the same genes on the chromosome 15 inherited from the mother are imprinted. When these paternal genes are missing, the brain and other parts of the body do not develop as expected. This is what causes the symptoms associated with PWS.

In 99% of the cases of PWS the deletion is sporadic. This means that it happens randomly and there is not an apparent cause. It does not run in the family. If a child has PWS due to a sporadic deletion in the paternal chromosome 15, the chance the parents could have another child with PWS is less than 1%. In fewer than 1% of the cases of PWS there is a chromosomal rearrangement in the family which causes the deletion. This chromosomal rearrangement is called a "translocation." If a parent has a translocation the risk of having a child with PWS is higher than 1%.

PWS can also develop if a child receives both chromosome 15s from his/her mother. This is seen in approximately 25% of the cases of PWS. "Maternal uniparental disomy". Maternal uniparental disomy for chromosome 15 leads to PWS because the genes on chromosome 15 that should have been inherited from the father are missing, and the genes on both the chromosome 15s inherited from the mother are imprinted.

PWS caused by maternal uniparental is sporadic. This means that it occurs randomly and there is not an apparent cause. If a child has PWS due to maternal uniparental disomy the chance the parents could have another child with PWS is less than 1%.

Approximately 3–4% of patients with PWS have a change (mutation) in a gene located on the q arm of chromosome 15. This mutation leads to incorrect imprinting. This mutation causes genes inherited from the father to be imprinted or silenced, which should not normally be imprinted. If a child has PWS due to a mutation that changes imprinting, the chance the parents could have another child with PWS is approximately 5%.

Infants with PWS have weak muscle tone (hypotonia). This hypotonia causes problems with sucking and eating. Infants with PWS may have problems gaining weight. Some infants with PWS are diagnosed with "failure to thrive" due to slow growth and development. During infancy, babies with PWS may also sleep more than normal and have problems controlling their temperature.

Some of the unique physical features associated with PWS can be seen during infancy. Genitalia that is smaller than normal is common. This may be more evident in males with PWS. Hands and feet may also be smaller than average. The unique facial features seen in some patients with PWS may be difficult to detect in infancy. These facial features are very mild and do not cause physical problems.

As early as six months, but more commonly at one to two years a compulsive desire to eat develops. This uncontrollable appetite is a classic feature of PWS. Individuals with PWS lack the ability to feel full or satiated. This uncontrollable desire to eat is thought to be related to a difference in the brain, which controls hunger. Over-eating (hyperpahgia), a lack of a desire to exercise, and a slow metabolism places individuals with

PWS at high risk for severe obesity. Some individuals with PWS may also have a reduced ability to vomit.

Behavior problems are a common feature of PWS. Some behavior problems develop from the desire to eat. Other reported problems include obsessive/compulsive behaviors, depression, and temper tantrums. Individuals with PWS may also pick their own skin (skin picking). This unusual behavior may be due to a reduced **pain** threshold.

Developmental delay, learning disabilities, and mental retardation are associated with PWS. Approximately 50% of individuals with PWS have developmental delay. The remaining 50% are described as having mild mental retardation. The **mental retardation** can occasionally be more severe. Infants and children with PWS are often delayed in development.

Puberty may occur early or late, but it is usually incomplete. In addition to the effects on sexual development and fertility, individuals do not undergo the normal adolescent growth spurt and may be short as adults. Muscles often remain underdeveloped and body fat is increased.

Diagnosis

During infancy the diagnosis of PWS may be suspected if poor muscle tone, feeding problems, small genitalia, or the unique facial features are present. If an infant has these features, testing for PWS should be performed. This testing should also be offered to children and adults who display features commonly seen in PWS (developmental delay, uncontrollable appetite, small genitalia, etc.). There are several different genetic tests that can detect PWS. All of these tests can be performed from a blood sample.

Methylation testing detects 99% of the cases of PWS. Methylation testing can detect the absence of the paternal genes that should be normally active on chromosome 15. Although methylation testing can accurately diagnose PWS, it can not determine if the PWS is caused by a deletion, maternal uniparental disomy, or a mutation that disrupts imprinting. This information is important for **genetic counseling**. Therefore, additional testing should be performed.

Chromosome analysis can determine if the PWS is the result of a deletion in the q arm of chromosome 15. Chromosome analysis, also called "karyotyping," involves staining the chromosomes and examining them under a microscope. In some cases the deletion of material from chromosome 15 can be easily seen. In other cases, further testing must be performed. FISH (fluorescence in-situ hybridization) is a special technique that detects small deletions that cause PWS.

More specialized DNA testing is required to detect maternal uniparental disomy or a mutation that disrupts imprinting. This DNA testing identifies unique DNA patterns in the mother and father. The unique DNA patterns are then compared with the DNA from the child with PWS.

PWS can be detected before birth if the mother undergoes **amniocentesis** testing or chorionic villus sampling (CVS). This testing is only recommended if the mother or father is known to have a chromosome rearrangement, or if they already have a child with PWS syndrome.

Treatment

There is currently not a cure for PWS. Treatment during infancy includes therapies to improve muscle tone. Some infants with PWS also require special nipples and feeding techniques to improve weight gain.

Treatment and management during childhood, adolescence, and adulthood is typically focused on weight control. Strict control of food intake is vital to prevent severe obesity. In many cases food must be made inaccessible. This may involve unconventional measures such as locking the refrigerator or kitchen cabinets. A lifelong restricted-calorie diet and regular **exercise** program are also suggested. Unfortunately, diet medications have not been shown to significantly prevent obesity in PWS. However, growth hormone therapy has been shown to improve the poor muscle tone and reduced height typically associated with PWS.

Special education may be helpful in treating developmental delays and behavior problems. Individuals with PWS typically excel in highly structured environments.

Prognosis

Life expectancy is normal and the prognosis good, if weight gain is well controlled.

Resources

BOOKS

Couch, Cheryl. *My Rag Doll*. Couch Publishing, October 2000.

PERIODICALS

Butler, Merlin G. and Travis Thompson. "Prader-WilliSyndrome: Clinical and Genetic Findings." *The Endocrinologist* 10 (2000): 3S–16S.

KEY TERMS

Amniocentesis—A procedure in which a needle is inserted through a pregnant woman's abdomen and into her uterus. Amniotic fluid is then removed from around the fetus and may be used for genetic testing.

Centromere—Major constriction in a chromosome.

Deletion—Removal of a piece of genetic material.

DNA—Deoxyribonucleic acid. Genes are made of sections of DNA.

FISH—(flourescence in-situ hybridization) Technique used to detect small deletions or rearrangements in chromosomes.

Gene—Segment of DNA that controls the development and function of the body. Genes are contained within chromosomes.

Hyperphagia—Over-eating.

Hypotonia—Low muscle tone.

Imprinting—Process that silences a gene or group of genes. The genes are silenced depending on if they are inherited through the egg or the sperm.

Maternal—From one's mother.

Maternal uniparental disomy—Chromosome abnormality in which both chromosomes in a pair are inherited from one's mother.

Methylation testing—DNA testing that detects if a gene is active or imprinted.

Mutation—A change in a gene.

Paternal—From one's father.

Translocation—Chromosome abnormality in which chromosomes are rearranged and placed together.

Uniparental disomy—Chromosome abnormality in which both chromosomes in a pair are inherited from the same parent.

State, Matthew W., and Elisabeth Dykens. "Genetics of Childhood Disorders: XV. Prader-Willi Syndrome: Genes, Brain and Behavior." *J. Am. Acad. Child. Adolesc. Psychiatry* 39, no. 6 (June 2000): 797–800.

ORGANIZATIONS

Alliance of Genetic Support Groups. 4301 Connecticut Ave. NW, Suite 404, Washington DC 20008. (202) 966-5557. Fax: (202) 966-8553. <http://www.geneticalliance.org>.

International Prader-Willi Syndrome Organization. <http://www.ipwsp.org>.

Prader-Willi syndrome

National Organization for Rare Disorders, Inc. P.O. Box 8923, New Fairfield, CT 06812. (800) 999-6673. < http://www.rarediseases.org >.

Prader-Willi Foundation. 223 Main Street, Port Washington, NY 11050. (800)253- 7993. < http://www.prader-willi.org >.

Prader-Willi Syndrome Association (USA). 5700 Midnight Pass Rd., Sarasota, FL 34242. (800)926-4797. < http://www.pwsusa.org >.

OTHER

Gene Clinics. < http://www.geneclinics.org/profiles/ pws/details.html >.

OMIM. < http://www.ncbi.nlm.nih.gov/htbin-port/ Omim/dispmim?176270 >.

Holly Ann Ishmael, M.S.

Praziquantel *see* **Antihelminthic drugs**

Precocious puberty

Definition

Sexual development before the age of eight in girls, and age 10 in boys.

Description

Not every child reaches **puberty** at the same time, but in most cases it's safe to predict that sexual development will begin at about age 11 in girls and 12 or 13 in boys. However, occasionally a child begins to develop sexually much earlier. Between four to eight times more common in girls than boys, precocious puberty occurs in one out of every 5,000 to 10,000 U.S. children.

Precocious puberty often begins before age 8 in girls, triggering the development of breasts and hair under the arms and in the genital region. The onset of ovulation and menstruation also may occur. In boys, the condition triggers the development of a large penis and testicles, with spontaneous erections and the production of sperm. Hair grows on the face, under arms and in the pubic area, and **acne** may become a problem.

While the early onset of puberty may seem fairly benign, in fact it can cause problems when hormones trigger changes in the growth pattern, essentially halting growth before the child has reached normal adult height. Girls may never grow above 5 ft (152 cm) and boys often stop growing by about 5 ft 2 in (157 cm).

The abnormal growth patterns are not the only problem, however. Children with this condition look noticeably different than their peers, and may feel rejected by their friends and socially isolated. Adults may expect these children to act more maturely simply because they look so much older. As a result, many of these children–especially boys–are much more aggressive than others their own age, leading to behavior problems both at home and at school.

Causes and symptoms

Puberty begins when the brain secretes a hormone that triggers the pituitary gland to release gonadotropins, which in turn stimulate the ovaries or testes to produce sex hormones. These sex hormones (especially estrogen in girls and testosterone in boys) are what causes the onset of sexual maturity.

The hormonal changes of precious puberty are normal–it's just that the whole process begins a few years too soon. Especially in girls, there is not usually any underlying problem that causes the process to begin too soon. However, some boys do inherit the condition; the responsible gene may be passed directly from father to son, or inherited indirectly from the maternal grandfather through the mother, who does not begin early puberty herself. This genetic condition in girls can be traced in only about 1% of cases.

In about 15% of cases, there is an underlying cause for the precocious puberty, and it is important to search for these causes. The condition may result from a benign tumor in the part of the brain that releases hormones. Less commonly, it may be caused by other types of brain tumors, central nervous system disorders, or adrenal gland problems.

Diagnosis

Physical exams can reveal the development of sexual characteristics in a young child. Bone x rays can reveal bone age, and **pelvic ultrasound** may show an enlarged uterus and rule out ovarian or adrenal tumors. Blood tests can highlight higher-than-normal levels of hormones. MRI or CAT scans should be considered to rule out intracranial tumors.

Treatment

Treatment aims to halt or reverse sexual development so as to stop the accompanying rapid growth that will limit a child's height. There are two possible approaches: either treat the underlying condition (such as an ovarian or intracranial tumor) or change the hormonal balance to stop sexual development. It may not be possible to treat the underlying condition;

for this reason, treatment is usually aimed at adjusting hormone levels.

There are several drugs that have been developed to do this:

- histrelin (Supprelin)
- nafarelin (Synarel)
- synthetic gonadotropin-releasing hormone agonist
- deslorelin
- ethylamide
- triptorelin
- leuprolide

Prognosis

Drug treatments can slow growth to 2–3 in (5–7.5 cm) a year, allowing these children to reach normal adult height, although the long-term effects aren't known.

Resources

ORGANIZATIONS

National Institute of Child Health and Human Development. Bldg 31, Room 2A32, MSC 2425, 31 Center Drive, Bethesda, MD 20892-2425. (800) 505-2742. <http://www.nichd.nih.gov/sids/sids.htm>.

Carol A. Turkington

Prednis *see* **Corticosteroids**

Preeclampsia and eclampsia

Definition

Preeclampsia and eclampsia are complications of **pregnancy**. In preeclampsia, the woman has dangerously high blood pressure, swelling, and protein in the urine. If allowed to progress, this syndrome will lead to eclampsia.

Description

Blood pressure is a measurement of the pressure of blood on the walls of blood vessels called arteries. The arteries deliver blood from the heart to all of the tissues in the body. Blood pressure is reported as two numbers. For example, a normal blood pressure is reported as 110/70 mm Hg (read as 110 over 70 millimeters of mercury; or just 110 over 70). These two numbers represent two measurements, the systolic pressure and the diastolic pressure. The systolic pressure (the first number in the example; 110/70 mm Hg) measures the peak pressure of the blood against the artery walls. This higher pressure occurs as blood is being pumped out of the heart and into the circulatory system. The pumping chambers of the heart (ventricles) squeeze to force the blood out of the heart. The diastolic pressure (the second number in the example 110/70 mm Hg) measures the pressure, during the filling of the ventricles. At this point, the atria contract to fill the ventricles. Because the ventricles are relatively relaaxed, and are not pumping blood into the arteries, pressure in the arteries is lower as well.

High blood pressure in pregnancy (**hypertension**) is a very serious complication. It puts both the mother and the fetus (developing baby) at risk for a number of problems. Hypertension can exist in several different forms:

- The preeclampsia-eclampsia continuum (also called pregnancy-induced hypertension or PIH). In this type of hypertension, high blood pressure is first noted sometime after week 20 of pregnancy and is accompanied by protein in the urine and swelling.

- Chronic hypertension. This type of hypertension usually exists before pregnancy or may develop before week 20 of pregnancy.

- Chronic hypertension with superimposed preeclampsia. This syndrome occurs when a woman with pre-existing chronic hypertension begins to have protein in the urine after week 20 of pregnancy.

- Late hypertension. This is a form of high blood pressure occurring after week 20 of pregnancy and is unaccompanied by protein in the urine and does not progress the way preeclampsia-eclampsia does.

Preeclampsia is most common among women who have never given birth to a baby (called nulliparas). About 7% of all nulliparas develop preeclampsia. The disease is most common in mothers under the age of 20, or over the age of 35. African-American women have higher rates of preeclampsia than do Caucasian women. Other risk factors include poverty, multiple pregnancies (twins, triplets, etc.), pre-existing chronic hypertension or **kidney disease**, diabetes, excess amniotic fluid, and a condition of the fetus called nonimmune hydrops. The tendency to develop preeclampsia appears to run in families. The daughters and sisters of women who have had preeclampsia are more likely to develop the condition.

Causes and symptoms

Experts are still trying to understand the exact causes of preeclampsia and eclampsia. It is generally accepted that preeclampsia and eclampsia are problematic because these conditions cause blood vessels to leak. The effects are seen throughout the body.

- General body tissues. When blood vessels leak, they allow fluid to flow out into the tissues of the body. The result is swelling in the hands, feet, legs, arms, and face. While many pregnant women experience swelling in their feet, and sometimes in their hands, swelling of the upper limbs and face is a sign of a more serious problem. As fluid is retained in these tissues, the woman may experience significant weight gain (two or more pounds per week).

- Brain. Leaky vessels can cause damage within the brain, resulting in seizures or **coma**.

- Eyes. The woman may experience problems seeing, and may have blurry vision or may see spots. The retina may become detached.

- Lungs. Fluid may leak into the tissues of the lungs, resulting in shortness of breath.

- Liver. Leaky vessels within the liver may cause it to swell. The liver may be involved in a serious complication of preeclampsia, called the HELLP syndrome. In this syndrome, red blood cells are abnormally destroyed, chemicals called liver enzymes are abnormally high, and cells involved in the clotting of blood (platelets) are low.

- Kidneys. The small capillaries within the kidneys can leak. Normally, the filtration system within the kidney is too fine to allow protein (which is relatively large) to leave the bloodstream and enter the urine. In preeclampsia, however, the leaky capillaries allow protein to be dumped into the urine. The development of protein in the urine is very serious, and often results in a low birth weight baby. These babies have a higher risk of complications, including **death**.

- Blood pressure. In preeclampsia, the volume of circulating blood is lower than normal because fluid is leaking into other parts of the body. The heart tries to make up for this by pumping a larger quantity of blood with each contraction. Blood vessels usually expand in diameter (dilate) in this situation to decrease the work load on the heart. In preeclampsia, however, the blood vessels are abnormally constricted, causing the heart to work even harder to pump against the small diameters of the vessels. This causes an increase in blood pressure.

The most serious consequences of preeclampsia and eclampsia include brain damage in the mother due to brain swelling and oxygen deprivation during seizures. Mothers can also experience blindness, kidney failure, liver rupture, and placental abruption. Babies born to preeclamptic mothers are often smaller than normal, which makes them more susceptible to complications during labor, delivery, and in early infancy. Babies of preeclamptic mothers are also at risk of being born prematurely, and can suffer the complications associated with **prematurity**.

Diagnosis

Diagnosing preeclampsia may be accomplished by noting painless swelling of the arms, legs, and/or face, in addition to abnormal weight gain. The patient's blood pressure is taken during every doctor's visit during pregnancy. An increase of 30 mm Hg in the systolic pressure, or 15 mm Hg in the diastolic pressure, or a blood pressure reading greater than 140/90 mm Hg is considered indicative of preeclampsia. A simple laboratory test in the doctor's office can indicate the presence of protein in a urine sample (a dipstick test). A more exact measurement of the amount of protein in the urine can be obtained by collecting urine for 24 hours, and then testing it in a laboratory to determine the actual quantity of protein present. A 24-hour urine specimen containing more than 500 mg of protein is considered indicative of preeclampsia.

Treatment

With mild preeclampsia, treatment may be limited to bed rest, with careful daily monitoring of weight, blood pressure, and urine protein via dipstick. This careful monitoring will be required throughout pregnancy, labor, delivery, and even for 2–4 days after the baby has been born. About 25% of all cases of eclampsia develop in the first few days after the baby's birth. If the diastolic pressure does not rise over 100 mm Hg prior to delivery, and no other symptoms develop, the woman can continue pregnancy until the fetus is mature enough to be delivered safely. Ultrasound tests can be performed to monitor the health and development of the fetus.

If the diastolic blood pressure continues to rise over 100 mm Hg, or if other symptoms like headache, vision problems, abdominal **pain**, or blood abnormalities develop, then the patient may require medications to prevent seizures. Magnesium sulfate is commonly given through a needle in a vein (intravenous, or IV). Medications that lower blood pressure

KEY TERMS

Capillary—The tiniest blood vessels with the smallest diameter. These vessels receive blood from the arterioles and deliver blood to the venules.

Diastolic—The phase of blood circulation in which the heart's pumping chambers (ventricles) are being filled with blood. During this phase, the ventricles are at their most relaxed, and the pressure against the walls of the arteries is at its lowest.

Placenta—The organ that provides oxygen and nutrition from the mother to the fetus during pregnancy. The placenta is attached to the wall of the uterus and leads to the fetus via the umbilical cord.

Placental abruption—An abnormal separation of the placenta from the uterus before the birth of the baby, with subsequent heavy uterine bleeding. Normally, the baby is born first and then the placenta is delivered within a half hour.

Systolic—The phase of blood circulation in which the heart's pumping chambers (ventricles) are actively pumping blood. The ventricles are squeezing (contracting) forcefully, and the pressure against the walls of the arteries is at its highest.

Urine dipstick test—A test using a small, chemically treated strip that is dipped into a urine sample; when testing for protein, an area on the strip changes color depending on the amount of protein (if any) in the urine.

Uterus—The muscular organ that contains the developing baby during pregnancy.

Ventricles—The two chambers of the heart that are involved in pumping blood. The right ventricle pumps blood into the lungs to receive oxygen. The left ventricle pumps blood into the circulation of the body to deliver oxygen to all of the body's organs and tissues.

Prognosis

The prognosis in preeeclampsia and eclampsia depends on how carefully a patient is monitored. Very careful, consistent monitoring allows quick decisions to be made, and improves the woman's prognosis. Still, the most common causes of death in pregnant women are related to high blood pressure.

About 33% of all patients with preeclampsia will have the condition again with later pregnancies. Eclampsia occurs in about 1 out of every 200 women with preeclampsia. If not treated, eclampsia is almost always fatal.

Prevention

More information on how preeclampsia and eclampsia develop is needed before recommendations can be made on how to prevent these conditions. Research is being done with patients in high risk groups to see if calcium supplementation, **aspirin**, or fish oil supplementation may help prevent preeclampsia. Most importantly, it is clear that careful monitoring during pregnancy is necessary to diagnose preeclampsia early. Although even carefully monitored patients may develop preeclampsia and eclampsia, close monitoring by practitioners will help decrease the complications of these conditions.

Resources

ORGANIZATIONS

American College of Obstetricians and Gynecologists. 409 12th Street, S.W., P.O. Box 96920.

Rosalyn Carson-DeWitt, MD

Pregnancy-induced high blood pressure *see* **Preeclampsia and eclampsia**

(**antihypertensive drugs**) are reserved for patients with very high diastolic pressures (over 110 mm Hg), because lowering the blood pressure will decrease the amount of blood reaching the fetus. This places the fetus at risk for oxygen deprivation. If preeclampsia appears to be progressing toward true eclampsia, then medications may be given in order to start labor. Babies can usually be delivered vaginally. After the baby is delivered, the woman's blood pressure and other vital signs will usually begin to return to normal quickly.

Pregnancy

Definition

The period from conception to birth. After the egg is fertilized by a sperm and then implanted in the lining of the uterus, it develops into the placenta and embryo, and later into a fetus. Pregnancy usually lasts 40 weeks, beginning from the first day of the woman's last menstrual period, and is divided into three trimesters, each lasting three months.

Description

Pregnancy is a state in which a woman carries a fertilized egg inside her body. Due to technological advances, pregnancy is increasingly occurring among older women in the United States.

First month

At the end of the first month, the embryo is about a third of an inch long, and its head and trunk–plus the beginnings of arms and legs–have started to develop. The embryo receives nutrients and eliminates waste through the umbilical cord and placenta. By the end of the first month, the liver and digestive system begin to develop, and the heart starts to beat.

Second month

In this month, the heart starts to pump and the nervous system (including the brain and spinal cord) begins to develop. The 1 in (2.5 cm) long fetus has a complete cartilage skeleton, which is replaced by bone cells by month's end. Arms, legs and all of the major organs begin to appear. Facial features begin to form.

Third month

By now, the fetus has grown to 4 in (10 cm) and weighs a little more than an ounce (28 g). Now the major blood vessels and the roof of the mouth are almost completed, as the face starts to take on a more recognizably human appearance. Fingers and toes appear. All the major organs are now beginning to form; the kidneys are now functional and the four chambers of the heart are complete.

Fourth month

The fetus begins to kick and swallow, although most women still can't feel the baby move at this point. Now 4 oz (112 g), the fetus can hear and urinate, and has established sleep-wake cycles. All organs are now fully formed, although they will continue to grow for the next five months. The fetus has skin, eyebrows, and hair.

Fifth month

Now weighing up to a 1 lb (454 g) and measuring 8–12 in (20–30 cm), the fetus experiences rapid growth as its internal organs continue to grow. At this point, the mother may feel her baby move, and she can hear the heartbeat with a stethoscope.

Sixth month

Even though its lungs are not fully developed, a fetus born during this month can survive with intensive care. Weighing 1–1.5 lbs (454–681 g), the fetus is red, wrinkly, and covered with fine hair all over its body. The fetus will grow very fast during this month as its organs continue to develop.

Seventh month

There is a better chance that a fetus born during this month will survive. The fetus continues to grow rapidly, and may weigh as much as 3 lb (1.3 kg) by now. Now the fetus can suck its thumb and look around its watery womb with open eyes.

Eighth month

Growth continues but slows down as the baby begins to take up most of the room inside the uterus. Now weighing 4–5 lbs (1.8–2.3 kg) and measuring 16–18 in (40–45 cm) long, the fetus may at this time prepare for delivery next month by moving into the head-down position.

Ninth month

Adding 0.5 lb (227 g) a week as the due date approaches, the fetus drops lower into the mother's abdomen and prepares for the onset of labor, which may begin any time between the 37th and 42nd week of gestation. Most healthy babies will weigh 6–9 lb (2.7–4 kg) at birth, and will be about 20 in. long.

Causes and symptoms

The first sign of pregnancy is usually a missed menstrual period, although some women bleed in the beginning. A woman's breasts swell and may become tender as the mammary glands prepare for eventual breastfeeding. Nipples begin to enlarge and the veins over the surface of the breasts become more noticeable.

Nausea and vomiting are very common symptoms and are usually worse in the morning and during the first trimester of pregnancy. They are usually caused by hormonal changes, in particular, increased levels of progesterone. Women may feel worse when their stomach is empty, so it is a good idea to eat several small meals throughout the day, and to keep things like crackers on hand to eat even before getting out of bed in the morning.

Many women also feel extremely tired during the early weeks. Frequent urination is common, and there

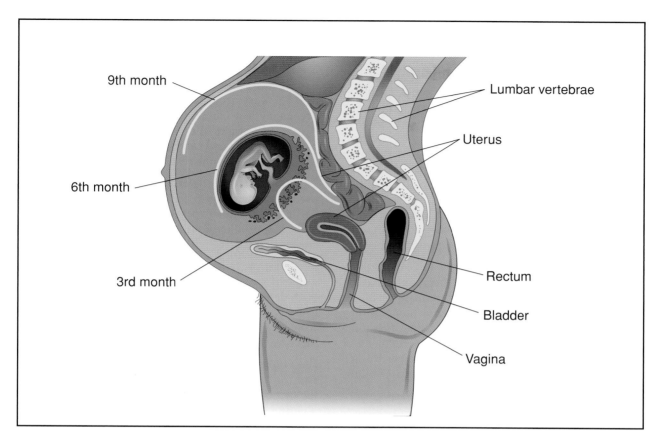

9th month

6th month

3rd month

Lumbar vertebrae

Uterus

Rectum

Bladder

Vagina

Pregnancy usually lasts 40 weeks in humans, beginning from the first day of the woman's last menstrual period, and is divided into three trimesters. The illustration above depicts the position of the developing fetus during each trimester. *(Illustration by Electronic Illustrators Group.)*

may be a creamy white discharge from the vagina. Some women crave certain foods, and an extreme sensitivity to smell may worsen the **nausea**. Weight begins to increase.

In the second trimester (13–28 weeks) a woman begins to look noticeably pregnant and the enlarged uterus is easy to feel. The nipples get bigger and darker, skin may darken, and some women may feel flushed and warm. Appetite may increase. By the 22nd week, most women have felt the baby move. During the second trimester, nausea and **vomiting** often fade away, and the pregnant woman often feels much better and more energetic. Heart rate increases as does the volume of blood in the body.

By the third trimester (29–40 weeks), many women begin to experience a range of common symptoms. Stretch marks may develop on abdomen, breasts, and thighs, and a dark line may appear from the navel to pubic hair. A thin fluid may be expressed from the nipples. Many women feel hot, sweat easily and often find it hard to get comfortable. Kicks from

an active baby may cause sharp pains, and lower backaches are common. More rest is needed as the woman copes with the added **stress** of extra weight. Braxton Hicks contractions may get stronger.

At about the 36th week in a first pregnancy (later in repeat pregnancies), the baby's head drops down low into the pelvis. This may relieve pressure on the upper abdomen and the lungs, allowing a woman to breathe more easily. However, the new position places more pressure on the bladder.

A healthy gain for most women is between 25 and 35 pounds. Women who are overweight should gain less; and women who are underweight should gain more. On average, pregnant women need an additional 300 calories a day. Generally, women will gain three to five pounds in the first three months, adding one to two pounds a week until the baby is born. An average, healthy full-term baby at birth weighs 7.5 lb (3.4 kg), and the placenta and fluid together weigh another 3.5 lb. The remaining weight that a woman gains during pregnancy is mostly due to water retention and fat stores. Her breasts, for instance, gain about 2 lb. in weight, and she gains another 4 lb due to the increased blood volume of pregnancy.

In addition to the typical, common symptoms of pregnancy, some women experience other problems that may be annoying, but which usually disappear after delivery. **Constipation** may develop as a result of food passing more slowly through the intestine. **Hemorrhoids** and **heartburn** are fairly common during late pregnancy. Gums may become more sensitive and bleed more easily; eyes may dry out, making contact lenses feel painful. **Pica** (a craving to eat substances other than food) may occur. Swollen ankles and **varicose veins** may be a problem in the second half of pregnancy, and chloasma may appear on the face.

Chloasma, also known as the "mask of pregnancy" or melasma, is caused by hormonal changes that result in blotches of pale brown skin appearing on the forehead, cheeks, and nose. These blotches may merge into one dark mask. It usually fades gradually after pregnancy, but it may become permanent or recur with subsequent pregnancies. Some women also find that the line running from the top to the bottom of their abdomen darkens. This is called the linea nigra.

While the above symptoms are all considered to be normal, there are some symptoms that could be a sign of a more dangerous underlying problem. A pregnant woman with any of the following signs should contact her doctor immediately:

- abdominal pain
- rupture of the amniotic sac or leaking of fluid from the vagina
- bleeding from the vagina
- no fetal movement for 24 hours (after the fifth month)
- continuous headaches
- marked, sudden swelling of eyelids, hands, or face during the last three months
- dim or blurry vision during last three months
- persistent vomiting

Diagnosis

Many women first discover they are pregnant after a positive home pregnancy test. Pregnancy urine tests check for the presence of human chorionic gonadotropin (hCG), which is produced by a placenta. The newest home tests can detect pregnancy on the day of the missed menstrual period.

Home pregnancy tests are more than 97% accurate if the result is positive, and about 80% accurate if the result is negative. If the result is negative and there is no menstrual period within another week, the pregnancy test should be repeated. While home pregnancy tests are very accurate, they are less accurate than a pregnancy test conducted at a lab. For this reason, women may want to consider having a second pregnancy test conducted at their doctor's office to be sure of the accuracy of the result.

Blood tests to determine pregnancy are usually used only when a very early diagnosis of pregnancy is needed. This more expensive test, which also looks for hCG, can produce a result within nine to 12 days after conception.

Once pregnancy has been confirmed, there are a range of screening tests that can be done to screen for **birth defects**, which affect about 3% of unborn children. Two tests are recommended for all pregnant women: alpha-fetoprotein (AFP) and the triple marker test.

Other tests are recommended for women at higher risk for having a child with a birth defect. This would include women over age 35, who had another child or a close relative with a birth defect, or who have been exposed to certain drugs or high levels of radiation. Women with any of these risk factors may want to consider **amniocentesis**, **chorionic villus sampling** (CVS) or ultrasound.

Other prenatal tests

There are a range of other prenatal tests that are routinely performed, including:

- PAP test
- gestational diabetes screening test at 24–28 weeks
- tests for sexually transmitted diseases
- urinalysis
- blood tests for anemia or blood type
- screening for immunity to various diseases, such as German measles

Treatment

Prenatal care is vitally important for the health of the unborn baby. A pregnant woman should be sure to eat a balanced, nutritious diet of frequent, small meals. Women should begin taking 400 mcg of **folic acid** several months before becoming pregnant, as folic acid has been shown to reduce the risk of spinal cord defects, such as **spina bifida**.

KEY TERMS

Alpha-fetoprotein—A substance produced by a fetus' liver that can be found in the amniotic fluid and in the mother's blood. Abnormally high levels of this substance suggests there may be defects in the fetal neural tube, a structure that will include the brain and spinal cord when completely developed. Abnormally low levels suggest the possibility of Down' syndrome.

Braxton Hicks' contractions—Short, fairly painless uterine contractions during pregnancy that may be mistaken for labor pains. They allow the uterus to grow and help circulate blood through the uterine blood vessels.

Chloasma—A skin discoloration common during pregnancy, also known as the "mask of pregnancy" or melasma, in which blotches of pale brown skin appear on the face. It is usually caused by hormonal changes. The blotches may appear in the forehead, cheeks, and nose, and may merge into one dark mask. It usually fades gradually after pregnancy, but it may become permanent or recur with subsequent pregnancies. Some women may also find that the line running from the top to the bottom of their abdomen darkens. This is called the linea nigra.

Embryo—An unborn child during the first eight weeks of development following conception (fertilization with sperm). For the rest of pregnancy, the embryo is known as a fetus.

Fetus—An unborn child from the end of the eights week after fertilization until birth.

Human chorionic gonadotropin (hCG)—A hormone produced by the placenta during pregnancy.

Placenta—The organ that develops in the uterus during pregnancy that links the blood supplies of the mother and baby.

Rhythm method—The oldest method of contraception with a very high failure rate, in which partners periodically refrain from having sex during ovulation. Ovulation is predicted on the basis of a woman's previous menstrual cycle.

Spina bifida—A congenital defect in which part of the vertebrae fail to develop completely, leaving a portion of the spinal cord exposed.

No medication (not even a nonprescription drug) should be taken except under medical supervision, since it could pass from the mother through the placenta to the developing baby. Some drugs, called teratogens, have been proven harmful to a fetus, but no drug should be considered completely safe (especially during early pregnancy). Drugs taken during the first three months of a pregnancy may interfere with the normal formation of the baby's organs, leading to birth defects. Drugs taken later on in pregnancy may slow the baby's growth rate, or they may damage specific fetal tissue (such as the developing teeth), or cause preterm birth.

To have the best chance of having a healthy baby, a pregnant woman should avoid:

- smoking
- alcohol
- street drugs
- large amounts of **caffeine**
- artificial sweeteners

Nutrition

Women should begin following a healthy diet even before they become pregnant. This means cutting back on high-calorie, high-fat, high-sugar snacks, and increasing the amount of fruits, vegetables and whole grains in her diet. Once she becomes pregnant, she should make sure to get at least six to 11 servings of breads and other whole grains, three to five servings of vegetables, two to four servings of fruits, four to six servings of milk and milk products, three to four servings of meat and protein foods, and six to eight glasses of water. She should limit caffeine to no more than one soft drink or cup of coffee per day.

Prognosis

Pregnancy is a natural condition that usually causes little discomfort provided the woman takes care of herself and gets adequate prenatal care. **Childbirth** education classes for the woman and her partner help prepare the couple for labor and delivery.

Prevention

There are many ways to avoid pregnancy. A woman has a choice of many methods of **contraception** which will prevent pregnancy, including (in order of least to most effective):

- spermicide alone
- natural (rhythm) method
- diaphragm or cap alone
- condom alone

- diaphragm with spermicide
- condom with spermicide
- intrauterine device (IUD)
- contraceptive pill
- sterilization (either a man or woman)
- avoiding intercourse

Resources

ORGANIZATIONS

Healthy Mothers, Healthy Babies National Coalition. 409 12th St., Washington, DC 20024. (202) 638-5577.

National Institute of Child Health and Human Development. 9000 Rockville Pike, Bldg. 31, Rm. 2A32, Bethesda, MD 20892. (301) 496-5133.

Positive Pregnancy and Parenting Fitness. 51 Saltrock Rd., Baltic, CT 06330. (203) 822-8573.

OTHER

Doulas of North America < http://www.dona.com >.
Planned Parenthood. < http://www.plannedparenthood.org >.
Pregnancy Information. < http://www.childbirth.org >.

Debra Gordon

Pregnancy test *see* **Human chorionic gonadotropin pregnancy test**

Preleukemia *see* **Myelodysplastic syndrome**

Premature atrial contractions *see* **Atrial ectopic beats**

Premature birth *see* **Prematurity**

Premature ejaculation

Definition

Premature ejaculation occurs when male sexual climax (orgasm) occurs before a man wishes it or too quickly during intercourse to satisfy his partner.

Description

Premature ejaculation is the most commonly reported sexual complaint of men and couples. The highest number of complaints is among teenage, young adult, and sexually inexperienced males. Increased risk is associated with sexual inexperience and lack of knowledge of normal male sexual responses.

Causes and symptoms

There are several reasons why a man may ejaculate prematurely. For some men, the cause is due to an innate reflex or psychological predisposition of the nervous system. Sometimes it can be caused by certain drugs, such as non-prescription cold medications. Psychological factors, such as **stress**, fear, or guilt can also play a role. Examples of psychological factors include guilt that the sexual activity is wrong or sinful, fear of getting caught, or stress from problems at work or home.

In general, symptoms are when a male reaches climax in less than two minutes or when it occurs before the male or couple want it to occur.

Diagnosis

There are no tests used to diagnose premature ejaculation. It is usually determined by the male involved based on his belief that he reached orgasm too quickly. General guidelines for premature ejaculation is if it occurs in two minutes or less, or prior to about 15 thrusts during sexual intercourse.

Treatment

In 1966, William H. Masters and Virginia E. Johnson published *Human Sexual Response,* in which they broke the first ground in approaching this topic from a new perspective. Their method was devised by Dr. James Seman and has been modified subsequently by Dr. Helen Singer Kaplan and others.

A competent and orthodox sex therapist will spend much more time focusing on the personal than the sexual relationship between the two people who come for treatment. Without emotional intimacy, sexual relations are superficial and sexual problems such as premature ejaculation are not always overcome.

With that foremost in mind, a careful plan is outlined that requires dedication, patience, and commitment by both partners. It necessarily begins by prohibiting intercourse for an extended period of time—at least a week, often a month. This is very important to the man because "performance anxiety" is the greatest enemy of performance. If he knows he cannot have intercourse he is able to relax and focus on the exercises. The first stage is called "sensate focus" and involves his concentration on the process of sexual arousal and climax. He should learn to recognize each step in the process, most particularly the moment just before the "point of no return." Ideally, this stage of treatment requires the man's partner to be devoted to his sensations. In order to regain equality, he should in turn spend separate time stimulating and pleasing his mate, without intercourse.

At this point the techniques diverge. The original "squeeze technique" requires that the partner become expert at squeezing the head of the penis at intervals to prevent orgasm. The modified procedure, described by Dr. Ruth Westheimer, calls upon the man to instruct the partner when to stop stimulating him to give him a chance to draw back. A series of stages follows, each offering greater stimulation as the couple gains greater control over his arousal. This whole process has been called "outercourse." After a period of weeks, they will have together retrained his response and gained satisfactory control over it. In addition, they will each have learned much about the other's unique sexuality and ways to increase each other's pleasure.

With either technique, the emphasis is on the mutual goal of satisfactory sexual relations for both partners.

However, the 1990s ushered in a new era in the treatment of premature ejaculation when physicians discovered that certain antidepression drugs had a side effect of delaying ejaculation. Clinical studies have shown that a class of antidepressants called selective seratonin reuptake inhibitors (SSRIs) can be very effective in prolonging the time to ejaculation. The individual drugs and the average amount of time they delay ejaculation are fluoxetine (Prozac), one to two minutes with doses of 20–40 milligrams per day (mg/day) and eight minutes with 60 mg/day; paroxetine (Paxil), three to 10 minutes with doses of 20–40 mg/day; and sertraline (Zoloft), two to five minutes with doses of 50–200 mg/day.

Alternative treatment

There are several alternative products, usually found in health food and **nutrition** stores, designed to be sprayed or rubbed on the penis to delay ejaculation. Although the products promise results, there are no valid clinical studies to support the claims. A device called a testicular restraint, sold through erotic mail-order magazines, sometimes helps men delay ejaculation. The Velcro-like device restrains the testicles from their natural tendency to move during sex. Testicular movement can cause premature ejaculation.

Prognosis

The "squeeze technique" has elicited a 95% success rate, whereby the patient is able to control ejaculation.

Treatment with SSRIs is effective in 85–90% of cases. However, the effectiveness begins to decrease after five weeks of daily administration. Although more studies are needed, this suggests the SSRIs are more effective when used on an as-needed basis.

Prevention

The best prevention is obtaining adequate information on normal sexual responses of males before having sex. It is also helpful to have sex in a comfortable, relaxed, private setting, free of guilt, stress, and fear.

Resources

PERIODICALS

"Lengthen Your Fuse." *Men's Health* November 1999: 56.
Rowland, David L., and Arthur L. Burnett. "Pharmacotherapy in the Treatment of Male Sexual Dysfunction." *The Journal of Sex Research* August 2000: 226+.

ORGANIZATIONS

American Association for Marriage and Family Therapy. 1133 15th St. NW, Suite 300, Washington, DC 20005-2710. (202) 452-0109. < http://www.aamft.org. >.
American Association of Sex Educators, Counselors, and Therapists. P.O. Box 5488, Richmond, VA 23220. < http://www.aasect.org. >.
Sexuality Information and Education Council of the U.S. 130 W. 42nd St., Ste. 350, New York, NY 10036. (212) 819-9770. < http://www.siecus.org. >.

Ken R. Wells

Premature labor

Definition

Premature labor is the term to describe contractions of the uterus that begin at weeks 20–36 of a **pregnancy**.

Description

The usual length of a human pregnancy is 38–42 weeks after the first day of the last menstrual period. Labor is a natural series of events that indicate that the birth process is starting. Premature labor is defined as contractions that occur after 20 weeks and before 37 weeks during the term of pregnancy. The baby is more likely to survive and be healthy if it remains in the uterus for the full term of the pregnancy. It is estimated that around 10% of births in the United States occur during the premature period. Premature birth is the greatest cause of newborn illness and death. In the United States, **prematurity** has a greater impact on African-Americans.

Causes and symptoms

The causes of premature labor cannot always be determined. Some research suggests that infection of the urinary or reproductive tract may stimulate premature labor and premature births. Multiple pregnancies (twins, triplets, etc.) are more likely to result in to premature labor. Smoking, alcohol use, drug **abuse**, and poor **nutrition** can increase the risk of premature labor and birth. Adolescent mothers are also at higher risk for premature delivery. Women whose mothers took diethylstilbestrol (DES) when they carried them are more likely to deliver prematurely, as are women who have had previous surgery on the cervix.

The symptoms of premature labor can include contractions of the uterus or tightening of the abdomen, which occurs every ten minutes or more frequently. These contractions usually increase in frequency, duration, and intensity, and may or may not be painful. Other symptoms associated with premature labor can include menstrual-like cramps, abdominal cramping with or without diarrhea, pressure or **pain** in the pelvic region, low backache, or a change in the color or amount of vaginal discharge. As labor progresses, the cervix or opening of the uterus will open (dilate) and the tissue around it will become thinner (efface). **Premature rupture of membranes** (when the water breaks) may also occur.

An occasional contraction can occur anytime during the pregnancy and does not necessarily indicate that labor is starting. Premature contractions are sometimes confused with Braxton Hicks contractions, which can occur throughout the pregnancy. Braxton Hicks contractions do not cause the cervix to open or efface, and are considered "false labor."

Diagnosis

The health care provider will conduct a physical examination and ask about the timing and intensity of the contractions. A vaginal examination is the only way to determine if the cervix has started to dilate or efface. Urine and blood samples may be collected to screen for infection. A vaginal culture (a cotton-tipped

---

KEY TERMS

Braxton Hicks contractions—Tightening of the uterus or abdomen that can occur throughout pregnancy. These contractions do not cause changes to the cervix and are sometimes called false labor or practice contractions.

Cervix —The opening at the bottom of the uterus, which dilates or opens in order for the fetus to pass into the vagina or birth canal during the delivery process.

Contraction—A tightening of the uterus during pregnancy. Contractions may or may not be painful and may or may not indicate labor.

---

swab is used to collect some fluid and cells from the vagina) may be done to look for a vaginal infection. A fetal heart monitor may be placed on the mother's abdomen to record the heartbeat of the fetus and to time the contractions. A fetal ultrasound may be performed to determine the age and weight of the fetus, the condition of the placenta, and to see if there is more than one fetus present. **Amniocentesis** will sometimes be performed. This is a procedure where a needle-like tube is inserted through the mother's abdomen to draw out some of the fluid surrounding the fetus. Analysis of the amniotic fluid can determine if the baby's lungs are mature. A baby with mature lungs is much more likely to survive outside the uterus.

Treatment

The goal of treatment is to stop the premature labor and prevent the fetus from being delivered before it is full term. A first recommendation may be for the woman with premature contractions to lie down with feet elevated and to drink juice or other fluids. If contractions continue or increase, medical attention should be sought. In addition to bed rest, medical care may include intravenous fluids. Sometimes, this extra fluid is enough to stop contractions. In some cases, oral or injectable drugs like terbutaline sulfate, ritodrine, magnesium sulfate, or nifedipine must be given to stop the contractions. These are generally very effective; however, as with any drug therapy, there are risks of side effects. Some women may need to continue on medication for the duration of the pregnancy. **Antibiotics** may be prescribed if a vaginal or urinary tract infection is detected. If the membranes have already ruptured, it may be difficult or impossible to stop premature labor. If infection of the membranes that cover the fetus (chorioamnionitis) develops, the baby must be delivered.

Prognosis

If premature labor is managed successfully, the pregnancy may continue normally for the delivery of a healthy infant. Once symptoms of preterm labor occur during the pregnancy, the mother and fetus need to be monitored regularly since it is likely that premature labor will occur again. If the preterm labor cannot be stopped or controlled, the infant will be delivered prematurely. These infants that are born prematurely have an increased risk of health problems including **birth defects**, lung problems, mental retardation, blindness, deafness, and developmental disabilities. If the infant is born too early, its body systems may not be mature enough for it to survive. Evaluating the infant's lung maturity is one of the keys to determining its chance of survival. Fetuses delivered further into pregnancy and those with more mature lungs are more likely to survive.

Prevention

Smoking, poor nutrition, and drug or alcohol abuse can increase the risk of premature labor and early delivery. Smoking and drug or alcohol use should be stopped. A healthy diet and prenatal vitamin supplements (prescribed by the health care provider) are important for the growth of the fetus and the health of the mother. Pregnant women are advised to see a health care provider early in the pregnancy and receive regular prenatal examinations throughout the pregnancy. The health care provider should be informed of any medications that the mother is receiving and any health conditions that exist before and during the pregnancy.

Resources

ORGANIZATIONS

March of Dimes Birth Defects Foundation. 1275 Mamaroneck Ave., White Plains, NY 10605. (914) 428-7100. resourcecenter@modimes.org. <http://www.modimes.org>.

OTHER

"Am I in Labor?" *The Virtual Hospital Page*. University of Iowa. <http://www.vh.org>.

Altha Roberts Edgren

Premature menopause

Definition

The average age at which American women go through **menopause** is 51 years. If menopause (hormonal changes at the end of the female reproductive years) occurs before age 40, it is said to be premature menopause. Possible causes include autoimmune problems and common cancer treatments.

Description

About half of all women will go through menopause before age 51 and the rest will go through it after. Most women will finish menopause between the ages of 42 and 58. A small number of women will find that their periods stop prematurely, before age 40.

Causes and symptoms

There are many possible causes of premature menopause. Women who have premature menopause often have **autoimmune disorders** like thyroid disease or **diabetes mellitus**. In these diseases, the body produces antibodies to one or more of its own organs. These antibodies interfere with the normal function of the organ. Just as antibodies might attack the thyroid or the pancreas (causing thyroid disease or diabetes), antibodies may attack the ovaries and stop the production of female hormones.

Cancer treatments like **chemotherapy** or radiation can cause premature menopause. The risk depends on the type and length of treatment and the age of the woman when she first begins radiation or chemotherapy.

If the ovaries are surgically removed (during a **hysterectomy**, for example) menopause will occur within a few days, no matter how old the woman is.

The symptoms of premature menopause are similar to those of menopause at any time. Menstrual periods stop and women may notice hot flashes, vaginal dryness, mood swings, and sleep problems. Sometimes the first symptom of premature menopause is **infertility**. A woman may find that she cannot become pregnant because she is not ovulating (producing eggs) anymore.

When menopause occurs after the ovaries are surgically removed, the symptoms begin within several days after surgery and tend to be more severe. This happens because the drop in the level of estrogen is dramatic, unlike the gradual drop that usually occurs.

Diagnosis

Premature menopause can be confirmed by blood tests to measure the levels of follicle stimulating hormone (FSH) and luteinizing hormone (LH). The levels of these hormones will be higher if menopause has occurred.

Because premature menopause is often associated with other hormonal problems, women who have premature menopause should be screened for diabetes, thyroid disease, and similar diseases.

Treatment

There is no treatment to reverse premature menopause. Hormone replacement therapy (HRT) can prevent the common symptoms of menopause and lower the long-term risk of **osteoporosis**. Women who have premature menopause should take HRT. Estrogen relieves the unpleasant symptoms of menopause, including the hot flashes and the vaginal dryness. Estrogen is especially important for women who go through premature menopause. The long-term health risks of menopause (osteoporosis and increased risk of heart disease) are even more likely to occur after premature menopause. However, women who have certain medical conditions (like **liver disease**, uterine cancer, or breast cancer) may not be candidates for estrogen.

If a woman still has her uterus after premature menopause, she will also need to take progesterone along with the estrogen. If her uterus has been removed, estrogen alone will be enough.

Women who wish to become pregnant after premature menopause now have the option of fertility treatments using donor eggs. This is similar to in vitro fertilization, but the eggs come from a donor instead of the woman who is trying to become pregnant.

Prevention

Premature menopause cannot be prevented.

Resources

BOOKS

Hall, Janet E. "Amenorrhea." In *Primary Care of Women*, edited by Karen J. Carlson and Stephanie A. Eisenstat. St. Louis: Mosby-Year Book, Inc., 1995.

Amy B. Tuteur, MD

Premature rupture of membranes

Definition

Premature rupture of membranes (PROM) is an event that occurs during **pregnancy** when the sac containing the developing baby (fetus) and the amniotic fluid bursts or develops a hole prior to the start of labor.

Description

During pregnancy, the unborn baby (fetus) is surrounded and cushioned by a liquid called amniotic fluid. This fluid, along with the fetus and the placenta, is enclosed within a sac called the amniotic membrane. The amniotic fluid is important for several reasons. It cushions and protects the fetus, allowing the fetus to move freely. The amniotic fluid also allows the umbilical cord to float, preventing it from being compressed and cutting off the fetus's supply of oxygen and nutrients. The amniotic membrane contains the amniotic fluid and protects the fetal environment from the outside world. This barrier protects the fetus from organisms (like bacteria or viruses) that could travel up the vagina and potentially cause infection.

Although the fetus is almost always mature at between 36–40 weeks and can be born without complication, a normal pregnancy lasts an average of 40 weeks. At the end of 40 weeks, the pregnancy is referred to as being "term." At term, labor usually begins. During labor, the muscles of the uterus contract repeatedly. This allows the cervix to begin to grow thinner (called effacement) and more open (dilatation). Eventually, the cervix will become completely effaced and dilated. In the most common sequence of events (about 90% of all deliveries), the amniotic membrane breaks (ruptures) around this time. The baby then leaves the uterus and enters the birth canal. Ultimately, the baby will be delivered out of the mother's vagina. In the 30 minutes after the birth of the baby, the placenta should separate from the wall of the uterus and be delivered out of the vagina.

Sometimes the membranes burst before the start of labor, and this is called premature rupture of membranes (PROM). There are two types of PROM. One occurs at a point in pregnancy before normal labor and delivery should take place. This is called preterm PROM. The other type of PROM occurs at 36–40 weeks of pregnancy.

PROM occurs in about 10% of all pregnancies. Only about 20% of these cases are preterm PROM. Preterm PROM is responsible for about 34% of all premature births.

Causes and symptoms

The causes of PROM have not been clearly identified. Some risk factors include **smoking**, multiple pregnancies (twins, triplets, etc.), and excess amniotic fluid (**polyhydramnios**). Certain procedures carry an increased risk of PROM, including **amniocentesis** (a diagnostic test involving extraction and examination of amniotic fluid) and cervical cerclage (a procedure in which the uterus is sewn shut to avoid **premature labor**). A condition called **placental abruption** is also associated with PROM, although it is not known which condition occurs first. In some cases of preterm PROM, it is believed that bacterial infection of the amniotic membrane causes it to weaken and then break. However, most cases of PROM and infection occur in the opposite order, with PROM occurring first followed by an infection.

The main symptom of PROM is fluid leaking from the vagina. It may be a sudden, large gush of fluid, or it may be a slow, constant trickle of fluid. The complications that may follow PROM include premature labor and delivery of the fetus, infections of the mother and/or the fetus, and compression of the umbilical cord (leading to oxygen deprivation in the fetus).

Labor almost always follows PROM, although the delay between PROM and the onset of labor varies. When PROM occurs at term, labor almost always begins within 24 hours. Earlier in pregnancy, labor can be delayed up to a week or more after PROM. The chance of infection increases as the time between PROM and labor increases. While this may cause doctors to encourage labor in the patient who has reached term, the risk of complications in a premature infant may cause doctors to try delaying labor and delivery in the case of preterm PROM.

The types of infections that can complicate PROM include amnionitis and endometritis. Amnionitis is an infection of the amniotic membrane. Endometritis is an infection of the innermost lining of the uterus. Amnionitis occurs in 0.5–1% of all pregnancies. In the case of PROM at term, amnionitis complicates about 3–15% of pregnancies. About 15–23% of all cases of preterm PROM will be complicated by amnionitis. The presence of amnionitis puts the fetus at great risk of developing an overwhelming infection (**sepsis**) circulating throughout its bloodstream. Preterm babies are the most susceptible to this life-threatening infection. One type of bacteria responsible for overwhelming infections in newborn babies is called group B streptococci.

Diagnosis

Depending on the amount of amniotic fluid leaking from the vagina, diagnosing PROM may be easy. Some doctors note that amniotic fluid has a very characteristic musty smell. A **pelvic exam** using a sterile medical instrument (speculum) may reveal a trickle of amniotic fluid leaving the cervix, or a pool of amniotic fluid collected behind the cervix. One of two easy tests can be performed to confirm that the liquid is amniotic fluid. A drop of the fluid can be placed on nitrazine paper. Nitrazine paper is made so that it turns from yellowish green to dark blue when it comes in contact with amniotic fluid. Another test involves smearing a little of the fluid on a slide, allowing it to dry, and then viewing it under a microscope. When viewed under the microscope, dried amniotic fluid will be easy to identify because it will look "feathery" like a fern.

Once PROM has been diagnosed, efforts are made to accurately determine the age of the fetus and the maturity of its lungs. Premature babies are at great risk if they have immature lungs. These evaluations can be made using amniocentesis and ultrasound measurements of the fetus' size. Amniocentesis also allows the practitioner to check for infection. Other indications of infection include a **fever** in the mother, increased heart rate of the mother and/or the fetus, high white blood cell count in the mother, foul smelling or pus-filled discharge from the vagina, and a tender uterus.

Treatment

Treatment of PROM depends on the stage of the patient's pregnancy. In PROM occurring at term, the mother and baby will be watched closely for the first 24 hours to see if labor will begin naturally. If no labor begins after 24 hours, most doctors will use medications to start labor. This is called inducing labor. Labor is induced to avoid a prolonged gap between PROM and delivery because of the increased risk of infection.

Preterm PROM presents more difficult treatment decisions. The younger the fetus, the more likely it may die or suffer serious permanent damage if delivered prematurely. Yet the risk of infection to the mother and/or the fetus increases as the length of time from PROM to delivery increases. Depending on the age of the fetus and signs of infection, the doctor must decide either to try to prevent labor and delivery until the fetus is more mature, or to induce labor and prepare to treat the complications of **prematurity**. However, the baby will need to be delivered to avoid serious risks to both it and the mother if infection is present, regardless of the risks of prematurity.

A variety of medications may be used in PROM:

- Medication to induce labor (oxytocin) may be used, either in the case of PROM occurring at term or in the case of preterm PROM and infection.

- Tocolytics may be given to halt or prevent the start of labor. These may be used in the case of preterm PROM, when there are no signs of infection. Delaying the start of labor may give the fetus time to develop more mature lungs.

- Steroids may be used to help the fetus' lungs mature early. Steroids may be given in preterm PROM if the fetus must be delivered early because of infection or labor that cannot be stopped.

- **Antibiotics** can be given to fight infections. Research is being done to determine whether antibiotics should be given prior to any symptoms of infection to avoid the development of infection.

Prognosis

The prognosis in PROM varies. It depends in large part on the maturity of the fetus and the development of infection.

KEY TERMS

Amniocentesis—A medical procedure during which a long, thin needle is inserted through the abdominal and uterine walls, and into the amniotic sac. A sample of amniotic fluid is withdrawn through the needle for examination.

Amniotic fluid—The fluid within the amniotic sac; the fluid surrounds, cushions, and protects the fetus.

Amniotic membrane—The thin tissue that creates the walls of the amniotic sac.

Cervical cerclage—A procedure in which the cervix is sewn closed; used in cases when the cervix starts to dilate too early in a pregnancy to allow the birth of a healthy baby.

Placenta—The organ that provides oxygen and nutrition from the mother to the fetus during pregnancy. The placenta is attached to the wall of the uterus, and leads to the fetus via the umbilical cord.

Prevention

The only controllable factor associated with PROM is smoking. Cigarette smoking should always be discontinued during a pregnancy.

Resources

ORGANIZATIONS

American College of Obstetricians and Gynecologists. 409 12th Street, S.W., P.O. Box 96920

Rosalyn Carson-DeWitt, MD

Premature ventricular contractions *see* **Ventricular ectopic beats**

Prematurity

Definition

The length of a normal **pregnancy** or gestation is considered to be 40 weeks (280 days) from the date of conception. Infants born before 37 weeks gestation are considered premature and may be at risk for complications.

Description

More than one out of every ten infants born in the United States is born prematurely. Advances in medical technology have made it possible for infants born as young as 23 weeks gestational age (17 weeks premature) to survive. These premature infants, however, are at higher risk for **death** or serious complications, which include heart defects, respiratory problems, blindness, and brain damage.

Causes and symptoms

The birth of a premature baby can be brought on by several different factors, including premature labor; placental abruption, in which the placenta detaches from the uterus; placenta previa, in which the placenta grows too low in the uterus; **premature rupture of membranes**, in which the amniotic sac is torn, causing the amniotic fluid to leak out; **incompetent cervix**, in which the opening to the uterus opens too soon; and maternal toxemia, or blood **poisoning**. While one of these conditions are often the immediate reason for a premature birth, its underlying cause is usually unknown. Prematurity is much more common in multiple pregnancy and for mothers who have a history of miscarriages or who have given birth to a premature infant in the past. One of the few, and most important, identifiable causes of prematurity is drug **abuse**, particularly **cocaine**, by the mother.

Infants born prematurely may experience major complications due to their low birth weight and the immaturity of their body systems. Some of the common problems among premature infants are **jaundice** (yellow discoloration of the skin and whites of the eyes), apnea (a long pause in breathing), and inability to breast or bottle feed. Body temperature, blood pressure, and heart rate may be difficult to regulate in premature infants. The lungs, digestive system, and nervous system (including the brain) are underdeveloped in premature babies, and are particularly vulnerable to complications. Some of the more common risks and complications of prematurity are described below.

Respiratory distress syndrome (RDS) is the most common problem seen in premature infants. Babies born too soon have immature lungs that have not developed **surfactant**, a protective film that helps air sacs in the lungs to stay open. With RDS, breathing is rapid and the center of the chest and rib cage pull inward with each breath. Extra oxygen can be supplied to the infant through tubes that fit into the nostrils of the nose, or by placing the baby under an oxygen hood. In more serious cases, the baby may have to have a breathing tube inserted and receive air from a respirator or ventilator. A surfactant drug can be given in some cases to coat the lung tissue. Extra oxygen may be need for a few days or weeks, depending on how small and premature the baby was at birth. Bronchopulmonary dysplasia is the development of scar tissue in the lungs, and can occur in severe cases of RDS.

Necrotizing enterocolitis (NEC) is a further complication of prematurity. In this condition, part of the baby's intestines are destroyed as a result of bacterial infection. In cases where only the innermost lining of the bowel dies, the infant's body can regenerate it over time; however, if the full thickness of a portion dies, it must be removed surgically and an opening (ostemy) must be made for the passage of wastes until the infant is healthy enough for the remaining ends to be sewn together. Because NEC is potentially fatal, doctors are quick to respond to its symptoms, which include lethargy, **vomiting**, a swollen and/or red abdomen, **fever**, and blood in the stool. Measures include taking the infant off mouth feedings and feeding him or her intravenously; administering **antibiotics**; and removing air and fluids from the digestive tract via a nasal tube. Approximately 70% of NEC cases can be successfully treated without surgery.

Intraventricular hemorrhage (IVH) is another serious complication of prematurity. It is a condition in which immature and fragile blood vessels within the brain burst and bleed into the hollow chambers (ventricles) normally reserved for cerebrospinal fluid and into the tissue surrounding them. Physicians grade the severity of IVH according to a scale of I–IV, with I being bleeding confined to a small area around the burst vessels and IV being an extensive collection of blood not only in the ventricles, but in the brain tissue itself. Grades I and II are not uncommon, and the baby's body usually reabsorbs the blood with no ill effects. However, more severe IVH can result in **hydrocephalus**, a potentially fatal condition in which too much fluid collects in the ventricles, exerting increased pressure on the brain and causing the baby's head to expand abnormally. To drain fluid and relieve pressure on the brain, doctors will either perform lumbar punctures, a procedure in which a needle is inserted into the spinal canal to drain fluids; install a reservoir, a tube that drains fluid from a ventricle and into an artificial chamber under or on top of the scalp; or install a ventricular shunt, a tube that drains fluid from the ventricles and into the abdomen, where it is reabsorbed by the body. Infants who are at high risk for IVH usually have an ultrasound taken of their brain in the first week after birth, followed by others if bleeding is detected. IVH cannot be prevented; however, close monitoring can ensure that procedures to reduce fluid in the brain are implemented quickly to minimize possible damage.

Apnea of prematurity is a condition in which the infant stops breathing for periods lasting up to 20 seconds. It is often associated with a slowing of the heart rate. The baby may become pale, or the skin color may change to a blue or purplish hue. Apnea occurs most commonly when the infant is asleep. Infants with serious apnea may need medications to stimulate breathing or oxygen through a tube inserted in the nose. Some infants may be placed on a ventilator or respirator with a breathing tube inserted into the airway. As the baby gets older, and the lungs and brain tissues mature, the breathing usually becomes more regular. A group of researchers in Cleveland reported in 2003, however, that children who were born prematurely are 3–5 times more likely to develop sleep-disordered breathing by age 10 than children who were full-term babies.

As the fetus develops, it receives the oxygen it needs from the mother's blood system. Most of the blood in the infant's system bypasses the lungs. Once the baby is born, its own blood must start pumping through the lungs to get oxygen. Normally, this bypass duct closes within the first few hours or days after birth. If it does not close, the baby may have trouble getting enough oxygen on its own. **Patent ductus arteriosus** is a condition in which the duct that channels blood between two main arteries does not close after the baby is born. In some cases, a drug, indomethacin, can be given to close the duct. Surgery may be required if the duct does not close on its own as the baby develops.

Retinopathy of prematurity is a condition in which the blood vessels in the baby's eyes do not develop normally, and can, in some cases, result in blindness. Premature infants are also more susceptible to infections. They are born with fewer antibodies, which are necessary to fight off infections.

Diagnosis

Many of the problems associated with prematurity depend on how early the baby is born and how much it weighs at birth. The most accurate way of determining the gestational age of an infant in utero is calculating from a known date of conception or using ultrasound imaging to observe development. When a baby is born, doctors can use the Dubowitz exam to estimate gestational age. This standardized test scores responses to 33 specific neurological stimuli to estimate the infant's neural development. Once the baby's gestational age and weight are determined, further tests and **electronic fetal monitoring** may need to be used to diagnose problems or to track the baby's condition. A blood pressure monitor may be wrapped around the arm or leg. Several types of monitors can be taped to the skin. A heart monitor or cardiorespiratory monitor may be attached to the baby's chest, abdomen, arms, or legs with adhesive patches to monitor breathing and heart rate. A thermometer probe may be taped on the skin to monitor body temperature. Blood samples may be taken from a vein or artery. X rays or ultrasound imaging may be used to examine the heart, lungs, and other internal organs.

Treatment

Treatment depends on the types of complications that are present. It is not unusual for a premature infant to be placed in a heat-controlled unit (an incubator) to maintain its body temperature. Infants that are having trouble breathing on their own may need oxygen either pumped into the incubator, administered through small tubes placed in their nostrils, or through a respirator or ventilator, which pumps air into a breathing tube inserted into the airway. The infant may require fluids and nutrients to be administered through an intravenous line in which a small needle is inserted into a vein in the hand, foot, arm, leg, or scalp. If the baby needs drugs or medications, they may also be administered through the intravenous line. Another type of line may be inserted into the baby's umbilical cord. This can be used to draw blood samples or to administer medications or nutrients. If heart rate is irregular, the baby may have heart monitor leads taped to the chest. Many premature infants require time and support with breathing and feeding until they mature enough to breathe and eat unassisted. Depending on the complications, the baby may require drugs or surgery.

A form of treatment that is being recommended by many mainstream practitioners as of 2003 is **massage therapy**. Research has shown that the risks of massaging preterm infants are minimal, and that the infants benefit from improved developmental scores, more rapid weight gain, and earlier discharge from the hospital. An additional benefit of massage therapy is closer bonding between the parents and their newborn child.

Prognosis

Advances in medical care have made it possible for many premature infants to survive and develop normally. However, whether or not a premature infant will survive is still intimately tied to his or her gestational age:

- 21 weeks or less: 0% survival rate
- 22 weeks: 0–10% survival rate
- 23 weeks: 10–35% survival rate
- 24 weeks: 40–70% survival rate
- 25 weeks: 50–80% survival rate
- 26 weeks: 80–90% survival rate
- 27 weeks: greater than 90% survival rate

Physicians cannot predict long-term complications of prematurity; some consequences may not become evident until the child is school-aged. Minor disabilities like learning problems, poor coordination, or short attention span may be the result of premature birth, but can be overcome with early intervention. The risks of serious long-term complications depend on many factors, including how premature the infant was at birth, weight at birth, and the presence or absence of breathing problems. Gender is a definite factor: a Swedish study published in 2003 found that boys are at greater risk of death or serious long-term consequences of prematurity than girls; for example, 60% of boys born at 24 weeeks' gestation die, compared to 38% mortality for girls. The development of infection or the presence of a birth defect can also affect long-term prognosis. Infections in premature and very low birth weight infants are a risk factor for later disorders of the nervous system; a study done at Johns Hopkins reported that 77 out of a group of 213 premature infants developed neurologic disorders. Severe disabilities like brain damage, blindness, and chronic lung problems are possible and may require ongoing care.

Prevention

Some of the risks and complications of premature delivery can be reduced if the mother receives good prenatal care, follows a healthy diet, avoids alcohol or drug consumption, and refrains from cigarette **smoking**. In some cases of **premature labor**, the mother may be placed on bed rest or given drugs that can stop labor contractions for days or weeks, giving the developing infant more time to develop before delivery. The physician may prescribe a steroid medication to be given to the mother before the delivery to help speed up the baby's lung development. The availability of neonatal intensive care unit, a special hospital unit equipped and trained to deal with premature infants, can also increase the chances of survival.

A new medication may help to prevent spontaneous premature births. Researchers at Wake Forest

---

KEY TERMS

Apnea—A long pause in breathing.

Dubowitz exam—A standardized test that scores responses to 33 specific neurological stimuli to estimate an infant's neural development and, hence, gestational age.

Intraventricular hemorrhage (IVH)—A condition in which blood vessels within the brain burst and bleed into the hollow chambers (ventricles) normally reserved for cerebrospinal fluid and into the tissue surrounding them.

Jaundice—Yellow discoloration of skin and whites of the eyes that results from excess bilirubin in the body's system.

Necrotizing enterocolitis (NEC)—A condition in which part of the intestines are destroyed as a result of bacterial infection.

Respiratory distress syndrome (RDS)—Condition in which a premature infant with immature lungs does not develop surfactant, a protective film that helps air sacs in the lungs to stay open. RDS is the most common problem seen in premature infants.

Retinopathy of prematurity—A condition in which the blood vessels in a premature infant's eyes do not develop normally, and can, in some cases, result in blindness.

Surfactant—A protective film that helps air sacs in the lungs to stay open. Premature infants may not have developed this protective layer before birth and are more susceptible to respiratory problems without it. Some surfactant drugs are available. These can be given through a respirator and will coat the lungs when the baby breathes the drug in.

University reported in June 2003 that a drug known as 17 alpha-hydroxyprogesterone caproate not only reduced the number of premature births in a group of women who received weekly injections of the drug compared to a placebo group, but also lowered the rates of necrotizing enterocolitis, intraventricular hemorrhage, and need for supplemental oxygen in their infants.

Resources

BOOKS

Beers, Mark H., MD, and Robert Berkow, MD., editors. "Premature Infant." In *The Merck Manual of Diagnosis and Therapy*. Whitehouse Station, NJ: Merck Research Laboratories, 2004.

PERIODICALS

Beachy, J. M. "Premature Infant Massage in the NICU." *Neonatal Network* 22 (May-June 2003): 39–45.

Holcroft, C. J., K. J. Blakemore, M. Allen, and E. M. Graham. "Association of Prematurity and Neonatal Infection with Neurologic Morbidity in Very Low Birth Weight Infants." *Obstetrics and Gynecology* 101 (June 2003): 1249–1253.

Ingemarsson, I. "Gender Aspects of Preterm Birth." *British Journal of Obstetrics and Gynecology* 110, Supplement 20 (April 2003): 34–38.

Meis, P. J., M. Klebanoff, E. Thom, et al. "Prevention of Recurrent Preterm Delivery by 17 Alpha-Hydroxyprogesterone Caproate." *New England Journal of Medicine* 348 (June 12, 2003): 2379–2385.

Rosen, C. L., E. K. Larkin, H. L. Kirchner, et al. "Prevalence and Risk Factors for Sleep-Disordered Breathing in 8- to 11-Year-Old Children: Association with Race and Prematurity." *Journal of Pediatrics* 142 (April 2003): 383–389.

Ward, R. M., and J. C. Beachy. "Neonatal Complications Following Preterm Birth." *British Journal of Obstetrics and Gynecology* 110, Supplement 20 (April 2003): 8–16.

ORGANIZATIONS

American Academy of Pediatrics (AAP). 141 Northwest Point Boulevard, Elk Grove Village, IL 60007. (847) 434-4000. < http://www.aap.org >.

National Institute of Child Health and Human Development (NICHD) Information Resource Center (IRC). P. O. Box 3006, Rockville, MD 20847. (800) 370-2943. < http://www.nichd.nih.gov >.

OTHER

Brazy, J. E. *For Parents of Preemies*. < http://www2.medsch.wisc.edu/childrenshosp/parents_of_preemies/index.html >.

Levison, Donna. "When Is It Too Early? A Guide to Help Prevent Premature Birth." *Health Net*. < http://www.health-net.com/preme.htm >.

"Survival of Extremely Premature Babies." *Dr. Plain Talk Health Care Information*. < http://www.drplaintalk.org >.

Altha Roberts Edgren
Rebecca J. Frey, PhD

Premenstrual dysphoric disorder

Definition

Premenstrual dysphoric disorder (PMDD) is a collection of physical and emotional symptoms that occurs 5 to 11 days before a woman's period begins, and goes away once menstruation starts. The most severe form of **premenstrual syndrome** (PMS) is PMDD.

Description

PMS is estimated to affect 70–90% of childbearing age. The more severe form of the disorder, PMDD, affects 3–5% of women of childbearing age. Up to 40% of women have PMDD symptoms that are so severe they interfere with their daily activities. It is more common in women in their late 20s and early 40s, who have at least one child and a history of depression, anxiety/tension, affective lability, or irritability/anger.

Causes and symptoms

Although the actual cause of PMDD is not known, it is believed to be related to hormonal changes that occur before menstruation. There are more than 150 signs and symptoms attributed to PMDD, and every woman experiences different ones at different times. There seem to be socioeconomic and genetic factors that precipitate PMDD. Twin studies have demonstrated a positive correlation with heritability and PMDD symptoms. Anti-anxiety medications have been shown to help improve symptoms associated with PMDD. The most common symptoms include **headache**, swelling of ankles, feet, and hands, backache, abdominal cramps, heaviness or **pain**, bloating and/or gas, **muscle spasms**, breast tenderness, weight gain, recurrent cold sores, **acne, nausea, constipation** or **diarrhea**, food cravings, **anxiety** or panic, confusion, difficulty concentrating and forgetfulness, poor judgment, and depression.

Diagnosis

PMDD is diagnosed when symptoms occur during the second half of the menstrual cycle (14 days or more after the first day of a woman's period), are absent for about seven days after the period ends, increase in severity as the cycle progresses, go away when the menstrual flow begins or shortly thereafter, and occur for at least three consecutive menstrual cycles. There are no tests to diagnose it. The diagnosis of PMDD emphasizes and requires psychologically important mood symptoms.

Treatment

Recently, the Food and Drug Administration approved the first prescription drug for the treatment of PMDD, Serafem (fluoxetine). Additionally, **nonsteroidal anti-inflammatory drugs**, such as ibuprofen

KEY TERMS

Antidepressant—A medication used to relieve the symptoms of clinical depression.

Beta blockers—Class of drug, including Corgard (nadolol), and Lanoxin (digoxin), that primarily work by blunting the action of adrenaline, the body's natural fight-or-flight chemical.

Nonsteroidal anti-inflammatory drugs—This class of drugs includes aspirin and ibuprofen, and primarily works by interfering with the formation of prostaglandins, enzymes implicated in pain and inflammation.

and **aspirin**, may help with bloating and pain; beta-blockers may help with migraines; anti-anxiety medications, such as buspirone or alpraxolam, may help with anxiety; and certain other antidepressants in addition to Serafem may help with depression.

Alternative treatment

Non-pharmaceutical treatments include a variety of lifestyle changes, such as following a healthy diet, **exercise**, **stress** relief therapies, and even such alternative therapies as **aromatherapy**. Certain **vitamins** and supplements may also help, such as vitamin B6, calcium, magnesium, and vitamin E. Certain herbs may also help with symptom relief, including vitex, black cohosh, valerian, kava kava, and **St. John's wort**.

Prognosis

The prognosis varies for each woman, and is largely dependent on how much work she is willing to do in terms of lifestyle changes. Additionally, planning for PMDD symptoms, joining a support group, and communicating with her spouse and family can help minimize the negative effects of PMDD and its impact on a woman's home and work environments.

Prevention

Some women may find their PMDD disappears periodically. Diet and **nutritional supplements** can have the greatest impact in preventing PMDD.

Resources

ORGANIZATIONS

Advancement of Women's Health Research. 1828 L Street, N.W., Suite 625 Washington, DC 20036. 202-223-8224. < http://www.womens-health.org >.

National Association for Premenstrual Syndrome. 7 Swift's Court, High Street, Seal, Kent TN15 0EG UK +44 (0) 1732 760011 < www.PMDD.org.uk >.

Premenstrual syndrome

Definition

Premenstrual syndrome (PMS) refers to symptoms that occur between ovulation and the onset of menstruation. The symptoms include both physical symptoms, such as breast tenderness, back **pain**, abdominal cramps, **headache**, and changes in appetite, as well as psychological symptoms of **anxiety**, depression, and unrest. Severe forms of this syndrome are referred to as **premenstrual dysphoric disorder (PMDD)**. These symptoms may be related to hormones and emotional disorders.

Description

Approximately 75% of all menstruating women experience some symptoms that occur before or during menstruation. PMS encompasses symptoms severe enough to interfere with daily life. About 3–seven% of women experience the more severe PMDD. These symptoms can last 4–10 days and can have a substantial impact on a woman's life.

The reason some women get severe PMS while others have none is not understood. PMS symptoms usually begin at about age 20–30 years. The disease may run in families and is also more prone to occur in women with a history of psychological problems. Overall however, it is difficult to predict who is most at risk for PMS.

Causes and symptoms

Because PMS is restricted to the second half of a woman's menstrual cycle, after ovulation, it is thought that hormones play a role. During a woman's monthly menstrual cycle, which lasts 24–35 days, hormone levels change. The hormone estrogen gradually rises during the first half of a woman's cycle, the preovulatory phase, and falls dramatically at ovulation. After ovulation, the postovulatory phase, progesterone levels gradually increase until menstruation occurs. Both estrogen and progesterone are secreted by the ovaries, which are responsible for producing the eggs.

The main role of these hormones is to cause thickening of the lining of the uterus (endometrium). However, estrogen and progesterone also affect other parts of the body, including the brain. In the brain and nervous system, estrogen can affect the levels of neurotransmitters, such as serotonin. Serotonin has long been known to have an effect on emotions, as well as eating behavior. It is thought that when estrogen levels go down during the postovulatory phase of the menstrual cycle, decreases in serotonin levels follow. Whether these changes in estrogen, progesterone, and serotonin are responsible for the emotional aspects of PMS is not known with certainty. However, most researchers agree that the chemical transmission of signals in the brain and nervous system is in some way related to PMS. This is supported by the fact that the times following **childbirth** and **menopause** are also associated with both depression and low estrogen levels.

Symptoms for PMS are varied and many, including both physical and emotional aspects that range from mild to severe. The physical symptoms include: bloating, headaches, food cravings, abdominal cramps, headaches, tension, and breast tenderness. Emotional aspects include mood swings, irritability, and depression.

Diagnosis

The best way to diagnose PMS is to review a detailed diary of a woman's symptoms for several months. PMS is diagnosed by the presence of physical, psychological, and behavioral symptoms that are cyclic and occur in association with the premenstrual period of time. PMDD, which is far less common, was officially recognized as a disease in 1987. Its diagnosis depends on the presence of at least five symptoms related to mood that disappear within a few days of menstruation. These symptoms must interfere with normal functions and activities of the individual. The diagnosis of PMDD has caused controversy in fear that it may be used against women, labeling them as being impaired by their menstrual cycles.

Treatment

There are many treatments for PMS and PMDD depending on the symptoms and their severity. For mild cases, treatment includes **vitamins, diuretics,** and pain relievers. Vitamins E and B$_6$ may decrease breast tenderness and help with **fatigue** and mood swings in some women. Diuretics that remove excess fluid from the body seem to work for some women. For more severe cases and for PMDD, treatments available include **antidepressant drugs,** hormone treatment, or (only in extreme cases) surgery to remove the ovaries. Hormone treatment usually involves **oral contraceptives.** This treatment, as well as removal of the ovaries, is used to prevent ovulation and the changes in hormones that accompany ovulation. Recent studies, however, indicate that hormone treatment has little effect over placebo.

Antidepressants

The most progress in the treatment of PMS and PMDD has been through the use of antidepressant drugs. The most effective of these include sertraline (Zoloft), fluoxetine (Prozac), and paroxetine (Paxil). They are termed **selective serotonin reuptake inhibitors** (SSRIs) and act by indirectly increasing the brain serotonin levels, thus stabilizing emotions. Some doctors prescribe antidepressant treatment for PMS throughout the cycle, while others direct patients to take the drug only during the latter half of the cycle. Antidepressants should be avoided by women wanting to become pregnant. A recent clinical study found that women who took sertraline had a significant improvement in productivity, social activities, and relationships compared with a placebo group. Side effects of sertraline were found to include **nausea, diarrhea,** and decreased libido.

Alternative treatment

There are alternative treatments that can both affect serotonin and hormone responses, as well as affect some of the physical symptoms of PMS.

Vitamins and minerals

Some women find relief with the use of vitamin and mineral supplements. Magnesium can reduce the fluid retention that causes bloating, while calcium may decrease both irritability and bloating. Magnesium and calcium also help relax smooth muscles and this may reduce cramping. Vitamin E may reduce breast tenderness, nervous tension, fatigue, and **insomnia.** Vitamin B$_6$ may decrease fluid retention, fatigue, irritability, and mood swings. Vitamin B$_5$ supports the adrenal glands and may help reduce fatigue.

Phytoestrogens and Natural Progesterone

The Mexican wild yam (*Dioscorea villosa*) contains a substance that may be converted to progesterone in the body. Because this substance is readily absorbed through the skin, it can be found as an ingredient in many skin creams. (Some products also have natural progesterone added to them.) Some herbalists believe that these products can have a progesterone-like effect on the body and decrease some of the symptoms of PMS.

The most important way to alter hormone levels may be by eating more phytoestrogens. These plant-derived compounds have an effect similar to estrogen in the body. One of the richest sources of phytoestrogens is soy products, such as tofu. Additionally, many supplements can be found that contain black cohosh (*Cimicifugaracemosa*) or dong quai (*Angelica sinensis*), which are herbs high in phytoestrogens. Red clover (*Trifolium pratense*), alfalfa (*Medicago sativa*), licorice (*Glycyrrhiza glabra*), hops (*Humulus lupulus*), and legumes are also high in phytoestrogens. Increasing the consumption of phytoestrogens is also associated with decreased risks of **osteoporosis**, **cancer**, and heart disease.

Antidepressant Alternatives

Many antidepressants act by increasing serotonin levels. An alternative means of achieving this is to eat more carbohydrates. For instance, two cups of cereal or a cup of pasta have enough carbohydrates to effectively increase serotonin levels. An herb known as **St. John's wort** (*Hypericum perforatum*) has stood up to scientific trials as an effective antidepressant. As with the standard antidepressants, however, it must be taken continuously and does not show an effect until used for 46 weeks. There are also herbs, such as skullcap (*Scutellaria lateriflora*) and kava (*Piper methysticum*), that can relieve the anxiety and irritability that often accompany depression. An advantage of these herbs is that they can be taken when symptoms occur rather than continually. Chaste tree (*Vitex agnuscastus*) in addition to helping rebalance estrogen and

progesterone in the body, also may relieve the anxiety and depression associated with PMS.

Prognosis

The prognosis for women with both PMS and PMDD is good. Most women who are treated for these disorders do well.

Prevention

Maintaining a good diet, one low in sugars and fats and high in phytoestrogens and complex carbohydrates, may prevent some of the symptoms of PMS. Women should try to **exercise** three times a week, keep in generally good health, and maintain a positive self image. Because PMS is often associated with **stress**, avoidance of stress or developing better means to deal with stress can be important.

Resources

PERIODICALS

Yonkers, Kimberly A., et al. "Symptomatic Improvement of Premenstrual Dysphoric Disorder with Sertraline Treatment: A Randomized Controlled Trial." *Journal of the American Medical Association* 278 (September 24, 1997): 983-989.

Cindy L. A. Jones, PhD

Prenatal surgery

Definition

Prenatal surgery is a surgical procedure performed on a fetus prior to birth.

Purpose

In most cases prenatal surgery is performed only when the fetus is not expected to survive delivery or live long after birth without prenatal intervention. The most common prenatal surgeries are for conditions in which the newborn will not be able to breathe on its own.

Most prenatal surgeries are performed for:

- urinary tract obstructions in males, usually caused by a narrowing of the urinary tract, in which urine backs up and injures the kidneys. About 10% of fetal urinary tract obstructions require prenatal surgery to prevent multiple abnormalities and depleted amniotic fluid.

- congenital diaphragmatic **hernia** (CDH), a condition in which the diaphragm—the muscle that separates the chest and the abdomen—does form completely. Without surgery about 50% of fetuses with CDH do not survive after birth because of underdeveloped lungs.

- congenital cystic adenomatoid malformation (CCAM), a condition in which one or more lobes of the lungs become fluid-filled sacs called cysts. Large CCAMs may prevent lung development, cause **heart failure**, or prevent the fetus from ingesting amniotic fluid.

- sacrococcygeal teratoma (SCT), tumors at the base of the tailbone. The most common tumor in newborns, occurring in one out of every 35,000–40,000 births, some prenatal SCTs are very large, hard, and full of blood vessels, and can **stress** the heart.

- twin-twin **transfusion** syndrome (TTTS), a condition in which, because of abnormal blood-vessel connections in the placenta, one twin pumps the circulating blood for both twins. Affecting up to 15% of twins sharing a placenta (monochorionic), TTTS can lead to a variety of problems including heart failure.

- twin:twin reverse arterial perfusion (TRAP) sequence, a condition in which one twin lacks a heart. Occurring in about 1% of monochorionic twins, the healthy twin pumps all of the blood and, if untreated, 50–75% of these normal twins die.

Other conditions that may be treated by prenatal surgery include:

- various congenital defects that block air passages and will prevent the newborn from breathing on its own

- various lung malformations

- omphalocele, a birth defect in which portions of the stomach, liver, and intestines protrude through an opening in the abdominal wall

- fetal gastroschisis—a birth defect in which the stomach and intestines protrude through improperly formed abdominal wall muscles and float in the amniotic fluid

- bowel obstructions, usually caused by a narrowing in the small intestine

- hypoplastic left heart syndrome, in which the blood flow through the left side of the heart is obstructed

- X-linked **severe combined immunodeficiency** syndrome

- **spina bifida** (myelomeningocele)—the second most common birth defect in the United States, affecting one out of every 2,000 newborns. It is a lesion or hole where the nerves of the spinal cord are not completely enclosed and is not considered to be life-threatening.

Precautions

Prenatal surgery involves:

- serious risks for the mother and fetus

- travel to a hospital that performs the procedure

- possibly having to stay near the hospital until delivery

- extended postoperative bed rest, sometimes until delivery

- a significant financial commitment.

Description

Prenatal surgery may be referred to as fetal surgery, antenatal surgery, or maternal-fetal surgery. There are only about 600 candidates for prenatal surgery in the United States each year. Of these, only about 10% actually undergo the procedure. Most prenatal surgeries are performed between 18 and 26 weeks of gestation. Some surgeries may not be covered by insurance.

Prenatal surgery usually requires a general anesthetic, although sometimes an epidural anesthetic to numb the abdominal region may be used. The fetus receives the anesthetic via the mother's blood. An anesthesiologist and a perinatologist monitor the heart rates of the mother and fetus during the procedure.

Prenatal surgeries include:

- inserting a device into the fetal bladder to drain urine into the amniotic sac for treating urinary tract obstruction

- draining or removing CCAMs

- destroying blood vessels leading to a large SCT

- amnioreduction for TTTS, in which a syringe through the mother's abdomen is used to remove fluid from the overfilled amniotic sac and replace it in the depleted sac of the twin pumping the blood. The procedure that may be repeated during the course of the pregnancy.

- destroying abnormal blood vessel connections in the placenta of TTTS twins

- severing the connections between TRAP sequence twins

- experimental hematopoietic-stem-cell transplants for X-linked severe combined **immunodeficiency** syndrome

- closing the lesion in spina bifida

Open surgeries

In open prenatal surgeries incisions are made through the mother's abdominal wall and the fetus is partially removed from the uterus or the entire uterus is removed through the mother's abdomen. Using ultrasound as a guide, the surgeon feels for the affected fetal part. The surgeon may knead and push on the uterus to move or flip the fetus away from the placenta, the disk-shaped organ within the uterus that supplies the fetal blood. A narrow tube is placed through a tiny hole in the uterine wall to drain and collect the amniotic fluid. Opening the uterus is the riskiest part of prenatal surgery. The first incision is made at a point away from the placenta to prevent damaging it. Following the procedure the fetus is replaced in the uterus and the incision is stitched. Prior to the final stitch the amniotic fluid is re-injected into the uterus. The uterus is repositioned in the mother's body cavity and her abdominal wall is closed.

The first successful open fetal surgery was performed in 1981 for a urinary tract obstruction. The first successful open fetal surgery for CDH was performed in 1989.

Prenatal open surgery for CCAM requires opening the fetus's chest. If a large cyst does not have a hard component, procedures called thoracoamniotic shunting or catheter decompression may be used to drain it. Otherwise the surgeon must remove part or all of the cyst. The first successful resection (removal) of a CCAM from a fetal lung was performed in 1990. The first resectioning of a fetal SCT was performed in 1992.

In prenatal surgery for spina bifida, An incision the size of a small fist is made in the uterus. The surgeon loosens and lifts the tissues of the spinal-canal lesion and stitches them closed. Between 1997 and 2004, more than 200 open surgeries were performed for spina bifida. As of 2005 the surgery was available only as part of a prospective randomized clinical trial.

Less invasive procedures

For urinary tract obstructions a needle may be used to insert a catheter through the mother's abdomen and uterus and into the fetal bladder where it drains the urine into the amniotic fluid. The catheter may have a wire mesh that expands in the bladder to prevent it from plugging up or dislodging.

The first successful fetoscopic temporary tracheal occlusion for CDH was performed in 1996. Small openings are made in the uterus and a tiny fiber-optic fetoscope is inserted to guide the operation. A needle-like instrument is used to place a balloon in the fetus's trachea to prevent lung fluid from escaping through the mouth, enabling the lungs to expand, grow, and push the abdominal organs out of the chest. The balloon is removed at birth.

Hypoplastic left heart syndrome is treated by passing a needle, guided by ultrasound, through the mother's abdominal wall, into the uterus, and the fetal heart. A catheter is passed through the needle across the fetus's aortic valve. A balloon is inflated, opening the valve and allowing blood to flow through the left side of the heart.

RADIOFREQUENCY ABLATION. Radiofrequency ablation (RFA) sometimes is used for SCT. Guided by ultrasound a needle is inserted through the mother's abdomen and uterus and into the tumor. Radiofrequency waves sent through the needle destroy the blood supply to the tumor with heat. This slows the tumor's growth and may enable the fetus to survive until delivery. The first RFA of a SCT was performed in 1998.

TRAP sequence also may be treated by RFA. A 3-mm needle targets the exact point where the blood enters the twin without a heart. Using an echocardiographic device, RFA is applied until the blood vessels and surrounding tissue are destroyed and the blood flow is halted. This procedure has eliminated the need for open surgery to treat TRAP sequence.

LASER TREATMENT. If TTTS does not respond to amnioreduction, laser treatment to halt the abnormal blood circulation may be attempted. A thin fetoscope is inserted through the mother's abdominal and uterine walls and into the amniotic cavity of the recipient twin to examine the surface placental blood vessels. The abnormal blood vessel connections are located and eliminated with a laser beam. The first successful fetoscopic laser treatment for TTTS was performed in 1999.

EXIT. Ex utero intrapartum treatment (EXIT) is a surgery performed for a congenital defect that blocks a fetal airway. The fetus is removed from the womb by **cesarean section** but the umbilical cord is left intact so that the mother's placenta continues to sustain the fetus. After the air passage is cleared, the umbilical cord is cut and the newborn can breathe on its own. The EXIT procedure is used for various types of airway obstruction including CCAM.

Preparation

The decision to perform prenatal surgery is made on the basis of detailed ultrasound imaging of the fetus—including echocardiograms that use ultrasound to obtain images of the heart—as well as other diagnostic tools. Consultations include a perinatologist, a neonatologist, a pediatric surgeon, a clinical nurse specialist, and a social worker. Since additional congenital defects preclude prenatal surgery, **amniocentesis** or chorionic villi sampling (CVS) are used to check for chromosomal abnormalities in the fetus.

Prior to surgery the mother must:

- arrange for postoperative bed rest to prevent preterm labor
- prepare for the possibility of remaining near the hospital until delivery
- receive betamethasone, a steroid, in two intramuscular injections 12–24 hours apart to accelerate fetal lung maturation
- wear a fetal/uterine monitor

The mother usually receives medications called tocolytics to prevent contractions and labor during and after surgery:

- terbutalin
- indocin suppositories before surgery and up to 48 hours after surgery
- magnesium sulfate for one to two days after surgery with careful monitoring
- nifedipine every four to six hours as the indocin is decreased, continuing until 37 weeks of gestation or delivery

Aftercare

In addition to usual post-surgical care, the mother:

- usually remains in the hospital for four to seven days
- lies on her side to help prevent contractions and ensure the best possible fetal circulation
- has a transparent dressing over the abdominal incision for fetal monitoring
- has continuous electronic fetal/uterine monitoring to check the fetal heart, the uterine response to tocolytics, and to watch for signs of preterm labor.

After discharge from the hospital the mother is on modified bed rest, lying on her side, until 37 weeks of gestation. This increases blood flow to the fetus and reduces pressure on the cervix to help prevent uterine contractions. She sees a perinatologist once a week and has at least one ultrasound per week.

Risks

Most prenatal surgeries are high risk and may be considered experimental. The greatest risk is that the placenta will be nicked during surgery, causing blood hemorrhaging, uterine contractions, and birth of a premature infant who may not survive. Preterm labor is the most common complication of prenatal surgery. Fetoscopic surgeries are less dangerous and traumatic than open fetal surgery and reduce the risk of **premature labor**. Subsequent children of a mother who has undergone prenatal surgery usually are delivered by cesarean section because of uterine scarring.

Maternal risks

Risks to the mother include:

- extensive blood loss
- complications from general anesthesia
- side effects—potentially fatal—from medications to control premature labor
- rupture of the uterine incision
- infection of the wound or uterus
- psychological stress
- inability to have additional children
- **death**.

Fetal risks

All fetuses that undergo surgery are born prematurely. Those born even six weeks early are at risk for walking and talking delays and learning disabilities. Infants born at 30 weeks of gestation or less are at risk for blindness, **cerebral palsy**, and brain hemorrhages.

About 25% of women undergoing prenatal surgery lose some amniotic fluid, often because of leakage at the uterine incision. Amniotic fluid is essential for lung development and protects the fetus from injury and infection. If all of the amniotic fluid is lost, the fetal lungs may not develop properly. Without the fluid cushion in which the fetus floats, the umbilical cord may be compressed, causing death.

Other risks to the fetus include:

- birth during surgery
- separation of the tissues surrounding the amniotic fluid sac and the uterus, causing early delivery or interference with blood flow to some fetal body part such as an arm or leg

KEY TERMS

Amniocentesis—Withdrawal of amniotic fluid through the mother's abdominal wall, using a needle and syringe, to test for fetal disorders.

Amniotic fluid—The watery fluid within the amniotic sac that surrounds the fetus.

Cesarean section—C-section; incision through the abdominal and uterine walls to deliver a baby.

Chorion—The outermost membrane of the sac enclosing the fetus.

Chorionic villus sampling (CVS)—The removal of fetal cells from the chorion for the diagnosis of genetic disorders.

Congenital cystic adenomatoid malformation (CCAM)—A condition in which one or more lobes of the fetal lungs develop into fluid-filled sacs called cysts.

Congenital diaphragmatic hernia (CDH)—A condition in which the fetal diaphragm—the muscle dividing the chest and abdominal cavity—does not close completely.

Echocardiography—Ultrasonic examination of the heart.

Ex utero intrapartum treatment (EXIT)—A cesarean section in which the infant is removed from the uterus but the umbilical cord is not cut until after surgery for a congenital defect that blocks an air passage.

Fetoscope—A fiber-optic instrument for viewing the fetus inside the uterus.

Monochorionic twins—Twins that share a single placenta.

Omphalocele—A congenital hernia in which a small portion of the fetal abdominal contents, covered by a membrane sac, protrudes into the base of the umbilical cord.

Placenta—The organ within the uterus that provides nourishment to the fetus.

Radiofrequency ablation (RFA)—A procedure in which radiofrequency waves are used to destroy blood vessels and tissues.

Sacrococcygeal teratoma (SCT)—A tumor occurring at the base of the fetus's tailbone.

Spina bifida—Myelomeningocele; a congenital defect in which the fetal backbone and spinal canal do not close completely, allowing the spinal cord and its surrounding membranes to protrude.

Tocolytic—A medication that inhibits uterine contractions.

Twin:twin reverse arterial perfusion (TRAP) sequence—A condition in which one fetus lacks a heart and the other fetus pumps the blood for both.

Twin-twin transfusion syndrome (TTTS)—A condition in monochorionic twins in which there is a connection between the two circulatory systems so that the donor twin pumps the blood to the recipient twin without a return of blood to the donor.

Ultrasound—A procedure that uses high-frequency sound waves to image a fetus.

- intrauterine infection requiring immediate birth of the fetus
- further damage to the spinal cord and nerves during surgery to treat spina bifida
- brain damage
- physical deformities
- death.

Normal results

Although fetal surgeries heal without scarring, it is difficult to predict their outcome because relatively few have been performed:

- Fetal surgery for CDH lessens the severity of the condition so that the fetus usually survives delivery and lives long enough to undergo corrective surgery.

- Thoracoamniotic shunting for CCAM usually results in infant survival.
- The infant survival rate following prenatal removal of solid CCAMs is about 50%.
- RFA to slow the growth of a tumor usually enables the fetus to survive delivery, after which the tumor can be removed.
- The infant survival rate following prenatal treatment for TTTS is about 70%. Since TTTS is a progressive disorder, early intervention may prevent later complications.

Spina bifida arises during the first month of fetal development. Fluid leaking from the spinal cord and exposure of the cord to amniotic fluid causes damage throughout gestation. Lesions higher up in the spinal cord can cause severe deformities, **paralysis**, and

mental retardation. Prenatal surgery may reduce the abnormalities, although it does not cure the condition. Babies who survive prenatal surgery appear to be 33–50% less likely to have **hydrocephalus**, a condition that requires surgically implanted tubes or shunts to remove fluid from the ventricles (cavities) of the brain. The surgery also appears to reverse hindbrain herniation, in which the back of the brain slips down into the spinal canal, causing breathing and swallowing problems and death in 15% of affected children. Children who had prenatal surgery to treat spina bifida appear to have better brain function than those who did not. However prenatal surgery does not prevent two of the most serious conditions associated with spina bifida: leg movement and bladder and bowel control. As of 2005 the long-term prognosis for these children was not known.

Resources

BOOKS

Bianchi, Diana W., et al. *Fetology: Diagnosis and Management of the Fetal Patient*. New York: McGraw-Hill, 2000.

Casper, Monica J. *The Making of an Unborn Patient: A Social Anatomy of Fetal Surgery*. New Brunswick, NJ: Rutgers University Press, 1998.

PERIODICALS

Hedrick, Holly L., et al. "History of Fetal Diagnosis and Therapy: Children's Hospital of Philadelphia Experience." *Fetal Diagnosis and Therapy* 18, no. 2 (March/April 2003): 65–82.

Jones, Maggie. "A Miracle, and Yet." *New York Times Magazine* July 15, 2001: 38–43.

Kalb, Claudia. "Treating the Tiniest Patients." *Newsweek* June 9, 2003.

Paek, Bettina W., et al. "Advances in Fetal Surgery." *Female Patient* 25, no. 6 (June 2000): 15–18.

ORGANIZATIONS

Fetal Treatment Center, University of California at San Francisco Children's Hospital. 505 Parnassus Ave., San Francisco, CA 94143. 800-RX-FETUS. < http://www.ucsfhealth.org/childrens/medical_services/surgical/fetal >.

Management of Myelomeningocele Study (MOMS). Catherine Shaer, M.D., The George Washington University Biostatistics Center, 6110 Executive Blvd., Suite 750, Rockville, MD 20852. 866-ASK-MOMS. < http://www.spinabifidamoms.com >.

OTHER

Bunch, Kathy. *Giving Baby a Chance, Before Birth*. WebMDHealth. 2001 [cited March 11, 2005]. < http://my.webmd.com/content/article/14/3606_466.htm?lastselectedguid = {5FE84E90-BC77-4056-A91C-9531713CA348} >.

Fetal Treatment. UCSF Children's Hospital. April 2002 [cited March 11, 2005]. < http://www.ucsfhealth.org/childrens/medical_services/surgical/fetal >.

Fetal Treatment: Patient Education. UCSF Children's Hospital. March 2003 [cited March 11, 2005]. < http://www.ucsfhealth.org/childrens/medical_services/surgical/fetal/moreinfo/patient_education.html >.

Mayo Clinic Staff. *Spina Bifida: Treatment*. Mayo Foundation for Medical Education and Research. December 8, 2003 [cited March 11, 2005]. < http://www.mayoclinic.com/invoke.cfm?objectid = CB5F085A-6152-42FC-8CFC55380EF705A2&dsection = 8 >.

Margaret Alic, Ph.D.

Prepregnancy counseling

Definition

Prepregnancy **pregnancy** counseling is advice supplied by an obstetrician, nurse, certified nurse-midwife, or **childbirth** educator about those steps a mother-to-be and father-to-be can take in preparation for pregnancy. Basically, it is a checklist for people to see if they are living lives that are most accommodating to having a healthy pregnancy. Prepregnancy counseling gives time for one to make changes before pregnancy.

Purpose

The purpose and goal of prepregnancy counseling is to help patients have full-term, healthy pregnancies and babies. The counseling and education are important because lifestyle habits such as **smoking** or alcohol usage can be hazardous to a developing fetus.

Precautions

Women who have diabetes should take special precautions before pregnancy. This counseling, usually provided by a team of professionals including a registered dietitian, diabetes educators, an obstetrician, and others, helps to prevent early pregnancy loss and congenital malformations in infants of diabetic mothers.

Women who have a history of genetic disease can opt to have **genetic testing**. Prepregnancy counseling can include referrals to those specialists.

Women who are over 40 have higher **cesarean section** rates. They are also more likely than younger women to have conditions such as high blood pressure, and are more likely to have babies with genetic problems, such as **Down syndrome**.

Women who are considering pregnancy should avoid exposure to hazards such as chemicals, illicit drugs, alcohol, and smoking. They should reduce their **caffeine** intake and be careful not to let their body temperatures rise to dangerous levels.

Description

Prepregnancy counseling involves communicating important aspects about **nutrition**, medication use, and lifestyle months in advance of getting pregnant. Issues include diet, nutrition, **exercise**, smoking, alcohol, drugs, emotional health, and referral to **genetic counseling** if a patient knows of a history of inherited disease.

Preparation

The mother-to-be should stop using birth control pills to allow for at least two regular menstrual cycles to occur before conception. This requires that she stop taking birth control pills several months before getting pregnant.

Other steps to prepare for pregnancy include:

Being at optimal weight. Women should not go on prepregnancy weight loss **diets** unless they are under the care of a physician because abrupt weight loss can affect the mother's menstrual cycle and reduce fertility.

Eating a balanced diet. This is achieved by taking a prenatal vitamin provided by a health care provider and focusing on nutrients that are important for a developing fetus. These include folate, or **folic acid**, which is important for the development of the baby's brain and spinal cord. Folate can be found in fortified cereals, citrus fruits, and green leafy vegetables. Calcium is important for baby and mother. It helps the baby's bones to develop normally and keeps the mother from suffering a calcium deficiency during pregnancy. Iron keeps the mother from developing anemia during pregnancy. Good sources of iron are green leafy vegetables, red meat, beans, and fortified cereal. Fiber helps mothers avoid **constipation**, a common occurrence during pregnancy. Good sources of fiber include beans, fruits, and vegetables.

Exercising on a regular basis. One should exercise for general overall health.

Undergoing routine physical and dental exams. These include having a physical and breast

---

examination and **Pap test**. Other tests might be recommended according to a woman's health and genetic history. They should also report any prescription drugs, over-the-counter medications, or natural **vitamins** and herbs they are taking. This is the time for a woman to make sure she is up to date on her immunizations. A dental exam, with x rays, can eliminate the need to have x rays while pregnant.

Getting psychological support. Mental support is also important in the prepregnancy stage. This can help a woman to relax and better prepare mentally and physically for what lies ahead.

Risks

About 10–15% of couples in the United States experience **infertility**. When couples should seek medical evaluation and an infertility work-up depends on their ages. Generally, it takes longer for older couples to conceive. Prepregnancy counseling might include a referral to such a specialist. While infertility is often treatable, treatment can be expensive, emotionally difficult, and time-consuming. About 10 percent of the time, doctors cannot detect a reason for the infertility.

There always is the risk that a pregnancy goes awry or a baby is born with a medical condition, regardless of whether or not a person has had prepregnancy counseling.

Normal results

The counseling can provide guidelines for people so that they can maximize their chances to have emotionally and physically healthy pregnancies and healthy babies.

Abnormal results

Many abnormal results, such as genetic conditions, **miscarriage**, **preeclampsia** (also known as toxemia), and preterm births, cannot be avoided even with prepregnancy counseling. Still, some abnormal results, such as miscarriages and preterm births, may occur when mothers and fathers lead unhealthy lifestyles despite their counseling.

Resources

ORGANIZATIONS

"About infertility and pregnancy." Ciberdiet.com. < http://www.cyberdiet.com/modules/ip/reproductive_years/preparation/nutritional_health.html >.

"General pre pregnancy guidelines." < http://parentsplace.com >.

"Preconception care of women with diabetes." American Diabetes Association. < http://journal.diabetes.org/FullText/Supplements/DiabetesCare/Supplement100/S65.htm >.

"Take a health inventory before pregnancy." UC Davis Health System. UC Davis Medical Center. 2315 Stockton Blvd. Sacramento, CA 95817. (916) 734-2011. < http:www.ucdmc.ucdavis.edu >.

Trish Booth, M.A., LCCE, FACCE, Childbirth Educator, Educational Process Consultant. 7507 Northfield Lane. Manlius, N.Y. 13104. (315) 682-2922.

Lisette Hilton

Presbyopia

Definition

The term presbyopia means "old eye" and is a vision condition involving the loss of the eye's ability to focus on close objects.

Description

Presbyopia is a condition that occurs as a part of normal **aging** and is not considered to be an eye disease. The process occurs gradually over a number of years. Symptoms are usually noticeable by age 40–45 and continue to develop until the process stabilizes some 10–20 years later. Presbyopia occurs without regard to other eye conditions.

Causes and symptoms

In the eye, the crystalline lens is located just behind the iris and the pupil. Tiny ciliary muscles pull and push the lens, adjusting its curvature, and thereby adjusting the eye's focal power to bring objects into focus. As individuals age, the lens becomes less flexible and elastic, and the muscles become less powerful. Because these changes result in inadequate adjustment of the lens of the eye for various distances, objects that are close will appear blurry. The major cause of presbyopia is loss of elasticity of the lens of the eye. Loss of ciliary muscle power, however, is also believed to contribute to the problem.

Symptoms of presbyopia result in the inability to focus on objects close at hand. As the lens hardens, it is unable to focus the rays of light that come from nearby objects. Individuals typically have difficulty reading small print, such as that in telephone directories and newspaper advertisements, and may need to hold reading materials at arm's length. Symptoms include headache and eyestrain when doing close work, blurry vision, and eye **fatigue**. Symptoms may be worse early in the morning or when individuals are fatigued. Dim lighting may also aggravate the problem.

Diagnosis

Presbyopia is officially diagnosed during an eye examination conducted by eye specialists, such as optometrists or ophthalmologists. After completing optometric college, doctors of optometry screen patients for eye problems and prescribe glasses and contact lenses. In contrast, ophthalmologists are medical doctors who specialize in eye diseases. They perform eye surgery, treat eye diseases, and also prescribe glasses and contact lenses.

A comprehensive **eye examination** requires at least 30 minutes. Part of the examination will assess vision while reading by using various strength lenses. If the pupils are dilated with drugs to permit a thorough examination of the retina, an additional hour is required. The cost of eye examinations can range from $40 to $250 depending on the complexity and site of the examination and the qualifications and reputation of the examiner. Some insurers cover the cost of routine eye examinations, while others do not. A thorough eye examination is recommended at regular intervals during the adult and aging years to monitor and diagnose eye conditions. However, individuals frequently self-diagnose presbyopia by trying on inexpensive mass-produced reading glasses until they find a pair that permits reading without strain.

Treatment

Presbyopia cannot be cured, but individuals can compensate for it by wearing reading, bifocal, or trifocal eyeglasses. A convex lens is used to make up for the lost automatic focusing power of the eye. Half-glasses can be worn, which leave the top open and uncorrected for distance vision. Bifocals achieve the same goal by allowing correction of other refractive errors (improper focusing of images on the retina of the eye).

In addition to glasses, contact lenses have also been found to be useful in the treatment of presbyopia. The two common types of contact lenses prescribed for this condition are bifocal and monovision contact lenses. Bifocal contact lenses are similar to bifocal glasses. The top portion of the lens serves as the distance lens while the lower serves as the near vision lens. To prevent rotation while in the eye, bifocal contacts use a specially manufactured type of lens. Good candidates for bifocal lenses are those patients who have a good tear film (moist eyes), good binocular vision (ability to focus both eyes together) and visual acuity in each eye, and no disease or abnormalities in the eyelids. The bifocal contact lens wearer must be motivated to invest the time it requires to maintain contact lenses and be involved in occupations that do not impose high visual demands. Further, bifocal contact lenses may limit binocular vision. Bifocal contact lenses are relatively expensive, in part due to the time it takes the patient to be accurately fitted.

An alternative to wearing eyeglasses or bifocal contact lenses is monovision contact lenses. Monovision fitting provides one contact lens that corrects for near vision and a second contact lens for the alternate eye that corrects for distance vision. If distance vision is normal, the individual wears only a single contact lens for near vision. Monovision works by having one eye focus for distant objects while the other eye becomes the reading eye. The brain learns to adapt to this and will automatically use the correct eye depending on the location of material in view. Advantages of monovision are patient acceptability, convenience, and lower cost.

Several problems exist with the use of contact lenses in the treatment of presbyopia. Some individuals experience **headache** and fatigue during the adjustment period or find the slight decrease in visual acuity unacceptable. Monovision contact lenses usually result in a small reduction in high-contrast visual acuity when compared with bifocal contact lenses.

Prognosis

The changes in vision due to aging usually start in a person's early 40s and continue for several decades. At some point, there is no further development of presbyopia, as the ability to accommodate is virtually gone.

Prevention

There is no known way to prevent presbyopia.

KEY TERMS

Accommodation—The ability of the eye to change its focus from near to distant objects.

Binocular vision—Using both eyes at the same time to see an image.

Ciliary muscles—The small muscles that permit the lens to change its shape in order to focus on near or distant objects.

Lens (or crystalline lens)—The eye structure behind the iris and pupil that helps focus light on the retina.

Visual acuity—Sharpness or clearness of vision.

Resources

ORGANIZATIONS

American Academy of Ophthalmology. 655 Beach Street, P.O. Box 7424, San Francisco, CA 94120-7424. < http://www.eyenet.org >.

American Optometric Association. 243 North Lindbergh Blvd., St. Louis, MO 63141. (314) 991-4100. < http://www.aoanet.org >.

Lighthouse National Center for Vision and Aging. 111 E. 59th St., New York, NY 10022. (800) 334-5497. < http://www.lighthouse.org >.

National Eye Institute. 2020 Vision Place, Bethesda, MD 20892-3655. (301) 496-5248. < http://www.nei.nih.gov >.

Elaine Souder, PhD

Presenile dementia *see* **Alzheimer's disease**

Pressure sores *see* **Bedsores**

Preterm labor *see* **Premature labor**

Priapism

Definition

Priapism is a rare condition that causes a persistent, and often painful, penile erection.

Description

Priapism is drug induced, injury related, or caused by disease, not sexual desire. As in a normal erection, the penis fills with blood and becomes erect. However, unlike a normal erection that dissipates after sexual activity ends, the persistent erection caused by priapism is maintained because the blood in the penile shaft does not drain. The shaft remains hard, while the tip of the penis is soft. If it is not relieved promptly, priapism can lead to permanent scarring of the penis and inability to have a normal erection.

Causes and symptoms

Priapism is caused by leukemia, **sickle cell disease**, or **spinal cord injury**. It has also been associated as a rare side effect to trazodone (Desyrel), a drug prescribed to treat depression. An overdose of self-injected chemicals to counteract **impotence** has also been responsible for priapism. The chemicals are directly injected into the penis, and at least a quarter of all men who have used this method of treatment for over three months develop priapism.

Diagnosis

A **physical examination** is needed to diagnose priapism. Further testing, including nuclear scanning or Doppler ultrasound, will diagnose the underlying cause of the condition.

Treatment

There are three methods of treatment. The most effective is the injection of medicines into the penis that allow the blood to escape. Cold packs may also be applied to alleviate the condition, but this method becomes ineffective after about eight hours. For the most serious cases and those that do not respond to the first two treatments, a needle can be used to remove the blood. The tissues may need to be flushed with saline or diluted medications by the same needle

method. That failing, there are more extensive surgical procedures available. One of them shuts off much of the blood supply to the penis so that it can relax. If the problem is due to a sickle cell crisis, treatment of the crisis with oxygen or **transfusion** may suffice.

Prognosis

If priapism is relieved within the first 12–24 hours, there is usually no residual damage. After that, permanent impotence may result, since the high pressure in the penis compromises blood flow and leads to tissue death (infarction).

Prevention

An antineoplastic drug (hydroxyurea) may prevent future episodes of priapism for patients with sickle cell disease.

Resources

BOOKS
Wertheimer, Neil. *Total Health for Men*. Emmaus, PA: Rodale Press, 1995.

PERIODICALS
Werthman, P., and J. Rajfer. "MUSE Therapy: Preliminary Clinical Observations." *Urology* 50 (November 1997): 809-811.

J. Ricker Polsdorfer, MD

Prickly heat

Definition

Also known as sweat retention syndrome or miliaria rubra, prickly heat is a common disorder of the sweat glands.

Description

The skin contains two types of glands: one produces oil and the other produces sweat. Sweat glands are coil-shaped and extend deep into the skin. They are capable of plugging up at several different depths, producing four distinct skin **rashes**.

- Miliaria crystallina is the most superficial of the occlusions. At this level, only the thin upper layer of skin is affected. Little blisters of sweat that cannot escape to the surface form. A bad **sunburn** as it just starts to blister can look exactly like this.

- Deeper plugging causes miliaria rubra as the sweat seeps into the living layers of skin, where it irritates and itches.

- Miliaria pustulosais (a complication of miliaria rubra) occurs when the sweat is infected with pyogenic bacteria and turns to pus.

- Deeper still is miliaria profunda. The skin is dry, and goose bumps may or may not appear.

There are two requirements for each of these phases of sweat retention: hot enough weather to induce sweating, and failure of the sweat to reach the surface.

Causes and symptoms

Best evidence as of 2001, suggests that bacteria form the plugs in the sweat glands. These bacteria are probably normal inhabitants of the skin, and why they suddenly interfere with sweat flow is still not known.

Infants are more likely to get miliaria rubra than adults. All the sweat retention rashes are also more likely to occur in hot, humid weather.

Besides **itching**, these conditions prevent sweat from cooling the body, which it is supposed to do by evaporating from the skin surface. Sweating is the most important cooling mechanism available in hot environments. If it does not work effectively, the body can rapidly become too hot, with severe and even lethal consequences. Before entering this phase of heat **stroke**, there will be a period of heat exhaustion symptoms–dizziness, thirst, weakness–when the body is still effectively maintaining its temperature. Then the temperature rises, often rapidly, to 104–5°F (40°C) and beyond. This is an emergency of the first order, necessitating immediate and rapid cooling. The best method is immersion in ice water.

Diagnosis

Rash and dry skin in hot weather are usually sufficient to diagnose these conditions.

Treatment

The rash itself may be treated with topical antipruritics (itch relievers). Preparations containing aloe, menthol, camphor, eucalyptus oil, and similar ingredients are available commercially. Even more effective, particularly for widespread itching in hot

---

KEY TERMS

Ambient—Surrounding.

Pyogenic—Capable of generating pus. *Streptococcus, Staphococcus* and bowel bacteria are the primary pyogenic organisms.

Syndrome—A collection of abnormalities that occur together often enough to suggest they have a common cause.

---

weather, are cool baths with corn starch and/or oatmeal (about 0.5 lb [224 g] of each per bathtub-full).

Dermatologists can peel off the upper layers of skin using a special ultraviolet light. This will remove the plugs and restore sweating, but is not necessary in most cases.

Much more important, however, is to realize that the body cannot cool itself adequately without sweating. Careful monitoring for symptoms of heat disease is important. If they appear, some decrease in the ambient temperature must be achieved by moving to the shade, taking a cool bath or shower, or turning up the air conditioner.

Prognosis

The rash disappears in a day with cooler temperatures, but the skin may not recover its ability to sweat for two weeks–the time needed to replace the top layers of skin with new growth from below.

Prevention

Experimental application of topical **antiseptics** like hexachlorophene almost completely prevented these rashes.

Resources

BOOKS

Berger, Timothy G. "Skin and Appendages." In *Current Medical Diagnosis and Treatment, 1996*, edited by Stephen McPhee, et al., 35 the ed. Stamford: Appleton & Lange, 1995.

J. Ricker Polsdorfer, MD

Primaquine *see* **Antimalarial drugs**

Primary biliary cirrhosis

Definition

Primary biliary **cirrhosis** is the gradual destruction of the biliary system for unknown reasons.

Description

Although the cause of this serious condition is not known, it has many features to suggest that it is an autoimmune disease. Autoimmunity describes the process whereby the body's defense mechanisms are turned against itself. The immune system is supposed to recognize and attack only dangerous foreign invaders like germs, but many times it attacks, for no apparent reason, the cells of the body itself. Autoimmune reactions occur in many different tissues of the body, creating a great variety of diseases.

Primary biliary cirrhosis progressively destroys the system that drains bile from the liver into the intestines. Bile is a collection of waste products excreted by the liver. As the disease progresses it also **scars** the liver, leading to cirrhosis. In some patients, the disease destroys the liver in as little as five years. In others, it may lie dormant for a decade or more.

Causes and symptoms

Ninety percent of patients with this disease are women between the ages of 35 and 60. The first sign of it may be an abnormal blood test on routine examination. **Itching** is a common early symptom, caused by a buildup of bile in the skin. Fatigue is also common in the early stages of the disease. Later symptoms include **jaundice** from the accumulation of bile and specific nutritional deficiencies–bruising from vitamin K deficiency, bone **pain** from vitamin D deficiency, night blindness from vitamin A deficiency, and skin **rashes**, possibly from vitamin E or essential fatty acid deficiency. All these vitamin problems are related to the absence of bile to assist in the absorption of nutrients from the intestines.

Diagnosis

Blood tests strongly suggest the correct diagnosis, but a liver biopsy is needed for confirmation. It is also usually necessary to x ray the biliary system to look for other causes of obstruction.

Treatment

Of the many medicines tried to relieve the symptoms and slow the progress of this disease, only one

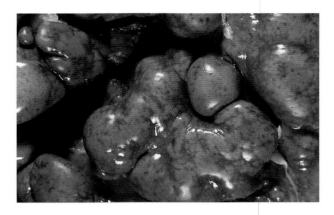

A close-up image indicating biliary cirrhosis of the liver. *(Custom Medical Stock Photo. Reproduced by permission.)*

KEY TERMS

Biopsy—Surgical removal of tissue for examination.

Cirrhosis—Scarring, usually referring to the liver.

Immunosuppression—Techniques to prevent transplant graft rejection by the body's immune system.

has had consistently positive results. Ursodeoxycholic acid, a chemical that dissolves gall stones, provides substantial symptomatic relief. It is still unclear if it slows liver damage.

Primary biliary cirrhosis is a major reason for liver transplantation. Patients do so well that this is becoming the treatment of choice. As experience, technique, and immunosuppression progressively improve, patients with this disease will come to transplant surgery earlier and earlier in their disease course.

Prognosis

So far, this disease has not returned in a transplanted liver.

Resources

ORGANIZATIONS

American Liver Foundation. 1425 Pompton Ave., Cedar Grove, NJ 07009. (800) 223-0179. < http://www.liverfoundation.org >.

J. Ricker Polsdorfer, MD

Primary degenerative dementia *see*
Alzheimer's disease

Primary polycythemia *see* **Polycythemia
vera**

Primary pulmonary hypertension *see*
Pulmonary hypertension

PRK *see* **Photorefractive keratectomy and
laser-assisted in-**

Pro time *see* **Prothrombin time**

Probenecid *see* **Gout drugs**

Procainamide *see* **Antiarrhythmic drugs**

Prochlorperazine *see* **Antinausea drugs**

Proctitis

Definition

Proctitis is an inflammation of the rectum.

Description

Proctitis affects mainly adolescents and adults. It is most common in men around age 30. Proctitis is caused by several different sexually transmitted diseases. Male homosexuals and people who practice anal intercourse are more likely to suffer from proctitis. Patients who have **AIDS** or who are immunocompromised are also more at risk.

Causes and symptoms

Proctitis is caused most often by **sexually transmitted diseases**, including **gonorrhea**, **syphilis**, herpes simplex (genital herpes), **candidiasis**, and chlamydia. It can also be caused by inflammatory bowel diseases, such as **Crohn's disease**, or **ulcerative colitis** (a chronic recurrent ulceration in the colon)–with which it is a very common component. Occasionally it is caused by an amoeba that causes **dysentery**.

Discharge of blood and mucus and intense **pain** in the area of the rectum and anus are all signs of proctitis. Patients feel the urge to have frequent bowel movements even when there is nothing present to eliminate. They may also have **constipation**, **diarrhea**, **fever**, and open sores around the anus. Other symptoms include cramping, lower back pain, difficulty urinating, and **impotence**.

Diagnosis

Proctitis is diagnosed by a patient history and physical examination. It is confirmed by a proctoscopy (examination of the rectum with an endoscope inserted through the anus). Proctoscopy usually shows a red, sore, inflamed lining of the rectum. Biopsies, smears, and lab cultures of rectal material are used to determine the exact cause of the inflammation so that the underlying cause can be treated appropriately.

Since the two problems often occur together, in the presence of proctitis, the large bowel should be examined for ulcerative colitis.

Treatment

Once the underlying cause of the inflammation is diagnosed, appropriate treatment begins. Antibiotics are given for bacterial infections. There is no cure for genital herpes, but the antiviral drug, acyclovir, is often prescribed to reduce symptoms. Corticosteroid suppositories or ointments such as hydrocortisone are used to lessen discomfort, and the patient is encouraged to take warm baths to ease painful symptoms. Ulcerative proctitis often responds well to corticosteroid **enemas** or foam, or to sulfasalazine and related drugs.

Alternative treatment

Depending on the cause of proctitis, alternative medicine has several types of treatments available. If proctitis is related to gonorrhea, syphilis, or chlamydia, appropriate antibiotic treatment is recommended. Supplementation with *Lactobacillus acidophilus* is also recommended during and following antibiotic therapy to help rebuild normal gut flora that is destroyed by **antibiotics**. If proctitis is herpes-related, antiviral herbs taken internally, as well as applied topically, can be be helpful. Sitz baths and compresses of herbal infusions (herbs steeped in hot water) and decoctions (herbal extracts prepared by boiling the herb in water) can be very effective. Among the herbs recommended are calendula (*Calendula officinalis*), comfrey (*Symphytum officinale*), and plantain (*Plantago major*). Proctitis related to candidiasis requires dietary alterations, especially elimination of sugar from the diet. Any immunocompromised person needs close medical attention. If proctitis is related to inflammatory bowel diseases, the resolution of the underlying condition should contribute to resolution of the proctitis. **Acupuncture** and homeopathic treatment can be very useful in resolving inflammatory bowel diseases.

KEY TERMS

Candidiasis—A common fungal infection caused by yeast that thrives in moist, warm areas of the body.

Chlamydia—A gonorrhea-like bacterial infection.

Proctoscopy—A procedure in which a thin tube containing a camera and a light is inserted into the rectum so that the doctor can visually inspect it.

Rectum—The final section of the large intestine.

Ulcerative colitis—Chronic ulceration of the colon and rectum.

Prognosis

Proctitis caused by bacteria is curable with antibiotics. **Genital herpes** is not curable. Although symptoms can be suppressed, proctitis may reoccur. Patients with AIDS are especially susceptible to candidiasis infections, which may be hard to control. Recovering from proctitis caused by inflammatory bowel diseases is variable and depends on successful management of those diseases. Severe proctitis can result in permanent narrowing of the anus.

Prevention

Proctitis is best prevented by using condoms and practicing safer sex to prevent acquiring sexually transmitted diseases. Avoiding anal intercourse also helps prevent damage to the rectum.

Resources

OTHER

ThriveOnline. "Proctitis." < http://thriveonline.oxygen.com >.

Tish Davidson, A.M.

Proctosigmoidoscopy *see* **Sigmoidoscopy**

Progesterone assay *see* **Sex hormones tests**

Progressive multifocal leukoencephalopathy

Definition

Progressive multifocal leukoencephalopathy (PML) is a rapidly progressive neuromuscular disease caused by opportunistic infection of brain cells (oligodendrocytes and astrocytes) by the JC virus (JCV).

Description

PML is an opportunistic infection associated with **AIDS** and certain cancers. It occurs in people with inadequate immune response and carries a poor prognosis. The incidence of PML, once quite rare, is rising as the numbers of people living with persistently compromised immune systems rises. An estimated 2–7% of people with HIV disease will develop PML. The infection also occurs among people undergoing long-term chemotherapy for **cancer**. PML is not considered a contagious disease. According to the Centers for Disease Control definition of AIDS, PML in the presence of HIV infection is sufficient to form a diagnosis of AIDS.

Causes and symptoms

Although at least 80% of the adults in the United States have been exposed to JC virus (as evidenced by the presence of antibodies to this virus), very few will develop PML. Little is certain about what causes JCV to produce active disease, but the virus persists in the kidneys of otherwise healthy people without making them ill. Recent evidence suggests that after prolonged compromise of the immune system, the virus changes into a form that can reach brain tissue and cause disease. In PML, the JCV infects and kills the cells (oligodendrocytes) that produce myelin, which is needed to form the sheath that surrounds and protects nerves.

About 45% of people with PML experience vision problems, most often a blindness affecting half of the visual field of each eye. Mental impairment affects about 38% of people with PML. Eventually, about 75% experience extreme weakness. Other symptoms include lack of coordination, **paralysis** on one side of the body (hemiparesis), and problems in speaking or using language.

Diagnosis

Diagnosis is difficult, but usually relies on a neurologist and radiologist assessing the white matter of the brain on a computed tomography scan or a magnetic resonance imaging (MRI). Tests of the cerebrospinal fluid can help distinguish between PML and other diseases, such as **multiple sclerosis** and acute hemorrhagic leukoencephalopathy. The rapid clinical progression in immunocompromised patients is another distinguishing factor.

KEY TERMS

Multifocal—Having many focal points. In progressive multifocal leukoencephalopathy, it means that damage caused by the disease occurs at multiple sites.

Opportunistic infection—A illness caused by infecting organisms that would not be able to produce disease in a person with a healthy immune system, but are able to take advantage of an impaired immune response.

Treatment

Currently, there is no known cure for PML, although it sometimes responds to treatment in patients with AIDS who are taking anti-HIV drugs (such as AZT, alpha-interferon, and peptide T). Although several agents have shown some potential in the last few years, such as the highly toxic cancer drug cytarabine, none are safe enough or sufficiently effective to be approved for PML.

Prognosis

PML is usually a very aggressive disease. The time between the onset of symptoms and death can be as little as one to six months. However, some patients infected with HIV have improved without receiving treatment specifically for PML.

Resources

PERIODICALS

Royal III, Walter. "Update on Progressive MultifocalLeukoencephalopathy." *The Hopkins HIV Report* 9 (March 1997).

Jill S. Lasker

Progressive supranuclear ophthalmoplegia *see* **Progressive supranuclear palsy**

Progressive supranuclear palsy

Definition

Progressive supranuclear palsy (PSP; also known as Steele-Richardson-Olszewski syndrome) is a rare disease that gradually destroys nerve cells in the parts of the brain that control eye movements, breathing, and muscle coordination. The loss of nerve cells causes palsy, or paralysis, that slowly gets worse as the disease progresses. The palsy affects ability to move the eyes, relax the muscles, and control balance.

Description

Progressive supranuclear palsy is a disease of middle age. Symptoms usually begin in the 60s, rarely before age 45 or after age 75. Men develop PSP more often than women do. It affects three to four people per million each year.

Causes and symptoms

PSP affects the brainstem, the basal ganglia, and the cerebellum. The brainstem is located at the top of the spinal cord. It controls the most basic functions needed for survival–the involuntary (unwilled) movements such as breathing, blood pressure, and heart rate. The brainstem has three parts: the medulla oblongata, the pons, and the midbrain. The parts affected by PSP are the pons, which controls facial nerves and the muscles that turn the eye outward, and the midbrain, the visual center. The basal ganglia are islands of nerve cells located deep within the brain. They are involved in the initiation of voluntary (willed) movement and control of emotion. Damage to the basal ganglia causes muscle stiffness (spasticity) and tremors. The cerebellum is located at the base of the skull. It controls balance and muscle coordination.

Vision is controlled by groups of cells called *nuclei* in the brainstem. In PSP, the nuclei continue to function, but the mechanisms that control the nuclei are destroyed. The term *supranuclear* means that the damage is done above (*supra*) the nuclei. Patients with PSP have difficulty with voluntary (willed) eye movement. At first, the difficulty only occurs in trying to look down. As the disease progresses, ability to move the eyes right and left is also affected. However, reflex or unwilled eye movements remain normal. Thus, when the patient's head is tilted upwards, the eyes move to look down. These reflex movements remain normal until late in the course of the disease. The upper eyelids may be pulled back, the eyebrows raised, and the brow wrinkled, causing a typical wide-eyed stare. Rate of blinking may decrease from the normal 20–30 per minute to three to five per minute. It becomes difficult to walk downstairs, to maintain eye contact during conversation, or to move the eyes up and down to read.

The earliest symptoms of PSP may be frequent falls or stiff, slow movements of the arms and legs. These symptoms may appear as much as five years before the characteristic vision problems. Walking becomes increasingly awkward, and some patients tend to lean and fall backward. Facial muscles may be weak, causing slurred speech and difficulty swallowing. Sleep may be disturbed and thought processes slowed. Although memory remains intact, the slowed speech and thought patterns and the rigid facial expression may be mistaken for senile **dementia** or **Alzheimer's disease**. Emotional responses may become exaggerated and inappropriate, and the patient may experience **anxiety**, depression, and agitation.

The cause of PSP is not known. Most people who develop PSP come from families with no history of the disease, so it does not seem to be inherited, except in certain rare instances. People who have PSP seem to lack the neurotransmitters dopamine and homovanillic acid in the basal ganglia. Neurotransmitters are chemicals that help carry electrical impulses along the nervous system. Transmitting structures in brain cells called neurofibrils become disorganized (neurofibrillary tangles). Neurofibrillary tangles are also found in Alzheimer's disease, but the pattern is somewhat different.

Diagnosis

PSP is sometimes mistaken for Parkinson's disease, which is also associated with stiffness, frequent falls, slurred speech, difficulty swallowing, and decreased spontaneous movement. The facial expression in Parkinson's, however, is blank or mask-like, whereas in PSP it is a grimace and wide-eyed stare. PSP does not cause the uncontrolled shaking (tremor) in muscles at rest that is associated with Parkinson's disease. Posture is stooped in Parkinson's disease, but erect in PSP. Speech is of low volume in both diseases, but is more slurred and irregular in rhythm in PSP.

Multiple strokes or abnormal accumulations of fluid within the skull (**hydrocephalus**) can also cause balance problems similar to PSP. **Magnetic resonance imaging** (MRI) scans of the brain may be needed to rule out these conditions. In advanced cases, MRI shows characteristic abnormalities in the brainstem described as "mouse ears."

Treatment

PSP cannot be cured. Drugs are sometimes given to relieve symptoms, but drug treatment is usually disappointing. Dopaminergic medications used in

---

KEY TERMS

Basal ganglia—Brain structure at the base of the cerebral hemispheres, involved in controlling movement.

Brainstem—Brain structure closest to the spinal cord, involved in controlling vital functions, movement, sensation, and nerves supplying the head and neck.

Cerebellum—The part of the brain involved in coordination of movement, walking, and balance.

Magnetic resonance imaging (MRI)—An imaging technique that uses a large circular magnet and radio waves to generate signals from atoms in the body. These signals are used to construct images of internal structures.

Parkinson's disease—A slowly progressive disease that destroys nerve cells. Parkinson's is characterized by shaking in resting muscles, a stooping posture, slurred speech, muscular stiffness, and weakness.

Parkinson's disease, such as levodopa (Sinemet), sometimes decrease stiffness and ease spontaneous movement. Anticholinergic medications, such as trihexyphenidyl (Artane), which restore function to neurotransmitters, or tricyclic drugs, such as amitriptyline (Elavil) may improve speech, walking, and inappropriate emotional responses.

Speech therapy may help manage the swallowing and speech difficulty in PSP. As the disease progresses, the difficulty in swallowing may cause the patient to choke and get small amounts of food in the lungs. This condition can cause aspiration **pneumonia**. The patient may also lose too much weight. In these cases, a feeding tube may be needed. The home environment should be modified to decrease potential injury from falls. Walkers can be weighted in front, to prevent backward falls and handrails can be installed in the bathroom. Because the patient cannot look down, low objects like throw rugs and coffee tables should be removed. Dry eyes from infrequent blinking can be treated with drops or ointments.

Prognosis

The patient's condition gradually deteriorates. After about seven years, balance problems and stiffness make it nearly impossible for the patient to walk. Persons with PSP become more and more immobile and unable to care for themselves. **Death** is not caused by the PSP itself. It is usually caused by pneumonia related to **choking** on secretions or by **starvation** related to swallowing difficulty. It usually occurs within 10 years, but if good general health and nutrition are maintained, the patient may survive longer.

Prevention

PSP cannot be prevented.

Resources

ORGANIZATIONS

American Academy of Neurology. 1080 Montreal Ave., St. Paul, MN 55116. (612) 695-1940. <http://www.aan.com>.

Society for Progressive Supranuclear Palsy, Inc. Suite #5065 Johns Hopkins Outpatient Center, 601 N. Caroline St., Baltimore, MD 21287. (800) 457-4777. <http://www.psp.org>.

Laurie Barclay, MD

Progressive systemic sclerosis *see* **Scleroderma**

Prolactin test

Definition

Prolactin is a hormone secreted by the anterior portion of the pituitary gland (sometimes called the "master gland"). Its role in the male has not been demonstrated, but in females, prolactin promotes **lactation**, or milk production, after **childbirth**.

Purpose

The prolactin test is used to diagnose pituitary dysfunction that might be caused by a tumor called an adenoma. In some circumstances, the test is also used to evaluate absence of menstrual periods (**amenorrhea**), or spontaneous production of milk (galactorrhea) by a woman who is not pregnant or lactating.

Precautions

Stress from trauma, illness, surgery, or even nervousness about a blood test can elevate prolactin levels. Drugs that may increase prolactin include phenothiazines, **oral contraceptives**, opiates, histamine antagonists, monoamine oxidase inhibitors

(MAO inhibitors), estrogen, and antihistamines. Drugs that can decrease values include levodopa and dopamine.

Description

Prolactin is also known as the lactogenic hormone or lactogen. It is essential for the development of the mammary glands for lactation during pregnancy, and for stimulating and maintaining lactation after childbirth. Like the human growth hormone, prolactin acts directly on tissues, and its levels rise in response to sleep and to physical or emotional stress. During sleep, prolactin levels can increase to the circulating levels found in pregnant women (as high as ten to twenty times the normal level).

Prolactin secretion is controlled by prolactin-releasing and prolactin-inhibiting chemicals (factors) secreted by an area of the brain called the hypothalamus. Another hormone, thyroid-releasing hormone, or TRH, can also stimulate prolactin.

Tumors of the pituitary, called adenomas, are the most common cause of excessive levels of prolactin. Depending on the type of cell involved, these tumors are also called prolactin-secreting pituitary acidophilic or chromophobic adenomas. Moderately high prolactin levels are found to a lesser extent in women with secondary amenorrhea, **galactorrhea**, low thyroid, anorexia, and a disorder known as polycystic ovary syndrome, a disease whose cause is not well-known.

Because high prolactin levels are more likely due to pituitary adenoma than other causes, the prolactin level is used to diagnose and monitor this type of tumor. Several stimulation and suppression tests, with TRH or levodopa, respectively, have been designed to differentiate pituitary adenoma from other causes of prolactin overproduction.

Preparation

This test requires a blood sample that should be drawn in the morning at least two hours after the patient wakes (samples drawn earlier may show sleep-induced peak levels). The patient need not restrict food or fluids nor limit physical activity, but should relax for approximately 30 minutes before the test.

Risks

Risks posed by this test are minimal, but may include slight bleeding from the blood-drawing site, **fainting** or lightheadedness after venipuncture,

KEY TERMS

Adenoma—A benign tumor

Amenorrhea—The absence or abnormal stoppage of menstrual periods.

Factor—Any of several substances necessary to produce a result or activity in the body. The term is used when the chemical nature of the substance is unknown. In endocrinology, when the chemical nature is known, factors are renamed hormones.

Galactorrhea—Excessive or spontaneous flow of milk.

Pituitary gland—A gland located at the base of the brain, and controlled by the hypothalamus. It controls most endocrine functions and is responsible for things such as kidney function, lactation, and growth and development.

or hematoma (blood accumulating under the puncture site).

Normal results

Reference ranges vary from laboratory to laboratory but are generally within the following values:

- adult male: 0–20 ng/ml
- adult female: 0–20 ng/ml
- pregnant female: 20–400 ng/ml

Abnormal results

Increased prolactin levels are found in galactorrhea, amenorrhea, prolactin-secreting pituitary tumor, infiltrative diseases of the hypothalamus, and metastatic **cancer** of the pituitary gland. Higher levels than normal are seen in stress which may be produced by **anorexia nervosa**, surgery, strenuous exercise, trauma, and in renal (kidney) failure.

Decreased prolactin levels are seen in Sheehan's syndrome, a condition of severe hemorrhage after obstetric delivery that causes decreased blood supply to the pituitary.

Resources

BOOKS

Pagana, Kathleen Deska. *Mosby's Manual of Diagnostic and Laboratory Tests.* St. Louis: Mosby, Inc., 1998.

Janis O. Flores

Prolactinoma *see* **Galactorrhea**

Prolapsed disk *see* **Herniated disk**

Prolonged QT syndrome

Definition

Prolonged QT syndrome, also known as long QT syndrome (LQTS), refers to a group of disorders that increase the risk for sudden **death** due to an abnormal heartbeat.

Description

Abnormal heartbeats (cardiac **arrhythmias**) are a primary cause of sudden death, especially in the young population. In the United States, an estimated 1 in 300,000 individuals per year die suddenly due to irregular heart rhythms. One of the better understood causes of these arrhythmias is LQTS.

The QT of LQTS refers to an interval between two points (Q and T) on the common electrocardiogram (ECG, EKG) used to record the electrical activity of the heart. This electrical activity, in turn, is the result of small molecules (ions such as sodium and potassium) passing in and out of channels in the membranes surrounding heart cells. A prolonged QT interval indicates an abnormality in electrical activity that leads to irregularities in heart muscle contraction. One of these irregularities is a specific pattern of very rapid contractions (tachycardia) of the lower chambers of the heart called torsade de pointes, a type of **ventricular tachycardia**. The rapid contractions, which are not effective in pumping blood to the body, result in a decreased flow of oxygen-rich blood to the brain. This can result in a sudden loss of consciousness (syncope) and death.

Causes and symptoms

Both inherited and acquired forms of LQTS have been identified. Most acquired forms are thought to be due to certain drugs including adrenaline (epinephrine), several **antihistamines** and **antibiotics**, specific heart medications, **diuretics**, and others. It has been proposed, but not yet documented, that individuals who experience LQTS after using one of these medications, may actually have a genetic defect that increases their tendency to cardiac arrhythmias. Severe weight loss such as is associated with **anorexia nervosa** can also disrupt ion balances in the heart and result in prolongation of the QT interval.

Three inherited forms of LQTS have been described to date. Jervell and Lange-Neilsen syndrome, named for the physicians who described the condition in 1957, is associated with congenital deafness and is inherited as an autosomal recessive trait. Romano-Ward syndrome, the most common inherited form of LQTS, was first described in the 1960's. It is inherited in an autosomal dominant pattern and is not associated with other physical impairments such as deafness. In 1995, a third type of LQTS was reported in to occur in association with bilateral **syndactyly**. Little is known about the inheritance of this form, except that reported cases have been sporadic with no associated family history of LQTS.

As of early 2001, six different genes had been associated with the inherited forms of LQTS, and mutations in at least four of these genes had been reported in a number of affected individuals and families. The genes involved in LQTS play important roles in the formation of ion channels in the cell membrane, and, thus, mutations in these genes disrupt normal cardiac rhythms.

LQTS usually presents with symptoms that constitute a life-threatening emergency. Sudden loss of consciousness or cardiac arrest can be brought on by emotional or physical **stress** in young, otherwise healthy individuals, both female and male. Fright, anger, surprise, sudden awakening as a result of loud sounds (alarm clock, telephone), as well as physical activities, especially swimming, have all been reported to precipitate an episode of cardiac arrhythmia in susceptible individuals. Sudden death often occurs. Although the information is preliminary, recent research has also suggested that a small number of SIDS (**sudden infant death syndrome**) cases may be due to mutations in one or more of the genes associated with LQTS.

Diagnosis

Problems exist in diagnosing LQTS. Although the method of diagnosis is the electrocardiogram, most young, healthy people do not routinely undergo this test, and, thus, their first, and possibly fatal, episode of LQTS comes without warning. In some cases, a non-fatal episode is mistakenly treated as a seizure, and, therefore, a follow-up assessment does not include an electrocardiogram. In addition, some cases of LQTS cannot be diagnosed by a routine electrocardiogram. That is, the QT interval is not found to be prolonged in routine testing. If LQTS is suspected either because of

a previous episode of syncope or because of a family member with LQTS, an **exercise** electrocardiogram should be performed. In all instances where an individual is diagnosed with LQTS, family members should be thoroughly evaluated, and a detailed family history should be taken noting any individuals with episodes of sudden loss of consciousness and any cases of unexplained sudden death. Because many of the genes involved in LQTS have been identified, **genetic testing** can offer a more reliable means of diagnosis of other family members at risk. The first step in determining if this type of testing is appropriate in any particular situation is to consult a genetic counselor or medical geneticist.

Treatment

A conventional treatment is the oral administration of beta-blockers, medications that decrease the input from the sympathetic nervous system to the heart. Although beta-blockers do not correct the abnormalities in the ion channels of the heart cells, they do appear to decrease the occurrence of cardiac arrhythmias. However, these medications are not helpful in all cases, and are actually contraindicated in some individuals. Potassium supplementation is also being explored as a treatment in certain cases. As the genetics of LQTS becomes better understood, it should be possible to tailor treatments that will be effective for each of the various gene mutations.

Alternative treatment

In some patients, severing of the sympathetic nerve to the heart has decreased the occurrence of arrhythmias. **Pacemakers** and defibrillators appear to hold promise as new forms of treatment. As devices of this type are developed that are smaller in size, they may come into more widespread use, either alone or in conjunction with specific medications.

Prognosis

LQTS is a life-long condition. Individuals who are not diagnosed and treated are at an increased risk of syncope and sudden death. Adequate treatment can decrease this risk. There is no cure. Individuals with one of the inherited forms of LQTS are at risk of passing the mutation and the disease to their offspring.

Prevention

The risk of cardiac arrhythmias due to acquired forms of LQTS can be decreased by avoiding the

KEY TERMS

Anorexia nervosa—A loss of appetite for food not explainable by local disease. It is thought to have a psychological basis.

Autosomal dominant—A pattern of inheritance in which only one of the two copies of an autosomal gene must be abnormal for a genetic condition or disease to occur. An autosomal gene is a gene that is located on one of the autosomes or non-sex chromosomes. A person with an autosomal dominant disorder has a 50% chance of passing it to each of their offspring.

Autosomal recessive—A pattern of inheritance in which both copies of an autosomal gene must be abnormal for a genetic condition or disease to occur. An autosomal gene is a gene that is located on one of the autosomes or non-sex chromosomes. When both parents have one abnormal copy of the same gene, they have a 25% chance with each pregnancy that their offspring will have the disorder.

Diuretic—An agent that increases the production of urine.

Electrocardiogram—A record of the electrical activity of the heart showing certain waves called P, Q, R, S, and T waves. The Q, R, S, T waves are associated with contraction of the ventricles, the lower two chambers of the heart.

Sympathetic nervous system—A division of the autonomic nervous sytem, the portion of the nervous system that controls involuntary bodily functions such as heart rate.

Syndactyly—A fusion of two or more toes or fingers.

medications and situations that trigger episodes. At present there is no genetic therapy to correct the gene mutations present in the inherited forms of LQTS, but individuals who are known to have an inherited form may also be able to lessen the risk of a life-threatening episode by avoiding such environmental triggers and by taking the appropriate medications.

Resources

BOOKS

Keating, Mark T., and Sanguinetti, Michael C. "Familial Cardiac Arrhythmias." In *The Metabolic & Molecular Bases of Inherited Disease*, edited by C.R. Scriver, et al. New York: McGraw-Hill Press, April 2001.

PERIODICALS

Towbin, Jeffrey A., and Vatta, Matteo. "Molecular Biology and the Prolonged QT Syndromes" *American Journal of Medicine* 110 (April 2001): 385–398.
Vizgirda, Vida M. "The Genetic Basis for Cardiac Dysrhythmias and the Long QT Syndrome" *J. Cardiovasc Nursing* 13, no.4 (1999): 34–45.

ORGANIZATIONS

Sudden Arrhythimia Death Syndromes Foundation. 540 Arapeen Drive, Suite 207, Salt Lake City Utah, 84108, (800) STOP SAD, < http://www.sads.org > or < http://www.ihc.com/research/longqt.html >.

OTHER

American Heart Association. < http://www.Americanheart.org/Heart_and_Stroke_A_Z_Guide/longqt.html >.
NORD (National Organization for Rare Disorders, Inc.). < http://www.rarediseases.org >.

Sallie Boineau Freeman, PhD

PROM *see* **Premature rupture of membranes**
Promethaz *see* **Antihistamines**

Prophylaxis

Definition

A prophylaxis is a measure taken to maintain health and prevent the spread of disease. Antibiotic prophylaxis is the focus of this article and refers to the use of **antibiotics** to prevent infections.

Purpose

Antibiotics are well known for their ability to treat infections. But some antibiotics also are prescribed to *prevent* infections. This usually is done only in certain situations or for people with particular medical problems. For example, people with abnormal heart valves have a high risk of developing heart valve infections after even minor surgery. This happens because bacteria from other parts of the body get into the bloodstream during surgery and travel to the heart valves. To prevent these infections, people with heart valve problems often take antibiotics before having any kind of surgery, including dental surgery.

Antibiotics also may be prescribed to prevent infections in people with weakened immune systems, such as people with **AIDS** or people who are having chemotherapy treatments for cancer. But even healthy people with strong immune systems may occasionally be given preventive antibiotics–if they are having certain kinds of surgery that carry a high risk of infection, or if they are traveling to parts of the world where they are likely to get an infection that causes **diarrhea**, for example.

In all of these situations, a physician should be the one to decide whether antibiotics are necessary. Unless a physician says to do so, it is not a good idea to take antibiotics to prevent ordinary infections.

Because the overuse of antibiotics can lead to resistance, drugs taken to prevent infection should be used only for a short time.

Description

Among the drugs used for antibiotic prophylaxis are amoxicillin (a type of penicillin) and fluoroquinolones such as ciprofloxacin (Cipro) and trovafloxacin (Trovan). These drugs are available only with a physician's prescription and come in tablet, capsule, liquid, and injectable forms.

Recommended dosage

The recommended dosage depends on the type of antibiotic prescribed and the reason it is being used. For the correct dosage, check with the physician or dentist who prescribed the medicine or the pharmacist who filled the prescription. Be sure to take the medicine exactly as prescribed. Do not take more or less than directed, and take the medicine only for as long as the physician or dentist says to take it.

Precautions

If the medicine causes **nausea**, **vomiting**, or diarrhea, check with the physician or dentist who prescribed it as soon as possible. Patients who are taking antibiotics before surgery should not wait until the day of the surgery to report problems with the medicine. The physician or dentist needs to know right away if problems occur.

For other specific precautions, see the entry on the type of drug prescribed such as penicillins or **fluoroquinolones**.

Side effects

Antibiotics may cause a number of side effects. For details, see entries on specific types of antibiotics. Anyone who has unusual or disturbing symptoms

---

KEY TERMS

AIDS—Acquired immunodeficiency syndrome. A disease caused by infection with the human immunodeficiency virus (HIV). In people with this disease, the immune system breaks down, opening the door to other infections and some types of cancer.

Antibiotic—A medicine used to treat infections.

Chemotherapy—Treatment of an illness with chemical agents. The term is usually used to describe the treatment of cancer with drugs.

Immune system—The body's natural defenses against disease and infection.

---

after taking antibiotics should get in touch with his or her physician.

Interactions

Whether used to treat or to prevent infection, antibiotics may interact with other medicines. When this happens, the effects of one or both of the drugs may change or the risk of side effects may be greater. Anyone who takes antibiotics for any reason should inform the physician about all the other medicines he or she is taking and should ask whether any possible interactions may interfere with drugs' effects. For details of **drug interactions**, see entries on specific types of antibiotics.

Nancy Ross-Flanigan

Proportionate dwarfism *see* **Pituitary dwarfism**

Proptosis *see* **Exophthalmos**

Prostaglandins *see* **Drugs used in labor**

▌Prostate biopsy

Definition

Prostate biopsy is a surgical procedure that involves removing a small piece of prostate tissue for microscopic examination.

Purpose

This test is usually done to determine whether the patient has prostate cancer. Occasionally, it may also be used to diagnose a condition called benign prostatic hyperplasia that causes enlargement of the prostate. In the United States, prostate cancer is the most common **cancer** among men over 50, and is the second leading cause of cancer deaths. According to statistics released in 2003, African American men in the United States are at much greater risk of developing **prostate cancer** after age 50 than Caucasian or Asian American men.

Prostate biopsy is recommended when a digital rectal examination (a routine screening test for prostate diseases) reveals a lump or some other abnormality in the prostate. In addition, if blood tests reveal that the levels of certain markers, such as PSA, are above normal, the doctor may order a biopsy.

Description

The prostate gland is one of the three male sex glands and lies just below the urinary bladder, in the area behind the penis and in front of the rectum. It secretes semen, the liquid portion of the ejaculate. The urethra carries the urine from the urinary bladder and the semen from the sex glands to the outside of the body.

Prostate biopsies can be performed in three different ways. They can be performed by inserting a needle through the perineum (the area between the base of the penis and the rectum), by inserting a needle through the wall of the rectum, or by cytoscopy. Before the procedure is performed, the patient may be given a sedative to help him relax. Patients undergoing cytoscopy may be given either **general anesthesia** or **local anesthesia**. The doctor will ask the patient to have an enema before carrying out the biopsy. The patient is also given **antibiotics** to prevent any possible infection.

Needle biopsy via the perineum

The patient lies either on one side or on his back with his knees up. The skin of the perineum is thoroughly cleansed with an iodine solution. A local anesthetic is injected at the site where the biopsy is performed. Once the area is numb, the doctor makes a small (1 in) incision in the perineum. The doctor places one finger in the rectum to guide the placement of the needle. The needle is then inserted into the prostate, a small amount of tissue is collected, and the needle is withdrawn. The needle is then re-inserted into another part of the prostate. Tissue may be taken from several areas. Pressure is then applied at the biopsy site to stop the bleeding. The procedure generally takes 15–30 minutes and is usually done in a physician's office or in a hospital operating room. Although it sounds painful, it typically causes only slight discomfort.

Needle biopsy via the rectum

This procedure is also done in the physician's office or in the hospital operating room, and is usually done without any anesthetic, although some doctors prefer to inject a local anesthetic, usually lidocaine. The patient is asked to lie on his side or on his back with his legs in stirrups. The doctor attaches a curved needle guide to his finger and then inserts the finger into the rectum. After firmly placing the needle guide in the rectum, the biopsy needle is pushed along the guide, through the wall of the rectum and into the prostate. The needle is rotated gently, prostate tissue samples are collected and the needle withdrawn. When an ultrasound probe is used to guide the needle, the procedure is called a transrectal ultrasound-guided biopsy, or TRUS.

Cytoscopy

For this procedure, the patient is given either a general or a local anesthetic. An instrument called a cytoscope (a thin-lighted tube with telescopic lenses) is passed through the urethra. By looking through the cytoscope, the doctor can see if there is any blockage in the urethra and remove it. Tissue samples from the urinary bladder or the prostate can be collected for microscopic examination.

This test is generally performed in an operating room or in a physician's office. An hour before the procedure, the patient is given a sedative to help him relax. An intravenous (IV) line will be placed in a vein in the arm to give medications and fluids if necessary. The patient is asked to lie on a special table with his knees apart and stirrups are used to support his feet and thighs. The genital area is cleansed with an antiseptic solution. If general anesthesia is being used, the patient is given the medication through the IV tube or inhaled gases or both. If a local anesthetic is being used, the anesthetic solution is gently instilled into the urethra.

After the area is numb, a cytoscope is inserted into the urethra and slowly pushed into the prostate. Tiny forceps or scissors are inserted through the cytoscope to collect small pieces of tissue that are used for biopsy. The cytoscope is then withdrawn. The entire procedure may take 30–45 minutes. Sometimes a catheter (tube) is left in the urinary bladder to help the urine drain out, until the swelling in the urethra has subsided.

Alternate procedures

Many different tests can be performed to diagnose prostate diseases and cancer. A routine screening test called digital **rectal examination** (DRE) can identify any lumps or abnormality with the prostate. Blood tests that measure the levels of certain protein markers, such as PSA, can indicate the presence of prostate cancer cells. X rays and other imaging techniques (such as computed tomography scans, magnetic resonance imaging, and ultrasonograms), where detailed pictures of areas inside the body are put together by a computer, can also be used to determine the extent and spread of the disease. However, a prostate biopsy and examination of the cells under a microscope remains the most definitive test for diagnosing and grading prostate cancer.

Preparation

Before scheduling the biopsy, the doctor should be made aware of all the medications that the patient is taking, if the patient is allergic to any medication, and if he has any bleeding problems. The patient may be given an antibiotic shortly before the test to reduce the risk of any infection afterwards. If the biopsy is done through the perineum, there are no special preparations. If it is being done through the rectum, the patient is asked to take an enema and is instructed on how to do it.

If a cytoscopy is being performed, the patient is asked to sign a consent form. The patient is also asked to take antibiotics before and for several days after the test to prevent infection due to insertion of the instruments. If a general anesthetic is going to be used, food and liquids will be restricted for at least eight hours before the test.

Aftercare

Following a needle biopsy, the patient may experience some **pain** and discomfort. He should avoid strenuous activities for the rest of the day. He may also notice some blood in his urine for two to three days after the test and some amount of rectal bleeding. If there is persistent bleeding, pain, or **fever**, and if the patient is unable to urinate for 24 hours, the doctor should be notified immediately.

When a cytoscopy is performed under a local anesthetic, the patient is asked to lie down for 30 minutes after the test and is then allowed to go. If general anesthesia is used, the patient is taken to the recovery room and kept there until he wakes up and is able to walk. He is allowed food and liquids after he wakes up. After general anesthesia, the patient may experience some tiredness and aching of the muscles throughout the body. If local anesthesia was administered, there is a brief burning sensation and a strong urge to urinate when the cytoscope is removed.

After the procedure, it is common to experience frequent urination with a burning sensation for a few days. Drinking a lot of fluids will help reduce the burning sensation and the chances of an infection. There may also be some blood in the urine. However, if **blood clots** are seen, or if the patient is unable to pass urine eight hours after the cytoscopy, the doctor should be notified. In addition, if the patient develops a high fever, and complains of chills or abdominal pain after the procedure, he should see the doctor right away. Although serious infections are rare, a few patients develop such severe illnesses as **meningitis** following a prostate biopsy.

Risks

Prostate biopsy performed with a needle is a low-risk procedure. The possible complications include some bleeding into the urethra, bleeding from the rectum, an infection, a temporarily lowered sperm count, or an inability to urinate. These complications are treatable and the doctor should be notified of them.

Cytoscopy is generally a very safe procedure. The most common complication is an inability to urinate due to a swelling of the urethra. A catheter (tube) may have to be inserted to help drain out the urine. If there is an infection after the procedure, antibiotics are given to treat it. In very rare instances, the urethra or the urinary bladder may be perforated because of the insertion of the instrument. If this complication occurs, surgery may be needed to repair the damage.

Normal results

If the prostate tissue samples show no sign of inflammation, and if no cancerous cells are detected, the results are normal.

Abnormal results

Analysis of the prostate tissue under the microscope reveals any abnormalities. In addition, the presence of cancerous cells can be detected. If a tumor is

KEY TERMS

Benign prostatic hyperplasia (BPH)—A noncancerous condition of the prostate that causes overgrowth of the prostate tissue, thus enlarging the prostate and obstructing urination.

Biopsy—The surgical removal and microscopic examination of living tissue for diagnostic purposes.

Computed tomography (CT) scan—A medical procedure in which a series of x rays are taken and put together by a computer in order to form detailed pictures of areas inside the body.

Digital rectal examination—A routine screening test that is used to detect any lumps in the prostate gland or any hardening or other abnormality of the prostate tissue. The doctor inserts a gloved and lubricated finger (digit) into the patient's rectum, which lies just behind the prostate. Typically, since a majority of tumors develop in the posterior region of the prostate, they can be detected through the rectum.

Magnetic resonance imaging (MRI)—A medical procedure used for diagnostic purposes where pictures of areas inside the body are created using a magnet linked to a computer.

Pathologist—A doctor who specializes in the diagnosis of disease by studying cells and tissues under a microscope.

Ultrasonogram—A procedure in which high-frequency sound waves that cannot be heard by human ears are bounced off internal organs and tissues. These sound waves produce a pattern of echoes that are then used by the computer to create sonograms or pictures of areas inside the body.

Urethra—The tube that carries the urine from the urinary bladder and (in males) the semen from the sex glands to the outside of the body.

present, the pathologist "grades" the tumor, in order to estimate how aggressive the tumor is. The most commonly used grading system is called the "Gleason system."

Normal prostate tissue has certain characteristic features that the cancerous tissue lacks. In the Gleason system, prostate cancers are graded by how closely they resemble normal prostate tissue. The system assigns a grade ranging from 1 to 5. The grades

assigned to two areas of cancer are added up for a combined score that is between 2 and 10. A score between 2 and 4 is called low and implies that the cancer is a slow-growing one. A Gleason score of 8 to 10 is high and indicates that the cancer is aggressive. The higher the Gleason score, the more likely it is that the cancer is fast-growing and may have already grown out of the prostate and spread to other areas (metastasized).

Resources

BOOKS

Beers, Mark H., MD, and Robert Berkow, MD., editors. "Prostate Cancer." In *The Merck Manual of Diagnosis and Therapy*. Whitehouse Station, NJ: Merck Research Laboratories, 2004.

PERIODICALS

Adamakis, I., D. Mitropoulos, K. Haritopoulos, et al. "Pain During Transrectal Ultrasonography Guided Prostate Biopsy: A Randomized Prospective Trial Comparing Periprostatic Infiltration with Lidocaine with the Intrarectal Instillation of Lidocaine-Prilocain Cream." *World Journal of Urology* 20 (December 2003): E-pub.

Hsieh, K., and P. C. Albertsen. "Populations at High Risk for Prostate Cancer." *Urological Clinics of North America* 30 (November 2003): 669–676.

Jones, J. S., and C. D. Zippe. "Rectal Sensation Test Helps Avoid Pain of Apical Prostate Biopsy." *Journal of Urology* 170 (December 2003): 2316–2318.

Meisel, F., C. Jacobi, R. Kollmar, et al. "Acute Meningitis after Transrectal Prostate Biopsy." [in German] *Der Urologe: Ausg. A* 42 (December 2003): 1611–1615.

Seitz, C., S. Palermo, and B. Djavan. "Prostate Biopsy." *Minerva Urologica Nefrologica* 55 (December 2003): 205–218.

Shetty, Sugandh, MD. "Transrectal Ultrasound of the Prostate (TRUS)." *eMedicine* March 1, 2004. <http://www.emedicine.com/med/topic3477.htm>.

ORGANIZATIONS

American Cancer Society. 1599 Clifton Rd., NE, Atlanta, GA 30329-4251. (800) 227-2345. <http://www.cancer.org>.

American Urologic Association. 1120 N. Charles St., Baltimore, MD 21201. (410) 223-4310.

National Prostate Cancer Coalition. 1300 19th Street NW, Suite 400, Washington, DC 20036. (202) 842-3600 ext. 214.

Prostate Cancer InfoLink. <http://www.comed.com/Prostate/index.html>.

Lata Cherath, PhD
Rebecca J. Frey, PhD

Prostate cancer

Definition

Prostate **cancer** is a disease in which cells in the prostate gland become abnormal and start to grow uncontrollably, forming tumors.

Description

Prostate cancer is a malignancy of one of the major male sex glands. Along with the testicles and the seminal vesicles, the prostate secretes the fluid that makes up semen. The prostate is about the size of a walnut and lies just behind the urinary bladder. A tumor in the prostate interferes with proper control of the bladder and normal sexual functioning. Often the first symptom of prostate cancer is difficulty in urinating. However, because a very common, non-cancerous condition of the prostate, benign prostatic hyperplasia (BPH), also causes the same problem, difficulty in urination is not necessarily due to cancer.

Cancerous cells within the prostate itself are generally not deadly on their own. However, as the tumor grows, some of the cells break off and spread to other parts of the body through the lymph or the blood, a process known as metastasis. The most common sites for prostate cancer to metastasize are the seminal vesicles, the lymph nodes, the lungs, and various bones around the hips and the pelvic region. The effects of these new tumors are what can cause **death**.

As of the early 2000s, prostate cancer is the most commonly diagnosed malignancy among adult males in Western countries. Although prostate cancer is often very slow growing, it can be aggressive, especially in younger men. Given its slow growing nature, many men with the disease die of other causes rather than from the cancer itself.

Prostate cancer affects African-American men twice as often as white men; the mortality rate among African-Americans is also two times higher. African-Americans have the highest rate of prostate cancer of any world population group.

Causes and symptoms

The precise cause of prostate cancer is not known as of the early 2000s. However, there are several known risk factors for disease including age over 55, African-American heritage, a family history of the disease, occupational exposure to cadmium or rubber, and a high fat diet. Men with high plasma testosterone levels may also have an increased risk for developing prostate cancer.

Frequently, prostate cancer has no symptoms and the disease is diagnosed when the patient goes for a routine screening examination. However, when the tumor is big or the cancer has spread to the nearby tissues, the following symptoms may be seen:

- weak or interrupted flow of the urine
- frequent urination (especially at night)
- difficulty starting urination
- inability to urinate
- **pain** or burning sensation when urinating
- blood in the urine
- persistent pain in lower back, hips, or thighs (bone pain)
- painful ejaculation

Diagnosis

Prostate cancer is curable when detected early. Yet the early stages of prostate cancer are often asymptomatic, so the disease often goes undetected until the patient has a routine **physical examination**. Diagnosis of prostate cancer can be made using some or all of the following tests.

Digital rectal examination (DRE)

In order to perform this test, the doctor puts a gloved, lubricated finger (digit) into the rectum to feel for any lumps in the prostate. The rectum lies just behind the prostate gland, and a majority of prostate tumors begin in the posterior region of the prostate. If the doctor does detect an abnormality, he or she may order more tests in order to confirm these findings.

Blood tests

Blood tests are used to measure the amounts of certain protein markers, such as prostate-specific antigen (PSA), found circulating in the blood. The cells lining the prostate generally make this protein and a small amount can be detected normally in the bloodstream. In contrast, prostate cancers produce a lot of this protein, significantly raising the circulating levels. A finding of a PSA level higher than normal for the patient's age group therefore suggests that cancer is present.

Transrectal ultrasound

A small probe is placed in the rectum and sound waves are released from the probe. These sound waves bounce off the prostate tissue and an image is created. Since normal prostate tissue and prostate tumors reflect the sound waves differently, the test is an efficient and accurate way to detect tumors. Though the insertion of the probe into the rectum may be slightly uncomfortable, the procedure is generally painless and takes only 20 minutes.

Prostate biopsy

If cancer is suspected from the results of any of the above tests, the doctor will remove a small piece of prostate tissue with a hollow needle. This sample is then checked under the microscope for the presence of cancerous cells. **Prostate biopsy** is the most definitive diagnostic tool for prostate cancer.

Prostate cancer can also be diagnosed based on the examination of the tissue removed during a transurethral resection of the prostate (TURP). This procedure is performed to help alleviate the symptoms of BPH, a benign enlargement of the prostate. Like a biopsy, this is a definitive diagnostic method for prostate cancer.

X rays and imaging techniques

A **chest x ray** may be ordered to determine whether the cancer has spread to the lungs. Imaging techniques (such as **computed tomography scans (CT)** and **magnetic resonance imaging** (MRI)), where a computer is used to generate a detailed picture of the prostate and areas nearby, may be done to get a clearer view of the internal organs. A bone scan may be used to check whether the cancer has spread to the bone.

Treatment

Once cancer is detected during the microscopic examination of the prostate tissue during a biopsy or TURP, doctors will determine two different numerical scores that will help define the patient's treatment and prognosis.

Tumor grading

Initially, the pathologist will grade the tumor based on his or her examination of the biopsy tissue. The pathologist scores the appearance of the biopsy sample using the Gleason system. This system uses a scale of one to five based on the sample's similarity or dissimilarity to normal prostate tissue. If the tissue is very similar to normal tissue, it is still well differentiated and given a low grading number, such as one or two. As the tissue becomes more and more abnormal (less and less differentiated), the grading number

increases, up to five. Less differentiated tissue is considered more aggressive and more likely to be the source of metastases.

The Gleason grading system is best predictive of the prognosis of a patient if the pathologist gives two scores to a particular sample—a primary and a secondary pattern. The two numbers are then added together and that is the Gleason score reported to the patient. Thus, the lowest Gleason score available is two (a primary and secondary pattern score of one each). A typical Gleason score is five (which can be a primary score of two and a secondary score of three or visa-versa). The highest score available is 10, with a pure pattern of very undifferentiated tissue, that is, of grade five. The higher the score, the more abnormal behavior of the tissue, the greater the chance for metastases, and the more serious the prognosis after surgical treatment. A study found that the ten-year cancer survival rate without evidence of disease for grade two, three, and four cancers is 94% of patients. The rate is 91% for grade five cancers, 78% for grade six, 46% for grade seven, and 23% for grade eight, nine, and ten cancers.

Cancer staging

The second numeric score determined by the doctor will be the stage of the cancer, which takes into account the grade of the tumor determined by the pathologist. Based on the recommendations of the American Joint Committee on Cancer (AJCC), two kinds of data are used for staging prostate cancer. Clinical data are based on the external symptoms of the cancer, while histopathological data is based on surgical removal of the prostate and examination of its tissues. Clinical data are most useful to make treatment decisions, while pathological data is the best predictor of prognosis. For this reason, the staging of prostate cancer takes into account both clinical and histopathologic information. Specifically, doctors look at tumor size (T), lymph node involvement (N), the presence of visceral (internal organ) involvement (metastasis = M), and the grade of the tumor (G).

The classification of tumor as T1 means the cancer that is confined to the prostate gland and the tumor that is too small to be felt during a DRE. T1 tumors are often found after examination of tissue removed during a TURP. The T1 definition is subdivided into those cancers that show less than 5% cancerous cells in the tissue sample (T1a) or more than 5% cancerous cells in the tissue sample (T1b). T1c means that the biopsy was performed based on an elevated PSA result. The second tumor classification is T2, where the tumor is large enough to be felt during the DRE.

T2a indicates that only the left or the right side of the gland is involved, while T2b means both sides of the prostate gland has tumor.

With a T3 tumor the cancer has spread to the connective tissue near the prostate (T3a) or to the seminal vesicles as well (T3b). T4 indicates that cancer has spread within the pelvis to tissue next to the prostate such as the bladder's sphincter, the rectum, or the wall of the pelvis. Prostate cancer tends to spread next into the regional lymph nodes of the pelvis, indicated as N1. Prostate cancer is said to be at the M1 stage when it has metastasized outside the pelvis in distant lymph nodes (M1a), bone (M1b) or organs such as the liver or the brain (M1c). Pain, weight loss, and **fatigue** often accompany the M1 stage.

The grade of the tumor (G) can assessed during a biopsy, TURP surgery, or after removal of the prostate. There are three grades recognized: G1, G2, and G3, indicating the tumor is well, moderately, or poorly differentiated, respectively. The G, LN, M descriptions are combined with the T definition to determine the stage of the prostate cancer.

Stage I prostate cancer comprises patients that are T1a, N0, M0, G1. Stage II includes a variety of condition combinations including T1a, N0, M0, G2, 3 or 4; T1b, N0, M0, Any G; T1c, N0, M0, Any G; T1, N0, M0, Any G or T2, N0, M0, Any G. The prognosis for cancers at these two stages is very good. For men treated with stage I or stage II disease, over 95% are alive after five years.

Stage III prostate cancer occurs when conditions are T3, N0, M0, any G. Stage IV is T4, N0, M0, any G; any T, N1, M0, any G; or any T, any N, M1, Any G. Although the cancers of Stage III are more advanced, the five year prognosis is still good, with 70% of men diagnosed at these stage still living. The spread of the cancer into the pelvis (T4), lymph (N1), or distant locations (M1) are very significant events, as the five year survival rate drops to 30% for Stage IV.

Treatment options

The doctor and the patient will decide on the treatment mode after considering many factors. For example, the patient's age, the stage of the disease, his general health, and the presence of any co-existing illnesses have to be considered. In addition, the patient's personal preferences and the risks and benefits of each treatment protocol are also taken into account before any decision is made.

SURGERY. For stage I and stage II prostate cancer, surgery is the most common method of treatment because it theoretically offers the chance of completely removing the cancer from the body. Radical **prostatectomy** involves complete removal of the prostate. The surgery can be done using a perineal approach, where the incision is made between the scrotum and the anus, or using a retropubic approach, where the incision is made in the lower abdomen. Perineal approach is also known as nerve-sparing prostatectomy, as it is thought to reduce the effect on the nerves and thus reduce the side effects of **impotence** and incontinence. However, the retropubic approach allows for the simultaneous removal of the pelvic lymph nodes, which can give important pathological information about the tumor spread.

The drawback to surgical treatment for early prostate cancer is the significant risk of side effects that impact the quality of life of the patient. Even using nerve-sparing techniques, studies run by the National Cancer Institute (NCI) found that 60–80% of men treated with radical prostatectomy reported themselves as impotent (unable to achieve an erection sufficient for sexual intercourse) two years after surgery. This side effect can be sometimes countered by prescribing **sildenafil citrate** (Viagra). Furthermore, 8% to 10% of patients were incontinent in that time span. Despite the side effects, the majority of men were reported as satisfied with their treatment choice. Additionally, there is some evidence that the skill and the experience of the surgeon are central factors in the ultimate side effects seen.

A second method of surgical treatment of prostate cancer is cryosurgery. Guided by ultrasound, surgeons insert up to eight cryoprobes through the skin and into close proximity with the tumor. Liquid nitrogen (temperature of -320.8 o F, or -196o C) is circulated through the probe, freezing the tumor tissue. In prostate surgery, a warming tube is also used to keep the urethra from freezing. Patients currently spend a day or two in the hospital following the surgery, but it could be an outpatient procedure in the near future. Recovery time is about one week. Side effects have been reduced in recent years, although impotence still affects almost all who have had cryosurgery for prostate cancer. Cryosurgery is considered a good alternative for those too old or sick to have traditional surgery or radiation treatments or when these more traditional treatments are unsuccessful. There is a limited amount of information about the long-term efficacy of this treatment for prostate cancer.

Radiation therapy

Radiation therapy involves the use of high-energy x rays to kill cancer cells or to shrink tumors. It can be used instead of surgery for stage I and II cancer. The radiation can either be administered from a machine outside the body (external beam radiation), or small radioactive pellets can be implanted in the prostate gland in the area surrounding the tumor, called brachytherapy or interstitial implantation. Pellets containing radioactive iodine (I-125), palladium (Pd 103), or iridium (Ir 192) can be implanted on an outpatient basis, where they remain permanently. The radioactive effect of the seeds last only about a year.

The side effects of radiation can include inflammation of the bladder, rectum, and small intestine as well as disorders of blood clotting (coagulopathies). Impotence and incontinence are often delayed side effects of the treatment. A study indicated that bowel control problems were more likely after radiation therapy when compared to surgery, but impotent and incontinence were more likely after surgical treatment. Long-term results with radiation therapy are dependent on stage. A review of almost 1000 patients treated with megavoltage irradiation showed 10 year survival rates to be significantly different by T-stage: T1 (79%), T2 (66%), T3 (55%), and T4 (22%). There does not appear to be a large difference in survival between external beam or interstitial treatments.

HORMONE THERAPY. Hormone therapy is commonly used when the cancer is in an advanced stage and has spread to other parts of the body, such as stage III or stage IV. Prostate cells need the male hormone testosterone to grow. Decreasing the levels of this hormone or inhibiting its activity will cause the cancer to shrink. Hormone levels can be decreased in several ways. Orchiectomy is a surgical procedure that involves complete removal of the testicles, leading to a decrease in the levels of testosterone. Another method tricks the body by administering the female hormone estrogen. When estrogen is given, the body senses the presence of a sex hormone and stops making the male hormone testosterone. However, there are some unpleasant side effects to hormone therapy. Men may have "hot flashes," enlargement and tenderness of the breasts, or impotence and loss of sexual desire, as well as **blood clots**, heart attacks, and strokes, depending on the dose of estrogen. Another side effect is **osteoporosis**, or loss of bone mass leading to brittle and easily fractured bones.

WATCHFUL WAITING. Watchful waiting means no immediate treatment is recommended, but doctors keep the patient under careful observation. This is often done using periodic PSA tests. This option is generally used in older patients when the tumor is not very aggressive and the patients have other, more life-threatening, illnesses. Prostate cancer in older men tends to be slow-growing. Therefore, the risk of the patient dying from prostate cancer, rather than from other causes, is relatively small.

Treatments for prostate cancer that are under investigation in the early 2000s include evaluation of combination therapies, such as postoperative radiation delivery, use of cytotoxic agents, and hormonal treatment using luteinizing hormone-releasing hormone (LHRH) agonists and/or antiandrogens to shut down the growth of the hormone-dependent tumors. Other drugs that are being tested as of 2003 are chemoprotective agents like amifostine (Ethyol), which are given to prostate cancer patients to counteract the harmful side effects of radiation treatment.

Alternative treatment

Alternative treatments that have been found helpful in coping with the emotional **stress** associated with prostate cancer include **meditation, guided imagery**, and relaxation techniques. **Acupuncture** is effective in relieving pain in some patients.

A variety of herbal products have been used to treat prostate cancer, including various compounds used in **traditional Chinese medicine** as well as single agents like Reishi mushrooms (*Ganoderma lucidum*). One herbal compound that was under investigation by the National Center for Complementary and Alternative Medicine (NCCAM) as a possible treatment for prostate cancer was PC-SPES, a mixture of eight herbs adapted from traditional Chinese medicine. In the summer of 2002, however, NCCAM put its studies of PC-SPES on hold when the Food and Drug Administration (FDA) determined that samples of the product were contaminated with undeclared prescription drug ingredients. PC-SPES was withdrawn from the American market in late 2002.

Prevention

Because the cause of the cancer is not known, there is no definite way to prevent prostate cancer. Given its common occurrence and the low cost of screening, the American Cancer Society (ACS) and the National Comprehensive Cancer Network (NCCN) recommends that all men over age 40 have an annual **rectal examination** and that men have an annual PSA test beginning at age 50. African-American men and men with a family history of prostate cancer, who have a higher than average risk, should begin annual PSA testing even earlier, starting at age 45.

However, mandatory screening for prostate cancer is controversial. Because the cancer is so slow

KEY TERMS

Antiandrogen—A substance that blocks the action of androgens, the hormones responsible for male characteristics. Used to treat prostate cancers that require male hormones for growth.

Benign prostatic hyperplasia (BPH)—A non-cancerous swelling of the prostate.

Brachytherapy—A method of treating cancers, such as prostate cancer, involving the implantation near the tumor of radioactive seeds.

Gleason grading system—A method of predicting the tendency of a tumor in the prostate to metastasize based on how similar the tumor is to normal prostate tissue.

Granulocyte/macrophage colony stimulating factor (GM-CSF)—A substance produced by cells of the immune system that stimulates the attack upon foreign cells. Used to treat prostate cancers as a genetically engineered component of a vaccine that stimulates the body to attack prostate tissue.

Histopathology—The study of diseased tissues at a minute (microscopic) level.

Luteinizing hormone releasing hormone (LHRH) agonist—A substance that blocks the action of LHRH, a hormone that stimulates the production of testosterone (a male hormone) in men. Used to treat prostate cancers that require testosterone for growth.

Orchiectomy—Surgical removal of the testes that eliminates the production of testosterone to treat prostate cancer.

Radical prostatectomy—Surgical removal of the entire prostate, a common method of treating prostate cancer.

Prostate-specific antigen—A protein made by the cells of the prostate that is increased by both BPH and prostate cancer.

Transurethral resection of the prostate (TURP)—Surgical removal of a portion of the prostate through the urethra, a method of treating the symptoms of an enlarged prostate, whether from BPH or cancer.

---

growing, and the side effects of the treatment can have significant impact on patient quality of life, some medical organizations question the wisdom of yearly exams. Some organizations have even noted that the effect of screening is discovering the cancer at an early stage when it may never grow to have any outward effect on the patient during their lifetime. Nevertheless, the NCI reports that the current aggressive screening methods have achieved a reduction in the death rate of prostate cancer of about 2.3% for African-Americans and about 4.6% for Caucasians since the mid-1990s, with a 20% increase in overall survival rate during that period.

A low-fat diet may slow the progression of prostate cancer. To reduce the risk or progression of prostate cancer, the American Cancer Society recommends a diet rich in fruits, vegetables and dietary fiber, and low in red meat and saturated fats.

Resources

BOOKS

Beers, Mark H., MD, and Robert Berkow, MD., editors. "Prostate Cancer." In *The Merck Manual of Diagnosis and Therapy.* Whitehouse Station, NJ: Merck Research Laboratories, 2004.

Carroll, Peter R., et al. "Cancer of the Prostate." In *Cancer Principles and Practice of Oncology,* edited by Vincent T. DeVita, et al. Philadelphia: Lippincott Williams & Wilkins, 2001.

Wainrib, Barbara R., and Sandra Haber. *Men, Women, and Prostate Cancer.* Oakland, CA: New Harbinger Productions, Inc., 2000.

PERIODICALS

Alimi, D., C. Rubino, E. Pichard-Leandri, et al. "Analgesic Effect of Auricular Acupuncture for Cancer Pain: A Randomized, Blinded, Controlled Trial." *Journal of Clinical Oncology* 21 (November 15, 2003): 4120–4126.

Chang, S. S. "Exploring the Effects of Luteinizing Hormone-Releasing Hormone Agonist Therapy on Bone Health: Implications in the Management of Prostate Cancer." *Urology* 62 (December 22, 2003): 29–35.

de la Fouchardiere, C., A. Flechon, and J. P. Droz. "Coagulopathy in Prostate Cancer." *Netherlands Journal of Medicine* 61 (November 2003): 347–354.

Dziuk, T., and N. Senzer. "Feasibility of Amifostine Administration in Conjunction with High-Dose Rate Brachytherapy." *Seminars in Oncology* 30 (December 2003): 49–57.

Hsieh, K., and P. C. Albertsen. "Populations at High Risk for Prostate Cancer." *Urological Clinics of North America* 30 (November 2003): 669–676.

Linares, L. A., and D. Echols. "Amifostine and External Beam Radiation Therapy and/or High-Dose Rate Brachytherapy in the Treatment of Localized Prostate Carcinoma: Preliminary Results of a Phase II Trial." *Seminars in Oncology* 30 (December 2003): 58–62.

Sliva, D. "*Ganoderma lucidum* (Reishi) in Cancer Treatment." *Integrative Cancer Therapies* 2 (December 2003): 358–364.

Spetz, A. C., E. L. Zetterlund, E. Varenhorst, and M. Hammar. "Incidence and Management of Hot Flashes in Prostate Cancer." *Journal of Supportive Oncology* 1 (November–December 2003): 263–273.

Wilson, S. S., and E. D. Crawford. "Prostate Cancer Update." *Minerva Urologica e Nefrologica* 55 (December 2003): 199–204.

ORGANIZATIONS

Association for the Cure of Cancer of the Prostate (CaPCure). 1250 Fourth St., Suite 360, Santa Monica, CA 90401. (800) 757-CURE. < http://www.capcure.org >.

National Cancer Institute. Building 31, Room 10A31 31 Center Drive, MSC 2580, Bethesda, MD 20892-2580. (800) 4-CANCER. < http://cancernet.nci.nih.gov >.

National Center for Complementary and Alternative Medicine (NCCAM) Clearinghouse. P. O. Box 7923, Gaithersburg, MD 20898. (888) 644-6226. < http://nccam.nih.gov >.

OTHER

FDA MedWatch Safety Alert for PC-SPES, SPES, updated September 20, 2002. < http://www.fda.gov/medwatch/ SAFETY/2002/safety02.htm#spes >.

National Center for Complementary and Alternative Medicine (NCCAM). *Recall of PC-SPES and SPES Dietary Supplements.* NCCAM Publication No. D149, September 2002. < http://nccam.nih.gov/health/alerts/ spes/index.htm >.

Lata Cherath, PhD
Michelle Johnson, M.S., J.D.
Rebecca J. Frey, PhD

Prostate gland removal *see* **Prostatectomy**

Prostate sonogram *see* **Prostate ultrasound**

Prostate-specific antigen test

Definition

Prostate-specific antigen, or PSA, is a protein produced by the prostate gland that may be found in elevated levels in the blood when a person develops certain diseases of the prostate, notably **prostate cancer**. PSA is *specific*, because it is present only in prostate tissue. It is not specific for prostate *cancer*, however, as it may also be elevated in men with benign enlargement of this organ. The PSA test has been called the "male PAP test."

Purpose

The blood test for PSA is used to screen older men to detect prostate **cancer** at an early stage, and also to monitor its response to treatment. After lung cancer, prostate cancer is the most common form of cancer in men in the United States. Any routine physical exam of a man aged 50 and older should include a digital rectal examination (DRE), in which the doctor's finger probes the surface of the prostate gland to detect any suspicious area of hardness or a tumor mass. If the examination suggests that a tumor may in fact be present or if the examiner is uncertain the logical next step is a PSA test. If the PSA test is positive, a sample of prostate tissue (biopsy) may be taken to confirm that cancer is present. If negative, the test may be repeated immediately to confirm the diagnosis, or repeated the next year. Many physicians today routinely do both a DRE and a PSA test each year on their older male patients, so that, if cancer does develop, it will be found at an early stage will be easier to treat. The combination of a DRE and a PSA test can detect approximately 80% of all prostate cancers.

At present, the PSA test is widely accepted as a way of telling whether a patient with definite cancer is responding to treatment. Because only the prostate produces PSA, its presence in the blood following complete removal of the prostate (radical **prostatectomy**) indicates that some cancer has been left behind.

Precautions

There is no physical reason not to do a PSA test. Although, the level of PSA usually is elevated in men with prostate cancer, it also may be abnormally high (though usually not *as* high) in men with non-cancerous enlargement of the prostate (benign prostatic hyperplasia or BPH). If thousands of men have the PSA test routinely each year, many of them will have unnecessary tests (such as biopsy or an ultrasound study) to confirm cancer. If a "false-positive" result is obtained, where the PSA level seems high but really is not, some men may even be treated for prostate cancer when no cancer is present. Both the American Cancer Society and the American Urological Association urge annual PSA testing to detect early cancers, but the National Cancer Institute does not.

Description

The PSA test is a radioimmunoassay. Any antigen causes the body to produce antibodies in an attempt to neutralize or eliminate the antigen, often a substance that harms body tissues. In the laboratory, a sample of the patient's blood is exposed to the antibody against PSA, so that the amount of antigen (PSA) can be measured. The results generally are available the next day.

KEY TERMS

Antibody—A substance formed in the body in reaction to some foreign material invading the body, or sometimes to diseased body tissue such as prostate cancer. An antibody also may be prepared in the laboratory and used to measure the amount of antigen in the blood.

Antigen—Either a foreign substance such as a virus or bacterium, or a protein produced by diseased or injured body tissue.

Biopsy—A procedure using a hollow needle to obtain a small sample of tissue, such as from the prostate. Often done to determine whether cancer is present.

BPH—Benign prostatic hyperplasia, a noncancerous disorder that causes the prostate to enlarge.

Preparation

No special measures are needed when doing a PSA test other than taking the usual precautions to prevent infection at the needle puncture site.

Normal results

Each laboratory has its own normal range for PSA. In fact, they may redefine the normal range whenever starting to use a new batch of test chemicals.

Abnormal results

Some experts believe that more than 90% of men with prostate cancer will have an elevated PSA level. Others claim that as many as one-third of cancers will be missed. The amount of PSA in the blood drops when cancer is successfully treated, but rises again if the tumor recurs, especially if it spreads to other parts of the body. A new variation of the PSA test shows how much of the material is bound to other protein in the blood and how much is "free." This procedure may be more accurate and could well indicate whether either prostate cancer or BPH is present.

Resources

ORGANIZATIONS

Prostate Health Council, American Foundation for Urologic Disease. 1128 N. Charles St., Baltimore, MD 21201.

OTHER

Prostate Health Council *Important Information About Prostate-Specific Antigen (PSA)*. American Foundation for Urologic Disease, 1128 N.Charles St., Baltimore, MD 21201.

David A. Cramer, MD

Prostate ultrasound

Definition

A prostate ultrasound is a diagnostic test used to detect potential problems with a man's prostate. An ultrasound test uses very high frequency sound waves that are passed through the body. The pattern of reflected sound waves, or "echoes," shows the outline of the prostate. This test can show whether the prostate is enlarged, and whether an abnormal growth that might be cancer is present.

Purpose

The prostate is a chestnut-shaped organ surrounding the beginning of the urethra in men. It produces a milky fluid that is part of the seminal fluid discharged during ejaculation. The prostate can become enlarged, particularly in men over age 50. Also, **cancer** of the prostate can develop, which tends to affect older men.

During a **physical examination**, a doctor may perform a digital **rectal examination**. In this examination, the doctor uses a gloved and lubricated finger inserted in the rectum to feel for any abnormalities. If this examination shows that the prostate is enlarged or a hard lump is present, an ultrasound may be done. Another reason a doctor might perform an ultrasound is if a blood test shows abnormal levels of a substance called prostate-specific antigen (PSA). Abnormal levels of PSA may indicate the presence of cancer.

If there is a suspicious lump, the doctor will want to take a sample of some of the tissue (prostate biopsy) to test it to see whether it is in fact cancer. Doing an ultrasound first will show the doctor what part of the prostate should be taken as a sample. Ultrasound can also show whether cancerous tissue is still only within the prostate or whether it has begun to spread to other locations. If **prostate cancer** is present and the doctor decides to treat it with a surgical freezing procedure, ultrasound is used as an aid in the procedure.

An ultrasound can reveal other types of prostate disease as well. For example, it can show if there is inflammation of the prostate (**prostatitis**). Sometimes it is used to learn why a man is unable to father children (**infertility**).

Precautions

A prostate ultrasound study is generally not performed on men who have recently had surgery on their lower bowel. This is because the test requires placing an ultrasound probe about the size of a finger into the rectum.

Description

Prostate ultrasound is generally done using a technique called the transrectal method. This procedure can be done in an outpatient clinic. The cylinder-shaped ultrasound probe is gently placed in the rectum as the patient lies on his left side with the knees bent. The probe is rocked back and forth to obtain images of the entire prostate. The procedure takes about 15–25 minutes to perform. After the test, the patient's doctor can be notified right away, and usually he or she will have a written report within 36 hours.

Preparation

To prepare for a prostate ultrasound, an enema is taken two to four hours before the exam. The patient should not urinate for one hour before the test. If biopsies may be done, the doctor will prescribe an antibiotic that usually is taken in four doses starting the night before the biopsy, the morning of the test, that evening, and the following morning.

Aftercare

There is some discomfort, but less than most patients expect. In fact, worrying ahead of time is usually the hardest part. Generally, the patient is allowed to leave after a radiologist or urologist has reviewed the results. There may be some mucus or a small amount of bleeding from the rectum after the ultrasound. Some patients notice a small amount of blood in the urine for up to two days after the test. Blood may also be present in the semen. As long as the amount of blood is small, there is no cause for concern.

Risks

There are no serious risks from a prostate ultrasound study. Infection is rare and probably is a result of biopsy rather than the sonogram itself. If the ultrasound probe is moved too vigorously, some bleeding may continue for a few days.

Normal results

Modern ultrasound techniques can display both the smooth-surfaced outer shell of the prostate and the core tissues surrounding the urethra. The entire volume of the prostate should be less than 20 milliliters, and its outline should appear as a smooth echo-reflecting (echogenic) rim. Some irregularities within the substance of the gland and calcium deposits are normal findings.

Abnormal results

An **enlarged prostate** with dimmed echoes may indicate either prostatitis or benign enlargement of the gland, called benign prostatic hypertrophy (BPH). A distinct lump of tissue more likely means cancer. Cancer also often appears as an irregular area within the gland that distorts the normal pattern of echoes. In either case, a biopsy should clarify the diagnosis.

Resources

ORGANIZATIONS

Prostate Health Council, American Foundation for Urologic Disease. 1128 N. Charles St., Baltimore, MD 21201. 800-242-AFUD.

David A. Cramer, MD

Prostatectomy

Definition

Prostatectomy refers to the surgical removal of part of the prostate gland (transurethral resection, a procedure performed to relieve urinary symptoms caused by benign enlargement), or all of the prostate (radical prostatectomy, the curative surgery most often used to treat **prostate cancer**).

Purpose

Benign disease

When men reach their mid-40s, the prostate gland begins to enlarge. This condition, benign prostatic hyperplasia (BPH) is present in more than half of men in their 60s and as many as 90% of those over 90. Because the prostate surrounds the urethra, the tube leading urine from the bladder out of the body, the enlarging prostate narrows this passage and makes urination difficult. The bladder does not empty completely each time a man urinates, and, as a result, he must urinate with greater frequency, night and day. In time, the bladder can overfill, and urine escapes from the urethra, resulting in incontinence. An operation called transurethral resection of the prostate (TURP) relieves symptoms of BPH by removing the prostate tissue that is blocking the urethra. No incision is needed. Instead a tube (retroscope) is passed through the penis to the level of the prostate, and tissue is either removed or destroyed, so that urine can freely pass from the body.

Malignant disease

Prostate **cancer** is the single most common form of non-skin cancer in the United States and the most common cancer in men over 50. Half of men over 70 and almost all men over the age of 90 have prostate cancer, and the American Cancer Society estimates that 198,000 new cases will be diagnosed in 2001. This condition does not always require surgery. In fact, many elderly men adopt a policy of "watchful waiting," especially if their cancer is growing slowly. Younger men often elect to have their prostate gland totally removed along with the cancer it contains—an operation called radical prostatectomy. The two main types of this surgery, radical retropubic prostatectomy and radical perineal prostatectomy, are performed only on patients whose cancer is limited to the prostate. If cancer has broken out of the capsule surrounding the prostate gland and spread in the area or to distant sites, removing the prostate will not prevent the remaining cancer from growing and spreading throughout the body.

Precautions

Potential complications of TURP include bleeding, infection, and reactions to general or **local anesthesia**. About one man in five will need to have the operation again within 10 years.

Open (incisional) prostatectomy for cancer should not be done if the cancer has spread beyond the prostate, as serious side effects may occur without the benefit of removing all the cancer. If the bladder is retaining urine, it is necessary to insert a catheter before starting surgery. Patients should be in the best possible general condition before radical prostatectomy. Before surgery, the bladder is inspected using an instrument called a cystoscope to help determine the best surgical technique to use, and to rule out other local problems.

Description

TURP

This procedure does not require an abdominal incision. With the patient under either general or spinal anesthesia, a cutting instrument or heated wire loop is inserted to remove as much prostate tissue as possible and seal blood vessels. The excised tissue is washed into the bladder, then flushed out at the end of the operation. A catheter is left in the bladder for one to five days to drain urine and blood. Advanced laser technology enables surgeons to safely and effectively burn off excess prostate tissue blocking the bladder opening with fewer of the early and late complications associated with other forms of prostate surgery. This procedure can be performed on an outpatient basis, but urinary symptoms do not improve until swelling subsides several weeks after surgery.

Radical prostatectomy

RADICAL RETROPUBIC PROSTATECTOMY. This is a useful approach if the prostate is very large, or cancer is suspected. With the patient under general or spinal anesthesia or an epidural, a horizontal incision is made in the center of the lower abdomen. Some surgeons begin the operation by removing pelvic lymph nodes to determine whether cancer has invaded them, but recent findings suggest there is no need to sample them in patients whose likelihood of lymph node metastases is less than 18%. A doctor who removes the lymph nodes for examination will not continue the operation if they contain cancer cells, because the surgery will not cure the patient. Other surgeons remove the prostate gland before examining the lymph nodes. A tube (catheter) inserted into the penis to drain fluid from the body is left in place for 14–21 days.

Originally, this operation also removed a thin rim of bladder tissue in the area of the urethral sphincter—a muscular structure that keeps urine from escaping from the bladder. In addition, the nerves supplying the penis often were damaged, and many men found themselves impotent (unable to achieve erections) after prostatectomy. A newer surgical method called potency-sparing radical prostatectomy preserves sexual potency in 75% of patients and fewer than 5% become incontinent following this procedure.

RADICAL PERINEAL PROSTATECTOMY. This procedure is just as curative as radical retropubic prostatectomy but is performed less often because it does not allow the surgeon to spare the nerves associated with erection or, because the incision is made above the rectum and below the scrotum, to remove lymph nodes. Radical perineal prostatectomy is sometimes used when the cancer is limited to the prostate and there is no need to spare nerves or when the patient's health might be compromised by the longer procedure. The perineal operation is less invasive than retropubic prostatectomy. Some parts of the prostate can be seen better, and blood loss is limited. The absence of an abdominal incision allows patients to recover more rapidly. Many urologic surgeons have not been trained to perform this procedure. Radical prostatectomy procedures last one to four hours, with radical perineal prostatectomy taking less time than radical retropubic prostatectomy. The patient remains in the hospital three to five days following surgery and can return to work in three to five weeks. Ongoing research indicates that laparoscopic radical prostatectomy may be as effective as open surgery in treatment of early-stage disease.

Cryosurgery

Also called **cryotherapy** or cryoablation, this minimally invasive procedure uses very low temperatures to freeze and destroy cancer cells in and around the prostate gland. A catheter circulates warm fluid through the urethra to protect it from the cold. When used in connection with ultrasound imaging, cryosurgery permits very precise tissue destruction. Traditionally used only in patients whose cancer had not responded to radiation, but now approved by Medicare as a primary treatment for prostate cancer, cryosurgery can safely be performed on older men, on patients who are not in good enough general health to undergo radical prostatectomy, or to treat recurrent

disease. Recent studies have shown that total cryosurgery, which destroys the prostate, is at least as effective as radical prostatectomy without the trauma of major surgery.

Preparation

As with any type of major surgery done under **general anesthesia**, the patient should be in optimal condition. Most patients having prostatectomy are in the age range when cardiovascular problems are frequent, making it especially important to be sure that the heart is beating strongly, and that the patient is not retaining too much fluid. Because long-standing prostate disease may cause kidney problems from urine "backing up," it also is necessary to be sure that the kidneys are working properly. If not, a period of catheter drainage may be necessary before doing the surgery.

Aftercare

Following TURP, a catheter is placed in the bladder to drain urine and remains in place for two to three days. A solution is used to irrigate the bladder and urethra until the urine is clear of blood, usually within 48 hours after surgery. Whether **antibiotics** should be routinely given remains an open question. Catheter drainage also is used after open prostatectomy. The bladder is irrigated only if **blood clots** block the flow of urine through the catheter. Patients are given intravenous fluids for the first 24 hours, to ensure good urine flow. Patients resting in bed for long periods are prone to blood clots in their legs (which can pass to the lungs and cause serious breathing problems). This can be prevented by elastic stockings and by periodically exercising the patient's legs. The patient remains in the hospital one to two days following surgery and can return to work in one to two weeks.

Risks

The complications and side effects that may occur during and after prostatectomy include:

- Excessive bleeding, which in rare cases may require blood transfusion.
- Incontinence when, during retropubic prostatectomy, the muscular valve (sphincter) that keeps urine in the bladder is damaged. Less common today, when care is taken not to injure the sphincter.
- Impotence, occurring when nerves to the penis are injured during the retropubic operation. Today's

KEY TERMS

BPH—Benign prostatic hypertrophy, a very common noncancerous cause of prostatic enlargement in older men.

Catheter—A tube that is placed through the urethra into the bladder in order to provide free drainage of urine and blood following either TURP or open prostatectomy.

Cryosurgery—In prostatectomy, the use of a very low-temperature probe to freeze and thereby destroy prostatic tissue.

Impotence—The inability to achieve and sustain penile erections.

Incontinence—The inability to retain urine in the bladder until a person is ready to urinate voluntarily.

Prostate gland—The gland surrounding the male urethra just below the base of the bladder. It secretes a fluid that constitutes a major portion of the semen.

Urethra—The tube running from the bladder to the tip of the penis that provides a passage for eliminating urine from the body.

"nerve-sparing" technique has drastically cut down on this problem.

• Some patients who receive a large volume of irrigating fluid after TURP develop high blood pressure, **vomiting**, trouble with their vision, and mental confusion. This condition is caused by a low salt level in the blood, and is reversed by giving salt solution.

• A permanent narrowing of the urethra called a stricture occasionally develops when the urethra is damaged during TURP.

• There is about a 34% chance that the cancer will recur within 10 years of the procedure. In addition, about 25% of patients experience what is known as biochemical recurrence, which means that the level of prostate-specific antigen (PSA) in the patient's blood serum begins to rise rapidly. Recurrence of the tumor or biochemical recurrence can be treated with **radiation therapy** or androgen deprivation therapy.

Normal results

In patients with BPH who have the TURP operation, urination should become much easier and less frequent, and dribbling or incontinence should cease.

In patients having radical prostatectomy for cancer, a successful operation will remove the tumor and prevent its spread to other areas of the body (metastasis). If examination of lymph nodes shows that cancer already had spread beyond the prostate at the time of surgery, other measures are available to control the tumor.

Resources

BOOKS

Beers, Mark H., MD, and Robert Berkow, MD., editors. "Prostate Cancer." Section 17, Chapter 233 In *The Merck Manual of Diagnosis and Therapy*. Whitehouse Station, NJ: Merck Research Laboratories, 2002.

Marks, Sheldon. *Prostate Cancer: A Family Guide to Diagnosis, Treatment and Survival*. Cambridge, MA: Fisher Books, 2000.

Wainrib, Barbara, et al. *Men, Women, and Prostate Cancer: A Medical and Psychological Guide for Women and the Men they Love*. Oakland, CA: New Harbinger Publications, 2000.

PERIODICALS

Augustin, H., and P. G. Hammerer. "Disease Recurrence After Radical Prostatectomy. Contemporary Diagnostic and Therapeutical Strategies." *Minerva Urologica e Nefrologica* 55 (December 2003): 251–261.

Gomella, L. G., I. Zeltser, and R. K. Valicenti. "Use of Neoadjuvant and Adjuvant Therapy to Prevent or Delay Recurrence of Prostate Cancer in Patients Undergoing Surgical Treatment for Prostate Cancer." *Urology* 62, Supplement 1 (December 29, 2003): 46–54.

Nelson, J. B., and H. Lepor. "Prostate Cancer: Radical Prostatectomy." *Urologic Clinics of North America* 30 (November 2003): 703–723.

Zimmerman, R. A., and D. G. Culkin. "Clinical Strategies in the Management of Biochemical Recurrence after Radical Prostatectomy." *Clinical Prostate Cancer* 2 (December 2003): 160–166.

ORGANIZATIONS

Cancer Research Institute. 681 Fifth Ave., New York, NY 10022. (800) 99CANCER. < http://www.cancerresearch.org >.

National Prostate Cancer Coalition. 1156 15th St., NW, Washington, DC 20005. (202) 463-9455. < http://www.4npcc.org >.

Prostate Health Council. American Foundation for Urologic Disease. 1128 N. Charles St., Baltimore, MD 21201-5559. (800) 828-7866. < http://www.afud.org >.

David A. Cramer, MD
Rebecca J. Frey, PhD

Prostatic acid phosphatase test *see* **Acid phosphatase test**

Prostatitis

Definition

Prostatitis is an inflammation of the prostate gland, a common condition in adult males. Often caused by infection, prostatitis may develop rapidly (*acute*) or slowly (*chronic*).

Description

Prostatitis may be the symptom-producing disease of the genitourinary tract for which men most often seek medical help. About 40% of visits to a specialist in genitourinary problems (urologist) are for prostatitis. Forms of prostate inflammation include acute and chronic bacterial prostatitis and inflammation not caused by bacterial infection. A painful condition called *prostatodynia*, which may be caused by abnormal nerves or muscles in the region, is also thought to be a form of prostatitis. The chronic bacterial form is sometimes experienced by men whose sex partners have a bacterial infection of the vagina, making this a sexually transmitted disease. Other cases occur when small stones form within the prostate and become infected. Sometimes infection is caused by poor hygiene, surgical procedures, or even swimming in polluted water.

The sexually transmitted disease **gonorrhea** may sometimes cause prostatitis, and **tuberculosis** may spread to the prostate. Parasites and fungi may infect the prostate gland. Some men whose prostatitis is not caused by any microorganism have microscopic collections of cells called *granulomas* in their prostate tissue. Whether viruses also may cause prostatitis is debatable.

Causes and symptoms

However the inflammation may begin, it causes blockages in the tiny glands within the prostate so that secretions build up, and the prostate swells. In acute cases, this swelling can occur very suddenly and cause considerable **pain**. When prostatitis develops gradually, trouble with the flow of urine may be the first symptom. Small stones may form, because the body attempts to neutralize bacteria by coating them with calcium. These stones may become infected themselves and make the condition worse.

Symptoms and signs that are typically experienced by men with prostatitis include:

- Difficulties in urinating. Most urinary problems are caused when the swollen prostate blocks the tube that carries urine from the bladder to the outside of the body (urethra). Patients feel the need to urinate more often than usual, often urgently. Urination is sometimes painful. It is hard to start the flow of urine and difficult to totally empty the bladder. Patients wake up at night to urinate. The stream may be weak or split. Dribbling after attempts to urinate may leave embarrassing wet spots on clothing. In severe prostatitis blood or sand-like particles (small calcium collections) may be passed in the urine.

- Pain. Besides pain when urinating, caused by prostate swelling, stimulation of nerves in the prostate gland may cause pain in the penis, one or both testicles, the lower stomach, the low back, and the area between the scrotum and the anus (perineum). Some patients experience pain during or after ejaculation, whenever they sit down or walk, or during bowel movements.

- Sex and fertility. The pain of prostatitis can make it impossible to enjoy sex. Men with prostatitis may be troubled by early release of sperm (premature ejaculation). Occasionally there is blood in the semen. Some of the drugs prescribed to ease the flow of the urine can dampen the desire to have sex. Because the normal prostate secretions make up part of the semen, prostatitis may lower fertility by severely lowering the number of sperm and making them less mobile.

- Psychological problems. A man with prostatitis who feels that nothing can be done and he "just has to live with it" may experience serious depression. Low sexual desire certainly contributes to depression.

A person with *acute prostatitis* may suddenly develop fever and chills, along with rapidly developing urinary symptoms and pain in the perineum or low back. This state is a medical emergency that demands immediate medical help.

Diagnosis

Most often the symptoms and physical findings are enough to form a diagnosis of prostatitis. When the examiner inserts a finger in the rectum, the swollen prostate can be felt; it may be extremely tender when probed. Squeezing the gland slightly will produce a few drops of fluid that may be *cultured* to learn whether bacteria are present. The fluid typically contains a large number of white blood cells, especially the cells used to fight off infection (*macrophages*). Note: too much pressure on the prostate can force bacteria into the blood and cause a serious general infection. Many patients with chronic bacterial prostatitis also have recurring urinary tract infections (diagnosed by examining and culturing urine samples). These infections can be an important clue to the diagnosis. If doubt remains, the urologist may insert a special instrument called a *cystoscope* through the penis to directly view the prostate from inside and see whether it looks inflamed.

Treatment

Acute prostatitis is first treated with **antibiotics**. Even though it may be difficult for drugs to actually get into the inflamed prostate, most patients do quickly get better. If intravenous antibiotics are needed or the bladder is retaining urine, a hospital stay may be necessary. Broad-spectrum antibiotics that work against most bacteria are used first. At the same time tests are done with samples of prostatic fluid to determine which bacterium is causing the infection, so that drugs can be prescribed to fight the specific germ. In chronic cases, the best results are obtained with a combination of the antibiotics trimethoprim and sulfamethoxazole. Oral antibiotics should be given for one to three months; longer, if necessary. If a fungus or some other organism is causing infection, special drugs are available. If chronic prostatitis continues despite all medical efforts and is seriously affecting the patient's life, the prostate may be removed surgically.

Nonbacterial prostatitis requires other measures to relieve urinary symptoms. These measures include drugs that fight inflammation (steroids or nonsteroids) and a type of drug called an alpha-blocker that reduces muscle tension. Reduced muscle tension eases urine flow, allowing the bladder to empty. A narrowed urethra may be widened by placing a collapsed balloon at the site of obstruction and expanding it. This procedure is called *balloon dilation*. The effects of such dilation are usually temporary. Some physicians believe that **stress** is an important factor in prostatitis, and therefore prescribe diazepam (Valium) or another tranquilizer. The type of prostatitis known as prostatodynia is usually treated with a combination of muscle relaxing drugs, heat, special exercises, and sometimes a tranquilizer.

There are a number of "tips" for relieving symptoms of prostatitis. They are especially helpful early on, before antibiotics have a chance to cure infection, or for patients with chronic or non-bacterial prostatitis:

- Hot sitz baths. Exposing the perineum to very hot water for 20 minutes or longer often relieves pain.
- Ice. When heat does not help, ice packs, or simply placing a small ice cube in the rectum, may relieve pain for hours.
- Water. A patient who has to urinate very often may want to cut back on his fluid intake but this will cause **dehydration** and increase the risk of bladder infection. Instead, it is best to drink plenty of water.
- Diet. Most doctors recommend cutting out–or cutting down on–caffeine (as in coffee or tea), alcohol, and spicy or acid foods. **Constipation** should be avoided because large, hard bowel movements may press on the swollen prostate and cause great pain. Bran cereals and whole-grain breads are helpful.
- Exercise. It is especially important for patients with chronic prostatitis to keep up their activity level. Simply walking often will help (unless walking happens to make the pain worse).
- Frequent ejaculation. Ejaculating two or three times a week often is recommended, especially when taking antibiotics.

Alternative treatment

A treatment popularized in the Philippines is called "prostate drainage." At regular intervals, a finger is inserted into the rectum, to exert pressure on the prostate at the same time that an antibiotic treatment is given. **Acupuncture** and Chinese herbal medicine also can be effective in treating prostatitis. **Nutritional supplements** that support the prostate, including zinc, **omega-3 fatty acids**, several amino acids, and anti-inflammatory nutrients and herbs, can help reduce pain and promote healing. Western herbal medicine recommends saw palmetto (*Serenoa repens*) to support the prostate gland. Hot and cold contrast sitz baths can help reduce inflammation.

Prognosis

Most patients with acute bacterial prostatitis are cured if they receive proper antibiotic treatment. Every effort should be made to get a cure at the acute stage because chronic prostatitis can be much more difficult to eliminate. If the acute illness is *not* controlled, complications such as a localized infection (prostatic **abscess**), kidney infection, or infection of the blood (septicemia) may develop. When chronic prostatitis cannot be cured, it still is possible to keep urinary symptoms under control and keep the patient active by using low doses of antibiotics and other measures. If a man with any form of prostatitis develops serious psychological problems, he should be referred to a psychiatric specialist.

Prevention

Potential sources of infection should be avoided. Good perineal hygiene should be maintained and sex

KEY TERMS

Culture—A test in which a sample of body fluid, such as prostatic fluid, is placed on materials specially formulated to grow microorganisms. A culture is used to learn what type of bacterium is causing infection.

Cystoscope—A viewing instrument that is passed up the urethra into the region of the prostate to get a good look at the organ "from the inside."

Ejaculation—The process by which semen (made up in part of prostatic fluid) is ejected by the erect penis.

Granuloma—A cluster of cells that form in tissue which has been inflamed for some time.

Perineum—An area close to the prostate, between the scrotum and anus.

should be avoided when one's partner has an active bacterial vaginal infection. If the kidneys, bladder, or other genitourinary organs are infected, prompt treatment may prevent the development of prostatitis. By far the best way of preventing chronic prostatitis is to treat an initial *acute* episode promptly and effectively.

Resources

ORGANIZATIONS

Prostate Health Council, American Foundation for Urologic Disease. 1128 N. Charles St., Baltimore, MD 21201. (800) 242-AFUD.

Prostatitis Foundation, Information Distribution Center. 2029 Ireland Grove Park, Bloomington, IL 61704. (309) 664-6222. < http://www.prostate.org >.

David A. Cramer, MD

Prosthetic joint infection *see* **Infectious arthritis**

Protease inhibitors

Definition

A protease inhibitor is a type of drug that cripples the enzyme protease. An enzyme is a substance that triggers chemical reactions in the body. The human **immunodeficiency** virus (HIV) uses protease in the final stages of its reproduction (replication) process.

Purpose

The drug is used to treat selected patients with HIV infection. Blocking protease interferes with HIV reproduction, causing it to make copies of itself that cannot infect new cells. The drug may improve symptoms and suppress the infection but does not cure it.

Precautions

Patients should not discontinue this drug even if symptoms improve without consulting a doctor.

These drugs do not necessarily reduce the risk of transmitting HIV to others through sexual contact, so patients should avoid sexual activities or use condoms.

Description

Protease inhibitors are considered one of the most potent medications for HIV developed so far.

This class of drugs includes indinavir (Crixivan), ritonavir (Norvir), nelfinavir (Viracept), amprenavir (Agenerase), lopinavir plus ritonavir (Kaletra), saquinavir (Fortovase), and a new drug called atazanavir (Reyataz). Reyataz received approval from the U.S. Food and Drug Administration (FDA) in mid-2003 and was the first protease inhibitor approved for once-daily dosing. Several weeks or months of drug therapy may be required before the full benefits are apparent.

The drug should be taken at the same time each day. Some types should be taken with a meal to help the body absorb them. Each of the types of protease inhibitor may have to be taken in a different way. In most cases, protease inhibitors are part of a combination therapy, used in conjunction with other classes of HIV drugs.

Risks

Common side effects include **diarrhea**, stomach discomfort, nausea, and mouth sores. Less often, patients may experience rash, muscle **pain**, **headache**, or weakness. Rarely, there may be confusion, severe skin reaction, or seizures. Some of these drugs can have interactions with other medication, and indinavir can be associated with kidney stones. Diabetes or high blood pressure may become worse when these drugs are taken. Reyatraz has been shown to have fewer side effects than some protease inhibitors, though it can interact with other medications, including certain heart medications and antidepressants.

Experts do not know whether the drugs pass into breast milk, so breastfeeding mothers should avoid them or should stop nursing until the treatment is completed.

Resources

PERIODICALS

"HIV Drugs Approved as of August 2003." *AIDS Treatment News* July 25, 2003: 4.

LoBuono, Charlotte. "FDA Gives Bod to First Once-daily Protease Inhibitor." *Drug Topics* July 21, 2003: 16.

Wilson, Billie Ann. "Understanding Strategies for Treating HIV."*Medical Surgical Nursing* 6 (April 1, 1997): 109–111.

ORGANIZATIONS

National AIDS Treatment Advocacy Project. 580 Broadway, Ste. 403, New York, NY 10012. (888) 266-2827. < http://www.natap.org >.

Carol A. Turkington
Teresa G. Odle

Protein-calorie malnutrition *see* **Protein-energy malnutrition**

▌Protein components test

Definition

Protein components tests measure the amounts and types of protein in the blood. Proteins are constituents of muscle, enzymes, hormones, transport proteins, hemoglobin, and other functional and structural elements of the body. Albumin and globulin make up most of the protein within the body and are measured in the total protein of the blood and other body fluids. Thus, the serum (blood) protein components test measures the total protein, as well as its albumin and globulin components in the blood.

Purpose

The protein components test is used to diagnose diseases that either affect proteins as a whole, or that involve a single type of protein. The test is also used to monitor the course of disease in certain cancers, intestinal and kidney protein-wasting states, immune disorders, liver dysfunction, and impaired **nutrition**.

Precautions

Drugs that may cause increased protein levels include the anabolic steroids, androgens (male hormones), growth hormone, insulin, and progesterone. Drugs that may decrease protein levels include estrogen, drugs poisonous to the liver, and oral contraceptives.

Description

Proteins are large molecules (complex organic compounds) that consist of amino acids, sugars, and lipids. There are two main types of proteins: those that are made of fiber and form the structural basis of body tissues, such as hair, skin, muscle, tendons, and cartilage; and globular proteins (generally water soluble), which interact with many hormones, various other proteins in the blood, including hemoglobin and antibodies, and all the enzymes (substances that promote biochemical reactions in the body).

Proteins are needed in the diet to supply the body with amino acids. Ingested proteins are broken down in the digestive system to amino acids, which are then absorbed and rebuilt into new body proteins. One of the most important functions of proteins in the body is to contribute to the osmotic pressure (the movement of water between the bloodstream and tissues). An example of this is seen in diseases that result in damage to the filtering units of the kidneys (**nephrotic syndrome**). A severe loss of protein from the bloodstream into the urine (proteinuria) results, lowering the protein content of the blood and resulting in fluid retention, or **edema**.

Albumin and globulin are two key components of protein. Albumin is made in the liver and constitutes approximately 60% of the total protein. The main function of albumin is to maintain osmotic pressure and to help transport certain blood constituents around the body via the bloodstream. Because albumin is made in the liver, it is one element that is used to monitor liver function.

Globulin is the basis for antibodies, glycoproteins (protein-carbohydrate compounds), lipoproteins (proteins involved in fat transport), and clotting factors. Globulins are divided into three main groups, the alpha-, beta-, and gammaglobulins. Alphaglobulins include enzymes produced by the lungs and liver, and haptoglobin, which binds hemoglobin together. The betaglobulins consist mostly of low-density lipoproteins (LDLs), substances involved in fat transport. All of the gammaglobulins are antibodies, proteins produced by the immune system in response to infection, during allergic reaction, and after organ transplants.

Both serum albumin and globulin are measures of nutrition. Malnourished patients, especially after surgery, demonstrate greatly decreased protein levels, while burn patients and those who have protein-losing syndromes show low levels despite normal synthesis. **Pregnancy** in the third trimester is also associated with reduced protein levels.

The relationship of albumin to globulin is determined by ratio, so when certain diseases cause the albumin levels to drop, the globulin level will be increased by the body in an effort to maintain a normal total protein level. For example, when the liver is unable to synthesize sufficient albumin in chronic **liver disease**, the albumin level will be low, but the globulin levels will be normal or higher than normal. In such cases, the protein components test is an especially valuable diagnostic aid because it determines the ratio of albumin to globulin, as well as the total protein level. It should be noted, however, that when globulin is provided as a calculation (total protein – albumin = globulin), the result is much less definitive than other methods of determining globulin.

Consequently, when the albumin/globulin ratio (A/G ratio) is less than 1.0, more precise tests should be ordered. These tests include protein electrophoresis, a method of separating the different blood proteins into groups. If the protein electrophoresis indicates a rise, or "spike" at the globulin level, an even more specific test for globulins, called **immuno-electrophoresis**, should be ordered to separate out the various globulins according to type. Some diseases characterized by dysproteinemia (derangement of the protein content of the blood), have typical electrophoretic globulin peaks.

Preparation

Unless this is requested by the physician, there is no need that the patient restrict food or fluids before the test.

Risks

Risks posed by this test are minimal, but may include slight bleeding from the blood-drawing site, **fainting** or lightheadedness after venipuncture, or hematoma (blood accumulating under the puncture site).

Normal results

Reference values vary from laboratory to laboratory, but can generally be found within the following ranges: Total protein: 6.4–8.3 g/dL; albumin: 3.5–5.0 g/dL; globulin: 2.3–3.4 g/dL.

KEY TERMS

Nephrotic syndromes—A collection of symptoms that result from damage to the filtering units of the kidney (glomeruli) causing severe loss of protein from the blood into the urine.

Abnormal results

Increased total protein levels are seen in **dehydration**, in some cases of chronic liver disease (like **autoimmune hepatitis** and **cirrhosis**), and in certain tropical diseases (for example, **leprosy**). Very low total protein levels (less than 4.0 g/dl) and low albumin cause the edema (water retention) usually seen in nephrotic syndromes. Decreased protein levels may be seen in pregnancy, chronic **alcoholism**, prolonged immobilization, heart failure, starvation, and malabsorption or **malnutrition**.

Increased albumin levels are found in dehydration. Decreased albumin levels are indicative of liver disease, protein-losing syndromes, malnutrition, inflammatory disease, and familial idiopathic (of unknown cause) dysproteinemia, a genetic disease in which the albumin is significantly reduced and globulins increased.

Increased globulin levels are found in multiple myeloma and Waldenström's macroglobulinemia, two cancers characterized by overproduction of gammaglobulin from proliferating plasma cells. Increased globulin levels are also found in chronic inflammatory diseases such as **rheumatoid arthritis**, acute and chronic infection, and cirrhosis. Decreased globulin levels are seen in genetic immune disorders and secondary immune deficiency.

Resources

BOOKS

Pagana, Kathleen Deska. *Mosby's Manual of Diagnostic and Laboratory Tests*. St. Louis: Mosby, Inc., 1998.

Janis O. Flores

Protein electrophoresis

Definition

Electrophoresis is a technique used to separate different elements (fractions) of a blood sample into individual components. Serum protein electrophoresis (SPEP) is a screening test that measures the major blood proteins by separating them into five distinct fractions: albumin, alpha$_1$, alpha$_2$, beta, and gamma proteins. Protein electrophoresis can also be performed on urine.

Purpose

Protein electrophoresis is used to evaluate, diagnose, and monitor a variety of diseases and conditions. It can be used for these purposes because the levels of different blood proteins rise or fall in response to such disorders as **cancer**, intestinal or kidney protein-wasting syndromes, disorders of the immune system, liver dysfunction, impaired nutrition, and chronic fluid-retaining conditions.

Precautions

Certain other diagnostic tests or prescription medications can affect the results of SPEP tests. The administration of a contrast dye used in some other tests may falsely elevate protein levels. Drugs that can alter results include **aspirin**, bicarbonates, chlorpromazine (Thorazine), **corticosteroids**, isoniazid (INH), and neomycin (Mycifradin).

Description

Proteins are major components of muscle, enzymes, hormones, hemoglobin, and other body tissues. Proteins are composed of elements that can be separated from one another by several different techniques: chemical methods, ultracentrifuge, or electrophoresis. There are two major types of electrophoresis: protein electrophoresis and **immunoelectrophoresis**. Immunoelectrophoresis is used to assess the blood levels of specific types of proteins called immunoglobulins. An immunoelectrophoresis test is usually ordered if a SPEP test has a "spike," or rise, at the immunoglobulin level. Protein electrophoresis is used to determine the total amount of protein in the blood, and to establish the levels of other types of proteins called albumin, alpha$_1$ globulin, alpha$_2$ globulin, and beta-globulin.

Blood proteins

ALBUMIN. Albumin is a protein that is made in the liver. It helps to retain elements like calcium, some hormones, and certain drugs in the circulation by binding to them to prevent their being filtered out by the kidneys. Albumin also acts to regulate the movement of water between the tissues and the bloodstream by attracting water to areas with higher concentrations of salts or proteins.

GLOBULINS. Globulins are another type of protein, larger in size than albumin. They are divided into three main groups: alpha, beta, and gamma.

- Alphaglobulins. These proteins include alpha$_1$ and alpha$_2$ globulins. Alpha$_1$ globulin is predominantly alpha$_1$ antitrypsin, an enzyme produced by the lungs and liver. Alpha$_2$ globulin, which includes serum haptoglobin, is a protein that binds hemoglobin to prevent its excretion by the kidneys. Various other alphaglobulins are produced as a result of inflammation, tissue damage, autoimmune disorders, or certain cancers.

- Betaglobulins. These include low-density substances involved in fat transport (lipoproteins), iron transport (transferrin), and blood clotting (plasminogen and complement).

- Gammaglobulins. All of the gammaglobulins are antibodies–proteins produced by the immune system in response to infection, allergic reactions, and organ transplants. If serum protein electrophoresis has demonstrated a significant rise at the **gammaglobulin** level, immunoelectrophoresis is done to identify the specific globulin that is involved.

Electrophoretic measurement of proteins

All proteins have an electrical charge. The SPEP test is designed to make use of this characteristic. There is some difference in method, but basically the sample is placed in or on a special medium (e.g., a gel), and an electric current is applied to the gel. The protein particles move through the gel according to the strength of their electrical charges, forming bands or zones. An instrument called a densitometer measures these bands, which can be identified and associated with specific diseases. For example, a decrease in albumin with a rise in the alpha$_2$ globulin usually indicates an acute reaction of the type that occurs in infections, **burns**, **stress**, or heart attack. On the other hand, a slight decrease in albumin, with a slight increase in gammaglobulin, and a normal alpha$_2$ globulin is more indicative of a chronic inflammatory condition, as might be seen in **cirrhosis** of the liver.

Protein electrophoresis is performed on urine samples to classify kidney disorders that cause protein loss. Here also certain band patterns are specific for disease. For example, the identification of a specific protein called the Bence Jones protein (by performing the **Bence Jones protein test**) during the procedure suggests **multiple myeloma**.

Preparation

The serum protein electrophoresis test requires a blood sample. It is not necessary for the patient to restrict food or fluids before the test. The urine protein electrophoresis test requires either an early morning urine sample or a 24-hour urine sample according to the physician's request. The doctor should check to see if the patient is taking any medications that may affect test results.

Risks

Risks posed by the blood test are minimal but may include slight bleeding from the puncture site, **fainting** or lightheadedness after the blood is drawn, or the development of a small bruise at the puncture site.

Normal results

The following values are representative, although there is some variation among laboratories and specific methods. These values are based on the agarose system.

- total protein: 5.9–8.0 g/dL
- albumin: 4.0–5.5 g/dL
- alpha$_1$ globulin: 0.15–0.25 g/dL
- alpha$_2$ globulin: 0.43–0.75 g/dL
- beta-globulin: 0.5–1.0 g/dL
- gammaglobulin: 0.6–1.3 g/dL

Abnormal results

Albumin levels are increased in **dehydration**. They are decreased in **malnutrition**, **pregnancy**, **liver disease**, inflammatory diseases, and such protein-losing syndromes as **malabsorption syndrome** and certain kidney disorders.

Alpha$_1$ globulins are increased in inflammatory diseases. They are decreased or absent in juvenile pulmonary **emphysema**, which is a genetic disease.

Alpha$_2$ globulins are increased in a kidney disorder called nephrotic syndrome. They are decreased in patients with an overactive thyroid gland (**hyperthyroidism**) or severe liver dysfunction.

Betaglobulin levels are increased in conditions of high cholesterol levels (**hypercholesterolemia**) and iron deficiency anemia. They are decreased in malnutrition.

Gammaglobulin levels are increased in chronic inflammatory disease (for example, rheumatoid

---

arthritis, systemic lupus erythematosus); cirrhosis; acute and chronic infection; and a cancerous disease characterized by uncontrolled multiplication of plasma cells in the bone marrow (multiple myeloma). Gammaglobulins are decreased in a variety of genetic immune disorders, and in secondary immune deficiency related to steroid use, leukemia, or severe infection.

Resources

BOOKS

Pagana, Kathleen Deska. *Mosby's Manual of Diagnosticand Laboratory Tests.* St. Louis: Mosby, Inc., 1998.

Janis O. Flores

Protein-energy malnutrition

Definition

Protein-energy **malnutrition** (PEM) is a potentially fatal body-depletion disorder. It is the leading cause of **death** in children in developing countries.

Description

PEM is also referred to as protein-calorie malnutrition. It develops in children and adults whose consumption of protein and energy (measured by calories) is insufficient to satisfy the body's nutritional needs. While pure protein deficiency can occur when a person's diet provides enough energy but lacks the protein minimum, in most cases the deficiency will be dual. PEM may also occur in persons who are unable to absorb vital nutrients or convert them to energy essential for healthy tissue formation and organ function.

Although PEM is not prevalent among the general population of the United States, it is often seen in elderly people who live in nursing homes and in children whose parents are poor. PEM occurs in one of every two surgical patients and in 48% of all other hospital patients.

Types of PEM

Primary PEM results from a diet that lacks sufficient sources of protein and/or energy. Secondary PEM is more common in the United States, where it usually occurs as a complication of AIDS, **cancer**, **chronic kidney failure**, inflammatory bowel disease, and other illnesses that impair the body's ability to absorb or use nutrients or to compensate for nutrient losses. PEM can develop gradually in a patient who has a chronic illness or experiences chronic semi-starvation. It may appear suddenly in a patient who has an acute illness.

Kwashiorkor

Kwashiorkor, also called wet protein-energy malnutrition, is a form of PEM characterized primarily by protein deficiency. This condition usually appears at the age of about 12 months when breastfeeding is discontinued, but it can develop at any time during a child's formative years. It causes fluid retention (**edema**); dry, peeling skin; and hair discoloration.

Marasmus

Primarily caused by energy deficiency, marasmus is characterized by stunted growth and wasting of muscle and tissue. Marasmus usually develops between the ages of six months and one year in children who have been weaned from breast milk or who suffer from weakening conditions like chronic **diarrhea**.

Causes and symptoms

Secondary PEM symptoms range from mild to severe, and can alter the form or function of almost every organ in the body. The type and intensity of symptoms depend on the patient's prior nutritional status and on the nature of the underlying disease and the speed at which it is progressing.

Mild, moderate, and severe classifications have not been precisely defined, but patients who lose 10–20% of their body weight without trying are usually said to have moderate PEM. This condition is also

characterized by a weakened grip and inability to perform high-energy tasks.

Losing 20% of body weight or more is generally classified as severe PEM. People with this condition can't eat normal-sized meals. They have slow heart rates and low blood pressure and body temperatures. Other symptoms of severe secondary PEM include baggy, wrinkled skin; constipation; dry, thin, brittle hair; lethargy; pressure sores and other **skin lesions**.

Kwashiorkor

People who have kwashiorkor often have extremely thin arms and legs, but liver enlargement and **ascites** (abnormal accumulation of fluid) can distend the abdomen and disguise weight loss. Hair may turn red or yellow. Anemia, diarrhea, and fluid and **electrolyte disorders** are common. The body's immune system is often weakened, behavioral development is slow, and mental retardation may occur. Children may grow to normal height but are abnormally thin.

Kwashiorkor-like secondary PEM usually develops in patients who have been severely burned, suffered trauma, or had **sepsis** (tissue-destroying infection) or another life-threatening illness. The condition's onset is so sudden that body fat and muscle mass of normal-weight people may not change. Some obese patients even gain weight.

Marasmus

Profound weakness accompanies severe marasmus. Since the body breaks down its own tissue to use as calories, people with this condition lose all their body fat and muscle strength, and acquire a skeletal appearance most noticeable in the hands and in the temporal muscle in front of and above each ear. Children with marasmus are small for their age. Since their immune systems are weakened, they suffer from frequent infections. Other symptoms include loss of appetite, diarrhea, skin that is dry and baggy, sparse hair that is dull brown or reddish yellow, mental retardation, behavioral retardation, low body temperature (**hypothermia**), and slow pulse and breathing rates.

The absence of edema distinguishes marasmus-like secondary PEM, a gradual wasting process that begins with weight loss and progresses to mild, moderate, or severe malnutrition (cachexia). It is usually associated with cancer, chronic obstructive pulmonary disease (COPD), or another chronic disease that is inactive or progressing very slowly.

Some individuals have both kwashiorkor and marasmus at the same time. This most often occurs when a person who has a chronic, inactive condition develops symptoms of an acute illness.

Hospitalized patients

Difficulty chewing, swallowing, and digesting food, pain, nausea, and lack of appetite are among the most common reasons that many hospital patients don't consume enough nutrients. Nutrient loss can be accelerated by bleeding, diarrhea, abnormally high sugar levels (glycosuria), **kidney disease**, malabsorption disorders, and other factors. **Fever**, infection, surgery, and benign or malignant tumors increase the amount of nutrients hospitalized patients need. So do trauma, **burns**, and some medications.

Diagnosis

A thorough **physical examination** and a health history that probes eating habits and weight changes, focuses on body-fat composition and muscle strength, and assesses gastrointestinal symptoms, underlying illness, and nutritional status is often as accurate as blood tests and urinalyses used to detect and document abnormalities.

Some doctors further quantify a patient's nutritional status by:

- comparing height and weight to standardized norms
- calculating body mass index (BMI)
- measuring skinfold thickness or the circumference of the upper arm

Treatment

Treatment is designed to provide adequate **nutrition**, restore normal body composition, and cure the condition that caused the deficiency. Tube feeding or intravenous feeding is used to supply nutrients to patients who can't or won't eat protein-rich foods.

In patients with severe PEM, the first stage of treatment consists of correcting fluid and electrolyte imbalances, treating infection with **antibiotics** that don't affect protein synthesis, and addressing related medical problems. The second phase involves replenishing essential nutrients slowly to prevent taxing the patient's weakened system with more food than it can handle. Physical therapy may be beneficial to patients whose muscles have deteriorated significantly.

Prognosis

Most people can lose up to 10% of their body weight without side effects, but losing more than 40% is almost always fatal. Death usually results from heart failure, an electrolyte imbalance, or low body temperature. Patients with certain symptoms, including semiconsciousness, persistent diarrhea, **jaundice**, and low blood sodium levels, have a poorer prognosis than other patients. Recovery from marasmus usually takes longer than recovery from kwashiorkor. The long-term effects of childhood malnutrition are uncertain. Some children recover completely, while others may have a variety of lifelong impairments, including an inability to properly absorb nutrients in the intestines and **mental retardation**. The outcome appears to be related to the length and severity of the malnutrition, as well as to the age of the child when the malnutrition occurred.

Prevention

Breastfeeding a baby for at least six months is considered the best way to prevent early-childhood malnutrition. Preventing malnutrition in developing countries is a complicated and challenging problem. Providing food directly during famine can help in the short-term, but more long-term solutions are needed, including agricultural development, public health programs (especially programs that monitor growth and development, as well as programs that provide nutritional information and supplements), and improved food distribution systems. Programs that distribute infant formula and discourage breastfeeding should be discontinued, except in areas where many mothers are infected with HIV.

Every patient being admitted to a hospital should be screened for the presence of illnesses and conditions that could lead to PEM. The nutritional status of patients at higher-than-average risk should be more thoroughly assessed and periodically reevaluated during extended hospital stays or nursing home residence.

Resources

ORGANIZATIONS

American College of Nutrition. 722 Robert E. Lee Drive, Wilmington, NC 20412-0927. (919) 152-1222.

American Institute of Nutrition. 9650 Rockville Pike, Bethesda, MD 20814-3990. (301) 530-7050.

Food and Nutrition Information Center. 10301 Baltimore Boulevard, Room 304, Beltsville, MD 20705-2351. < http://www.nalusda.gov/fnic >.

Maureen Haggerty

Protein-modified diet *see* **Diets**

Prothrombin time

Definition

The prothrombin time test belongs to a group of blood tests that assess the clotting ability of blood. The test is also known as the pro time or PT test.

Purpose

The PT test is used to monitor patients taking certain medications as well as to help diagnose clotting disorders.

Diagnosis

Patients who have problems with delayed blood clotting are given a number of tests to determine the cause of the problem. The prothrombin test specifically evaluates the presence of factors VIIa, V, and X, prothrombin, and fibrinogen. Prothrombin is a protein in the liquid part of blood (plasma) that is converted to thrombin as part of the clotting process. Fibrinogen is a type of blood protein called a globulin; it is converted to fibrin during the clotting process. A drop in the concentration of any of these factors will cause the blood to take longer to clot. The PT test is used in combination with the **partial thromboplastin time** (PTT) test to screen for **hemophilia** and other hereditary clotting disorders.

Monitoring

The PT test is also used to monitor the condition of patients who are taking warfarin (Coumadin). Warfarin is a drug that is given to prevent clots in the deep veins of the legs and to treat **pulmonary embolism**. It interferes with blood clotting by lowering the liver's production of certain clotting factors.

Description

A sample of the patient's blood is obtained by venipuncture. The blood is collected in a tube that contains sodium citrate to prevent the clotting process from starting before the test. The blood cells are separated from the liquid part of blood (plasma). The PT test is performed by adding the patient's plasma to a protein in the blood (thromboplastin) that converts prothrombin to thrombin. The mixture is then kept in a warm water bath at 37°C for one to two minutes. Calcium chloride is added to the mixture in order to counteract the sodium citrate and allow clotting to proceed. The test is timed from the addition of the calcium chloride until the plasma clots. This time is called the prothrombin time.

Preparation

The doctor should check to see if the patient is taking any medications that may affect test results. This precaution is particularly important if the patient is taking warfarin, because there are a number of medications that can interact with warfarin to increase or decrease the PT time.

Aftercare

Aftercare consists of routine care of the area around the puncture mark. Pressure is applied for a few seconds and the wound is covered with a bandage.

Risks

The primary risk is mild **dizziness** and the possibility of a bruise or swelling in the area where the blood was drawn. The patient can apply moist warm compresses.

Normal results

The normal prothrombin time is 11–15 seconds, although there is some variation depending on the source of the thromboplastin used in the test. (For this reason, laboratories report a normal control value along with patient results.) A prothrombin time within this range indicates that the patient has normal amounts of clotting factors VII and X.

Abnormal results

A prolonged PT time is considered abnormal. The prothrombin time will be prolonged if the concentration of any of the tested factors is 10% or more below normal plasma values. A prolonged prothrombin time indicates a deficiency in any of factors VII, X, V, prothrombin, or fibrinogen. It may mean that the patient has a vitamin K deficiency, a **liver disease**, or disseminated intravascular coagulation (DIC). The prothrombin time of patients receiving warfarin therapy will also be prolonged—usually in the range of one and one half to two times the normal PT time. A PT time that exceeds approximately two and a half times the control value (usually 30 seconds or longer) is grounds for concern, as abnormal bleeding may occur.

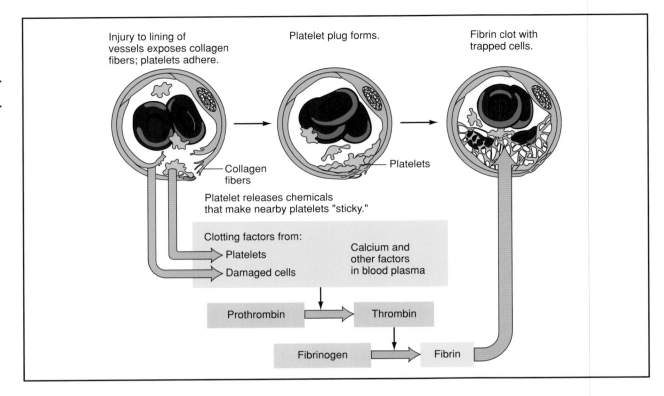

Injury to lining of vessels exposes collagen fibers; platelets adhere.

Platelet plug forms.

Fibrin clot with trapped cells.

Collagen fibers

Platelets

Platelet releases chemicals that make nearby platelets "sticky."

Clotting factors from:

Platelets

Damaged cells

Calcium and other factors in blood plasma

Prothrombin → Thrombin

Fibrinogen → Fibrin

The blood clotting process. *(Illustration by Hans & Cassady.)*

Resources

BOOKS

Berktow, Robert, et al., editors. *Merck Manual of Medical Information.* Whitehouse Station, NJ: Merck Research Laboratories, 2004.

John T. Lohr, PhD

Proton pump inhibitors

Definition

The proton pump inhibitors are a group of drugs that reduce the secretion of gastric (stomach) acid. They act by binding with the enzyme $H+$, $K(+)$-*ATPase, hydrogen/potassium adenosine triphosphatase*, which is sometimes referred to as the proton pump. This enzyme causes parietal cells of the stomach lining to produce acid.

Although they perform much the same functions as the histamine H-2 receptor blockers, the proton pump inhibitors reduce stomach acid more and over a longer period.

Purpose

Proton pump inhibitors are used to treat ulcers; gastroesophageal reflux disease (GERD), a condition in which backward flow of acid from the stomach causes **heartburn** and injury of the food pipe (esophagus); and conditions in which the stomach produces too much acid, such as Zollinger-Ellison syndrome. Omeprazole is used in combination with other medications to treat recurrent ulcers caused by helicobacter pylori infections.

Two of the proton pump inhibitors, lansoprazole and omeprazole, have been used to improve pancreatic enzyme absorption in **cystic fibrosis** patients with intestinal malabsorption.

Proton pump inhibitors may be used to protect against the ulcerogenic effects of non-steroidal anti-inflammatory drugs and to help heal ulcers caused by these drugs.

Description

There are five drugs in this class: esomeprazole (Nexium), lansoprazole (Prevacid), omeprazole (Prilosec), pantoprazole (Protonix), and rabeprazole (Aciphex). They act in a similar manner, and their cautions and adverse effects are similar.

The products are generally formulated as enteric-coated granules. Absorption does not start until the granules have left the stomach and reached the intestine, so the onset of action is delayed about an hour, subject to gastric emptying time. Since they act slowly, proton pump inhibitors are not a suitable alternative to **antacids** which have a rapid effect.

Although these drugs are eliminated from the body relatively quickly, usually within 90 minutes of absorption, they all work for over 24 hours after a dose. This is because the factor that determines duration of action is how long it takes the body to replace the H+, K(+)-ATPase. There is some build up over time. For example, a single dose of lansoprazole reduces stomach acid by 71%, but after a week of regular dosing, the acid reduction rises to 80%.

For treatment of recurrent ulcers, the proton pump inhibitors are part of combination therapy that uses an antibiotic (occasionally two **antibiotics**) and proton pump inhibitor. There are a number of regimens, and while they may vary in the selection of specific drugs, or even types of drugs used, usually they include a proton pump inhibitor. The cure rates are all within similar ranges for these regimens.

Recommended dosage

Dose varies with the indication. The following are commonly prescribed doses:

- Esomeprazole: 20 to 40 mg once a day.
- Lansoprazole: 15 to 30 mg once a day.
- Omeprazole: 20 to 40 mg once a day.
- Pantoprazole: 40 mg once or twice a day.
- Rabeprazole: 20 mg once a day. In hypersecretory conditions, doses as high as 60 mg twice daily have been reported.

In the above examples, the lower dose is usually adequate for GERD, while the higher dose may be required for ulcer therapy or hypersecretory conditions.

Precautions

Proton pump inhibitors should not be given to any patient who has shown a reaction to any of the components of the drug or a related drug. Proton pump inhibitors should also not be given to patients with severe **liver disease**.

Omeprazole is **pregnancy** category C, while esomeprazole, lansoprazole, rabeprazole, and pantoprazole are category B. As of 2005, there are no adequate and well-controlled studies concerning the effects of these drugs on pregnant women. These drugs should be used during pregnancy only if the potential benefit justifies the risk to the fetus. Because the proton pump inhibitors are excreted into breast milk, they should not be used by women who are breastfeeding their babies.

The proton pump inhibitors may mask the symptoms of **stomach cancer**.

Side effects

The proton pump inhibitors are relatively safe drugs. The most commonly observed adverse effects are **constipation**, **diarrhea**, **dizziness**, **headache**, skin itch, and skin rash. Less often, the following adverse effects have been reported: abdominal **pain** with cramps, appetite changes, and **nausea**.

The following adverse effects are extremely rare but have been reported with this class of drugs:

- acute pancreatitis
- anxiety
- cough
- depression

KEY TERMS

Antacid—A substance that counteracts or neutralizes acidity, usually of the stomach. Antacids have a rapid onset of action compared to histamine H-2 receptor blockers and proton pump inhibitors, but they have a short duration of action and require frequent dosing.

Cystic fibrosis—A hereditary disease that appears in early childhood, involves functional disorder of digestive glands, and is marked especially by faulty digestion due to a deficiency of pancreatic enzymes, by difficulty in breathing due to mucus accumulation in airways, and by excessive loss of salt in the sweat.

Enteric coat—A coating put on some tablets or capsules to prevent their disintegration in the stomach. The contents of coated tablets or capsules will be released only when the dose reaches the intestine. This may be done to protect the drug from stomach acid, to protect the stomach from drug irritation, or to delay the onset of action of the drug.

GERD—A chronic condition in which the lower esophageal sphincter allows gastric acids to reflux into the esophagus, causing heartburn, acid indigestion, and possible injury to the esophageal lining.

Malabsorption—Defective or inadequate absorption of nutrients from the intestinal tract.

Parietal cells—Cells of the gastric glands that secret hydrochloric acid.

Recurrent ulcer—Stomach ulcers that return after apparently complete healing. These ulcers appear to be caused by helicobacter pylori infections and can generally be successfully treated with a combination of antibiotics and gastric acid reducing compounds, particularly the proton pump inhibitors.

- drug toxin-related hepatitis
- erythema multiforme
- flu-like symptoms
- myalgia
- Stevens-Johnson syndrome
- thrombocytopenia
- toxic epidermal necrolysis
- ulcerative colitis

- upper respiratory hypersensitivity reaction
- upper respiratory infection
- vomiting

Interactions

Proton pump inhibitors should not be used in conjunctions with the anti-retroviral (anti-AIDS) drug atazanavir (Rayataz). The conjunction may reduce the effectiveness of the atazanavir. Proton pump inhibitors should not be used in combination with the anti-fungal drugs itraconazole or ketoconazole. This combination may reduce the effectiveness of the anti-fungal drugs.

Resources

BOOKS

Green, Steven M. *Tarascon Pocket Pharmacopoeia*. Deluxe labcoat pocket edition. Lompoc, CA: Tarascon Publishing, 2005.

Physicians' Desk Reference 2005. Montvale, NJ: Thomson Healthcare, 2004.

Yamada, Tadataka, et al., eds. *Textbook of Gastroenterology*. 4th ed. Philadelphia, PA: Lippincott Williams & Wilkins, 2003.

PERIODICALS

Peura, D. A. "Prevention of nonsteroidal anti-inflammatory drug-associated gastrointestinal symptoms and ulcer complications." *American Journal of Medicine* 117, Suppl. 5A (September 6, 2004): 63S–71S.

Vanderhoff, Bruce T., and Rundsarah M. Tahboub. "Proton Pump Inhibitors: An Update." *American Family Physician* 66 (2002): 273–80.

Van Pinxteren, B., et al. "Short-term treatment of gastro-esophageal reflux disease." *Journal of General Internal Medicine* 18, no. 9 (September 2003): 755–63.

Zed, P. J., et al. "Meta-analysis of proton pump inhibitors in treatment of bleeding peptic ulcers." *Annals of Pharmacotherapy* 35, no. 12 (December 2001): 1528–34.

ORGANIZATION

International Foundation for Functional Gastrointestinal Disorders. PO Box 170864, Milwaukee, WI 53217-8076. (414)964-1799. <www.iffgd.org>.

Samuel D. Uretsky, Pharm.D.

Pruritis *see* **Itching**

PSA test *see* **Prostate-specific antigen test**

PSDD *see* **Premenstrual disphoric disorder**

Pseudoephedrin *see* **Decongestants**

Pseudogout

Definition

Pseudogout is a form of arthritis that causes **pain**, redness, and inflammation in one or more joints.

Description

Pseudogout is also known by another name: calcium pyrophosphate dihydrate deposition disease (CPPD), the basis of which is derived from the calcium deposits that collect in the joint. The deposits or crystals, as they are sometimes called, cause pain and inflammation in the joint. According to the Arthritis Foundation, this can eventually weaken the cartilage, which serves as padding between the bones, "allowing bone to rub against bone." Pseudogout typically affects the large joints, such as the knees, wrists, and ankles. In general, it occurs with equal frequency in men and women.

Most often seen in older adults, pseudogout can also affect younger patients, especially those with diseases that put them at a greater risk of developing it, such as **hemochromatosis**, **hypercalcemia**, **hypothyroidism**, ochronosis, or Wilson's disease. Some people, according to an article for the American College of Rheumatology, experience attacks of pseudogout "following joint surgery or other surgery. Because many older people have calcium crystal deposits in their joints, any kind of insult to the joint can trigger the release of the calcium crystals, which then induce a painful inflammatory response." Pseudogout affects about 3% of elderly people. Not all will experience severe attacks. By their nineties, 50% of people will have joint deposits. Although researchers have noticed that some people with pseudogout also have a family history of the disease, it is not clear what role genetics might play in its development.

Causes and symptoms

As the Arthritis Foundation points out, it is unclear what causes the crystals to form, but some speculation exists that "an abnormality in the cartilage cells or connective tissue could be responsible" for their development. Acute pain and fluid accumulation that leads to joint swelling are typical symptoms of pseudogout. When the crystals move into a joint, the Arthritis Foundation categorizes the pain as "sudden and severe." Many patients report that joint motion is limited. Statistically speaking, in 50% of the cases, the patient will run a **fever**. Half of all the acute pseudogout attacks will involve a knee. The experts at MedlinePlus identify "chronic (long term) arthritis" as a symptom that can be present at the time of an acute pseudogout attack. The word "acute" implies short term; therefore, acute attacks of pseudogout will come and go, but chronic arthritis may remain. In addition, progressive degenerative arthritis is sometimes seen in numerous joints.

Diagnosis

Pseudogout and **gout** have similar symptoms, which can be confusing. However, uric acid is associated with gout, whereas calcium pyrophosphate crystals are associated with pseudogout. After a patient's detailed medical history is obtained, a diagnosis can be made based on the symptoms and medical tests.

Using a needle, the physician can take a sample of the synovial fluid from the swollen or painful joint to ascertain the presence of calcium pyrophosphate crystals. The fluid will also contain white blood cells, which can be counted to assist in the diagnosis. Synovial fluid is the lubricating fluid that's secreted by the membranes that line the joints.

X rays may also be taken to confirm the presence of crystals. The x-rays may also show joint damage or that crystals have led to a condition called chondrocalcinosis, which is calcification of the cartilage. Other possible causes such as gout, **rheumatoid arthritis**, or infection must be ruled out too. Blood tests can also help to confirm the diagnosis. Indeed, as the experts at MedlinePlus indicated, "careful workup, with analysis of crystals found in the joints, should ultimately lead to the correct diagnosis."

Treatment

There are a variety of treatment options. It if the patients have an adequate support system, such as family and friends willing to help, it makes it easier for patients to recover faster. Patients are often advised to avoid putting pressure on the affected joint. In some cases, it is appropriate for the patient to engage in special isometric exercises designed to help their specific condition heal faster. Once the inflammation and pain subsides, exercises are sometimes suggested to regain range of motion.

Medications can be prescribed to ease the pain, which typically fall into the nonsteroidal anti-inflammatory

KEY TERMS

hemochromatosis—This disease refers to when a person's body absorbs too much iron.

hypercalcemia—This disease refers to when a person's bones absorb too much calcium.

hypothyroidism—This disease refers to when a person's thyroid gland is underactive.

ochronosis—People with this rare hereditary condition tend to develop arthritis in adulthood.

Wilson's disease—Wilson's disease causes the body to retain copper, which ultimately can lead to liver damage.

category. For example, ibuprofen (Motrin) and naproxen (Aleve) are **nonsteroidal anti-inflammatory drugs** (NSAIDs) that are used quite often, because they are generally well tolerated and highly effective. However, in the article Dr. Schumacher wrote for the American College of Rheumatology he cautions patients by stating that, "people with poor kidney function, a history of stomach ulcers, and those who are on blood thinners often cannot take NSAIDs." Indomethacin (Indocin) is also a first-line drug that is commonly used to treat pseudogout that falls into this category.

When no infection is present, steroids, such as prednisone, may be prescribed. Much of the literature discussing treatment options also suggests a medication called colchicine, which is only available as a generic. It is generally prescribed in low doses and should not be used by anyone with significant bone marrow dysfunction or renal insufficiency. Patients should talk with their physicians regarding any other reasons why colchicine may not be suitable for them.

In order to relieve some of the pressure, the excess fluid around the joint can be removed (or aspirated, as it is sometimes called) with a needle.

Treatment options to reduce inflammation are valuable, "because they may slow the progression of joint degeneration that often accompanies pseudogout," according to Dr. Schumacher in his American College of Rheumatology article. If joint degeneration does occur, surgery is available to replace or repair damaged joints; however, it is better for patients to engage in preventative measures that will help them avoid the need for surgery. As the old saying goes, "an ounce of prevention is worth a pound of cure."

Prognosis

With regard to an acute attack of pseudogout, the prognosis is usually very good. The symptoms usually go away within two weeks. However, over time, joint degeneration can occur.

Prevention

There are not specific techniques applicable to every patient to prevent the formulation of the crystals; however, some patients with certain diseases are at greater risk of developing them. Diagnoses and treatment of underlying disorders is one of the most important aspects of managing crystal-induced arthopathies. Once a causative crystal is identified and a diagnosis has been established, long-term management and prevention can be devised.

Resources

PERIODICALS

Schumacher, H. R. "Crystal-induced arthritis: an overview." *American Journal of Medicine* 100 (1996): 46S–52S.

OTHER

Arthritis Foundation "Calcuim pyrophosphate dehydrate crystal deposition disease (CPPD) pseudogout." *Arthritis Foundation* 2004. The Arthritis Foundation. 29 Mar. 2005 < http://www.arthritis.org/ DiseaseCenter/cppd.asp >.

Medline Plus "Pseudogout." *U.S. National Library of Medicine* July 2004. U.S. National Library of Medicine and the National Institutes of Health. 29 Mar. 2005 < http://www.nlm.nih.gov/medlineplus/ency/ article000421.htm >.

Schumacher, H. R. "Pseudogout." *American College of Rheumatology* April 2004. American College of Rheumatology. 29 Mar. 2005 < http://www. rheumatology.org/public/factsheets/ pseudogout_new.asp >.

Lee Ann Paradise

Pseudohermaphroditism *see* **Intersex states**

Pseudomembraneous enterocolitis *see* **Antibiotic-associated colitis**

Pseudomonas aeruginosa infection *see* **Pseudomonas infections**

Pseudomonas infections

Definition

A pseudomonas infection is caused by a bacterium, *Pseudomonas aeruginosa*, and may affect any part of the body. In most cases, however, pseudomonas infections strike only persons who are very ill, usually hospitalized.

Description

P. aeruginosa is a rod-shaped organism that can be found in soil, water, plants, and animals. Because it rarely causes disease in healthy persons, but infects those who are already sick or who have weakened immune systems, it is called an opportunistic pathogen. Opportunistic pathogens are organisms that do not ordinarily cause disease, but multiply freely in persons whose immune systems are weakened by illness or medication. Such persons are said to be immunocompromised. Patients with **AIDS** have an increased risk of developing serious pseudomonas infections. Hospitalized patients are another high-risk group, because *P. aeruginosa* is often found in hospitals. Infections that can be acquired in the hospital are sometimes called nosocomial diseases.

Of the two million nosocomial infections each year, 10% are caused by *P. aeruginosa*. The bacterium is the second most common cause of nosocomial pneumonia and the most common cause of intensive care unit (ICU) pneumonia. Pseudomonas infections can be spread within hospitals by health care workers, medical equipment, sinks, disinfectant solutions, and food. These infections are a very serious problem in hospitals for two reasons. First, patients who are critically ill can die from a pseudomonas infection. Second, many *Pseudomonas* bacteria are resistant to certain **antibiotics**, which makes them difficult to treat.

P. aeruginosa is able to infect many different parts of the body. Several factors make it a strong opponent. These factors include:

- the ability to stick to cells
- minimal food requirements
- resistance to many antibiotics
- production of proteins that damage tissue
- a protective outer coat

Infections that can occur in specific body sites include:

- Heart and blood. *P. aeruginosa* is the fourth most common cause of bacterial infections of the blood (**bacteremia**). Bacteremia is common in patients with blood **cancer** and patients who have pseudomonas infections elsewhere in the body. *P. aeruginosa* infects the heart valves of intravenous drug abusers and persons with artificial heart valves.

- Bones and joints. Pseudomonas infections in these parts of the body can result from injury, the spread of infection from other body tissues, or bacteremia. Persons at risk for pseudomonas infections of the bones and joints include diabetics, intravenous drug abusers, and bone surgery patients.

- Central nervous system. *P. aeruginosa* can cause inflammation of the tissues covering the brain and spinal cord (**meningitis**) and brain abscesses. These infections may result from brain injury or surgery, the spread of infection from other parts of the body, or bacteremia.

- Eye and ear. *P. aeruginosa* can cause infections in the external ear canal–so-called "swimmer's ear"– that usually disappear without treatment. The bacterium can cause a more serious ear infection in elderly patients, possibly leading to hearing problems, facial **paralysis**, or even **death**. Pseudomonas infections of the eye usually follow an injury. They can cause ulcers of the cornea that may cause rapid tissue destruction and eventual blindness. The risk factors for pseudomonas eye infections include: wearing soft extended-wear contact lenses; using topical corticosteroid eye medications; being in a **coma**; having extensive **burns**; undergoing treatment in an ICU; and having a tracheostomy or endotracheal tube.

- Urinary tract. Urinary tract infections can be caused by catheterization, medical instruments, and surgery.

- Lung. Risk factors for *P. aeruginosa* **pneumonia** include: cystic fibrosis; chronic lung disease; immunocompromised condition; being on antibiotic therapy or a respirator; and congestive heart failure. Patients with **cystic fibrosis** often develop pseudomonas infections as children and suffer recurrent attacks of pneumonia.

- Skin and soft tissue. Even healthy persons can develop a pseudomonas skin rash following exposure to the bacterium in contaminated hot tubs, water parks, whirlpools, or spas. This skin disorder is called pseudomonas or "hot tub" **folliculitis**, and is often confused with **chickenpox**. Severe skin infection may occur in patients with *P. aeruginosa* bacteremia. The bacterium is the second most common cause of burn wound infections in hospitalized patients.

Causes and symptoms

P. aeruginosa can be sudden and severe, or slow in onset and cause little **pain**. Risk factors for acquiring a pseudomonas infection include: having a serious illness; being hospitalized; undergoing an invasive procedure such as surgery; having a weakened immune system; and being treated with antibiotics that kill many different kinds of bacteria (broad-spectrum antibiotics).

Each of the infections listed above has its own set of symptoms. *Pseudomonas* bacteremia resembles other bacteremias, producing **fever**, tiredness, muscle pains, joint pains, and chills. Bone infections are marked by swelling, redness, and pain at the infected site and possibly fever. *Pseudomonas* meningitis causes fever, **headache**, irritability, and clouded consciousness. Ear infection is associated with pain, ear drainage, facial paralysis, and reduced hearing. Pseudomonas infections of the eye cause ulcers that may spread to cover the entire eye, pain, reduced vision, swelling of the eyelids, and pus accumulation within the eye.

P. aeruginosa pneumonia is marked by chills, fever, productive **cough**, difficult breathing, and blue-tinted skin. Patients with cystic fibrosis with pseudomonas lung infections experience coughing, decreased appetite, weight loss, tiredness, **wheezing**, rapid breathing, fever, blue-tinted skin, and abdominal enlargement. Skin infections can cause a range of symptoms from a mild rash to large bleeding ulcers. Symptoms of pseudomonas folliculitis include a red itchy rash, headache, dizziness, earache, sore eyes, nose, and throat, breast tenderness, and stomach pain. Pseudomonas wound infections may secrete a blue-green colored fluid and have a fruity smell. Burn wound infections usually occur one to two weeks after the burn and cause discoloration of the burn scab, destruction of the tissue below the scab, early scab loss, bleeding, swelling, and a blue-green drainage.

Diagnosis

Diagnosis and treatment of pseudomonas infections can be performed by specialists in infectious disease. Because *P. aeruginosa* is commonly found in hospitals, many patients carry the bacterium without having a full-blown infection. Consequently, the mere presence of *P. aeruginosa* in patients does not constitute a diagnostic finding. Cultures, however, can be easily done for test purposes. The organism grows readily in laboratory media; results are usually available in two to three days. Depending on the location of the infection, body fluids that can be tested for *P. aeruginosa* include blood, urine, cerebrospinal fluid, sputum, pus, and drainage from an infected ear or eye. X rays and other imaging techniques can be used to assess infections in deep organ tissues.

Treatment

Medications

Because *P. aeruginosa* is commonly resistant to antibiotics, infections are usually treated with two antibiotics at once. Pseudomonas infections may be treated with combinations of ceftazidime (Ceftaz, Fortraz, Tazicef), ciprofloxacin (Cipro), imipenem (Primaxin), gentamicin (Garamycin), tobramycin (Nebcin), ticarcillin-clavulanate (Timentin), or piperacillin-tazobactam (Zosyn). Most antibiotics are administered intravenously or orally for two to six weeks. Treatment of an eye infection requires local application of antibiotic drops.

Surgery

Surgical treatment of pseudomonas infections is sometimes necessary to remove infected and damaged tissue. Surgery may be required for brain abscesses, eye infections, bone and joint infections, ear infections, heart infections, and wound infections. Infected **wounds** and burns may cause permanent damage requiring arm or leg amputation.

Prognosis

Most pseudomonas infections can be successfully treated with antibiotics and surgery. In immunocompromised persons, however, *P. aeruginosa* infections have a high mortality rate, particularly following bacteremia or infections of the lower lung. Mortality rates range from 15 to 20% of patients with severe ear infections to 89% of patients with infections of the left side of the heart.

Prevention

Most hospitals have programs for the prevention of nosocomial infections. Patients with cystic fibrosis may be given periodic doses of antibiotics to prevent episodes of pseudomonas pneumonia.

Minor skin infections can be prevented by avoiding hot tubs with cloudy water; avoiding public swimming pools at the end of the day; removing wet swimsuits as soon as possible; bathing after sharing a hot tub or using a public pool; cleaning hot tub filters

KEY TERMS

Bacteremia—Bacterial infection of the blood.

"Hot tub" folliculitis—A skin infection caused by *P. aeruginosa* that often follows bathing in a hot tub or public swimming pool.

Immunocompromised—Having a weak immune system due to disease or the use of certain medications.

Nosocomial infection—An infection that is acquired in the hospital.

Opportunistic—Causing disease only under certain conditions, as when a person is already sick or has a weak immune system.

Pathogen—Any microorganism that produces disease.

every six weeks; and using appropriate amounts of chlorine in the water.

Resources

OTHER

Centers for Disease Control. < http://www.cdc.gov/nccdphp/ddt/ddthome.htm >.

Belinda Rowland, PhD

Pseudomonas pseudomallei infection *see* **Melioidosis**

Pseudost *see* **Strabismus**

Pseudotuberculosis *see* **Sarcoidosis**

▍Pseudoxanthoma elasticum

Definition

Pseudoxanthoma elascticum (PXE) is an inherited connective tissue disorder in which the elastic fibers present in the skin, eyes, and cardiovascular system gradually become calcified and inelastic.

Description

PXE was first reported in 1881 by Rigal, but the defect in elastic fibers was described in 1986 by Darier, who gave the condition its name. PXE is also known as Grönblad-Strandberg-Touraine syndrome and systemic elastorrhexis.

The course of PXE varies greatly between individuals. Typically it is first noticed during adolescence as yellow-orange bumps on the side of the neck. Similar bumps may appear at other places where the skin bends a lot, like the backs of the knees and the insides of the elbows. The skin in these areas tends to get thick, leathery, inelastic, and acquire extra folds. These skin problems have no serious consequences, and for some people, the disease progresses no further.

Bruch's membrane, a layer of elastic fibers in front of the retina, becomes calcified in some people with PXE. Calcification causes cracks in Bruch's membrane, which can be seen through an ophthalmoscope as red, brown, or gray streaks called angioid streaks. The cracks can eventually (e.g., in 10–20 years) cause bleeding, and the usual resultant scarring leads to central vision deterioration. However, peripheral vision is unaffected.

Arterial walls and heart valves contain elastic fibers that can become calcified. This leads to a greater susceptibility to the conditions that are associated with hardening of the arteries in the normal **aging** population—high blood pressure, **heart attack**, **stroke**, and arterial obstruction—and, similarly, **mitral valve prolapse**. Heart disease and **hypertension** associated with PXE have been reported in children as young as four to 13 years of age. Although often appearing at a younger age, the overall incidence of these conditions is only slightly higher for people with PXE than it is in the general population.

Arterial inelasticity can lead to bleeding from the gastrointestinal tract and, rarely, acute vomiting of blood.

PXE is rare and occurs in about 1 in every 160,000 people in the general population. It is likely, though, that PXE is underdiagnosed, because of the presence of mild symptoms in some affected persons and the lack of awareness of the condition among primary care physicians.

Causes and symptoms

PXE is caused by changes in the genetic material, called mutations, that are inherited in either a dominant or recessive mode. A person with the recessive form of the disease (which is most common) must possess two copies of the PXE gene to be affected, and, therefore, must have received one from each parent. In the dominant form, one copy of the defective gene is sufficient to cause the disease. In some cases, a person with the dominant form inherits the abnormal gene from a parent with PXE. More commonly, the mutation arises as a spontaneous change in the genetic material of the affected person. These cases are called "sporadic" and do not affect parents or siblings, although each child of a person with sporadic PXE has a 50% risk to inherit the condition.

Both males and females develop PXE, although the skin findings seem to be somewhat more common in females.

The actual genetic causes of this condition were not discovered until 2000. The recessive, dominant, and sporadic forms of PXE all appear to be caused by different mutations or deletions in a single gene called ABCC6 (also known as MRP6), located on chromosome 16. Although the responsible gene has been identified, how it causes PXE is still unknown.

Genetic researchers have since identified mutations in a number of persons with PXE, most of whom have been found to have the recessive type. Affected individuals in these families had mutations in both copies of the gene and parents, who are obligate carriers, had a mutation in only one copy. Contrary to the usual lack of symptoms in carriers of recessive genes, some carriers of recessive PXE have been found to have cardiovascular symptoms typical of PXE.

Although the recessive type is the most common, there are also familial and sporadic cases that have been found to be caused by dominant mutations in the ABCC6 gene.

A wide range in the type and severity of symptoms exists between people with PXE. The age of onset also varies, although most people notice initial symptoms during adolescence or early adulthood. Often, the first symptoms to appear are thickened skin with yellow bumps in localized areas such as the folds of the groin, arms, knees, and armpits. These changes can also occur in the mucous membranes, most often in the inner portion of the lower lip. The appearance of the skin in PXE has been likened to a plucked chicken or Moroccan leather.

Angioid streaks in front of the retina are present in most people with PXE and an ophthalmologic examination can be used as an initial screen for the condition. Persons with PXE often complain of sensitivity to light. Because of the progressive breakdown of Bruch's membrane, affected persons are at increased risk for bleeding and scarring of the retina, which can lead to decreased central vision but does not usually cause complete blindness.

Calcium deposits in the artery walls contribute to early-onset **atherosclerosis**, and another condition called claudication, inadequate blood flow that results in **pain** in the legs after exertion. Abnormal bleeding, caused by calcification of the inner layer of the arteries, can occur in the brain, retina, uterus, bladder, and joints but is most common in the gastrointestinal tract.

Diagnosis

The presence of calcium in elastic fibers, as revealed by microscopic examination of biopsied skin, unequivocally establishes the diagnosis of PXE.

Treatment

PXE cannot be cured, but **plastic surgery** can treat PXE skin lesions, and **laser surgery** is used to prevent or slow the progression of vision loss. Excessive blood loss due to bleeding into the gastrointestinal tract or other organ systems may be treated by **transfusion**. Mitral valve prolapse (protrusion of one or both cusps of the mitral heart valve back into the atrium during heart beating) can be corrected by surgery, if necessary.

Measures should be taken to prevent or lessen cardiovascular complications. People with PXE should control their cholesterol and blood pressure, and maintain normal weight. They should exercise for cardiovascular health and to prevent or reduce claudication later in life. They should also avoid the use of tobacco, thiazide **antihypertensive drugs**, blood thinners like coumadin, and **nonsteroidal anti-inflammatory drugs** like **aspirin** and ibuprofen. In addition, they should avoid strain, heavy lifting, and contact sports, since these activities could trigger retinal and gastrointestinal bleeding.

People with PXE should have regular eye examinations by an ophthalmologist and report any eye problems immediately. Regular check-ups with a physician are also recommended, including periodic blood pressure readings.

Some people have advocated a calcium-restricted diet, but it is not yet known whether this aids the problems brought about by PXE. It is known, however, that calcium-restriction can lead to bone disorders.

Prognosis

The prognosis is for a normal life span with an increased chance of cardiovascular and circulatory

KEY TERMS

Angioid streaks—Gray, orange, or red wavy branching lines in Bruch's membrane.

Bruch's membrane—A membrane in the eye between the choroid membrane and the retina.

Carrier—A person who possesses a gene for an abnormal trait without showing signs of the disorder. The person may pass the abnormal gene on to offspring.

Claudication—Pain in the lower legs after exercise caused by insufficient blood supply.

Connective tissue—A group of tissues responsible for support throughout the body; includes cartilage, bone, fat, tissue underlying skin, and tissues that support organs, blood vessels, and nerves throughout the body.

Deletion—The absence of genetic material that is normally found in a chromosome. Often, the genetic material is missing due to an error in replication of an egg or sperm cell.

Dominant trait—A genetic trait in which one copy of the gene is sufficient to yield an outward display of the trait; dominant genes mask the presence of recessive genes; dominant traits can be inherited from a single parent.

Elastic fiber—Fibrous, stretchable connective tissue made primarily from proteins, elastin, collagen, and fibrillin.

Gene—A building block of inheritance, which contains the instructions for the production of a particular protein, and is made up of a molecular sequence found on a section of DNA. Each gene is found on a precise location on a chromosome.

Mitral valve—The heart valve that prevents blood from flowing backwards from the left ventricle into the left atrium. Also known as bicuspid valve.

Mutation—A permanent change in the genetic material that may alter a trait or characteristic of an individual, or manifest as disease, and can be transmitted to offspring.

Recessive trait—An inherited trait or characteristic that is outwardly obvious only when two copies of the gene for that trait are present.

problems, hypertension, gastrointestinal bleeding, and impaired vision. However, now that the gene for PXE has been identified, the groundwork for research to provide effective treatment has been laid. Studying the

role of the ABCC6 protein in elastic fibers may lead to drugs that will ameliorate or arrest the problems caused by PXE.

Genetic tests are now available that can provide knowledge needed to both diagnose PXE in symptomatic persons and predict it prior to the onset of symptoms in persons at risk. Prenatal diagnosis of PXE, by testing fetal cells for mutations in the ABCC6 gene, can be done in early pregnancy by procedures such as **amniocentesis** or chorionic villus sampling. For most people, PXE is compatible with a reasonably normal life, and prenatal diagnosis is not likely to be highly desired.

Genetic testing to predict whether an at-risk child will develop PXE may be helpful for medical management. A child who is found to carry a mutation can be monitored more closely for eye problems and bleeding, and can begin the appropriate lifestyle changes to prevent cardiovascular problems.

Resources

PERIODICALS

Ringpfeil, F., et al. "Pseudoxanthoma Elasticum: Mutations in the MRP6 Gene Encoding a Transmembrane AFP-binding Cassette (ABC) Transporter." *Proceedings of the National Academy of Sciences* 97 (May 2000): 6001–6.

Sherer, D.W., et al. "Pseudoxanthoma Elasticum: An Update." *Dermatology* 199 (1999): 3–7.

ORGANIZATIONS

National Association for Pseudoxanthoma Elasticum. 3500 East 12th Avenue, Denver, CO 80206. (303) 355-3866. Fax: (303) 355-3859. Pxenape@estreet.com. < http://www.napxe.org >.

PXE International, Inc. 23 Mountain Street, Sharon, MA 02067. (781) 784-3817. Fax: (781) 784-6672. PXEInter@aol.com. < http://www.pxe.org/ >.

Barbara J. Pettersen

Psittacosis *see* **Parrot fever**

Psoas abscess *see* **Abscess**

Psoriasis

Definition

Named for the Greek word *psōra* meaning "itch," psoriasis is a chronic, non-contagious disease characterized by inflamed lesions covered with silvery-white scabs of dead skin.

Description

Psoriasis, which affects at least four million Americans, is slightly more common in women than in men. Although the disease can develop at any time, 10–15% of all cases are diagnosed in children under 10, and the average age at the onset of symptoms is 28. Psoriasis is most common in fair-skinned people and extremely rare in dark-skinned individuals.

Normal skin cells mature and replace dead skin every 28–30 days. Psoriasis causes skin cells to mature in less than a week. Because the body can't shed old skin as rapidly as new cells are rising to the surface, raised patches of dead skin develop on the arms, back, chest, elbows, legs, nails, folds between the buttocks, and scalp.

Psoriasis is considered mild if it affects less than 5% of the surface of the body; moderate, if 5–30% of the skin is involved, and severe, if the disease affects more than 30% of the body surface.

Types of psoriasis

Dermatologists distinguish different forms of psoriasis according to what part of the body is affected, how severe symptoms are, how long they last, and the pattern formed by the scales.

PLAQUE PSORIASIS. Plaque psoriasis (psoriasis vulgaris), the most common form of the disease, is characterized by small, red bumps that enlarge, become inflamed, and form scales. The top scales flake off easily and often, but those beneath the surface of the skin clump together. Removing these scales exposes tender skin, which bleeds and causes the plaques (inflamed patches) to grow.

Plaque psoriasis can develop on any part of the body, but most often occurs on the elbows, knees, scalp, and trunk.

SCALP PSORIASIS. At least 50 of every 100 people who have any form of psoriasis have scalp psoriasis. This form of the disease is characterized by scale-capped plaques on the surface of the skull.

NAIL PSORIASIS. The first sign of nail psoriasis is usually pitting of the fingernails or toenails. Size, shape, and depth of the marks vary, and affected nails may thicken, yellow, or crumble. The skin around an affected nail is sometimes inflamed, and the nail may peel away from the nail bed.

GUTTATE PSORIASIS. Named for the Latin word *gutta,* which means "a drop," guttate psoriasis is characterized by small, red, drop-like dots that enlarge rapidly and may be somewhat scaly. Often found on the arms, legs, and trunk and sometimes in the scalp, guttate psoriasis can clear up without treatment or disappear and resurface in the form of plaque psoriasis.

PUSTULAR PSORIASIS. Pustular psoriasis usually occurs in adults. It is characterized by blister-like lesions filled with non-infectious pus and surrounded by reddened skin. Pustular psoriasis, which can be limited to one part of the body (localized) or can be widespread, may be the first symptom of psoriasis or develop in a patient with chronic plaque psoriasis.

Generalized pustular psoriasis is also known as Von Zumbusch pustular psoriasis. Widespread, acutely painful patches of inflamed skin develop suddenly. Pustules appear within a few hours, then dry and peel within two days.

Generalized pustular psoriasis can make life-threatening demands on the heart and kidneys.

Palomar-plantar pustulosis (PPP) generally appears between the ages of 20 and 60. PPP causes large pustules to form at the base of the thumb or on the sides of the heel. In time, the pustules turn brown and peel. The disease usually becomes much less active for a while after peeling.

Acrodermatitis continua of Hallopeau is a form of PPP characterized by painful, often disabling, lesions on the fingertips or the tips of the toes. The nails may become deformed, and the disease can damage bone in the affected area.

INVERSE PSORIASIS. Inverse psoriasis occurs in the armpits and groin, under the breasts, and in other areas where skin flexes or folds. This disease is characterized by smooth, inflamed lesions and can be debilitating.

ERYTHRODERMIC PSORIASIS. Characterized by severe scaling, **itching**, and **pain** that affects most of the body, erythrodermic psoriasis disrupts the body's chemical balance and can cause severe illness. This particularly inflammatory form of psoriasis can be the first sign of the disease, but often develops in patients with a history of plaque psoriasis.

PSORIATIC ARTHRITIS. About 10% of partients with psoriasis develop a complication called **psoriatic arthritis**. This type of arthritis can be slow to develop and mild, or it can develop rapidly. Symptoms of psoriatic arthritis include:

- joint discomfort, swelling, stiffness, or throbbing
- swelling in the toes and ankles
- pain in the digits, lower back, wrists, knees, and ankles
- eye inflammation or pink eye (conjunctivitis)

Causes and symptoms

The cause of psoriasis is unknown, but research suggests that an immune-system malfunction triggers the disease. Factors that increase the risk of developing psoriasis include:

- family history
- stress
- exposure to cold temperatures
- injury, illness, or infection
- steroids and other medications
- race

Trauma and certain bacteria may trigger psoriatic arthritis in patients with psoriasis.

Diagnosis

A complete medical history and examination of the skin, nails, and scalp are the basis for a diagnosis of psoriasis. In some cases, a microscopic examination of skin cells is also performed.

Blood tests can distinguish psoriatic arthritis from other types of arthritis. **Rheumatoid arthritis**, in particular, is diagnosed by the presence of a particular antibody present in the blood. That antibody is not present in the blood of patients with psoriatic arthritis.

Treatment

Age, general health, lifestyle, and the severity and location of symptoms influence the type of treatment used to reduce inflammation and decrease the rate at which new skin cells are produced. Because the course of this disease varies with each individual, doctors must experiment with or combine different treatments to find the most effective therapy for a particular patient.

Mild-moderate psoriasis

Steroid creams and ointments are commonly used to treat mild or moderate psoriasis, and steroids are sometimes injected into the skin of patients with a limited number of lesions. In mid-1997, the United States Food and Drug Administration (FDA) approved the use of tazarotene (Tazorac) to treat mild-to-moderate plaque psoriasis. This water-based gel has chemical properties similar to vitamin A.

Brief daily doses of natural sunlight can significantly relieve symptoms. **Sunburn** has the opposite effect.

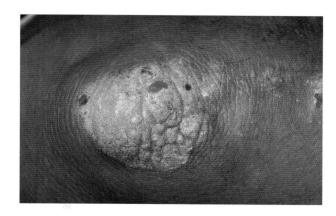

Psoriasis, a chronic skin disorder, may appear on any area of the body, including the elbow, as shown above. *(Photo Researchers, Inc. Reproduced by permission.)*

Moisturizers and bath oils can loosen scales, soften skin, and may eliminate the itch. So can adding a cup of oatmeal to a tub of bath water. Salicylic acid (an ingredient in **aspirin**) can be used to remove dead skin or increase the effectiveness of other therapies.

Moderate psoriasis

Administered under medical supervision, ultraviolet light B (UVB) is used to control psoriasis that covers many areas of the body or that has not responded to topical preparations. Doctors combine UVB treatments with topical medications to treat some patients and sometimes prescribe home **phototherapy**, in which the patient administers his or her own UVB treatments.

Photochemotherapy (PUVA) is a medically supervised procedure that combines medication with exposure to ultraviolet light (UVA) to treat localized or widespread psoriasis. An individual with widespread psoriasis that has not responded to treatment may enroll in one of the day treatment programs conducted at special facilities throughout the United States. Psoriasis patients who participate in these intensive sessions are exposed to UVB and given other treatments for six to eight hours a day for two to four weeks.

Severe psoriasis

Methotrexate (MTX) can be given as a pill or as an injection to alleviate symptoms of severe psoriasis or psoriatic arthritis. Patients who take MTX must be carefully monitored to prevent liver damage.

Psoriatic arthritis can also be treated with non steroidal anti-inflammatory drugs (NSAID), like acetaminophen (Tylenol) or aspirin. Hot compresses and warm water soaks may also provide some relief for painful joints.

Other medications used to treat severe psoriasis include etrentiate (Tegison) and isotretinoin (Accutane), whose chemical properties are similar to those of vitamin A. Most effective in treating pustular or erythrodermic psoriasis, Tegison also relieves some symptoms of plaque psoriasis. Tegison can enhance the effectiveness of UVB or PUVA treatments and reduce the amount of exposure necessary.

Accutane is a less effective psoriasis treatment than Tegison, but can cause many of the same side effects, including nosebleeds, inflammation of the eyes and lips, bone spurs, hair loss, and **birth defects**. Tegison is stored in the body for an unknown length of time, and should not be taken by a woman who is pregnant or planning to become pregnant. A woman should use reliable birth control while taking Accutane and for at least one month before and after her course of treatment.

Cyclosporin emulsion (Neoral) is used to treat stubborn cases of severe psoriasis. Cyclosporin is also used to prevent rejection of transplanted organs, and Neoral, approved by the FDA in 1997, should be particularly beneficial to psoriasis patients who are young children or African-Americans, or those who have diabetes.

Other conventional treatments for psoriasis include:

- Capsaicin (*Capsicum frutecens*), an ointment that can stop production of the chemical that causes the skin to become inflamed and halts the runaway production of new skin cells. Capsaicin is available without a prescription, but should be used under a doctor's supervision to prevent **burns** and skin damage.
- Hydrocortisone creams, topical ointments containing a form of vitamin D called calcitriol, and coal-tar shampoos and ointments can relieve symptoms. Hydrocortisone creams have been associated with such side effects as **folliculitis** (inflammation of the hair follicles), while coal-tar preparations have been associated with a heightened risk of skin cancer.

Alternative treatment

Non-traditional psoriasis treatments include:

- Soaking in warm water and German chamomile (*Matricaria recutita*) or bathing in warm salt water.
- Drinking as many as three cups a day of hot tea made with one or a combination of the following herbs: burdock (*Arctium lappa*) root, dandelion

(*Taraxacum mongolicum*) root, Oregon grape (*Mahonia aquifolium*), sarsaparilla (*Smilax officinalis*), and balsam pear (*Momardica charantia*).

- Taking two 500-mg capsules of evening primrose oil (*Oenothera biennis*) a day. Pregnant women should not use evening primrose oil, and patients with **liver disease** or **high cholesterol** should use it only under a doctor's supervision.
- Eating a diet that includes plenty of fish, turkey, celery (for cleansing the kidneys), parsley, lettuce, lemons (for cleansing the liver), limes, fiber, and fruit and vegetable juices.
- Eating a diet that eliminates animal products high in saturated fats, since they promote inflammation.
- Drinking plenty of water (at least eight glasses) each day.
- Taking **nutritional supplements** including **folic acid**, lecithin, vitamin A (specific for the skin), vitamin E, selenium, and zinc.
- Regularly imagining clear, healthy skin.

Other helpful alternative approaches include identifying and eliminating food allergens from the diet, enhancing the fuction of the liver, augmenting the hydrochloric acid in the stomach, and completing a **detoxification** program. Constitutional homeopathic treatment, if properly prescribed, can also help resolve psoriasis.

Prognosis

Most cases of psoriasis can be controlled, and most people who have psoriasis can live normal lives.

Some people who have psoriasis are so self conscious and embarrassed about their appearance that they become depressed and withdrawn. The Social Security Administration grants disability benefits to about 400 psoriasis patients each year, and a comparable number die from complications of the disease.

Prevention

A doctor should be notified if:

- psoriasis symptoms appear or reappear after treatment

- pustules erupt on the skin and the patient experiences **fatigue**, muscle aches, and **fever**

- unfamiliar, unexplained symptoms appear.

Resources

ORGANIZATIONS

American Academy of Dermatology. 930 N. Meacham Road, P.O. Box 4014, Schaumburg, IL 60168-4014. (847) 330-0230. Fax: (847) 330-0050. <http://www.aad.org>.

American Skin Association, Inc. 150 E. 58th St., 3rd floor, New York, NY 10155-0002. (212) 688-6547.

National Psoriasis Foundation. 6600 S.W. 92nd Ave., Suite 300, Portland, OR 97223. (800) 723-9166. <http://www.psoriasis.org>.

Maureen Haggerty

Psoriatic arthritis

Definition

Psoriatic arthritis is a form of arthritic joint disease associated with the chronic skin scaling and fingernail changes seen in **psoriasis**.

Description

Physicians recognize a number of different forms of psoriatic arthritis. In some patients, the arthritic symptoms will affect the small joints at the ends of the fingers and toes. In others, symptoms will affect joints on one side of the body but not on the other. In addition, there are patients whose larger joints on both sides of the body simultaneously become affected, as in rheumatoid arthritis. Some people with psoriatic arthritis experience arthritis symptoms in the back and spine; in rare cases, called psoriatic arthritis mutilans, the disease destroys the joints and bones, leaving patients with gnarled and club-like hands and feet. In many patients, symptoms of psoriasis precede the arthritis symptoms; a clue to possible joint disease is pitting and other changes in the fingernails.

Most people develop psoriatic arthritis at ages 35–45, but it has been observed earlier in adults and children. Both the skin and joint symptoms will come and go; there is no clear relationship between the severity of the psoriasis symptoms and arthritis **pain** at any given time. It is unclear how common psoriatic arthritis is. Recent surveys suggest that between 1 in 5 people and 1 in 2 people with psoriasis may also have some arthritis symptoms.

Causes and symptoms

The cause of psoriatic arthritis is unknown. As in psoriasis, genetic factors appear to be involved. People with psoriatic arthritis are more likely than others to have close relatives with the disease, but they are just as likely to have relatives with psoriasis but no joint disease. Researchers believe genes increasing the susceptibility to developing psoriasis may be located on chromosome 6p and chromosome 17, but the specific genetic abnormality has not been identified. Like psoriasis and other forms of arthritis, psoriatic arthritis also appears to be an autoimmune disorder, triggered by an attack of the body's own immune system on itself.

Symptoms of psoriatic arthritis include dry, scaly, silver patches of skin combined with joint pain and destructive changes in the feet, hands, knees, and spine. Tendon pain and nail deformities are other hallmarks of psoriatic arthritis.

Diagnosis

Skin and nail changes characteristic of psoriasis with accompanying arthritic symptoms are the hallmarks of psoriatic arthritis. A blood test for rheumatoid factor, antibodies that suggest the presence of **rheumatoid arthritis**, is negative in nearly all patients with psoriatic arthritis. X rays may show characteristic damage to the larger joints on either side of the body as well as fusion of the joints at the ends of the fingers and toes.

Treatment

Treatment for psoriatic arthritis is meant to control the skin lesions of psoriasis and the joint inflammation of arthritis. **Nonsteroidal anti-inflammatory drugs**, gold salts, and sulfasalazine are standard arthritis treatments, but have no effect on psoriasis. Antimalaria drugs and systemic corticosteroids should be avoided because they can cause dermatitis or exacerbate psoriasis when they are discontinued.

Several treatments are useful for both the **skin lesions** and the joint inflammation of psoriatic arthritis. Etretinate, a vitamin A derivative; methotrexate, a potent suppressor of the immune system; and ultraviolet light therapy have all been successfully used to treat psoriatic arthritis.

KEY TERMS

Psoriasis—A common recurring skin disease that is marked by dry, scaly, and silvery patches of skin that appear in a variety of sizes and locations on the body.

Psoriatic arthritis mutilans—A severe form of psoriatic arthritis that destroys the joints of the fingers and toes and causes the bones to fuse, leaving patients with gnarled and club-like hands and feet.

Rheumatoid arthritis—A systemic disease that primarily affects the joints, causing inflammation, changes in structure, and loss of function.

Rheumatoid factor—A series of antibodies that signal the presence of rheumatoid arthritis. May also be present in Sjögren's syndrome and systemic lupus erythematosus, among others.

Alternative treatment

Food allergies/intolerances are believed to play a role in most **autoimmune disorders**, including psoriatic arthritis. Identification and elimination of food allergens from the diet can be helpful. Constitutional homeopathy can work deeply and effectively with this condition, if the proper prescription is given. **Acupuncture**, Chinese herbal medicine, and western herbal medicine can all be useful in managing the symptoms of psoriatic arthritis. Nutritional supplements can contribute added support to the healing process. Alternative treatments recommended for psoriasis and rheumatoid arthritis may also be helpful in treating psoriatic arthritis.

Prognosis

The prognosis for most patients with psoriatic arthritis is good. For many the joint and other arthritis symptoms are much milder than those experienced in rheumatoid arthritis. One in five people with psoriatic arthritis, however, face potentially crippling joint disease. In some cases, the course of the arthritis can be far more mutilating than in rheumatoid arthritis.

Prevention

There are no preventive measures for psoriatic arthritis.

Resources

ORGANIZATIONS

American Academy of Dermatology. 930 N. Meacham Road, P.O. Box 4014, Schaumburg, IL 60168-4014. (847) 330-0230. Fax: (847) 330-0050. < http://www.aad.org >.

The American College of Rheumatology. 1800 Century Place, Suite 250, Atlanta, GA 30345. (404) 633-3777. < http://www.rheumatology.org >.

Richard H. Camer

PSP *see* **Progressive supranuclear palsy**

Psychiatric confinement

Definition

Psychiatric confinement is the use of restraints to detain a person in need of care and further evaluation.

Purpose

The purpose of restraint and confinement are crucial since they have a medico legal implication. The primary purpose for such intervention is typically an urgent or emergent condition that could cause danger to the affected person or others, or cause severe disability to the extent whereby the affected person is unable to care for his/herself.

Precautions

Clinicians utilizing this form of patient and public safety should perform a comprehensive mental status examination and document the findings. This approach can potentially provide clear records establishing the specific presenting problems and symptoms that can lead to ambiguities and potential legal action.

Description

Confinement with restraints can be categorized as urgent or emergent. Emergent causes can include patients exhibiting abnormal vital signs (breathing, pulse rate, temperature, blood pressure), threatening or violent behavior, and those who present with signs and symptoms of alcohol or illicit drug intoxication. Urgent use of confinement is indicated in patients showing suicidal thoughts, extreme **anxiety**, homicidal tendencies, violence, or a danger to self or the public at large.

Preparation

Those categorized as emergent should be prepared for further testing that can include blood chemistry and psychological assessment and evaluation. Initially the patient is restrained with four point leather restraints (both arms and both legs) and placed in a quiet room with a sitter. For those with urgent needs, restraint is initiated and initial management is directed to assess for an underlying medical cause and address psychological needs.

Aftercare

Further assessment, testing, and evaluation is necessary for a definitive diagnosis and devising an appropriate treatment plan.

Risks

A deficiency in record-keeping can lead to legal problems. The criteria and specifications for confinement should be clearly indicated. Meticulous clinical examination and documentation is essential for a definitive diagnosis. Persons who are confined due to **substance abuse** problems may have legal issues. As of 2001 there is proposed legislation concerning the misuse of restraints for psychiatric inpatients, which in the past has been responsible for numerous wrongful deaths. There are currently no federal laws that regulate the use of inpatient restraints nor any requirements for reporting injuries or **death**.

Resources

PERIODICALS

Reeves,R., et al. "Medicolegal Errors in the ED Related to the Involuntary Confinement of Psychiatric Patients." *American Journal of Emergency Medicine* November 1998.

Laith Farid Gulli, M.D.
Catherine Seeley
Keith Tatarelli, J.D.

Psychoanalysis

Definition

Psychoanalysis is a form of psychotherapy used by qualified psychotherapists to treat patients who have a range of mild to moderate chronic life problems. It is related to a specific body of theories about the relationships between conscious and unconscious mental processes, and should not be used as a synonym for psychotherapy in general. Psychoanalysis is done one-on-one with the patient and the analyst; it is not appropriate for group work.

Purpose

Psychoanalysis is the most intensive form of an approach to treatment called psychodynamic therapy. Psychodynamic refers to a view of human personality that results from interactions between conscious and unconscious factors. The purpose of all forms of psychodynamic treatment is to bring unconscious mental material and processes into full consciousness so that the patient can gain more control over his or her life.

Classical psychoanalysis has become the least commonly practiced form of psychodynamic therapy because of its demands on the patient's time, as well as on his or her emotional and financial resources. It is, however, the oldest form of psychodynamic treatment. The theories that underlie psychoanalysis were worked out by Sigmund Freud (1856–1939), a Viennese physician, during the early years of the twentieth century. Freud's discoveries were made in the context of his research into hypnosis. The goal of psychoanalysis is the uncovering and resolution of the patient's internal conflicts. The treatment focuses on the formation of an intense relationship between the therapist and patient, which is analyzed and discussed in order to deepen the patient's insight into his or her problems.

Psychoanalytic psychotherapy is a modified form of psychoanalysis that is much more widely practiced. It is based on the same theoretical principles as psychoanalysis, but is less intense and less concerned with major changes in the patient's character structure. The focus in treatment is usually the patient's current life situation and the way problems relate to early conflicts and feelings, rather than an exploration of the unconscious aspects of the relationship that has been formed with the therapist.

Not all patients benefit from psychoanalytic treatment. Potential patients should meet the following prerequisites:

• The capacity to relate well enough to form an effective working relationship with the analyst. This relationship is called a therapeutic alliance.

• At least average intelligence and a basic understanding of psychological theory.

CARL GUSTAV JUNG (1875–1961)

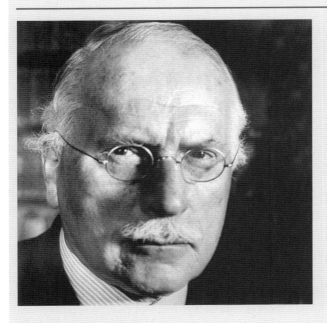

(Library of Congress.)

Carl Gustav Jung was born in Kesswil, Switzerland, on July 26, 1875, to a Protestant clergyman who moved his family to Basel when Jung was four. While growing up,

Jung exhibited an interest in many diverse areas of study but finally decided to pursue medicine at the University of Basel and the University of Zurich, earning his degree in 1902. He also studied psychology in Paris. In 1903, Jung married Emma Rauschenbach, his companion and collaborator. The couple had five children.

Jung's professional career began in 1900 at the University of Zurich where he worked as an assistant to Eugene Blueler in the psychiatric clinic. During his internship, he and some co-workers used an experiment that revealed groups of ideas in the unconscious psyche which he named *complexes*. Jung sent his publication *Studies in Word Association* (1904) to Sigmund Freud after finding his own beliefs confirmed by Freud's work. Jung and Freud became friends and collaborators until 1913 when Jung's ideas began to conflict with Freud's. During the time following this split, Jung published *Two Essays on Analytical Psychology* (1916, 1917) and *Psychological Types* (1921). Jung's later work developed from the concepts in his *Two Essays* publication and he became known as a founder of modern depth psychology.

In 1944, Jung gave up his psychological practice and his explorations after he suffered a severe heart attack. Jung received honorary doctorates from numerous universities and in 1948 he founded the C. G. Jung Institute in Zurich. Jung died on June 6, 1961.

• The ability to tolerate frustration, sadness, and other painful emotions.

• The capacity to distinguish between reality and fantasy.

People considered best suited to psychoanalytic treatment include those with depression, character disorders, neurotic conflicts, and chronic relationship problems. When the patient's conflicts are long-standing and deeply entrenched in his or her personality, psychoanalysis may be preferable to psychoanalytic psychotherapy, because of its greater depth.

Precautions

Psychoanalysis is not usually considered suitable for patients suffering from severe depression or such psychotic disorders as **schizophrenia**, although some analysts have successfully treated patients with psychoses. It is also not appropriate for people with addictions or substance dependency, disorders of aggression or impulse control, or acute crises; some of these people may benefit from psychoanalysis after the crisis has been resolved.

Description

In both psychoanalysis and psychoanalytic psychotherapy, the therapist does not tell the patient how to solve problems or offer moral judgments. The focus of treatment is exploration of the patient's mind and habitual thought patterns. Such therapy is termed "non-directed." It is also "insight-oriented," meaning that the goal of treatment is increased understanding of the sources of one's inner conflicts and emotional problems. The basic techniques of psychoanalytical treatment include:

Therapist neutrality

Neutrality means that the analyst does not take sides in the patient's conflicts, express feelings about the patient, or talk about his or her own life. Therapist neutrality is intended to help the patient stay focused on issues rather than be concerned with the therapist's reactions. In psychoanalysis, the patient lies on a couch facing away from the therapist. In psychodynamic psychotherapy, however, the patient and therapist usually sit in comfortable chairs facing each other.

Free association

Free association means that the patient talks about whatever comes into mind without censoring or editing the flow of ideas or memories. Free association allows the patient to return to earlier or more childlike emotional states ("regress"). Regression is sometimes necessary in the formation of the therapeutic alliance. It also helps the analyst to understand the recurrent patterns of conflict in the patient's life.

Therapeutic alliance and transference

Transference is the name that psychoanalysts use for the patient's repetition of childlike ways of relating that were learned in early life. If the therapeutic alliance has been well established, the patient will begin to transfer thoughts and feelings connected with siblings, parents, or other influential figures to the therapist. Discussing the transference helps the patient gain insight into the ways in which he or she misreads or misperceives other people in present life.

Interpretation

In psychoanalytic treatment, the analyst is silent as much as possible, in order to encourage the patient's free association. However, the analyst offers judiciously timed interpretations, in the form of verbal comments about the material that emerges in the sessions. The therapist uses interpretations in order to uncover the patient's resistance to treatment, to discuss the patient's transference feelings, or to confront the patient with inconsistencies. Interpretations may be either focused on present issues ("dynamic") or intended to draw connections between the patient's past and the present ("genetic"). The patient is also often encouraged to describe dreams and fantasies as sources of material for interpretation.

Working through

"Working through" occupies most of the work in psychoanalytic treatment after the transference has been formed and the patient has begun to acquire insights into his or her problems. Working through is a process in which the new awareness is repeatedly tested and "tried on for size" in other areas of the patient's life. It allows the patient to understand the influence of the past on his or her present situation, to accept it emotionally as well as intellectually, and to use the new understanding to make changes in present life.

Working through thus helps the patient to gain some measure of control over inner conflicts and to resolve them or minimize their power.

Although psychoanalytic treatment is primarily verbal, medications are sometimes used to stabilize patients with severe **anxiety**, depression, or other mood disorders during the analysis.

The cost of either psychoanalysis or psychoanalytic psychotherapy is prohibitive for most patients without insurance coverage. A full course of psychoanalysis usually requires three to five weekly sessions with a psychoanalyst over a period of three to five years. A course of psychoanalytic psychotherapy involves one to three meetings per week with the therapist for two to five years. Each session or meeting typically costs between $80 and $200, depending on the locale and the experience of the therapist. The increasing reluctance of most HMOs and other managed care organizations to pay for long-term psychotherapy is one reason that these forms of treatment are losing ground to short-term methods of treatment and the use of medications to control the patient's emotional symptoms. It is also not clear as of 2003 that long-term psychoanalytically oriented approaches are more beneficial than briefer therapy methods for many patients. On the other hand, patients who can benefit from a psychoanalytic approach but cannot afford private fees may wish to contact the American Psychoanalytic Association, which maintains a list of analysts in training who offer treatment for reduced fees.

Preparation

Some patients may need evaluation for possible medical problems before entering psychoanalysis because numerous diseases—including virus infections and certain vitamin deficiencies—have emotional side effects or symptoms. The therapist will also want to know whether the patient is taking any prescription medications that may affect the patient's feelings or ability to concentrate. In addition, it is important to make sure that the patient is not abusing drugs or alcohol.

Risks

The primary risk to the patient is related to the emotional **pain** resulting from new insights and changes in long-standing behavior patterns. In some patients, psychoanalysis produces so much anxiety that they cannot continue with this treatment method. In other cases, the therapist's lack of skill or

KEY TERMS

Free association—A technique used in psychoanalysis in which the patient allows thoughts and feelings to emerge without trying to organize or censor them.

Interpretation—A verbal comment made by the analyst in response to the patient's free association. It is intended to help the patient gain new insights.

Neurosis—A mental and emotional disorder that affects only part of the personality and is accompanied by a significantly less distorted perception of reality than in psychosis.

Psychodynamic—An approach to psychotherapy based on the interplay of conscious and unconscious factors in the patient's mind. Psychoanalysis is one type of psychodynamic therapy.

Regression—The process in which the patient reverts to earlier or less mature feelings and behaviors.

Therapeutic alliance—The working relationship between a therapist and a patient that is necessary to the success of therapy.

Transference—The process that develops during psychoanalytic work during which the patient redirects feelings about early life figures toward the analyst.

Working through—The repeated testing of insights, which takes up most of the work in psychoanalysis after the therapeutic alliance has been formed.

differences in cultural background may prevent the formation of a solid therapeutic alliance.

Normal results

Psychoanalysis and psychoanalytic psychotherapy both have the goal of basic changes in the patient's personality structure and level of functioning, although psychoanalysis typically aims at more extensive and more profound change. In general, this approach to treatment is considered successful if the patient has shown:

- reduction in intensity or number of symptoms
- some resolution of basic emotional conflicts
- increased independence and self-esteem
- improved functioning and adaptation to life

Attempts to compare the effectiveness of psychoanalytical treatment to other modes of therapy are difficult to evaluate. Some aspects of Freudian theory have been questioned since the 1970s on the grounds of their limited applicability to women and to people from non-Western cultures. In particular, some psychiatrists with cross-cultural experience maintain that psychoanalysis presupposes a highly individualistic Western concept of human personhood that is alien to traditional Asian and African societies. There is, however, general agreement that psychoanalytic approaches work well for certain types of patients, specifically those with neurotic conflicts.

Resources

PERIODICALS

Blass, R. B. "On Ethical Issues at the Foundation of the Debate Over the Goals of Psychoanalysis." *International Journal of Psychoanalysis* 84 (August 2003): 929–943.

Gabbard, G. O., and D. Westen. "Rethinking Therapeutic Action." *International Journal of Psychoanalysis* 84 (August 2003): 823–841.

Lombardi, R. "Mental Models and Language Registers in the Psychoanalysis of Psychosis: An Overview of a Thirteen-Year Analysis." *International Journal of Psychoanalysis* 84 (August 2003): 843–863.

Roland, A. "Psychoanalysis Across Civilizations: A Personal Journey." *Journal of the American Academy of Psychoanalysis and Dynamic Psychiatry* 31 (Summer 2003): 275–295.

ORGANIZATIONS

American Psychoanalytic Association. 309 East 49th Street, New York, NY 10017. (212) 752-0450. < http://www.apsa-co.org >.

Rebecca J. Frey, PhD

Psychological tests

Definition

Psychological tests are written, visual, or verbal evaluations administered to assess the cognitive and emotional functioning of children and adults.

Purpose

Psychological tests are used to assess a variety of mental abilities and attributes, including achievement and ability, personality, and neurological functioning.

Achievement and ability tests

For children, academic achievement, ability, and intelligence tests may be used as a tool in school placement, in determining the presence of a learning disability or a developmental delay, in identifying giftedness, or in tracking intellectual development. Intelligence testing may be used with adults to determine vocational ability (e.g., in career counseling) or to assess adult intellectual ability in the classroom.

Personality tests

Personality tests are administered for a wide variety of reasons, from diagnosing psychopathology (e.g., personality disorder, depressive disorder) to screening job candidates. They may be used in an educational or vocational setting to determine personality strengths and weaknesses, or in the legal system to evaluate parolees.

Neuropsychological tests

Patients who have experienced a traumatic brain injury, brain damage, or organic neurological problems (for example, **dementia**) are administered neuropsychological tests to assess their level of functioning and identify areas of mental impairment. They may also be used to evaluate the progress of a patient who has undergone treatment or **rehabilitation** for a neurological injury or illness. In addition, certain neuropsychological measures may be used to screen children for developmental delays and/or learning disabilities.

Precautions

Psychological testing requires a clinically trained examiner. All psychological tests should be administered, scored, and interpreted by a trained professional, preferably a psychologist or psychiatrist with expertise in the appropriate area.

Psychological tests are only one element of a psychological assessment. They should never be used alone as the sole basis for a diagnosis. A detailed history of the test subject and a review of psychological, medical, educational, or other relevant records are required to lay the groundwork for interpreting the results of any psychological measurement.

Cultural and language differences in the test subject may affect test performance and may result in inaccurate test results. The test administrator should be informed before psychological testing begins if the test taker is not fluent in English and/or belongs to a minority culture. In addition, the subject's motivation and motives may also affect test results.

Description

Psychological tests are formalized measures of mental functioning. Most are objective and quantifiable; however, certain projective tests may involve some level of subjective interpretation. Also known as inventories, measurements, questionnaires, and scales, psychological tests are administered in a variety of settings, including preschools, primary and secondary schools, colleges and universities, hospitals, outpatient healthcare settings, social agencies, prisons, and employment or human resource offices. They come in a variety of formats, including written, verbal, and computer administered.

Achievement and ability tests

Achievement and ability tests are designed to measure the level of an individual's intellectual functioning and cognitive ability. Most achievement and ability tests are standardized, meaning that norms were established during the design phase of the test by administering the test to a large representative sample of the test population. Achievement and ability tests follow a uniform testing protocol, or procedure (i.e., test instructions, test conditions, and scoring procedures) and their scores can be interpreted in relation to established norms. Common achievement and ability tests include the **Wechsler intelligence test** (WISC-III and WAIS) and the **Stanford-Binet intelligence scales**.

Personality tests

Personality tests and inventories evaluate the thoughts, emotions, attitudes, and behavioral traits that comprise personality. The results of these tests determine an individual's personality strengths and weaknesses, and may identify certain disturbances in personality, or psychopathology. Tests such as the *Minnesota multiphasic personality inventory MMPI-2)* and the *Millon clinical multiaxial Inventory III (MMPI-III)*, are used to screen individuals for specific psychopathologies or emotional problems.

Another type of personality test is the projective personality assessment. A projective test asks a subject to interpret some ambiguous stimuli, such as a series of inkblots. The subject's responses provide insight into his or her thought processes and personality traits. For example, the Rorschach inkblot test and the **Holtzman ink blot test** (HIT) use a series of inkblots that the test

KEY TERMS

Norms—A fixed or ideal standard; normative or mean score for a particular age group.

Psychopathology—A mental disorder or illness, such as schizophrenia, personality disorder, or major depressive disorder.

Quantifiable—Can be expressed as a number. The results of quantifiable psychological tests can be translated into numerical values, or scores.

Representative sample—A random sample of people that adequately represent the test taking population in age, gender, race, and socioeconomic standing.

Standardization—The process of determining established norms and procedures for a test to act as a standard reference point for future test results.

Normal results

All psychological and neuropsychological assessments should be administered, scored, and interpreted by a trained professional. When interpreting test results for test subjects, the test administrator will review with subjects: what the test evaluates, its precision in evaluation, any margins of error involved in scoring, and what the individual scores mean in the context of overall test norms and the background of the test subject.

Resources

ORGANIZATIONS

American Psychological Association (APA). 750 First St. NE, Washington, DC 20002-4242. (202) 336-5700. < ttp://www.apa.org >.

Paula Anne Ford-Martin

subject is asked to identify. Another projective assessment, the **Thematic apperception test** (TAT), asks the subject to tell a story about a series of pictures. Some consider projective tests to be less reliable than objective personality tests. If the examiner is not well-trained in psychometric evaluation, subjective interpretations may affect the evaluation of these tests.

Neuropsychological tests

Many insurance plans cover all or a portion of diagnostic neuropsychological or psychological testing. As of 1997, Medicare reimbursed for psychological and neuropsychological testing. Billing time typically includes test administration, scoring and interpretation, and reporting.

Preparation

Prior to the administration of any psychological test, the administrator should provide the test subject with information on the nature of the test and its intended use, complete standardized instructions for taking the test (including any time limits and penalties for incorrect responses), and information on the confidentiality of the results. After these disclosures are made, informed consent should be obtained from the test subject before testing begins (except in cases of legally mandated testing, where consent is not required of the subject).

Psychosis

Definition

Psychosis is a symptom or feature of mental illness typically characterized by radical changes in personality, impaired functioning, and a distorted or non-existent sense of objective reality.

Description

Patients suffering from psychosis have impaired reality testing; that is, they are unable to distinguish personal subjective experience from the reality of the external world. They experience **hallucinations** and/or **delusions** that they believe are real, and may behave and communicate in an inappropriate and incoherent fashion. Psychosis may appear as a symptom of a number of mental disorders, including mood and **personality disorders**. It is also the defining feature of **schizophrenia**, schizophreniform disorder, **schizoaffective disorder**, delusional disorder, and the psychotic disorders (i.e., brief psychotic disorder, shared psychotic disorder, psychotic disorder due to a general medical condition, and substance-induced psychotic disorder).

Causes and symptoms

Psychosis may be caused by the interaction of biological and psychosocial factors depending on the disorder in which it presents; psychosis can also be caused by purely social factors, with no biological component.

Biological factors that are regarded as contributing to the development of psychosis include genetic abnormalities and substance use. With regard to chromosomal abnormalities, studies indicate that 30% of patients diagnosed with a psychotic disorder have a microdeletion at chromosome 22q11. Another group of researchers has identified the gene G72/G30 at chromosome 13q33.2 as a susceptibility gene for childhood-onset schizophrenia and psychosis not otherwise specified.

With regard to **substance abuse**, several different research groups reported in 2004 that cannabis (**marijuana**) use is a risk factor for the onset of psychosis.

Migration is a social factor that influences people's susceptibility to psychotic disorders. Psychiatrists in Europe have noted the increasing rate of schizophrenia and other psychotic disorders among immigrants to almost all Western European countries. Black immigrants from Africa or the Caribbean appear to be especially vulnerable. The stresses involved in migration include family breakup, the need to adjust to living in large urban areas, and social inequalities in the new country.

Schizophrenia, schizophreniform disorder, and schizoaffective disorder

Psychosis in schizophrenia and perhaps schizophreniform disorder appears to be related to abnormalities in the structure and chemistry of the brain, and appears to have strong genetic links; but its course and severity can be altered by social factors such as **stress** or a lack of support within the family. The cause of schizoaffective disorder is less clear cut, but biological factors are also suspected.

Delusional disorder

The exact cause of delusional disorder has not been conclusively determined, but potential causes include heredity, neurological abnormalities, and changes in brain chemistry. Some studies have indicated that delusions are generated by abnormalities in the limbic system, the portion of the brain on the inner edge of the cerebral cortex that is believed to regulate emotions. Delusional disorder is also more likely to develop in persons who are isolated from others in their society by language difficulties and/or cultural differences.

Brief psychotic disorder

Trauma and stress can cause a short-term psychosis (less than a month's duration) known as brief psychotic disorder. Major life-changing events such as the **death** of a family member or a natural disaster have been known to stimulate brief psychotic disorder in patients with no prior history of mental illness.

Psychotic disorder due to a general medical condition

Psychosis may also be triggered by an organic cause, termed a psychotic disorder due to a general medical condition. Organic sources of psychosis include neurological conditions (for example, epilepsy and cerebrovascular disease), metabolic conditions (for example, porphyria), endocrine conditions (for example, hyper- or **hypothyroidism**), renal failure, electrolyte imbalance, or **autoimmune disorders**.

Substance-induced psychotic disorder

Psychosis is also a known side effect of the use, **abuse**, and withdrawal from certain drugs. So-called recreational drugs, such as hallucinogenics, PCP, amphetamines, **cocaine**, marijuana, and alcohol, may cause a psychotic reaction during use or withdrawal. Certain prescription medications such as steroids, anticonvulsants, chemotherapeutic agents, and antiparkinsonian medications may also induce psychotic symptoms. Toxic substances such as carbon monoxide have also been reported to cause substance-induced psychotic disorder.

Shared psychotic disorder

Shared psychotic disorder, also known as *folie à deux* or psychosis by association, is a relatively rare delusional disorder involving two (or more) people with close emotional ties. In the West, shared psychosis most commonly develops between two sisters or between husband and wife, while in Japan the most common form involves a parent and a son or daughter. Shared psychosis occasionally involves an entire nuclear family.

Psychosis is characterized by the following symptoms:

• Delusions. Those delusions that occur in schizophrenia and its related forms are typically bizarre (i.e., they could not occur in real life). Delusions occurring in delusional disorder are more plausible, but still patently untrue. In some cases, delusions may be accompanied by feelings of **paranoia**.

- Hallucinations. Psychotic patients see, hear, smell, taste, or feel things that aren't there. Schizophrenic hallucinations are typically auditory or, less commonly, visual; but psychotic hallucinations can involve any of the five senses.

- Disorganized speech. Psychotic patients, especially those with schizophrenia, often ramble on in incoherent, nonsensical speech patterns.

- Disorganized or catatonic behavior. The catatonic patient reacts inappropriately to his/her environment by either remaining rigid and immobile or by engaging in excessive motor activity. Disorganized behavior is behavior or activity that is inappropriate for the situation, or unpredictable.

Diagnosis

Patients with psychotic symptoms should undergo a thorough **physical examination** and history to rule out such possible organic causes as seizures, **delirium**, or alcohol withdrawal, and such other psychiatric conditions as dissociation or panic attacks. If a psychiatric cause such as schizophrenia is suspected, a mental health professional will typically conduct an interview with the patient and administer one of several clinical inventories, or tests, to evaluate mental status. This assessment takes place in either an outpatient or hospital setting.

Psychotic symptoms and behaviors are considered psychiatric emergencies, and persons showing signs of psychosis are frequently taken by family, friends, or the police to a hospital emergency room. A person diagnosed as psychotic can be legally hospitalized against his or her will, particularly if he or she is violent, threatening to commit **suicide**, or threatening to harm another person. A psychotic person may also be hospitalized if he or she has become malnourished or ill as a result of failure to feed, dress appropriately for the climate, or otherwise take care of him- or herself.

Treatment

Psychosis that is symptomatic of schizophrenia or another psychiatric disorder should be treated by a psychologist and/or psychiatrist. An appropriate course of medication and/or psychosocial therapy is employed to treat the underlying primary disorder. If the patient is considered to be at risk for harming himself or others, inpatient treatment is usually recommended.

Treatment of shared psychotic disorder involves separating the affected persons from one another as well as using antipsychotic medications and psychotherapy.

Antipsychotic medication such as thioridazine (Mellaril), haloperidol (Haldol), chlorpromazine (Thorazine), clozapine (Clozaril), sertindole (Serlect), olanzapine (Zyprexa), or risperidone (Risperdal) is usually prescribed to bring psychotic symptoms under control and into remission. Possible side effects of antipsychotics include **dry mouth**, drowsiness, muscle stiffness, and **tardive dyskinesia** (involuntary movements of the body). Agranulocytosis, a potentially serious but reversible health condition in which the white blood cells that fight infection in the body are destroyed, is a possible side effect of clozapine. Patients treated with this drug should undergo weekly blood tests to monitor white blood cell counts for the first six months, then every two weeks.

After an acute psychotic episode has subsided, antipsychotic drug maintenance treatment is typically employed and psychosocial therapy and living and vocational skills training may be attempted.

Prognosis

Prognosis for brief psychotic disorder is quite good; for schizophrenia, less so. Generally, the longer and more severe a psychotic episode, the poorer the prognosis is for the patient. Early diagnosis and treatment are critical to improving outcomes for the patient across all psychotic disorders.

Approximately 10% of America's permanently disabled population is comprised of schizophrenic individuals. The mortality rate of schizophrenic individuals is also high—approximately 10% of schizophrenics commit suicide, and 20% attempt it. However, early diagnosis and long-term follow up care can improve the outlook for these patients considerably. Roughly 60% of patients with schizophrenia will show substantial improvement with appropriate treatment.

Resources

BOOKS

American Psychiatric Association. *Diagnostic and Statistical Manual of Mental Disorders.*4th ed., revised. Washington, D.C.: American Psychiatric Association, 2000.

Beers, Mark H., MD, and Robert Berkow, MD., editors. "Psychiatric Emergencies." In *The Merck Manual of Diagnosis and Therapy*. Whitehouse Station, NJ: Merck Research Laboratories, 2004.

Beers, Mark H., MD, and Robert Berkow, MD., editors. "Schizophrenia and Related Disorders." In *The Merck Manual of Diagnosis and Therapy*. Whitehouse Station, NJ: Merck Research Laboratories, 2004.

KEY TERMS

Brief psychotic disorder—An acute, short-term episode of psychosis lasting no longer than one month. This disorder may occur in response to a stressful event.

Delirium—An acute but temporary disturbance of consciousness marked by confusion, difficulty paying attention, delusions, hallucinations, or restlessness. Delirium may be caused by drug intoxication, high fever related to infection, head trauma, brain tumors, kidney or liver failure, or various metabolic disturbances.

Delusional disorder—Individuals with delusional disorder suffer from long-term, complex delusions that fall into one of six categories: persecutory, grandiose, jealousy, erotomanic, somatic, or mixed.

Delusions—An unshakable belief in something untrue which cannot be explained by religious or cultural factors. These irrational beliefs defy normal reasoning and remain firm even when overwhelming proof is presented to refute them.

Hallucinations—False or distorted sensory experiences that appear to be real perceptions to the person experiencing them.

Paranoia—An unfounded or exaggerated distrust of others, sometimes reaching delusional proportions.

Porphyria—A disease of the metabolism characterized by skin lesions, urine problems, neurologic disorders, and/or abdominal pain.

Schizoaffective disorder—Schizophrenic symptoms occurring concurrently with a major depressive and/or manic episode.

Schizophrenia—A debilitating mental illness characterized by delusions, hallucinations, disorganized speech and behavior, and inappropriate or flattened affect (a lack of emotions) that seriously hampers the afflicted individual's social and occupational functioning. Approximately 2 million Americans suffer from schizophrenia.

Schizophreniform disorder—A short-term variation of schizophrenia that has a total duration of one to six months.

Shared psychotic disorder—Also known as *folie à deux*, shared psychotic disorder is an uncommon disorder in which the same delusion is shared by two or more individuals.

Tardive dyskinesia—Involuntary movements of the face and/or body which are a side effect of the long-term use of some older antipsychotic (neuroleptic) drugs. Tardive dyskinesia affects 15-20% of patients on long-term neuroleptic treatment.

PERIODICALS

Addington, A. M., M. Gornick, A. L. Sporn, et al. "Polymorphisms in the 13q33.2 Gene G72/G30 Are Associated with Childhood-Onset Schizophrenia and Psychosis Not Otherwise Specified." *Biological Psychiatry* 55 (May 15, 2004): 976–980.

Hutchinson, G., and C. Haasen. "Migration and Schizophrenia: The Challenges for European Psychiatry and Implications for the Future." *Social Psychiatry and Psychiatric Epidemiology* 39 (May 2004): 350–357.

Sharon, Idan, MD, and Roni Sharon. "Shared Psychotic Disorder." *eMedicine* June 4, 2004. < http://www.emedicine.com/med/topic3352.htm > .

Sim, M. G., E. Khong, and G. Hulse. "Cannabis and Psychosis." *Australian Family Physician* 33 (April 2004): 229–232.

Tolmac, J., and M. Hodes. "Ethnic Variation among Adolescent Psychiatric In-Patients with Psychotic Disorders." *British Journal of Psychiatry* 184 (May 2004): 428–431.

Verdoux, H., and M. Tournier. "Cannabis Use and Risk of Psychosis: An Etiological Link?" *Epidemiologia e psichiatria sociale* 13 (April-June 2004): 113–119.

Williams, N. M., and M. J. Owen. "Genetic Abnormalities of Chromosome 22 and the Development of Psychosis." *Current Psychiatry Reports* 6 (June 2004): 176–182.

ORGANIZATIONS

American Psychiatric Association. 1400 K Street NW, Washington DC 20005. (888) 357-7924. < http://www.psych.org >.

American Psychological Association (APA). 750 First St. NE, Washington, DC 20002-4242. (202) 336-5700. < http://www.apa.org > .

National Alliance for the Mentally Ill (NAMI). Colonial Place Three, 2107 Wilson Blvd., Ste. 300, Arlington, VA 22201-3042. (800) 950-6264. < http://www.nami.org >.

National Institute of Mental Health (NIMH). 6001 Executive Boulevard, Room 8184, MSC 9663, Bethesda, MD 20892-9663. (301) 443-4513. < http://www.nimh.nih.gov >.

OTHER

The Schizophrenia Page. < http://www.schizophrenia.com >.

Paula Anne Ford-Martin
Rebecca Frey, PhD

Psychosocial disorders

Definition

A psychosocial disorder is a mental illness caused or influenced by life experiences, as well as maladjusted cognitive and behavioral processes.

Description

The term psychosocial refers to the psychological and social factors that influence mental health. Social influences such as peer pressure, parental support, cultural and religious background, socioeconomic status, and interpersonal relationships all help to shape personality and influence psychological makeup. Individuals with psychosocial disorders frequently have difficulty functioning in social situations and may have problems effectively communicating with others.

In the American Psychiatric Association it distinguishes 16 different subtypes (or categories) of mental illness. Although psychosocial variables arguably have some degree of influence on all subtypes of mental illness, the major categories of mental disorders thought to involve significant psychosocial factors include:

- Substance-related disorders. Disorders related to alcohol and drug use, **abuse**, dependence, and withdrawal.

- **Schizophrenia** and other psychotic disorders. These include the schizoid disorders (schizophrenia, schizophreniform, and **schizoaffective disorder**), delusional disorder, and psychotic disorders.

- Mood disorders. Affective disorders such as depression (major, dysthymic) and bipolar disorders.

- **Anxiety** disorders. Disorders in which a certain situation or place triggers excessive fear and/or anxiety symptoms (i.e., **dizziness**, racing heart), such as **panic disorder**, **agoraphobia**, social phobia, **obsessive-compulsive disorder**, **post-traumatic stress disorder**, and generalized anxiety disorders.

- **Somatoform disorders**. Somatoform disorders involve clinically significant physical symptoms that cannot be explained by a medical condition (e.g., somatization disorder, conversion disorder, **pain** disorder, **hypochondriasis**, and body dysmorphic disorder).

- Factitious disorders. Disorders in which an individual creates and complains of symptoms of a nonexistent illness in order to assume the role of a patient (or sick role).

- Sexual and gender identity disorders. Disorders of sexual desire, arousal, and performance. It should be noted that the categorization of **gender identity disorder** as a mental illness has been a point of some contention among mental health professionals.

- Eating disorders. Anorexia and bulimia nervosa.

- **Adjustment disorders**. Adjustment disorders involve an excessive emotional or behavioral reaction to a stressful event.

- Personality disorders. Maladjustments of personality, including paranoid, schizoid, schizotypal, antisocial, borderline, histrionic, narcissistic, avoidant, dependent, and obsessive-compulsive personality disorder (not to be confused with the anxiety disorder OCD).

- Disorders usually first diagnosed in infancy childhood, or adolescence. Some learning and developmental disorders (i.e., **ADHD**) may be partially psychosocial in nature.

Causes and symptoms

It is important to note that the causes of mental illness are diverse and not completely understood. The majority of psychological disorders are thought to be caused by a complex combination of biological, genetic (hereditary), familial, and social factors or biopsychosocial influences. In addition, the role that each of these play can differ from person to person, so that a disorder such as depression that is caused by genetic factors in one person may be caused by a traumatic life event in another.

The symptoms of psychosocial disorders vary depending on the diagnosis in question. In addition to disorder-specific symptoms, individuals with psychosocial dysfunction usually have difficulty functioning normally in social situations and may have trouble forming and maintaining close interpersonal relationships.

Diagnosis

Patients with symptoms of psychosocial disorders or other mental illness should undergo a thorough **physical examination** and patient history to rule out an organic cause for the illness (such as a neurological disorder). If no organic cause is suspected, a psychologist or other mental healthcare professional will meet with the patient to conduct an interview and take a detailed social and medical history. If the patient is a minor, interviews with a parent or guardian may also be part of the diagnostic process. The physician may also administer one or more **psychological tests** (also called clinical inventories, scales, or assessments).

Treatment

Counseling is typically a front-line treatment for psychosocial disorders. A number of counseling or talk therapy approaches exist, including psychotherapy, cognitive therapy, behavioral therapy, and **group therapy**. Therapy or counseling may be administered by social workers, nurses, licensed counselors and therapists, psychologists, or psychiatrists.

Psychoactive medication may also be prescribed for symptom relief in patients with mental disorders considered psychosocial in nature. For disorders such as major depression or **bipolar disorder**, which may have psychosocial aspects but also have known organic causes, drug therapy is a primary treatment approach. In cases such as personality disorder that are thought to not have biological roots, psychoactive medications are usually considered a secondary, or companion treatment to psychotherapy.

Many individuals are successful in treating psychosocial disorders through regular attendance in self-help groups or 12-step programs such as Alcoholics Anonymous. This approach, which allows individuals to seek advice and counsel from others in similar circumstances, can be extremely effective.

In some cases, treating mental illness requires hospitalization of the patient. This hospitalization, also known as inpatient treatment, is usually employed in situations where a controlled therapeutic environment is critical for the patient's recovery (e.g., **rehabilitation** treatment for **alcoholism** or other drug addictions), or when there is a risk that the patient may harm himself (**suicide**) or others. It may also be necessary when the patient's physical health has deteriorated to a point where life-sustaining treatment is necessary, such as with severe **malnutrition** associated with **anorexia nervosa**.

KEY TERMS

Affective disorder—An emotional disorder involving abnormal highs and/or lows in mood.

Bipolar disorder—An affective mental illness that causes radical emotional changes and mood swings, from manic highs to depressive lows. The majority of bipolar individuals experience alternating episodes of mania and depression.

Bulimia—An eating disorder characterized by binge eating and inappropriate compensatory behavior such as vomiting, misusing laxatives, or excessive exercise.

Cognitive processes—Thought processes (i.e., reasoning, perception, judgment, memory).

Learning disorders—Academic difficulties experienced by children and adults of average to above-average intelligence that involve reading, writing, and/or mathematics, and which significantly interfere with academic achievement or daily living.

Schizophrenia—A debilitating mental illness characterized by delusions, hallucinations, disorganized speech and behavior, and flattened affect (i.e., a lack of emotions) that seriously hampers normal functioning.

Alternative treatment

Therapeutic approaches such as **art therapy** that encourage self-discovery and empowerment may be useful in treating psychosocial disorders. Art therapy, the use of the creative process to express and understand emotion, encompasses a broad range of humanistic disciplines, including visual arts, dance, drama, music, film, writing, literature, and other artistic genres. This use of the creative process is believed to provide the patient/artist with a means to gain insight to emotions and thoughts they might otherwise have difficulty expressing. After the artwork is created, the patient/artist continues the therapeutic journey by interpreting its meaning under the guidance of a trained therapist.

Prognosis

According to the National Institute of Mental Health, more than 90% of Americans who commit suicide have a diagnosable mental disorder, so swift and appropriate treatment is important. Because of the diversity of types of mental disorders influenced by psychosocial factors, and the complexity of diagnosis and treatment, the prognosis for psychosocial disorders is highly variable. In some cases, they can be effectively managed with therapy and/or medication. In others, mental illness can cause long-term disability.

Prevention

Patient education (i.e., therapy or self-help groups) can encourage patients to take an active part in their treatment program and to recognize symptoms of a relapse of their condition. In addition, educating friends and family members on the nature of the psychosocial disorder can assist them in knowing how and when to provide support to the patient.

Resources

PERIODICALS

Epperly, Ted D., and Kevin E. Moore. "Health Issues in Men: Part II. Common Psychosocial Disorders." *American Family Physician* 62 (July 2000): 117-24.

ORGANIZATIONS

National Institute of Mental Health. 6001 Executive Boulevard, Rm. 8184, MSC 9663, Bethesda, MD 20892-9663. (301) 443-4513.

OTHER

Satcher, David. *Mental Health: A Report of the Surgeon General.* Washington, DC: Government Printing Office, 1999.

Paula Anne Ford-Martin

Psychosurgery

Definition

Psychosurgery involves severing or otherwise disabling areas of the brain to treat a personality disorder, behavior disorder, or other mental illness. Modern psychosurgical techniques target the pathways between the limbic system (the portion of the brain on the inner edge of the cerebral cortex) that is believed to regulate emotions, and the frontal cortex, where thought processes are seated.

Purpose

Lobotomy is a psychosurgical procedure involving selective destruction of connective nerve fibers or tissue. It is performed on the frontal lobe of the brain and its purpose is to alleviate mental illness and chronic **pain** symptoms. The bilateral cingulotomy, a modern psychosurgical technique which has replaced the lobotomy, is performed to alleviate mental disorders such as major depression, bipolar disorder, or **obsessive-compulsive disorder** (OCD), which have not responded to psychotherapy, behavioral therapy, electroshock, or pharmacologic treatment. Bilateral cingulotomies are also performed to treat chronic pain in **cancer** patients.

Precautions

Psychosurgery should be considered only after all other non-surgical psychiatric therapies have been fully explored. Much is still unknown about the biology of the brain and how psychosurgery affects brain function.

Description

Psychosurgery, and lobotomy in particular, reached the height of use just after World War II. Between 1946 and 1949, the use of the lobotomy grew from 500 to 5,000 annual procedures in the United States. At that time, the procedure was viewed as a possible solution to the overcrowded and understaffed conditions in state-run mental hospitals and asylums. Known as prefrontal or transorbital lobotomy, depending on the surgical technique used and area of the brain targeted, these early operations were performed with surgical knives, electrodes, suction, or ice picks, to cut or sweep out portions of the frontal lobe.

Today's psychosurgical techniques are much more refined. Instead of going in "blind" to remove large sections on the frontal lobe, as in these early operations, neurosurgeons use a computer-based process called stereotactic magnetic resonance imaging to guide a small electrode to the limbic system (brain structures involved in autonomic or automatic body functions and some emotion and behavior). There an electrical current **burns** in a small lesion [usually 0.5 in (1.3 cm) in size]. In a bilateral cingulotomy, the cingulate gyrus, a small section of brain that connects the limbic region of the brain with the frontal lobes, is targeted. Another surgical technique uses a non-invasive tool known as a gamma knife to focus beams of radiation at the brain. A lesion forms at the spot where the beams converge in the brain.

Preparation

Candidates for cingulotomies or other forms of psychosurgery undergo a rigorous screening process

KEY TERMS

Gamma knife—A surgical tool that focuses beams of radiation at the head, which converge in the brain to form a lesion.

Lesion—Any discontinuity of tissue. Often a cut or wound.

Limbic system—A portion of the brain on the inner edge of the cerebral cortex that is thought to regulate emotions.

Psychosurgery—Brain surgery performed to alleviate chronic psychological conditions such as obsessive-compulsive disorder (OCD), depression, and bipolar disorder.

Stereotactic technique—A technique used by neurosurgeons to pinpoint locations within the brain. It employs computer imaging to create an external frame of reference.

Resources

ORGANIZATIONS

Massachusetts General Hospital. Functional and Stereotactic Neurosurgery Cingulotomy Unit. Fruit St., Boston, MA 02114. (617) 726-2000. < http://neurosurgery.mgh.harvard.edu/cingulot.htm >.

National Alliance for the Mentally Ill (NAMI). Colonial Place Three, 2107 Wilson Blvd., Ste. 300, Arlington, VA 22201-3042. (800) 950-6264. < http://www.nami.org >.

National OCD Headquarters. P.O. Box 70, Milford, CT 06460. (203) 878-5669.

Paula Anne Ford-Martin

Psyllium preparations *see* **Laxatives**

PT *see* **Prothrombin time**

Pterygium *see* **Pinguecula and pterygium**

Ptomaine poisoning *see* **Food poisoning**

to ensure that all possible non-surgical psychiatric treatment options have been explored. Psychosurgery is only performed with the patient's informed consent.

Aftercare

Ongoing behavioral and medication therapy is often required in OCD patients who undergo cingulotomy. All psychosurgery patients should remain under a psychiatrist's care for follow-up evaluations and treatment.

Risks

As with any type of brain surgery, psychosurgery carries the risk of permanent brain damage, though the advent of non-invasive neurosurgical techniques, such as the gamma knife, has reduced the risk of brain damage significantly.

Normal results

In a 1996 study at Massachusetts General Hospital, over one-third of patients undergoing cingulotomy demonstrated significant improvements after the surgery. And, in contrast to the bizarre behavior and personality changes reported with lobotomy patients in the 1940s and 1950s, modern psychosurgery patients have demonstrated little post-surgical losses of memory or other high level thought processes.

Ptosis

Definition

Ptosis is the term used for a drooping upper eyelid. Ptosis, also called blepharoptosis, can affect one or both eyes.

Description

The eyelids serve to protect and lubricate the outer eye. The upper eyelid is lifted by a muscle called the levator muscle. Inside the back part of the lid is a tarsal plate which adds rigidity to the lid. The levator muscle is attached to the tarsal plate by a flat tendon called the levator aponeurosis. When the muscle cannot lift the eyelid or lifts it only partially, the person is said to have a ptosis.

There are two types of ptosis, acquired and congenital. Acquired ptosis is more common. Congenital ptosis is present at birth. Both congenital and acquired ptosis can be, but are not necessarily, hereditary.

Causes and symptoms

Ptosis may occur because the levator muscle's attachment to the lid is weakening with age. Acquired ptosis can also be caused by a number of different things, such as disease that impairs the nerves, diabetes, injury, tumors, inflammation, or

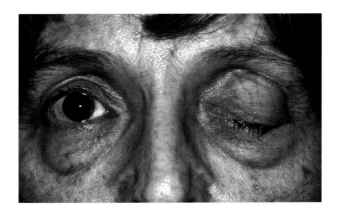

A close-up view of a drooping upper eyelid (ptosis) on an elderly woman's face. Ptosis is normally due to a weakness of the levator muscle of the upper eyelid or to interference with the nerve supply to the muscle. *(Photograph by Dr. P. Marazzi, Photo Researchers, Inc. Reproduced by permission.)*

aneurysms. Congenital ptosis may be caused by a problem with nerve innervation or a weak muscle. Drooping eyelids may also be the result of diseases such as **myotonic dystrophy** or **myasthenia gravis**.

The primary symptom of ptosis is a drooping eyelid. Adults will notice a loss of visual field because the upper portion of the eye is covered. Children who are born with a ptosis usually tilt their head back in an effort to see under the obstruction. Some people raise their eyebrows in order to lift the lid slightly and therefore may appear to be frowning.

Diagnosis

Diagnosis of ptosis is usually made by observing the drooping eyelid. Finding the cause of the condition will require testing for any of the illnesses or injuries known to have this effect. Some possible tests include x rays and blood tests.

Treatment

Ptosis is usually treated surgically. Surgery can generally be done on an outpatient basis under local anesthetic. For minor drooping, a small amount of the eyelid tissue can be removed. For more pronounced ptosis the approach is to surgically shorten the levator muscle or connect the lid to the muscles of the eyebrow. Or, the aponeurosis can be reattached to the tarsal plate if it has separated. Correcting the ptosis is usually done only after determining the cause of the condition. For example, myasthenia gravis must be ruled out before performing any surgery. As with any surgery, there are risks, and they should be discussed with the surgeon.

Children with ptosis need not have surgery immediately, however their vision must be checked periodically to prevent lazy eye (**amblyopia**).

"Ptosis crutches" are also available. These can be attached to the frame of eyeglasses to hold up the eyelid. These devices are uncomfortable and usually not well tolerated.

Prognosis

After diagnosing the cause of a drooping eyelid, then correcting the condition, most people have no further problems related to the ptosis. The correction, however, may still not make the eyes symmetrical. Patients should have reasonable expectations and discuss the outcome with their doctor prior to surgery.

Prevention

Ptosis cannot be prevented.

Resources

ORGANIZATIONS

American Academy of Ophthalmology. 655 Beach Street, P.O. Box 7424, San Francisco, CA 94120-7424. < http://www.eyenet.org >.

American Medical Association. 515 N. State St., Chicago, IL 60612. (312) 464-5000. < http://www.ama-assn.org >.

American Optometric Association. 243 North Lindbergh Blvd., St. Louis, MO 63141. (314) 991-4100. < http://www.aoanet.org >.

U.S. Department of Health and Human Services. 200 Independence Ave., SW, Washington, DC 20201, (202) 619-0257

Dorothy Elinor Stonely

PTSD *see* **Post-traumatic stress disorder**

PTT *see* **Partial thromboplastin time**

Puberty

Definition

Puberty is the period of human development during which physical growth and sexual maturation occurs.

Description

Beginning as early as age eight in girls–and two years later, on average, in boys–the hypothalamus (part of the brain) signals hormonal change that stimulates the pituitary. In turn, the pituitary releases its own hormones called gonadotrophins that stimulate the gonads and adrenals. From these glands come a flood of sex hormones–androgens and testosterone in the male, estrogens and progestins in the female–that regulate the growth and function of the sex organs. It is interesting to note that the gonadotrophins are the same for males and females, but the sex hormones they induce are different.

In the United States, the first sign of puberty occurs on average at age 11 in girls, with menstruation and fertility following about two years later. Boys lag behind by about two years. Puberty may not begin until age 16 in boys and continue in a desultory fashion on past age 20. In contrast to puberty, adolescence is more of a social/cultural term referring to the interval between childhood and adulthood.

Diagnosis

Puberty has been divided into five Sexual Maturity Rating (SMR) stages by two doctors, W. Marshall and J. M. Tanner. These ratings are often referred to as Tanner Stages 1–5. Staging is based on pubic hair growth, on male genital development, and female breast development. Staging helps determine whether development is normal for a given age. Both sexes also grow axillary (arm pit) hair and pimples. Males develop muscle mass, a deeper voice, and facial hair. Females redistribute body fat. Along with the maturing of the sex organs, there is a pronounced growth spurt averaging 3–4 in (8–10 cm) and culminating in full adult stature. Puberty can be precocious (early) or delayed. It all depends upon the sex hormones.

Puberty falling outside the age limits considered normal for any given population should prompt a search for the cause. As health and **nutrition** have improved over the past few generations, there has been a gradual decrease in the average age for the normal onset of puberty.

- Excess hormone stimulation is the cause for precocious puberty. It can come from the brain in the form of gonadotrophins or from the gonads and adrenals. Overproduction may be caused by functioning tumors or simple overactivity. Brain overproduction can also be the result of brain infections or injury.

- Likewise, delayed puberty is due to insufficient hormone. If the pituitary output is inadequate, so will be the output from the gonads and adrenals. On the other hand, a normal pituitary will overproduce if it senses there are not enough hormones in the circulation.

- There are several congenital disorders (polyglandular deficiency syndromes) that include failure of hormone output. These children do not experience normal puberty, but it may be induced by giving them the proper hormones at the proper time.

- Finally, there are in females abnormalities in hormone production that produce male characteristics–so called virilizing syndromes. Should one of these appear during adolescence, it will disturb the normal progress of puberty. Notice that virilizing requires abnormal hormones in the female, while feminizing results from absent hormones in the male. Each embryo starts out life as female. Male hormones transform it if they are present.

Delayed or **precocious puberty** requires measurement of the several hormones involved to determine which are lacking or which are in excess. There are blood tests for each one. If a tumor is suspected, imaging of the suspect organ needs to be done with x rays, **computed tomography scans** (CT scans), or magnetic resonance imaging (MRI).

Treatment

Puberty is a period of great **stress**, both physically and emotionally. The psychological changes and challenges of puberty are made infinitely greater if its timing is off.

In precocious puberty, the offending gland or tumor may require surgical attention, although there are several drugs now that counteract hormone effects. If delayed, puberty can be stimulated with the correct hormones. Treatment should not be delayed because necessary bone growth is also affected.

Prognosis

Properly administered hormones can restore the normal growth pattern.

KEY TERMS

Adrenals—Glands on top of the kidneys that produce four different types of hormones.

Computed tomography scan (CT)—A method of creating images of internal organs using x rays.

Embryo—The life in the womb during the first two months.

Hormone—A chemical produced in one place that has an effect somewhere else in the body.

Hypothalamus—Part of the brain located deep in the center of the skull and just above the pituitary.

Gonads—Glands that make sex hormones and reproductive cells–testes in the male, ovaries in the female.

Magnetic resonance imaging (MRI)—A method of creating images of internal organs. Magnetic resonance imaging (MRI) uses magnet fields and radio-frequency signals.

Pituitary—The "master gland" of the body, controlling many of the others by releasing stimulating hormones.

Syndrome—A collection of abnormalities that occur often enough to suggest they have a common cause.

Resources

BOOKS

Fauci, Anthony S., et al., editors. *Harrison's Principles of Internal Medicine.* New York: McGraw-Hill, 1997.

J. Ricker Polsdorfer, MD

Pubic lice *see* **Lice infestation**

Puerperal infection

Definition

The term puerperal infection refers to a bacterial infection following **childbirth**. The infection may also be referred to as puerperal or postpartum fever. The genital tract, particularly the uterus, is the most commonly infected site. In some cases infection can spread to other points in the body. Widespread infection, or **sepsis**, is a rare, but potentially fatal complication.

Description

Puerperal infection affects an estimated 1–8% of new mothers in the United States. Given modern medical treatment and **antibiotics**, it very rarely advances to the point of threatening a woman's life. An estimated 2–4% of new mothers who deliver vaginally suffer some form of puerperal infection, but for cesarean sections, the figure is five-10 times that high.

Deaths related to puerperal infection are very rare in the industrialized world. It is estimated three in 100,000 births result in maternal **death** due to infection. However, the death rate in developing nations may be 100 times higher.

Postpartum **fever** may arise from several causes, not necessarily infection. If the fever is related to infection, it often results from endometritis, an inflammation of the uterus. Urinary tract, breast, and wound infections are also possible, as well as septic **thrombophlebitis**, a blood clot-associated inflammation of veins. A woman's susceptibility to developing an infection is related to such factors as cesarean section, extended labor, **obesity**, anemia, and poor prenatal **nutrition**.

Causes and symptoms

The primary symptom of puerperal infection is a fever at any point between birth and 10 days postpartum. A temperature of 100.4°F (38°C) on any two days during this period, or a fever of 101.6°F (38.6 °C) in the first 24 hours postpartum, is cause for suspicion. An assortment of bacterial species may cause puerperal infection. Many of these bacteria are normally found in the mother's genital tract, but other bacteria may be introduced from the woman's intestine and skin or from a healthcare provider.

The associated symptoms depend on the site and nature of the infection. The most typical site of infection is the genital tract. Endometritis, which affects the uterus, is the most prominent of these infections. Endometritis is much more common if a small part of the placenta has been retained in the uterus. Typically, several species of bacteria are involved and may act synergistically–that is, the bacteria's negative effects are multiplied rather than simply added together. Synergistic action by the bacteria can result in a stubborn infection such as an **abscess**. The major symptoms of a genital tract infection include fever, malaise, abdominal **pain**, uterine tenderness, and abnormal vaginal discharge. If these symptoms do not respond to antibiotic therapy, an abscess or blood clot may be suspected.

Other causes of postpartum fever include urinary tract infections, wound infections, septic thrombophlebitis, and **mastitis**. Mastitis, or breast infection, is indicated by fever, malaise, achy muscles, and reddened skin on the affected breast. It is usually caused by a clogged milk duct that becomes infected. Infections of the urinary tract are indicated by fever, frequent and painful urination, and back pain. An **episiotomy** and a **cesarean section** carry the risk of a wound infection. Such infections are suggested by a fever and pus-like discharge, inflammation, and swelling at wound sites.

Diagnosis

Fever is not an automatic indicator of puerperal infection. A new mother may have a fever owing to prior illness or an illness unconnected to childbirth. However, any fever within 10 days postpartum is aggressively investigated. Physical symptoms such as pain, malaise, loss of appetite, and others point to infection.

Many doctors initiate antibiotic therapy early in the fever period to stop an infection before it advances. A pelvic examination is done and samples are taken from the genital tract to identify the bacteria involved in the infection. The pelvic examination can reveal the extent of infection and possibly the cause. Blood samples may also be taken for blood counts and to test for the presence of infectious bacteria. A **urinalysis** may also be ordered, especially if the symptoms are indicative of a urinary tract infection.

If the fever and other symptoms resist antibiotic therapy, an ultrasound examination or computed tomography scan (CT scan) is done to locate potential abscesses or **blood clots** in the pelvic region. **Magnetic resonance imaging** (MRI) may be useful as well, in addition to a heparin challenge test if blood clots are suspected. If a lung infection is suspected, a **chest x ray** may also be ordered.

Treatment

Antibiotic therapy is the backbone of puerperal infection treatment. Initial antibiotic therapy may consist of clindamycin and gentamicin, which fight a broad array of bacteria types. If the fever and other symptoms do not respond to these antibiotics, a third, such as ampicillin, is added. Other antibiotics may be used depending on the identity of the infective bacteria and the possibility of an allergic reaction to certain antibiotics.

Antibiotics taken together are effective against a wide range of bacteria, but may not be capable of clearing up the infection alone, especially if an abscess

---

KEY TERMS

Abscess—A pus-filled area with definite borders.

Blood clot—A dense mat formed by certain components of the blood stream to prevent blood loss.

Cesarean section—Incision through the abdomen and uterus to facilitate delivery.

Computed tomography scan (CT scan)—Cross-sectional x rays of the body are compiled to create a three-dimensional image of the body's internal structures.

Episiotomy—Incision of the vulva (external female genitalia) during vaginal delivery to prevent tissue tearing.

Heparin—A blood component that controls the amount of clotting. It can be used as a drug to reduce blood clot formation.

Heparin challenge test—A medical test to evaluate how readily the blood clots.

Magnetic resonance imaging (MRI)—An imaging technique that uses a large circular magnet and radio waves to generate signals from atoms in the body. These signals are used to construct images of internal structures.

Postpartum—Referring to the time period following childbirth.

Prophylactic—Measures taken to prevent disease.

Sepsis—The presence of viable bacteria in the blood or body tissues.

Septic—Referring to the presence of infection.

Thrombophlebitis—An inflammation of veins accompanied by the formation of blood clots.

Ultrasound examination—A medical test in which high frequency sound waves are directed at a particular internal area of the body. As the sound waves are reflected by internal structures, a computer uses the data to construct an image of the structures.

Warfarin—A drug that reduces the ability of the blood to clot.

---

or blood clot is present. Heparin is combined with the antibiotic therapy in order to break apart blood clots. Heparin is used for five-seven days, and may be followed by warfarin for the following month. If the infection is complicated, it may be necessary to surgically drain the infected site. Infected episiotomies can be opened and allowed to drain, but abscesses and blood clots may require surgery.

Prognosis

Antibiotic therapy and other treatment measures are virtually always successful in curing puerperal infections.

Prevention

Careful attention to antiseptic procedures during childbirth is the basic underpinning of preventing infection. With some procedures, such as cesarean section, a doctor may administer prophylactic antibiotics as a preemptive strike against infectious bacteria.

Resources

PERIODICALS

Hamadeh, Ghassan, Cindy Dedmon, and Paul D. Mozley. "Postpartum Fever." *American Family Physician* 52, no. 2 (August 1995): 531.

Julia Barrett

Pulmonary alveolar proteinosis

Definition

Pulmonary alveolar proteinosis (PAP) is a rare disease of the lungs.

Description

In this disease, also called alveolar proteinosis or phospholipidosis, gas exchange in the lungs is progressively impaired by the accumulation of phospholipids, compounds widely found in other living cells of the body. The alveoli are filled with this substance that renders them less effective in protecting the lung. This may explain why infections are often associated with the disease.

Pulmonary alveolar proteinosis most commonly affects people ages 20–50, although it has been reported in children and the elderly. The incidence is 5 out of every 1 million people. The disease is more common among males.

Causes and symptoms

The cause of this disease is unknown. In some people, however, it appears to result from infection,

immune deficiency, or from exposure to silica, aluminum oxide, and a variety of dusts and fumes.

Symptoms include mild **shortness of breath** associated with a nonproductive or minimally productive **cough**, weight loss, and **fatigue**. Acute symptoms such as **fever** or progressive shortness of breath suggest a complicating infection.

Diagnosis

Physical examination may reveal clubbing of the fingers or a bluish coloration of the skin as a result of decreased oxygen.

A **chest x ray** may show alveolar disease. An arterial blood gas reveals low oxygen levels in the blood. **Bronchoscopy** with transtracheal biopsy shows alveolar proteinosis. Specific diagnosis requires a **lung biopsy**.

Treatment

Treatment consists of periodic whole-lung lavage, a washing out of the phospholipids from the lung with a special tube placed in the trachea. This is performed under **general anesthesia**.

Prognosis

In some, spontaneous remission occurs, while in others progressive **respiratory failure** develops. Disability from respiratory insufficiency is common, but **death** rarely occurs. Repeated lavage may be necessary. Lung transplant is a last resort option.

Prevention

There is no known prevention for this very rare disorder.

Resources

ORGANIZATIONS

American Association for Respiratory Care. 11030 Ables Lane, Dallas, Texas 75229. (972) 243-2272. <http://www.aarc.org>.

American Lung Association. 1740 Broadway, New York, NY 10019. (800) 586-4872. <http://www.lungusa.org>.

Lorraine Steefel, RN

Pulmonary artery catheterization

Definition

Pulmonary artery catheterization is a diagnostic procedure in which a small catheter is inserted through a neck, arm, chest, or thigh vein and maneuvered into the right side of the heart, in order to measure pressures at different spots in the heart.

Purpose

Pulmonary artery catheterization is performed to:
- evaluate **heart failure**
- monitor therapy after a **heart attack**
- check the fluid balance of a patient with serious burns, kidney disease, or after heart surgery
- check the effect of medications on the heart

Precautions

Pulmonary artery catheterization is a potentially complicated and invasive procedure. The doctor must decide if the value of the information obtained will outweigh the risk of catheterization.

Description

Pulmonary artery catheterization, sometimes called Swan-Ganz catheterization, is usually performed at the bedside of a patient in the intensive care unit. A catheter is threaded through a vein in the arm, thigh, chest, or neck until it passes through the right side of the heart. This procedure takes about 30 minutes. **Local anesthesia** is given to reduce discomfort.

Once the catheter is in place, the doctor briefly inflates a tiny balloon at its end. This temporarily blocks the blood flow and allows the doctor to make a pressure measurement in the pulmonary artery system. Pressure measurements are usually recorded for the next 48–72 hours in different parts of the heart. During this time, the patient must stay in bed so the catheter stays in place. Once the pressure measurements are no longer needed, the catheter is removed.

Preparation

Before and during the test, the patient will be connected to an electrocardiograph, which makes a recording of the electrical stimuli that cause the heart to contract. The insertion site is sterilized and prepared. The catheter is often sutured to the skin to prevent dislodgment.

Aftercare

The patient is observed for any sign of infection or complications from the procedure.

Risks

Pulmonary artery catheterization is not without risks. Possible complications from the procedure include:
- infection at the site where the catheter was inserted
- pulmonary artery perforation
- blood clots in the lungs
- irregular heartbeat

Normal results

Normal pressures reflect a normally functioning heart with no fluid accumulation. These normal pressure readings are:
- right atrium: 1–6 mm of mercury (mm Hg)
- right ventricle during contraction (systolic): 20–30 mm Hg
- right ventricle at the end of relaxation (end diastolic): less than 5 mm Hg

- pulmonary artery during contraction (systolic): 20–30 mm Hg
- pulmonary artery during relaxation (diastolic): about 10 mm Hg
- mean pulmonary artery: less than 20 mm Hg
- pulmonary artery wedge pressure: 6–12 mm Hg
- left atrium: about 10 mm Hg

Abnormal results

Abnormally high right atrium pressure can indicate:

- pulmonary disease
- right side heart failure
- fluid accumulation
- compression of the heart after hemorrhage (cardiac tamponade)
- right heart valve abnormalities
- pulmonary **hypertension** (high blood pressure)

Abnormally high right ventricle pressure may indicate:

- pulmonary hypertension (high blood pressure)
- pulmonary valve abnormalities
- right ventricle failure
- defects in the wall between the right and left ventricle
- congestive heart failure
- serious heart inflammation

Abnormally high pulmonary artery pressure may indicate:

- diversion of blood from a left-to-right cardiac shunt
- pulmonary artery hypertension
- chronic obstructive pulmonary disease or emphysema
- blood clots in the lungs
- fluid accumulation in the lungs
- left ventricle failure

Abnormally high pulmonary artery wedge pressure may indicate:

- left ventricle failure
- mitral valve abnormalities
- cardiac insufficiency
- compression of the heart after hemorrhage

Resources

BOOKS

"Pulmonary Artery Catheterization." In *The Patient's Guide to Medical Tests*, ed. Barry L. Zaret, et al., Boston: Houghton Mifflin, 1997.

Tish Davidson, A.M.

Pulmonary edema

Definition

Pulmonary **edema** is a condition in which fluid accumulates in the lungs, usually because the heart's left ventricle does not pump adequately.

Description

The build-up of fluid in the spaces outside the blood vessels of the lungs is called pulmonary edema. Pulmonary edema is a common complication of heart disorders, and most cases of the condition are associated with **heart failure**. Pulmonary edema can be a chronic condition, or it can develop suddenly and quickly become life threatening. The life-threatening type of pulmonary edema occurs when a large amount of fluid suddenly shifts from the pulmonary blood vessels into the lung, due to lung problems, **heart attack**, trauma, or toxic chemicals. It can also be the first sign of coronary heart disease.

In heart-related pulmonary edema, the heart's main chamber, the left ventricle, is weakened and does not function properly. The ventricle does not completely eject its contents, causing blood to back up and cardiac output to drop. The body responds by increasing blood pressure and fluid volume to compensate for the reduced cardiac output. This, in turn, increases the force against which the ventricle must expel blood. Blood backs up, forming a pool in the pulmonary blood vessels. Fluid leaks into the spaces between the tissues of the lungs and begins to accumulate. This process makes it more difficult for the lungs to expand. It also impedes the exchange of air and gases between the lungs and blood moving through lung blood vessels.

Causes and symptoms

Most cases of pulmonary edema are caused by failure of the heart's main chamber, the left ventricle. It can be brought on by an acute heart attack, severe **ischemia**, volume overload of the heart's left ventricle, and mitral stenosis. Non-heart-related pulmonary edema is caused by lung problems like **pneumonia**, an excess of intravenous fluids, some types of **kidney disease**, bad **burns**, **liver disease**, nutritional problems, and **Hodgkin's disease**. Non-heart-related pulmonary edema can also be caused by other conditions where the lungs do not drain properly, and conditions where the respiratory veins are blocked.

Early symptoms of pulmonary edema include:

- shortness of breath upon exertion
- sudden respiratory distress after sleep
- difficulty breathing, except when sitting upright
- coughing

In cases of severe pulmonary edema, these symptoms will worsen to:

- labored and rapid breathing
- frothy, bloody fluid containing pus coughed from the lungs (sputum)
- a fast pulse and possibly serious disturbances in the heart's rhythm (atrial fibrillation, for example)
- cold, clammy, sweaty, and bluish skin
- a drop in blood pressure resulting in a thready pulse

Diagnosis

A doctor can usually diagnose pulmonary edema based on the patient's symptoms and a physical exam. Patients with pulmonary edema will have a rapid pulse, rapid breathing, abnormal breath and heart sounds, and enlarged neck veins. A **chest x ray** is often used to confirm the diagnosis. Arterial blood gas testing may be done. Sometimes **pulmonary artery catheterization** is performed to confirm that the patient has pulmonary edema and not a disease with similar symptoms (called **adult respiratory distress syndrome** or "noncardiogenic pulmonary edema").

Treatment

Pulmonary edema requires immediate emergency treatment. Treatment includes: placing the patient in a sitting position, oxygen, assisted or mechanical ventilation (in some cases), and drug therapy. The goal of treatment is to reduce the amount of fluid in the lungs,

KEY TERMS

Edema—Swelling caused by accumulation of fluid in body tissues.

Ischemia—A condition in which the heart muscle receives an insufficient supply of blood and slowly starves.

Left ventricle—The large chamber on the lower left side of the heart. The left ventricle sends blood to the aorta and the rest of the body.

Mitral stenosis—Narrowing or constricting of the mitral valve, which separates the left atrium from the left ventricle.

Pulmonary—Referring to the lungs and respiratory system.

improve gas exchange and heart function, and, where possible, to correct the underlying disease.

To help the patient breathe better, he/she is placed in a sitting position. High concentrations of oxygen are administered. In cases where respiratory distress is severe, a mechanical ventilator and a tube down the throat (tracheal intubation) will be used to improve the delivery of oxygen. Non-invasive pressure support ventilation is a new treatment for pulmonary edema in which the patient breathes against a continuous flow of positive airway pressure, delivered through a face or nasal mask. Non-invasive pressure support ventilation decreases the effort required to breath, enhances oxygen and carbon dioxide exchange, and increases cardiac output.

Drug therapy could include morphine, nitroglycerin, **diuretics**, angiotensin-converting enzyme (ACE) inhibitors, and **vasodilators**. Vasopressors are used for cardiogenic **shock**. Morphine is very effective in reducing the patient's **anxiety**, easing breathing, and improving blood flow. Nitroglycerin reduces pulmonary blood flow and decreases the volume of fluid entering the overloaded blood vessels. Diuretics, like furosemide (Lasix), promote the elimination of fluids through urination, helping to reduce pressure and fluids in the blood vessels. ACE inhibitors reduce the pressure against which the left ventricle must expel blood. In patients who have severe **hypertension**, a vasodilator such as nitroprusside sodium (Nipride) may be used. For cardiogenic shock, an adrenergic agent (like dopamine hydrochloride [Intropin], dobutamine hydrochloride [Dobutrex], or epinephrine) or a bipyridine (like amrinone lactate [Inocor] or milrinone lactate [Primacor]) are given.

Prognosis

Most patients with pulmonary edema who seek immediate treatment can be treated quickly and effectively.

Prevention

Cardiogenic pulmonary edema can sometimes be prevented by treating the underlying heart disease. These treatments, can including maintaining a healthy diet, taking appropriate medications correctly, and avoiding excess alcohol and salt.

Resources

PERIODICALS

Sacchetti, Alfred D., and Russel H. Harris. "Acute Cardiogenic Pulmonary Edema: What's the Latest in Emergency Treatment?" *Postgraduate Medicine* 103, no. 2 (February 1998): 145-166.

Lori De Milto

Pulmonary embolism

Definition

Pulmonary **embolism** is an obstruction of a blood vessel in the lungs, usually due to a blood clot, which blocks a coronary artery.

Description

Pulmonary embolism is a fairly common condition that can be fatal. According to the American Heart Association, an estimated 600,000 Americans develop pulmonary embolism annually; 60,000 die from it. As many as 25,000 Americans are hospitalized each year for pulmonary embolism, which is a relatively common complication in hospitalized patients. Even without warning symptoms, pulmonary embolism can cause sudden **death**. Treatment is not always successful.

Pulmonary embolism is difficult to diagnose. Less than 10% of patients who die from pulmonary embolism were diagnosed with the condition. It occurs when emboli block a pulmonary artery, usually due to a blood clot that breaks off from a large vein and travels to the lungs. More than 90% of cases of pulmonary embolism are complications of deep vein thrombosis, **blood clots** from the leg or pelvic veins. Emboli can

also be comprised of fat, air, or tumor tissue. When emboli block the main pulmonary artery, pulmonary embolism can quickly become fatal.

Causes and symptoms

Pulmonary embolism is caused by emboli that travel through the blood stream to the lungs and block a pulmonary artery. When this occurs, circulation and oxygenation of blood is compromised. The emboli are usually formed from blood clots but are occasionally comprised of air, fat, or tumor tissue. Risk factors include: prolonged bed rest, surgery, **childbirth**, **heart attack**, **stroke**, congestive **heart failure**, **cancer**, **obesity**, a broken hip or leg, **oral contraceptives**, sickle cell anemia, congenital **coagulation disorders**, chest trauma, certain congenital heart defects, and old age.

Common symptoms of pulmonary embolism include:

- labored breathing, sometimes accompanied by chest pain.
- a rapid pulse.
- a **cough** that produces bloody sputum.
- a low **fever**.
- fluid build-up in the lungs.

  Less common symptoms include:
- coughing up a lot of blood
- pain caused by movement
- leg swelling
- bluish skin
- fainting
- swollen neck veins

In some cases there are no symptoms.

Diagnosis

Pulmonary embolism can be diagnosed through the patient's history, a physical exam, and diagnostic tests including **chest x ray**, lung scan, pulmonary angiography, electrocardiography, arterial blood gas measurements, and leg vein ultrasonography or **venography**.

A chest x ray can be normal or show fluid or other signs and rule out other diseases. The lung scan shows poor flow of blood in areas beyond blocked arteries. The patient inhales a small amount of radiopharmaceutical and pictures of airflow into the lungs are taken with a gamma camera. Then a different

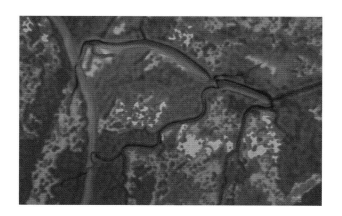

An angiography of a pulmonary embolism. *(Custom Medical Stock Photo. Reproduced by permission.)*

radiopharmaceutical is injected into an arm vein and lung blood flow is scanned. A normal result essentially rules out pulmonary embolism. A lung scan can be performed in a hospital or an outpatient facility and takes about 45 minutes.

Pulmonary **angiography** is the most reliable test for diagnosing pulmonary embolism but it is not used often, because it carries some risk and is expensive, invasive, and not readily available in many hospitals. Pulmonary angiography is a radiographic test which involves injection of a pharmaceutical "contrast agent" to show up the pulmonary arteries. A cinematic camera records the blood flow through the lungs of the patient, who lies on a table. Pulmonary angiography is usually performed in a hospital's radiology department and takes 30 minutes to one hour.

An electrocardiograph shows the heart's electrical activity and helps distinguish pulmonary embolism from a heart attack. Electrodes covered with conducting jelly are placed on the patient's chest, arms, and legs. Impulses of the heart's activity are traced on paper. The test takes about 10 minutes and can be performed in a physician's office or hospital lab.

Arterial blood gas measurements can be helpful, but they are rarely diagnostic for pulmonary embolism. Blood is taken from an artery instead of a vein, usually in the wrist and it is analyzed for oxygen, carbon dioxide and acid levels.

Venography is used to look for the most likely source of pulmonary embolism, deep vein thrombosis. It is very accurate, but it is not used often, because it is painful, expensive, exposes the patient to a fairly high dose of radiation, and can cause complications. Venography identifies the location, extent, and degree of attachment of the blood clots and enables the condition of the deep leg veins to be assessed. A contrast solution is injected into a foot vein through a catheter. The physician observes the movement of the solution through the vein with a fluoroscope while a series of x rays are taken. Venography takes between 30–45 minutes and can be done in a physician's office, a laboratory, or a hospital. Radionuclide venography, in which a radioactive isotope is injected, is occasionally used, especially if a patient has had reactions to contrast solutions. Most commonly performed are ultrasound and Doppler studies of leg veins.

Treatment

Patients with pulmonary embolism are hospitalized and generally treated with clot-dissolving and clot-preventing drugs. **Oxygen therapy** is often needed to maintain normal oxygen concentrations. For people who can't take anticoagulants and in some other cases, surgery may be needed to insert a device that filters blood returning to the heart and lungs. The goal of treatment is to maintain the patient's cardiovascular and respiratory functions while the blockage resolves, which takes 10–14 days, and to prevent the formation of other emboli.

Thrombolytic therapy to dissolve blood clots is the aggressive treatment for very severe pulmonary embolism. Streptokinase, urokinase, and recombinant tissue plasminogen activator (TPA) are thrombolytic agents. Heparin is the injectable anticoagulant (clot-preventing) drug of choice for preventing formation of blood clots. Warfarin, an oral anticoagulant, is usually continued when the patient leaves the hospital and doesn't need heparin any longer.

Prognosis

About 10% of patients with pulmonary embolism die suddenly within the first hour of onset of the condition. The outcome for all other patients is generally good; only 3% of patients who are properly diagnosed and treated die. In cases of undiagnosed pulmonary embolism, about 30% of patients die.

Prevention

Pulmonary embolism risk can be reduced in certain patients through judicious use of antithrombotic drugs such as heparin, venous interruption, gradient elastic stockings and/or intermittent pneumatic compression of the legs.

Resources

ORGANIZATIONS

American Heart Association. 7320 Greenville Ave. Dallas, TX 75231. (214) 373-6300 or (800) 242-8721. inquire@heart.org < http://www.americanheart.org >.

Lori De Milto

Pulmonary fibrosis

Definition

Pulmonary fibrosis is scarring in the lungs.

Description

Pulmonary fibrosis develops when the alveoli, tiny air sacs that transfer oxygen to the blood, become damaged and inflamed. The body tries to heal the damage with **scars**, but these scars collapse the alveoli and make the lungs less elastic. If the cycle of inflammation and scarring continues, the lungs become increasingly unable to deliver oxygen to the blood. Changes in the lungs can also increase the blood pressure in the pulmonary artery. This condition, called pulmonary **hypertension**, makes the heart work harder and it may fail.

Pulmonary fibrosis can result from many different lung diseases including **sarcoidosis**, drug reactions, autoimmune diseases, environmental **allergies** such as Farmer's lung, and exposure to toxic dusts and gases.

Pulmonary fibrosis that develops without a known cause is called idiopathic pulmonary fibrosis. This disease is equally common in men and women. It is usually diagnosed between the ages of 40 and 60.

Causes and symptoms

The causes and risk factors vary with the underlying disease. They may include genetics, environmental factors, and infections.

The first symptom of pulmonary fibrosis is usually shortness of breath—at first, during **exercise**, but later also while resting. Patients may also have a dry **cough**, a rapid heartbeat, or enlargement of the fingertips and ends of the toes. Some people feel tired or have a **fever**, weight loss, muscle or joint pains. In late stages of the disease, the lack of oxygen in the blood can give the skin and mucus membranes a blue tinge known as **cyanosis**.

Diagnosis

Pulmonary fibrosis is often referred to a lung specialist. Several tests are usually needed to diagnose this disease and determine its cause. They include a physical examination, detailed history of the symptoms, chest x rays, lung function tests, and blood tests, including a measurement of the amount of oxygen in the blood. Computed tomography (CT scan) may give a more detailed picture of the lungs. **Bronchoscopy** may be done to examine the air passages and analyze the cells found deep in the lungs.

Lung biopsies are necessary to diagnose some diseases. Lung biopsies can be done through a needle inserted into the chest through the skin, during bronchoscopy, or as a surgical procedure under **general anesthesia**.

Treatment

The treatment of pulmonary fibrosis depends on the underlying cause. Many diseases are treated by suppressing inflammation with **corticosteroids**. Stronger immune suppressants such as cyclophosphamide (Cytoxan) or azathioprine (Imuran) may also be tried. Some patients need supplemental oxygen. A lung transplant may be an option for incurable diseases. Approximately 60–80% of patients live for at least two years after the transplant.

There is no good treatment for idiopathic pulmonary fibrosis. Only 10–20% of patients with this disease respond to corticosteroids.

Alternative treatment

Anxiety and fear can make breathing difficulties worse. Some patients find that activities such as **yoga**, prayer or **meditation**, **music therapy**, or **biofeedback** help to relax them.

KEY TERMS

Alveoli—Tiny air sacs in the lungs where oxygen and carbon dioxide are exchanged with the blood.

Autoimmune disease—A disease that develops when the immune system attacks normal cells or organs.

Bronchoscopy Scan—The examination of the air passages through a flexible or rigid tube inserted into the nostril (or mouth). Sometimes cells are collected by washing the lungs with a small amount of fluid.

Computed tomography(CT)—A special x-ray technique that produces a cross sectional image of the organs inside the body.

Corticosteroids—A class of drugs, related to hormones naturally found in the body, that suppress the immune system. One example is prednisone, sold under many brand names including Deltasone.

End-stage lung disease—The final stages of lung disease, when the lung can no longer keep the blood supplied with oxygen. End-stage lungs in pulmonary fibrosis have large air spaces separated by bands of inflammation and scarring.

Farmer's lung—An allergic reaction to moldy hay, most often seen in farmers, that results in lung disease.

Immune suppressant drug—Any drug that dampens immune responses and decreases inflammation.

Inflammation—The body's reaction to an irritant, characterized by the accumulation of immune cells, redness, and swelling.

Lung function tests—Tests of how much air the lungs can move in and out, and how quickly and efficiently this can be done. Lung function tests are usually done by breathing into a device that measures air flow.

Mucous membranes—The moist coverings that line the mouth, nose, intestines, and other internal organs.

Pulmonary artery—The blood vessel that delivers blood from the heart to the lungs.

Sarcoidosis—A disease of unknown origin that results in clumps of immune cells and inflammation in organs throughout the body.

Prognosis

The prognosis depends on the specific disease. Some cases may stop progressing or improve, particularly if the cause can be identified and treated. Others may develop quickly or slowly into end-stage lung disease. The course of idiopathic pulmonary fibrosis is very difficult to predict; however, average survival is approximately five to seven years.

Prevention

There is no known prevention for idiopathic pulmonary fibrosis.

Some ways to prevent other causes of pulmonary fibrosis are:

- avoid exposure to particle dust such as asbestos, coal dust, and silica

- avoid exposure to chemical fumes

- do not smoke

Resources

BOOKS

Kobzik, Lester. "Diffuse Interstitial (Infiltrative,Restrictive) Diseases." In *Robbins Pathologic Basis of Disease*, edited by Ramzi S. Cotran, Vinay Kumar, and Tucker Collins, 6th ed. Philadelphia: W.B. Saunders, 2000, pp. 727-740.

Toews, Galen B. "Interstitial Lung Disease." In*Cecil Textbook of Medicine*, edited by Lee Goldman and J. Claude Bennett, 21st ed. Philadelphia: W.B. Saunders, 2000,pp. 409-419.

PERIODICALS

Mason, Robert J., Marvin I. Schwarz, Gary W. Hunninghake, and Robert A. Musson. "Pharmacologic Therapy for Idiopathic Pulmonary Fibrosis: Past, Present, and Future." *American Journal of Respiratory and Critical CareMedicine* 160 (1999): 1771-1777.

Michaelson, Jeffrey E., Samuel M. Aguayo, and Jesse Roman. "Idiopathic Pulmonary Fibrosis: A Practical Approach for Diagnosis and Management." *Chest* 118, no. 3 (September2000): 788-94.

ORGANIZATIONS

The American Lung Association. 1740 Broadway, New York. NY 10019. (212) 315-8700. < http://www.lungusa.org >.

Pulmonary Fibrosis Association. P.O. Box 75004, Seattle, WA 98125-0004. (206) 417-0949. < http://pulmonaryfibrosisassn.com >.

Pulmonary Fibrosis Foundation. 1075 Santa Fe Drive, Denver, Colorado 80204. (720) 932-7850. < http://pulmonaryfibrosis.org >.

OTHER

"Bronchoscopy with Transtracheal Biopsy " *Health Encyclopedia.* 2001. [cited May 2, 2001]. < http://www.merck-medco.com/medco/index.jsp >.

Chronic Lung Disease Information Resource. The Cheshire Medical Center. May 5, 2001. < http://www.cheshire-med.com/programs/pulrehab/rehinfof.html >.

"Lung Needle Biopsy." *Health Encyclopedia.* 2001. [cited May 2, 2001]. < http://www.merck-medco.com/medco/index.jsp >.

"Open Lung Biopsy " *Health Encyclopedia.* 2001. [cited May 2, 2001]. < http://www.merck-medco.com/medco/index.jsp >.

Anna Rovid Spickler, D.V.M., Ph.D.

Pulmonary fibrosis *see* **Idiopathic infiltrative lung diseases**

Pulmonary function test

Definition

Pulmonary function tests are a group of procedures that measure the function of the lungs, revealing problems in the way a patient breathes. The tests can determine the cause of **shortness of breath** and may help confirm lung diseases, such as **asthma**, **bronchitis** or **emphysema**. The tests also are performed before any major **lung surgery** to make sure the person won't be disabled by having a reduced lung capacity.

Purpose

Pulmonary function tests can help a doctor diagnose a range of respiratory diseases which might not otherwise be obvious to the doctor or the patient. The tests are important since many kinds of lung problems can be successfully treated if detected early.

The tests are also used to measure how a lung disease is progressing, and how serious the lung disease has become. Pulmonary function tests also can be used to assess how a patient is responding to different treatments.

One of the most common of the pulmonary function tests is spirometry (from the Greco-Latin term meaning "to measure breathing"). This test, which can be given in a hospital or doctor's office, measures how much and how fast the air is moving in and out of the lungs. Specific measurements taken during the test include the volume of air from start to finish, the fastest flow that is achieved, and the volume of air exhaled in the first second of the test.

A peak flow meter can determine how much a patient's airways have narrowed. A test of blood gases is a measurement of the concentration of oxygen and carbon dioxide in the blood, which shows how efficient the gas exchange is in the lungs.

Another lung function test reveals how efficient the lungs are in absorbing gas from the blood. This is measured by testing the volume of carbon monoxide a person breathes out after a known volume of the gas has been inhaled.

Precautions

Pulmonary function tests shouldn't be given to patients who have had a recent **heart attack**, or who have certain other types of heart disease. It is crucial that the patient cooperate with the health care team if accurate results are to be obtained.

Description

The patient places a clip over the nose and breathes through the mouth into a tube connected to a machine known as a spirometer. First the patient breathes in deeply, and then exhales as quickly and forcefully as possible into the tube. The exhale must last at least six seconds for the machine to work properly. Usually the patient repeats this test three times, and the best of the three results is considered to be the measure of the lung function. The results will help a doctor figure out which type of treatment to pursue.

Preparation

The patient should not eat a heavy meal before the test, nor smoke for four to six hours beforehand. The patient's doctor will issue specific instructions about whether or not to use specific medications, including **bronchodilators** or inhalers, before the test. Sometimes, medication may be administered as part of the test.

Risks

The risk is minimal for most people, although the test carries a slight risk of a collapsed lung in some patients with lung disease.

Normal results

Normal results are based on a person's age, height, and gender. Normal results are expressed as a percentage

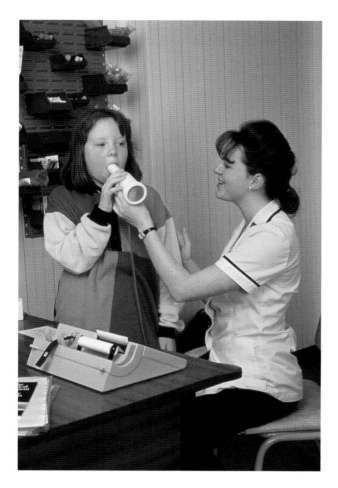

This young girl is undergoing a pulmonary function test in order to measure the functionality of her lungs. *(Custom Medical Stock Photo. Reproduced by permission.)*

Resources

BOOKS

Ruppel, Gregg L. *Manual of Pulmonary Function Testing.* St. Louis: Mosby, 1997.

Carol A. Turkington

Pulmonary heart disease *see* **Cor pulmonale**

Pulmonary hypertension

Definition

Pulmonary **hypertension** is a rare lung disorder characterized by increased pressure in the pulmonary artery. The pulmonary artery carries oxygen-poor blood from the lower chamber on the right side of the heart (right ventricle) to the lungs where it picks up oxygen.

Description

Pulmonary hypertension is present when the blood pressure in the circulation of the lungs is measured at greater than 25 mm of mercury (Hg) at rest or 30 mm Hg during **exercise**. Pulmonary hypertension can be either primary or secondary:

- Primary pulmonary hypertension. The cause of pulmonary hypertension is unknown. It is rare, affecting one people per-million. The illness most often occurs in young adults, especially women.

- Secondary pulmonary hypertension. Secondary pulmonary hypertension is increased pressure of the blood vessels of the lungs as a result of other medical conditions.

Regardless of whether pulmonary hypertension is primary or secondary, the disorder results in thickening of the pulmonary arteries and narrowing of these blood vessels. In response, the right side of the heart works harder to move the blood through these arteries and it becomes enlarged. Eventually overworking the right side of the heart may lead to right-sided **heart failure**, resulting in **death**.

Causes and symptoms

While the cause of primary pulmonary hypertension is uncertain, researchers think that in most people who develop the disease, the blood vessels are sensitive to certain factors that cause them to narrow. Diet suppressants, **cocaine**, and **pregnancy** are some of the

KEY TERMS

Emphysema—A disease in which the small air sacs in the lungs become damaged, causing shortness of breath. In severe cases it can lead to respiratory or heart failure.

of the predicted lung capacity. The prediction takes into account the patient's age, height, and sex.

Abnormal results

Abnormal results mean that the person's lung capacity is less than 80% of the predicted value. Such findings usually mean that there is some degree of chest or lung disease.

KEY TERMS

Hypertension—The medical term for abnormally high blood pressure.

Perfusion lung scan—A scan that shows the pattern of blood flow in the lungs.

Pulmonary—Having to do with the lungs.

Pulmonary function test—A test that measures how much air the lungs hold and the air flow in and out of the lungs.

Right-heart cardiac catherization—A medical procedure during which a physician threads a catheter into the right side of the heart to measure the blood pressure in the right side of the heart and the pulmonary artery. The right heart's pumping ability can also be evaluated.

factors that are thought to trigger constriction or narrowing of the pulmonary artery. In about 6–10% of cases, primary pulmonary hypertension is inherited.

Secondary pulmonary hypertension can be associated with breathing disorders such as emphysema and **bronchitis**, or diseases such as **scleroderma**, systemic lupus erythematosus (SLE) or congenital heart disease involving heart valves, and pulmonary thromboembolism.

Symptoms of pulmonary hypertension include shortness of breath with minimal exertion, general fatigue, dizziness, and **fainting**. Swelling of the ankles, bluish lips and skin, and chest **pain** are among other symptoms of the disease.

Diagnosis

Pulmonary hypertension is rarely detected during routine physical examinations and, therefore, often progresses to later stages before being diagnosed. In addition to listening to heart sounds with a stethoscope, physicians also use electrocardiogram, pulmonary function tests, perfusion lung scan, and/or right-heart **cardiac catheterization** to diagnose pulmonary hypertension.

Treatment

The aim of treatment for pulmonary hypertension is to treat the underlying cause, if it is known. For example, thromboendarterectomy is a surgical procedure performed to remove a blood clot on the lung

that is causing the pulmonary hypertension. Lung transplants are another surgical treatment.

Some patients are helped by taking medicines that make the work of the heart easier. Anticoagulants, drugs that thin the blood, decrease the tendency of the blood to clot and allow blood to flow more freely. **Diuretics** decrease the amount of fluid in the body and reduce the amount of work the heart has to do. Calcium channel blockers relax the smooth muscle in the walls of the heart and blood vessels and improve the ability of the heart to pump blood.

One effective medical treatment that dilates blood vessels and seems to help prevent blood clots from forming is epoprostenol (prostacyclin). Prostacyclin is given intravenously to improve survival, exercise duration, and well-being. It is sometimes used as a bridge to help people who are waiting for a lung transplant. In other cases it is used for long-term treatment.

Some people require supplemental oxygen through nasal prongs or a mask if breathing becomes difficult.

Prognosis

Pulmonary hypertension is chronic and incurable with an unpredictable survival rate. Length of survival has been improving, with some patients able to live 15–20 years or longer with the disorder.

Prevention

Since the cause of primary pulmonary hypertension is still unknown, there is no way to prevent or cure this disease. A change in lifestyle may assist patients with daily activities. For example, relaxation exercises help to reduce **stress**. Good health habits such as a healthy diet, not **smoking**, and getting plenty of rest should be maintained.

Resources

ORGANIZATIONS

American Association for Respiratory Care. 11030 Ables Lane, Dallas, TX 75229. (972) 243-2272. < http://www.aarc.org >.

Pulmonary Hypertension Association. P.O. Box 24733, Speedway, IN 46224-0733. (800) 748-7274. < http://www.phassociation.org >.

OTHER

"Primary Pulmonary Hypertensiton." *National Heart, Lung, and Blood Institute.* < http://www.nhlbi.nih.gov/nhlbi/lung/other/gp/pph.txt >.

Lorraine Steefel, RN

Pulmonary incompetence *see* **Pulmonary valve insufficiency**

Pulmonary regurgitation *see* **Pulmonary valve insufficiency**

Pulmonary stenosis *see* **Pulmonary valve stenosis**

Pulmonary valve insufficiency

Definition

Pulmonary valve insufficiency is a disorder involving a defect of the valve located in the pulmonary artery.

Description

This disorder is also known as pulmonary valve regurgitation or pulmonary incompetence. The pulmonary valve is the structure in the pulmonary artery consisting of three flaps, which open and close during each heartbeat. The flaps keep blood from flowing back into the heart from the pulmonary artery–the artery that supplies blood to the lungs. With pulmonary valve insufficiency, the flaps may allow the blood to flow backward, resulting in a distinct murmur. The disorder may be congenital, but also often occurs in patients with severe **pulmonary hypertension**.

Causes and symptoms

There are generally few to no symptoms with pulmonary valve insufficiency. It may be initially noticed as a murmur in a routine exam of the heart and chest with a stethoscope. The most common causes of the disorder are severe pulmonary **hypertension**, or the presence of high pressure in the arteries and veins of the lungs. Pulmonary hypertension is usually caused by chronic lung disease, lung **blood clots**, and sometimes other diseases, such as **endocarditis**, an inflammation of the lining of the heart and valves. Previous surgery for **congenital heart disease** may also cause pulmonary valve insufficiency.

Diagnosis

The pitch and location of the murmur will help a physician determine if the cause is pulmonary valve insufficiency. An electrocardiogram (EKG) can detect flow changes. **Echocardiography** with color Doppler can usually detect regurgitation of blood in the area. This exam is done with ultrasound imaging. A **chest x ray** may show prominence of the pulmonary artery. In some cases, angiocardiography, or x ray of the arteries and vessels with injection of a dye, may be ordered.

KEY TERMS

Congenital—Used to describe a condition or defect present at birth.

Endocarditis—Inflammation of the lining of the heart and valves.

Prophylaxis—Preventive. Antibiotic prophylaxis is the use of antibiotics to prevent a possible infection.

Pulmonary—Refers to the lungs and the breathing system and function.

Pulmonary hypertension—High blood pressure in the veins and arteries of the lungs.

Treatment

On its own, pulmonary valve insufficiency is seldom severe enough to require treatment. **Antibiotics** are usually recommended before dental work to reduce the possibility of bacterial endocarditis. Management of the primary condition, such as medications to manage pulmonary hypertension, may help control pulmonary valve insufficiency.

Alternative treatment

Since there are few or no symptoms and the disorder is a structural defect, alternative treatment may have only limited usefulness. Proper diet, **exercise**, and **stress reduction** may help control hypertension. Coenzyme Q10 and hawthorn (*Crataegus laevigata*) are two important nutrients to nourish the heart. Antioxidant supplements (including **vitamins** A, C, and E, selenium, and zinc) can help keep the tissues of the whole body, including the heart, in optimal condition.

Prognosis

Patients with this disorder may never experience limitations from pulmonary valve insufficiency. The disorder may only show up if complicated by pulmonary hypertension. There is an increased incidence of bacterial endocarditis in patients with pulmonary valve insufficiency. Endocarditis can progress rapidly and be fatal.

Prevention

Pulmonary valve insufficiency resulting from chronic lung diseases can be prevented by behaviors and interventions to prevent those primary diseases. Bacterial endocarditis resulting from pulmonary valve insufficiency can usually be prevented with the use of antibiotic **prophylaxis** in preparation for dental procedures or other procedures which may introduce bacteria into the bloodstream.

Resources

ORGANIZATIONS

American Heart Association. 7320 Greenville Ave. Dallas, TX 75231. (214) 373-6300 or (800) 242-8721. inquire@heart.org < http://www.americanheart.org >.

National Heart, Lung and Blood Institute. P.O. Box 30105, Bethesda, MD 20824-0105. (301) 251-1222. < http:// www.nhlbi.nih.gov >.

Teresa Odle

Pulmonary valve stenosis

Definition

Pulmonary valve stenosis is a congenital heart defect in which blood flow from the heart to the pulmonary artery is blocked.

Description

Pulmonary valve stenosis is an obstruction in the pulmonary valve, located between the right ventricle and the pulmonary artery. Normally, the pulmonary valve opens to let blood flow from the right ventricle to the lungs. When the pulmonary valve is malformed, it forces the right ventricle to pump harder to overcome the obstruction. In its most severe form, pulmonary valve stenosis can be life-threatening.

Patients with pulmonary valve stenosis are at increased risk for getting valve infections and must take antiobiotics to help prevent this before certain dental and surgical procedures. Pulmonary valve stenosis is also called pulmonary stenosis.

Causes and symptoms

Pulmonary valve stenosis is caused by a congenital malformation in which the pulmonary valve does not open properly. In most cases, scientists don't know why it occurs. In cases of mild or moderate stenosis, there are often no symptoms. With more severe obstruction, symptoms include a bluish skin tint and signs of **heart failure**.

Diagnosis

Diagnosis of pulmonary valve stenosis begins with the patient's medical history and a physical exam. Tests to confirm the diagnosis include **chest x ray**, echocardiogram, electrocardiogram, and catherization. An electrocardiograph shows the heart's activity. Electrodes covered with conducting jelly are placed on the patient. The electrodes send impulses that are traced on a recorder. **Echocardiography** uses sound waves to create an image of the heart's chambers and valves. The technician applies gel to a wand (transducer) and presses it against the patient's chest. The returning sound waves are converted into an image displayed on a monitor. Catherization is an invasive procedure used to diagnose, and in some cases treat, heart problems. A thin tube, called a catheter, is inserted into a blood vessel and threaded up into the heart, enabling physicians to see and sometimes correct the problems.

Treatment

Patients with mild to moderate pulmonary valve stenosis, and few or no symptoms, do not require treatment. In more severe cases, the blocked valve will be opened surgically, either through **balloon valvuloplasty** or surgical valvulotomy. For initial treatment, balloon valvuloplasty is the procedure of choice. This is a catherization procedure in which a special catheter containing a deflated balloon is inserted in a blood vessel and threaded up into the heart. The catheter is positioned in the narrowed heart valve and the balloon is inflated to stretch the valve open.

In some cases, surgical valvulotomy may be necessary. This is open heart surgery performed with a heart-lung machine. The valve is opened with an incision and in some cases, hypertrophied muscle in the right ventricle is removed. Rarely does the pulmonary valve need to be replaced.

Alternative treatment

Pulmonary valve stenosis can be life threatening and always requires a physician's care. In mild to

KEY TERMS

Congenital—Present at birth.

Pulmonary—Relating to the opening leading from the right large chamber of the heart into the lung artery.

Stenosis—A narrowing or constriction, in this case of various heart valves. Stenosis reduces or cuts off the flow of blood.

Valve—Tissue between the heart's upper and lower chambers that controls blood flow.

moderate cases of pulmonary valve stenosis, general lifestyle changes, including dietary modifications, **exercise**, and **stress reduction**, can contribute to maintaining optimal wellness.

Prognosis

Patients with the most severe form of pulmonary valve stenosis may die in infancy. The prognosis for children with more severe stenosis who undergo balloon valvuloplasty or surgical valvulotomy is favorable. Patients with mild to moderate pulmonary stenosis can lead a normal life, but they require regular medical care.

Prevention

Pulmonary valve stenosis cannot be prevented.

Resources

ORGANIZATIONS

American Heart Association. 7320 Greenville Ave. Dallas, TX 75231. (214) 373-6300. < http://www.americanheart.org >.

Children's Health Information Network. 1561 Clark Drive, Yardley, PA 19067. (215) 493-3068. < http://www.tchin.org >.

Congenital Heart Anomalies Support, Education & Resources, Inc. 2112 North Wilkins Road, Swanton, OH 43558. (419) 825-5575. < http://www.csun.edu/~hfmth006/chaser >.

Texas Heart Institute. Heart Information Service. P.O. Box 20345, Houston, TX 77225-0345. < http://www.tmc.edu/thi >.

Lori De Milto

Punctures *see* **Wounds**

Purple coneflower *see* **Echinacea**

Purpura hemorrhagica *see* **Idiopathic thrombocytopenic purpura**

Pustule *see* **Skin lesions**

Pyelography *see* **Intravenous urography**

Pyelonephritis

Definition

Pyelonephritis is an inflammation of the kidney and upper urinary tract that usually results from non-contagious bacterial infection of the bladder (**cystitis**).

Description

Acute pyelonephritis is most common in adult females but can affect people of either sex and any age. Its onset is usually sudden, with symptoms that often are mistaken as the results of straining the lower back. Pyelonephritis often is complicated by systemic infection. Left untreated or unresolved, it can progress to a chronic condition that lasts for months or years, leading to scarring and possible loss of kidney function.

Causes and symptoms

The most common cause of pyelonephritis is the backward flow (reflux) of infected urine from the bladder to the upper urinary tract. Bacterial infections also may be carried to one or both kidneys through the bloodstream or lymph glands from infection that began in the bladder. Kidney infection sometimes results from urine that becomes stagnant due to obstruction of free urinary flow. A blockage or abnormality of the urinary system, such as those caused by stones, tumors, congenital deformities, or loss of bladder function from nerve disease, increases a person's risk of pyelonephritis. Other risk factors include diabetes mellitus, pregnancy, chronic bladder infections, a history of analgesic abuse, paralysis from **spinal cord injury**, or tumors. Catheters, tubes, or surgical procedures may also trigger a kidney infection.

The bacteria most likely to cause pyelonephritis are those that normally occur in the feces. *Escherichia coli* causes about 85% of acute bladder and kidney infections in patients with no obstruction or history of surgical procedures. *Klebsiella, Enterobacter, Proteus,* or *Pseudomonas* are other common causes of infection. Once these organisms enter the urinary tract, they cling to the tissues that line the tract and multiply in them.

Symptoms of acute pyelonephritis typically include fever and chills, burning or frequent urination, aching **pain** on one or both sides of the lower back or abdomen, cloudy or bloody urine, and **fatigue**. The patient also may have **nausea**, **vomiting**, and **diarrhea**. The flank pain may be extreme. The symptoms of chronic pyelonephritis include weakness, loss of appetite, hypertension, anemia, and protein and blood in the urine.

Diagnosis

The diagnosis of pyelonephritis is based on the patient's history, a **physical examination**, and the results of laboratory and imaging tests. During the physical examination, the doctor will touch (palpate) the patient's abdomen carefully in order to rule out **appendicitis** or other causes of severe abdominal pain.

Laboratory tests

In addition to collecting urine samples for **urinalysis** and urine culture and sensitivity tests, the doctor will take a sample of the patient's blood for a blood cell count. If the patient has pyelonephritis, the urine tests will show the presence of white blood cells, and bacteria in the urine. Bacterial counts of 100,000 organisms or higher per milliliter of urine point to a urinary tract infection. The presence of antibody-coated bacteria (ACB) in the urine sample distinguishes kidney infection from bladder infection, because bacteria in the kidney trigger an antibody response that coats the bacteria. The blood cell count usually indicates a sharp increase in the number of white blood cells.

Imaging studies

The doctor may order ultrasound imaging of the kidney area if he or she suspects that there is an obstruction blocking the flow of urine. X rays may demonstrate scarring of the kidneys and ureters resulting from long-standing infection.

Treatment

Treatment of acute pyelonephritis may require hospitalization if the patient is severely ill or has complications. Therapy most often involves a two- to three-week course of **antibiotics**, with the first few days of treatment given intravenously. The choice of antibiotic is based on laboratory sensitivity studies. The antibiotics used most often include ciprofloxacin

---

KEY TERMS

Bacteremia—The presence of bacteria in the bloodstream.

Cystitis—Inflammation of the bladder, usually caused by bacterial infection.

Reflux—The backward flow of a fluid in the body. Pyelonephritis is often associated with the reflux of urine from the bladder to the upper urinary tract.

(Cipro), ampicillin (Omnipen), or trimethoprim-sulfamethoxazole (Bactrim, Septra). Several advances in antibiotic therapy have been made in recent years. In 2003, the U.S. Food and Drug Administration (FDA) approved Cipro extended release tablets (Cipro XR) that could be taken once daily for acute uncomplicated pyelonephritis. A study in Europe also showed that a shorter course than that normally used in the United States could eradicate the bacteria that cause the disease. The primary objective of antimicrobial therapy is the permanent eradication of bacteria from the urinary tract. The early symptoms of pyelonephritis usually disappear within 48 to 72 hours of the start of antibacterial treatment. Repeat urine cultures are done in order to evaluate the effectiveness of the medication.

Chronic pyelonephritis may require high doses of antibiotics for as long as six months to clear the infection. Other medications may be given to control **fever**, nausea, and pain. Patients are encouraged to drink extra fluid to prevent **dehydration** and increase urine output. Surgery sometimes is necessary if the patient has complications caused by **kidney stones** or other obstructions, or to eradicate infection. Urine cultures are repeated as part of the follow-up of patients with chronic pyelonephritis. These repeat tests are necessary to evaluate the possibility that the patient's urinary tract is infected with a second organism as well as to assess the patient's response to the antibiotic. Some persons are highly susceptible to reinfection, and a second antibiotic may be necessary to treat the organism.

Prognosis

The prognosis for most patients with acute pyelonephritis is quite good if the infection is caught early and treated promptly. The patient is considered cured if the urine remains sterile for a year. Untreated or recurrent kidney infection can lead to bacterial invasion of the bloodstream (bacteremia), **hypertension**, chronic pyelonephritis with scarring of the kidneys, and permanent kidney damage. In 2003, a report on long-term follow-up of adults with acute pyelonephritis looked at kidney scarring and resulting complications. Kidney damage that causes complications is rare after 10 to 20 years, even though many women showed renal scarring.

Prevention

Persons with a history of urinary tract infections should urinate frequently, and drink plenty of fluids at the first sign of infection. Women should void after intercourse which may help flush bacteria from the bladder. Girls should be taught to wipe their genital area from front to back after urinating to avoid getting fecal matter into the opening of the urinary tract.

Resources

PERIODICALS

Jancin, Bruce. "Short-course Cipro for Pyelonephritis: Unapproved Regimen Shows Promise." *OB GYN News* November 1, 2003: 5.

Mangan, Doreen. "The FDA has Approved Ciprofloxacin Extended Release Tavlets (Cipro XR), a Once-daily Formulation, for the Treatment of Complicated Urinary Tract Infections (cUTIs) and Acute Pyelonephritis (AUP), or Kidney Infection." *RN* November 2003: 97.

Raz, Paul, et al. "Long-term Follow-up of Women Hospitalized for Acute Pyelonephritis." *Clinical Infectious Diseases* (October 15, 2003):1014–1017.

ORGANIZATIONS

American Foundation for Urologic Disease. 1128 N. Charles St., Baltimore, MD 21201. (401) 468-1800. < http://www.afud.org >.

Kathleen D. Wright, RN
Teresa G. Odle

Pyloric stenosis

Definition

Pyloric stenosis refers to a narrowing of the passage between the stomach and the small intestine. The condition, which affects infants during the first several weeks of life, can be corrected effectively with surgery.

Description

Frequent **vomiting** may be an indication of pyloric stenosis. The pylorus is the passage between the stomach and the small intestine. During the digestive process food passes through the pylorus, which is located near the bottom of the stomach, on its way to the intestines. In pyloric stenosis, the muscular wall of the passage becomes abnormally thickened. This causes the pylorus to become too narrow, which prevents food from emptying out of the stomach in a normal fashion. The partially digested contents of the stomach are forced upwards into the mouth. As a result, a baby with pyloric stenosis often vomits after feedings.

The condition affects one in 4,000 infants. Most are diagnosed between three and five weeks old, though some babies may show symptoms during the first or second week of life. Infants with a family history of pyloric stenosis are more at risk for the condition, which tends to occur less often in females, blacks, and Asians. Pyloric stenosis is also referred to as hypertrophic pyloric stenosis.

Causes and symptoms

The cause of pyloric stenosis is not known. The main symptom is vomiting after feedings. These episodes of vomiting usually get worse over time, happening more often and becoming more forceful (forceful vomiting is often called "projectile" vomiting). Other symptoms include increased appetite, weight loss, infrequent bowel movements, belching, and **diarrhea**. Due to **dehydration**, the infant may also have fewer wet diapers.

Diagnosis

The clinician will examine the baby and talk with the parents about their infant's symptoms. If a child has the condition, the doctor should be able to feel a hard mass (about 2 cm wide and olive shaped) in the area above the bellybutton. If the doctor cannot detect the mass, ultrasonography will be done to confirm the diagnosis. A blood test may also be performed to see if the infant is dehydrated, in which case intravenous fluids can be used to correct the problem.

Treatment

Pyloric stenosis can be cured with a surgical procedure called a pyloromyotomy. In this operation, the surgeon makes an incision in the baby's abdomen. Then a small cut is made in the thickened muscle of the pylorus and it is spread apart. In this manner, the passage can be widened without removing any tissue. (The procedure may be performed with the aid of a laparoscope.) After surgery, the pylorus will heal itself. The thickening gradually goes away and the passage resumes a normal shape. The whole procedure (including anesthesia) takes about an hour.

Most babies go home one or two days after surgery. Any mild discomfort can be controlled with Tylenol. The infant may still vomit occasionally after surgery, but this is not usually a cause for alarm. However, if vomiting occurs three or more times a day, or for several consecutive days, the baby's pediatrician should be notified.

Alternative treatment

None known.

Prognosis

Surgery is often a complete cure. Most infants do not experience complications or long-term effects.

Prevention

It is not known how to prevent pyloric stenosis.

Resources

BOOKS

Behrman, Richard E., et al., *Nelson Textbook of Pediatrics.* Philadelphia: WB Saunders, 2000.

PERIODICALS

Yoshizawa J, et al. Ultrasonographic Features of Normalizationof the Pylorus after Pyloromyotomy for Hypertrophic Pyloric Stenosis. *"Journal of PediatricSurgery"* 36 (April 2001): 582-6.

ORGANIZATIONS

American Academy of Family Physicians. 11400 Tomahawk Creek Parkway, Leawood, KS 66211-2672. (913) 906-6000. < http://www.aafp.org/ > . fp@aafp.org.

American Academy of Pediatrics. 141 Northwest Point Boulevard, Elk Grove Village, IL 60007-1098. (847) 434-4000. < http://www.aap.org >.

Greg Annussek

Pyloroplasty

Definition

Pyloroplasty is an elective surgical procedure in which the lower portion of the stomach, the pylorus, is cut and resutured, to relax the muscle and widen the opening into the intestine. Pyloroplasty is a treatment for high-risk patients for gastric or peptic ulcer disease. A peptic ulcer is a well-defined sore on the stomach where the lining of the stomach or duodenum has been eaten away by stomach acid and digestive juices.

Purpose

The end of the pylorus is surrounded by a strong band of muscle (pyloric sphincter), through which stomach contents are emptied into the duodenum (the first part of the small intestine). Pyloroplasty widens this opening into the duodenum.

A pyloroplasty is performed to treat complications of gastric ulcer disease, or when conservative treatment is unsatisfactory. The longitudinal cut made in the pylorus is closed transversely, permitting the muscle to relax. By establishing an enlarged outlet from the stomach into the intestine, the stomach empties more quickly. A pyloroplasty is often done is conjunction with a **vagotomy**, a procedure in which the nerves that stimulate stomach acid production and gastric motility (movement) are cut. As these nerves are cut, gastric emptying may be delayed, and the pyloroplasty compensates for that effect.

Preparation

As with any surgical procedure, the patient will be required to sign a consent form after the procedure is explained thoroughly. Blood and urine studies, along with various x rays may be ordered as the doctor deems necessary. Food and fluids will be prohibited after midnight before the procedure. Cleansing **enemas** may be ordered to empty the intestine. If **nausea** or **vomiting** are present, a suction tube to empty the stomach may be used.

Aftercare

Post-operative care for the patient who has had a pyloroplasty, as for those who have had any major surgery, involves monitoring of blood pressure, pulse, respiration, and temperature. Breathing tends to be shallow because of the effect of anesthesia and the patient's reluctance to breathe deeply and experience **pain** that is caused by the abdominal incision. The patient is shown how to support the operative site while breathing deeply and coughing, and given pain medication as necessary. Fluid intake and output is measured, and the operative site is observed for color and wound drainage. Fluids are given intravenously for 24–48 hours, until the patient's diet is gradually advanced as bowel activity resumes. The patient is generally allowed to walk approximately eight hours after surgery and the average hospital stay, dependent upon overall recovery status, ranges from six to eight days.

Risks

Potential complications of this abdominal surgery include:

- excessive bleeding
- surgical wound infection
- incisional **hernia**
- recurrence of gastric ulcer
- chronic **diarrhea**
- malnutrition

Normal results

Complete healing is expected without complications. Four to six weeks should be allowed for recovery from the surgery.

Abnormal results

The doctor should be made aware of any of the following problems after surgery:

- increased pain, swelling, redness, drainage, or bleeding in the surgical area
- headache, muscle aches, **dizziness**, or **fever**
- increased abdominal pain or swelling, **constipation**, nausea or vomiting, rectal bleeding, or black, tarry stools

Resources

OTHER

"Peptic ulcer surgery."*ThriveOnline*. April 20, 1988. < http://thriveonline.oxygen.com >.

Kathleen D. Wright, RN

Pylorus repair *see* **Pyloroplasty**

Pyorrhea *see* **Periodontal disease**

Pyrazinamide *see* **Antituberculosis drugs**

Pyridoxine deficiency *see* **Vitamin B$_6$ deficiency**

Pyrimethamine *see* **Antimalarial drugs**

Pyruvate kinase deficiency

Definition

Pyruvate kinase deficiency (PKD) is part of a group of disorders called hereditary nonspherocytic hemolytic **anemias**. Hereditary nonspherocytic anemias are rare genetic conditions that affect the red blood cells. PKD is caused by a deficiency in the enzyme, pyruvate kinase. Although PKD is the second most common of the hereditary nonspherocytic anemias, it is still rare, with the incidence estimated to be 51 cases per million in the Caucasian population.

Description

In PKD, there is an functional abnormality with the enzyme, pyruvate kinase. Usually, pyruvate kinase acts as a catalyst in the glycolysis pathway, and is considered an essential component in this pathway. Glycolysis is the method by which cells produce their own energy. A problem with any of the key components in glycolysis can alter the amount of energy produced. In the red blood cells, glycolysis is the only method available to produce energy. Without the proper amount of energy, the red blood cells do not function normally. Since pyruvate kinase is one of the key components in glycolysis, when there is a problem with this enzyme in the red blood cells, there is a problem with the production of energy, causing the red blood cells not to function properly.

There are four different forms of the pyruvate kinase enzyme in the human body. These forms, called isozymes, all perform the same function but each isozyme of pyruvate kinase is structurally different and works in different tissues and organs. The four isozymes of pyruvate kinase are labeled M1, M2, L, and R. The isozyme M1 is found in the skeletal muscle and brain, isozyme M2 can be found in most fetal and adult tissues, isozyme L works in the liver, and isozyme R works in the red blood cells. In PKD, only the pyruvate kinase isozyme found in red blood cells, called PKR, is abnormal. Therefore, PKD only affects the red blood cells and does not directly affect the energy production in the other organs and tissues of the body.

In general, PKD not does appear to affect one gender more than another or be more common in certain regions. However, there are studies of an Amish group in Pennsylvania where a severe form of PKD is more common. As previously mentioned, the three mutations found in the PKLR gene have been linked to individuals of specific decents. Caucasians of northern and central European decent are more likely to have the 1529A mutations, individuals of southern European descent usually have the 1456T mutation, and individuals of Asian descent are more likely to have the 1468T mutation.

Causes and symptoms

There are two PK genes and each gene produces two of the four isozymes of pyruvate kinase. The M1 and M2 isozymes are produced by the pyruvate kinase gene called PKM2 and pyruvate kinase isozymes, L and R, are products of the pyruvate kinase gene, PKLR. The PKLR gene is located on chromosome 1, on the q arm (the top half of the chromosome), in region 21 (written as 1q21). As of 2001, there have been over 125 different mutations described in the PKLR gene that have been detected in individuals with PKD.

PKD is mainly inherited in an autosomal recessive manner. There have been a few families where it appeared that PKD was inherited in either an autosomal dominant manner or where the carriers of PKD exhibited mild problems with their red blood cells. As with all autosomal recessive conditions, affected individuals have a mutation in both pair of genes. Most individuals with PKD are compound heterozygotes, meaning that each PKLR gene in a pair contains a different mutation. There are individuals who have the same mutation on each PKLR gene, but these individuals tend to be children of parents who are related to each other.

There are three mutations in the PKLR gene called, 1529A, 1456T, and 1468T, that are seen more frequently in individuals with PKD than the other mutations. The mutation 1529A is most frequently seen in Caucasians of northern and central European descent and is the most common mutation seen in PKD. The mutation 1456T is more common in individuals of southern European descent and the mutation 1468T is more common in individuals of Asian descent.

In general, the more severe the PKD, the earlier in life symptoms tend to be detected. Individuals with the more severe form of PKD often show symptoms soon after birth, but most individuals with PKD begin to exhibit symptoms during infancy or childhood. In individuals with the more mild form of PKD, the condition is sometimes not diagnosed until late adulthood, after an acute illness, or during a **pregnancy** evaluation.

For most of the mutations seen in the PKLR gene, no correlation between the specific mutation and the severity of the disorder has been observed. However, for two of the mutations, there has been speculation on their effect on the severity of PKD. When the mutation 1456T has been seen in the homozygous state (when both PKLR genes contain the same mutation), those rare individuals experienced very mild symptoms of PKD. Also, there have been individuals who were homozygous for the 1529A mutation. These individuals had a very severe form of PKD. Therefore, it is thought that the 1456T mutation is associated

KEY TERMS

Anemia—When the amount of red blood cells is less than normal.

Catalyst—A substance that causes the next step in a pathway or reaction to occur, but is not physically changed by the process.

Compound heterozygotes—Individuals who have one gene in a pair with one mutation and the other gene in the pair has a different mutation.

Enzyme—A protein produced by cells that acts as a catalyst to allow a change or function to occur.

Glycolysis—The pathway in which a cell breaks down glucose into energy.

Hemolytic anemia—Anemia that results from red blood cells being destroyed sooner than normal.

Heterozygote/Heterozygotes—Are individuals who have one gene in a pair that has a mutation while the other gene in the pair is unaffected.

Homozygote/Homozygotes—Are individuals who have both genes in a pair with the same mutation.

Homozygous—When both genes in a pair have the same mutation.

Isozyme/Isoenzyme—Are a group of enzymes that perform the same function, but are different from one another in their structure or how they move.

Mutation—A change in the gene that causes it to alter its function

Nonspherocytic—Literally means not sphere-shaped. Often in inherited hemolytic anemias, the red blood cells are sphere-shaped. In Nonspherocytic Hemolytic Anemias, the red blood cells are not sphere-shaped.

with a milder form of the disease and the 1529A mutation is associated with a more severe form of the disease. It is not known how these mutations affect the severity of PKD when paired with different mutations.

Symptoms of PKD are similar to those symptoms seen in individuals who have long-term **hemolytic anemia**. The more common symptoms include variable degrees of **jaundice** (a yellowish pigment of the skin), slightly to moderately enlarged spleen (splenomegaly), and increased incidence of **gallstones**. Other physical effects of PKD can include smaller head size and the forehead appearing prominent and rounded (called frontal bossing). If a child with PKD has their spleen removed, their growth tends to improve. Even within

the same family, individuals can have different symptoms and severity of PKD.

In individuals with PKD, the red blood cells are taken out of their circulation earlier than normal (shorten life-span). Because of this, individuals with PKD will have hemolytic anemia. Additionally, the anemia or other symptoms of PKD may worsen during a sudden illness or pregnancy.

Diagnosis

A diagnosis of PKD can be made by measuring the amount of pyruvate kinase in red blood cells. Individuals with PKD tend to have 5–25% of the normal amount of pyruvate kinase. Carriers of PKD also can have less pyruvate kinase in their red blood cells, approximately 40–60% of the normal value. However, there is an overlap between the normal range of pyruvate kinase and the ranges seen with carriers of PKD. Therefore, measuring the amount of pyruvate kinase in the red blood cells is not a good method of detecting carriers of PKD. If the mutations causing PKD in a family are known, it may be possible to perform mutation analysis to determine carrier status of an individual and to help diagnose individuals with PKD.

Treatment

In the severest cases, individuals with PKD will require multiple blood transfusions. In some of those cases, the spleen may be removed (**splenectomy**). Red blood cells are normally removed from circulation by the spleen. By removing an individual's spleen (usually a child), the red blood cells are allowed to stay in circulation longer than normal; thereby, reducing the severity of the anemia. After a splenectomy, or once an individual with PKD is older, the number of transfusions tends to decrease.

Prognosis

The prognosis of PKD is extremely variable. Early intervention and treatment of symptoms frequently improves the individual's health. Without treatment, individuals may experience severe complications that may become lethal. Individuals with a mild form of PKD may appear to have no symptoms at all.

Resources

PERIODICALS

Beutler, Ernest, and Terri Gelbart. "Estimating the Prevalence of Pyruvate Kinase Deficiency from the

Gene Frequency in the General White Population." *Blood* 95 (June 2000): 3585-3588.

Kugler, W., et. al. "Eight Novel Mutations and Consequences of mRNA and Protein Level in Pyruvate Kinase Deficient Patients with Nonspherocytic Hemolytic Anemia." *Human Mutation* 15 (2000): 261-272.

ORGANIZATIONS

NIH/National Heart, Lung, and Blood Institute. 31 Center Drive.

OTHER

"Entry 266200: Pyruvate Kinase Deficiency of Erythrocyte." *OMIM—Online Mendelian Inheritance in Man.* < http://www.ncbi.nih.gov/htbin-post/Omim/dispmim?266200 >.

Sharon A. Aufox, MS, CGC

Pyschogenic disorder *see* **Somatoform disorders**

Q

Q fever

Definition

Q fever is an illness caused by a type of bacteria, *Coxiella burnetii*, resulting in a **fever** and rash.

Description

C. burnetii lives in many different kinds of animals, including cattle, sheep, goats, ticks, cats, rabbits, birds, and dogs. In sheep and cattle, for example, the bacteria tends to accumulate in large numbers in the female's uterus (the organ where lambs and calves develop) and udder. Other animals have similar patterns of bacterial accumulation within the females. As a result, *C. burnetii* can cause infection through contaminated milk, or when humans come into contact with the fluids or tissues produced when a cow or sheep gives birth. Also, the bacteria can survive in dry dust for months; therefore, if the female's fluids contaminate the ground, humans may become infected when they come in contact with the contaminated dust.

Persons most at risk for Q fever include anybody who works with cattle or sheep, or products produced from them. These include farm workers, slaughterhouse workers, workers in meat-packing plants, veterinarians, and wool workers. Since September 2001, however, Q fever has become an additional concern because of its potential as an agent of bioterrorism.

Q fever has been found all over the world, except in some areas of Scandinavia, Antarctica, and New Zealand.

Causes and symptoms

C. burnetii causes infection when a human breathes in tiny droplets, or drinks milk, containing the bacteria. After three to 30 days, symptoms of the illness appear.

The usual symptoms of Q fever include fever, chills, heavy sweating, **headache**, **nausea and vomiting**, **diarrhea**, **fatigue**, and **cough**. Also, a number of other problems may present themselves, including inflammation of the liver (hepatitis); inflammation of the sac containing the heart (**pericarditis**); inflammation of the heart muscle itself (**myocarditis**); inflammation of the coverings of the brain and spinal cord, or of the brain itself (meningoencephalitis); and **pneumonia**.

Chronic Q fever occurs most frequently in patients with other medical problems, including diseased heart valves, weakened immune systems, or **kidney disease**. Such patients usually have about a year's worth of vague symptoms, including a low fever, enlargement of the spleen and/or liver, and fatigue. Testing almost always reveals that these patients have inflammation of the lining of the heart (**endocarditis**).

Diagnosis

Q fever is diagnosed by demonstrating that the patient's immune system is making increasing numbers of antibodies (special immune cells) against markers (antigens) that are found on *C. burnetii*.

Treatment

Doxycycline and quinolone **antibiotics** are effective for treatment of Q fever. Treatment usually lasts for two weeks. Rifampin and doxycycline together are given for chronic Q fever. Chronic Q fever requires treatment for at least three years.

Minocycline has been found to be useful in treating post-Q fever fatigue. The dosage is 100 mg per day for three months.

Prognosis

Death is rare from Q fever. Most people recover completely, although some patients with endocarditis will require surgery to replace their damaged heart valves.

Prevention

Q fever can be prevented by the appropriate handling of potentially infective substances. For example, milk should always be pasteurized, and people who work with animals giving birth should carefully dispose of the tissues and fluids associated with birth. Industries which process animal materials (meat, wool) should take care to prevent the contamination of dust within the plant.

Vaccines are available for workers at risk for Q fever.

Resources

BOOKS

Beers, Mark H., MD, and Robert Berkow, MD, editors. "Biological Warfare and Terrorism." In *The Merck Manual of Diagnosis and Therapy.* Whitehouse Station, NJ: Merck Research Laboratories, 2004.

Beers, Mark H., MD, and Robert Berkow, MD, editors. "Q Fever." In *The Merck Manual of Diagnosis and Therapy.* Whitehouse Station, NJ: Merck Research Laboratories, 2004.

PERIODICALS

Arashima, Y., K. Kato, T. Komiya, et al. "Improvement of Chronic Nonspecific Symptoms by Long-Term Minocycline Treatment in Japanese Patients with *Coxiella burnetii* Infection Considered to Have Post-Q Fever Fatigue Syndrome." *Internal Medicine* 43 (January 2004): 1–2.

Gami, A. S., V. S. Antonios, R. L. Thompson, et al. "Q Fever Endocarditis in the United States." *Mayo Clinic Proceedings* 79 (February 2004): 253–257.

Madariaga, M. G., J. Pulvirenti, M. Sekosan, et al. "Q Fever Endocarditis in HIV-Infected Patient." *Emerging Infectious Diseases* 10 (March 2004): 501–504.

Wortmann, G. "Pulmonary Manifestations of Other Agents: Brucella, Q Fever, Tularemia and Smallpox." *Respiratory Care Clinics of North America* 10 (March 2004): 99–109.

ORGANIZATIONS

Centers for Disease Control and Prevention. 1600 Clifton Rd., NE, Atlanta, GA 30333. (800) 311-3435, (404) 639-3311. < http://www.cdc.gov >.

Rosalyn Carson-DeWitt, MD
Rebecca J. Frey, PhD

Qigong

Definition

Qigong (pronounced "chee-gung," also spelled *chi kung*) is translated from the Chinese to mean "energy cultivation" or "working with the life energy." Qigong is an ancient Chinese system of postures, exercises, breathing techniques, and meditations. Its techniques are designed to improve and enhance the body's *qi.* According to traditional Chinese philosophy, qi is the fundamental life energy responsible for health and vitality.

Purpose

Qigong may be used as a daily routine to increase overall health and well-being, as well as for disease prevention and longevity. It can be used to increase energy and reduce **stress.** In China, qigong is used in conjunction with other medical therapies for many chronic conditions, including **asthma, allergies, AIDS, cancer,** headaches, **hypertension,** depression, mental illness, strokes, heart disease, and **obesity**.

Qigong is presently being used in Hong Kong to relieve depression and improve the overall psychological and social well-being of elderly people with chronic physical illnesses.

Description

Origins

Qigong originated before recorded history. Scholars estimate qigong to be as old as 5,000–7,000 years old. Tracing the exact historical development of qigong is difficult, because it was passed down in secrecy among monks and teachers for many generations. Qigong survived through many years before paper was invented, and it also survived the Cultural Revolutions in China of the 1960s and 1970s, which banned many traditional practices.

Qigong has influenced and been influenced by many of the major strands of Chinese philosophy. The Taoist philosophy states that the universe operates within laws of balance and harmony, and that people must live within the rhythms of nature—ideas that pervade qigong. When Buddhism was brought from India to China around the seventh century A.D., **yoga** techniques and concepts of mental and spiritual awareness were introduced to qigong masters. The Confucian school was concerned with how people should live their daily lives, a concern of qigong as well. The martial arts were highly influenced by qigong, and many of them, such as **t'ai chi** and kung fu, developed directly from it. **Traditional Chinese medicine** also shares many of the central concepts of qigong, such as the patterns of energy flow in the body. **Acupuncture** and **acupressure** use the same points on the body that qigong seeks to stimulate. In China, qigong masters have been renowned physicians and healers. Qigong is often prescribed by Chinese physicians as part of the treatment.

Due to the political isolation of China, many Chinese concepts have been shrouded from the Western world. Acupuncture was "discovered" by American doctors only in the 1970s, although it had been in use for thousands of years. With an increased exchange of information, more Americans have gained access to the once-secret teachings of qigong. In 1988, the First World Conference for Academic Exchange of Medical Qigong was held in Beijing, China, where many studies were presented to attendees from around the world. In 1990, Berkeley, California, hosted the First International Congress of Qigong. In the past decade, more Americans have begun to discover the beneficial effects of qigong, which motivate an estimated 60 million Chinese to practice it every day.

Basic concepts

In Chinese thought, qi, or chi, is the fundamental life energy of the universe. It is invisible but present in air, water, food and sunlight. In the body, qi is the unseen vital force that sustains life. We are all born with inherited amounts of qi, and we also get acquired qi from the food we eat and the air we breathe. In qigong, the breath is believed to account for the largest quantity of acquired qi, because the body uses air more than any other substance. The balance of our physical, mental, and emotional levels also affect qi levels in the body.

Qi travels through the body along channels called meridians. There are 12 main meridians, corresponding to the 12 principal organs as defined by the traditional Chinese system: the lung, large intestines, stomach, spleen, heart, small intestine, urinary bladder, kidney, liver, gallbladder, pericardium, and the "triple warmer," which represents the entire torso region. Each organ has qi associated with it, and each organ interacts with particular emotions on the mental level. Qigong techniques are designed to improve the balance and flow of energy throughout the meridians, and to increase the overall quantity and volume of qi. In qigong philosophy, mind and body are not separated as they often are in Western medicine. In qigong, the mind is present in all parts of the body, and the mind can be used to move qi throughout the body.

Yin and yang are also important concepts in qigong. The universe and the body can be described by these two separate but complementary principles, which are always interacting, opposing, and influencing each other. One goal of qigong is to balance yin and yang within the body. Strong movements or techniques are balanced by soft ones, leftward movements by rightward, internal techniques by external ones, and so on.

Practicing qigong

There are thousands of qigong exercises. The specific ones used may vary depending on the teacher, school, and objective of the practitioner. Qigong is used for physical fitness, as a martial art, and most frequently for health and healing. Internal qigong is performed by those wishing to increase their own energy and health. Some qigong masters are renowned for being able to perform external qigong, by which the energy from one person is passed on to another for healing. This transfer may sound suspect to Western logic, but in the world of qigong there are some amazing accounts of healing and extraordinary capabilities demonstrated by qigong masters. Qigong masters generally have deep knowledge of the concepts of Chinese medicine and healing. In China, there are hospitals that use medical qigong to heal patients, along with herbs, acupuncture, and other techniques. In these hospitals, qigong healers use external qigong and also design specific internal qigong exercises for patients' problems.

There are basic components of internal qigong sessions. All sessions require warm-up and concluding exercises. Qigong consists of postures, movements, breathing techniques, and mental exercises. Postures may involve standing, sitting, or lying down. Movements include stretches, slow motions, quick thrusts, jumping, and bending. Postures and movements are designed to strengthen, stretch, and tone the body to improve the flow of energy. One sequence of postures and movements is known as the "Eight Figures for Every Day." This sequence is designed to quickly and effectively work the entire body, and is commonly performed daily by millions in China.

Breathing techniques include deep abdominal breathing, chest breathing, relaxed breathing, and holding breaths. One breathing technique is called the "Six Healing Sounds." This technique uses particular breathing sounds for each of six major organs. These sounds are believed to stimulate and heal the organs.

Meditations and mind exercises are used to enhance the mind and move qi throughout the body. These exercises are often visualizations that focus on different body parts, words, ideas, objects, or energy flowing along the meridians. One mental **exercise** is called the "Inner Smile," during which the practitioner visualizes joyful, healing energy being sent sequentially to each organ in the body. Another mental exercise is called the "Microscopic Orbit Meditation," in which the practitioner intently meditates on increasing and connecting the flow of qi throughout major channels.

Discipline is an important dimension of qigong. Exercises are meant to be performed every morning and evening. Sessions can take from 15 minutes to hours. Beginners are recommended to practice between 15–30 minutes twice a day. Beginners may take classes once or twice per week, with practice outside of class. Classes generally cost between $10–$20 per session.

Preparations

Qigong should be practiced in a clean, pleasant environment, preferably outdoors in fresh air. Loose and comfortable clothing is recommended. Jewelry should be removed. Practitioners can prepare for success at qigong by practicing at regular hours each day to promote discipline. Qigong teachers also recommend that students prepare by adopting lifestyles that promote balance, moderation, proper rest,

and healthy **diets**, all of which are facets of qigong practice.

Precautions

Beginners should learn from an experienced teacher, as performing qigong exercises in the wrong manner may cause harm. Practitioners should not perform qigong on either full or completely empty stomachs. Qigong should not be performed during extreme weather, which may have negative effects on the body's energy systems. Menstruating and pregnant women should perform only certain exercises.

Side effects

Side effects may occur during or after qigong exercises for beginners, or for those performing exercises incorrectly. Side effects may include **dizziness**, **dry mouth**, **fatigue**, headaches, **insomnia**, rapid heartbeat, **shortness of breath**, heaviness or **numbness** in areas of the body, emotional instability, **anxiety**, or decreased concentration. Side effects generally clear up with rest and instruction from a knowledgeable teacher.

Research and general acceptance

Western medicine generally does not endorse any of the traditional Chinese healing systems that utilize the concept of energy flow in the body, largely because this energy has yet to be isolated and measured scientifically. New research is being conducted using sophisticated equipment that may verify the existence of energy channels as defined by the Chinese system. Despite the lack of scientific validation, the results of energy techniques including qigong and acupuncture have gained widespread interest and respect. One California group of qigong practitioners now conducts twice-yearly retreats to improve their skills and energy level. Furthermore, qigong masters have demonstrated to Western observers astounding control over many physical functions, and some have even shown the ability to increase electrical voltage measured on their skin's surface. Most of the research and documentation of qigong's effectiveness for medical conditions has been conducted in China, and is slowly becoming more available to English readers. Papers from the World Conferences for Academic Exchange of Medical Qigong are available in English, and address many medical studies and uses of qigong. A video is now available that presents the basic concepts of medical qigong as well as specific exercise prescriptions for the treatment of **breast cancer**. The exercise

---

KEY TERMS

Martial arts—Group of diverse activities originating from the ancient fighting techniques of the Orient.

Meridians—Channels or conduits through which Qi travels in the body.

Qi—Basic life energy, according to traditional Chinese medicine.

Yin/Yang—Universal characteristics used to describe aspects of the natural world.

---

prescriptions consist of movements, postures, visualizations, and positive affirmations.

In terms of mainstream research in the United States, the first ongoing long-term study of qigong began in 1999 at the Center for Alternative and Complementary Medicine Research in Heart Disease at the University of Michigan; it focuses on the speed of healing of graft **wounds** in patients undergoing coronary bypass surgery. The National Center for Complementary and Alternative Medicine (NCCAM) has been funding studies of qigong since 2000. The first such study was conducted by a researcher in Arizona with patients using heart devices (**pacemakers**, etc.).

The breathing techniques of qigong are being studied intensively by Western physicians as of 2003 as a form of therapy for anxiety-related problems and for disorders involving the vocal cords. Qigong is also being used in the **rehabilitation** of patients with severe asthma or chronic obstructive pulmonary disease (COPD).

Training and certification

In China, qigong has been subject to much government regulation, from banning to increased requirements for teachers. In the United States at this time, qigong has not been regulated. Different schools may provide teacher training, but there are no generally accepted training standards. Qigong teachings may vary, depending on the founder of the school, who is often an acknowledged Chinese master. The organizations listed below can provide further information to consumers.

Resources

BOOKS

Pelletier, Kenneth R., MD. *The Best Alternative Medicine, Part I: Sound Mind, Sound Body: Qi Gong.* New York: Simon & Schuster, 2002.

PERIODICALS

Baker, S. E., C. M. Sapienza, and S. Collins. "Inspiratory Pressure Threshold Training in a Case of Congenital Bilateral Abductor Vocal Fold Paralysis." *International Journal of Pediatric Otorhinolaryngology* 67 (April 2003): 413–416.

Biggs, Q. M., K. S. Kelly, and J. D. Toney. "The Effects of Deep Diaphragmatic Breathing and Focused Attention on Dental Anxiety in a Private Practice Setting." *Dental Hygiene* 77 (Spring 2003): 105–113.

Emerich, K. A. "Nontraditional Tools Helpful in the Treatment of Certain Types of Voice Disturbances." *Current Opinion in Otolaryngology and Head and Neck Surgery* 11 (June 2003): 149–153.

Golden, Jane. "Qigong and Tai Chi as Energy Medicine." *Share Guide* (November-December 2001): 37.

Johnson, Jerry Alan. "Medical Qigong for Breast Disease." *Share Guide* (November-December 2001): 109.

Ram, F. S., E. A. Holloway, and P. W. Jones. "Breathing Retraining for Asthma." *Respiratory Medicine* 97 (May 2003): 501–507.

Tsang, H. W., C. K. Mok, Y. T. Au Yeung, and S. Y. Chan. "The Effect of Qigong on General and Psychosocial Health of Elderly with Chronic Physical Illnesses: A Randomized Clinical Trial." *International Journal of Geriatric Psychiatry* 18 (May 2003): 441–449.

ORGANIZATIONS

Chinese National Chi Kung Institute. PO Box 31578. San Francisco, CA 94131. (800) 824-2433.

International Chi Kung/Qi Gong Directory. 2730 29th Street. Boulder, CO 80301. (303) 442-3131.

National Center for Complementary and Alternative Medicine (NCCAM) Clearinghouse. P.O. Box 7923, Gaithersburg, MD 20898-7923. (888) 644-6226. < http://nccam.nih.gov >.

Qigong Human Life Research Foundation. PO Box 5327. Cleveland, OH 44101. (216) 475-4712.

OTHER

Qigong Magazine. PO Box 31578. San Francisco, CA 94131. (800) 824-2433.

Qi: The Journal of Traditional Eastern Health and Fitness. PO Box 221343. Chantilly, VA 22022. (202) 378 3859.

Douglas Dupler, MA
Rebecca J. Frey, PhD

Quadriplegia *see* **Paralysis**

Quarantine *see* **Isolation**

Quinidine *see* **Antiarrhythmic drugs**

Quinine *see* **Antimalarial drugs**

R

Rabbit fever *see* **Tularemia**

Rabies

Definition

Rabies is an acute viral disease of the central nervous system that affects humans and other mammals but is most common in carnivores (flesh-eaters). It is sometimes referred to as a **zoonosis**, or disease of animals that can be communicated to humans. Rabies is almost exclusively transmitted through saliva from the bite of an infected animal. Another name for the disease is *hydrophobia*, which literally means "fear of water," a symptom shared by half of all people infected with rabies. Other symptoms include **fever**, depression, confusion, painful **muscle spasms**, sensitivity to touch, loud noise, and light, extreme thirst, painful swallowing, excessive salivation, and loss of muscle tone. If rabies is not prevented by immunization, it is almost always fatal.

Description

Cases of rabies in humans are very infrequent in the United States and Canada, averaging one or two a year (down from over 100 cases annually in 1900), but the worldwide incidence is estimated to be between 30,000 and 50,000 cases each year. These figures are based on data collected by the World Health Organization (WHO) in 1997 and updated in 2002. Rabies is most common in developing countries in Africa, Latin America, and Asia, particularly India. Dog bites are the major origin of infection for humans in developing countries, but other important host animals may include the wolf, mongoose, raccoon, jackal, and bat. A group of researchers in India found that monkeys as well as dogs were frequent vectors of rabies. The team also reported that the male:female ratio of rabies patients in India is 4:1.

Most deaths from rabies in the United States and Canada result from bat bites; the most recent fatality was a 66-year-old man in California who died in September 2003. The **death** of a nine-year-old girl in Quebec in the fall of 2000 was the first case of human rabies in Canada since 1985. Public health officials eventually determined that the girl had been bitten while she was sleeping by a silver-haired bat that had gotten into the family's home.

On October 18, 2004, a Wisconsin teenager was diagnosed with full-blown rabies after suffering from a minor bat bite on September 12, 2004. Miraculously, she was cured of rabies after doctors induced **coma** and administered four **antiviral drugs** to her. Since the therapy was only given and successful for one case, its curative properties needs to be corroborated by other cases before it will be considered a viable treatment option. The case and the physicians' findings will be published in a medical journal.

People whose work frequently brings them in contact with animals are considered to be at higher risk than the general population. This would include those in the fields of veterinary medicine, animal control, wildlife work, and laboratory work involving live rabies virus. People in these occupations and residents of or travelers to areas where rabies is a widespread problem should consider being immunized.

In late 2002, rabies re-emerged as an important public health issue. Dr. Charles E. Rupprecht, director of the World Health Organization (WHO) Collaborating Center for Rabies Reference and Research, has listed several factors responsible for the increase in the number of rabies cases worldwide:

- Rapid evolution of the rabies virus. Bats in the United States have developed a particularly infectious form of the virus.

- Increased diversity of animal hosts for the disease.

- Changes in the environment that are bringing people and domestic pets into closer contact with infected wildlife.

- Increased movement of people and animals across international borders. In one recent case, a man who had contracted rabies in the Philippines was not diagnosed until he began to feel ill in the United Kingdom.

- Lack of advocacy about rabies.

Causes and symptoms

Rabies is caused by a rod- or bullet-shaped virus that belongs to the family Rhabdoviridae. The rabies virus is a member of a genus of viruses called lyssaviruses, which include several related viruses that infect insects as well as mammals. The rabies virus is usually transmitted via an animal bite, however, cases have also been reported in which the virus penetrated the body through infected saliva, moist tissues such as the eyes or lips, a scratch on the skin, or the transplantation of infected tissues. Inhalation of the virus in the air, as might occur in a highly populated bat cave, is also thought to occur.

From the bite or other area of penetration, the virus multiplies as it spreads along nerves that travel away from the spinal cord and brain (efferent nerves) and into the salivary glands. The rabies virus may lie dormant in the body for several weeks or months, but rarely much longer, before symptoms appear. Initially, the area around the bite may burn and be painful. Early symptoms may also include a **sore throat**, low-grade fever, **headache**, loss of appetite, **nausea and vomiting**, and **diarrhea**. Painful spasms develop in the muscles that control breathing and swallowing. The individual may begin to drool thick saliva and may have dilated or irregular pupils, increased tears and perspiration, and low blood pressure.

Later, as the disease progresses, the patient becomes agitated and combative and may exhibit increased mental confusion. The affected person usually becomes sensitive to touch, loud noises, and bright lights. The victim also becomes extremely thirsty, but is unable to drink because swallowing is painful. Some patients begin to dread water because of the painful spasms that occur. Other severe symptoms during the later stage of the disease include excessive salivation, **dehydration**, and loss of muscle tone. Death usually occurs three to 20 days after symptoms have developed. Unfortunately, recovery is very rare.

Diagnosis

After the onset of symptoms, blood tests and **cerebrospinal fluid (CSF) analysis** tests will be conducted. CSF will be collected during a procedure called a lumbar puncture in which a needle is used to withdraw a sample of CSF from the area around the spinal cord. The CSF tests do not confirm diagnosis but are useful in ruling out other potential causes for the patient's altered mental state.

The two most common diagnostic tests are the fluorescent antibody test and isolation of the rabies virus from an individual's saliva or **throat culture**. The fluorescent antibody test involves taking a small sample of skin (biopsy) from the back of the neck of the patient. If specific proteins, called antibodies, that are produced only in response to the rabies virus are present, they will bind with the fluorescent dye and become visible. Another diagnostic procedure involves taking a corneal impression in which a swab or slide is pressed lightly against the cornea of the eye to determine whether viral material is present.

Treatment

Until the most recent successful cure of a late-term rabies case can be validated with further success and validation from the medical community, the historic treatment options for rabies prevention immediately following a bite remains the most viable treatment. Because of the extremely serious nature of a rabies infection, the need for rabies immunizations will be carefully considered for anyone who has been bitten by an animal, based on a personal history and results of diagnostic tests.

If necessary, treatment includes the following:

- The wound is washed thoroughly with medicinal soap and water. Deep puncture **wounds** should be flushed with a catheter and soapy water. Unless absolutely necessary, a wound should not be sutured.

- Tetanus toxoid and **antibiotics** will usually be administered.

- Rabies **vaccination** may or not be given, based on the available information. If the individual was bitten by a domestic animal and the animal was captured, the animal will be placed under observation in quarantine for ten days. If the animal does not develop rabies within four to seven days, then no immunizations are required. If the animal is suspected of being rabid, it is killed, and the brain is examined for evidence of rabies infection. In cases involving bites from domestic animals where the animal is not available for examination, the decision for vaccination is made based on the prevalence of rabies within the region where the bite occurred. If the bite was from a wild animal and the animal was captured, it is generally killed because the incubation period of rabies is unknown in most wild animals.

• If necessary, the patient is vaccinated immediately, generally through the administration of human rabies immune globulin (HRIG) for passive immunization, followed by human diploid cell vaccine (HDCV) or rabies vaccine adsorbed (RVA) for active immunization. Passive immunization is designed to provide the individual with antibodies from an already immunized individual, while active immunization involves stimulating the individual's own immune system to produce antibodies against the rabies virus. Both rabies vaccines are equally effective and carry a lower risk of side effects than some earlier treatments. Unfortunately, however, in underdeveloped countries, these newer vaccines are usually not available. Antibodies are administered to the patient in a process called passive immunization. To do this, the HRIG vaccine is administered once, at the beginning of treatment. Half of the dose is given around the bite area, and the rest is given in the muscle. Inactivated viral material (antigenic) is then given to stimulate the patient's own immune system to produce antibodies against rabies. For active immunization, either the HDCV or RVA vaccine is given in a series of five injections. Immunizations are typically given on days one, three, seven, 14, and 28.

In those rare instances in which rabies has progressed beyond the point where immunization would be effective, the groundbreaking treatment involving a drug-induced coma and the administration of four different antiviral drugs will most likely be a radical treatment option. The traditional approach prior to October 2004 was to provide as much relief from **pain** and suffering as possible through medical intervention while waiting to see if survival was possible. The patient would be given medication to prevent seizures, relieve some of the **anxiety**, and relieve painful muscle spasms. Pain relievers would also be given. In the later stages, aggressive supportive care would be provided to maintain breathing and heart function. Survival via the traditional treatment is rare but can occur.

Prognosis

If preventative treatment is sought promptly, rabies need not be fatal. Immunization is almost always effective if started within two days of the bite. Chance of effectiveness declines, however, the longer vaccination is put off. It is, however, important to start

---

KEY TERMS

Active immunization—Treatment that provides immunity by challenging an individual's own immune system to produce antibody against a particular organism, in this case the rabies virus.

Antibody—A specific protein produced by the immune system in response to a specific foreign protein or particle called an antigen.

Biopsy—The removal of a small sample of tissue for diagnostic purposes.

Efferent nerves—Nerves that convey impulses away from the central nervous system to the periphery.

Fluorescent antibody test (FA test)—A test in which a fluorescent dye is linked to an antibody for diagnostic purposes.

Lumbar puncture—A procedure that involves withdrawing a small sample of cerebrospinal fluid from the back around the spinal cord.

Lyssavirus—A genus of viruses that includes the rabies virus and related viruses that infect insects as well as mammals.

Passive immunization—Treatment that provides immunity through the transfer of antibodies obtained from an immune individual.

Rhabdovirus—A type of virus named for its rod- or bullet-like shape. The rabies virus belongs to a family of viruses called Rhabdoviridae.

Vector—An animal or insect that carries a disease-producing organism.

Zoonosis—Any disease of animals that can be transmitted to humans. Rabies is an example of a zoonosis.

---

immunizations, even if it has been weeks or months following a suspected rabid animal bite, because the vaccine can be effective even in these cases. If immunizations do not prove effective or are not received, rabies is nearly always fatal with a few days of the onset of symptoms.

As of October 2004, the medical community awaits the publication of findings by the doctors that administered a life-saving treatment that cured a Wisconsin teenager of full-blown rabies. Further test cases will prove whether or not this treatment option will be a historic development in the search for a cure for rabies.

Prevention

One promising preventive strategy that has been used since the early 2000s is the distribution of wildlife baits containing an oral vaccine against rabies. This strategy has been used in Germany to vaccinate wild foxes, which are frequent carriers of the disease in Europe. In the United States, veterinary researchers at Kansas State University have developed an oral vaccine for fruit bats; early trials of the vaccine have given promising results.

The following precautions should be observed in environments where humans and animals may likely come into contact.

- Domesticated animals, including household pets, should be vaccinated against rabies. If a pet is bitten by an animal suspected to have rabies, its owner should contact a veterinarian immediately and notify the local animal control authorities. Domestic pets with current vaccinations should be revaccinated immediately; unvaccinated dogs, cats, or ferrets are usually euthanized (put to sleep). Further information about domestic pets and rabies is available on the American Veterinary Medical Association (AVMA) web site.

- Wild animals should not be touched or petted, no matter how friendly they may appear. It is also important not to touch an animal that appears ill or passive, or whose behavior seems odd, such as failing to show the normal fear of humans. These are all possible signs of rabies. Many animals, such as raccoons and skunks, are nocturnal and their activity during the day should be regarded as suspicious.

- People should not interfere in fights between animals.

- Because rabies is transmitted through saliva, a person should wear rubber gloves when handling a pet that has had an encounter with a wild animal.

- Garbage or pet food should not be left outside the house or camp site because it may attract wild or stray animals.

- Windows and doors should be screened. Some victims of rabies have been attacked by infected animals, particularly bats, that entered through unprotected openings.

- State or county health departments should be consulted for information about the prevalence of rabies in an area. Some areas, such as New York City, have been rabies-free, only to have the disease reintroduced at a later time.

- Preventative vaccination against rabies should be considered if one's occupation involves frequent contact with wild animals or non-immunized domestic animals.

- Bites from mice, rats, or squirrels rarely require rabies prevention because these rodents are typically killed by any encounter with a larger, rabid animal, and would, therefore, not be carriers.

- Travelers should ask about the prevalence of the disease in countries they plan to visit.

Resources

BOOKS

Beers, Mark H., MD, and Robert Berkow, MD., editors. "Central Nervous System Viral Diseases: Rabies (Hydrophobia)." Section 13, Chapter 162 In *The Merck Manual of Diagnosis and Therapy*. Whitehouse Station, NJ: Merck Research Laboratories, 2004.

PERIODICALS

Chhabra, M., R. L. Ichhpujani, K. N. Tewari, and S. Lal. "Human Rabies in Delhi." *Indian Journal of Pediatrics* 71 (March 2004): 217–220.

Deshaies, D., P. A. Pilon, L. Valiquette, and J. Carsley. "A Public Health Intervention at the Time of a Case of Rabies in Quebec." [in French] *Canadian Journal of Public Health* 95 (March-April 2004): 138–141.

Fooks, A. R., N. Johnson, S. M. Brookes, et al. "Risk Factors Associated with Travel to Rabies Endemic Countries." *Journal of Applied Microbiology* 94, Supplement (2003): 31S–36S.

"Human Death Associated with Bat Rabies—California, 2003." *Morbidity and Mortality Weekly Report* 53 (January 23, 2004): 33–35.

Messenger, S. L., J. S. Smith, L. A. Orciari, et al. "Emerging Pattern of Rabies Deaths and Increased Viral Infectivity." *Emerging Infectious Diseases* 9 (February 2003): 151–154.

Peters, C., R. Isaza, D. J. Heard, et al. "Vaccination of Egyptian Fruit Bats (*Rousettus aegyptiacus*) with Monovalent Inactivated Rabies Vaccine." *Journal of Zoo and Wildlife Medicine* 35 (March 2004): 55–59.

Rosenthal, Elisabeth. "Girl is first to survive rabies without a shot." *The New York Times* November 25, 2004: A28.

Smith, J., L. McElhinney, G. Parsons, et al. "Case Report: Rapid Ante-Mortem Diagnosis of a Human Case of Rabies Imported Into the UK from the Philippines." *Journal of Medical Virology* 69 (January 2003): 150–155.

Stringer, C. "Post-Exposure Rabies Vaccination." *Nursing Standard* 17 (February 5-11, 2003): 41–42.

Thulke, H. H., T. Selhorst, T. Muller, et al. "Assessing Anti-Rabies Baiting—What Happens on the Ground?" *BMC Infectious Diseases* 4 (March 9, 2004): 9.

Weiss, R. A. "Cross-Species Infections." *Current Topics in Microbiology and Immunology* 278 (2003): 47–71.

ORGANIZATIONS

American Veterinary Medical Association (AVMA). 1931 North Meacham Road, Suite 100, Schaumburg, IL 60173-4360. < http://www.avma.org >.

Centers for Disease Control and Prevention. 1600 Clifton Rd., NE, Atlanta, GA 30333. (800) 311-3435, (404) 639-3311. <http://www.cdc.gov>.

Institut Pasteur. 25-28, rue du Dr. Roux, 75015 Paris, France. +33 (0) 1 45 68 80 00. <http://www.pasteur.fr/haut_ext.html>.

OTHER

CDC. "Epidemiology of Rabies." <http://www.cdc.gov/ncidod/dvrd/rabies/Epidemiology/Epidemiology.htm>.

National Association of State Public Health Veterinarians, Inc. "Compendium of Animal Rabies Prevention and Control, 2003." *Morbidity and Mortality Weekly Report Recommendations and Reports* 52 (March 21, 2003) (RR-5): 1–6.

Janet Byron Anderson
Rebecca J. Frey, PhD

Radial keratotomy

Definition

Radial keratotomy (RK) is a type of eye surgery used to correct **myopia** (nearsightedness). It works by changing the shape of the cornea–the transparent part of the eye that covers the iris and the pupil.

Purpose

About 25–30% of all people in the world are nearsighted and need eyeglasses or contact lenses for distance vision to be clear. For a number of reasons, some people don't like wearing corrective lenses. Some feel unattractive in eyeglasses. Others worry about not being able to see without their glasses in an emergency, such as a house fire or a burglary. Both glasses and contact lenses can be scratched, broken, or lost. In addition, contact lenses require special care and can irritate the eyes.

Radial keratotomy was introduced in North America in 1978. Since then doctors have improved the technique, and its results have become more predictable. Radial keratotomy is one of several surgical techniques to correct nearsightedness, reducing or eliminating the need for corrective lenses. It is most successful in patients with a low to moderate amount of nearsightedness–people whose eyes require up to -5.00 diopters of correction. A diopter (D) is a unit of measure of focusing power. Minus lenses correct nearsightedness.

Precautions

Not every nearsighted person is a good candidate for radial keratotomy. This type of surgery cannot help people whose nearsightedness is caused by keratoconus, a rare condition in which the cornea is cone shaped. The procedure usually is not done on patients under 18, because their eyes are still growing and changing shape. It is important that visual status is stable. Women who are pregnant, have just given birth, or are breast-feeding should not have the surgery because hormonal changes may cause temporary changes in the cornea. In addition, anyone with **glaucoma** or with any disease that interferes with healing (e.g., **rheumatoid arthritis**, lupus erythematosus, or uncontrolled diabetes) should not have RK.

Radial keratotomy weakens the cornea, making it vulnerable to injuries even long after the surgery. Getting hit in the head after having RK can cause the cornea to tear and can lead to blindness. For this reason, the procedure is not recommended for people who engage in sports that could result in a blow to the head (i.e., karate or racquetball).

It is important to keep in mind that RK is a permanent procedure and that success cannot be guaranteed. An experienced eye surgeon can estimate how likely it is that the surgery will help a particular patient, but that is just an estimate. There is no way to know for sure whether the surgery will improve eyesight enough to eliminate the need for corrective lenses. Vision usually improves after RK, but it is not always perfect. Anyone who decides to have RK should be prepared to accept less-than-perfect vision after surgery, which may necessitate the continued use of glasses or contact lenses. This surgery does not eliminate the need for reading glasses. Actually, someone who didn't need reading glasses before surgery because their myopia allowed near vision to be clear may find themselves needing reading glasses. Patients must ask about this prior to surgery.

Anyone considering RK should also be aware that certain professions, including branches of the military, are not open to people who have had the procedure.

A reputable ophthalmologist will discuss the risks of the procedure and should tell anyone considering it that perfect vision can't be guaranteed. Patients should be wary of any doctor who tries too hard to "sell" them on RK.

Description

In a person with clear vision, light passes through the cornea and the lens of the eye and focuses on a

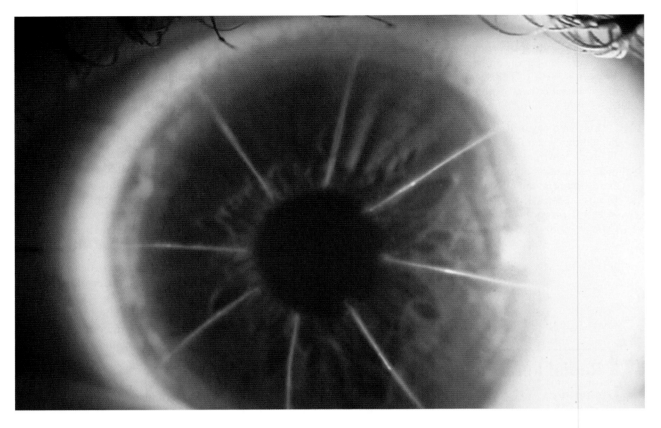

Radial keratotomy scars on the cornea of an eye. *(Photograph by Bob Masini, Phototake NYC. Reproduced by permission.)*

membrane lining the back of the eye called the retina. In a person with myopia, the eyeball is usually too long, so light focuses in front of the retina. Radial keratotomy reduces myopia by flattening the cornea. This reduces the focusing power of the cornea allowing light to focus further back onto the retina (or at least closer to it), forming a clearer image.

A surgeon performing RK uses a very small diamond-blade knife to makes four to eight radial incisions around the edge of the cornea. These slits are made in a pattern that resembles the spokes of wheel. As the cornea heals, its center flattens out.

Radial keratotomy is usually performed in an ophthalmologist's office. Before the surgery begins, the patient may be given medicine to help him or her relax. A local anesthetic–usually in the form of eye drops–is used to numb the eye, but the patient remains conscious during the procedure. The surgeon looks through a surgical microscope while making the slits. The treatment usually takes no more than 30 minutes.

Some ophthalmologists will perform RK on both eyes at once but others prefer to do one eye at a time. It once was thought that surgeons could use the results of the first eye to predict how the well the procedure would work on the second eye. However, a study published in 1997 found that this was not the case. The authors of the study cautioned that there might be other reasons not to operate on both eyes at once, such as increased risk of infection and other complications.

The cost for RK depends on the surgeon, but usually ranges from \$1,000–\$1,500 per eye. Medical insurance usually does not cover RK, because it is considered an elective procedure–one that people choose to have done.

Preparation

Before beginning the procedure, the surgeon marks an area in the center of the cornea called the optical zone. This is the part of the cornea that one sees through (it is the area over the pupil). No cuts are made in this region. The surgeon also measures the cornea's thickness, to decide how deep the slits should be.

Aftercare

After the surgery is over, the anesthetic wears off. Some patients feel slight **pain** and are given eye drops and medications to relieve their discomfort. For several days after the surgery, the eye that was treated may feel scratchy and look red. This is normal. The eye may also water, burn slightly, and be sensitive to light.

As with any type of surgery, it is important to guard against infection. Patients are given eye drops to protect against infection and may be told to use them for several weeks after the surgery. Because RK weakens the cornea it is important to protect the head and eyes.

The cornea heals slowly, and full recovery can take several months (another reason not to have the surgery done on both eyes at the same time). While the cornea is healing, patients may experience these problems:

- Variations in vision. Eyesight may be better in the morning than in the evening or vice versa.

- Temporary pain.

- Increased glare.

- Starburst or halo effects. Rays or rings of light around lights at night.

- Hyperopic shift. As the cornea flattens, vision may become more farsighted (hyperopic). For this reason, the surgeon may initially undercorrect the patient. This gradual shift may occur over several years.

If RK does not completely correct a person's nearsightedness, glasses or contact lenses may be needed. In general, people who were able to wear contact lenses before the procedure can still wear them afterward. Even patients whose nearsightedness was corrected may still need glasses for reading. This is especially true for middle-aged and older patients. The lens of the eye stiffens with age, making reading glasses necessary (**presbyopia**). Radial keratotomy does not correct this problem.

The surgeon who performs the RK procedure will tell the patient how often to return for follow-up visits. Often, two to four visits are needed, including one the day after surgery. It is also important to know what side effects should be reported immediately to the surgeon (e.g., pain or **nausea**).

Risks

Complications from RK are rare, but they can occur. These include:

- cataract a clouding of the lens of the eye, resulting in partial or total loss of vision

- serious infection

- lasting pain

KEY TERMS

Cornea—The transparent part of the eye that covers the iris and the pupil.

Diopter (D)—Unit describing the amount of focusing power of a lens.

Iris—The colored part of the eye.

Laser-assisted in situ keratomileusis (LASIK)—A type of refractive eye surgery using a laser and another instrument to change the shape of the cornea.

Local anesthetic—Used to numb an area where surgery or another procedure is to be done, without causing the patient to lose consciousness.

Myopia—Nearsightedness. People with myopia cannot see distant objects clearly.

Ophthalmologist—A physician who specializes in treating eyes.

Photorefractive keratectomy (PRK)—A type of refractive eye surgery using a laser to change the shape of the cornea.

Pupil—The part of the eye that looks like a black circle in the center of the iris. It is actually an opening through which light passes.

Retina—A membrane lining the back of the eye onto which light is focused to form images.

- rips along an incision, especially after being hit in the head or eye

- loss of vision

- chance of overcorrection (hyperopic shift)

The chances of complications are reduced when the surgery is done by an ophthalmologist with a lot of experience in RK. Younger patients also tend to heal faster.

Normal results

The desired result of radial keratotomy is a reduction in myopia. A major study by the National Eye Institute, reported in 1994, tracked the success of RK in 374 patients who had had the procedure done 10 years earlier. The study found that:

- 85% had at least 20/40 vision (the acuity considered good enough to drive without glasses)

- 70% did not need glasses or contact lenses for distance vision

- 53% had 20/20 vision without glasses
- 30% still needed glasses or contact lenses to see clearly
- 1–3% had worse vision than before they had RK
- 40% had a hyperopic shift.

As with all surgeries, RK has risks. These risks include having worse vision than before the surgery; halos; glare; and although rare, blindness. Some aftereffects, such as halos or glare may last for years. Other refractive surgeries, such as photorefractive keratectomy (PRK) and laser-assisted in situ keratomileusis (LASIK) use lasers to change the shape of the cornea and they may produce fewer side effects. It is important to speak with an experienced eye surgeon who has done many refractive surgeries to fully understand the options and risks involved before making a decision.

Resources

ORGANIZATIONS

American Academy of Ophthalmology. 655 Beach Street, P.O. Box 7424, San Francisco, CA 94120-7424. <http://www.eyenet.org>.

American Optometric Association. 243 North Lindbergh Blvd., St. Louis, MO 63141. (314) 991-4100. <http://www.aoanet.org>.

American Society of Cataract & Refractive Surgery. 4000 Legato Road, Suite 850, Fairfax, VA 22033. (703) 591-2220. <http://www.ascrs.org>.

Nancy Ross-Flanigan

▌Radiation injuries

Definition

Radiation injuries are caused by ionizing radiation emitted by sources such as the sun, x-ray and other diagnostic machines, tanning beds, and radioactive elements released in nuclear power plant accidents and detonation of nuclear weapons during war and as terrorist acts.

Description

Ionizing radiation is made up of unstable atoms that contain an excess amount of energy. In an attempt to stabilize, the atoms emit the excess energy into the atmosphere, creating radiation. Radiation can either be electromagnetic or particulate.

The energy of electromagnetic radiation is a direct function of its frequency. The high–energy, high–frequency waves that can penetrate solids to various depths cause damage by separating molecules into electrically charged pieces, a process known as ionization. X rays are a type of electromagnetic radiation. Atomic particles come from radioactive isotopes as they decay to stable elements. Electrons are called beta particles when they radiate. Alpha particles are the nuclei of helium atoms—two protons and two neutrons—without the surrounding electrons. Alpha particles are too large to penetrate a piece of paper unless they are greatly accelerated in electric and magnetic fields. Both beta and alpha particles are types of particulate radiation. When over-exposure to ionizing radiation occurs, there is chromosomal damage in deoxyribonucleic acid (DNA). DNA is very good at repairing itself; both strands of the double helix must be broken to produce genetic damage.

Because radiation is energy, it can be measured. There are a number of units used to quantify radiation energy. Some refer to effects on air, others to effects on living tissue. The roentgen, named after Wilhelm Conrad Roentgen, who discovered x rays in 1895, measures ionizing energy in air. A rad expresses the energy transferred to tissue. The rem measures tissue response. A roentgen generates about a rad of effect and produces about a rem of response. The gray and the sievert are international units equivalent to 100 rads and rems, respectively. A curie, named after French physicists who experimented with radiation, is a measure of actual radioactivity given off by a radioactive element, not a measure of its effect. The average annual human exposure to natural background radiation is roughly 3 milliSieverts (mSv).

Any amount of ionizing radiation will produce some damage, however, there is radiation everywhere, from the sun (cosmic rays) and from traces of radioactive elements in the air (radon) and the ground (uranium, radium, carbon-14, potassium-40 and many others). Earth's atmosphere protects us from most of the sun's radiation. Living at 5,000 feet altitude in Denver, Colorado, doubles exposure to radiation, and flight in a commercial airliner increases it 150-fold by lifting us above 80% of that atmosphere. Because no amount of radiation is perfectly safe and because radiation is ever present, arbitrary limits have been established to provide some measure of safety for those exposed to unusual amounts. Less than 1% of them reach the current annual permissible maximum of 20 mSv.

A 2001 ruling by the Federal Court of Australia indicated that two soldiers died from **cancer** caused by minimal exposure to radiation while occupying Hiroshima in 1945. The soldiers were exposed to less than 5 mSv of radiation. The international recommendation for workers is safety level of up to 20 mSv. The ruling and its support by many international agencies suggests that even extremely low doses of radiation can be potentially harmful.

Ultraviolet (UV) radiation exposure from the sun and tanning beds

UV radiation from the sun and tanning beds and lamps can cause skin damage, premature **aging**, and skin cancers. **Malignant melanoma** is the most dangerous of skin cancers and there is a definite link between type UVA exposure used in tanning beds and its occurrence. UVB type UV radiation is associated with **sunburn**, and while not as penetrating as UVA, it still damages the skin with over exposure. Skin damage accumulates over time, and effects do not often manifest until individuals reach middle age. Light-skinned people who most often burn rather than tan are at a greater risk of skin damage than darker-skinned individuals that almost never burn. The U.S. Food and Drug Administration (FDA) and the Centers for Disease Control (CDC) discourage the use of tanning beds and sun lamps and encourage the use of sunscreen with at least an SPF of 15 or greater.

Over exposure during medical procedures

Ionizing radiation has many uses in medicine, both in diagnosis and in treatment. X rays, CT scanners, and fluoroscopes use it to form images of the body's insides. Nuclear medicine uses radioactive isotopes to diagnose and to treat medical conditions. In the body, radioactive elements localize to specific tissues and give off tiny amounts of radiation. Detecting that radiation provides information on both anatomy and function. During the past 10 years, skin injuries caused by too much exposure during a medical procedure have been documented. In 1995, the FDA issued a recommendation to physicians and medical institutions to record and monitor the dosage of radiation used during medical procedures on patients in order to minimize the amount of skin injuries. The FDA suggested doses of radiation not exceed 1 Grey (Gy). (A Grey is roughly equivalent to a sievert.) As of 2001, the FDA was preparing further guidelines for fluoroscopy, the procedure most often associated with medical-related radiation skin injuries such as **rashes** and more serious **burns** and tissue death. Injuries occurred most often during **angioplasty** procedures using fluoroscopy.

CT scans of children have also been problematic. Oftentimes the dosage of radiation used for an adult isn't decreased for a child, leading to radiation over exposure. Children are more sensitive to radiation and a February 2001 study indicates 1,500 out of 1.6 million children under 15 years of age receiving CT scans annually will develop cancer. Studies show that decreasing the radiation by half for CT scans of children will effectively decrease the possibility of over exposure while still providing an effective diagnostic image. The benefits to receiving the medical treatment utilizing radiation is still greater than the risks involved, however, more stringent control over the amount of radiation used during the procedures will go far to minimize the risk of radiation injury to the patient.

Radiation exposure from nuclear accidents, weaponry, and terrorist acts

Between 1945 and 1987, there were 285 nuclear reactor accidents, injuring over 1,550 people and killing 64. The most striking example was the meltdown of the graphite core nuclear reactor at Chernobyl in 1986, which spread a cloud of radioactive particles across the entire continent of Europe. Information about radiation effects is still being gathered from that disaster, however 31 people were killed in the immediate accident and 1,800 children have thus far been diagnosed with **thyroid cancer**. In a study published in May 2001 by the British Royal Society, children born to individuals involved in the cleanup of Chernobyl and born after the accident are 600% more likely to have genetic mutations than children born before the accident. These findings indicate that exposure to low doses of radiation can cause inheritable effects.

Since the terrorist attack on the World Trade Center and the Pentagon on September 11, 2001, the possibility of terrorist-caused nuclear accidents has been a growing concern. All 103 active nuclear power plants in the United States are on full alert, but they are still vulnerable to sabotage such as bombing or attack from the air. A no-fly zone of 12 miles below 18,000 feet has been established around nuclear power plants by the Federal Aviation Administration (FAA). There is also growing concern over the security of spent nuclear fuel—more than 40,000 tons of spent fuel is housed in buildings at closed plants around the country. Unlike the active nuclear reactors that are enclosed in concrete-reinforced buildings, the spent fuel is stored in non-reinforced buildings. Housed in cooling pools, the spent fuel could emit dangerous levels of radioactive material if exploded or used in makeshift weaponry. Radioactive medical and industrial waste could also be used to make "dirty

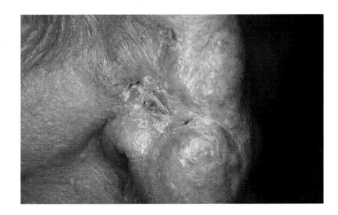

This person's nose is inflamed and scaly due to radiation exposure. *(Custom Medical Stock Photo. Reproduced by permission.)*

bombs." Since 1993, the Nuclear Regulatory Commission (NRC) has reported 376 cases of stolen radioactive materials.

Causes and symptoms

Radiation can damage every tissue in the body. The particular manifestation will depend upon the amount of radiation, the time over which it is absorbed, and the susceptibility of the tissue. The fastest growing tissues are the most vulnerable, because radiation as much as triples its effects during the growth phase. Bone marrow cells that make blood are the fastest growing cells in the body. A fetus in the womb is equally sensitive. The germinal cells in the testes and ovaries are only slightly less sensitive. Both can be rendered useless with very small doses of radiation. More resistant are the lining cells of the body—skin and intestines. Most resistant are the brain cells, because they grow the slowest.

The length of exposure makes a big difference in what happens. Over time the accumulating damage, if not enough to kill cells outright, distorts their growth and causes scarring and/or cancers. In addition to leukemias, cancers of the thyroid, brain, bone, breast, skin, stomach, and lung all arise after radiation. Damage depends, too, on the ability of the tissue to repair itself. Some tissues and some types of damage produce much greater consequences than others.

There are three types of radiation injuries.

- External irradiation: as with x-ray exposure, all or part of the body is exposed to radiation that either is absorbed or passes through the body.

- Contamination: as with a nuclear accident, the environment and its inhabitants are exposed to radiation.

People are affected internally, externally, or with both internal and external exposure.

- Incorporation: dependent on contamination, the bodies of individuals affected incorporate the radiation chemicals within cells, organs, and tissues and the radiation is dispersed throughout the body.

Immediately after sudden irradiation, the fate of those affected depends mostly on the total dose absorbed. This information comes mostly from survivors of the atomic bomb blasts over Japan in 1945.

- Massive doses incinerate immediately and are not distinguishable from the heat of the source.

- A sudden whole body dose over 50 Sv produces such profound neurological, heart, and circulatory damage that patients die within the first two days.

- Doses in the 10–20 Sv range affect the intestines, stripping their lining and leading to death within three months from **vomiting**, **diarrhea**, **starvation**, and infection.

- Victims receiving 6–10 Sv all at once usually escape an intestinal death, facing instead bone marrow failure and death within two months from loss of blood coagulation factors and the protection against infection provided by white blood cells.

- Between 2–6 Sv gives a fighting chance for survival if victims are supported with blood transfusions and **antibiotics**.

- One or two Sv produces a brief, non-lethal sickness with vomiting, loss of appetite, and generalized discomfort.

Treatment

It is clearly important to have some idea of the dose received as early as possible, so that attention can be directed to those victims in the 2–10 Sv range that might survive with treatment. Blood transfusions, protection from infection in damaged organs, and possibly the use of newer stimulants to blood formation can save many victims in this category.

Local radiation exposures usually damage the skin and require careful wound care, removal of dead tissue, and **skin grafting** if the area is large. Again **infection control** is imperative.

One of the best known, and perhaps even mainstream, treatments of radiation injury is the use of *Aloe vera* preparations on damaged areas of skin. It has demonstrated remarkable healing properties even for chronic ulcerations resulting from radiation exposure.

Alternative treatment

There is considerable interest these days in benevolent chemicals called "free radical scavengers." How well they work is yet to be determined, but population studies strongly suggest that certain **diets** are better than others, and that those diets are full of free radical scavengers, otherwise known as antioxidants. The recommended ingredients are beta-carotene, **vitamins** E and C, and selenium, all available as commercial preparations. Beta-carotene is yellow-orange and is present in yellow and orange fruits and vegetables. Vitamin C can be found naturally in citrus fruits. **Traditional Chinese medicine** (TCM) and **acupuncture**, botanical medicine, and homeopathy all have contributions to make to recovery from the damage of radiation injuries. The level of recovery will depend on the exposure. Consulting practitioners trained in these modalities will result in the greatest benefit.

Resources

PERIODICALS

Grunwald, Michael, and Peter Behr. "Are Nuclear Plants Secure? Industry Called Unprepared for Sept. 11-Style Attack." *The Washington Post* November 3, 2001, p. A01.

Vergano, Dan. " 'Dirty' Bombs Latest Fear." *USA Today* November 3, 2001.

Jacqueline L. Longe

Radiation sickness *see* **Radiation injuries**

Radiation therapy

Definition

Radiation therapy, sometimes called radiotherapy, x-ray therapy radiation treatment, cobalt therapy, electron beam therapy, or irradiation uses high energy, penetrating waves or particles such as x rays, gamma rays, proton rays, or neutron rays to destroy **cancer** cells or keep them from reproducing.

Purpose

The purpose of radiation therapy is to kill or damage cancer cells. Radiation therapy is a common form of cancer therapy. It is used in more than half of all cancer cases. Radiation therapy can be used:

- alone to kill cancer
- before surgery to shrink a tumor and make it easier to remove
- during surgery to kill cancer cells that may remain in surrounding tissue after the surgery (called intraoperative radiation)
- after surgery to kill cancer cells remaining in the body
- to shrink an inoperable tumor in order to and reduce **pain** and improve quality of life.
- in combination with **chemotherapy**

For some kinds of cancers such as early-stage **Hodgkin's disease**, non-Hodgkin's lymphoma, and certain types of prostate, or brain cancer, radiation therapy alone may cure the disease. In other cases, radiation therapy used in conjunction with surgery, chemotherapy, or both, increases survival rates over any of these therapies used alone.

Precautions

Radiation therapy does not make the person having the treatments radioactive. In almost all cases, the benefits of this therapy outweigh the risks. However radiation therapy can have has serious consequences, so anyone contemplating it should be sure understand why the treatment team believes it is the best possible treatment option for their cancer. Radiation therapy is often not appropriate for pregnant women, because the radiation can damage the cells of the developing baby. Women who think they might be pregnant should discuss this with their doctor.

Description

Radiation therapy is a local treatment. It is painless. The radiation acts only on the part of the body that is exposed to the radiation. This is very different from chemotherapy in which drugs circulate throughout the whole body. There are two main types of radiation therapy. In external radiation therapy a beam of radiation is directed from outside the body at the cancer. In internal radiation therapy, called brachytherapy or implant therapy, where a source of radioactivity is surgically placed inside the body near the cancer.

How radiation therapy works

The protein that carries the code controlling most activities in the cell is called deoxyribonucleic acid or DNA. When a cell divides, its DNA must also double and divide. High-energy radiation kills cells by damaging their DNA, thus blocking their ability to grow and increase in number.

One of the characteristics of cancer cells is that they grow and divide faster than normal cells. This makes them particularly vulnerable to radiation. Radiation also damages normal cells, but because normal cells are growing more slowly, they are better able to repair radiation damage than are cancer cells. In order to give normal cells time to heal and reduce side effects, radiation treatments are often given in small doses over a six or seven week period.

External radiation therapy

External radiation therapy is the most common kind of radiation therapy. It is usually done during outpatient visits to a hospital clinic and is usually covered by insurance.

Once a doctor, called a radiation oncologist, determines the proper dose of radiation for a particular cancer, the dose is divided into smaller doses called fractions. One fraction is usually given each day, five days a week for six to seven weeks. However, each radiation plan is individualized depending on the type and location of the cancer and what other treatments are also being used. The actual administration of the therapy usually takes about half an hour daily, although radiation is administered for only from one to five minutes at each session. It is important to attend every scheduled treatment to get the most benefit from radiation therapy.

Recently, trials have begun to determine if there are ways to deliver radiation fractions so that they kill more cancer cells or have fewer side effects. Some trials use smaller doses given more often. Up-to-date information on voluntary participation in clinical trials and where they are being held is available by entering the search term "radiation therapy" at the following web sites:

- National Cancer Institute. < http://cancertrials.nci.nih.gov > or (800) 4-CANCER.
- National Institutes of Health Clinical Trials. < http://clinicaltrials.gov >
- Center Watch: A Clinical Trials Listing. < http://www.centerwatch.com > .

The type of machines used to administer external radiation therapy and the material that provides the radiation vary depending on the type and location of the cancer. Generally, the patient puts on a hospital gown and lies down or sits in a special chair. Parts of the body not receiving radiation are covered with special shields that block the rays. A technician then directs a beam of radiation to a pre-determined spot on the body where the cancer is located. The patient must stay still during the administration of the radiation so that no other parts of the body are affected. As an extra precaution in some treatments, special molds are made to make sure the body is in the same position for each treatment. However, the treatment itself is painless, like having a bone x-rayed.

Internal radiation therapy

Internal radiation therapy is called brachytherapy, implant therapy, interstitial radiation, or intracavitary radiation. With internal radiation therapy, a bit of radioactive material is sealed in an implant (sometimes called a seed or capsule). The implant is then placed very close to the cancer. The advantage of internal radiation therapy is that it concentrates the radiation near the cancer and lessens the chance of damage to normal cells. Many different types of radioactive materials can be used in the implant, including cesium, iridium, iodine, phosphorus, and palladium.

How the implant is put near the cancer depends on the size and location of the cancer. Internal radiation therapy is used for some cancers of the head, neck, thyroid, breast, female reproductive system, and prostate. Most people will have the radioactive capsule implanted by a surgeon while under either general or **local anesthesia** at a hospital or surgical clinic.

Patients receiving internal radiation therapy do become temporarily radioactive. They must remain in the hospital during the time that the implant stays in place. The length of time is determined by the type of cancer and the dose of radioactivity to be delivered. During the time the implant is in place, the patient will have to stay in bed and remain reasonably still.

While the implant is in place, the patient's contact with other people will be limited. Healthcare workers will make their visits as brief as possible to avoid exposure to radiation, and visitors, especially children and pregnant women, will be limited.

The implant usually can be removed in a simple procedure without an anesthetic. As soon as the implant is out of the body, the patient is no longer radioactive, and restrictions on being with other people are lifted. Generally people can return to a level of activity that feels comfortable to them as soon as the implant is removed. Occasionally the site of the implant is sore for some time afterwards. This discomfort may limit specific activities.

In some cases, an implant is left permanently inside the body. People who have permanent implants need to stay in the hospital and away from other people for the first few days. Gradually the radioactivity of the implant decreases, and it is safe to be around other people.

Radioimmunotherapy

Radioimmunotherapy is a promising way to treat cancer that has spread (metastasized) to multiple locations throughout the body. Antibodies are immune system proteins that specifically recognize and bind to only one type of cell. They can be designed to bind only with a certain type of cancer cell. To carry out radioimmunotherapy, antibodies with the ability to bind specifically to a patient's cancer cells are attached to radioactive material and injected into the patient's bloodstream. When these man-made antibodies find a cancer cell, they bind to it. Then the radiation kills the cancer cell. This process is still experimental, but because it can be used to selectively attack only cancer cells, it holds promise for eliminating cancers that have spread beyond the primary tumor.

Radiation used to treat cancer

PHOTON RADIATION. Early radiation therapy used x rays like those used to take pictures of bones, or gamma rays. X rays and gamma rays are high energy rays composed of massless particles of energy (like light) called photons. The distinction between the two is that gamma rays originate from the decay of radioacive substances (like radium and cobalt-60), while x rays are generated by devices that excite electrons (such as cathode ray tubes and linear accelerators). These high energy rays act on cells by disrupting the electrons of atoms within the molecules inside cells, disrupting cell functions, and most importantly stop their ability to divide and make new cells.

PARTICLE RADIATION. Particle radiation is radiation delivered by particles that have mass. Proton therapy has been used since the early 1990s. Proton rays consist of protons, a type of positively charged atomic particle, rather than photons, which have neither mass nor charge. Like x rays and gamma rays, proton rays disrupt cellular activity. The advantage of using proton rays is that they can be shaped to conform to the irregular shape of the tumor more precisely than x rays and gamma rays. They allow delivery of higher radiation doses to tumors without increasing damage to the surrounding tissue.

Neutron therapy is another type of particle radiation. Neutron rays are very high-energy rays. They are composed of neutrons, which are particles with mass but no charge. The type of damage they cause to cells is much less likely to be repaired than that caused by x rays, gamma rays, or proton rays.

Neutron therapy can treat larger tumors than conventional radiation therapy. Conventional radiation therapy depends on the presence of oxygen to work. The center of large tumors lack sufficient oxygen to be susceptible to damage from conventional radiation. Neutron radiation works in the absence of oxygen, making it especially effective for the treatment of inoperable **salivary gland tumors**, bone cancers, and some kinds of advanced cancers of the pancreas, bladder, lung, prostate, and uterus.

Recent advances in radiation therapy

A newer mode of treating brain cancers with radiation therapy is known as stereotactic radiosurgery. As of the early 2000s, this approach is limited to treating cancers of the head and neck because only these parts of the body can be held completely still throughout the procedure. Stereotactic radiosurgery allows the doctor to deliver a single high-level dose of precisely directed radiation to the tumor without damaging nearby healthy brain tissue. The treatment is planned with the help of three-dimensional computer-aided analysis of CT and MRI scans. The patient's head and neck are held steady in a skeletal fixation device during the actual treatment. Stereotactic radiosurgery can be used in addition to standard surgery to treat a recurrent **brain tumor**, or in place of surgery if the tumor cannot be reached by standard surgical techniques.

Two major forms of stereotactic radiosurgery are in use as of 2003. The gamma knife is a stationary machine that is most useful for small tumors, blood vessels, or similar targets. Because it does not move, it can deliver a small, highly localized and precise beam of radiation. Gamma knife treatment is done all at once in a single hospital stay. The second type of radiosurgery uses a movable linear accelerator-based machine that is preferred for larger tumors. This treatment is delivered in several small doses given over several weeks. Radiosurgery that is performed with divided doses is known as fractionated radiosurgery. The total dose of radiation is higher with a linear accelerator-based machine than with gamma knife treatment.

Another advance in intraoperative radiotherapy (IORT) is the introduction of mobile devices that allow the surgeon to use radiotherapy in early-stage disease and to operate in locations where it would be difficult to transport the patient during surgery for radiation treatment. Mobile IORT units have been used successfully as of 2003 in treating early-stage **breast cancer** and **rectal cancer**.

Radiation sensitizers are another recent innovation in radiation therapy. Sensitizers are medications that are given to make cancer cells easier to kill by radiation than normal calls. Gemcitabine (Gemzar) is one of the drugs most commonly used for this purpose.

Preparation

Before radiation therapy, the size and location of the patient's tumor are determined very precisely using **magnetic resonance imaging** (MRI) and/or **computed tomography scans** (CT scans). The correct radiation dose, the number of sessions, the interval between sessions, and the method of application are calculated by a radiation oncologist based on the tumor type, its size, and the sensitivity of the nearby tissues.

The patient's skin is be marked with a semi-permanent ink to help the radiation technologist achieve correct positioning for each treatment. Molds may be built to hold tissues in exactly the right place each time.

Aftercare

Many patients experience skin burn, **fatigue**, **nausea**, and **vomiting** after radiation therapy regardless of the where radiation is applied. After treatment, the skin around the site of the treatment may also become sore. Affected skin should be kept clean and can be treated like **sunburn**, with skin lotion or vitamin A and D ointment. Patients should avoid perfume and scented skin products and protect affected areas from the sun.

Nausea and vomiting are most likely to occur when the radiation dose is high or if the abdomen or another part of the digestive tract is irradiated. Sometimes nausea and vomiting occur after radiation to other regions, but in these cases the symptoms usually disappear within a

---

KEY TERMS

Anemia—Insufficient red blood cells in the body.

Antibody—Protein molecule that recognizes and binds specifically to a foreign substance in the body in order to eliminate it.

Chemotherapy—Injecting drugs into the body where they circulate and kill cancer cells.

Computed tomography (CT or CAT) scan—Using x rays taken from many angles and computer modeling, CT scans help locate and size tumors and provide information on whether they can be surgically removed.

Fractionation—A procedure for dividing a dose of radiation into smaller treatment doses.

Gamma rays—Short wavelength, high energy electromagnetic radiation emitted by radioactive substances.

Hodgkin's disease—Cancer of the lymphatic system, characterized by lymph node enlargement and the presence of a large polyploid cells called Reed-Sternberg cells.

Magnetic resonance imaging (MRI)—MRI uses magnets and radio waves to create detailed cross-sectional pictures of the interior of the body.

Stereotactic—Characterized by precise positioning in space. When applied to radiosurgery, stereotactic refers to a system of three-dimensional coordinates for locating the target site.

---

few hours after treatment. Nausea and vomiting can be treated with **antacids**, Compazine, Tigan, or Zofran.

Fatigue frequently starts after the second week of therapy and may continue until about two weeks after the therapy is finished. Patients may need to limit their activities, take naps, and get extra sleep at night.

Patients should see their oncologist (cancer doctor) at least once within the first few weeks after their final radiation treatment. They should also see an oncologist every six to twelve months for the rest of their lives so they can be checked to see if the tumor has reappeared or spread.

Risks

Radiation therapy can cause anemia, nausea, vomiting, **diarrhea**, hair loss, skin burn, sterility, and rarely **death**. However, the benefits of radiation therapy almost always exceed the risks. Patients should discuss the risks with their doctor and get a second opinion about their treatment plan.

Normal results

The outcome of radiation treatment varies depending on the type, location, and stage of the cancer. For some cancers such as Hodgkin's disease, about 75% of the patients are cured. **Prostate cancer** also responds well to radiation therapy. Radiation to painful bony metastases is usually a dramatically effective form of pain control. Other cancers may be less sensitive to the benefits of radiation.

Resources

PERIODICALS

Goer, D. A., C. W. Musslewhite, and D. M. Jablons. "Potential of Mobile Intraoperative Radiotherapy Technology." *Surgical Oncology Clinics of North America* 12 (October 2003): 943–954.

Lawrence, T. S. "Radiation Sensitizers and Targeted Therapies." *Oncology (Huntington)* 17 (December 2003): 23–28.

Merrick, H. W. IIIrd, L. L. Gunderson, and F. A. Calvo. "Future Directions in Intraoperative Radiation Therapy." *Surgical Oncology Clinics of North America* 12 (October 2003): 1099–1105.

Nag, S., and K. S. Hu. "Intraoperative High-Dose-Rate Brachytherapy." *Surgical Oncology Clinics of North America* 12 (October 2003): 1079–1097.

Witt, M. E., M. Haas, M. A. Marrinan, and C. N. Brown. "Understanding Stereotactic Radiosurgery for Intracranial Tumors, Seed Implants for Prostate Cancer, and Intravascular Brachytherapy for Cardiac Restenosis" *Cancer Nursing* 26 (December 2003): 494–502.

ORGANIZATIONS

American Cancer Society. 1599 Clifton Rd. NE, Atlanta GA 30329-4251. (800) ACS-2345. < http://www.cancer.org >.

International Radiosurgery Support Association (IRSA). 3005 Hoffman Street, Harrisburg, PA 17110. (717) 260-9808. < http://www.irsa.org >.

National Association for Proton Therapy. 7910 Woodmont Ave., Suite 1303, Bethesda, MD 20814. (301) 913-9360. < http://www.proton-therapy.org/Default.htm >.

OTHER

Radiation Therapy and You. A Guide to Self-Help During Treatment. National Cancer Institute CancerNet Information Service. < http://cancernet.nci.nih.gov >.

Lorraine Lica, PhD
Rebecca J. Frey, PhD

Radiation treatments *see* **Radiation therapy**

Radical neck dissection

Definition

Radical neck dissection is an operation used to remove cancerous tissue in the head and neck.

Purpose

The purpose of radical neck dissection is to remove lymph nodes and other structures in the head and neck that are likely or proven to be malignant. Variations on neck dissections exist depending on the extent of the **cancer**. A radical neck dissection removes the most tissue. It is done when the cancer has spread widely in the neck. A modified neck dissection removes less tissue, and a selective neck dissection even less.

Precautions

This operation should not be done if cancer has metastasized (spread) beyond the head and neck, or if the cancer has invaded the bones of the cervical vertebrae (the first seven vertebrae of the spinal column) or the skull. In these cases, the surgery will not effectively contain the cancer.

Description

Cancers of the head and neck (sometimes inaccurately called throat cancer) often spread to nearby tissues and into the lymph nodes. Removing these structures is one way of controlling the cancer.

Of the 600 hundred lymph nodes in the body, about 200 are in the neck. Only a small number of these are removed during a neck dissection. In addition, other structures such as muscles, veins, and nerves may be removed during a radical neck dissection. These include the sternocleidomastoid muscle (one of the muscles that functions to flex the head), internal jugular (neck) vein, submandibular gland (one of the salivary glands), and the spinal accessory nerve (a nerve that helps control speech, swallowing and certain movements of the head and neck). The goal is always to remove all the cancer but to save as many components surrounding the nodes as possible.

Radical neck dissections are done in a hospital under **general anesthesia** by a head and neck surgeon. An incision is made in the neck, and the skin is pulled back to reveal the muscles and lymph nodes. The surgeon is guided in what to remove by tests done

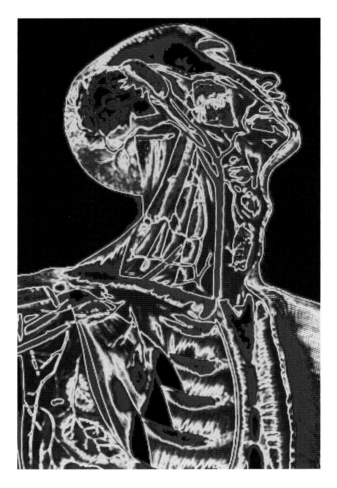

A digitized illustration of the human head and chest showing nasal passages, sinuses, trachea, vascular nerves, as well as ribs and parts of the lungs. *(Custom Medical Stock Photo. Reproduced by permission.)*

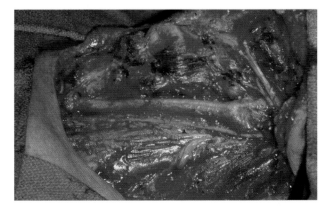

A specimen taken from radical neck surgery. *(Custom Medical Stock Photo. Reproduced by permission.)*

prior to surgery and by examination of the size and texture of the lymph nodes.

Preparation

Radical neck dissection is a major operation. Extensive tests are done before the operation to try to determine where and how far the cancer has spread. These may include lymph node biopsies, CT (computed tomography) scans, MRI scans, and barium swallows. In addition, standard pre-operative blood and **liver function tests** are performed, and the patient will meet with an anesthesiologist before the operation. The patient should tell the anesthesiologist about all drug **allergies** and all medication (prescription, non-prescription, or herbal) that he or she is taking.

Aftercare

A person who has had a radical neck dissection will stay in the hospital several days after the operation, and sometimes longer if surgery to remove the primary tumor was done at the same time. Drains are inserted under the skin to remove the fluid that accumulates in the neck area. Once the drains are removed and the incision appears to be healing well, patients are usually discharged from the hospital, but will require follow-up doctor visits. Depending on how many structures are removed, a person who has had a radical neck dissection may require physical therapy to regain use of the arm and shoulder.

Risks

The greatest risk in a radical neck dissection is damage to the nerves, muscles, and veins in the neck. Nerve damage can result in **numbness** (either temporary or permanent) to different regions on the neck and loss of function (temporary or permanent) to parts of the neck, throat, and shoulder. The more extensive the neck dissection, the more function the patient is likely to lose. As a result, it is common following radical neck dissection for a person to have stooped shoulders, limited ability to lift the arm, and limited head and neck rotation and flexion due to the removal of nerves and muscles. Other risks are the same as for all major surgery: potential bleeding, infection, and allergic reaction to anesthesia.

Normal results

Normal lymph nodes are small and show no cancerous cells under the microscope.

KEY TERMS

Barium swallow—Barium is used to coat the throat in order to take x-ray pictures of the tissues lining the throat.

Computed tomography (CT or CAT) scan—Using x rays taken from many angles and computer modeling, CT scans help size and locate tumors and provide information on whether they can be surgically removed.

Lymphatic system—Primary defense against infection in the body. The tissues, organs, and channels (similar to veins) that produce, store, and transport lymph and white blood cells to fight infection.

Lymph nodes—Small, bean-shaped collections of tissue found in lymph vessels. They produce cells and proteins that fight infection and filter lymph. Nodes are sometimes called lymph glands.

Malignant—Cancerous. Cells tend to reproduce without normal controls on growth and form tumors or invade other tissues.

Metastasize—Spread of cells from the original site of the cancer to other parts of the body where secondary tumors are formed.

Magnetic resonance imaging (MRI)—MRI uses magnets and radio waves to create detailed cross-sectional pictures of the interior of the body.

Abnormal results

Abnormal lymph nodes may be enlarged and show malignant cells when examined under the microscope.

Resources

ORGANIZATIONS

American Cancer Society. 1599 Clifton Road NE, Atlanta, GA 30329. (800) ACS-2345). < http:// www.cancer.org >.

Cancer Information Service. National Cancer Institute, Building 31, Room 10A19, 9000 Rockville Pike, Bethesda, MD 20892. (800) 4-CANCER. < http:// www.nci.nih.gov/cancerinfo/index.html >.

OTHER

The Voice Center at Eastern Virginia Medical School. February 17, 2001. [cited June 7, 2001]. < http:// www.voice-center.com >.

John T. Lohr, PhD
Tish Davidson, A.M.

Radioactive implants

Definition

Radioactive implants are devices that are placed directly within cancerous tissue or tumors, in order to deliver **radiation therapy** intended to kill cancerous cells. The practice of internal radiation therapy also is referred to as brachytherapy.

Purpose

With the use of radioactive implants, the tumor is subjected to radioactive activity over a longer period of time, as compared to external beam therapy.

Precautions

The patient is required to remain in his or her bed or room during the treatment. During the period of greatest radioactivity (24–72 hours), health care providers will limit the amount of time spent with the patient to that required for essential care. Some radiation exposure to family members has been noted with certain radiation implants. However, a study in 2003 found that exposure to family members of **prostate cancer** patients, an increasingly more commonly treated group of patients to receive implants, is low.

Description

Interstitial radiation therapy places the sources of radiation directly into the tumor and surrounding tissue. Most commonly used in tumors of the head, neck, prostate, and breast, it also may be used in combination with external radiation therapy. The implant may be permanent or removable. A permanent implant of radioactive seeds, such as gold or iodine, is placed directly into the organ. Over several weeks or months, the seeds slowly deliver radiation to the tumor. More commonly used is the removable implant that requires an operation under **general anesthesia** to place narrow, hollow stainless steel needles through the tumor. Teflon tubes are inserted through the needles, and the needles are then removed. After the patient returns to his or her room, radioactive seeds are inserted into the tubes in a procedure called afterloading. Once the desired dosage is reached, the tubes and seeds are removed.

The planning and procedures used for treatment with radioactive implants is becoming increasingly accurate and sophisticated as technology develops. Special imaging tools and computer software help physicians and radiation therapists visualize implant

KEY TERMS

Ageusia—The loss of taste perception.

Alopecia—The loss of hair, or baldness.

Dysgeusia—Unpleasant alteration of taste sensation, often with a metallic taste.

Hypogeusia—Diminshed taste perception.

placements. Further, improved radiologic imaging techniques help physicians track the progress of this and other **cancer** therapies.

Intracavity radiation often is used for gynecologic cancers. Under general or spinal anesthesia, hollow applicators are placed directly inside the affected organ. Correct positioning is confirmed by x rays, and once the patient has returned to his or her room, a small plastic tube containing the radioactive isotope is inserted into the hollow applicator. The treatment is delivered over 48–72 hours, after which time the applicator and radioactive sources are removed. Very high doses of radiation can be delivered to the tumor, while the rapid removal of the radioactive dose limits damage to the surrounding structures.

Abnormal results

Normal cells are subjected to the effects of radiation; any tissue near the radiation site may be damaged or destroyed. Some side effects are acute and temporary, while others develop over time and may be permanent. Skin reactions, such as redness, **itching**, flaking, or stripping of the top layer, usually are temporary; long-term effects can include scarring, and changes in texture. Radiation recall is a delayed skin side effect in which the area that had been exposed to radiation becomes irritated or blistered after the patient receives certain **chemotherapy**.

Following treatment for tumors of the head and neck region, the lining of the mouth and throat can become inflamed or irritated, resulting in a condition known as mucositis or **stomatitis**. Injury to the salivary glands can decrease saliva production, resulting in a condition known as xerostomia, or **dry mouth**. There also may be alteration in the patient's taste buds, resulting in decrease or loss of taste sensation (hypogeusia or ageusia), or the presence of unpleasant taste, sometimes described as metallic (dysgeusia). Patients may experience **nausea and vomiting** as a result of the effect of radiation on the brain. Hair loss (**alopecia**) may result from radiation's effect on hair follicles.

Radiation's effect on the rapidly growing cells of the gastrointestinal tract may result in **diarrhea** or abdominal cramping. Pelvic radiation can affect the bowel, bladder, or sexual function. Radiation also can affect production of blood cell components in the bone marrow.

Resources

PERIODICALS

"Brachytherapy Software Receives FDA Approval." *Urology Times* August 2003: 48.

"Radiation Exposure Among Family Members of Prostate Brachytherapy Patients Appears to be Low." *Urology Times* September 2003: 12.

ORGANIZATIONS

American Cancer Society. 1599 Clifton Rd., NE, Atlanta, GA 30329-4251. (800) 227-2345. < http://www.cancer.org >.

National Cancer Institute. Building 31, Room 10A31, 31 Center Drive, MSC 2580, Bethesda, MD 20892-2580. (800) 422-6237. < http://www.nci.nih.gov >.

Kathleen D. Wright, RN
Teresa G. Odle

Radioactive iodine uptake test *see* **Thyroid nuclear medicine scan**

Radioallergosorbent test (RAST) *see* **Allergy tests**

Radiotherapy *see* **Radiation therapy**

Raloxifene *see* **Bone disorder drugs**

Range-of-motion exercises *see* **Exercise**

Rape and sexual assault

Definition

The various definitions of rape range from the broad (coercing a person to engage in any sexual act) to the specific (forcing a woman to submit to sexual intercourse). The United States Code includes the crime of rape under the more comprehensive term "sexual abuse." Two types of sexual assault are defined in the code: sexual **abuse** and aggravated sexual abuse. Sexual abuse includes acts in which an individual is forced to engage in sexual activity by use of threats or other fear tactics, or instances in which an individual is physically unable to decline. Aggravated sexual abuse occurs when an individual is forced to submit to sexual acts by use of physical force; threats of **death**, injury, or kidnapping; or substances that render that individual unconscious or impaired.

Description

Many misconceptions exist about rape and sexual assault. It is often assumed that rape victims are all women who have been attacked by a total stranger and forced into having sexual intercourse. In reality, sexual assault can take many forms—it may be violent or nonviolent; the victim may be male or female, child or adult; the offender may be a stranger, relative, friend, authority figure, or spouse.

The number of sexual assaults reported depends on how those abuses are defined. The United States Code uses two terms to distinguish between different sexual activities:

- Sexual act: contact between penis and vagina or penis and anus that involves penetration; contact between the mouth and genitals or anus; penetration of the vagina or anus with an object; or direct touching (not through clothing) of the genitals of an individual under the age of 16.

- Sexual contact: intentional touching of the genitals, breasts, buttocks, anus, inner thigh, or groin with no sexual penetration.

National statistics

According to the Federal Bureau of Investigation's *Uniform Crime Reports*, there were 95,136 forcible rapes reported to United States law enforcement agencies in 2002. Sixty-five out of every 100,000 women were reported to be victims of rape that year, up 4.7% from 2001 but down 3.9% from 1998. The actual number of rapes and sexual assaults, however, is in reality much larger; estimates of unreported rape range between 2 and 10 times the number reported to law enforcement. The National Violence Against Women Survey, jointly sponsored by the Centers for Disease Control and Prevention (CDC) and the National Institute of Justice (NIJ) and conducted in the mid-1900s, found that one in six women (18%) and one in 33 men (3%) has experienced an attempted or completed rape. The survey estimated that approximately 17,722,672 women and 2,782,440 men in the United States have been raped or have had rape attempted as a child or adult, and that 302,091 women and 92,748 men were raped in the 12 months prior to the study.

There are numerous reasons why the majority of sexual assaults are never reported. Often the victim

What To Do If You Are Raped

Don't bathe
Don't blame yourself
Retain all evidence
Get examined
Consider the "morning-after" pill

fears retaliation from the offender. He or she may be afraid of family, friends, the community, or the media learning about the offense. There may be a concern about being judged or blamed by others. The victim may think that no one will believe the assault occurred.

THE VICTIMS. The 2000 "Victim, Incident, and Offender Characteristics," published by the National Center for Juvenile Justice (NCJJ), analyzed sexual assault data collected by law enforcement agencies over a five-year span. The following characteristics were found to be significant among victims of sexual assault:

- Age: Over two-thirds of reported victims of sexual assault were juveniles under the age of 18. Twelve to 18 year olds represented the largest group of victims at 33%; 20% were between the ages of six and 11; children less than five years old and adults between 18 and 24 years of age each constituted 14% of victims; 12% were between the ages of 25 and 34; and 7% were over the age of 34. Persons over the age of 54 represented 1% of all victims. One out of every seven victims surveyed in the study were under the age of six.

- Gender: Females were more than six times more likely to be a victim of sexual assault then males; more than 86% of victims were females. The great majority (99%) of the victims of forcible rapes were women, while men constituted the majority (54%) of the victims of forcible sodomy (oral or anal intercourse). Females are most likely to be the victim of sexual assault at age 14, while males are at most risk at age four.

- Location: The residence of the victim was the most commonly noted location of sexual assault (70%). Other common locations included schools, hotels/motels, fields, woods, parking lots, roadways, and commercial/office buildings.

- Weapons: A personal weapon (hands, feet, or fists) was used in 77% of cases. No weapon was noted in 14% of assaults; other weapons (knifes, clubs, etc.) were used in 6% of cases. Firearms were involved in only 2% of assaults.

THE OFFENDERS. Similar statistics were gathered by the NCJJ regarding the perpetrators of rape and sexual assault. These characteristics included:

- Age: Over 23% of offenders were under the age of 18; juveniles were more likely to be perpetrators of forcible sodomy and fondling. The remaining 77% of offenders were adults and were responsible for 67% of juvenile victims. For younger juvenile victims (under the age of 12), juvenile offenders were responsible for approximately 40% of assaults.

- Gender: The great majority of all reported offenders were male (96%). The number of female offenders rose for victims under the age of six (12%), in contrast to 6% for victims aged six through 12, 3% for victims aged 12 through 17, and 1% for adult victims.

- Relationship with offender: Approximately 59% of offenders were acquaintances of their victims, compared to family members (27%) or strangers (14%). Family members were more likely to be perpetrators against juveniles (34%) than against adults (12%). In contrast, strangers accounted for 27% of adult victims and 7% of juveniles.

- Past offenses: In 19% of juvenile cases, the victim was not the only individual to be assaulted by the offender, compared to only 4% of adult cases.

Consequences

Victims of sexual assault may sustain a range of injuries; male victims are more likely than females to suffer severe physical trauma. The National Women's Study, funded by the National Institute of Drug Abuse, found that more than 70% of rape victims report no physical injuries as a result of their assault; only 4% sustain serious injuries that require hospitalization. At least 49% of victims, however, state that they feared severe injuries or death during their assault. Fatalities occur in approximately 0.1% of rape cases.

Sexually transmitted diseases (STDs) are a source of concern for many victims of sexual assault. The most commonly transmitted diseases are **gonorrhea** (caused by *Neisseria gonorrhoeae*), chlamydia (caused by *Chlamydia trachomatis*), **trichomoniasis**) (caused by *Trichomonas vaginalis*), and **genital warts** (caused by human papillomavirus). **Syphilis** (caused by *Treponema pallidum*) and human **immunodeficiency** virus (HIV) are also noted among some sexual assault victims. The transmission rate of STDs is estimated to be between 3.6% and 30% of rapes.

According to the National Women's Study, approximately 5% of adult female rape victims become pregnant as a result of their assault, leading

---

Common Misconceptions Of Males Perpetrating Date Rape

Since I took her out and paid for the date, she should have sex with me.
When she says no, she really means yes.
If she's aroused, she wants to have sex.
She wouldn't go parking with me if she didn't want to have sex.
If she didn't wan to have sex, why did she let me go as far as she did?
If she gets me erect, then it's her responsibility to do something about it.
She's slept with other people, so she should sleep with me.
We've had sex before, and she didn't say no then.

---

to 32,100 pregnancies a year among women 18 years of age or older. Approximately 50% of pregnant rape victims had an abortion, 6% put the child up for adoption, and 33% kept the child (the remaining pregnancies resulted in **miscarriage**).

MENTAL HEALTH PROBLEMS. Also known as rape trauma syndrome, **post-traumatic stress disorder** (PTSD) is a mental health disorder that describes a range of symptoms often experienced by someone who has undergone a severely traumatic event. Approximately 31% of rape victims develop PTSD as a result of their assault; victims are more than six times more likely to develop PTSD than women who have not been victimized.

The symptoms of PTSD include:

- recurrent memories or flashbacks of the incident
- nightmares
- insomnia
- mood swings
- difficulty concentrating
- panic attacks
- emotional numbness
- depression
- **anxiety**

Persons who have been sexually assaulted have also been noted to have increased risk for developing other mental health problems. Over those who have not been victimized, rape victims are:

- three times more likely to have a major depressive episode
- four times more likely to have contemplated suicide
- thirteen times more likely to develop alcohol dependency problems
- twenty-six times more likely to develop drug abuse problems

Treatment

Once a victim of sexual assault reports the crime to local authorities, calls a rape crisis hotline, or arrives at the emergency room to be treated for injuries, a multidisciplinary team is often formed to address his or her physical, psychological, and judicial needs. This team usually includes law enforcement officers, physicians, nurses, mental health professionals, victim advocates, and/or prosecutors.

The victim of sexual assault may continue to feel fear and anxiety for some time after the incident, and in some instances this may significantly impact his or her personal or professional life. Follow-up counseling should therefore be provided for the victim, particularly if symptoms of PTSD become evident.

Forensic medical examination

Because rape is a crime, there are certain requirements for medical evaluation of the patient and for record keeping. The forensic medical examination is an invaluable tool for collecting evidence against a perpetrator that may be admissible in court. Since the great majority of victims know their assailant, the purpose of the medical examination is often not to establish identity but to establish nonconsensual sexual contact. The Sexual Assault Nurse Examiner program is an effective model that is used in many United States hospitals and clinics to collect and document evidence, evaluate and treat for STDs and **pregnancy**, and refer victims to follow-up medical care and counseling. The "Sexual Assault Nurse Examiner Development and Operation Guide," prepared by the Sexual Assault Resource Service, describes the ideal protocol for collecting evidence from a sexual assault victim. This includes:

- performing the medical examination within 72 hours of the assault
- taking a history of the assault
- documenting the general health of the victim, including menstrual cycle, potential **allergies**, and pregnancy status
- assessment for trauma and taking photographic evidence of injuries
- taking fingernail clippings or scrapings
- taking samples for sperm or seminal fluid
- combing head/pubic hair for foreign hairs, fibers, and other substances
- collection of bloody, torn, or stained clothing
- taking samples for **blood typing** and DNA screening

Prevention

STD Prevention

While the concern of sexual assault victims of contracting an STD is often high, the actual risk of transmission is relatively low; the CDC estimates that the risk of contracting gonorrhea from an offender is between 6% and 12%, chlamydia between 4% and 17%, syphilis between 0.5% and 3%, and HIV less than 1%. Nonetheless, post-exposure **prophylaxis** (preventative treatment) against certain STDs is often provided for the victim. Treatment with zidovudine, for example, is recommended for individuals who are at a high risk of exposure to HIV. The CDC recommends the following prophylactic regimen be provided for victims of sexual assaults in which vaginal, oral, or anal penetration took place:

- a single dose of ceftriaxone, an antibiotic effective against *Neisseria gonorrhoeae*
- a single dose of metronidazole, an antibiotic effective against *Trichomonas vaginalis*
- a single dose of azithromycin or doxycycline, **antibiotics** effective against *Chlamydia trachomatis*
- inoculation with the post-exposure **hepatitis B** vaccine

In some instances, cultures may be taken during the medical examination and at time points afterward to test for gonorrhea or chlamydia. It is important that the victim receive information regarding the symptoms of STDs and be counseled to return for further examination if any of these symptoms occur.

Pregnancy prevention

Female victims at risk for becoming pregnant after an assault should be counseled on the availability of **emergency contraception**. According to the Food and Drug Administration (FDA), emergency **contraception** is not effective if there is no pregnancy but works to prevent pregnancy from occurring by delaying or preventing ovulation, by affecting the transport of sperm, and/or by thinning the inner layer of the uterus (endometrium) so that implantation is prevented. It is therefore not a form of abortion.

A number of options are available for women if they choose to use emergency contraceptives to prevent pregnancy following a sexual assault. The Yupze regimen uses two oral contraceptive pills that contain both of the hormones estrogen and progestin. The risk of pregnancy is reduced by 75% after use of the Yupze regimen, reducing the average number of pregnancies after unprotected sex from eight in 100 to two in 100.

KEY TERMS

Aggravated sexual abuse—When an individual is forced to submit to sexual acts by use of physical force; threats of death, injury, or kidnapping; or substances that render that individual unconscious or impaired.

Forcible sodomy—Forced oral or anal intercourse.

Forensic—Pertaining to or used during legal proceedings.

Post-traumatic stress disorder (PTSD)—Also known as rape trauma syndrome; a mental health disorder that describes a range of symptoms often experienced by someone who has undergone a severely traumatic event.

Sexual abuse—When an individual is forced to engage in sexual activity by use of threats or other fear tactics, or instances in which an individual is physically unable to refuse.

Sexual assault nurse examiner (SANE)—A registered nurse who is trained to collect and document evidence from a sexual assault victim, evaluate and treat for STDs and pregnancy, and refer victims to follow-up medical care and counseling.

Yupze regimen—A form of emergency contraception in which two oral contraceptive pills that contain both of the hormones estrogen and progestin are taken to prevent pregnancy.

Progestin-only **oral contraceptives** are also available and reduce the risk of pregnancy by 89% to 95%.

Resources

BOOKS

American Psychiatric Association. *Diagnostic and Statistical Manual of Mental Disorders*, 4th ed., revised. Washington, DC: American Psychiatric Association, 2000.

Beers, Mark H., MD, and Robert Berkow, MD., editors. "Medical Examination of the Rape Victim." Section 18, Chapter 244 In *The Merck Manual of Diagnosis and Therapy*. Whitehouse Station, NJ: Merck Research Laboratories, 2004.

Beers, Mark H., MD, and Robert Berkow, MD., editors. "Psychosexual Disorders." Section 15, Chapter 192 In *The Merck Manual of Diagnosis and Therapy*. Whitehouse Station, NJ: Merck Research Laboratories, 2004.

Federal Bureau of Investigation. *Uniform Crime Reports: Crime in the United States—2002*. Washington, DC: Government Printing Office, 2003.

PERIODICALS

Brewin, C. R., and E. A. Holmes. "Psychological Theories of Posttraumatic Stress Disorder." *Clinical Psychology Review* 23 (May 2003): 339–376.

Bushman, B. J., A. M. Bonacci, M. van Dijk, and R. F. Baumeister. "Narcissism, Sexual Refusal, and Aggression: Testing a Narcissistic Reactance Model of Sexual Coercion." *Journal of Personal and Social Psychology* 84 (May 2003): 1027–1040.

Frazier, P. A. "Perceived Control and Distress Following Sexual Assault: A Longitudinal Test of a New Model." *Journal of Personal and Social Psychology* 84 (June 2003): 1257–1269.

Koss, M. P., K. J. Bachar, and C. Q. Hopkins. "Restorative Justice for Sexual Violence: Repairing Victims, Building Community, and Holding Offenders Accountable." *Annals of the New York Academy of Science* 989 (June 2003): 384–396.

Reynolds, Matthew W., Jeffery Peipert, and Beverly Collins. "Epidemiologic Issues of Sexually Transmitted Diseases in Sexual Assault Victims." *Obstetrical and Gynecological Survey* 55 (January 2000): 51–57.

ORGANIZATIONS

American Psychiatric Association (APA). 1400 K Street, NW, Washington, DC 20005. (888) 357-7924. < http://www.psych.org >.

Federal Bureau of Investigation. J. Edgar Hoover Building, 935 Pennsylvania Avenue, NW, Washington, DC 20535-0001. (202) 324-3000. < http://www.fbi.gov >.

Rape, Abuse, and Incest National Network. 635-B Pennsylvania Ave. SE, Washington, DC 20003. (800) 656-HOPE.

United States Department of Justice, Office for Victims of Crime. 810 7th Street NW, Washington, DC 20531.

OTHER

Kilpatrick, Dean G., Anna Whalley, and Christine Edmunds. "Sexual Assault." In *2000 National Victim Assistance Academy Textbook*, edited by Anne Seymour, Morna Murray, Jane Sigmon, Christine Edmunds, Mario Gaboury, and Grace Coleman. October 2000.

Ledray, Linda E. "Sexual Assault Nurse Examiner Development and Operation Guide." *Sexual Assault Resource Service*. August 1999.

"National Crime Victim's Rights Week: Resource Guide." *U.S. Department of Justice, Office for Victims of Crime.* April 2001.

"Rape Fact Sheet: Prevalence and Incidence." *Centers for Disease Control and Prevention*. February 10, 2000.

Snyder, Howard N. "Sexual Assault of Young Children as Reported to Law Enforcement: Victim, Incident, and Offender Characteristics." *National Center for Juvenile Justice*. July 2000.

Stéphanie Dionne
Rebecca J. Frey, PhD

Rashes

Definition

The popular term for a group of spots or red, inflamed skin that is usually a symptom of an underlying condition or disorder. Often temporary, a rash is only rarely a sign of a serious problem.

Description

A rash may occur on only one area of the skin, or it could cover almost all of the body. Also, a rash may or may not be itchy. Depending on how it looks, a rash may be described as:

- blistering (raised oval or round collections of fluid within or beneath the outer layer of skin)

- macular (flat spots)

- nodular (small, firm, knotty rounded mass)

- papular (small solid slightly raised areas)

- pustular (pus-containing skin blister).

Causes and symptoms

There are many theories as to the development of skin rashes, but experts are not completely clear what causes some of them. Generally a skin rash is an intermittent symptom, fading and reappearing. Rashes may accompany a range of disorders and conditions, such as:

- Infectious illness. A rash is symptom of many different kinds of childhood infectious illnesses, including **chickenpox** and **scarlet fever**. It may be triggered by other infections, such as **Rocky Mountain spotted fever** or **ringworm**.

- Allergic reactions. One of the most common symptoms of an allergic reaction is an itchy rash. **Contact dermatitis** is a rash that appears after the skin is exposed to an allergen, such as metal, rubber, some cosmetics or lotions, or some types of plants (e.g. poison ivy). Drug reactions are another common allergic cause of rash; in this case, a rash is only one of a variety of possible symptoms, including **fever**, seizures, **nausea and vomiting**, **diarrhea**, heartbeat irregularities, and breathing problems. This rash usually appears soon after the first dose of the course of medicine is taken.

- **Autoimmune disorders**. Conditions in which the immune system turns on the body itself, such as **systemic lupus erythematosus** or purpura, often have a characteristic rash.

- nutritional disorders. For example, **scurvy**, a disease caused by a lack of Vitamin C, has a rash as one of its symptoms.

- **cancer**. A few types of cancer, such as chronic lymphocytic leukemia, can be the underlying cause of a rash.

Rashes in infancy

Rashes are extremely common in infancy, and are usually not serious at all and can be treated at home.

Diaper rash is caused by prolonged skin contact with bacteria and the baby's waste products in a damp diaper. This rash has red, spotty sores and there may be an ammonia smell. In most cases the rash will respond within three days to drying efforts. A diaper rash that does not improve in this time may be a yeast infection requiring prescription medication. A doctor should be consulted if the rash is solid, bright red, causes fever, or the skin develops blisters, **boils**, or pus.

Infants also can get a rash on cheeks and chin caused by contact with food and stomach contents. This rash will come and go, but usually responds to a good cleaning after meals. About a third of all infants develop "acne" usually after the third week of life in response to their mothers' hormones before birth. This rash will disappear between weeks and a few months. Heat rash is a mass of tiny pink bumps on the back of the neck and upper back caused by blocked sweat glands. The rash usually appears during hot, humid weather, although a baby with a fever can also develop the rash.

A baby should see a doctor immediately if the rash:

- appears suddenly and looks purple or blood-colored

- looks like a burn

- appears while the infant seems to be sick

Diagnosis

A physician can make a diagnosis based on the medical history and the appearance of the rash, where it appears, and any other accompanying symptoms.

Treatment

Treatment of rashes focuses on resolving the underlying disorder and providing relief of the **itching** that often accompanies them. Soothing lotions or oral **antihistamines** can provide some relief, and **topical antibiotics** may be administered if the patient, particularly a child, has caused a secondary infection by scratching.

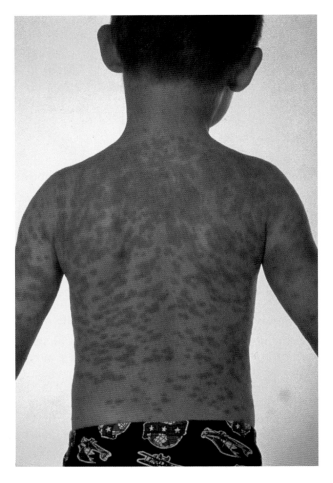

An unidentified rash on young boy's back. *(Custom Medical Stock Photo. Reproduced by permission.)*

The rash triggered by **allergies** should disappear as soon as the allergen is removed; drug rashes will fade when the patient stops taking the drug causing the allergy. For the treatment of diaper rash, the infant's skin should be exposed to the air as much as possible; ointments are not needed unless the skin is dry and cracked. Experts also recommend switching to cloth diapers and cleaning affected skin with plain water.

Prognosis

Most rashes that have an acute cause, such as an infection or an allergic reaction, will disappear as soon as the infection or irritant is removed from the body's system. Rashes that are caused by chronic conditions, such as autoimmune disorders, may remain indefinitely or fade and return periodically.

Prevention

Some rashes can be prevented, depending on the triggering factor. A person known to be allergic to certain drugs or substances should avoid those things in order to prevent a rash. Diaper rash can be prevented by using cloth diapers and keeping the diaper area very clean, breast feeding, and changing diapers often.

Resources

ORGANIZATIONS

American Academy of Dermatology. 930 N. Meacham Road, P.O. Box 4014, Schaumburg, IL 60168-4014. (847) 330-0230. Fax: (847) 330-0050. < http://www.aad.org >.

Carol A. Turkington

Rat-bite fever

Definition

Rat-bite **fever** refers to an infection which develops after having been bitten or scratched by an infected animal.

Description

Rat-bite fever occurs most often among laboratory workers who handle lab rats in their jobs, and among people who live in poor conditions, with rodent infestation. Children are particularly likely to be bitten by rodents infesting their home, and are therefore most likely to contract rat-bite fever. Other animals that can carry the types of bacteria responsible for this illness include mice, squirrels, weasels, dogs, and cats. One of the causative bacteria can cause the same illness if it is ingested, for example in unpasteurized milk.

Causes and symptoms

There are two variations of rat-bite fever, caused by two different organisms. In the United States, the bacteria *Streptobacillus moniliformis* is the most common cause (causing streptobacillary rat-bite fever). In other countries, especially Africa, *Spirillum minus* causes a different form of the infection (called spirillary rat-bite fever).

Streptobacillary rat-bite fever occurs up to 22 days after the initial bite or scratch. The patient becomes ill with fever, chills, **nausea and vomiting**, **headache**, and **pain** in the back and joints. A rash made up of tiny pink bumps develops, covering the palms of the hands and the soles of the feet. Without treatment, the patient is at risk of developing serious infections of the lining of the heart (**endocarditis**), the sac containing the heart (**pericarditis**), the coverings of the brain and spinal cord (**meningitis**), or lungs (**pneumonia**). Any tissue or organ throughout the body may develop a pocket of infection and pus, called an **abscess**.

Spirillary rat-bite fever occurs some time after the initial injury has already healed, up to about 28 days after the bite or scratch. Although the wound had appeared completely healed, it suddenly grows red and swollen again. The patient develops a fever. Lymph nodes in the area become swollen and tender, and the patient suffers from fever, chills, and headache. The skin in the area of the original wound sloughs off. Although rash is less common than with streptobacillary rat-bite fever, there may be a lightly rosy, itchy rash all over the body. Joint and muscle pain rarely occur. If left untreated, the fever usually subsides, only to return again in repeated two- to four-day cycles. This can go on for up to a year, although, even without treatment, the illness usually resolves within four to eight weeks.

Diagnosis

In streptobacillary rat-bite fever, found in the United States, diagnosis can be made by taking a sample of blood or fluid from a painful joint. In a laboratory, the sample can be cultured, to allow the growth of organisms. Examination under a microscope will then allow identification of the bacteria *Streptobacillus moniliformis*.

In spirillary rat-bite fever, diagnosis can be made by examining blood or a sample of tissue from the wound for evidence of *Spirillum minus*.

Treatment

Shots of procaine penicillin G or penicillin V by mouth are effective against both streptobacillary and spirillary rat-bite fever. When a patient is allergic to

---

KEY TERMS

Abscess—A pocket of infection; a collection of pus.

Endocarditis—An inflammation of the lining of the heart.

Meningitis—An inflammation of the tissues covering the brain and spinal cord.

Pasteurization—A process during which milk is heated up and maintained at a particular temperature long enough to kill bacteria.

Pericarditis—An inflammation of the sac containing the heart.

---

the **penicillins**, erythromycin may be given by mouth for streptobacillary infection, or tetracycline by mouth for spirillary infection.

Prognosis

With treatment, prognosis is excellent for both types of rat-bite fever. Without treatment, the spirillary form usually resolves on its own, although it may take up to a year to do so.

The streptobacillary form, found in the United States, however, can progress to cause extremely serious, potentially fatal complications. In fact, before **antibiotics** were available to treat the infection, streptobacillary rat-bite fever frequently resulted in **death**.

Prevention

Prevention involves avoiding contact with those animals capable of passing on the causative organisms. This can be an unfortunately difficult task for people whose economic situations do not allow them to move out of rat-infested buildings. Because streptobacillary rat-bite fever can occur after drinking contaminated milk or water, only pasteurized milk, and water from safe sources, should be ingested.

Resources

ORGANIZATIONS

Centers for Disease Control and Prevention. 1600 Clifton Rd., NE, Atlanta, GA 30333. (800) 311-3435, (404) 639-3311. < http://www.cdc.gov >.

Rosalyn Carson-DeWitt, MD

Rational-emotive therapy *see* **Cognitive-behavioral therapy**

Raynaud's disease

Definition

Raynaud's disease refers to a disorder in which the fingers or toes (digits) suddenly experience decreased blood circulation. It is characterized by repeated episodes of color changes of the skin of digits on cold exposure or emotional **stress**.

Description

Raynaud's disease can be classified as one of two types: primary (or idiopathic) and secondary (also called Raynaud's phenomenon). Primary Raynaud's disease has no predisposing factor, is more mild, and causes fewer complications. About half of all cases of Raynaud's disease are of this type. Women are five times more likely than men to develop primary Raynaud's disease. The average age of diagnosis is between 20 and 40 years. Approximately three out of ten people with primary Raynaud's disease eventually progress to secondary Raynaud's disease after diagnosis. About 15% of individuals improve.

Secondary Raynaud's disease is the same as primary Raynaud's disease, but occurs in individuals with a predisposing factor, usually a form of collagen vascular disease. What is typically identified as primary Raynaud's is later identified as secondary once a predisposing disease is diagnosed. This occurs in approximately 30% of patients. As a result, the secondary type is often more complicated and severe, and is more likely to worsen.

Several related conditions that predispose persons to secondary Raynaud's disease include **scleroderma**, **systemic lupus erythematosus**, **rheumatoid arthritis** and **polymyositis**. **Pulmonary hypertension** and some nervous system disorders such as herniated discs and tumors within the spinal column, strokes, and **polio** can progress to Raynaud's disease. Finally, injuries due to mechanical trauma caused by vibration (such as that associated with chain saws and jackhammers), repetitive motion (**carpal tunnel syndrome**), electrical shock, and exposure to extreme cold can led to the development of Raynaud's disease. Some drugs used to control high blood pressure or migraine headaches have been known to cause Raynaud's disease.

The prevalence of Reynaud's Phenomena in the general population varies 4–15%. Females are seven times more likely to develop Raynaud's diseases than are men. The problem has not been correlated with coffee consumption, dietary habits, occupational history (excepting exposure to vibration) and exposure to most drugs. An association between Raynaud's disease and migraine headaches and has been reported. Secondary Raynaud's disease is common among individuals systemic lupus erythematosus in tropical countries.

Causes and symptoms

There is significant familial aggregation of primary Raynaud's disease. However, no causative gene has been identified.

Risk factors for Raynaud's disease differ between males and females. Age and **smoking** seem to be associated with Raynaud's disease only in men, while the associations of marital status and alcohol use with Raynaud's disease are usually only observed in women. These findings suggest that different mechanisms influence the expression of Raynaud's disease in men and women.

Both primary and secondary Raynaud's disease signs and symptoms are thought to be due to arterioles over-reacting to stimuli. Cold normally causes the tiny muscles in the walls of arteries to contract, thus reducing the amount of blood that can flow through them. In people with Raynaud's disease, the extent of constriction is extreme, thus severely restricting blood flow. Attacks or their effects may be brought on or worsened by **anxiety** or emotional distress.

There are three distinct phases to an episode of Raynaud's disease. When first exposed to cold, small arteries respond with intense contractions (vasoconstriction). The affected fingers or toes (in rare instances, the tip of the nose or tongue) become pale and white because they are deprived of blood and, thus, oxygen. In response, capillaries and veins expand (dilate). Because these vessels are carrying deoxygenated blood, the affected area then becomes blue in color. The area often feels cold and tingly or numb. After the area begins to warm up, the arteries dilate. Blood flow is significantly increased. This changes the color of the area to a bright red. During this phase, persons often describe the affected area as feeling warm and throbbing painfully.

Raynaud's disease may initially affect only the tips of fingers or toes. As the disease progresses, it may eventually involve all of one or two digits. Ultimately, all the fingers or toes may be affected. About one person in ten, will experience a complication called sclerodactyly. In sclerodactyly, the skin over the involved digits becomes tight, white, thick, smooth and shiny. In approximately 1% of cases of

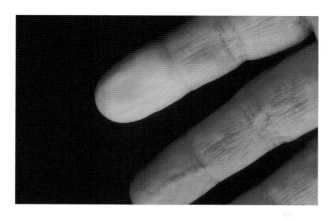

A close-up view of a patient's fingers afflicted with Raynaud's disease. While this disorder may initially only affect the tips of the fingers and toes, eventually blood circulation of the entire finger or toe is affected. *(Custom Medical Stock Photo. Reproduced by permission.)*

Raynaud's disease, deep sores (ulcers) may develop in the skin. In rare cases of frequent, repetitive bouts of severe **ischemia** (decreased supply of oxygenated blood to tissues or organs), tissue loss, or **gangrene** may result and **amputation** may be required.

Diagnosis

Primary Raynaud's disease is diagnosed following the Allen Brown criteria. There are four components. The certainty of the diagnosis and severity of the disease increase as more criteria are met. The first is that at least two of the three color changes must occur during attacks provoked by cold and or stress. The second is that episodes must periodically occur for at least two years. The third is that attacks must occur in both the hands and the feet in the absence of vascular occlusive disease. The last is that there is no other identifiable cause for the Raynaud's episodes.

A cold stimulation test may also be performed to help to confirm a diagnosis of Raynaud's disease. The temperature of affected fingers or toes is taken. The hand or foot is then placed completely into a container of ice water for 20 seconds. After removal from the water, the temperature of the affected digits is immediately recorded. The temperature is retaken every five minutes until it returns to the pre-immersion level. Most individuals recover normal temperature within 15 minutes. People with Raynaud's disease may require 20 minutes or more to reach their pre-immersion temperature.

Laboratory testing is performed frequently. However, these results are often inconclusive for several reasons. Provocative testing such as the ice

emergence just described, is difficult to interpret because there is considerable overlap between normal and abnormal results. The **antinuclear antibody test** of blood is usually negative in Raynaud's disease. Capillary beds under finger nails usually appear normal. Erythrocyte sedimentation rates are often abnormal in people with connective tissue diseases. Unfortunately, this finding is not consistent in people with Raynaud's disease.

Treatment

There is no known way to prevent the development of Raynaud's disease. Further, there is no known cure for this condition. Therefore, avoidance of the trigger is the best supportive management available. Most cases of primary Raynaud's disease can be controlled with proper medical care and avoidance.

Many people are able to find relief by simply adjusting their lifestyles. Affected individuals need to stay warm, and keep their hands and feet well covered in cold weather. Layered clothing, scarves, heavy coats, heavy socks, and mittens under gloves are suggested because gloves alone allow heat to escape. It is also recommended that patients cover or close the space between their sleeves and mittens. Indoors, they should wear socks and comfortable shoes. Smokers should quit as nicotine will worsen the problem. Avoid the use of vibrating tools as well.

People with severe cases of Raynaud's disease may need to be treated with medications to help keep the arterioles relaxed and dilated. Medications such as calcium-channel blockers, reserpine or nitroglycerin may be prescribed to relax artery walls and improve blood flow.

Alternative Treatment

Because episodes of Raynaud's disease have also been associated with stress and emotional upset, the condition may be improved by learning to manage stress. Regular **exercise** is known to decrease stress and lower anxiety. Hypnosis, relaxation techniques, and visualization are also useful methods to help control emotions.

Biofeedback training is a technique during which a patient is given continuous information on the temperature of his or her digits, and then taught to voluntarily control this temperature. Some alternative practitioners believe that certain dietary supplements and herbs may be helpful in decreasing the vessel spasm of Raynaud's disease. Suggested supplements include vitamin E (found in fruits, vegetables, seeds,

KEY TERMS

Arteriole—The smallest type of artery.

Artery—A blood vessel that carries blood away from the heart to peripheral tissues.

Gangrene—Death of a tissue, usually caused by insufficient blood supply and followed by bacterial infection of the tissue.

Idiopathic—Of unknown origin.

Polymyositis—An inflammation of many muscles.

Pulmonary hypertension—A severe form of high blood pressure caused by diseased arteries in the lung.

Rheumatoid arthritis—Chronic, autoimmune disease marked by inflammation of the membranes surrounding joints.

Scleroderma—A relatively rare autoimmune disease affecting blood vessels and connective tissue that makes skin appear thickened.

Systemic lupus erythematosus—A chronic inflammatory disease that affects many tissues and parts of the body including the skin.

and nuts), magnesium (found in seeds, nuts, fish, beans, and dark green vegetables), and fish oils. The circulatory herbs cayenne, ginger and prickly ash may help enhance circulation to affected areas.

Prognosis

The prognosis for most people with Raynaud's disease is very good. In general, primary Raynaud's disease has the best prognosis, with a relatively small chance (1%) of serious complications. Approximately half of all affected individuals do well by taking simple precautions, and never require medication. The prognosis for people with secondary Raynaud's disease (or phenomenon) is less predictable. This prognosis depends greatly on the severity of other associated conditions such as scleroderma, lupus, or Sjögren syndrome.

Prevention

There is no way to prevent the development of Raynaud's disease. Once an individual realizes that he or she suffers from this disorder, however, steps can be taken to reduce the frequency and severity of episodes.

Resources

BOOKS

Rosenwasser, Lanny J. "The Vasaculitic Syndromes." In *Cecil Textbook of Medicine.* Lee Goldman, et al., editors. Philadelphia: Saunders, 2000, pp. 1524-1527.

PERIODICALS

Fraenkel, L., et al. "Different Factors Influencing the Expression of Raynaud's Phenomenon in Men and Women." *Arthritis and Rheumatology* 42, no. 2 (February 1999): 306-310.

Voulgari, P. V., et al. "Prevalence of Raynaud's Phenomenon in a Healthy Greek Population." *Annals of Rheumatic Disease* 59, no. 3 (March 2000): 206-210.

ORGANIZATIONS

American Heart Association. 7320 Greenville Ave., Dallas, TX 75231-4596. (214) 373-6300 or (800) 242-8721. inquire@heart.org. < http://www.americanheart.org >.

Irish Raynaud's and Scleroderma Society. PO Box 2958 Foxrock, Dublin 18, Ireland (01) 235 0900. irss@indigo.ie.

National Heart, Lung, and Blood Institute. PO Box 30105, Bethesda, MD 20824-0105. (301) 592-8573. nhlbiinfo@rover.nhlbi.nih.gov. < http://www.nhlbi.nih.gov >.

National Organization for Rare Disorders (NORD). PO Box 8923, New Fairfield, CT 06812-8923. (203) 746-6518 or (800) 999-6673. Fax: (203) 746-6481. < http://www.rarediseases.org >.

Raynaud's & Scleroderma Association (UK). 112 Crewe Road, Alsager, Cheshire, ST7 2JA. UK (44) (0) 1270 872776. webmaster@raynauds.demon.co.uk. < http://www.raynauds.demon.co.uk >.

OTHER

Arthritis Foundation. < http//www.arthritis-foundation .com/ >.

British Sjögren's Syndrome Association. < http://ourworld .copmpuserve.com/homepages/BSSAssociation >.

Raynaud's & Scleroderma Association. < http://www.Raunaud's.demon.co,uk/ >.

Rodriguez, J., and S. Wasson. "Raynaud's Disease." Wayne State University School of Medicine. < http://www.med.wayne.edu/raynauds/ >.

L. Fleming Fallon, Jr., MD, PhD, DrPH

RDS *see* **Respiratory distress syndrome**

Reactive airway disease *see* **Asthma**

Reactive polycythemia *see* **Secondary polycythemia**

Reading disorder *see* **Learning disorders**

Recompression treatment

Definition

Recompression treatment is the use of elevated pressure to treat conditions within the body after it has been subjected to a rapid decrease in pressure. It also includes hyperbaric **oxygen therapy**.

Purpose

Recompression treatment is used to overcome the adverse effects of **gas embolism** and **decompression sickness** (sometimes called the bends) in underwater divers who breathe compressed air. It is also approved for treatment of severe **smoke inhalation**, **carbon monoxide poisoning**, gas **gangrene**, radiation tissue damage, thermal **burns**, extreme blood loss, crush injuries, and **wounds** that won't heal.

Precautions

Hyperbaric oxygen therapy delivers greater amounts of oxygen more quickly to the body than breathing room air (which is only 21% oxygen) at regular pressure. Unmonitored, increased oxygen can produce toxic effects. Treatments must follow safe time-dose limits and may only be administered by a doctor.

Description

Recompression treatment is performed in a **hyperbaric chamber**, a sealed compartment in which the patient breathes normal air or "enhanced" air with up to 100% oxygen while exposed to controlled pressures up to three times normal atmospheric pressure. The patient may receive the oxygen through a face mask, a hood or tent around the head, or an endotracheal tube down the windpipe if the patient is already on a ventilator. When used to treat decompression sickness or gas **embolism**, the increased pressure reduces the size of gas bubbles in the patient's body. The increased oxygen concentration speeds the diffusion of the nitrogen within the bubbles out of the patient's body. As gas bubbles deflate, the trauma of gas embolism and decompression sickness begins to resolve. Treatment for diving emergencies typically involves one session, lasting four to six hours, at three atmospheres of pressure.

When used to treat other conditions, the increased pressure allows oxygen and other gases to dissolve more rapidly into the blood and thus be carried to oxygen-starved tissues to enhance healing. Elevated oxygen levels can also purge toxins such as carbon monoxide from the body. In addition, when body tissues are super-saturated with oxygen, the destruction of some bacteria is enhanced and the spread of certain toxins is halted. This makes hyperbaric oxygen therapy useful in treating gas gangrene and infections that cause tissue necrosis (death). Hyperbaric oxygen therapy also promotes the growth of new blood vessels.

Preparation

Oxygen is often administered to a patient as first aid while he or she is being transported to a hyperbaric chamber. The treatment begins with chamber compression; as the pressure of the chamber atmosphere increases, the temperature also rises and the patient's ears may fill as they would during an airplane landing. Swallowing and yawning are ways to relieve the inner ear pressure. Once the desired pressure is achieved, the patient is given pure oxygen to breathe. Because treatment is lengthy, patients are encouraged to sleep or listen to music. In larger chambers, patients may also read or watch videos.

Aftercare

Depending on the reason for treatment and the treatment outcome, the patient may be taken to a hospital for further care, or examined and released.

Risks

There is minimal risk when recompression treatment is administered by a competent physician. However, some common side effects are sinus **pain**, temporary changes in vision, and **fatigue**.

Normal results

With prompt and appropriate recompression treatment, most patients show marked improvement in their blood oxygen levels and tissue circulation, as well as other signs of healing. Divers treated for gas embolism or decompression sickness may recover with no lasting effects.

Abnormal results

When recompression treatment is not begun promptly or not conducted at adequate time-dose levels, patients with decompression sickness may develop bone necrosis. This significant destruction of bone, most commonly found in the hip and shoulder, produces chronic pain and severe disability. Another result of delayed or inadequate treatment may be permanent neurological damage. When decompression sickness involves the spinal cord, partial **paralysis** may occur.

Resources

ORGANIZATIONS

American College of Hyperbaric Medicine. P.O. Box 25914-130, Houston, Texas 77265. (713) 528-0657. <http://www.hyperbaricmedicine.org>.

Divers Alert Network. The Peter B. Bennett Center, 6 West Colony Place, Durham, NC 27705. (800) 446-2671. <http://www.diversalertnetwork.org>.

Undersea and Hyperbaric Medical Society. 10531 Metropolitan Ave., Kensington, MD 20895. (301) 942-2980. <http://www.uhms.org>.

Bethany Thivierge

Reconstructive surgery *see* **Plastic, cosmetic, and reconstructive surgery**

Rectal cancer

Definition

The rectum is the portion of the large bowel that lies in the pelvis, terminating at the anus. **Cancer** of the rectum is the disease characterized by the development of malignant cells in the lining or epithelium of the rectum. Malignant cells have changed such that they lose normal control mechanisms governing growth. These cells may invade surrounding local tissue or they may spread throughout the body and invade other organ systems.

Description

The rectum is the continuation of the colon (part of the large bowel) after it leaves the abdomen and descends into the pelvis. It is divided into equal thirds: the upper, mid, and lower rectum.

The pelvis and other organs in the pelvis form boundaries to the rectum. Behind, or posterior to the rectum is the sacrum (the lowest portion of the spine, closest to the pelvis). Laterally, on the sides, the rectum is bounded by soft tissue and bone. In front, the rectum is bounded by different organs in the male and female. In the male, the bladder and prostate are present. In the female, the vagina, uterus, and ovaries are present.

The upper rectum receives its blood supply from branches of the inferior mesenteric artery from the abdomen. The lower rectum has blood vessels entering from the sides of the pelvis. Lymph, a protein-rich fluid that bathes the cells of the body, is transported in small channels known as lymphatics. These channels run with the blood supply of the rectum. Lymph nodes are small filters through which the lymph flows on its way back to the blood stream. Cancer spreads elsewhere in the body by invading the lymph and vascular systems.

When a cell or cells lining the rectum become malignant, they first grow locally and may invade partially or totally through the wall of the rectum. The tumor here may invade surrounding tissue or the organs that bound it, a process known as local invasion. In this process, the tumor penetrates and may invade the lymphatics or the capillaries locally and gain access to the circulation in this way. As the malignant cells work their way to other areas of the body, they again become locally invasive in the new area to which they have spread. These tumor deposits, originating in the primary tumor in the rectum, are then known as metastasis. If metastases are found in the regional lymph nodes, they are known as regional metastases. If they are distant from the primary tumor, they are known as distant metastases. The patient with distant metastases may have widespread disease, also referred to as systemic disease. Thus the cancer originating in the rectum begins locally and, given time, may become systemic.

By the time the primary tumor is originally detected, it is usually larger than 1 cm (about 0.39 in) in size and has over one million cells. This amount of growth is estimated to take about three to seven years. Each time the cells double in number, the size of the tumor quadruples. Thus like most cancers, the part that is identified clinically is later in the progression than would be desired. Screening becomes a very important endeavor to aid in earlier detection of this disease.

Passage of red blood with the stool, (noticeable bleeding with defecation), is much more common in rectal cancer than that originating in the colon because the tumor is much closer to the anus. Other symptoms (**constipation** and/ or **diarrhea**) are caused by obstruction and, less often, by local invasion of the tumor into pelvic organs or the sacrum. When the tumor has spread to distant sites, these metastases may cause dysfunction of the organ they have spread to. Distant metastasis usually occurs in the liver, less often to the lung(s), and rarely to the brain.

There are about 36,500 cases of rectal cancer diagnosed per year in the United States. Together, colon and rectal cancers account for 10% of cancers in men and 11% of cancers in women. It is the second most common site-specific cancer affecting both men and women. Nearly 57,000 people died from colon and rectal cancer in the United States in 2003. In recent years the incidence of this disease is decreasing very slightly, as has the mortality rate. It is difficult to tell if the decrease in mortality reflects earlier diagnosis, less **death** related to the actual treatment of the disease, or a combination of both factors.

Cancer of the rectum is felt to arise sporadically in about 80% of those who develop the disease. About 20% of cases probably arise from genetic predisposition; some people have a family history of rectal cancer occurring in a first-degree relative. Development of rectal cancer at an early age suggests a genetically transmitted form of the disease as opposed to the sporadic form.

Causes and symptoms

Causes of rectal cancer are probably environmental in sporadic cases (80%), and genetic in the heredity-predisposed (20%) cases. Since malignant cells have a changed genetic makeup, this means that in 80% of cases, the environment spontaneously induces change. Those born with a genetic predisposition are either destined to get the cancer, or it will take less environmental exposure to induce the cancer. Exposure to agents in the environment that may induce mutation is the process of carcinogenesis and is caused by agents known as carcinogens. Specific carcinogens have been difficult to identify; dietary factors, however, seem to be involved.

Rectal cancer is more common in industrialized nations. Dietary factors may be the reason. **Diets** high in fat, red meat, total calories, and alcohol seem to add to increased risk. Diets high in fiber are associated with a decreased risk. High-fiber diets may be related to less exposure of the rectal epithelium to carcinogens from the environment as the transit time through the bowel is faster with a high-fiber diet than with a low-fiber diet.

Age plays a definite role in rectal cancer risk. Rectal cancer is rare before age 40. This incidence increases substantially after age 50 and doubles with each succeeding decade.

There also is a slight increase of risk for rectal cancer in the individual who smokes.

Patients who suffer from an inflammatory disease of the colon known as **ulcerative colitis** are also at increased risk.

On chromosome 5 is the APC gene associated with familial adenomatous polyposis (FAP) syndrome. There are multiple mutations that occur at this site, yet they all cause a defect in tumor suppression that results in early and frequent development of **colon cancer**. This is transmitted to 50% of offspring and each of those affected will develop colon or rectal cancer, usually at an early age. Another syndrome, hereditary non-polyposis colon cancer (HNPCC), is related to mutations in any of four genes responsible for DNA mismatch repair. In patients with colon or rectal cancer, the p53 gene is mutated 70% of the time.

When the p53 gene is mutated and ineffective, cells with damaged DNA escape repair or destruction, allowing the damaged cell to multiply. Continued replication of the damaged DNA may lead to tumor development. Though these syndromes (FAP and HNPCC) have a very high incidence of colon or rectal cancer, family history without the syndromes is also a substantial risk factor. When considering first-degree relatives, history of one with colon or rectal cancer raises the baseline risk from 2% to 6%; the presence of a second raises the risk to 17%.

The development of polyps of the colon or rectum commonly precedes the development of rectal cancer. Polyps are growths of the rectal lining. They can be unrelated to cancer, pre-cancerous, or malignant. Polyps, when identified, are removed for diagnosis. If the polyp, or polyps, are benign, the patient should undergo careful surveillance for the development of more polyps or the development of colon or rectal cancer.

Symptoms of rectal cancer most often result from the local presence of the tumor and its capacity to invade surrounding pelvic structure:

- bright red blood present with stool

- abdominal distention (stretching from internal pressure), bloating, inability to have a bowel movement

- narrowing of the stool, so-called ribbon stools

- pelvic pain

- unexplained weight loss

- persistent chronic **fatigue**

- rarely, urinary infection or passage of air in urine in males (late symptom)

- rarely, passage of feces through vagina in females(late symptom)

If the tumor is large and obstructing the rectum, the patient will not be evacuating stool normally and will get bloated and have abdominal discomfort. The tumor itself may bleed and, since it is near the anus, the patient may see bright red blood on the surface of the stool. Blood alone (without stool) may also be passed. Thus, **hemorrhoids** are often incorrectly blamed for bleeding, delaying the diagnosis. If anemia develops, which is rare, the patient will experience chronic fatigue. If the tumor invades the bladder in the male or the vagina in the female, stool will get where it does not belong and cause infection or discharge. (This condition is also rare.) Patients with widespread disease lose weight secondary to the chronic illness.

Diagnosis

Screening evaluation of the colon and rectum are accomplished together. Screening involves physical exam, simple laboratory tests, and the visualization of the lining of the rectum and colon. X rays (indirect visualization) and endoscopy (direct visualization) are used to visualize the organs' lining.

The **physical examination** involves the performance of a digital rectal exam (DRE). At the time of this exam, the physician checks the stool on the examining glove with a chemical to see if any occult (invisible), blood is present. At home, after having a bowel movement, the patient is asked to swipe a sample of stool obtained with a small stick on a card. After three such specimens are on the card, the card is then easily chemically tested for occult blood. These exams are accomplished as an easy part of a routine yearly physical exam.

Proteins are sometimes produced by cancers and these may be elevated in the patients blood. When this occurs the protein produced is known as a tumor marker. There is a tumor marker for cancer of the colon and rectum; it is known as carcinoembryonic antigen, (CEA). Unfortunately, this may be made by other adenocarcinomas as well, or it may not be produced by a particular colon or rectal cancer. Therefore, screening by chemical analysis for CEA has not been helpful. CEA has been helpful in patients treated for colon or rectal cancer if their tumor makes the protein. It is used in a follow-up role, not a screening role.

Direct visualization of the lining of the rectum is accomplished using a scope or endoscope. The physician introduces the instrument into the rectum and is able to see the epithelium of the rectum directly. A simple rigid tubular scope may be used to see the rectal epithelium; however, screening of the colon is done at the same time. The lower colon may be visualized using a fiberoptic flexible scope in a procedure known as flexible **sigmoidoscopy**. When the entire colon is visualized, the procedure is known as total **colonoscopy**. Each type of endoscopy requires pre-procedure preparation (evacuation) of the rectum and colon.

The American Cancer Society has recommended the following screening protocol for colon and rectal cancers those over age 50:

- yearly fecal occult blood test

- flexible sigmoidoscopy at age 50

- flexible sigmoidoscopy repeated every 5 years

- double contrast **barium enema** every five years

- colonoscopy every 10 years

If there are predisposing factors such as positive family history, history of polyps, or a familial syndrome, screening evaluations should start sooner.

Evaluation of patients with symptoms

When patients visit their physician because they are experiencing symptoms that could possibly be related to colon or rectal cancer, the entire colon and rectum must be visualized. Even if a rectal lesion is identified, the entire colon must be screened to rule out a syndromous polyp or cancer of the colon. The combination of a flexible sigmoidoscopy and double contrast barium enema may be performed, but the much preferred evaluation of the entire colon and rectum is that of complete colonoscopy. Colonoscopy allows direct visualization, photography, as well as the opportunity to obtain a biopsy, (a sample of tissue), of any abnormality visualized. If, for technical reasons the entire colon is not visualized endoscopically, a double contrast barium enema should complement the colonoscopy. A patient who is identified to have a problem in one area of the colon or rectum is at greater risk to have a similar problem in area of the colon or rectum. Therefore the entire colon and rectum need to be visualized during the evaluation.

The diagnosis of rectal cancer is actually made by the performance of a biopsy of any abnormal lesion in the rectum. Many rectal cancers are within reach of the examiner's finger. Identifying how close to the anus the cancer has developed is very important in planning the treatment. Another characteristic ascertained by exam is whether the tumor is mobile or fixed to surrounding structure. Again, this will have implications related to primary treatment. As a general rule, it is easier to identify and adequately obtain tissue for evaluation in the rectum as opposed to the colon. This is because the lesion is closer to the anus.

If the patient has advanced disease, areas where the tumor has spread, such as the liver, may require biopsy. Such biopsies are usually obtained using a special needle under **local anesthesia**.

Once a diagnosis of rectal cancer has been established by biopsy, in addition to the physical exam, an **endorectal ultrasound** will be performed to assess the extent of the disease. For rectal cancer, endorectal ultrasound is the most preferred method for staging both depth of tumor penetration and local lymph node status. Endorectal ultrasound:

- differentiates areas of invasion within large rectal adenomas that seem benign

- determines the depth of tumor penetration into the rectal wall

- determines the extent of regional lymph node invasion

- can be combined with other tests (chest x rays and **computed tomography scans**, or CT scans) to determine the extent of cancer spread to distant organs, such as the lungs or liver

The resulting rectal cancer staging allows physicians to determine the need for—and order of—radiation, surgery, and **chemotherapy**. In 2003, it was reported that **magnetic resonance imaging** (MRI) also may be useful in staging rectal cancer. MRI may help physicians determine if a tumor can be resected and risk of cancer recurrence.

Treatment

Once the diagnosis has been confirmed by biopsy and the endorectal ultrasound has been performed, the clinical stage of the cancer is assigned. The treating physicians use staging to plan the specific treatment protocol for the patient. In addition, the stage of the cancer at the time of presentation gives a statistical likelihood of the treatment outcome (prognosis).

Clinical staging

Rectal cancer first invades locally and then progresses to spread to regional lymph nodes or to other organs. Stage is derived using the characteristics of the primary tumor, its depth of penetration through the rectum, local invasion into pelvic structure, and the presence or absence of regional or distant metastases. A CT scan of the pelvis is helpful in staging because tumor invasion into the sacrum or pelvic sidewalls may mean surgical therapy is not initially possible. On this basis, clinical staging is used to begin treatment. The pathologic stage is defined when the results of analyzing the surgical specimen are available. (typically stage I and II).

Rectal cancer is assigned stages I through IV, based on the following general criteria:

- Stage I: the tumor is confined to the epithelium or has not penetrated through the first layer of muscle in the rectal wall.

- Stage II: the tumor has penetrated through to the outer wall of the rectum or has gone through it, possibly invading other local tissue or organs.

- Stage III: Any depth or size of tumor associated with regional lymph node involvement.

- Stage IV: any of previous criteria associated with distant metastasis.

Surgery

The first, or primary, treatment modality utilized in the treatment of rectal cancer is surgery. Stage I, II, and even suspected stage III disease are treated by surgical removal of the involved section of the rectum along with the complete vascular and lymphatic supply. Most Stage II and Stage III rectal cancers (based on endorectal ultrasound, CT scan, and **chest x ray**) are treated with radiation and possibly chemotherapy prior to surgery.

When determining primary treatment for rectal cancer, the surgeon's ability to reconnect the ends of the rectum. The pelvis is a confining space that makes the performance of the hook-up more difficult to do safely when the tumor is in the lower rectum. The upper rectum does not usually present a substantial problem to the surgeon restoring bowel continuity after the cancer has been removed. Mid-rectal tumors, (especially in males where the pelvis is usually smaller than a woman's), may present technical difficulties in hooking the proximal bowel to the remaining rectum. Technical advances in stapling instrumentation have largely overcome these difficulties. If the anastomosis (hook-up) leaks postoperatively, infection can occur. In the past, this was a major cause of complications in resection of rectal cancers. Today, utilizing the stapling instrumentation, a hook-up at the time of original surgery is much safer. If the surgeon feels that the hook-up is compromised or may leak, a **colostomy** may be performed. A colostomy is performed by bringing the colon through the abdominal wall and sewing it to the skin. In these cases the stool is diverted away from the hook-up, allowing it to heal and preventing the infectious complications associated with leak. Later, when the hook-up has completely healed, the colostomy can be taken down and bowel continuity restored.

Stapling devices have allowed the surgeon to get closer to the anus and still allow the technical performance of a hook-up, but there are limits. It is generally felt that there should be at least three centimeters of normal rectum below the tumor or the risk of recurrence locally will be excessive. In addition, if there is no residual native rectum, the patient will not have normal sensation or control and will have problems with uncontrollable soilage, (incontinence). For these reasons, patients presenting with low rectal tumors may undergo total removal of the rectum and anus. This procedure is known as an abdominal-perineal resection. A permanent colostomy is performed in the lower left abdomen.

Radiation

As mentioned, for many late stage II or stage III tumors, **radiation therapy** can shrink the tumor prior to surgery. The other roles for radiation therapy are as an aid to surgical therapy in locally advanced disease that has been removed, and in the treatment of certain distant metastases. Especially when utilized in combination with chemotherapy, radiation used postoperatively has been shown to reduce the risk of local recurrence in the pelvis by 46% and death rates by 29%. Such combined therapy is recommended in patients with locally advanced primary tumors that have been removed surgically. Radiation has been helpful in treating effects of distant metastases, particularly in the brain. In very few cases, radiation alone may be the curative treatment for rectal cancer.

Chemotherapy

Adjuvant chemotherapy, (treating the patient who has no evidence of residual disease but who is at high risk for recurrence), is considered in patients whose tumors deeply penetrate or locally invade (late stage II and stage III). If the tumor was not locally advanced, this form of chemotherapeutic adjuvant therapy may be recommended without radiation. This therapy is identical to that of colon cancer and leads to similar results. Standard therapy is treatment with 5-fluorouracil, (5-FU) combined with leucovorin for a period of six to 12 months. 5-FU is an antimetabolite and leucovorin improves the response rate. Another agent, levamisole, (which seems to stimulate the immune system), may be substituted for leucovorin. These protocols reduce rate of recurrence by about 15% and reduce mortality by about 10%. The regimens have some toxicity but usually are tolerated fairly well.

Similar chemotherapy is administered for stage IV disease or if a cancer progresses and metastasis develops. Results show response rates of about 20%. A response is a temporary regression of the cancer in response to the chemotherapy. Unfortunately, these patients eventually succumb to the disease. Clinical trials have now shown that the results can be improved with the addition of another agent to this regimen. Irinotecan does not seem to increase toxicity but has improved response rates to 39%, added two to three months to disease free survival, and prolonged overall survival by a little more than two months.

Alternative treatment

Most alternative therapies have not been studied in clinical trials. Large doses of **vitamins**, fiber, and green tea are among therapies tried. A 2003 report on a large Harvard University study showed that people who took multivitamins for at least 15 years had a 34% reduction in risk of rectal cancer. Before initiating any alternative therapies, the patient should consult his or her physician to be sure that these therapies do not complicate or interfere with the recommended therapy.

Prognosis

Prognosis is the long-term outlook or survival after therapy. Overall, about 50% of patients treated for colon and rectal cancer survive the disease. As expected, the survival rates are dependent upon the stage of the cancer at the time of diagnosis, making early detection crucial.

About 15% of patients present with stage I disease, or are diagnosed with Stage I disease when they initially visit a doctor, and 85-90% survive. Stage II represents 20-30% of cases and 65-75% survive; 30-40% comprise the stage III presentation, of which 55% survive. The remaining 20-25% present with stage IV disease and are rarely cured.

Prevention

There is not an absolute method for preventing colon or rectal cancer. An individual can lessen risk or identify the precursors of colon and rectal cancer. The patient with a familial history can enter screening and surveillance programs earlier than the general population. High-fiber diets and vitamins, avoiding **obesity**, and staying active lessen the risk. In fact, a 2003 report said that vigorous **exercise** (to the point of sweating or feeling out of breath) lowered risk of rectal cancer by nearly 40% compared to those who exercised less. Avoiding cigarettes and alcohol may be helpful. By controlling these environmental factors, an individual can lessen risk and to this degree prevent the disease.

By undergoing appropriate screening when uncontrollable genetic risk factors have been identified, an individual may be rewarded by the identification of benign polyps that can be treated as opposed

to having these growths degenerate into a malignancy.

KEY TERMS

Adenocarcinoma—Type of cancer beginning in glandular epithelium.

Adjuvant therapy—Treatment involving radiation, chemotherapy (drug treatment), or hormone therapy, or a combination of all three given after the primary treatment for the possibility of residual microscopic disease.

Anastomosis—Surgical re-connection of the ends of the bowel after removal of a portion of the bowel.

Anemia—The condition caused by too few circulating red blood cells, often manifest in part by fatigue.

Carcinogens—Substances in the environment that cause cancer, presumably by inducing mutations, with prolonged exposure.

Defecation—The act of having a bowel movement.

Epithelium—Cells composing the lining of an organ.

Lymphatics—Channels that are conduits for lymph.

Lymph nodes—Cellular filters through which lymphatics flow.

Malignant—Cells that have been altered such that they have lost normal control mechanisms and are capable of local invasion and spread to other areas of the body.

Metastasis—Site of invasive tumor growth that originated from a malignancy elsewhere in the body.

Mutation—A change in the genetic makeup of a cell that may occur spontaneously or be environmentally induced.

Occult blood—Presence of blood that cannot be appreciated visually.

Polyps—Localized growths of the epithelium that can be benign, pre-cancerous, or harbor malignancy.

Resect—To remove surgically.

Sacrum—Posterior bony wall of the pelvis.

Systemic—Referring to throughout the body.

Resources

BOOKS

Abelhoff, Martin, MD, James O. Armitage MD, Allen S. Lichter MD, and John E. Niederhuber MD. *Clinical Oncology Library*. Philadelphia: Churchill Livingstone, 1999.

Jorde, Lynn B., PhD, John C. Carey MD, Michael J. Bamshad MD, and Raymond L. White, PhD. *Medical Genetics*. 2nd ed. St. Louis: Mosby, 1999.

PERIODICALS

"Colon Cancer; Facts to Know." *NWHRC Health Center* December 15, 2003.

"Endoscopy and MRI Are Important in Staging Rectal Cancer." *Clinical Oncology Week* October 6, 2003: 56.

Greenlee, Robert T., PhD, MPH, Mary Beth Hill-Harmon, MSPH, Taylor Murray, and Michael Thun, MD, MS. "Cancer Statistics 2001." *CA: A Cancer Journal for Clinicians*, 51, no. 1 (January-February 2001).

Saltz, Leonard, et al. "Irinotecan plus Fluorouracil and Leucovorin for Metastatic Colorectal Cancer." *The New England Journal of Medicine* 343, no. 13 (September 28, 2000).

Splete, Heidi. "Multivitamins May Lower Risk of Rectal Cancer: Drops 34% at 15 Years." *Family Practice News* December 1, 2003: 33.

"Vigourous Physical Activity May Reduce the Risk of Rectal Cancer." *Environmental Nutrition* October 2003: 8.

ORGANIZATIONS

American Cancer Society. 1599 Clifton Road NE, Atlanta, GA 30329. (800)ACS-2345. Lt;http://www.cancer.org >.

Cancer Information Service of the NCI. 9000 Rockville Pike, Building 31, Suite 10A18, Bethesda, MD 20892. (800) 4-CANCER. < http://wwwicic.nci.nih.gov >.

OTHER

Colon Cancer Alliance. < http://www.ccalliance.org >.

National Cancer Institute Clinical Trials. < http://www.cancertrials.nci.nih.gov >.

Richard A. McCartney, MD
Teresa G. Odle

Rectal examination

Definition

Rectal examination or digital rectal examination (DRE) is performed by means of inserting a gloved, lubricated finger into the rectum and palpating (feeling) for lumps.

Purpose

DRE is used as a screening tool to locate **rectal cancer** and **prostate cancer**. It is also used as a diagnostic test to find non-cancerous abnormalities within the rectum like **hemorrhoids**, anal fissures, or congenital deformities that can cause chronic **constipation**.

Precautions

There are no precautions when performing DRE, aside from routine sanitary procedures.

Description

DRE is performed in most instances as an annual routine procedure in colorectal **cancer** screening. Digital palpitation of the rectum can often find abnormal growths which may require further testing or commonplace hemorrhoids. It is a critical initial clinical test and is important in the assessment of the size and location of tumors.

This procedure is often not performed routinely on patients over 70, even though this population is at high risk for colorectal cancer. It also is not done as often in elderly women as in elderly men.

DRE has also been used as a screening tool for prostate cancer. It seems to be very effective for larger masses found in the prostate and correlated well with higher prostate-specific antigens.

Of less predictive value was DRE in routine rectovaginal examinations of women under the age of 50. These instances of DRE did not locate colorectal cancer or any other abnormality.

More gastroenterologists are recommending that pediatricians and family physicians perform DRE on pediatric patients exhibiting chronic constipation before those patients are referred to intestinal specialists. The pediatrician or family physician could identify fecal compaction and treat it themselves, and then only refer patients who have a specific abnormality to gastroenterologists.

Preparation

The physician must conduct DRE using a gloved hand. Some sort of lubricant should be used so that penetration of the rectum is easier and does not create the damage that the procedure is seeking.

Aftercare

There is no aftercare after a DRE is performed.

Risks

There are no risks to DRE and it is virtually painless.

Normal results

The physician finds a normal rectal canal with no abnormalities.

Abnormal results

Growths, tears, anal fissures, or congenital structural defects can be found inside the rectum with DRE.

Resources

PERIODICALS

Kirchner, Jeffrey T. "Digital Rectal Examination in Children with Constipation." *American Family Physician* 60, no. 5 (October 1, 1999): 1530.

Schroder, Fritz H. "Evaluation of the Digital Rectal Examination as a Screening Test for Prostate Cancer." *JAMA, The Journal of the American Medical Association* 281, no. 7 (February 7, 1999) 594.

OTHER

Practice Parameters for the Treatment of Rectal Carcinoma American Society of Colon and Rectal Surgeons May 7, 2001. < http://www.asco.org/prof/me/html/abstracts/gasc/m_969.htm >.

Janie F. Franz

Rectal polyps

Definition

Rectal polyps are tissue growths that arise from the wall of the rectum and protrude into it. They may be either benign or malignant (cancerous).

Description

The rectum is the last segment of the large intestine, ending in the anus, the opening to the exterior of the body. Rectal polyps are quite common. They occur in 7–50% of all people, and in two thirds of people over age 60.

Rectal polyps can be either benign or malignant, large or small. There are several different types of polyps. The type is determined by taking a sample of the polyp and examining it microscopically. Most polyps are benign. They are of concern, however, because 90% of colon and rectal cancers arise from polyps that are initially benign. For this reason, rectal polyps are usually removed when they are discovered.

Causes and symptoms

The cause of most rectal polyps is unknown, however a diet high in animal fat and red meat, and low in fiber, is thought to encourage polyp formation. Some types of polyps are hereditary. In an inherited disease called **familial polyposis**, hundreds of small, malignant and pre-malignant polyps are produced before the age of 40. Also, inflammatory bowel disease may cause growth of polyps and pseudo-polyps. Juvenile polyps (polyps in children) are usually benign and often outgrow their blood supply and disappear at **puberty**.

Most rectal polyps produce no symptoms and are discovered on routine digital or endoscopic examination of the rectum. Rectal bleeding is the most common complaint when symptoms do occur. Abdominal cramps, **pain**, or obstruction of the intestine occur with some large polyps. Certain types of polyps cause mucous-filled or watery **diarrhea**.

Diagnosis

Rectal polyps are commonly found by **sigmoido-scopy** (visual inspection with an instrument consisting of a tube and a light) or **colonoscopy**. If polyps are found in the rectum, a complete examination of the large intestine is done, as multiple polyps are common. Polyps do not show up on regular x rays, but they do appear on **barium enema** x rays.

Treatment

Normally polyps are removed when they are found. Polypectomy is the name for the surgery that removes these growths. Polypectomy is performed at a hospital, outpatient surgical facility or in a doctor's office, depending on the number and type of polyps to be removed, and the age and health of the patient. The procedure can be done by a surgeon, gastroenterologist, or family practitioner.

Before the operation, a colonoscopy (examination of the intestine with an endoscope) is performed, and standard pre-operative blood and urine studies are done. The patient is also given medicated **enemas** to cleanse the bowel.

The patient is given a sedative and a narcotic pain killer. A colonoscope is inserted into the rectum. The polyps are located and removed with a wire snare, ultrasound, or laser beam. After they are removed, the polyps are examined to determine if they are malignant or benign. When polyps are malignant, it may be necessary to remove a portion of the rectum or colon to completely remove cancerous tissue.

Alternative treatment

In addition to a diet low in animal fat and high in fiber, nutritionists recommend anitoxidant supplements (including **vitamins** A, C, and E, selenium, and zinc) to reduce rectal polyps.

Prognosis

For most people, the removal of polyps is an uncomplicated procedure. Benign polyps that are left in place can give rise to **rectal cancer**. People who have had rectal polyps once are more likely to have them again and should have regular screening examinations.

Prevention

Eating a diet low in red meat and animal fat, and high in fiber, is thought to help prevent rectal polyps.

Resources

ORGANIZATIONS

American Cancer Society. 1599 Clifton Rd., NE, Atlanta, GA 30329-4251. (800) 227-2345. < http://www.cancer.org >.

National Cancer Institute. Building 31, Room 10A31, 31 Center Drive, MSC 2580, Bethesda, MD 20892-2580. (800) 422-6237. < http://www.nci.nih.gov >.

Tish Davidson, A.M.

Rectal prolapse

Definition

Rectal prolapse is protrusion of rectal tissue through the anus to the exterior of the body. The rectum is the final section of the large intestine.

Description

Rectal prolapse can be either partial or complete. In partial prolapse, only the mucosa layer (mucous membrane) of the rectum extends outside the body. The projection is generally 0.75–1.5 in (2–4 cm) long. In complete prolapse, called procidentia, the full thickness of the rectum protrudes for up to 4.5 in (12 cm).

Rectal prolapse is most common in people over age 60, and occurs much more frequently in women than in men. It is also more common in psychiatric patients. Prolapse can occur in normal infants, where it is usually transient. In children it is often an early sign of **cystic fibrosis** or is due to neurological or anatomical abnormalities.

Although rectal prolapse in adults may initially reduce spontaneously after bowel movements, it eventually becomes permanent. Adults who have had prior rectal or vaginal surgery, who have chronic **constipation**, regularly depend on **laxatives**, have **multiple sclerosis** or other neurologic diseases, **stroke**, or **paralysis** are more likely to experience rectal prolapse.

Causes and symptoms

Rectal prolapse in adults is caused by a weakening of the sphincter muscle or ligaments that hold the rectum in place. Weakening can occur because of **aging**, disease, or in rare cases, surgical trauma. Prolapse is brought on by straining to have bowel movements, chronic laxative use, or severe **diarrhea**.

Symptoms of rectal prolapse include discharge of mucus or blood, **pain** during bowel movements, and inability to control bowel movements (**fecal incontinence**). Patients may also feel the mass of tissue protruding from the anus. With large prolapses, the patient may lose the normal urge to have a bowel movement.

Diagnosis

Prolapse is initially diagnosed by taking a patient history and giving a **rectal examination** while the patient is in a squatting position. It is confirmed by **sigmoidoscopy** (inspection of the colon with a viewing instrument called a endoscope) **Barium enema** x rays and other tests are done to rule out neurologic (nerve) disorders or disease as the primary cause of prolapse.

Treatment

In infants, conservative treatment, consisting of strapping the buttocks together between bowel movements and eliminating any causes of bowel straining, usually produces a spontaneous resolution of prolapse. For partial prolapse in adults, excess tissue is surgically tied off with special bands causing the tissue to wither in a few days.

Complete prolapse requires surgery. Different surgical techniques are used, but all involve anchoring the rectum to other parts of the body, and using plastic mesh to reinforce and support the rectum. In patients too old, or ill, to tolerate surgery, a wire or plastic loop can be inserted to hold the sphincter closed and prevent prolapse. Treatment should be undertaken as soon as prolapse is diagnosed, since the longer the condition exists, the more difficult it is to reverse.

Alternative treatment

Alternative therapies can act as support for conventional threatment, especially if surgery is required. **Acupuncture**, homeopathy, and botanical medicine can all be used to assist in resolution of the prolapse or in recovery from surgery.

Prognosis

Successful resolution of rectal prolapse involves prompt treatment and the elimination of any underlying causes of prolapse. Infants and children usually recover completely without complications. Recovery in adults depends on age, general health, and the extent of the prolapse.

KEY TERMS

Rectum—The part of the large intestine that ends at the anal canal.

Prevention

Reducing constipation by eating a diet high in fiber, drinking plenty of fluids, and avoiding straining during bowel movements help prevent the onset of prolapse. Exercises that strengthen the anal sphincter may also be helpful.

Resources

OTHER

"Rectal Prolapse." *ThriveOnline.* < http:// thriveonline.oxygen.com >.

Tish Davidson, A.M.

Recurrent fever *see* **Relapsing fever**

Recurrent miscarriage

Definition

Recurrent **miscarriage** is defined as three or more miscarriages of a fetus before 20 weeks of gestation (i.e., before the fetus can live outside the womb).

Description

Also referred to as spontaneous abortion, miscarriage occurs in 15–20% of all conceptions. The majority of miscarriages occur during the first trimester. The number of previous miscarriages does not affect subsequent full-term pregnancies.

Causes and symptoms

Recurrent miscarriage can be caused by several factors, including fetal, placental, or maternal abnormalities.

- In over half of all miscarriages, the fetus is abnormal. The abnormality can either be genetic or developmental. The fetus is very sensitive to ionizing radiation. Tobacco and even moderate alcohol consumption are known to cause fetal damage that may lead to miscarriage. There is some evidence that over four cups of coffee a day, because of the **caffeine**, adversely affect **pregnancy**, as well.

- Placental abnormalities, including abnormal implantation in the placental wall and premature separation of the placenta, can cause miscarriage.

- Maternal abnormalities include insufficient hormones (usually progesterone) to support the pregnancy, an **incompetent cervix** (mouth of the womb does not stay closed), or a deformed uterus (womb). A deformed uterus can be caused by diethylstilbestrol (DES) given to the mother's mother during her pregnancy. Some immunologic abnormalities may cause the mother to reject the fetus as if it were an infection or a transplant. Maternal blood clotting abnormalities may cut-off blood supply to the fetus, causing miscarriage.

- Maternal **diabetes mellitus** causes miscarriage if the diabetes is poorly controlled. Maternal infections may occasionally lead to miscarriage. There is some evidence that conceptions that take place between old eggs (several days after ovulation) or old sperm (that start out several days before ovulation) may be more likely to miscarry.

Symptoms of miscarriage include pink or brown colored discharge for several weeks, which develops into painful cramping and increased vaginal bleeding; dilation of the cervix; and expulsion of the fetus.

Diagnosis

A pelvic examination can detect a deformed uterus, and frequent examinations during pregnancy can detect an incompetent cervix. Blood tests can detect the presence of immunologic or blood-clotting problems in the mother. **Genetic testing** can also determine if chromosomal abnormalities may be causing the miscarriages.

Treatment

If a uterus is deformed, it may be surgically repaired. If a cervix is incompetent, it can be surgically fortified, until the fetus matures, by a procedure known as circlage (tying the cervix closed). Supplemental progesterone may also help sustain a pregnancy. Experimental treatment of maternal immunologic abnormalities with white cell immunization (injecting the mother with white cells from the father) has been successful in some cases of recurrent

miscarriage. Clotting abnormalities can be treated with **anticoagulant drugs**, such as heparin and **aspirin**, to keep blood flowing to the fetus.

Prognosis

If there is no underlying disease or abnormality present, the rate of successful pregnancy after several miscarriages approaches normal. Seventy to eighty-five percent of women with three or more miscarriages will go on to complete a healthy pregnancy.

Resources

BOOKS

Cunningham, F. Gary, et al., editor. *Williams Obstetrics.* Stamford: Appleton & Lange, 1997.

J. Ricker Polsdorfer, MD

Red blood cell indices

Definition

Red blood cell indices are measurements that describe the size and oxygen-carrying protein (hemoglobin) content of red blood cells. The indices are used to help in the differential diagnosis of anemia. They are also called red cell absolute values or erythrocyte indices.

Purpose

Anemia includes a variety of conditions with the same outcome: a person's blood cannot carry as much oxygen as it should. A healthy person has an adequate number of correctly sized red blood cells that contain enough hemoglobin to carry sufficient oxygen to all the body's tissues. An anemic person has red blood cells that are either too small or too few in number. As a result, the heart and lungs must work harder to make up for the lack of oxygen delivered to the tissues by the blood.

Anemia is caused by many different diseases or disorders. The first step in finding the cause is to determine what type of anemia the person has. Red blood cell indices help to classify the **anemias**.

Precautions

Certain prescription medications may affect the test results. These drugs include zidovudine (Retrovir), phenytoin (Dilantin), and azathioprine (Imuran).

Description

Overview

Anemia has several general causes: blood loss; a drop in production of red blood cells; or a rise in the number of red blood cells destroyed. Blood loss can result from severe hemorrhage or a chronic slow bleed, such as the result of an accident or an ulcer. Lack of iron, vitamin B_{12}, or **folic acid** in the diet, as well as certain chronic diseases, lower the number of red blood cells produced by the bone marrow. Inherited disorders affecting hemoglobin, severe reactions to blood transfusions, prescription medications, or poisons can cause red blood cells to burst (hemolyze) well before the end of their usual 120-day lifespan.

Anemia of any type affects the results of one or more of the common blood tests. These tests are the **hematocrit**, hemoglobin, and red blood cell count. The hematocrit is a measure of red blood cell mass, or how much space in the blood is occupied by red blood cells. The **hemoglobin test** is a measure of how much hemoglobin protein is in the blood. The red blood cell count (RBC) measures the number of red blood cells present in the blood. Red blood cell indices are additional measurements of red blood cells based on the relationship of these three test results.

The relationships between the hematocrit, the hemoglobin level, and the RBC are converted to red blood cell indices through mathematical formulas. These formulas were worked out and first applied to the classification of anemias by Maxwell Wintrobe in 1934.

The indices include these measurements: mean corpuscular volume (MCV); mean corpuscular hemoglobin (MCH); mean corpuscular hemoglobin concentration (MCHC); and red cell distribution width (RDW). They are usually calculated by an automated instrument as part of a complete **blood count** (CBC). Indices are covered by insurance when medically necessary. Results are available the same day that the blood is drawn or the following day.

Mean corpuscular volume (MCV)

MCV is the index most often used. It measures the average volume of a red blood cell by dividing the hematocrit by the RBC. The MCV categorizes red blood cells by size. Cells of normal size are called normocytic, smaller cells are microcytic, and larger cells are macrocytic. These size categories are used to classify anemias. Normocytic anemias have normal-sized cells and a normal MCV; microcytic anemias have small cells and a decreased MCV; and macrocytic anemias have large cells and an increased MCV. Under a microscope, stained red blood cells with a high MCV appear larger than cells with a normal or low MCV.

Mean corpuscular hemoglobin concentration (MCHC)

The MCHC measures the average concentration of hemoglobin in a red blood cell. This index is calculated by dividing the hemoglobin by the hematocrit. The MCHC categorizes red blood cells according to their concentration of hemoglobin. Cells with a normal concentration of hemoglobin are called normochromic; cells with a lower than normal concentration are called hypochromic. Because there is a physical limit to the amount of hemoglobin that can fit in a cell, there is no hyperchromic category.

Just as MCV relates to the size of the cells, MCHC relates to the color of the cells. Hemoglobin contains iron, which gives blood its characteristic red color. When examined under a microscope, normal red blood cells that contain a normal amount of hemoglobin stain pinkish red with a paler area in the center. These normochromic cells have a normal MCHC. Cells with too little hemoglobin are lighter in color with a larger pale area in the center. These hypochromic cells have a low MCHC. Anemias are categorized as hypochromic or normochromic according to the MCHC index.

Mean corpuscular hemoglobin (MCH)

The average weight of hemoglobin in a red blood cell is measured by the MCH. The formula for this index is the sum of the hemoglobin multiplied by 10 and divided by the RBC. MCH values usually rise or fall as the MCV is increased or decreased.

Red cell distribution width (RDW)

The RDW measures the variation in size of the red blood cells. Usually red blood cells are a standard size. Certain disorders, however, cause a significant variation in cell size.

Obtaining the blood sample

The RBC indices test requires 0.17–24 oz (5–7 ml) of blood. A healthcare worker ties a tourniquet on the person's upper arm, locates a vein in the inner elbow region, and inserts a needle into that vein. Vacuum action draws the blood through the needle into an attached tube. Collection of the sample takes only a few minutes.

Preparation

The doctor should check to see if the patient is taking any medications that may affect test results. The patient does not need to fast before the test.

Aftercare

Aftercare consists of routine care of the area around the puncture mark. Pressure is applied for a few seconds and the wound is covered with a bandage.

Risks

The primary risk is mild **dizziness** and the possibility of a bruise or swelling in the area where the blood was drawn. The patient can apply moist warm compresses.

Normal results

Normal results for red blood cell indices are as follows:

- MCV 82–98 fl (femtoliters)
- MCHC 31–37 g/dl
- MCH 26–34 pg (picograms)
- RDW 11.5–14.5%.

Abnormal results

The category into which a person's anemia is placed based on the indices provides a significant clue as to the cause of the anemia, but further testing is needed to confirm a specific diagnosis.

KEY TERMS

Anemia—A variety of conditions in which a person's blood can't carry as much oxygen as it should due to a decreased number or size of red blood cells.

Hypochromic—A descriptive term applied to a red blood cell with a decreased concentration of hemoglobin.

Macrocytic—A descriptive term applied to a larger than normal red blood cell.

Mean corpuscular hemoglobin (MCH)—A measurement of the average weight of hemoglobin in a red blood cell.

Mean corpuscular hemoglobin concentration (MCHC)—The measurement of the average concentration of hemoglobin in a red blood cell.

Mean corpuscular volume (MCV)—A measure of the average volume of a red blood cell.

Microcytic—A descriptive term applied to a smaller than normal red blood cell.

Normochromic—A descriptive term applied to a red blood cell with a normal concentration of hemoglobin.

Normocytic—A descriptive term applied to a red blood cell of normal size.

Red blood cell indices—Measurements that describe the size and hemoglobin content of red blood cells.

Red cell distribution width (RDW)—A measure of the variation in size of red blood cells.

The most common causes of macrocytic anemia (high MCV) are vitamin B_{12} and folic acid deficiencies. Lack of iron in the diet, **thalassemia** (a type of hereditary anemia), and chronic illness are the most common causes of microcytic anemia (low MCV). Normocytic anemia (normal MCV) can be caused by kidney and **liver disease**, bone marrow disorders, or excessive bleeding or hemolysis of the red blood cells.

Lack of iron in the diet and thalassemia are the most common causes of hypochromic anemia (low MCHC). Normocytic anemias are usually also normochromic and share the same causes (normal MCHC).

The RDW is increased in anemias caused by deficiencies of iron, vitamin B_{12}, or folic acid. Abnormal hemoglobins, such as in sickle cell anemia, can change the shape of red blood cells as well as cause them to hemolyze. The abnormal shape and the cell fragments resulting from hemolysis increase the RDW. Conditions that cause more immature cells to be released into the bloodstream, such as severe blood loss, will increase the RDW. The larger size of immature cells creates a distinct size variation.

Resources

BOOKS

Pagana, Kathleen Deska, and Timothy James Pagana, editors. *Mosby's Manual of Diagnostic and Laboratory Tests.* St. Louis: Mosby, Inc., 1998.

Nancy J. Nordenson

Red blood cell test *see* **Hemoglobin test**

Reflex sympathetic dystrophy

Definition

Reflex sympathetic dystrophy is the feeling of **pain** associated with evidence of minor nerve injury.

Description

Historically, reflex sympathetic dystrophy (RSD) was noticed during the civil war in patients who suffered pain following gunshot **wounds** that affected the median nerve (a major nerve in the arm). In 1867 the condition was called causalgia form the Greek term meaning "burning pain." Causalgia refers to pain associated with major nerve injury. The exact causes of RSD are still unclear. Patients usually develop a triad of phases. In the first phase, pain and sympathetic activity is increased. Patients will typically present with swelling (**edema**), stiffness, pain, increased vascularity (increasing warmth), hyperhydrosis, and x-ray changes demonstrating loss of **minerals** in bone (demineralization). The second phase develops three to nine months later, It is characterized by increased stiffness and changes in the extremity that include a decrease in warmth and atrophy of the skin and muscles. The late phase commencing several months to years later presents with a pale, cold, painful, and atrophic extremity. Patients at this stage will also have **osteoporosis**.

It has been thought that each phase relates to a specific nerve defect that involves nerve tracts from the periphery spinal cord to the brain. Both sexes are affected, but the number of new cases is higher in women, adolescents, and young adults. RDS has been associated with other terms such as Sudeck's atrophy, post-traumatic osteoporosis, causalgia, shoulder-hand syndrome, and reflex neuromuscular dystrophy.

Causes and symptoms

The exact causes of RSD at present is not clearly understood. There are several theories such as sympathetic overflow (over activity), abnormal circuitry in nerve impulses through the sympathetic system, and as a post-operative complication for both elective and traumatic surgical procedures. Patients typically develop pain, swelling, temperature, color changes, and skin and muscle wasting.

Diagnosis

The diagnosis is simple and confirmed by a local anesthetic block along sympathetic nerve paths in the hand or foot, depending on whether an arm or leg is affected. A test called the **erythrocyte sedimentation rate** (ESR) can be performed to rule out diseases with similar presentation and arising from other causes.

Treatment

The preferred method to treat RSD includes sympathetic block and physical therapy. Pain is improved as motion of the affected limb improves. Patients may also require tranquilizers and mild **analgesics**. Patients who received repeated blocks should consider surgical symathectomy (removal of the nerves causing pain).

Prognosis

The prognosis for treatment during phase one is favorable. As the disease progresses undetected into phase two or three the prognosis for recovery is poor.

Prevention

There is no known prevention since the cause is not clearly understood.

KEY TERMS

Atrophy—Abnormal changes in a cell that lead to loss of cell structure and function.

Osteoporosis—Reduction in the quantity of bone.

Resources

BOOKS

Goetz, Christopher G., et al, editors. *Textbook of Clinical Neurology*. 1st ed. W. B. Saunders Company, 1999.

Ruddy, Shaun, et al, editors. *Kelly's Textbook of Rheumatology*. 6th ed. W. B. Saunders Company, 2001.

OTHER

Reflex Sympathetic Dystrophy Syndrome Association of America. < http://www.rsds.org/fact.html >.

Laith Farid Gulli, M.D.
Robert Ramirez, B.S.

Reflex tests

Definition

Reflex tests are simple physical tests of nervous system function.

Purpose

A reflex is a simple nerve circuit. A stimulus, such as a light tap with a rubber hammer, causes sensory neurons (nerve cells) to send signals to the spinal cord. Here, the signals are conveyed both to the brain and to nerves that control muscles affected by the stimulus. Without any brain intervention, these muscles may respond to an appropriate stimulus by contracting.

Reflex tests measure the presence and strength of a number of reflexes. In so doing, they help to assess the integrity of the nerve circuits involved. Reflex tests are performed as part of a neurological exam, either a "mini-exam" done to quickly confirm integrity of the spinal cord, or a more complete exam performed to diagnose the presence and location of **spinal cord injury** or neuromuscular disease.

Deep tendon reflexes are responses to muscle stretch. The familiar "knee-jerk" reflex is an example; this reflex tests the integrity of the spinal cord in the lower back region. The usual set of deep tendon reflexes tested, involving increasingly higher regions of the spinal cord, are:

- ankle
- knee
- abdomen
- forearm
- biceps
- triceps

Another type of reflex test is called the Babinski test, which involves gently stroking the sole of the foot to assess proper development of the spine and cerebral cortex.

Precautions

Reflex tests are entirely safe, and no special precautions are needed.

Description

The examiner positions the patient in a comfortable position, usually seated on the examination table with legs hanging free. The examiner uses a rubber mallet to strike different points on the patient's body, and observes the response. The examiner may position, or hold, one of the limbs during testing, and may require exposure of the ankles, knees, abdomen, and arms. Reflexes can be difficult to elicit if the patient is paying too much attention to the stimulus. To compensate for this, the patient may be asked to perform some muscle contraction, such as clenching teeth or grasping and pulling the two hands apart. When performing the Babinski reflex test, the doctor will gently **stroke** the outer soles of the patient's feet with the mallet while checking to see whether or not the big toe extends out as a result.

Normal results

The strength of the response depends partly on the strength of the stimulus. For this reason, the examiner will attempt to elicit the response with the smallest stimulus possible. Learning the range of normal responses requires some clinical training. Responses should be the same for both sides of the body. A normal response to the Babinski reflex test depends upon the age of the person being examined. In children under the age of one and a half years, the big toe will extend out with or without the other toes. This is due to the fact that the fibers in the spinal cord and cerebral cortex have not been completely covered in myelin, the protein and lipid sheath that aids in processing neural signals. In adults and children over the age of one and a half years, the myelin sheath should be completely formed, and, as a result, all the toes will curl under (planter flexion reflex).

Abnormal results

Weak or absent response may indicate damage to the nerves outside the spinal cord (**peripheral** neuropathy), damage to the motor neurons just before or just after they leave the spinal cord (motor neuron disease), or muscle disease. Excessive response may indicate spinal cord damage above the level controlling the hyperactive response. Different responses on the two sides of the body may indicate early onset of progressive disease, or localized nerve damage, as from trauma. An adult or older child who responds to the Babinski with an extended big toe may have a lesion in the spinal cord or cerebral cortex.

Resources

OTHER

Rathe, Richard. "The Neurological Exam." *A Healthy Me Page*. July 2, 1997. < http://www.ahealthyme.com >.

Richard Robinson

Reflexology

Definition

Reflexology is a therapeutic method of relieving **pain** by stimulating predefined pressure points on the feet and hands. This controlled pressure alleviates the source of the discomfort. In the absence of any particular malady or abnormality, reflexology may be as effective for promoting good health and for preventing illness as it may be for relieving symptoms of **stress**, injury, and illness.

Reflexologists work from maps of predefined pressure points that are located on the hands and feet. These pressure points are reputed to connect directly through the nervous system and affect the bodily organs and glands. The reflexologist manipulates the pressure points according to specific techniques of reflexology therapy. By means of this touching therapy, any part of the body that is the source of pain, illness, or potential debility can be strengthened through the application of pressure at the respective foot or hand location.

Purpose

Reflexology promotes healing by stimulating the nerves in the body and encouraging the flow of blood. In the process, reflexology not only quells the sensation of pain, but relieves the source of the pain as well.

Anecdotally, reflexologists claim success in the treatment of a variety of conditions and injuries. One

EUNICE INGHAM (1889–1974)

Eunice D. Ingham was born on February 24, 1889. A physical therapist by occupation, she was a colleague of Dr. Shelby Riley, who along with Dr. W. H. Fitzgerald actively developed zone therapy, a similar but distinct therapy from reflexology. Unlike reflexology, zone therapy does not connect the zones with the body as a whole. In the 1930s, Ingham discovered an unmistakable pattern of reflexes on the human foot; she subsequently devoted the rest of her life to publicizing the message of reflexology until shortly before her death on December 10, 1974.

Ingham traveled and lectured widely about reflexology, initially to audiences of extremely desperate or aging patients who had lost hope in finding relief. Because of their sometimes astonishing improvement, reflexology became better known and respected among the medical community and gained credibility for its therapeutic value. Ingham described her theories of reflexology in her 1938 book, entitled *Stories the Feet Can Tell*, which included a map of the reflex points on the feet and the organs that they parallel. The book was translated into seven languages, although it was erroneously published as *Zone Therapy* in some countries, an error which led to misunderstanding about the true nature of reflexology and inaccurately linked it to zone therapy.

condition is **fibromyalgia**. People with this disease are encouraged to undergo reflexology therapy to alleviate any of a number of chronic bowel syndromes associated with the condition. Frequent brief sessions of reflexology therapy are also recommended as an alternative to drug therapy for controlling the muscle pain associated with fibromyalgia and for relieving difficult breathing caused by tightness in the muscles of the patient's neck and throat.

Reflexology applied properly can alleviate allergy symptoms, as well as stress, back pain, and chronic **fatigue**. The techniques of reflexology can be performed conveniently on the hand in situations where a session on the feet is not practical, although the effectiveness of limited hand therapy is less pronounced than with the foot pressure therapy.

Description

Origins

Reflexology is a healing art of ancient origin. Although its origins are not well documented, there are reliefs on the walls of a Sixth Dynasty Egyptian tomb (c. 2450 B.C.) that depict two seated men receiving massage on their hands and feet. From Egypt, the practice may have entered the Western world during the conquests of the Roman Empire. The concepts of reflexology have also been traced to pre-dynastic China (possibly as early as 3000 B.C.) and to ancient Indian medicine. The Inca civilization may have subscribed to the theories of reflexology and passed on the practice of this treatment to the Native Americans in the territories that eventually entered the United States.

In recent times, Sir Henry Head first investigated the concepts underlying reflexology in England in the 1890s. Therapists in Germany and Russia were researching similar notions at approximately the same time, although with a different focus. Less than two decades later, a physician named William H. Fitzgerald presented a similar concept that he called zone analgesia or zone therapy. Fitzgerald's zone analgesia was a method of relieving pain through the application of pressure to specific locations throughout the entire body. Fitzgerald divided the body into 10 vertical zones, five on each side, that extended from the head to the fingertips and toes, and from front to back. Every aspect of the human body appears in one of these 10 zones, and each zone has a reflex area on the hands and feet. Fitzgerald and his colleague, Dr. Edwin Bowers, demonstrated that by applying pressure on one area of the body, they could anesthetize or reduce pain in a corresponding part. In 1917, Fitzgerald and Bowers published *Relieving Pain at Home*, an explanation of zone therapy.

Later, in the 1930s, a physical therapist, Eunice D. Ingham, explored the direction of the therapy and made the startling discovery that pressure points on the human foot were situated in a mirror image of the corresponding organs of the body with which the respective pressure points were associated. Ingham documented her findings, which formed the basis of reflexology, in *Stories the Feet Can Tell*, published in 1938. Although Ingham's work in reflexology was inaccurately described as zone therapy by some, there are differences between the two therapies of pressure analgesia. Among the more marked differences, reflexology defines a precise correlation between pressure points and afflicted areas of the body. Furthermore, Ingham divided each foot and hand into 12 respective pressure zones, in contrast to the 10 vertical divisions that encompass the entire body in Fitzgerald's zone therapy.

In 1968 two siblings, Dwight Byers and Eusebia Messenger, established the National Institute of Reflexology. By the early 1970s the institute had grown and was renamed the International Institute of Reflexology.

In a typical reflexology treatment, the therapist and patient have a preliminary discussion prior to therapy, to enable the therapist to focus more accurately on the patient's specific complaints and to determine the appropriate pressure points for treatment.

A reflexology session involves pressure treatment that is most commonly administered in foot therapy sessions of approximately 40–45 minutes in duration. The foot therapy may be followed by a brief 15-minute hand therapy session. No artificial devices or special equipment are associated with this therapy. The human hand is the primary tool used in reflexology. The therapist applies controlled pressure with the thumb and forefinger, generally working toward the heel of the foot or the outer palm of the hand. Most reflexologists apply pressure with their thumbs bent; however, some also use simple implements, such as the eraser end of a pencil. Reflexology therapy is not massage, and it is not a substitute for medical treatment.

Reflexology is a complex system that identifies and addresses the mass of 7,000 nerve endings that are contained in the foot. Additional reflexology addresses the nerves that are located in the hand. This is a completely natural therapy that affords relief without the use of drugs. The Reflexology Association of America (RAA) formally discourages the use of oils or other preparations in performing this hands-on therapy.

Preparations

In order to realize maximum benefit from a reflexology session, the therapist as well as the patient should be situated so as to afford optimal comfort for both. Patients in general receive treatment in a reclining position, with the therapist positioned as necessary—to work on the bare feet, or alternately on the bare hands.

A reflexology patient removes both shoes and socks in order to receive treatment. No other preparation is involved. No prescription drugs, creams, oils, or lotions are used on the skin.

Precautions

Reflexology is extremely safe. It may even be self-administered in a limited form whenever desired. The qualified reflexologist offers a clear and open disclaimer that reflexology does not constitute medical treatment in any form, nor is reflexology given as a substitute for medical advice or treatment. The ultimate purpose of the therapy is to promote wellness; fundamentally it is a form of preventive therapy.

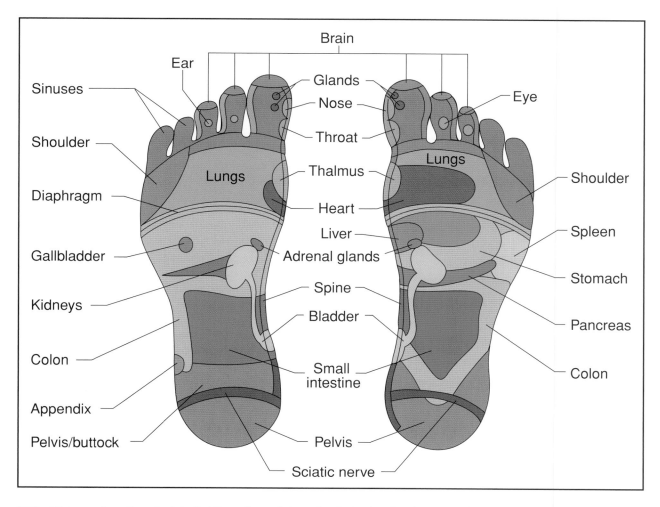

Ear
Brain
Glands
Sinuses
Nose
Eye
Throat
Shoulder
Thalmus
Lungs
Lungs
Shoulder
Diaphragm
Heart
Liver
Spleen
Gallbladder
Adrenal glands
Stomach
Spine
Kidneys
Bladder
Pancreas
Colon
Colon
Small intestine
Appendix
Pelvis/buttock
Pelvis
Sciatic nerve

Reflexology employs the principle that the reflex points on the feet, when hand pressure is applied, will reflexively stimulate energy to a related muscle or organ in the body and promote healing. *(Illustration by Electronic Illustrators Group.)*

People with serious and long-term medical problems are urged to seek the advice of a physician. Diabetes patients in particular are urged to approach this therapy cautiously. Likewise pregnant women are cautioned emphatically to avoid reflexology during the early phases of **pregnancy** altogether, as accidentally induced labor and subsequent premature delivery can result from reflexology treatment.

A consultation with a reflexologist is recommended in order to determine the safety and appropriateness of reflexology therapy for a specific health problem or condition.

Side effects

Because reflexology is intended to normalize the body functions, the therapy does not cause a condition to worsen. Most patients find that pain diminishes over the course of the therapy. It has been noted, however, that some patients experience greater discomfort in the second session than in the first session, because a significant easing of pain and tension is generally associated with the initial therapy session. As a result, when pressure is reapplied to the tender points of the foot during the second session, the sensitivity has been heightened. This increase in sensitivity may cause minor additional discomfort for the patient.

Research and general acceptance

Although only one controlled trial of reflexology therapy, done in 1993, has been documented in medical journals, this therapy is practiced worldwide at different levels of medical care. In Russia, for example, only licensed physicians may legally perform reflexology treatment. In contrast, the practice is a commonplace homestyle remedy in the Netherlands. The Internet "Home of Reflexology" lists at least 66 professional organizations worldwide, including New Zealand and Malaysia. Associations include the following:

- Academy of Reflexology Austria
- Association of Finnish Reflexologists
- Chinese Society of Reflexologists
- Hellenic Association of Reflexologists
- Indian Society for Promotion of Reflexology
- International Council of Reflexologists (HQ: San Diego, USA)
- Israeli Reflexology Association
- New Zealand Reflexology Association
- Polish Instytut of Reflexology (Polish Language)
- Reflexology Association of America
- Reflexology Association of Australia
- Rwo-Shr Health Institute International (Malaysia)
- The South African Reflexology Society

Regulatory status

Ongoing legislative debate ensued during the 1990s regarding the legal status of the reflexology trade. The reflexology community, along with legislators and other bodywork practitioners, engaged in reassessment of the reflexology business and its relationship to **massage therapy** and massage parlors. Organizations and individuals brought judicial appeals of certain court cases that threatened the legitimate licensing of reflexologists as practitioners of alternative medicine. Such professional reflexology interests as the RAA documented in detail the disparities between reflexology and massage, citing the purpose of reflexology, which is to stimulate internal body functions (glands and organs) as opposed to the topical muscular and joint relief associated with massage. In a status update in 1998 the Association reported that 19 states had laws requiring the licensing of massage/reflexology therapists. Licensing laws established educational requirements and required candidates to pass written, oral, and/or practical examinations.

Also at issue was a trend among municipalities to license massage parlors (and reflexologists) under the business codes affecting the adult entertainment business. B. and K. Kunz reported that judicial decisions in two states—Tennessee and New Mexico—had excluded the practice of reflexology practice from the laws pertaining to massage parlors. Those courts held

---

KEY TERMS

Pressure points—Specific locations on the feet and hands that correspond to nerve endings that connect to the organs and glands of the human body via the spinal cord.

Zone therapy—Also called zone analgesia, a method of relieving pain by applying pressure to specific points on the body. It was developed in the early twentieth century by Dr. William Fitzgerald.

---

that reflexology is a business separate and distinct from massage parlors, and deserving of its own respective licensing standards. In Sacramento, California, reflexologists petitioned successfully to become licensed as practitioners of somatic therapy rather than as providers of adult entertainment. Likewise, in the Canadian province of Ontario, a nonprofit organization to register reflexology practitioners was established in order to define a distinct classification for therapists separate from erotic body rubbers, which was the original classification given to reflexologists. Other states where court proceedings or legislative attempts to legitimize reflexology have stalled include Pennsylvania, Florida, New Jersey, and New York

Training and certification

Training programs

Reflexology is taught by means of a series of seminars, classes, and training films. Certification is earned after a six month program that includes 200 hours of training. The certification training breaks down as follows: 28 hours of preliminary seminar training; 14 hours of advanced seminar training; 58 hours of self-directed study; and 100 hours of practical experience, including administering reflexology to a minimum of 15 people.

Specific aspects of the training include instruction in the assessment of the pressure points on the feet and hands through a study of human anatomy. Students also learn to give reflexology sessions to patients along with specific techniques for working with the hands.

Certification and advanced certification

As part if its function, the independently organized American Reflexology Certification Board (ARCB) certifies the competency of reflexology practitioners on an individual basis. The ARCB does not evaluate schools and teachers. Prerequisites for individual certification include completion of educational requirements and passing a standard qualifying examiniation. Successful candidates receive the title of Board Certified Reflexologist.

Minimum qualifications to take the certification examination include attendance at an advanced seminar within two years prior to taking the examination. In addition, the applicant must have attended preliminary seminars for two full days—in addition to the required day of advanced seminar training—and the applicant is required to have a minimum of six months of practical experience in administering the therapy. Applicants are examined by means of both written tests and practical demonstrations.

Continuing education certification is available. Advanced training focuses on mastering the ability to perform hand reflexology. The therapist also receives instruction in new and advanced techniques of basic reflexology. Some reflexology training classes may be applied toward degree programs in other disciplines, depending on the specific course of study and the certification of the respective training institutions involved.

The RAA provides published standards of practice for reflexologists.

Resources

ORGANIZATIONS

International Institute of Reflexology. P.O. Box 12642. St. Petersburg, FL 33733-2642. (727) 343-4811. Fax: (727) 381-2807. E-mail: fteflex@concentric.net.

Reflexology Association of America. 4012 Rainbow St. KPMB#585. Las Vegas, NV 89103-2059.

Gloria Cooksey

Refsum's syndrome *see* **Lipidoses**

Regional anesthetic *see* **Anesthesia, local**

Regional enteritis *see* **Crohn's disease**

Rehabilitation

Definition

Rehabilitation is a treatment or treatments designed to facilitate the process of recovery from injury, illness, or disease to as normal a condition as possible.

Purpose

The purpose of rehabilitation is to restore some or all of the patient's physical, sensory, and mental capabilities that were lost due to injury, illness, or disease. Rehabilitation includes assisting the patient to compensate for deficits that cannot be reversed medically. It is prescribed after many types of injury, illness, or disease, including amputations, arthritis, **cancer**, cardiac disease, neurological problems, orthopedic injuries, spinal cord injuries, **stroke**, and traumatic brain injuries. The Institute of Medicine has estimated that as many as 14% of all Americans may be disabled at any given time.

Precautions

Rehabilitation should be carried out only by qualified therapists. Exercises and other physical interventions must take into account the patient's deficit. An example of a deficit is the loss of a limb.

Description

A proper and adequate rehabilitation program can reverse many disabling conditions or can help patients cope with deficits that cannot be reversed by medical care. Rehabilitation addresses the patient's physical, psychological, and environmental needs. It is achieved by restoring the patient's physical functions and/or modifying the patient's physical and social environment. The main types of rehabilitation are physical, occupational, and speech therapy.

Each rehabilitation program is tailored to the individual patient's needs and can include one or more types of therapy. The patient's physician usually coordinates the efforts of the rehabilitation team, which can include physical, occupational, speech, or other therapists; nurses; engineers; physiatrists (physical medicine); psychologists; orthotists (makes devices such as braces to straighten out curved or poorly shaped bones); prosthetists (a therapist who makes artificial limbs or protheses); and vocational counselors. Family members are often actively involved in the patient's rehabilitation program.

Physical therapy

Physical therapy helps the patient restore the use of muscles, bones, and the nervous system through the use of heat, cold, massage, whirlpool baths, ultrasound, **exercise**, and other techniques. It seeks to relieve **pain**, improve strength and mobility, and train the patient to perform important everyday tasks. Physical therapy may be prescribed to rehabilitate a

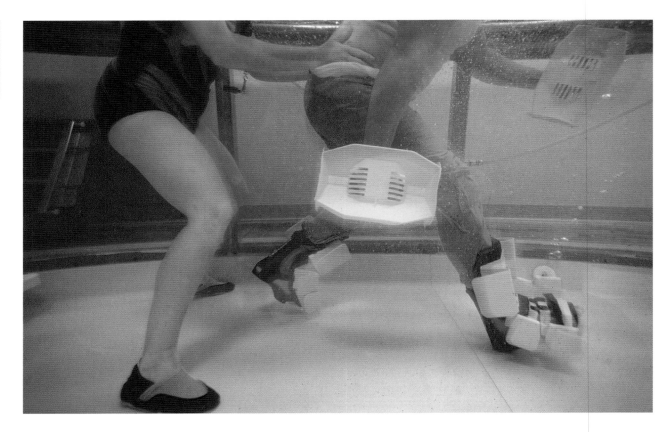

A patient (holding paddles) is undergoing a hydrotherapy treatment. *(Photograph by Will & Deni McIntyre, Photo Researchers, Inc. Reproduced by permission.)*

patient after amputations, arthritis, **burns**, cancer, cardiac disease, cervical and lumbar dysfunction, neurological problems, orthopedic injuries, pulmonary disease, spinal cord injuries, stroke, traumatic brain injuries, and other injuries/illnesses. The duration of the physical therapy program varies depending on the injury/illness being treated and the patient's response to therapy.

Exercise is the most widely used and best known type of physical therapy. Depending on the patient's condition, exercises may be performed by the patient alone or with the therapist's help, or with the therapist moving the patient's limbs. Exercise equipment for physical therapy could include an exercise table or mat, a stationary bicycle, walking aids, a wheelchair, practice stairs, parallel bars, and pulleys and weights.

Heat treatment, applied with hot-water compresses, infrared lamps, short-wave radiation, high frequency electrical current, ultrasound, paraffin wax, or warm baths, is used to stimulate the patient's circulation, relax muscles, and relieve pain. Cold treatment is applied with ice packs or cold-water soaking. Soaking in a whirlpool can ease muscle spasm pain

and help strengthen movements. Massage aids circulation, helps the patient relax, relieves pain and **muscle spasms**, and reduces swelling. Very low strength electrical currents applied through the skin stimulate muscles and make them contract, helping paralyzed or weakened muscles respond again.

Occupational therapy

Occupational therapy helps the patient regain the ability to do normal everyday tasks. This may be achieved by restoring old skills or teaching the patient new skills to adjust to disabilities through adaptive equipment, orthotics, and modification of the patient's home environment. Occupational therapy may be prescribed to rehabilitate a patient after **amputation**, arthritis, cancer, cardiac disease, head injuries, neurological injuries, orthopedic injuries, pulmonary disease, spinal cord disease, stroke, and other injuries/ illnesses. The duration of the occupational therapy program varies depending on the injury/illness being treated and the patient's response to therapy.

Occupational therapy includes learning how to use devices to assist in walking (artificial limbs,

KEY TERMS

Orthotist—A health care professional who is skilled in making and fitting orthopedic appliances.

Physiatrist—A physician who specializes in physical medicine.

Prosthetist—A health care professional who is skilled in making and fitting artificial parts (prosthetics) for the human body.

canes, crutches, walkers), getting around without walking (wheelchairs or motorized scooters), or moving from one spot to another (boards, lifts, and bars). The therapist will visit the patient's home and analyze what the patient can and cannot do. Suggestions on modifications to the home, such as rearranging furniture or adding a wheelchair ramp, will be made. Health aids to bathing and grooming could also be recommended.

Speech therapy

Speech therapy helps the patient correct **speech disorders** or restore speech. Speech therapy may be prescribed to rehabilitate a patient after a brain injury, cancer, neuromuscular diseases, stroke, and other injuries/illnesses. The duration of the speech therapy program varies depending on the injury/illness being treated and the patient's response to therapy.

Performed by a speech pathologist, speech therapy involves regular meetings with the therapist in an individual or group setting and home exercises. To strengthen muscles, the patient might be asked to say words, smile, close his mouth, or stick out his tongue. Picture cards may be used to help the patient remember everyday objects and increase his vocabulary. The patient might use picture boards of everyday activities or objects to communicate with others. Workbooks might be used to help the patient recall the names of objects and practice reading, writing, and listening. Computer programs are available to help sharpen speech, reading, recall, and listening skills.

Other types of therapists

Inhalation therapists, audiologists, and registered dietitians are other types of therapists. Inhalation therapists help the patient learn to use respirators and other breathing aids to restore or support breathing. Audiologists help diagnose the patient's **hearing loss** and recommend solutions. Dietitians provide dietary advice to help the patient recover from or avoid specific problems or diseases.

Rehabiltation centers

Rehabilitation services are provided in a variety of settings including clinical and office practices, hospitals, skilled-care nursing homes, sports medicine clinics, and some health maintenance organizations. Some therapists make home visits. Advice on choosing the appropriate type of therapy and therapist is provided by the patient's medical team.

Resources

ORGANIZATIONS

National Rehabilitation Association. 633 S. Washington St., Alexandria, VA 22314. (703) 836-0850.
National Rehabilitation Information Center. 8455 Colesville Road, Suite 935, Silver Spring, MD 20910. (800) 34-NARIC.
Rehabilitation International. 25 East 21st St., New York, NY 10010. (212) 420-1500.

Lori De Milto

Rehydration *see* **Intravenous rehydration**

Reiki

Definition

Reiki is a form of therapy that uses simple hands-on, no-touch, and visualization techniques, with the goal of improving the flow of life energy in a person. Reiki (pronounced *ray-key*) means "universal life energy" in Japanese, and Reiki practitioners are trained to detect and alleviate problems of energy flow on the physical, emotional, and spiritual level. Reiki touch therapy is used in much the same way to achieve similar effects that traditional **massage therapy** is used—to relieve **stress** and **pain**, and to improve the symptoms of various health conditions.

Purpose

Reiki claims to provide many of the same benefits as traditional massage therapy, such as reducing stress, stimulating the immune system, increasing energy, and relieving the pain and symptoms of health conditions. Practitioners have reported success in helping patients with acute and chronic illnesses, from **asthma** and arthritis to trauma and recovery from surgery. Reiki is a gentle and safe technique,

MIKAO USUI (1865–1926)

Mikao Usui, born in the Gifu Prefecture (Japan), was an ethereal child who sought to unravel the mysteries of the universe. As an adult he developed an interest in the metaphysical healing talent of Buddha. Usui became determined to regenerate the healing secrets of Buddha in order to improve the lot of humanity. He traveled to many temples and spoke with holy people, but all said that the secret of Buddha's powers were lost to the world due to lack of use.

Eventually the abbot of a Zen monastery encouraged Usui to study the ancient writings containing the secrets on healing. Usui learned two new languages, Chinese and Sanskrit, in order to understand the writings better, and from his reading he obtained the formula for healing. The Sutras in particular provided the enlightenment that he sought.

Usui next set out to obtain the power to heal. It is widely believed that he developed that ability after spending 21 days in retreat and in fasting on the holy Mountain of Kori-yama, where he had a vision of light and received the knowledge of the symbols of reiki and their use in healing. He officially formulated Usui Reiki therapy in 1922 and touted as many as one million followers during his lifetime.

Prior to the transition (death) of Usui, he imparted the secrets of healing to 16 teachers in order that the secrets would not be lost again.

and has been used successfully in some hospitals. It has been found to be very calming and reassuring for those suffering from severe or fatal conditions. Reiki can been used by doctors, nurses, psychologists and other health professionals to bring touch and deeper caring into their healing practices.

Description

Origins

Reiki was developed in the mid-1800s by Dr. **Mikao Usui**, a Japanese scholar of religion. According to the story that has been passed down among reiki teachers, Usui was a Christian who was intrigued by the idea that Christ could heal sick people by touching them with his hands. Searching for clues that would explain the secrets of healing with hands, Usui made a long pilgrimage around the world, visiting many ancient religious sects and studying ancient books. Some reiki teachers claim that Usui found clues

leading back nearly 10,000 years to healing arts that originated in ancient Tibet. During his intense studies, Usui claimed he had a spiritual experience, which enabled him to heal with his own hands by becoming aware of and tapping into the universal life force. After that, he dedicated his life to helping the sick and poor. His reputation grew as he healed sick people for many years in Kyoto, Japan. Before his death, Usui passed on his healing insights using universal life energy to Dr. Chujiru Hayashi, a close acquaintance. Hayashi, in turn, passed on the healing techniques in 1938 to Hawayo Takata, a Japanese woman from Hawaii, whom he had cured of life-threatening illness using reiki methods. Takata became a firm believer and proponent of reiki, and during the 1970s formed an initiation program for training reiki masters to preserve Usui's teachings. Before she died, she prepared her granddaughter, Phyllis Lei Furumoto, to continue the lineage. Takata had personally trained 21 practitioners before she died at the age of 80 in 1980. Along with other reiki masters authorized by Takata, Furumoto formed the reiki Alliance. A faction led by Barbara Ray, formed the American Reiki Association, which was known as Radiance Technique Association International. Today, there are over 1,000 reiki masters practicing around the world, whose methods can all be traced back directly to Dr. Usui.

The basic philosophy of reiki

The basic concept underlying reiki is that the body has an energy field that is central to its health and proper functioning, and this energy travels in certain pathways that can become blocked or weakened. This idea of energy flow in the body is also a central concept in **Ayurvedic medicine** and **traditional Chinese medicine**, including **acupuncture**.

Reiki practitioners believe that everyone has the potential to access the universal life energy, but that over time most people's systems become blocked and the energy becomes weakened in them. A reiki practitioner is trained to be able to detect these blockages, and practitioners will use their hands, thoughts, and own energy fields to improve the energy flow in a patient. Reiki is one of the more esoteric alternative medical practices, because no one is sure exactly how it works on the physiological level. Practitioners claim that it works on very subtle energy levels, or possibly works on the *chakra* system. The chakras are the system of seven energy centers along the middle of the body believed to be connected with the nervous and endocrine systems, as defined by **yoga** and Ayurvedic medicine. Reiki masters claim that healing energy can even be sent to a person from far away, noting that reiki works on the same principles that enables praying to work for some patients, although a practitioner needs advanced training to be able to send energy from afar.

According to the original principles of Usui, patients must also have a proper attitude for reiki to work most effectively. Patients must take responsibility for their own health, and must want to be healed. Furthermore, when energy is received from a reiki healer, patients must be willing to give back energy to others, and to compensate the healer in some way, as well. Finally, Usui claimed that a healing attitude was free from worry and fear, was filled with gratitude for life and for others, and placed emphasis on each person finding honest and meaningful work in their lives—all this, in order to complete the picture of overall health.

A reiki session

Reiki sessions can take various forms, but most commonly resemble typical bodywork appointments, where the receiver lies clothed on his or her back on a flat surface or massage table. A session generally lasts from an hour to an hour and a half. Reiki is a simple procedure, consisting of calm and concentrated touching, with the practitioner focusing on healing and giving energy to specific areas on the receiver's body. Practitioners place their hands over positions on the body where the organs and endocrine glands reside, and the areas that correspond to the chakra centers. Practitioners also use mental visualization to send healing energy to areas of the receiver's body that need it. In special cases or with injuries, a no-touch technique is used, where the practitioner's hands are sometimes held just above the body without touching it. Advanced practitioners rely on intuition and experience to determine which areas of a body need the most energy healing.

The practitioner's hands are held flat against the receiver's body, with the fingertips touching. There can be over 20 positions on both sides of the body where the hands are placed. The positions begin at the crown of the head and move towards the feet. The receiver usually turns over once during the session. The practitioner's hands are held in each position for a usually five minutes, to allow the transfer of energy and the healing process to take place. In each position, the hands are kept stationary, unlike typical massage where the hands move, and both the giver and receiver attempt to maintain an attitude of awareness, openness, and caring.

Reiki practitioners recommend that those receiving reiki for the first time go through a series of three to four initial treatments over the course of about a week, to allow for cleansing and the initial readjustment of energy. Reiki sessions can cost from $30–100 per session. Insurance coverage is rare, and consumers should consult their individual policies as to whether or not such therapies are included.

Self-treatment with reiki

Although reiki practitioners believe that formal training is necessary to learn the proper methods of energy channeling and healing, individuals can still use some of the basic positions of reiki to relieve stress and to stimulate healing on themselves or another. The positions can be performed anywhere and for however long they are needed. Positions generally move from the top of the body down, but positions can be used wherever there is pain or stress. Mental attitude is important during reiki; the mind should be cleared of all stressful thoughts and concentrated on compassion, love, and peace as forms of energy that are surrounding, entering, and healing the body.

The following positions are illustrated in *Reiki: Energy Medicine:*

- Position one: Hands are placed on the top of the head, with the wrists near the ears and the fingertips touching on the crown of the head. Eyes should be closed. Hold for five minutes or more, until the mind feels clear and calm.

- Position two: Cup the hands slightly and place the palms over the closed eyes, with the fingers resting on the forehead.

- Position three: Place the hands on the sides of the head, with the thumbs behind the ear and the palms over the lower jaws, with the fingers covering the temples.

- Position four: Place one hand on the back of the neck, at the base of the skull, and put the other hand on the head just above it, parallel to it.

- Position five: Wrap the hands around the front of the throat, and rest them there gently with the heels of the hands touching in front.

- Position six: Place each hand on top of a shoulder, close to the side of neck, on top of the trapezius muscle.

- Position seven: Form a T-shape with the hands over the chest, with the left hand covering the heart and the right hand above it, covering the upper part of the chest.

- Position eight: The hands are placed flat against the front of the body with fingertips touching. Hold for five minutes or so, and repeat four or five times, moving down a hand-width each time until the pelvic region is reached, which is covered with a v-shape of the hands. Then, for the final position, repeat this technique on the back, beginning as close to the shoulders as the hands can reach, and ending by forming a T-shape with the hands at the base of the spine.

Side effects

Reiki generally has no side effects, as it is a very low impact and gentle procedure. Some receivers report **tingling** or sensations of heat or cold during treatment. Others have reported sadness or **anxiety** during treatment, which practitioners claim are buried or repressed emotions being released by the new energy flow.

Research and general acceptance

Reiki has been used in major clinics and hospitals as part of alternative healing practice, and doctors, dentists, nurses and other health professionals have been trained to use its gentle touch techniques as part of their practice. To date, the little scientific research that has been conducted with reiki implies that its techniques bring about the *relaxation response*, in which stress levels decrease, and immune response increases. Reiki practitioners claim that the most important measurement of their technique is whether the individual feels better after treatment. They also claim that science cannot measure the subtle energy changes that they are attempting to bring about.

As of the early 2000s, there are differences of opinion within the mainstream medical community regarding the acceptability of reiki. On the one hand, medical professionals in Canada have proposed strategies to limit the popularity of reiki as well as several other alternative therapies by resisting the integration of these therapies with mainstream treatments and by opposing government research in complementary and alternative medicine. On the other hand, the U. S. National Center for Complementary and Alternative Medicine (NCCAM) is conducting a series of clinical trials to evaluate the efficacy of reiki. As of the summer of 2004, there are four NCCAM trials for reiki, measuring its effectiveness in treating such disorders as **fibromyalgia**, neuropathy, **prostate cancer**, and advanced **AIDS**.

Training and certification

Reiki practitioners undergo a series of *attunements*, which are sessions with reiki masters that teach the basic methods of energy healing. Several organizations provide resources for reiki training. Reiki practitioners believe these attunements are necessary for correct technique. The masters teach each person how to activate the universal life energy in themselves before they can pass it on to others. These initiations often are held during weekend workshops. Trainees can achieve up to four levels of attunements, until they reach the level of master themselves. The certification process is not a formal one; masters approve students when they feel satisfied with their progress.

Resources

PERIODICALS

Hallett, A. "Narratives of Therapeutic Touch." *Nursing Standard* 19 (September 15, 2004): 33–37.

Kelner, M., B. Wellman, H. Boon, and S. Welch. "Responses of Established Healthcare to the Professionalization of Complementary and Alternative Medicine in Ontario." *Social Science and Medicine* 59 (September 2004): 915–930.

ORGANIZATIONS

International Association of Reiki Professionals. P.O. Box 481, Winchester, MA 01890. < http://www.iarp.org >.

International Center for Reiki Training. 21421 Hilltop Street, Unit #28, Southfield, MI 48034. (800) 332-8112 or (248) 948-8112. Fax: (248) 948-9534. < http://www.reiki.org >.

National Center for Complementary and Alternative Medicine (NCCAM) Clearinghouse. P. O. Box 7923. Gaitherburg, MD 20898. (888) 644-6226. Fax: (866) 464-3616. < http://nccam.nih.gov >.

OTHER

American Reiki Masters Association (ARMA). PO Box 130, Lake City, FL 32056-0130. (904) 755-9638.

Global Reiki Healing Network. < http://www.reiki.org >.

NCCAM Reiki Clinical Trials. < http://nccam.nih.gov/clinicaltrials/reiki.htm >.

Reiki Alliance. P.O. Box 41, Cataldo, ID 83810-1041, phone (208) 682-3535.

Douglas Dupler, MA
Rebecca J. Frey, PhD

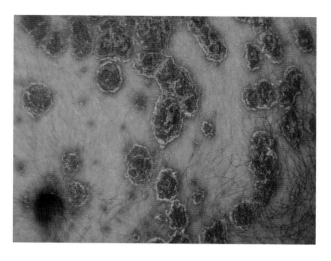

Keratoderma, a skin condition characterized by horny patches, is one symptom of Reiter's syndrome. *(Photograph by Milton Reisch, M.D., Corbis Images. Reproduced by permission.)*

Reiter's syndrome

Definition

Reiter's syndrome (RS), which is also known as arthritis urethritica, venereal arthritis, reactive arthritis, and polyarteritis enterica, is a form of arthritis that affects the eyes, urethra, and skin, as well as the joints. It was first described by Hans Reiter, a German physician, during World War I.

Description

Reiter's syndrome is marked by a cluster of symptoms in different organ systems of the body that may or may not appear simultaneously. The disease may be acute or chronic, with spontaneous remissions or recurrences.

RS primarily affects sexually active males between ages 20–40, particularly males who are HIV positive. Most women and children who develop RS acquire the disease in its intestinal form.

Causes and symptoms

The cause of Reiter's syndrome was unknown as of early 1998, but scientists think the disease results from a combination of genetic vulnerability and various disease agents. Over 80% of Caucasian patients and 50–60% of African Americans test positive for HLA-B27, which suggests that the disease has a genetic component. In sexually active males, most cases of RS follow infection with *Chlamydia trachomatis* or *Ureaplasma urealyticum*. Other patients develop the symptoms following gastrointestinal infection with *Shigella*, *Salmonella*, *Yersinia*, or *Campylobacter* bacteria.

The initial symptoms of RS are inflammation either of the urethra or the intestines, followed by acute arthritis four to 28 days later. The arthritis usually affects the fingers, toes, and weight-bearing joints in the legs. Other symptoms include:

- inflammation of the urethra, with painful urination and a discharge from the penis
- mouth ulcers
- inflammation of the eye
- keratoderma blennorrhagica, these are patches of scaly skin on the palms, soles, trunk, or scalp of RS patients

Diagnosis

Patient history

Diagnosis of Reiter's syndrome can be complicated by the fact that different symptoms often occur several weeks apart. The patient does not usually draw a connection between the arthritis and previous sexual activity. The doctor is likely to consider Reiter's syndrome when the patient's arthritis occurs together with or shortly following inflammation of the eye and the genitourinary tract lasting a month or longer.

Laboratory tests

There is no specific test for diagnosing RS, but the physician may have the urethral discharge cultured to rule out **gonorrhea**. Blood tests of RS patients are typically positive for the HLA-B27 genetic marker, with an elevated white blood cell (WBC) count and an increased sedimentation rate of red blood cells. The patient may also be mildly anemic.

Diagnostic imaging

X rays do not usually reveal any abnormalities unless the patient has had recurrent episodes of the disease. Joints that have been repeatedly inflamed may show eroded areas, signs of **osteoporosis**, or bony spurs when x rayed.

Treatment

There is no specific treatment for RS. Joint inflammation is usually treated with **nonsteroidal anti-inflammatory drugs** (NSAIDs.) Skin eruptions and eye inflammation can be treated with **corticosteroids**. Gold treatments may be given for eroded bone.

Patients with chronic arthritis are also given physical therapy and advised to **exercise** regularly.

Prognosis

The prognosis varies. Most patients recover in three to four months, but about 50% have recurrences for several years. Some patients develop complications that include inflammation of the heart muscle, stiffening inflammation of the vertebrae, **glaucoma**, eventual blindness, deformities of the feet, or accumulation of fluid in the lungs.

Prevention

In males, Reiter's syndrome can be prevented by sexual abstinence or the use of condoms.

Resources

BOOKS

Berktow, Robert, editor. "Musculoskeletal and Connective Tissue Disorders: Reiter's Syndrome (RS)." In *The Merck Manual of Diagnosis and Therapy*. 16th ed. Rahway, NJ: Merck Research Laboratories, 1992.

Hellman, David B. "Arthritis & Musculoskeletal Disorders." In *Current Medical Diagnosis and Treatment, 1998*, edited by Stephen McPhee, et al., 37th ed. Stamford: Appleton & Lange, 1997.

Rebecca J. Frey, PhD

Relapsing fever

Definition

Relapsing **fever** refers to two similar illnesses, both of which cause high fevers. The fevers resolve, only to recur again within about a week.

Description

Relapsing fever is caused by spiral-shaped bacteria of the genus *Borrelia*. This bacterium lives in rodents and in insects, specifically ticks and body lice. The form of relapsing fever acquired from ticks is slightly different from that acquired from body lice.

In tick-borne relapsing fever (TBRF), rodents (rats, mice, chipmunks, and squirrels) which carry *Borrelia* are fed upon by ticks. The ticks then acquire the bacteria, and are able to pass it on to humans. TBRF is most common in sub-Saharan Africa, parts of the Mediterranean, areas in the Middle East, India, China, and the south of Russia. Also, *Borrelia* causing TBRF exist in the western regions of the United States, particularly in mountainous areas. The disease is said to be endemic to these areas, meaning that the causative agents occur naturally and consistently within these locations.

In louse-borne relapsing fever (LBRF), lice acquire *Borrelia* from humans who are already infected. These lice can then go on to infect other humans. LBRF is said to be epidemic, as opposed to endemic, meaning that it can occur suddenly in large numbers in specific communities of people. LBRF occurs in places where poverty and overcrowding predispose to human infestation with lice. LBRF has flared during wars, when conditions are crowded and good hygiene is next to impossible. At this time, LBRF is found in areas of east and central Africa, China, and in the Andes Mountains of Peru.

Causes and symptoms

In TBRF, humans contract *Borrelia* when they are fed upon by ticks. Ticks often feed on humans at night, so many people who have been bitten are unaware that they have been. The bacteria is passed on to humans through the infected body fluids of the tick.

In LBRF, a louse must be crushed or smashed in order for *Borrelia* to be released. The bacteria then enter the human body through areas where the person may have scratched him or herself.

Both types of relapsing fever occur some days after having acquired the bacteria. About a week after becoming infected, symptoms begin. The patient spikes a very high fever, with chills, sweating, terrible **headache**, **nausea**, **vomiting**, severe **pain** in the muscles and joints, and extreme weakness. The patient may become dizzy and confused. The eyes may be bloodshot and very sensitive to light. A **cough** may develop. The heart rate is greatly increased, and the liver and spleen may be swollen. Because the substances responsible for blood clotting may be disturbed during the illness, tiny purple marks may appear on the skin, which are evidence of minor bleeding occurring under the skin. The patient may suffer from a **nosebleed**, or may cough up bloody sputum. All of these symptoms last for about three days in TBRF, and about five days in LBRF.

With or without treatment, a crisis may occur as the bacteria are cleared from the blood. This crisis, called a Jarisch-Herxheimer reaction, results in a new spike in fever, chills, and an initial rise in blood pressure. The blood pressure then falls drastically, which may deprive tissues and organs of appropriate blood flow (**shock**). This reaction usually lasts for about a day.

Recurrent episodes of fever with less severe symptoms occur after about a week. In untreated infections, fevers recur about three times in TBRF, and only once or twice in LBRF.

Diagnosis

Diagnosis of relapsing fever is relatively easy, because the causative bacteria can be found by examining a sample of blood under the microscope. The characteristically spiral-shaped bacteria are easily identifiable. The blood is best drawn during the period of high fever, because the bacteria are present in the blood in great numbers at that time.

Treatment

Either tetracycline or erythromycin is effective against both forms of relapsing fever. The medications are given for about a week for cases of TBRF; LBRF requires only a single dose. Children and pregnant women should receive either erythromycin or penicillin.

KEY TERMS

Endemic—Refers to a particular organism which consistently exists in a particular location under normal conditions.

Epidemic—Refers to a condition suddenly acquired by a large number of people within a specific community, and which spreads rapidly throughout that community.

Shock—A state in which the blood pressure is so low that organs and tissues are not receiving an appropriate flow of blood.

Because of the risk of the Jarish-Herxheimer reaction, patients must be very carefully monitored during the initial administration of antibiotic medications. Solutions containing salts must be given through a needle in the vein (intravenously) to keep the blood pressure from dropping too drastically. Patients with extreme reactions may need medications to improve blood circulation until the reaction resolves.

Prognosis

In epidemics of LBRF, **death** rates among untreated victims have run as high as 30%. With treatment, and careful monitoring for the development of the Jarish-Herxheimer reaction, prognosis is good for both LBRF and TBRF.

Prevention

Prevention of TBRF requires rodent control, especially in and near homes. Careful use of insecticides on skin and clothing is important for people who may be enjoying outdoor recreation in areas known to harbor the disease-carrying ticks.

Prevention of LBRF is possible, but probably more difficult. Good hygiene and decent living conditions would prevent the spread of LBRF, but these may be difficult for those people most at risk for the disease.

Resources

ORGANIZATIONS

Centers for Disease Control and Prevention. 1600 Clifton Rd., NE, Atlanta, GA 30333. (800) 311-3435, (404) 639-3311. < http://www.cdc.gov >.

Rosalyn Carson-DeWitt, MD

Relapsing polychondritis

Definition

Relapsing polychondritis is a disease characterized by autoimmune-like episodic or progressive inflammation of cartilage and other connective tissue, such as the nose, ears, throat, joints, kidneys, and heart.

Description

Cartilage is a tough, flexible tissue that turns into bone in many places in the body. Bones all start out as cartilage in the fetus. Consequently, children have more cartilage than adults. Cartilage persists in adults in the linings of joints, the ears, the nose, the airway and the ribs near the breast bone. All these sites are attacked by relapsing polychondritis, which usually occurs equally in middle-aged males and females. It is frequently diagnosed along with **rheumatoid arthritis**, **systemic lupus erythematosus**, and other connective tissue diseases.

Causes and symptoms

The most common first symptom of relapsing polychondritis is **pain** and swelling of the external ear. Usually, both ears turn red or purple and are tender to the touch. The swelling can extend into the ear canal and beyond, causing ear infections, **hearing loss**, balance disturbances with vertigo and **vomiting**, and eventually a droopy ear. The nose is often afflicted as well and can deteriorate into a flattened nose bridge called saddle nose. Inflammation of the eye occurs less frequently, but can lead to blindness.

As relapsing polychondritis advances, it causes more dangerous symptoms such as deterioration of the cartilage that holds the windpipe open. Progressive disease can destroy the integrity of the airway and compromise breathing. Destruction of the rib cartilage can collapse the chest, again hindering breathing. Joints everywhere are involved in episodes of arthritis, with pain and swelling. Other tissues besides cartilage are also involved, leading to a variety of problems with the skin and other tissues. Occasionally, the aorta or heart valves are damaged.

The disease may occur in episodes with complete remission between, or it may smolder along for years, causing progressive destruction.

Diagnosis

A characteristic array of symptoms and physical findings will yield a diagnosis of relapsing polychondritis. Laboratory tests are sometime helpful. Biopsies of the affected cartilage may confirm the diagnosis. Further diagnostic tests are done to confirm other associated conditions such as rheumatoid arthritis. It is important to evaluate the airway, although only 10% of patients will die from airway complications.

Treatment

Mild inflammations can be treated with **aspirin** or **nonsteroidal anti-inflammatory drugs** (NSAIDs) such as ibuprofen. **Corticosteroids** (most often prednisone) are usually prescribed for more advanced conditions and do improve the disease. They may have to be continued over long periods of time, in which case their usage must be closely watched to avoid complications. Immune suppression with cyclophosphamide, azathioprine, cyclosporine, or dapsone is reserved for more aggressive cases. A collapsed chest or airway may require surgical support, and a heart valve or aorta may need repair or replacing.

Prognosis

There is no known cure for relapsing polychondritis. It can only be combated with each onset of inflammation and deterioration of cartilaginous tissue. As the disease progresses over a period of years, the mortality rate increases. At five years duration, relapsing polychondritis has a 30% mortality rate.

Resources

BOOKS

Gilliland, Bruce C. "Relapsing Polychondritis and Other Arthritides." In *Harrison's Principles of Internal Medicine*, edited by Anthony S. Fauci, et al. New York: McGraw-Hill, 1997.

J. Ricker Polsdorfer, MD

Renal artery occlusion

Definition

Renal artery occlusion is a blockage of the major arteries that supply blood to the kidneys caused by thrombosis or **embolism**.

Description

Renal artery occlusion occurs when the flow of blood from the arteries leading to the kidneys becomes blocked by a blood clot or cholesterol emboli. The lack of oxygenation can lead to necrosis (tissue death) and ultimately, **chronic kidney failure**.

Causes and symptoms

Renal arterial occlusion occurs when a thrombus or embolism (blood clot or cholesterol plaque) breaks free and blocks the arteries leading to one or both kidneys.

Symptoms of an acute renal arterial occlusion may include:

- **hypertension**
- fever
- sudden **pain** in the lower back or flank
- nausea and vomiting
- protein and/or blood in the urine

An individual with renal arterial occlusion may have no overt symptoms, particularly if only one kidney is affected or if the blockage is only partial. Health problems from secondary complications such as chronic kidney failure may be the first indication that something is wrong.

Diagnosis

The high blood pressure that is sometimes associated with a renal artery blockage may be the first sign

---

> ### KEY TERMS
>
> **Angioplasty**—A non-surgical procedure that uses a balloon-tipped catheter to open a blocked artery.
>
> **Artherosclerotic plaque**—A deposit of fatty and calcium substances that accumulate in the lining of the artery wall, restricting blood flow.
>
> **Atrophy**—Cell or tissue wasting or death.
>
> **Chronic kidney failure**—End-stage renal disease (ESRD); chronic kidney failure is diagnosed as ESRD when kidney function falls to 5–10% of capacity.
>
> **Embolism**—Blood vessel obstruction by a blood clot or other substance (i.e., air).
>
> **Thrombus**—Formation of a blood clot within the vascular system. A thrombus becomes an embolism if it breaks away and blocks a blood vessel.

that it is present, particularly if the hypertension is not responding to standard treatment. Urine and blood tests may or may not be useful in diagnosing this condition. Blood tests may show an elevated plasma creatinine level. If kidney tissue infarction (cell death caused by a lack of blood supply) has occurred, lactic dehydrogenase (LDH) may also be present in the urine and blood.

An arteriogram, an x-ray study of the arteries that uses a radiopaque substance, or dye, to make the arteries visible under x ray, may also be performed. This test is used with caution in patients with impaired kidney function, as the contrast medium can cause further kidney damage. In patients with whom this is not an issue, a spiral computed tomography (CT) scan with contrast medium may also be used.

Treatment

Occlusions may be treated with anticoagulant (blood thinning) or thrombolytic (clot destroying) drugs. If the blockage is significant, surgical intervention or **angioplasty** may be required. Between 1996 and 2000, the number of these procedures performed on Medicare patients more than doubled, said a 2004 report.

Alternative treatment

Renal arterial occlusion is a serious and potentially life-threatening condition, and should always be treated by a healthcare professional familiar with the disorder.

Prognosis

The outcome of renal arterial occlusion depends on the speed with which it is treated. Once the blood supply is minimized or cut off to the kidney, tissue death soon results, ultimately leading to chronic kidney failure (end-stage renal disease).

Prevention

Atherosclerosis may encourage the formation of cholesterol emboli, a potential cause of renal artery occlusion. Strategies for avoiding vascular disease include eating right, maintaining a desirable weight, quitting **smoking**, managing **stress**, and exercising regularly. People prone to emboli from **blood clots** can take blood thinning drugs to prevent potential emboli from loding in the renal artery.

Resources

PERIODICALS

Bloch, M. J., and T. Pickering. "Renal Vascular Disease: Medical Management, Angioplasty, and Stenting." *Seminars in Nephrology* 20, no. 5 (September 2000): 474-88.

"Explosive Growth Seen in Renal Artery Interventional Procedures." *Heart Disease Weekly* September 26, 2004: 20.

Truelove, Christiane. "First for Pulmonary Embolism." *Med Ad News* August 2004: 82.

ORGANIZATIONS

American Kidney Fund (AKF). Suite 1010, 6110 Executive Boulevard, Rockville, MD 20852. (800) 638-8299. < http://www.arbon.com/kidney/ >.

National Institute of Diabetes and Digestive and Kidney Diseases (NIDDK). Natcher Building, 6AS-13K, 45 Center Drive, Bethesda, MD 20892-6600. < http://www.niddk.nih.gov >.

National Kidney Foundation. 30 East 33rd Street, New York, NY 10016. (800)622-9020. < http://www.kidney.org >.

Paula Anne Ford-Martin
Teresa G. Odle

Renal artery stenosis

Definition

Renal artery stenosis is a blockage or narrowing of the major arteries that supply blood to the kidneys.

Description

Renal artery stenosis occurs when the flow of blood from the arteries leading to the kidneys is constricted by tissue or artherosclerotic plaque. This narrowing of the arteries diminishes the blood supply to the kidneys, which can cause them to atrophy and may ultimately lead to kidney failure. It may also cause **renovascular hypertension**, or high blood pressure related to renal artery blockage.

Causes and symptoms

The two main causes of renal artery stenosis are **atherosclerosis** and fibromuscular disease. Fibromuscular diseases such as fibromuscular dysplasia cause growth of fibrous tissues on the arterial wall. Stenosis may also occur when scar tissue forms in the renal artery after trauma to the kidney.

Renal arterial stenosis has no overt symptoms. Eventually, untreated renal arterial stenosis causes secondary complications such as **chronic kidney failure**, which may be characterized by frequent urination, anemia, **edema**, headaches, **hypertension**, lower back **pain**, and other signs and symptoms.

Diagnosis

The high blood pressure that is sometimes associated with renal artery stenosis may be the first sign that it is present, particularly if the hypertension is not responding to standard treatment. Presence of a *bruit*, a swooshing sound from the artery that indicates an obstruction, may be heard through a stethoscope.

An arteriogram, an x-ray study of the arteries that uses a radiopaque substance, or dye, to make the arteries visible under x ray, may also be performed. This test is used with caution in patients with impaired kidney function, as the contrast medium may cause further kidney damage.

Treatment

Treatment for renal artery stenosis is either surgical, pharmaceutical, or with **angioplasty** or stenting. Angioplasty involves guiding a balloon catheter down into the renal artery and inflating the balloon to clear the blockage. A stent may be inserted into the artery to widen the opening. Some patients may be candidates for surgical revascularization, which involves restoring blood flow with an arterial bypass. Drugs known as angiotension-converting enzyme (ACE) inhibitors may be prescribed for some patients. The chosen treatment approach depends on the cause of the stenosis and factors such as the patient's kidney function and blood pressure control.

Alternative treatment

Renal artery stenosis is a serious and potentially life-threatening condition, and should always be treated by a healthcare professional familiar with the disorder.

Prognosis

Untreated renal artery stenosis can cause hypertension (high blood pressure) and may ultimately lead to chronic kidney failure (end-stage renal disease).

Prevention

Maintaining a heart healthy lifestyle can help to prevent cases of renal arterial stenosis attributable to artherosclerosis. Strategies for avoiding vascular disease include eating right, maintaining a desirable weight, quitting **smoking**, managing **stress**, and exercising regularly.

Resources

PERIODICALS

Bloch, M. J., and T. Pickering. "Renal Vascular Disease: Medical Management, Angioplasty, and Stenting." *Seminars in Nephrology* 20, no. 5 (September 2000): 474-88.

Fenves, A. Z., and C. V. Ram. "Fibromuscular Dysplasia of the Renal Arteries." *Current Hypertension Reports* 1, no. 6 (December 1999): 546-9.

ORGANIZATIONS

American Kidney Fund (AKF). Suite 1010, 6110 Executive Boulevard, Rockville, MD 20852. (800)638-8299. < http://www.arbon.com/kidney/ >.

National Institute of Diabetes and Digestive and Kidney Diseases (NIDDK). Natcher Building, 6AS-13K, 45 Center Drive, Bethesda, MD 20892-6600. < http://www.niddk.nih.gov >.

National Kidney Foundation. 30 East 33rd Street, New York, NY 10016. (800)622-9020. < http://www.kidney.org >.

Paula Anne Ford-Martin

Renal calculi *see* **Kidney stones**

Renal failure *see* **Acute kidney failure; Chronic kidney failure**

Renal nuclear medicine scan *see* **Kidney nuclear medicine scan**

Renal tubular acidosis

Definition

Renal tubular acidosis (RTA) is a condition characterized by too much acid in the body due to a defect in kidney function.

Description

Chemical balance is critical to the body's functioning. Therefore, the body controls its chemicals very strictly. The acid-base balance must be between a pH of 7.35 and 7.45 or trouble will start. Every other chemical in the body is affected by the acid-base balance. The most important chemicals in this system are sodium, chloride, potassium, calcium, ammonium, carbon dioxide, oxygen, and phosphates.

The lungs rapidly adjust acid-base balance by the speed of breathing, because carbon dioxide dissolved in water is an acid–carbonic acid. Faster breathing eliminates more carbon dioxide, decreases the carbonic acid in the blood and increases the pH. Holding your breath does the opposite. Blood acidity from carbon dioxide controls the rate of breathing, not oxygen.

The kidneys also regulate acid-base balance somewhat more slowly than the lungs. They handle all the chemicals, often trading one for another that is more or less acidic. The trading takes place between the blood and the urine, so that extra chemicals end up passing out of the body. If the kidneys do not effectively eliminate acid, it builds up in the blood, leading to a condition called **metabolic acidosis**. These conditions are called renal tubular acidosis.

Causes and symptoms

There are three types of renal tubular acidosis. They include:

- Distal renal tubular acidosis (type 1) may be a hereditary condition or may be triggered by an autoimmune disease, lithium therapy, **kidney transplantation**, or chronic obstruction.

- Proximal renal tubular acidosis (type 2) is caused by hereditary diseases, such as **Fanconi's syndrome**, fructose intolerance, and Lowe's syndrome. It can also develop with **vitamin D deficiency**, kidney transplantation, **heavy metal poisoning**, and treatment with certain drugs.

- Type 4 renal tubular acidosis is not hereditary, but is associated with **diabetes mellitus**, sickle cell anemia, an autoimmune disease, or an obstructed urinary tract.

Symptoms vary with the underlying mechanism of the defect and the readjustment of chemicals required to compensate for the defect.

- Distal RTA results in high blood acidity and low blood potassium levels. Symptoms include mild **dehydration**; muscle weakness or **paralysis** (due to potassium deficiency); **kidney stones** (due to excess calcium in the urine); and bone fragility and pain.

- Proximal RTA also results in high blood acidity and low blood potassium levels. Symptoms include mild dehydration.

- Type 4 RTA is characterized by high blood acidity and high blood potassium levels; it rarely causes symptoms unless potassium levels rise so high as to cause heart **arrhythmias** or muscle paralysis.

Diagnosis

RTA is suspected when a person has certain symptoms indicative of the disease or when routine tests show high blood acid levels and low blood potassium levels. From there, more testing of blood and urine chemicals will help determine the type of RTA present.

Treatment

The foundation of treatment for RTA types 1 and 2 is replacement of alkali (base) by drinking a bicarbonate solution daily. Potassium may also have to be replaced, and other chemicals added to maintain balance. In type 4 RTA acidity will normalize if

---

KEY TERMS

Autoimmune disease—Type of diseases characterized by antibodies that attack the body's own tissues.

Fanconi's syndrome—A disorder of the kidneys characterized by glucose in the urine.

Lowe's syndrome—A rare inherited disorder that is distinguished by congenital cataracts, glaucoma, and severe mental retardation.

Rickets—A deficiency disease that affects the bone development of growing bodies, usually causing soft bones.

---

potassium is reduced. This is done by changing the diet and by using diuretic medicines that promote potassium excretion in the urine.

Prognosis

Careful balancing of body chemicals will usually produce good results. If there is an underlying disease responsible for the kidney malfunction, it may be the determining factor in the prognosis.

Prevention

Relatives of patients with the possibly hereditary forms of renal tubular acidosis should be tested.

Resources

BOOKS

Chesney, Russell W. "Specific Renal Tubular Disorders." In *Cecil Textbook of Medicine*, edited by J. Claude Bennett and Fred Plum. Philadelphia: W. B. Saunders Co., 1996.

J. Ricker Polsdorfer, MD

Renal ultrasound *see* **Abdominal ultrasound**

Renal vein thrombosis

Definition

Renal vein thrombosis develops when a blood clot forms in the renal vein, which carries blood from the kidneys back to the heart. The disorder is not common.

Description

Renal vein thrombosis occurs in both infants and adults. Onset of the disorder can be rapid (acute) or gradual. The number of people who suffer from renal vein thrombosis is difficult to determine, as many people do not show symptoms, and the disorder is diagnosed only by specific tests. Ninety percent of childhood cases occur in children under one year old, and 75% occur in infants under one month of age. In adult women, oral contraceptive use increases the risk of renal vein thrombosis.

Causes and symptoms

In children, renal vein thrombosis almost always occurs rapidly after an episode of severe **dehydration**. Severe dehydration decreases blood volume and causes the blood to clot more readily.

In adults, renal vein thrombosis can be caused by injury to the abdomen or back, as a result of malignant kidney tumors growing into the renal vein, or as a result of kidney diseases that cause degenerative changes in the cells of the renal tubules (**nephrotic syndrome**).

Acute onset of renal vein thrombosis at any age causes **pain** in the lower back and side, **fever**, bloody urine, decreased urine output, and sometimes kidney failure. In adults, when the onset of the disorder is gradual, there is a slow decrease in kidney function, and protein appears in the urine. Many adults with renal vein thrombosis show few symptoms.

Diagnosis

Renal **venography**, where a contrast material (dye) is injected into the renal vein before x rays are taken, is one of the best ways to detect renal vein thrombosis. Other useful tests to detect a clot include **computed tomography scans** (CT scans), **magnetic resonance imaging** (MRI), and ultrasound.

Treatment

One of the major goals of treatment is to prevent the blood clot in the renal vein from detaching and moving into the lungs, where it can cause serious complications as a **pulmonary embolism**. The enzyme streptokinase may be given to help dissolve the renal clot. Anticoagulant medications are usually prescribed to prevent clots from recurring. Rarely, when there is a complete blockage of the renal vein in infants, the kidney must be surgically removed.

Prognosis

Most cases of renal vein thrombosis resolve without any permanent damage. **Death** from renal vein thrombosis is rare, and is often caused by the blood clot detaching and lodging in the heart or lungs.

Prevention

There is no specific prevention for renal vein thrombosis. Preventing dehydration reduces the risk that it will occur.

Resources

ORGANIZATIONS

National Kidney Foundation. 30 East 33rd St., New York, NY 10016. (800) 622-9010. < http://www.kidney.org >.

OTHER

"Renal Vein Thrombosis." *HealthAnswers.com.* < http://www.healthanswers.com/database/ami/converted/ooo513.html >.

Tish Davidson, A.M.

Rendu-Osler-Weber disease *see* **Hereditary hemorrhagic telangiectasia**

Renin assay *see* **Plasma renin activity**

▌ Renovascular hypertension

Definition

Renovascular **hypertension** is a secondary form of high blood pressure caused by a narrowing of the renal artery.

Description

Primary hypertension, or high blood pressure, affects millions of Americans. It accounts for over 90% of all cases of hypertension and develops without apparent causes. It is helpful for the clinician to know if a secondary disease is present and may be contributing to the high pressure. If clinical tests indicate this is so, the term used for the rise in blood pressure is secondary hypertension.

Renal hypertension is the most common form of secondary hypertension and affects no more than one percent of all adults with primary hypertension. There are two forms of renovascular hypertension.

In atherosclerotic renovascular hypertension disease, plaque is deposited in the renal artery. The deposits narrow the artery, disrupting blood flow. Atherosclerotic renovascular hypertension is most often seen in men over age 45 and accounts for two-thirds of the cases of renovascular hypertension. In most patients, it affects the renal arteries to both kidneys.

Renovascular hypertension caused by fibromuscular dysplasia occurs mainly in women under age 45. It is also the cause of hypertension in 10% of children with the disorder. In fibromuscular dysplasia, cells from the artery wall overgrow and cause a narrowing of the artery channel.

The risk of having hypertension is related to age, lifestyle, environment, and genetics. **Smoking**, **stress**, **obesity**, a diet high in salt, exposure to heavy metals, and an inherited predisposition toward hypertension all increase the chances that a person will develop both primary and renovascular hypertension.

Causes and symptoms

Narrowing of the renal artery reduces the flow of blood to the kidney. In response, the kidney produces the protein renin. Renin is released into the blood stream. Through a series of steps, renin is converted into an enzyme that causes sodium (salt) retention and constriction of the arterioles. In addition to atherosclerotic and fibromuscular dysplasia, narrowing of the renal artery can be caused by compression from an injury or tumor, or by **blood clots**.

Renovascular hypertension is suspected when hypertension develops suddenly in patients under 30 or over 55 years of age or abruptly worsens in any patient. Symptoms are often absent or subtle.

Diagnosis

No single test for renovascular hypertension is definitive. About half of patients with renovascular hypertension have a specific cardiovascular sound that is heard when a doctor listens to the upper abdomen with a stethoscope. Other diagnostic tests give occasional false positive and false negative results. Most tests are expensive, and some involve serious risks.

Imaging studies are used to diagnose renovascular hypertension. In **intravenous urography**, a dye is injected into the kidney, pictures are made, and the kidneys compared. In renal arteriography, contrast material is inserted into the renal artery and cinematic x rays (showing motion within the kidney) are taken. Studies of kidney function are performed. Tests are done to measure renin production. The results of these tests taken together are used to diagnose renovascular hypertension.

Treatment

Renovascular hypertension may not respond well to anti-hypertensive drugs. Percutaneous transluminal **angioplasty** (PTA), where a balloon catheter is used to dilate the renal artery and remove the blockage, is effective in improving the condition of about 90% of patients with fibromuscular dysplasia. One year later, 60% remain cured. It is less successful in patients with **atherosclerosis**, where renovascular hypertension recurs in half the patients. Where kidney damage occurs, surgery to repair or bypass the renal artery blockage is often effective. In some cases, the damaged kidney must be removed.

Alternative treatment

Alternative treatment stresses eliminating the root causes of hypertension. With renovascular hypertension, as with primary hypertension, the root causes generally cannot be totally reversed by any method. Lifestyle changes are recommended. These include stopping smoking, eating a diet low in animal fats and salt, avoiding exposure to heavy metals, stress control through **meditation**, and anger management. Herbal medicine practitioners recommend garlic (*Allium sativum*) to help lower blood pressure. Constitutional homeopathy and **acupuncture** also can be helpful in lowering blood pressure.

Prognosis

PTA is effective in many younger patients with fibromuscular dysplasia. Older patients are less responsive to this treatment. Surgery is also more risky and less successful in older patients.

Prevention

Renovascular hypertension is possibly preventable through lifestyles that prevent atherosclerosis and primary hypertension. It is unknown how to prevent fibromuscular hyperplasia

Resources

ORGANIZATIONS

American Heart Association. 7320 Greenville Ave. Dallas, TX 75231. (214) 373-6300. < http:// www.americanheart.org >.

Tish Davidson, A.M.

Respiratory acidosis

Definition

Respiratory acidosis is a condition in which a build-up of carbon dioxide in the blood produces a shift in the body's pH balance and causes the body's system to become more acidic. This condition is brought about by a problem either involving the lungs and respiratory system or signals from the brain that control breathing.

Description

Respiratory acidosis is an acid imbalance in the body caused by a problem related to breathing. In the lungs, oxygen from inhaled air is exchanged for carbon dioxide from the blood. This process takes place between the alveoli (tiny air pockets in the lungs) and the blood vessels that connect to them. When this exchange of oxygen for carbon dioxide is impaired, the excess carbon dioxide forms an acid in the blood. The condition can be acute with a sudden onset, or it can develop gradually as lung function deteriorates.

Causes and symptoms

Respiratory acidosis can be caused by diseases or conditions that affect the lungs themselves, such as **emphysema**, chronic **bronchitis**, **asthma**, or severe **pneumonia**. Blockage of the airway due to swelling, a foreign object, or vomit can induce respiratory acidosis. Drugs like anesthetics, sedatives, and **narcotics** can interfere with breathing by depressing the respiratory center in the brain. Head injuries or brain tumors can also interfere with signals sent by the brain to the lungs. Such neuromuscular diseases as **Guillain-Barré syndrome** or **myasthenia gravis** can impair the muscles around the lungs making it more difficult to breathe. Conditions that cause chronic **metabolic alkalosis** can also trigger respiratory acidosis.

The most notable symptom will be slowed or difficult breathing. **Headache**, drowsiness, restlessness, tremor, and confusion may also occur. A rapid heart rate, changes in blood pressure, and swelling of blood vessels in the eyes may be noted upon examination. This condition can trigger the body to respond with symptoms of metabolic alkalosis, which may include **cyanosis**, a bluish or purplish discoloration of the skin due to inadequate oxygen intake. Severe cases of respiratory acidosis can lead to **coma** and **death**.

KEY TERMS

pH—A measurement of acid or alkali (base) of a solution based on the amount of hydrogen ions available. Based on a scale of 14, a pH of 7.0 is neutral. A pH below 7.0 is an acid; the lower the number, the stronger the acid. A pH above 7.0 is a base; the higher the number, the stronger the base. Blood pH is slightly alkali with a normal range of 7.36–7.44.

Diagnosis

Respiratory acidosis may be suspected based on symptoms. A blood sample to test for pH and arterial blood gases can be used to confirm the diagnosis. In this type of acidosis, the pH will be below 7.35. The pressure of carbon dioxide in the blood will be high, usually over 45 mmHg.

Treatment

Treatment focuses on correcting the underlying condition that caused the acidosis. In patients with chronic lung diseases, this may include use of a bronchodilator or steroid drugs. Supplemental oxygen supplied through a mask or small tubes inserted into the nostrils may be used in some conditions, however, an oversupply of oxygen in patients with lung disease can make the acidosis worse. **Antibiotics** may be used to treat infections. If the acidosis is related to an overdose of narcotics, or a **drug overdose** is suspected, the patient may be given a dose of naloxone, a drug that will block the respiratory-depressing effects of narcotics. Use of mechanical ventilation like a respirator may be necessary. If the respiratory acidosis has triggered the body to compensate by developing metabolic alkalosis, symptoms of that condition may need to be treated as well.

Prognosis

If the underlying condition that caused the respiratory acidosis is treated and corrected, there may be no long term effects. Respiratory acidosis may occur chronically along with the development of lung disease or **respiratory failure**. In these severe conditions, the patient may require the assistance of a respirator or ventilator. In extreme cases, the patient may experience coma and death.

Prevention

Patients with chronic lung diseases and those who receive sedatives and narcotics need to be monitored closely for development of respiratory acidosis.

Resources

BOOKS

"Fluid, Electrolyte, and Acid-Base Disorders." In *Family Medicine Principles and Practices.* 5th ed. New York: Springer-Verlag, 1998.

Altha Roberts Edgren

Respiratory alkalosis

Definition

Respiratory alkalosis is a condition where the amount of carbon dioxide found in the blood drops to a level below normal range. This condition produces a shift in the body's pH balance and causes the body's system to become more alkaline (basic). This condition is brought on by rapid, deep breathing called hyperventilation.

Description

Respiratory alkalosis is an alkali imbalance in the body caused by a lower-than-normal level of carbon dioxide in the blood. In the lungs, oxygen from inhaled air is exchanged for carbon dioxide from the blood. This process takes place between the alveoli (tiny air pockets in the lungs) and the blood vessels that connect to them. When a person hyperventilates, this exchange of oxygen for carbon dioxide is speeded up, and the person exhales too much carbon dioxide. This lowered level of carbon dioxide causes the pH of the blood to increase, leading to alkalosis.

Causes and symptoms

The primary cause of respiratory alkalosis is hyperventilation. This rapid, deep breathing can be caused by conditions related to the lungs like **pneumonia**, lung disease, or **asthma**. More commonly, hyperventilation is associated with **anxiety**, **fever**, **drug overdose**, **carbon monoxide poisoning**, or serious infections. Tumors or swelling in the brain or nervous system can also cause this type of respiration. Other stresses to the body, including **pregnancy**, liver failure,

---

high elevations, or **metabolic acidosis** can also trigger hyperventilation leading to respiratory alkalosis.

Hyperventilation, the primary cause of respiratory alkalosis, is also the primary symptom. This symptom is accompanied by **dizziness**, light headedness, agitation, and **tingling** or numbing around the mouth and in the fingers and hands. Muscle twitching, spasms, and weakness may be noted. Seizures, irregular heart beats, and tetany (**muscle spasms** so severe that the muscle locks in a rigid position) can result from severe respiratory alkalosis.

Diagnosis

Respiratory alkalosis may be suspected based on symptoms. A blood sample to test for pH and arterial blood gases can be used to confirm the diagnosis. In this type of alkalosis, the pH will be elevated above 7.44. The pressure of carbon dioxide in the blood will be low, usually under 35 mmHg.

Treatment

Treatment focuses on correcting the underlying condition that caused the alkalosis. Hyperventilation due to anxiety may be relieved by having the patient breath into a paper bag. By rebreathing the air that was exhaled, the patient will inhale a higher amount of carbon dioxide than he or she would normally. **Antibiotics** may be used to treat pneumonia or other infections. Other medications may be required to treat fever, seizures, or irregular heart beats. If the alkalosis is related to a drug overdose, the patient may require treatment for **poisoning**. Use of mechanical ventilation

---

like a respirator may be necessary. If the respiratory alkalosis has triggered the body to compensate by developing metabolic acidosis, symptoms of that condition may need to be treated, as well.

Prognosis

If the underlying condition that caused the respiratory alkalosis is treated and corrected, there may be no long-term effects. In severe cases of respiratory alkalosis, the patient may experience seizures or heart beat irregularities that may be serious and life threatening.

Resources

BOOKS

"Fluid, Electrolyte, and Acid-Base Disorders." In *Family Medicine Principles and Practices.* 5th ed. New York: Springer-Verlag, 1998.

Altha Roberts Edgren

Respiratory distress syndrome

Definition

Respiratory distress syndrome (RDS) of the newborn, also known as infant RDS, is an acute lung disease present at birth, which usually affects premature babies. Layers of tissue called hyaline membranes keep the oxygen that is breathed in from passing into the blood. The lungs are said to be "airless." Without treatment, the infant will die within a few days after birth, but if oxygen can be provided, and the infant receives modern treatment in a neonatal intensive care unit, complete recovery with no after-effects can be expected.

Description

If a newborn infant is to breathe properly, the small air sacs (alveoli) at the ends of the breathing tubes must remain open so that oxygen in the air can get into the tiny blood vessels that surround the alveoli. Normally, in the last months of **pregnancy**, cells in the alveoli produce a substance called **surfactant**, which keep the surface tension inside the alveoli low so that the sacs can expand at the moment of birth, and the infant can breathe normally. Surfactant is produced starting at about 34 weeks of pregnancy and, by the time the fetal lungs mature at 37 weeks, a normal amount is present.

If an infant is born prematurely, enough surfactant might not have formed in the alveoli causing the lungs to collapse and making it very difficult for the baby to get enough air (and the oxygen it contains). Sometimes a layer of fibrous tissue called a hyaline membrane forms in the air sacs, making it even harder for oxygen to get through to the blood vessels. RDS in newborn infants used to be called hyaline membrane disease.

Causes and symptoms

RDS nearly always occurs in premature infants, and the more premature the birth, the greater is the chance that RDS will develop. RDS also is seen in some infants whose mothers are diabetic. Paradoxically, RDS is less likely in the presence of certain states or conditions which themselves are harmful: abnormally slow growth of the fetus; high blood pressure, a condition called **preeclampsia** in the mother; and early rupture of the birth membranes.

Labored breathing (the "respiratory distress" of RDS) may begin as soon as the infant is born, or within a few hours. Breathing becomes very rapid, the nostrils flare, and the infant grunts with each breath. The ribs, which are very flexible in young infants, move inwards each time a breath is taken. Before long the muscles that move the ribs and diaphragm, so that air is drawn into the lungs, become fatigued. When the oxygen level in the blood drops severely the infant's skin turns bluish in color. Tiny, very premature infants may not even have signs of trouble breathing. Their lungs may be so stiff that they cannot even start breathing when born.

There are two major complications of RDS. One is called **pneumothorax**, which means "air in the chest." When the infant itself or a breathing machine applies pressure on the lungs in an attempt to expand them, a lung may rupture, causing air to leak into the chest cavity. This air causes the lung to collapse further, making breathing even harder and interfering with blood flow in the lung arteries. The blood pressure can drop suddenly, cutting the blood supply to the brain. The other complication is called intraventricular hemorrhage; this is bleeding into the cavities (ventricles) of the brain, which may be fatal.

Diagnosis

When a premature infant has obvious trouble breathing when born or within a few hours of birth,

RDS is an obvious possibility. If premature birth is expected, or there is some condition that calls for delivery as soon as possible, the amount of surfactant in the amniotic fluid will indicate how well the lungs have matured. If little surfactant is found in an amniotic fluid sample taken by placing a needle in the uterus (**amniocentesis**), there is a definite risk of RDS. Often this test is at regular intervals so that the infant can be delivered as soon as the lungs are mature. If the membranes have ruptured, surfactant can easily be measured in a sample of vaginal fluid.

The other major diagnostic test is a **chest x ray**. Collapsed lung tissue has a typical appearance, and the more lung tissue is collapsed, the more severe the RDS. An x ray also can demonstrate pneumothorax (air or gas in the area around the lung), if this complication has occurred. The level of oxygen in the blood can be measured by taking a blood sample from an artery, or, more easily, using a device called an oximeter, which is clipped to an earlobe. Pneumothorax may have occurred if the infant suddenly becomes worse while on ventilation; x rays can help make the diagnosis.

Treatment

If only a mild degree of RDS is present at birth, placing the infant in an oxygen hood may be enough. It is important to guard against too much oxygen, as this may damage the retina and cause loss of vision. Using an oximeter to keep track of the blood oxygen level, repeated artery punctures or heel sticks can be avoided. In more severe cases a drug very like natural surfactant (Exosurf Neonatal or Survanta), can be dripped into the lungs through a fine tube (endotracheal tube) placed in the infant's windpipe (trachea). Typically the infant will be able to breathe more easily within a few days at the most, and complications such as lung rupture are less likely to occur. The drug is continued until the infant starts producing its own surfactant. There is a risk of bleeding into the lungs from surfactant treatment; about 10% of the smallest infants are affected.

Infants with severe RDS may require treatment with a ventilator, a machine that takes over the work of the lungs and delivers air under pressure. In tiny infants who do not breathe when born, ventilation through a tracheal tube is an emergency procedure. Assisted ventilation must be closely supervised, as too much pressure can cause further lung damage. A gentler way of assisting breathing, continuous positive airway pressure or CPAP, delivers an oxygen mixture through nasal prongs or a tube placed through the nose rather than an endotracheal tube. CPAP may be tried before resorting to a ventilator, or after an infant placed on a ventilator begins to improve. Drugs that stimulate breathing may speed the recovery process.

Pneumothorax is an emergency that must be treated right away. Air may be removed from the chest using a needle and syringe. A tube then is inserted into the lung cavity, and suction applied.

Prognosis

If an infant born with RDS is not promptly treated, lack of an adequate oxygen supply will damage the body's organs and eventually cause them to stop functioning altogether. **Death** is the result. The central nervous system in particular–made up of the brain and spinal cord–is very dependent on a steady oxygen supply and is one of the first organ systems to feel the effects of RDS. On the other hand, if the infant's breathing is supported until the lungs mature and make their own surfactant, complete recovery within three to five days is the rule.

If an air leak causes pneumothorax, immediate removal of air from the chest will allow the lungs to re-expand. Bleeding into the brain is a very serious condition that worsens the outlook for an infant with RDS.

Prevention

The best way of preventing RDS is to delay delivery until the fetal lungs have matured and are producing enough surfactant–generally at about 37 weeks of pregnancy. If delivery cannot be delayed, the mother may be given a steroid hormone, similar to a natural substance produced in the body, which crosses the barrier of the placenta and helps the fetal lungs to produce surfactant. The steroid should be given at least 24 hours before the expected time of delivery. If the infant does develop RDS, the risk of bleeding into the brain will be much less if the mother has been given a dose of steroid.

If a very premature infant is born without symptoms of RDS, it may be wise to deliver surfactant to its lungs. This may prevent RDS, or make it less severe if it does develop. An alternative is to wait until the first symptoms of RDS appear and then immediately give surfactant. Pneumothorax may be prevented by frequently checking the blood oxygen content, and limiting oxygen treatment under pressure to the minimum needed.

Resources

ORGANIZATIONS

American Lung Association. 1740 Broadway, New York, NY 10019. (800) 586-4872. < http://www.lungusa.org > .

KEY TERMS

Alveoli—The small air sacs located at the ends of the breathing tubes of the lung, where oxygen normally passes from inhaled air to blood vessels.

Amniotic fluid—The fluid bathing the fetus, which may be sampled using a needle to determine whether the fetus is making enough surfactant.

Endotracheal tube—A metal or plastic tube inserted in the windpipe which may be attached to a ventilator. It also may be used to deliver medications such as surfactant.

Hyaline membranes—A fibrous layer that settles in the alveoli in RDS, and prevents oxygen from escaping from inhaled air to the bloodstream.

Pneumothorax—Air in the chest, often a result of the lung rupturing when oxygen is delivered under too high a pressure.

Preeclampsia—A disease of pregnancy in which the mother's blood pressure is elevated; associated with both maternal and fetal complications, and sometimes with fetal death.

Steroid—A natural body substance that often is given to women before delivering a very premature infant to stimulate the fetal lungs to produce surfactant, hopefully preventing RDS (or making it less severe).

Surfactant—A material normally produced in the fetal lungs in the last months of pregnancy, which helps the air sacs to open up at the time of birth so that the newborn infant can breathe freely.

Ventilator—A machine that can breathe for an infant having RDS until its lungs are producing enough surfactant and are able to function normally.

National Respiratory Distress Syndrome Foundation. P.O. Box 723, Montgomeryville, PA 18936.

David A. Cramer, MD

Respiratory failure

Definition

Respiratory failure is nearly any condition that affects breathing function or the lungs themselves and can result in failure of the lungs to function properly. The main tasks of the lungs and chest are to get oxygen from the air that is inhaled into the bloodstream, and, at the same to time, to eliminate carbon dioxide (CO_2) from the blood through air that is breathed out. In respiratory failure, the level of oxygen in the blood becomes dangerously low, and/or the level of CO_2 becomes dangerously high. There are two ways in which this can happen. Either the process by which oxygen and CO_2 are exchanged between the blood and the air spaces of the lungs (a process called "gas exchange") breaks down, or the movement of air in and out of the lungs (ventilation) does not take place properly.

Description

Respiratory failure often is divided into two main types. One of them, called hypoxemic respiratory failure, occurs when something interferes with normal gas exchange. Too little oxygen gets into the blood (hypoxemia), and all organs and tissues in the body suffer as a result. One common type of hypoxemic failure, occurring in both adults and prematurely born infants, is **respiratory distress syndrome**, a condition in which fluid or tissue changes prevent oxygen from passing out of the air sacs of the lungs into the circulating blood. Hypoxemia also may result from spending time at high altitudes (where there is less oxygen in the air); various forms of lung disease that separate oxygen from blood in the lungs; severe anemia ("low blood"); and blood vessel disorders that shunt blood away from the lungs, thus precluding the lungs from picking up oxygen.

The other main type of respiratory failure is ventilatory failure, occurring when, for any reason, breathing is not strong enough to rid the body of CO_2. Then CO_2 builds up in the blood (hypercapnia). Ventilatory failure can result when the respiratory center in the brainstem fails to drive breathing; when muscle disease keeps the chest wall from expanding when breathing in; or when a patient has **chronic obstructive lung disease** that makes it very difficult to exhale air with its CO_2. Many of the specific diseases and conditions that cause respiratory failure cause both too little oxygen in the blood (hypoxemia) and abnormal ventilation.

Causes and symptoms

Several different abnormalities of breathing function can cause respiratory failure. The major categories, with specific examples of each, are:

- Obstruction of the airways. Examples are chronic **bronchitis** with heavy secretions; **emphysema**; **cystic fibrosis**; **asthma** (a condition in which it is very hard to get air in and out through narrowed breathing tubes).

- Weak breathing. This can be caused by drugs or alcohol, which depress the respiratory center; extreme **obesity**; or **sleep apnea**, where patients stop breathing for long periods while sleeping.

- Muscle weakness. This can be caused by a muscle disease called myasthenia; **muscular dystrophy**; **polio**; a **stroke** that paralyzes the respiratory muscles; injury of the spinal cord; or Lou Gehrig's disease.

- Lung diseases, including severe **pneumonia**. **Pulmonary edema**, or fluid in the lungs, can be the source of respiratory failure. Also, it can often be a result of heart disease; respiratory distress syndrome; **pulmonary fibrosis** and other scarring diseases of the lung; radiation exposure; burn injury when smoke is inhaled; and widespread lung **cancer**.

- An abnormal chest wall (a condition that can be caused by **scoliosis** or severe injury of the chest wall).

A majority of patients with respiratory failure are short of breath. Both low oxygen and high carbon dioxide can impair mental functions. Patients may become confused and disoriented and find it impossible to carry out their normal activities or do their work. Marked CO_2 excess can cause headaches and, in time, a semi-conscious state, or even **coma**. Low blood oxygen causes the skin to take on a bluish tinge. It also can cause an abnormal heart rhythm (arrhythmia). **Physical examination** may show a patient who is breathing rapidly, is restless, and has a rapid pulse. Lung disease may cause abnormal sounds heard when listening to the chest with a stethoscope: **wheezing** in asthma, "crackles" in obstructive lung disease. A patient with ventilatory failure is prone to gasp for breath, and may use the neck muscles to help expand the chest.

Diagnosis

The symptoms and signs of respiratory failure are not specific. Rather, they depend on what is causing the failure and on the patient's condition before it developed. Good general health and some degree of "reserve" lung function will help see a patient through an episode of respiratory failure. The key diagnostic determination is to measure the amount of oxygen, carbon dioxide, and acid in the blood at regular intervals. A sudden low oxygen level in the lung tissue may cause the arteries of the lungs to narrow. This, in turn, causes the resistance in these vessels to increase, which can be measured using a special catheter. A high blood level of CO_2 may cause increased pressure in the fluid surrounding the brain and spinal cord; this, too, can be measured.

Treatment

Nearly all patients are given oxygen as the first treatment. Then the underlying cause of respiratory failure must be treated. For example, **antibiotics** are used to fight a lung infection, or, for an asthmatic patient, a drug to open up the airways is commonly prescribed.

A patient whose breathing remains very poor will require a ventilator to aid breathing. A plastic tube is placed through the nose or mouth into the windpipe and is attached to a machine that forces air into the lungs. This can be a lifesaving treatment and should be continued until the patient's own lungs can take over the work of breathing. It is very important to use no more pressure than is necessary to provide sufficient oxygen; otherwise ventilation may cause further lung damage. Drugs are given to keep the patient calm, and the amount of fluid in the body is carefully adjusted so that the heart and lungs can function as normally as possible. Steroids, which combat inflammation, may sometimes be helpful but they can cause complications, including weakening the breathing muscles.

The respiratory therapist has a number of methods available to help patients overcome respiratory failure. They include:

- Suctioning the lungs through a small plastic tube passed through the nose, in order to remove secretions from the airways that the patient cannot **cough** up.

- Postural drainage, in which the patient is propped up at an angle or tilted to help secretions drain out of the lungs. The therapist may clap the patient on the chest or back to loosen the secretions, or a vibrator may be used for the same purpose.

- Breathing exercises often are prescribed after the patient recovers. They make the patient feel better and help to strengthen the muscles that aid breathing. One useful method is for the patient to suck on a tube attached to a clear plastic hosing containing a ball so as to keep the ball lifted. Regular deep breathing exercises are simpler and often just as helpful. Another technique is to have the patient breathe out against pursed lips to increase pressure in the airways and keep them from collapsing.

KEY TERMS

Chronic obstructive lung disease—A common form of lung disease in which breathing, and therefore gas exchange, is labored and increasingly difficult.

Gas exchange—The process by which oxygen is extracted from inhaled air into the bloodstream, and, at the same time, carbon dioxide is eliminated from the blood and exhaled.

Hypoxemia—An abnormally low amount of oxygen in the blood, the major consequence of respiratory failure, when the lungs no longer are able to perform their chief function of gas exchange.

Pulmonary fibrosis—An end result of many forms of lung disease (especially chronic inflammatory conditions). Normal lung tissue is converted to scarred, "fibrotic" tissue that cannot carry out gas exchange.

Prognosis

The outlook for patients with respiratory failure depends chiefly on its cause. If the underlying disease can be effectively treated, with the patient's breathing supported in the meantime, the outlook is usually good.

Care is needed not to expose the patient to polluting substances in the atmosphere while recovering from respiratory failure; this could tip the balance against recovery. When respiratory failure develops slowly, pressure may build up in the lung's blood vessels, a condition called **pulmonary hypertension**. This condition may damage the vessels, worsen hypoxemia, and cause the heart to fail. If it is not possible to provide enough oxygen to the body, complications involving either the brain or the heart may prove fatal.

If the kidneys fail or the diseased lungs become infected, the prognosis is worse. In some cases, the primary disease causing the lungs to fail is irreversible. The patient, family, and physician together then must decide whether to prolong life by ventilator support. Occasionally, **lung transplantation** is a possibility, but it is a highly complex procedure and is not widely available

Prevention

Because respiratory failure is not a disease itself, but the end result of many lung disorders, the best prevention is to treat any lung disease promptly and effectively. It is also important to make sure that any patient who has had lung disease is promptly treated for any respiratory infection (even of the upper respiratory tract). Patients with lung problems should also avoid exposure to pollutants, as much as is possible. Once respiratory failure is present, it is best for a patient to receive treatment in an intensive care unit, where specialized personnel and all the needed equipment are available. Close supervision of treatment, especially mechanical ventilation, will help minimize complications that would compound the problem.

Resources

ORGANIZATIONS

National Heart, Lung and Blood Institute. P.O. Box 30105, Bethesda, MD 20824-0105. (301) 251-1222. < http:// www.nhlbi.nih.gov >.

National Respiratory Distress Syndrome Foundation. P.O. Box 723, Montgomeryville, PA 18936.

David A. Cramer, MD

Respiratory syncytial virus infection

Definition

Respiratory syncytial virus (RSV) is a virus that can cause severe lower respiratory infections in children under the age of two, and milder upper respiratory infections in older children and adults. RSV infection is also called **bronchiolitis**, because it is marked in young children by inflammation of the bronchioles. Bronchioles are the narrow airways that lead from the bronchi to the tiny air sacs (alveoli) in the lungs. The result is **wheezing**, difficulty breathing, and sometimes fatal **respiratory failure**.

Description

RSV infection is caused by a group of viruses found worldwide. There are two different subtypes of the virus with numerous different strains. Taken together, these viruses account for a significant number of deaths in infants.

RSV infection is primarily a disease of winter or early spring, with waves of illness sweeping through a community. The rate of RSV infection is estimated to be 11.4 cases in every 100 children during their first year of life. In the United States, RSV infection occurs most frequently in infants between the ages of two months and six months.

RSV infection shows distinctly different symptoms, depending on the age of the infected person. In children under two, the virus causes a serious lower respiratory infection in the lungs. In older children and healthy adults, it causes a mild upper respiratory infection often mistaken for the **common cold**.

Although anyone can get this disease, infants suffer the most serious symptoms and complications. Breast feeding seems to provide partial protection from the virus. Conditions in infants that increase their risk of infection include:

- premature birth
- lower socio-economic environment
- congenital heart disease
- chronic lung diseases, such as cystic fibrosis
- immune system deficiencies, including HIV infection
- immunosuppressive therapy given to organ transplant patients

Many older children and adults get RSV infection, but the symptoms are so similar to the common cold that the true cause is undiagnosed. People of any age with weakened immune systems, either from such diseases as **AIDS** or leukemia, or as the result of **chemotherapy** or corticosteroid medications, are more at risk for serious RSV infections. So are people with chronic lung disease.

Causes and symptoms

Respiratory syncytial virus is spread through close contact with an infected person. It has been shown that if a person with RSV infection sneezes, the virus can be carried to others within a radius of 6 f (1.8 m). This group of viruses is hardy. They can live on the hands for up to half an hour and on toys or other inanimate objects for several hours.

Scientists have yet to understand why RSV viruses attack the lower respiratory system in infants and the upper respiratory system in adults. In infants, RSV begins with such cold symptoms as a low **fever**, runny nose, and **sore throat**. Soon, other symptoms appear that suggest an infection which involves the lower airways. Some of these symptoms resemble those of **asthma**. RSV infection is suggested by:

- wheezing and high-pitched, whistling breathing
- rapid breathing (more than 40 breaths per minute)
- shortness of breath
- labored breathing out (exhalations)
- bluish tinge to the skin (cyanosis)
- croupy, seal-like, barking **cough**
- high fever

Breathing problems occur in RSV infections because the bronchioles swell, making it difficult for air to get in and out of the lungs. If the child is having trouble breathing, immediate medical care is needed. Breathing problems are most common in infants under one year of age; they can develop rapidly.

Diagnosis

Physical examination and imaging studies

RSV infection is usually diagnosed during a **physical examination** by the pediatrician or primary care doctor. The doctor listens with a stethoscope for wheezing and other abnormal lung sounds in the patient's chest. The doctor will also take into consideration whether there is a known outbreak of RSV infection in the area. Chest x rays give some indication of whether the lungs are hyperinflated from an effort to move air in and out. X rays may also show the presence of a secondary bacterial infection, such as **pneumonia**.

Laboratory tests

A blood test can also detect RSV infection. This test measures the level of antibodies the body has formed against the virus. The blood test is less reliable in infants than in older children because antibodies in the infant's blood may have come from the mother during **pregnancy**. If infants are hospitalized, other tests such as an arterial **blood gas analysis** are done to determine if the child is receiving enough oxygen.

Treatment

Home care

Home treatment for RSV infection is primarily supportive. It involves taking steps to ease the child's breathing. **Dehydration** can be a problem, so children should be encouraged to drink plenty of fluids. **Antibiotics** have no effect on viral illnesses. In time, the body will make antibodies to fight the infection and return itself to health.

Home care for keeping a child with RSV comfortable and breathing more easily includes:

- Use a cool mist room humidifier to ease congestion and sore throat.
- Raise the baby's head by putting books under the head end of the crib.
- Give **acetaminophen** (Tylenol, Pandol, Tempra) for fever. **Aspirin** should not be given to children because of its association with **Reye's syndrome**, a serious disease.
- For babies too young to blow their noses, suction away any mucus with an infant nasal aspirator.

Hospital treatment

In the United States, RSV infections are responsible for 90,000 hospitalizations and 4,500 deaths each year. Children who are hospitalized receive oxygen and humidity through a mist tent or vaporizer. They also are given intravenous fluids to prevent dehydration. Mechanical ventilation may be necessary. Blood gases are monitored to assure that the child is receiving enough oxygen.

Medications

Bronchiodilators, such as albuterol (Proventil, Ventilin), may be used to keep the airways open. Ribavirin (Virazole) is used for desperately ill children to stop the growth of the virus. Ribavirin is both expensive and has toxic side effects, so its use is restricted to the most severe cases.

Alternative treatment

Alternative medicine has little to say specifically about bronchiolitis, especially in very young children. Practitioners emphasize that people get viral illnesses because their immune systems are weak. Prevention focuses on strengthening the immune system by eating a healthy diet low in sugars and high in fresh fruits and vegetables, reducing **stress**, and getting regular, moderate **exercise**. Like traditional practitioners, alternative practitioners recommend breastfeeding infants so that the child may benefit from the positive state of health of the mother. Inhaling a steaming mixture of lemon oil, thyme oil, eucalyptus, and tea tree oil (**aromatherapy**) may make breathing easier.

Prognosis

RSV infection usually runs its course in seven to 14 days. The cough may linger weeks longer. There are no medications that can speed the body's production of antibodies against the virus. Opportunistic bacterial infections that take advantage of a weakened

respiratory system may cause ear, sinus, and throat infections or pneumonia.

Hospitalization and **death** are much more likely to occur in children whose immune systems are weakened or who have underlying diseases of the lungs and heart. People do not gain permanent immunity to respiratory syncytial virus and can be infected many times. Children who suffer repeated infections seem to be more likely to develop asthma in later life.

Prevention

As of 1998 there are no vaccines against RSV. Respiratory syncytial virus infection is so common that prevention is impossible. However, steps can be taken to reduce a child's contact with the disease. People with RSV symptoms should stay at least six feet away from young children. Frequent handwashing, especially after contact with respiratory secretions, and the correct disposal of used tissues help keep the disease from spreading. Parents should try to keep their children under 18 month old away from crowded environments–for example, shopping malls during holiday seasons–where they are likely to come in contact with older people who have only mild symptoms of the disease. Child care centers should regularly disinfect surfaces that children touch.

Resources

PERIODICALS
Hemming, Val, et al. "Bracing for the Cold and Flu Season." *Patient Care* 31 (September 1997): 47-54.

Tish Davidson, A.M.

Restless legs syndrome

Definition

Restless legs syndrome (RLS) is characterized by unpleasant sensations in the limbs, usually the legs, that occur at rest or before sleep and are relieved by activity such as walking. These sensations are felt deep within the legs and are described as creeping, crawling, aching, or fidgety.

Description

Restless legs syndrome, also known as Ekbom syndrome, Wittmaack-Ekbom syndrome, *anxietas tibiarum*, or *anxietas tibialis*, affects up to 10–15% of the population. Some studies show that RLS is more common among elderly people. Almost half of patients over age 60 who complain of **insomnia** are diagnosed with RLS. In some cases, the patient has another medical condition with which RLS is associated. In idiopathic RLS, no cause can be found. In familial cases, RLS may be inherited from a close relative, most likely a parent.

Causes and symptoms

Most people experience mild symptoms. They may lie down to rest at the end of the day and, just before sleep, will experience discomfort in their legs that prompts them to stand up, massage the leg, or walk briefly. Eighty-five percent of RLS patients either have difficulty falling asleep or wake several times during the night, and almost half experience daytime **fatigue** or sleepiness. It is common for the symptoms to be intermittent. They may disappear for several months and then return for no apparent reason. Two-thirds of patients report that their symptoms become worse with time. Some older patients claim to have had symptoms since they were in their early 20s, but were not diagnosed until their 50s. Suspected under-diagnosis of RLS may be attributed to the difficulty experienced by patients in describing their symptoms.

More than 80% of patients with RLS experience periodic limb movements in sleep (PLMS). These random movements of arms or legs may result in further sleep disturbance and daytime fatigue. Most patients have restless feelings in both legs, but only one leg may be affected. Arms may be affected in nearly half of patients.

There is no known cause for the disorder, but recent research has focused on several key areas. These include:

- Central nervous system (CNS) abnormalities. Several types of drugs have been found to reduce the symptoms of RLS. Based on an understanding of how these drugs work, theories have been developed to explain the cause of the disorder. Levodopa and other drugs that correct problems with signal transmission within the central nervous system (CNS) can reduce the symptoms of RLS. It is therefore suspected that the source of RLS is a problem related to signal transmission systems in the CNS.

- Iron deficiency. The body stores iron in the form of ferritin. There is a relationship between low levels of iron (as ferritin) stored in the body and the occurrence of RLS. Studies have shown that older people with RLS often have low levels of ferritin. Supplements of iron sulfate have been shown to significantly reduce RLS symptoms for these patients.

Diagnosis

A careful history enables the physician to distinguish RLS from similar types of disorders that cause night time discomfort in the limbs, such as **muscle cramps**, burning feet syndrome, and damage to nerves that detect sensations or cause movement (polyneuropathy).

The most important tool the doctor has in diagnosis is the history obtained from the patient. There are several common medical conditions that are known to either cause or to be closely associated with RLS. The doctor may link the patient's symptoms to one of these conditions, which include anemia, diabetes, disease of the spinal nerve roots (lumbosacral radiculopathy), Parkinson's disease, late-stage **pregnancy**, kidney failure (uremia), and complications of stomach surgery. In order to identify or eliminate such a primary cause, blood tests may be performed to determine the presence of serum iron, ferritin, folate, vitamin B$_{12}$, creatinine, and thyroid-stimulating hormones. The physician may also ask if symptoms are present in any close family members, since it is common for RLS to run in families and this type is sometimes more difficult to treat.

In some cases, sleep studies such as **polysomnography** are undertaken to identify the presence of PLMS that are reported to affect 70–80% of people who suffer from RLS. The patient is often unaware of these movements, since they may not cause him to wake. However, the presence of PLMS with RLS can leave the person more tired, because it interferes with deep sleep. A patient who also displays evidence of some neurologic disease may undergo **electromyography** (EMG). During EMG, a very small, thin needle is inserted into the muscle and electrical activity of the muscle is recorded. A doctor or technician usually performs this test at a hospital outpatient department.

Treatment

The first step in treatment is to treat existing conditions that are known to be associated with RLS and that will be identified by blood tests. If the patient is anemic, iron (iron sulfate) or vitamin supplements (folate or vitamin B_{12}) will be prescribed. If **kidney disease** is identified as a cause, treatment of the kidney problem will take priority.

Prescription drugs

In some people whose symptoms cannot be linked to a treatable associated condition, drug therapy may be necessary to provide relief and restore a normal sleep pattern. Prescription drugs that are normally used for RLS include:

- **Benzodiazepines** and low-potency opioids. These drugs are prescribed for use only on an "as needed" basis, for patients with mild RLS. Benzodiazepines appear to reduce nighttime awakenings due to PLMS. The benzodiazepine most commonly used to treat RLS is clonazepam (Klonopin, Rivotril). The main disadvantage of this drug type is that it causes daytime drowsiness. It also causes unsteadiness that may lead to accidents, especially for an elderly patient. Opioids are narcotic **pain** relievers. Those commonly used for mild RLS are low potency opioids, such as codeine (Tylenol #3) and propoxyphene (Darvocet). Studies have shown that these can be successfully used in the treatment of RLS on a long-term basis without risk of **addiction**. However, **narcotics** can cause **constipation** and difficulty urinating.

- Levodopa (L-dopa) and carbidopa (Sinemet). Levodopa is the drug most commonly used to treat moderate or severe RLS. It acts by supplying a chemical called dopamine to the brain. It is often taken in conjunction with carbidopa to prevent or decrease side effects. Although it is effective against RLS, levodopa may also causes a worsening of symptoms during the afternoon or early evening in 50–80% of patients. This phenomenon is known as "restless legs augmentation," and if it occurs, the physician will probably discontinue Levodopa for a brief period while an alternate drug is used. Levodopa can often be reintroduced after a short break.

- Pergolide (Permax). Pergolide acts on the same part of the brain as Levodopa. It is less likely than

Levodopa to cause daytime worsening of symptoms (occurs in about 25% of patients). However, it is not recommended as the first choice in drug therapy since it causes a high rate of minor side effects. Pergolide is often used only if Levodopa has been discontinued.

- High potency opioids. If the symptoms of RLS are difficult to treat with the above medication, higher dose opioids will be used. These include **methadone** (Dolophine), oxycodone, and clonidine (Catapres, Combipres, Dixarit). A significant disadvantage of these drugs is risk of addiction.

- Anticonvulsants. Some cases of RLS may be improved by **anticonvulsant drugs**, such as carbamazepine (Tegretol).

- Combination therapy. Some patients respond well to combinations of drugs such as a benzodiazepine and Levodopa.

Many drugs have been investigated for treatment of RLS, but it seems as though the perfect therapy has not yet been found. However, careful monitoring of side effects and good communication between patient and doctor can result in a flexible program of therapy that minimizes side effects and maximizes effectiveness.

Alternative treatment

It is likely that the best alternative therapy will combine both conventional and alternative approaches. Levodopa may be combined with a therapy that relieves pain, relaxes muscles, or focuses in general on the nervous system and the brain. Any such combined therapy that allows a reduction in dosage of levodopa is advantageous, since this will reduce the likelihood of unacceptable levels of drug side effects. Of course, the physician who prescribes the medication should monitor any combined therapy. Alternative methods may include:

- **Acupuncture**. Patients who also suffer from **rheumatoid arthritis** may especially benefit from acupuncture to relieve RLS symptoms. Acupuncture is believed to be effective in arthritis treatment and may also stimulate those parts of the brain that are involved in RLS.

- Homeopathy. Homeopaths believe that disorders of the nervous system are especially important because the brain controls so many other bodily functions. The remedy is tailored to the individual patient and is based on individual symptoms as well as the general symptoms of RLS.

- **Reflexology**. Reflexologists claim that the brain, head, and spine all respond to indirect massage of specific parts of the feet.

- Nutritional supplements. Supplementation of the diet with vitamin E, calcium, magnesium, and **folic acid** may be helpful for people with RLS.

Some alternative methods may treat the associated condition that is suspected to cause restless legs. These include:

- Anemia or low ferritin levels. Chinese medicine will emphasize stimulation of the spleen as a means of improving blood circulation and vitamin absorption. Other treatments may include acupuncture and herbal therapies, such as ginseng (*Panax ginseng*) for anemia-related fatigue.

- Late-stage pregnancy. There are few conventional therapies available to pregnant women, since most of the drugs prescribed are not recommended for use during pregnancy. Pregnant women may benefit from alternative techniques that focus on body work, including **yoga**, reflexology, and acupuncture.

Prognosis

RLS usually does not indicate the onset of other neurological disease. It may remain static, although two-thirds of patients get worse with time. The symptoms usually progress gradually. Treatment with Levodopa is effective in moderate to severe cases that may include significant PLMS. However, this drug produces significant side effects, and continued successful treatment may depend on carefully monitored use of combination drug therapy. The prognosis is usually best if RLS symptoms are recent and can be traced to another treatable condition that is associated with RLS. Some associated conditions are not treatable. In these cases, such as for rheumatoid arthritis, alternative therapies such as acupuncture may be helpful.

Prevention

Diet is key in preventing RLS. A preventive diet will include an adequate intake of iron and the B **vitamins**, especially B_{12} and folic acid. Strict vegetarians should take vitamin supplements to obtain sufficient vitamin B_{12}. Ferrous gluconate may be easier on the digestive system than ferrous sulfate, if iron supplements are prescribed. Some medications may cause symptoms of RLS. Patients should check with their doctor about these possible side effects, especially if symptoms first occur after starting a new medication. **Caffeine**, alcohol, and nicotine use should be minimized or eliminated. Even a hot bath before bed has been shown to prevent symptoms for some sufferers.

Resources

PERIODICALS

Silber, Michael H. "Concise Review for Primary-Care Physicians. Restless Legs Syndrome." *Mayo Clinical Proceedings* 72 (March 1997): 261-264.

ORGANIZATIONS

Restless Legs Syndrome Foundation. 1904 Banbury Road, Raleigh, NC 27608-4428. (919) 781-4428. <http://www.rls.org>.

Ann M. Haren

Restrictive cardiomyopathy

Definition

Cardiomyopathy is an ongoing disease process that damages the muscle wall of the lower chambers of the heart. Restrictive cardiomyopathy is a form of cardiomyopathy in which the walls of the heart become rigid.

Description

Restrictive cardiomyopathy is the least common type of cardiomyopathy in the United States. The stiffened heart walls cannot stretch properly to allow enough blood to fill the ventricles between heartbeats. As the stiffening worsens, **heart failure** occurs. The blood backs up into the blood vessels, causing fluid buildup in tissues (congestion and **edema**).

Causes and symptoms

Restrictive cardiomyopathy can be caused by a number of diseases. Often, the cause is unknown. The rigidity of the heart walls may be caused by fibrosis, the replacement of muscle cells with tough, fibrous tissue. In some disorders, proteins and other substances are deposited in the heart wall. **Amyloidosis** is the accumulation of a protein material, called amyloid, in the tissue of the heart wall and other organs. In **hemochromatosis**, there is too much iron in the body and some of the excess iron can build up in the heart. **Sarcoidosis** causes the formation of many small lesions, called granulomas, in the heart wall and other tissues of the body. These granulomas contain inflammatory white blood cells and other cells that decrease the flexibility of the heart.

People with restrictive cardiomyopathy usually feel tired and weak, and have **shortness of breath**, especially during **exercise**. If blood is backing up in the circulation they may also experience edema (large amounts of fluid in tissues) of the legs and feet.

Diagnosis

The diagnosis is usually based on a **physical examination**, **echocardiography**, and other tests as needed. The physician listens to the heart with a stethoscope to detect abnormal heart rhythms and heart sounds.

Echocardiography uses sound waves to make images of the heart. These images provide information about the structures of the heart and its heart valves. Echocardiography can also be used to find out how much blood the heart is pumping. It determines the amount of blood in the ventricle, called the ventricular volume, and the amount of blood the ventricle pumps each time it beats, called the ejection fraction. A healthy heart pumps at least one half the amount of blood in the left ventricle with each heartbeat.

Computed tomography scan (CT scan) and **magnetic resonance imaging** (MRI) are imaging tests that can also provide information about the structure of the heart. However, these tests are rarely needed for diagnosis.

Cardiac catheterization may be needed to confirm a diagnosis or cause. In cardiac catheterization, a small tube called a catheter is inserted into an artery and passed into the heart. It is used to measure pressure in the heart and the amount of blood

pumped by the heart. A small tissue sample (biopsy) of the heart muscle can be removed through the catheter for microscopic examination. Fibrous tissue or deposits in the heart muscle can be identified in this biopsy.

Treatment

There is no effective treatment for restrictive cardiomyopathy. Treatment of a causative disease may reduce or stop the damage to the heart, but existing damage cannot be reversed. Medications may be used to lessen the workload on the heart and to control the heart rhythm. Drugs normally used to treat other types of cardiomyopathy and heart failure may cause problems for patients with restrictive cardiomyopathy. For example, medicines that reduce the heart's workload may lower blood pressure too much.

A heart transplant may be necessary for patients who develop severe heart failure.

Prognosis

The prognosis for patients with restrictive cardiomyopathy is poor. If the disease process causing the problem can be treated, the damage to the heart muscle may be stopped. Also, medicines may relieve symptoms. However, for most patients, restrictive cardiomyopathy eventually causes heart failure. A heart transplant may be necessary when heart failure becomes too severe to treat with medicines.

Prevention

Obtaining early treatment for diseases that might cause restrictive cardiomyopathy might prevent or slow the development of heart wall stiffness. Anyone experiencing symptoms of shortness of breath, tiredness, and weakness should see a physician.

Resources

ORGANIZATIONS

American Heart Association. 7320 Greenville Ave. Dallas, TX 75231. (214) 373-6300. <http://www.americanheart.org>.

National Heart, Lung and Blood Institute. P.O. Box 30105, Bethesda, MD 20824-0105. (301) 251-1222. <http://www.nhlbi.nih.gov>.

Texas Heart Institute. Heart Information Service. P.O. Box 20345, Houston, TX 77225-0345. <http://www.tmc.edu/thi>.

Toni Rizzo

Reticulocyte count

Definition

A reticulocyte count is a blood test performed to assess the body's production of immature red blood cells (reticulocytes). A reticulocyte count is usually performed when patients are evaluated for anemia and response to its treatment. It is sometimes called a retic count.

Purpose

Diagnosis

A reticulocyte count provides information about the rate at which the bone marrow is producing red cells. A normal count means that the production is adequate; a decreased count means it is not. This information helps determine whether a lack of red cells in an anemic person is caused by a bone marrow problem, by excessive bleeding, or by red cell destruction.

Monitoring

The test is also used to monitor the response of bone marrow response to treatment for anemia. The reticulocyte count rises within days if the treatment is successful. It is also used following bone marrow transplant to evaluate the new marrow's cell production.

Description

Reticulocytes were first described as transitional forms of red blood cells by Wilhelm H. Erb in 1865. A red cell begins in the bone marrow as a large bluish cell filled with ribonucleic acid (RNA). As the cell matures, it shrinks. Its color gradually changes from blue to pink as its load of oxygen-carrying protein (hemoglobin) increases and the RNA decreases. The center of the cell (nucleus) becomes clumped. It is expelled three days before the cell leaves the bone marrow. The cell is now a reticulocyte. On its fourth and final day of maturation, the reticulocyte enters the bloodstream. One day later, it is a mature red blood cell.

The first step in a retic count is drawing the patient's blood sample. About 17 oz (5 ml) of blood is withdrawn from a vein into a vacuum tube. The procedure, which is called a venipuncture, takes about five minutes.

After the sample is collected, the blood is mixed with a dye (methylene blue) in a test tube. The RNA remaining in the reticulocytes picks up a deep blue stain. Drops of the mixture are smeared on slides and examined under a microscope. Reticulocytes appear as cells containing dark blue granules or a blue network. The laboratory technologist counts 1,000 red cells, keeping track of the number of reticulocytes. The number of reticulocytes is reported as a percentage of the total red cells. When the red cell count is low, the percentage of reticulocytes is inaccurately high, suggesting that more reticulocytes are present than there are in reality. The percentage is mathematically corrected for greater accuracy. This figure is called the corrected reticulocyte count or reticulocyte index.

Reticulocyte counts can also be done on automated instruments, such as flow cytometers, using fluorescent stains. These instruments are able to detect small changes in the reticulocyte count because they count a larger number of cells (10,000–50,000).

Preparation

The doctor should make a note of any prescription medications that the patient is taking. Some drugs lower the red blood cell count.

Aftercare

Aftercare consists of routine care of the area around the puncture mark. Pressure is applied for a few seconds and the wound is covered with a bandage.

Risks

The primary risk is mild **dizziness** and the possibility of a bruise or swelling in the area where the blood was drawn. The patient can apply moist warm compresses.

Normal results

Adults have reticulocyte counts of 0.5–2.5%. Women and children usually have higher reticulocyte counts than men.

Abnormal results

A low reticulocyte count indicates that the bone marrow is not producing a normal number of red blood cells. Low production may be caused by a lack of vitamin B_{12}, **folic acid**, or iron in the diet; or by an illness affecting the bone marrow (for example, **cancer**). Further tests are needed to diagnose the specific cause.

The reticulocyte count rises when the bone marrow makes more red cells in response to blood loss or treatment of anemia.

Resources

PERIODICALS

Rowan, R. M., et al. "The Reticulocyte Count: Progress Towards the Resurrection of a Useful Clinical Test." *Clinical and Laboratory Haematology* 18, no. 1 (1996): 3-8.

Nancy J. Nordenson

Retinal artery occlusion

Definition

Retinal artery occlusion refers to the closure of the central retinal artery and usually results in complete loss of vision in one eye. Occlusion of its branches causes loss of vision in only a portion of the field of vision.

Description

Retinal artery occlusion (RAO) occurs when the central retinal artery, the main source of blood supply to the retina, or one of its branches becomes blocked.

Causes and symptoms

The main causes of RAO are the following:

- embolism (the sudden obstruction of a blood vessel by a blood clot)
- atherosclerotic disease that results in the progressive narrowing of the arteries over time
- endarteritis (the chronic inflammation of the inner layer of arteries)
- angiospasm (a spasmodic contraction of a blood vessel with increase in blood pressure)

The most common symptom of RAO is an acute, painless loss of vision in one eye. The degree of loss depends on the location of the occlusion. If the occlusion occurs in the central artery of the retina, damage usually results in complete loss of vision in the affected eye. If occlusion occurs in a branch artery, vision loss will be partial and may even go unnoticed if only a section of the peripheral vision is affected.

People affected by RAO typically have high blood pressure, heart disease, or diabetes as an underlying condition. Other conditions that may increase the risk of RAO include **high cholesterol** and **glaucoma**. Incidence is slightly more common in men and in people age 60 or older.

Diagnosis

RAO is diagnosed by examination of the retina with an ophtalmoscope.

Treatment

Central retinal artery occlusion (CRAO) is an emergency. If treatment begins within an hour, the patient has the highest possibility of regaining vision in the affected eye, although complete restoration is unlikely.

A common treatment is inhalation of carbon dioxide so as to dilate the retinal vessels and move the occlusion from the central retinal artery to a branch artery. This movement reduces the area of the retina affected and may restore a certain amount of vision. Eyeball massage may also be performed, also in

KEY TERMS

Angiospasm—Spasmodic contraction of a blood vessel with increase in blood pressure.

Arterioles—Small blood vessels that carry arterial (oxygenated) blood.

Atherosclerotic disease—The progressive narrowing and hardening of the arteries over time.

Central retinal artery—A branch of the ophthalmic artery that supplies blood to the retina and branches to form the arterioles of the retina.

Embolism—The sudden obstruction of a blood vessel by a blood clot.

Endarteritis—Chronic inflammation of the inner layer of arteries.

Hyperbaric oxygenation—Administration of oxygen in a compression chamber at an ambient pressure greater than 1 atmosphere, in order to increase the amount of oxygen in organs and tissues.

Occlusion—Momentary complete closure of some area or channel of the body.

Ophthalmic artery—The artery supplying the eye and adjacent structures with blood.

Ophthalmoscope—An instrument used for viewing the inside of the eye that consists of a concave mirror with a hole in the middle through which the physician examines the eye, and a light source that is reflected into the eye by the mirror.

Retina—Light sensitive layer of the eye, that consists of four major layers: the outer neural layer, containing nerve cells and blood vessels, the photoreceptor layer, a single layer that contains the light sensing rods and cones, the pigmented retinal epithelium (PRE) and the choroid, consisting of connective tissue and capillaries.

an effort to remove the occlusion. The physician may also consider puncturing the eyeball.

Drug therapy includes the use of carbonic anhydrase inhibitors to reduce the internal eye pressure and enhance movement of the occlusion. Both of the treatments would be used within the first 24 hours of noticeable vision loss.

Alternative treatment

Hyperbaric **oxygen therapy** may be beneficial if started within 90 minutes of the onset of symptoms.

Some studies indicate a 40% improvement of visual acuity using this method.

Prognosis

The prognosis for central retinal visual acuity is poor with only about one-third of patients recovering useful vision. The longest delay in getting treatment that has been associated with significant visual recovery was approximately 72 hours.

Branch retinal artery occlusions (BRAO) have a recovery rate of 80% where vision is restored to 20/40 or better.

Prevention

Individuals affected by underlying conditions such as high blood pressure, heart disease, diabetes, glaucoma, and elevated cholesterol should treat their conditions appropriately to minimize the possibility of a retinal artery occlusion.

Resources

ORGANIZATIONS

American Academy of Ophthalmology. P.O. Box 7424, San Francisco, CA 94120-7424. (415) 561-8500. Fax: (415) 561-8533. < http://www.eyenet.org/ >.

American Diabetes Association. 1701 North Beauregard Street, Alexandria, VA 22311. (800) DIABETES. < http://www.diabetes.org/ >.

American Heart Association National Center. 7272 Greenville Avenue, Dallas, Texas 75231. (877) 242-4277. < http://www.americanheart.org/ >.

CliniWeb International. < http://www.ohsu.edu/cliniweb/ C11/C11.768.html >.

Gary Gilles

Retinal detachment

Definition

Retinal detachment is movement of the transparent sensory part of the retina away from the outer pigmented layer of the retina. In other words, the moving away of the retina from the outer wall of the eyeball.

Description

There are three layers of the eyeball. The outer, tough, white sclera. Lining the sclera is the choroid, a

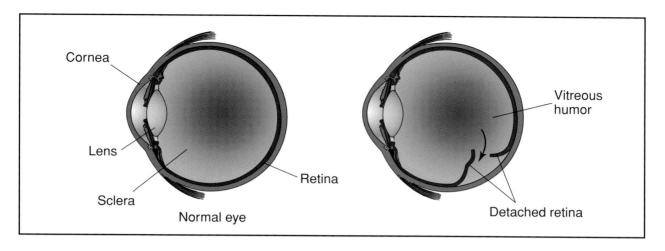

Retinal detachment refers to the movement of the retina away from the inner wall of the eyeball, resulting in a sudden defect in vision. Persons suffering from diabetes have a high incidence of developing retinal disease. *(Illustration by Electronic Illustrators Group.)*

thin membrane that supplies nutrients to part of the retina. The innermost layer is the retina.

The retina is the light-sensitive membrane that receives images and transmits them to the brain. It is made up of several layers. One layer contains the photoreceptors. The photoreceptors, the rods and cones, send the visual message to the brain. Between the photoreceptor layer (also called the sensory layer) and the choroid is the pigmented epithelium.

The vitreous is a clear gel-like substance that fills up most of the inner space of the eyeball. It lies behind the lens and is in contact with the retina.

A retinal detachment occurs between the two outermost layers of the retina–the photoreceptor layer and the outermost pigmented epithelium. Because the choroid supplies the photoreceptors with nutrients, a detachment can basically starve the photoreceptors. If a detachment is not repaired within 24–72 hours, permanent damage may occur.

Causes and symptoms

Several conditions may cause retinal detachment:

- Scarring or shrinkage of the vitreous can pull the retina inward.
- Small tears in the retina allow liquid to seep behind the retina and push it forward.
- Injury to the eye can simply knock the retina loose.
- Bleeding behind the retina, most often due to diabetic retinopathy or injury, can push it forward.

- Retinal detachment may be spontaneous. This occurs more often in the elderly or in very near-sighted (myopic) eyes.
- Cataract surgery causes retinal detachment 2% of the time.
- Tumors can cause the retina to detach.

Retinal detachment will cause a sudden defect in vision. It may look as if a curtain or shadow has just descended before the eye. If most of the retina is detached, there may be only a small hole of vision remaining. If just a part of the retina is involved, there will be a blind spot that may not even be noticed. It is often associated with *floaters*–little dark spots that float across the eye and can be mistaken for flies in the room. There may also be *flashes* of light. Anyone experiencing a sudden onset of flashes and/or floaters should contact their eye doctor immediately, as this may signal a detachment.

Diagnosis

If the eye is clear–that is, if there is no clouding of the liquids inside the eye–the detachment can be seen by looking into the eye with a hand-held instrument called an ophthalmoscope. To evaluate the blood vessels in the retina, a fluorescent dye (fluorescein) may be injected into a vein and photographed with ultraviolet light as it passes through the retina. Further studies may include computed tomography scan (CT scan), **magnetic resonance imaging** (MRI), or ultrasound study. Other lenses may be used to examine the back of the eyes. One example is binocular indirect ophthalmoscopy. The doctor dilates the patient's eyes with

KEY TERMS

Cauterize—To damage with heat or cold so that tissues shrink. It is an effective way to stop bleeding.

Diabetic retinopathy—Disease that damages the blood vessels in the back of the eye caused by diabetes.

Saline—A salt solution equivalent to that in the body–0.9% salt in water.

eyedrops and then examines the back of the eyes with a handheld lens.

Treatment

Reattaching the retina to the inner surface of the eye requires making a scar that will hold it in place and then bringing the retina close to the scarred area. The scar can be made from the outside, through the sclera, using either a laser or a freezing cold probe (cryopexy). Bringing the retina close to the scar can be done in two ways. A tiny belt tightened around the eyeball will bring the sclera in until it reaches the retina. This procedure is called scleral buckling and may be done under **general anesthesia**. Using this procedure permits the repair of retinal detachments without entering the eyeball. Sometimes, the eye must be entered to pump in air or gas, forcing the retina outward against the sclera and its scar. This is called pneumatic retinopexy and can generally be done under **local anesthesia**.

If all else fails, and especially if there is disease in the vitreous, the vitreous may have to be removed in a procedure called **vitrectomy**. This can be done through tiny holes in the eye, through which equally tiny instruments are placed to suck out the vitreous and replace it with saline, a salt solution. The procedure must maintain pressure inside the eye so that the eye does not collapse.

Prognosis

Retinal reattachment has an 80–90% success rate.

Prevention

In diseases such as diabetes, with a high incidence of retinal disease, routine eye examinations can detect early changes. Early treatment can prevent both progressing to detachment and blindness from other events like hemorrhage. The most common problem is weakness of blood vessels that causes them to break down and bleed. When enough vessels have been damaged, new vessels grow to replace them. These new vessels may grow into the vitreous, producing blind spots and scarring. The scarring can in turn pull the retina loose. Other diseases can cause the tiny holes and tears in the retina through which fluid can leak. Preventive treatment uses a laser to cauterize the blood vessels, so that they do not bleed and the holes, so they do not leak.

Good control of diabetes can help prevent diabetic eye disease. Blood pressure control can prevent **hypertension** from damaging the retinal blood vessels. Eye protection can prevent direct injury to the eyes. Regular eye exams can also detect changes that the patient may not be aware of. This is important for patients with high **myopia** who may be more prone to detachment.

Resources

ORGANIZATIONS

American Academy of Ophthalmology. 655 Beach Street, P.O. Box 7424, San Francisco, CA 94120-7424. < http://www.eyenet.org >.

American Optometric Association. 243 North Lindbergh Blvd., St. Louis, MO 63141. (314) 991-4100. < http://www.aoanet.org >.

J. Ricker Polsdorfer, MD

Retinal hemorrhage

Definition

Retinal hemorrhage is the abnormal bleeding of the blood vessels in the retina, the membrane in the back of the eye.

Description

The retina is the part of the eye that converts light into nerve signals that are processed by the brain into visual images. The retina is the inside surface of the back of the eye, consisting of millions of densely arranged, light-sensitive cells called rods and cones. Blood flow to the retina is maintained by the retinal vein and artery, and a dense network of small blood vessels (capillaries) supplies the area with circulation. These blood vessels can become damaged by injury and disease and may bleed (hemorrhage) and cause temporary or permanent loss of visual accuracy.

Because the cells of the retina are so dense and sensitive, even small injuries to the blood vessels can translate into vision problems. Diseases that affect the health of the circulatory system, such as diabetes and high blood pressure, also affect the blood vessels of the eye. Damage to the blood vessels in the retina, including hemorrhage, is termed retinopathy.

Causes and symptoms

Retinal hemorrhages can be caused by injuries, usually forceful blows to the head during accidents and falls, as well as by adverse health conditions. In infants, retinal hemorrhage is frequently associated with **child abuse** and has been termed **shaken baby syndrome**. A condition called retinopathy of **prematurity** occurs in prematurely born infants or infants with low birth weights. When children are born prematurely, the blood vessels in the eye may not have had time to fully develop and may become damaged easily, leaking or hemorrhaging. The condition must be determined by an opthalmologist, as the symptoms are not readily observable.

Diabetic retinopathy is a common eye problem associated with diabetes. Diabetes, by stressing the circulatory system, can cause damage, including hemorrhaging, to the small blood vessels of the retina. Non-proliferative retinopathy occurs when the damaged or leaking blood vessels do not spread. Symptoms of this disorder include vision spots, floaters (floating areas of blurred vision), decreased or loss of vision, or loss of fine vision for detailed activities such as reading. Proliferative retinopathy occurs when new blood vessels begin to form in damaged areas of the retina, and may lead to spots, floaters, decreased vision, or sudden loss of vision. Sudden vision loss may occur if one of the newly formed blood vessels ruptures. Due to increased pressure in the area, the retina may detach from the back of the eye, a serious condition and a cause of blindness.

People with high blood pressure (**hypertension**) may develop hypertensive retinopathy, in which blood vessels in the retina become damaged from increased blood pressure. Symptoms are typically not pronounced, but blurred or decreased vision may be caused by the disorder.

Central serous retinopathy is a condition in which the vessels behind the retina leak and cause fluid to collect in small blisters behind the retina. Symptoms include sudden blurry areas in the vision, blind spots, distorted vision areas, and loss of vision. This condition is most common in males between 20 and 50 years of age.

Diagnosis

Diagnosis of retinopathy is performed by an opthalmologist, particularly one who specializes in disorders of the retina (retinal specialist). The opthalmologist may perform an opthalmoscopy, using an instrument called an opthalmoscope to examine the inside of the eye. For a detailed view of the blood vessels of the retina, a fluorescein **angiography** test might be performed, in which a florescent dye is injected into the patient's bloodstream and photographs record the status of the blood vessels in the retina. Vision tests, patient history, and blood tests might also be ordered by the diagnosing physician.

Treatment

Laser surgery by an opthalmologist is a common treatment for retinal hemorrhages, in which a laser beam is used to remove or seal off damaged or bleeding blood vessels in the retina. Some vision loss occurs with this technique. For retinal hemorrhages associated with diabetes and high blood pressure, treating the overall condition is required.

Alternative treatment

Alternative treatment of retinal hemorrhages focuses on providing nutrients to strengthen and heal the injured blood vessels. **Nutritional supplements** include antioxidant **vitamins** A, C, and E; vitamin B-complex including B_6 and B_{12}; the mineral zinc; and essential fatty acids including omega-3 from fish oil and flaxseed oil. Herbal supplements include bilberry, grape seed extract, pine bark extract (pycnogenol), and lutein.

Prognosis

For retinal hemorrhages associated with retinopathy of prematurity, nearly 85 percent of cases heal without treatment. Diabetic retinopathy is the leading cause of blindness for those between 20 and 65 years old in the U.S. Diabetic retinopathy typically takes years to develop in people with diabetes, but occurs in nearly 80 percent of those with diabetes for over 20 years and who are treated with insulin. Regular monitoring and treatments can slow the degeneration of the eye, while advanced cases of the disorder lead to blindness. **Retinopathies** requiring laser treatment have a partial loss of vision due to the surgery. For hypertensive retinopathy, most vision problems go away when high blood pressure is treated and lowered. The majority of cases of central sirous retinopathy disappear after three to four months, and full vision generally returns within six months, although recurrence of the disorder is common.

Prevention

The first step in sound prevention is for people with vision problems, including visual spots, flashes or floaters in the vision, and loss or distortion of visual accuracy, to see an opthalmologist as soon as possible. To prevent complications of retinal hemorrhages in infants, the prevention includes regular prenatal care and monitoring of infants with high risks of the disorder (born prematurely or with weight less than four pounds and six ounces). For diabetic retinopathy, control of blood sugar and blood pressure fluctuations is necessary, as well as frequently scheduled eye exams by an opthalmologist. For retinal hemorrhages associated with hypertension, controlling high blood pressure through diet, **exercise**, and **stress reduction** is recommended. Central sirous retinopathy has been associated with high **stress** levels, so preventative care for this disorder includes stress management practices.

Resources

BOOKS

Abel, Robert. *The Eye Care Revolution: Prevent and Reverse Common Vision Problems.* Kensington, 1999.

Anshel, Jeffrey. *Smart Medicine for Your Eyes.* Avery Publishing, 1999.

Cassel, Gary H. *The Eye Book: A Compete Guide to Eye Disorders and Health.* Johns Hopkins University Press, 1998.

Grossman, Marc. *Natural Eye Care: An Encyclopedia.* McGraw Hill, 1999.

ORGANIZATIONS

American Academy of Ophthalmology. P.O. Box 7424, San Francisco, CA 94120. (415) 561-8500. < http:// www.aao.org >.

National Eye Institute. 2020 Vision Place, Bethesda, MD 20892-3655. (301) 496-5248. < http:// www.nei.nih.gov >.

Douglas Dupler

▮ Retinal vein occlusion

Definition

Retinal vein occlusion refers to the closure of the central retinal vein that drains the retina or to that of one of its branches.

Description

Retinal vein occlusion (RVO) occurs when the central retinal vein, the blood vessel that drains the retina, or one of its branches becomes blocked. RVO may be categorized by the anatomy of the occluded vein and the degree of **ischemia** produced. The two major RVO types are central retinal vein occlusion (CRVO) and branch retinal vein occlusion (BRVO). CRVO has been diagnosed in patients as young as nine months to patients of 90 years. The age of affected individuals is usually low to mid 60s. Approximately 90% of patients are over 50 at the time of diagnosis, with 57% of them being male and 43% being female. BRVO accounts for some 30% of all vein occlusions.

Causes and symptoms

CRVO is a painless loss of vision that can be caused by a swollen optic disk, the small area in the retina where the optic nerve enters the eye, by dilated retinal veins, and by retinal hemorrhages. CRVO is also called venous stasis retinopathy, or hemorrhagic retinopathy.

In BRVO, the superotemporal branch vein is the most often affected vessel. Retinal hemorrhages follows, often occurring at the crossing of two vessels near the optic disk. Initially the hemorrhage may be extensive and underlie the fovea.

The exact cause of RVO is not yet identified, but the following mechanisms been proposed:

- external compression between the central connective strand and the cribriform plate

- venous disease

- blood clot formation

Conditions associated with RVO risk include:

- hypertension
- hyperlipidemia
- diabetes mellitus
- hyperviscosity
- hypercoagulability
- **glaucoma**
- trauma

Diagnosis

A complete physical evaluation is recommended for CRVO and BRVO, including complete blood tests, and glucose tolerance test (for non-diabetics). In the case of a **head injury** when bleeding around the optic nerve is a possibility, an MRI may be performed.

Treatment

Following a patient with RVO is vital. Patients should be seen at least monthly for the first three months to monitor for signs of other complications, such as the abnormal formation of blood vessels (neovascularization) in the iris of the eye or glaucoma.

The treatment for retinal vein occlusion varies for each case and should be given based on the doctor's best recommendation. Although treatments for occlusion itself are limited, surgical treatment of the occlusion provides an option.

Treatments may include anticoagulants with heparin, bishydroxycoumarin, and streptokinase. When the blood is highly viscous, dilution of the blood may be useful. Ideally, an alternate pathway is needed to allow venous drainage. Recent reports published in 1999 suggest that use of a laser to create a retinal choroidal hole may be useful to treat CRVO. Laser therapy depends on the type of occlusion. The management of laser therapy should be controlled by an ophthalmologist.

Alternative treatment

There are no documented alternative treatment methods.

Prognosis

The outlook for people with RVO is fairly good whether it is treated early or not. With no treatment at all, approximately 60% of all patients recover 20/40 vision or better within a year.

Prevention

Retinal vein occlusion is difficult to prevent because the exact cause is still uncertain. Ethnic factors may play a role since in the UK the disease is rare in Asians and West Indians.

KEY TERMS

Anticoagultants—Drugs that act by lowering the capacity of the blood to coagulate, thus facilitating removal of blood clots.

Central retinal vein—Central blood vessel and its branches that drains the retina.

Cribriform plate—The horizontal bone plate perforated with several holes for the passage of olfactory nerve filaments from the nasal cavity.

Fovea—A small area of the retina responsible for acute vision.

Glaucoma—A group of eye diseases characterized by an increase in eyeball pressure.

Hyperlipidemia—A general term for elevated concentrations of any or all of the lipids in the plasma.

Iris—The contractile diaphragm located in the fluid in front of the lens of the eye and is perforated by the eye pupil.

Ischemia—A state of low oxygen in a tissue usually due to organ dysfunction.

Neovascularization—Abnormal or excessive formation of blood vessels as in some retinal disorders.

Occlusion—Momentary complete closure of some area or channel of the body.

Optic disk—The small area in the retina where the optic nerve enters the eye that is not sensitive to light. Also called the blind spot.

Retina—Light sensitive layer of the eye, that consists of four major layers: the outer neural layer, containing nerve cells and blood vessels, the photoreceptor layer, a single layer that contains the light sensing rods and cones, the pigmented retinal epithelium (PRE) and the choroid, consisting of connective tissue and capillaries.

Resources

BOOKS

Spaide, Richard F., MD. *Diseases of the Retina and Vitreous.* New York: W.B. Saunders Co., 1999.

Michael Sherwin Walston
Ronald Watson, PhD

Retinitis pigmentosa

Definition

Retinitis pigmentosa (RP) refers to a group of inherited disorders that slowly lead to blindness due to abnormalities of the photoreceptors (primarily the rods) in the retina.

Description

The retina lines the interior surface of the back of the eye. The retina is made up of several layers. One layer contains two types of photoreceptor cells referred to as the rods and cones. The cones are responsible for sharp, central vision and color vision and are primarily located in a small area of the retina called the fovea. The area surrounding the fovea contains the rods, which are necessary for peripheral vision and night vision (scotopic vision). The number of rods increases in the periphery. The rod and cone photoreceptors convert light into electrical impulses and send the message to the brain via the optic nerve. Another layer of the retina is called the retinal pigmented epithelium (RPE).

In RP, the photoreceptors (primarily the rods) begin to deteriorate and lose their ability to function. Because the rods are primarily affected, it becomes harder to see in dim light, thus causing a loss of night vision. As the condition worsens, peripheral vision disappears, which results in tunnel vision. The ability to see color is eventually lost. In the late stages of the disease, there is only a small area of central vision remaining. Ultimately, this too is lost.

There are many forms of retinitis pigmentosa. Sometimes the disorder is classified by the age of onset or the inheritance pattern. RP can also accompany other conditions. This entry discusses "non-syndromic" RP, the type that is not associated with other organ or tissue dysfunction.

Approximately 100,000 Americans have RP. It is estimated to affect about one in every 4,000 Americans and Europeans. For other parts of the world, there are no published data. Nor is there any known ethnic difference in the occurrence of RP.

Causes and symptoms

Retinitis pigmentosa is an inherited disease that has many different modes of inheritance. It is known to be caused by more than 100 different genetic mutations. RP, with any inheritance pattern, may be either familial (multiple family members affected) or isolated (only one affected person). In the non-sex-linked, or autosomal, form, it can either be a dominant or recessive trait. In the sex-linked form, called x-linked recessive, it is a recessive trait. This x-linked form is more severe than the autosomal forms. Two rare forms of RP are the digenic and mitochondrial forms.

Isolated RP cases represent 10–40% of all cases. Some of these cases may be the result of new gene mutations (changes in the genes). Other isolated cases are those in which the person has a relative with a mutation in the gene, but the relative is not affected by the condition.

Autosomal dominant RP (AdRP) occurs in about 15–25% of affected individuals. At least 12 different genes have been identified as causing AdRP. People with AdRP will usually have an affected parent. The risk for affected siblings or children is 50%.

Autosomal recessive RP (ArRP) occurs in about 5–20% of affected individuals. More than 16 genes have been identified that cause this type of RP. In ArRP, each parent of the affected person is a carrier of an abnormal gene that causes RP. Neither of these carrier parents is affected. There is a two-thirds chance that an unaffected sibling is a carrier of RP. All of the children of an affected person would be a carrier of the ArRP gene.

Five to 15% of individuals with RP have x-linked recessive RP (XLRP). Six different genes have been identified as the cause of this type of RP. Usually in this type of inheritance, males are affected carriers, while females are unaffected carriers or have a milder form of the disease. The mother may be a carrier of the mutation on the X-chromosome. It is also possible that a new mutation can occur for the first time in an affected person. For families with one affected male, there is a mathematical formula called the Baysean analysis that can be applied to the family history. It takes into account the number of unaffected males to determine whether a female is likely to be a carrier or not. If a mother is a carrier, her children have a 50% chance of inheriting the RP gene. For affected males,

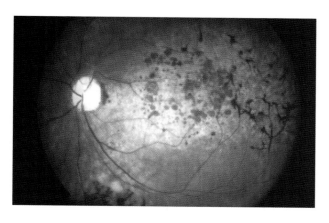

A fundus camera image showing the degeneration of the retina due to retinitis pigmentosa. The pattern of dark spots across the retina corresponds to the extent of loss of vision. *(Custom Medical Stock Photo. Reproduced by permission.)*

all of their daughters will be carriers but none of their sons will be affected.

The digenic form of RP occurs when the affected person has inherited one copy of an altered ROM1 gene from one parent and one copy of an altered peripherin/RDS gene from the other parent. The parents are asymptomatic. Mitochondrial inheritance occurs when the gene mutation is in a mitochondrial gene. People with this type of RP have progressive **hearing loss** and mild myopathy. Both of these types of RP are very rare.

The first symptoms, a loss of night vision followed by a loss of peripheral vision, usually begin in early adolescence or young adulthood. Occasionally, the loss of the ability to see color occurs before the loss of peripheral vision. Another possible symptom is seeing twinkling lights or small flashes of lights.

Diagnosis

When a person complains of a loss of night vision, a doctor will examine the interior of the eye with an ophthalmoscope to determine if there are changes in the retina. For people with advanced RP, the condition is characterized by the presence of clumps of black pigment in the inner retina (intraretinal). However, the appearance of the retina is not enough for an RP diagnosis since there are other disorders that may give the retina a similar appearance. There are also other reasons someone may have night blindness. Consequently, certain electrodiagnostic tests must be performed. An electroretinogram (ERG) determines the functional status of the photoreceptors by exposing the retina to light. The ERG uses a contact lens in

the eye, and the output is measured on a special instrument called an oscilloscope. The functional assessments of visual fields, visual acuity, or color vision may also be performed.

The diagnosis of RP can be established when the following criteria are met:

- rod dysfunction measured by dark adaptation test or ERG,
- progressive loss in photoreceptor function,
- loss of peripheral (side) vision,
- both eyes affected (bilaterality).

Molecular **genetic testing** is available on a research basis. Prenatal diagnosis for this condition has not yet been achieved.

Treatment

There are no medications or surgery to treat RP. However, researchers continue to seek possible treatments. In 2004, scientists injected stem cells to the back of mouse eyes and stopped retinal degeneration. Scientists are also exploring the possibility of retinal transplantation. Some doctors believe **vitamins** A and E will slightly slow the progression of the disease in some people. However, large doses of certain vitamins may be toxic and affected individuals should speak to their doctors before taking supplements.

If a person with RP must be exposed to bright sunlight, some doctors recommend wearing dark sunglasses to reduce the effect on the retina. Affected people should talk to their eye doctors about the correct lenses to wear outdoors.

Because there is no cure for RP, the affected person should be monitored for visual function and counseled about low-vision aids (for example, field-expansion devices). **Genetic counseling** is also appropriate. A three-generation family history with attention to other relatives with possible RP can help to clarify the inheritance pattern. For some people however, the inheritance pattern cannot be discerned.

Prognosis

There is no known cure for RP, which will eventually lead to blindness. The more severe forms will lead to blindness sooner than milder forms.

Resources

PERIODICALS

"Grant Boosts RP Research Into Transplantation." *Ophthalmology TImes* August 1, 2004: 6.

"Stem Cells Delivered Into Back of Eye Hold Promise for People With Retinitis Pigmentosa, Other Retinal Degenerations; Potential Treatment for Untreatable Blindness Shows Promise in Mice." *Ascribe Health News Service* September 15, 2004.

ORGANIZATIONS

American Academy of Ophthalmology. PO Box 7424, San Francisco, CA 94120-7424. (415) 561-8500. < http://www.eyenet.org >.

American Association of the Deaf-Blind. 814 Thayer Ave., Suite 302, Silver Spring, MD 20910. (301) 588-6545.

American Optometric Association. 243 North Lindbergh Blvd., St. Louis, MO 63141. (314) 991-4100. < http://www.aoanet.org >.

Foundation Fighting Blindness. Executive Plaza 1, Suite 800, 11350 McCormick Rd., Hunt Valley, MD 21031. (888) 394-3937. < http://www.blindness.org >.

National Retinitis Pigmentosa Foundation. 11350 McCormick Rd., Executive Plaza 1, Suite 800, Hung Valley, MD 21031-1014. (800) 683-5555. < http://www.blindness.org >.

Prevent Blindness America. 500 East Remington Rd., Schaumburg, IL 60173. (800) 331-2020. < http://www.prevent-blindness.org >.

OTHER

Genetic Alliance. < http://www.geneticalliance.org >.

National Federation of the Blind. < http://www.nfb.org >.

"OMIM—Online Mendelian Inheritance in Man." National Center for Biotechnology Information. < http://www.ncbi.nlm.nih.gov/Omim/searchomim.html >.

Retinitis Pigmentosa International. < http://www.rpinternational.org >.

Amy Vance, MS, CGC
Dorothy Elinor Stonely
Teresa G. Odle

Retinoblastoma

Definition

Retinoblastoma is a malignant tumor of the retina that occurs predominantly in young children.

Description

The eye has three layers, the sclera, the choroid, and the retina. The sclera is the outer protective white coating of the eye. The choroid is the middle layer and contains blood vessels that nourish the eye. The front portion of the choroid is colored and is called the iris. The opening in the iris is called the pupil. The pupil is responsible for allowing light into the eye and usually appears black. When the pupil is exposed to bright light it contracts (closes), and when it is exposed to low light conditions it dilates (opens) so that the appropriate amount of light enters the eye. Light that enters through the pupil hits the lens of the eye. The lens then focuses the light onto the retina, the innermost of the three layers. The job of the retina is to transform the light into information that can be transmitted to the optic nerve, which will transmit this information to the brain. It is through this process that people are able to see the world around them.

Occasionally a tumor, called a retinoblastoma, will develop in the retina of the eye. Usually this tumor forms in young children but it can occasionally occur in adults. Most people with retinoblastoma develop only one tumor (unifocal) in only one eye (unilateral). Some, however, develop multiple tumors (multifocal) in one or both eyes. When retinoblastoma occurs independently in both eyes, it is then called bilateral retinoblastoma.

Occasionally, children with retinoblastoma develop trilateral retinoblastoma. Trilateral retinoblastoma results from the development of an independent **brain tumor** that often forms in a part of the brain called the pineal gland. In order for retinoblastoma to be classified as trilateral retinoblastoma, the tumor must have developed independently and not as the result of the spread of the retinal **cancer**. The prognosis for trilateral retinoblastoma is quite poor.

The retinal tumor which characterizes retinoblastoma is malignant, meaning that it can metastasize (spread) to other parts of the eye and eventually other parts of the body. In most cases, however, retinoblastoma is diagnosed before it spreads past the eye to other parts of the body (intraocular) and the prognosis is quite good. The prognosis is poorer if the cancer has spread beyond the eye (extraocular).

Retinoblastoma can be inherited or can arise spontaneously. Approximately 40% of people with retinoblastoma have an inherited form of the condition and approximately 60% have a sporadic (not inherited) form. Individuals with multiple independent tumors, bilateral retinoblastoma, or trilateral retinoblastoma are more likely to be affected with the inherited form of retinoblastoma.

Approximately 1 in 15,000 to 1 in 30,000 infants in Western countries are born with retinoblastoma, making it the most common childhood **eye cancer**. It is, however, a relatively rare childhood cancer and accounts for approximately 3% of childhood cancers. The American Academy of Ophthalmology estimates that 300–350 cases of retinoblastoma occur in the United States each year.

Retinoblastoma is found mainly in children under the age of five but can occasionally be seen in older children and adults. Retinoblastoma is found in individuals of all ethnic backgrounds and is found equally frequently in males and females. The incidence of bilaterial retinoblastoma in the United States is thought to be slightly higher among black children than among either Caucasian or Asian American children.

Causes and symptoms

Causes

Retinoblastoma is caused by changes in or absence of a gene called RB1. RB1 is located on the long arm of chromosome 13. Cells of the body, with the exception of the egg and sperm cells, contain 23 pairs of chromosomes. All of the cells of the body excluding the egg and the sperm cells are called the somatic cells. The somatic cells contain two of each chromosome 13 and therefore two copies of the RB1 gene. Each egg and sperm cell contains only one copy of chromosome and therefore only one copy of the RB1 gene.

RB1 produces a tumor suppressor protein that normally helps to regulate the cell cycle of cells such as those of the retina. A normal cell of the retina goes through a growth cycle during which it produces new cells. Genes such as tumor suppressor genes tightly regulate this growth cycle.

Cells that lose control of their cell cycle and replicate out of control are called cancer cells. These undergo many cell divisions, often at a quicker rate than normal cells, and do not have a limited lifespan. A group of adjacent cancer cells can form a mass called a tumor. Malignant (cancerous) tumors can spread to other parts of the body. A malignant tumor of the retina (retinoblastoma) can result when just one retinal cell looses control of it cell cycle and replicates out of control.

Normally the tumor suppressor protein produced by RB1 prevents a retinal cell from becoming cancerous. Each RB1 gene produces tumor suppressor protein. Only one functioning RB1 gene in a retinal cell is necessary to prevent the cell from becoming cancerous. If both RB1 genes in a retinal cell become non-functional, then a retinal cell can become cancerous and retinoblastoma can result. An RB1 gene is non-functional when it is changed or missing (deleted) and no longer produces normal tumor suppressor protein.

Approximately 40% of people with retinoblastoma have inherited a non-functional or deleted RB1 gene from either their mother or father. Therefore, they have a changed/deleted RB1 gene in every somatic cell. A person with an inherited missing or non-functional RB1 gene will develop a retinal tumor if the remaining RB1 gene becomes changed or deleted in a retinal cell. The remaining RB1 gene can become non-functional when exposed to environmental triggers such as chemicals and radiation. In most cases, however, the triggers are unknown. Approximately 90% of people who inherit a changed or missing RB1 gene will develop retinoblastoma.

People with an inherited form of retinoblastoma are more likely to have a tumor in both eyes (bilateral) and are more likely to have more than one independent tumor (multifocal) in one or both eyes. The average age of onset for the inherited form of retinoblastoma is one year, which is earlier than the sporadic form of retinoblastoma. Although most people with the inherited form of retinoblastoma develop bilateral tumors, approximately 15% of people with a tumor in only one eye (unilateral) are affected with an inherited form of retinoblastoma.

A person with an inherited missing or non-functional RB1 gene has a 50% chance of passing on this abnormal gene to his or her offspring. The chance that their children will inherit the changed/deleted gene and actually develop retinoblastoma is approximately 45%.

Some people with retinoblastoma have inherited a non-functioning or missing RB1 gene from either their mother or father even though their parents have never developed retinoblastoma. It is possible that one parent has a changed or missing RB1 gene in every somatic cell but has not developed retinoblastoma because their remaining RB1 gene has remained functional. It is also possible that the parent had developed a retinal tumor that was destroyed by the body. In other cases, one parent has two normal RB1 genes in every somatic cell, but some of their egg or sperm cells contain a changed or missing RB1 gene. This is called gonadal mosaicism.

Retinoblastoma can also result when both RB1 genes become spontaneously changed or deleted in a retinal cell but the RB1 genes are normal in all the other cells of the body. Approximately 60% of people with retinoblastoma have this type of disease, called sporadic retinoblastoma. A person with sporadic retinoblastoma does not have a higher chance of having children with the disease. Their relatives do not have a higher risk of developing retinoblastoma themselves or having children who develop retinoblastoma. Sporadic retinoblastoma is usually unifocal and has an average age of onset of approximately two years.

Symptoms

The most common symptom of retinoblastoma is leukocoria. Leukocoria results when the pupil reflects a white color rather than the normal black or red color that is seen on a flash photograph. It is often most obvious in flash photographs; since the pupil is exposed to a lot of light and the duration of the exposure is so short, the pupil does not have time to constrict. Children with retinoblastoma can also have problems seeing and this can cause them to appear cross-eyed (**strabismus**). People with retinoblastoma may also experience red, painful, and irritated eyes, inflamed tissue around the eye, enlarged pupils, and possibly different-colored eyes.

Diagnosis

Children who have symptoms of retinoblastoma are usually first evaluated by their pediatrician. The pediatrician will often perform a red reflex test to diagnose or confirm leukocoria. Prior to this test the doctor inserts medicated eye drops into the child's eyes so that the pupils will remain dilated and not contract when exposed to bright light. The doctor then examines the eyes with an ophthalmoscope, which shines a bright light into the eyes and allows the doctor to check for leukocoria. Leukocoria can also be diagnosed by taking a flash Polaroid photograph of a patient who has been in a dark room for three to five minutes.

If the pediatrician suspects retinoblastoma on the basis of these evaluations, he or she will most likely refer the patient to an ophthalmologist (eye doctor) who has experience with retinoblastoma. The ophthalmologist will examine the eye using an indirect ophthalmoscope. The opthalmoscope shines a bright light into the eye, which helps the doctor to visualize the retina. This evaluation is usually done under general anesthetic, although some very young or older patients may not require it. Prior to the examination, medicated drops are put into the eyes to dilate the pupils, and anesthetic drops may also be used. A metal clip is used to keep the eyes open during the evaluation. During the examination, a cotton swab or a metal instrument with a flattened tip is used to press on the outer lens of the eye so that a better view of the front areas of the retina can be obtained. Sketches or photographs of the tumor as seen through the ophthalmoscope are taken during the procedure.

An ultrasound evaluation is used to confirm the presence of the tumor and to evaluate its size. Computed axial tomography (CT scan) is used to determine whether the tumor has spread outside of the eye and to the brain. Sometimes **magnetic resonance imaging** (MRI) is also used to look at the eyes, eye sockets, and the brain to see if the cancer has spread.

In most cases the cancer has not spread beyond the eye, and other evaluations are unnecessary. If the cancer appears to have spread beyond the eye, then other assessments such as a blood test, spinal tap (lumbar puncture), and/or **bone marrow biopsy** may be recommended. During a spinal tap, a needle is inserted between the vertebrae of the spinal column and a small sample of the fluid surrounding the spinal cord is obtained. In a bone marrow biopsy, a small amount of tissue (bone marrow) is taken from inside the hip or breast bone for examination.

Genetic testing

Establishing whether someone is affected with an inherited or non-inherited form of retinoblastoma can help to ascertain whether other family members such as siblings, cousins, and offspring are at increased risk for developing retinoblastoma. It can also sometimes help guide treatment choices, since patients with an inherited form of retinoblastoma may be at increased risk for developing recurrent tumors or other types of cancers, particularly when treated with radiation. It is helpful for the families of a child diagnosed with retinoblastoma to meet with a genetic specialist such as a genetic counselor and/or geneticist. These specialists can help to ascertain the chances that the retinoblastoma is inherited and facilitate **genetic testing** if desired.

If a patient with unilateral or bilateral retinoblastoma has a relative or relatives with retinoblastoma, it can be assumed that they have an inherited form of retinoblastoma. However, it cannot be assumed that a patient without a family history of the disease has a sporadic form.

Even when there is no family history, most cases of bilateral and trilateral retinoblastoma are inherited, as are most cases of unilateral, multifocal retinoblastoma. However, only 15% of unilateral, unifocal retinoblastoma cases are inherited.

The only way to establish whether someone has an inherited form of retinoblastoma is to see if the retinoblastoma gene is changed or deleted in the blood cells obtained from a blood sample. Approximately 5–8% of individuals with retinoblastoma possess a chromosomal abnormality involving the RB1 gene that can be detected by looking at their chromosomes under the microscope. The chromosomes can be seen by obtaining a blood sample. If this type of chromosomal abnormality is detected in a child, then analysis of the parents' chromosomes should be performed. If one of the parents possesses a chromosomal abnormality, then they are at higher risk for having other offspring with retinoblastoma. Chromosome testing would be recommended for the blood relatives of the parent with the abnormality.

Usually, however, a chromosomal abnormality is not detected in a child with retinoblastoma. In this case, specialized DNA tests that look for small RB1 gene changes need to be performed on the blood cells. DNA testing can be difficult, time consuming, and expensive, since there are many possible RB1 gene changes that can cause the gene to become nonfunctional.

If a sample of tumor is available, then it is recommended that DNA testing be performed on the tumor cells prior to DNA testing of the blood cells. This testing can usually identify the gene changes/deletions in the RB1 genes that caused the tumor to develop. In some cases, RB1 gene changes/deletions are not found in the tumor cells (as of 2001, approximately 20% of RB1 gene changes or deletions are not detectable). In these cases, DNA testing of the blood cells will not be able to ascertain whether someone is affected with an inherited or non-inherited form of retinoblastoma.

If the changes in both RB1 genes are detected in the tumor cell, then these same changes can be looked for in the blood cells. If an RB1 gene is deleted or changed in all of the blood cells tested, the patient can be assumed to have been born with a changed/deleted RB1 gene in all of their cells. This person has a 50% chance of passing the RB1 gene change/deletion on to his or her children. Most of the time, this change/deletion has been inherited from a parent. Occasionally the gene change/deletion occurred spontaneously in the original cell that was formed when the egg and sperm came together at conception (de novo).

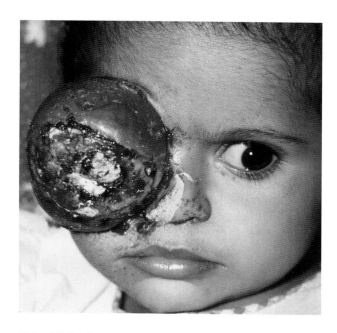

This child's right eye is completely covered with a tumor associated with retinoblastoma. (Custom Medical Stock Photo. Reproduced by permission.)

If an RB1 gene change/deletion is found in all of the blood cells tested, both parents should undergo blood testing to check for the same RB1 gene change/deletion. If the RB1 gene change/deletion is identified in one of the parents, it can be assumed that the retinoblastoma was inherited and that siblings have a 50% chance of inheriting the altered gene. More distant blood relatives of the parent with the identified RB1 gene change/deletion may also be at risk for developing retinoblastoma. Siblings and other relatives could undergo DNA testing to see if they have inherited the RB1 gene change/deletion.

If the RB1 gene change/deletion is not identified in either parent, then the results can be more difficult to interpret. In this case, there is a 90–94% chance that the retinoblastoma was not inherited.

In some cases, a person with retinoblastoma will have an RB1 gene change/deletion detected in some of their blood cells and not others. It can be assumed that this person did not inherit the retinoblastoma from either parent. Siblings and other relatives would therefore not be at increased risk for developing retinoblastoma. Offspring would be at increased risk since some of the egg or sperm cells could have the changed/deleted RB1 gene. The risks to offspring would probably be less than 50%.

In families where there are multiple family members affected with retinoblastoma, blood samples from multiple family members are often analyzed and compared through DNA testing. Ninety-five percent of the time, this type of analysis is able to detect patterns in the DNA that are associated with a changed RB1 gene in that particular family. When a pattern is detected, at-risk relatives can be tested to establish whether they have inherited an RB1 gene change/deletion.

PRENATAL TESTING. If chromosome or DNA testing identifies an RB1 gene/deletion in someone's blood cells, then prenatal testing can be performed on this person's offspring. An **amniocentesis** or **chorionic villus sampling** can be used to obtain fetal cells which can be analyzed for the RB1 gene change/deletion or chromosomal abnormality.

Treatment

A number of different classification (staging) systems are used to establish the severity of retinoblastoma and aid in choosing an appropriate treatment plan. The most widely used staging system is the Reese-Ellsworth system. This system is used to classify intraocular tumors and predict which tumors are favorable enough that sight can be maintained. The Reese-Ellsworth classification system is divided into:

- Group I (very favorable for maintenance of sight): small solitary or multiple tumors, less than 6.4 mm in size (1 inch = 25.4 mm), located at or below the equator of the eye

- Group II (favorable for maintenance of sight): solitary or multiple tumors, 6.4–16 mm in size, located at or behind the equator of the eye

- Group III (possible for maintenance of sight): any tumor located in front of the equator of the eye, or a solitary tumor larger than 16 mm in size and located behind the equator of the eye

- Group IV (unfavorable for maintenance of sight): multiple tumors, some larger than 16 mm in size, or any tumor extending in front of the outer rim of the retina (ora serrata)

- Group V (very unfavorable for maintenance of sight): large tumors involving more than half of the retina, or vitreous seeding, in which small pieces of tumor are broken off and floating around the inside of the eye

When choosing a treatment plan, the first important criteria to ascertain is whether the cancer is localized within the eye (intralocular) or has spread to other parts of the body (extralocular). An intraocular retinoblastoma may only involve the retina or could involve other parts of the eye. An extraocular retinoblastoma could involve only the tissues around the eye or could result from the spread of cancer to the brain or other parts of the body.

It is also important to establish whether the cancer is unilateral (one eye) or bilateral (both eyes), multifocal or unifocal. In order for the tumors to be considered multifocal, they must have arisen independently and not as the result of the spread of cancer cells. It is also important to check for trilateral retinoblastoma.

Treatments

The treatment chosen depends on the size and number of tumors, whether the cancer is unilateral or bilateral, and whether the cancer has spread to other parts of the body. The goal of treatment is to cure the cancer and prevent as much loss of vision as possible. Since the late 1990s, doctors treating patients with retinoblastoma have tended to avoid enucleation and external beam **radiation therapy** whenever possible, in favor of **chemotherapy** to reduce the tumor in addition to focal therapies. Improved methods of chemoreduction have led to increasing success in saving patients' eyes, often with some visual function.

TREATMENT OF INTRAOCULAR TUMORS. Surgical removal of the affected eye (enucleation) is used when the tumor(s) are so large and extensive that preservation of sight is not possible. This surgery is performed under general anesthetic and usually takes less than an hour. Most children who have undergone this surgery can leave the hospital on the same day. A temporary ball is placed in the eye socket after the surgery. Approximately three weeks after the operation, a plastic artificial eye (prosthesis) that looks like the normal eye is inserted into the eye socket.

Radiation therapy is often used for treatment of large tumors when preservation of sight is possible. External beam radiation therapy involves focusing a beam of radiation on the eye. If the tumor has not spread extensively, the radiation beam can be focused on the cancerous retinal cells. If the cancer is extensive, radiation treatment of the entire eye may be necessary. External beam radiation is performed on an outpatient basis and usually occurs over a period of three to four weeks. Some children may need sedatives prior to the treatment. This type of therapy can result in a temporary loss of a patch of hair on the back of the head and a small area of "sun-burned" skin. Long-term side effects of radiation treatment can include **cataracts**, vision problems, bleeding from the retina, and decreased growth of the bones on the side of the head. People with an inherited form of retinoblastoma have an increased risk of developing other cancers as a result of this therapy. Some consideration should therefore be given to alternative treatment therapies for those with an inherited form of retinoblastoma.

Photocoagulation therapy is often used in conjunction with radiation therapy but may be used alone to treat small tumors that are located on the back of the eye. Photocoagulation involves using a laser to destroy the cancer cells. This type of treatment is done under local or **general anesthesia** and is usually not associated with post-procedural **pain**.

Thermotherapy is also often used in conjunction with radiation therapy or drug therapy (chemotherapy). Thermotherapy involves the use of heat to help shrink tumor cells. The heat is either used on the whole eye or localized to the tumor area. It is done under local or general anesthesia and is usually not painful.

Cryotherapy is a treatment often used in conjunction with radiation therapy but can also be used alone on small tumors located on the front part of the retina. Cryotherapy involves the use of intense cold to destroy cancer cells and can result in harmless, temporary swelling of the external eye and eyelids that can last for up to five days. Eye drops or ointment are sometimes provided to reduce the swelling.

Brachytherapy involves the application of radioactive material to the outer surface of the eye at the base of the tumor. It is generally used for tumors of medium size. A patient undergoing this type of procedure is usually hospitalized for three to seven days. During that time, he or she undergoes one surgery to attach the radioactive material and one surgery to remove it. Eye drops are often administered for three to four weeks following the operation to prevent inflammation and infection. The long-term side effects of this treatment can include cataracts and damage to the retina, which can lead to impaired vision.

Intravenous treatment with one or more drugs (chemotherapy) is often used for treatment of both large and small tumors. Chemotherapy is sometimes used to shrink tumors prior to other treatments such as radiation therapy or brachytherapy. Occasionally, it is also used alone to treat very small tumors.

TREATMENT OF INTRAOCULAR AND UNILATERAL RETINOBLASTOMA. Often, by the time that unilateral retinoblastoma is diagnosed, the tumor is so large that useful vision cannot be preserved. In these cases removal of the eye (enucleation) is the treatment of choice. Other therapies are unnecessary if enucleation is used to treat intraocular unilateral retinoblastoma. If the tumor is small enough, other therapies such as external beam radiation therapy, photocoagulation,

cryotherapy, thermotherapy, chemotherapy, and brachytherapy may be considered.

TREATMENT OF INTRAOCULAR AND BILATERAL RETINOBLASTOMA. If vision can be preserved in both eyes, radiation therapy of both eyes may be recommended. Smaller, more localized tumors can sometimes be treated by local therapies such as cryotherapy, photocoagulation therapy, thermotherapy or brachytherapy. Some centers may use chemotherapy in place of radiation therapy when the tumors are too large to be treated by local therapies or are found over the optic nerve of the eye. Many centers are moving away from radiation treatment and toward chemotherapy because it is less likely to induce future tumors. Enucleation is performed on the more severely affected eye if sight cannot be preserved in both.

EXTRAOCULAR RETINOBLASTOMA. There is no proven effective therapy for the treatment of extraocular retinoblastomas. Commonly, radiation treatment of the eyes and chemotherapy is provided.

Alternative treatment

There are no alternative or complementary therapies specific to the treatment of retinoblastoma. Since most people diagnosed with retinoblastoma are small children, most drug-based alternative therapies designed to treat general cancer would not be recommended. Many specialists would, however, **stress** the importance of establishing a well-balanced diet, including certain fruits, vegetables, and vitamin supplements, to ensure that the body is strengthened in its fight against cancer. Some advocate the use of visualization strategies, in which patients would visualize the immune cells of their body attacking and destroying the cancer cells.

Prognosis

Individuals with intraocular retinoblastoma who do not have trilateral retinoblastoma usually have a good survival rate with a 90% chance of disease-free survival for five years. Those with extraocular retinoblastoma have less than a 10% chance of disease-free survival for the same amount of time. Trilateral retinoblastoma generally has a very poor prognosis. Patients with trilateral retinoblastoma who receive treatment have an average survival rate of approximately eight months, while those who remain untreated have an average survival rate of approximately one month. Patients with trilateral retinoblastoma who are asymptomatic at the time of diagnosis may have a better prognosis then those who experience symptoms.

Patients with an inherited form of unilateral retinoblastoma have a 70% chance of developing retinoblastoma in the other eye. Retinoblastoma reoccurs in the other eye in approximately 5% of people with a non-inherited form of retinoblastoma, so it is advisable for even these patients to be closely monitored. People with an inherited form of retinoblastoma who have not undergone radiation treatment have approximately a 26% chance of developing cancer in another part of the body within 50 years of the initial diagnosis. Those with an inherited form who have undergone radiation treatment have a 58% chance of developing a secondary cancer by 50 years after the initial diagnosis. Most of the secondary cancers are skin cancers, bone tumors (osteosarcomas), and soft-tissue **sarcomas**. Soft-tissue sarcomas are malignant tumors of the muscle, nerves, joints, blood vessels, deep skin tissues, or fat. The prognosis for retinoblastoma patients who develop secondary cancers, however, is very poor as of the early 2000s.

Survivors of retinoblastoma are likely to have visual field defects after their cancer treatment is completed, most commonly scotomas, which are areas of lost or depressed vision within an area of normal vision. The size and type of these visual defects are determined by the size and type of the original tumor and the form of therapy used to treat it.

Prevention

Although retinoblastoma cannot be prevented, appropriate screening and surveillance should be applied to all at-risk individuals to ensure that the tumor(s) are diagnosed at an early stage. The earlier the diagnosis, the more likely that an eye can be salvaged and vision maintained.

Screening of people diagnosed with retinoblastoma

Children who have been diagnosed with retinoblastoma should receive periodic dilated retinal examinations until the age of five. Young children will need to undergo these evaluations under anesthetic. After five years of age, periodic eye examinations are recommended. It may be advisable for patients with bilateral retinoblastoma or an inherited form of retinoblastoma to undergo periodic screening for the brain tumors found in trilateral retinoblastoma. There are no specific screening protocols designed to detect non-ocular tumors. All lumps and complaints of bone pain, however, should be thoroughly evaluated.

Screening of relatives

When a child is diagnosed with retinoblastoma, it is recommended that parents and siblings receive a dilated retinal examination by an ophthalmologist who is experienced in the diagnosis and treatment of the disease. It is also recommended that siblings continue to undergo periodic retinal examinations under anesthetic until they are three years of age. From three to seven years of age, periodic eye examinations are recommended. The retinal examinations can be avoided if DNA testing indicates that the patient has a non-inherited form of retinoblastoma or if the sibling has not inherited the RB1 gene change/deletion. Any relatives who are found through DNA testing to have inherited an RB1 gene change/deletion should undergo the same surveillance procedures as siblings.

The children of someone diagnosed with retinoblastoma should also undergo periodic retinal examinations under anesthetic. Retinal surveillance should be performed unless DNA testing proves that their child does not possess the RB1 gene change/deletion. If desired, prenatal detection of tumors using ultrasound may also be performed. During the ultrasound procedure, a hand-held instrument is placed on the maternal abdomen or inserted vaginally. The ultrasound produces sound waves that are reflected back from the body structures of the fetus, producing a picture that can be seen on a video screen. If a tumor is detected through this evaluation, the affected baby may be delivered a couple of weeks earlier. This can allow for earlier intervention and treatment.

Resources

BOOKS

Beers, Mark H., MD, and Robert Berkow, MD., editors. "Retinoblastoma." In *The Merck Manual of Diagnosis and Therapy*. Whitehouse Station, NJ: Merck Research Laboratories, 2004.

PERIODICALS

Abramson, D. H., M. R. Melson, and C. Servodidio. "Visual Fields in Retinoblastoma Survivors." *Archives of Ophthalmology* 122 (September 2004): 1324–1330.

Aerts, I., H. Pacquement, F. Doz, et al. "Outcome of Second Malignancies after Retinoblastoma: A Retrospective Analysis of 25 Patients Treated at the Institut Curie." *European Journal of Cancer* 40 (July 2004): 1522–1529.

Lohmann, D. R., and B. L. Gallie. "Retinoblastoma: Revisiting the Model Prototype of Inherited Cancer." *American Journal of Medical Genetics, Part*

Amniocentesis—Prenatal testing performed at 16 to 20 weeks of pregnancy that involves inserting a needle through the abdomen of a pregnant mother and obtaining a small sample of fluid from the amniotic sack, which contains the fetus. Often is used to obtain a sample of the fetus' cells for biochemical or DNA testing.

Benign tumor—An abnormal proliferation of cells that does not spread to other parts of the body.

Bilateral—Affecting both eyes.

Brachytherapy—Cancer treatment that involves the application of radioactive material to the site of the tumor.

Cryotherapy—Cancer treatment in which the tumor is destroyed by exposure to intense cold.

Chromosome—A microscopic structure found within each cell of the body, made of a complex of proteins and DNA.

Chorionic villus sampling (CVS)—Prenatal testing performed at 10 to 12 weeks of pregnancy, which involves inserting a catheter through the vagina of a pregnant mother or inserting a needle through the abdomen of the mother and obtaining a sample of placenta. Often is used to obtain a sample of the fetus' cells for biochemical or DNA testing.

DNA (deoxyribonucleic acid)—The hereditary material that makes up genes; influences the development and functioning of the body.

DNA testing—Testing for a change or changes in a gene or genes.

Enucleation—Surgical removal of the eye.

Equator—Imaginary line encircling the eyeball and dividing the eye into a front and back half.

Extraocular retinoblastoma—Cancer that has spread from the eye to other parts of the body.

Gene—A building block of inheritance, made up of a compound called DNA (deoxyribonucleic acid) and containing the instructions for the production of a particular protein. Each gene is found in a specific location on a chromosome.

Intraocular retinoblastoma—Cancer that is limited to the eye and has not spread to other parts of the body.

Malignant tumor—An abnormal proliferation of cells that can spread to other sites.

Multifocal—More than one tumor present.

Ophthalmologist—Physician specializing in the diseases of the eye.

Optic nerve—The part of the eye which contains nerve fibers that transmit signals from the eye to the brain.

Oncologist—A physician specializing in the diagnosis and treatment of cancer

Photocoagulation—Cancer treatment in which the tumor is destroyed by an intense beam of laser light.

Prenatal testing—Testing for a disease such as a genetic condition in an unborn baby.

Protein—A substance produced by a gene that is involved in creating the traits of the human body, such as hair and eye color, or is involved in controlling the basic functions of the human body, such as control of the cell cycle.

Retina—The light-sensitive layer of the eye that receives images and sends them to the brain.

Scotoma—An area of lost or depressed vision within the visual field surrounded by an area of normal vision. Survivors of retinoblastoma frequently develop scotomas.

Somatic cells—All the cells of the body with the exception of the egg and sperm cells.

Tumor—A growth of tissue resulting from the uncontrolled proliferation of cells.

Tumor-suppressor gene—Gene involved in controlling normal cell growth and preventing cancer.

Unifocal—Only one tumor present in one eye.

Unilateral—Affecting only one eye.

Vitreous—The transparent gel that fills the back part of the eye.

Vitreous seeding—When small pieces of tumor have broken off and are floating around the vitreous.

C: Seminars in Medical Genetics 129 (August 15, 2004): 23–28.

Provenzale, J. M., S. Gururangan, and G. Klintworth. "Trilateral Retinoblastoma: Clinical and Radiologic Progression." AJR: American Journal of Roentgenology 183 (August 2004): 505–511.

Shields, C. L., A. Mashayeki, J. Cater, et al. "Chemoreduction for Retinoblastoma. Analysis of Tumor Control and Risks for Recurrence in 457 Tumors." American Journal of Ophthalmology 138 (September 2004): 329–337.

Shields, C. L., and J. A. Shields. "Diagnosis and Management of Retinoblastoma." Cancer Control 11 (September-October 2004): 317–327.

ORGANIZATIONS

American Academy of Ophthalmology (AAO). P. O. Box 7424, San Francisco, CA 94120-7424. (415) 561-8500. Fax: (415) 561-8533. < http://www.aao.org >.

Institute for Families with Blind Children. PO Box 54700, Mail Stop 111, Los Angeles, CA 90054-0700. (213) 669-4649.

National Retinoblastoma Parents Group. PO Box 317, Watertown, MA 02471. (800) 562-6265. Fax: (617) 972-7444. napvi@perkins.pvt.k12.ma.us.

Retinoblastoma International. 4650 Sunset Blvd., Mail Stop #88, Los Angeles, CA 90027. (323) 669-2299. info@retinoblastoma.net. < http://www.retinoblastoma.net/rbi/index_rbi.htm >.

Retinoblastoma Society. Saint Bartholomew's Hospital, London, UK EC1A 7BE. Phone: 020 7600 3309 Fax: 020 7600 8579. < http://ds.dial.pipex.com/rbinfo >.

OTHER

Abramson, David, and Camille Servodidio. "A Parent's Guide to Understanding Retinoblastoma." June 20, 2001. < http://www.retinoblastoma.com/guide/guide.html >.

Kid's Eye Cancer. June 20, 2001. < http://www.kidseyecancer.org >.

Lohmann, Dietmar, N. Bornfeld, B. Horsthemke, and E. Passarge. "Retinoblastoma." Gene Clinics. July 17, 2000. [cited June 20, 2001]. < http://www.geneclinics.org/profiles/retinoblastoma >.

McCusick, Victor. "Retinoblastoma; RB1." Online Mendelian Inheritance in Man. February 14, 2001. [cited June 20, 2001. < http://www.ncbi.nlm.nih.gov/Omim >.

"Retinoblastoma" CancerNet. < http://cancernet.nci.nih.gov/Cancer_Types/Retinoblastoma.shtml >.

Solutions by Sequence. June 20, 2001. < http://www.solutionsbysequence.com >.

Lisa Andres, MS, CGC
Rebecca J. Frey, PhD

Retinol deficiency *see* **Vitamin A deficiency**

Retinopathies

Definition

Retinopathy is a noninflammatory disease of the retina. There are many causes and types of retinopathy.

Description

The retina is the thin membrane that lines the back of the eye and contains light-sensitive cells (photoreceptors). Light enters the eye and is focused onto the retina. The photoreceptors send a message to the brain via the optic nerve. The brain then "interprets" the electrical message sent to it, resulting in vision. The macula is a specific area of the retina responsible for central vision. The fovea is about 1.5 mm in size and located in the macula. The fovea is responsible for sharp vision. When looking at something, the fovea should be directed at the object.

Retinopathy, or damage to the retina, has various causes. A hardening or thickening of the retinal arteries is called arteriosclerotic retinopathy. High blood pressure in the arteries of the body can damage the retinal arteries and is called hypertensive retinopathy. The spreading of a **syphilis** infection to the retinal blood vessels cases syphilitic retinopathy, and diabetes damages the retinal vessels resulting in a condition called diabetic retinopathy. Sickle cell anemia also affects the blood vessels in the eyes. Exposure to the sun (or looking at the sun during an eclipse) can cause damage (solar retinopathy), as well as certain drugs (for example, chloroquine, thioridazine, and large doses of tamoxifen). The arteries and veins can become blocked, thus resulting in a retinal artery or vein occlusion. These are just some of the causes of the various retinopathies.

Retinopathies are divided into two broad categories, *simple* or *nonproliferative* retinopathies and *proliferative* retinopathies. The simple retinopathies include the defects identified by bulging of the vessel walls, by bleeding into the eye, by small clumps of dead retinal cells called cotton wool exudates, and by closed vessels. This form of retinopathy is considered mild. The proliferative, or severe, forms of retinopathies include the defects identified by newly grown blood vessels, by scar tissue formed within the eye, by closed-off blood vessels that are badly damaged, and by the retina breaking away from the mesh of blood vessels that nourish it (**retinal detachment**).

While each disease has its own specific effect on the retina, a general scenario for many of the retinopathies is as follows (note: not all retinopathies necessarily affect the blood vessels). Blood flow to the retina is disrupted, either by blockage or breakdown of the various vessels. This can lead to bleeding (hemorrhage) and fluids, cells, and proteins leaking into the area (exudates). There can be a lack of oxygen to surrounding tissues (hypoxia) or decreased blood flow (**ischemia**). Chemicals produced by the body then can cause new blood vessels to grow (neovascularization), however, these new vessels generally leak and cause more problems. Neovascularization even can grow on the colored part of the eye (iris). The retina can swell and vision will be affected.

Diabetic retinopathy is the leading cause of blindness in people ages 20 to 74. Diabetic retinopathy will occur in 90% of persons with type 1 diabetes (insulin-dependent, or insulin requiring) and 65% of persons with type II diabetes (non-insulin-dependent, or not requiring insulin) by about 10 years after the beginning of diabetes. In the United States, new cases of blindness most often are caused by diabetic retinopathy. Among these new cases of blindness, 12% are people between the ages of 20 to 44 years, and 19% are people between the ages of 45 to 64 years.

Causes and symptoms

There are many causes of retinopathy. Some of the more common ones are listed below.

Diabetic retinopathy

Diabetes is a complex disorder characterized by an inability of the body to properly regulate the levels of sugar and insulin (a hormone made by the pancreas) in the blood. As diabetes progresses, the blood vessels that feed the retina become damaged in different ways. The damaged vessels can have bulges in their walls (aneurysms); they can leak blood into the surrounding jelly-like material (vitreous) that fills the inside of the eyeball; they can become completely closed; or new vessels can begin to grow where there would not normally be blood vessels. However, although these new blood vessels are growing in the eye, they cannot nourish the retina and they bleed easily, releasing blood into the inner region of the eyeball, which can cause dark spots and cloudy vision.

Diabetic retinopathy begins prior to any outward signs of disease being noticed. Once symptoms are noticed, they include poorer than normal vision, fluctuating or distorted vision, cloudy vision, dark spots, episodes of temporary blindness, or permanent blindness.

Hypertensive retinopathy

High blood pressure can affect the vessels in the eyes. Some blood vessels can narrow. The blood vessels can thicken and harden (arteriosclerosis). There will be flame-shaped hemorrhages and macular swelling (**edema**). This edema may cause distorted or decreased vision.

Sickle cell retinopathy

Sickle cell anemia occurs mostly in blacks and is a hereditary disease that affects the red blood cells. The

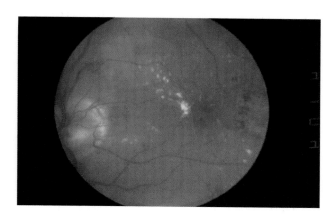

A slit lamp view of a human eye with diabetic retinopathy. *(Custom Medical Stock Photo. Reproduced by permission.)*

sickle-shaped blood cell reduces blood flow. People will not have visual symptoms early in the disease. However, patients need to be followed closely in case neovascularization occurs.

Retinal vein and artery occlusion

Retinal vein occlusion generally occurs in the elderly. There is usually a history of other systemic disease, such as diabetes or high blood pressure. The central retinal vein (CRV), or the retinal veins branching off of the CRV, can become compressed, thus stopping the drainage of blood from the retina. This may occur if the central retinal artery hardens.

Symptoms of retinal vein occlusion include a sudden, painless loss of vision or field of vision in one eye. There may be a sudden onset of floating spots (floaters) or flashing lights. Vision may be unchanged or decrease dramatically.

Retinal artery occlusion generally is the result of an **embolism** that dislodges from somewhere else in the body and travels to the eye. Transient loss of vision may precede an occlusion. Symptoms of a central retinal artery or branch occlusion include a sudden, painless loss of vision or decrease in visual field. Ten percent of the cases of a retinal artery occlusion occur because of giant cell arteritis (a chronic vascular disease).

Solar retinopathy

Looking directly at the sun or watching an eclipse can cause damage. There may be a loss of the central visual field or decreased vision. The symptoms can occur hours to days after the incident.

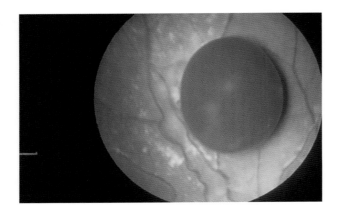

A close-up view of a human eye following retinal hemorrhage.
(Custom Medical Stock Photo. Reproduced by permission.)

Drug-related retinopathies

Certain medications can affect different areas of the retina. Doses of 20–40 mg a day of tamoxifen usually do not cause a problem, but much higher doses may cause irreversible damage.

Patients taking chloroquine for lupus, **rheumatoid arthritis**, or other disorders may notice a decrease in vision. If so, discontinuing medication will stop, but not reverse, any damage. However, patients should never discontinue medication without the advice of their physician.

Patients taking thioridazine may notice a decrease in vision or color vision.

These drug-related retinopathies generally only affect patients taking large doses. However, patients need to be aware if any medication they are taking will affect the eyes. Patients should inform their doctors of any visual effects.

Diagnosis

The damaged retinal blood vessels and other retinal changes are visible to an eye doctor when an examination of the retina (fundus exam) is done. This can be done using a hand-held instrument called an ophthalmoscope or another instrument called a binocular indirect ophthalmoscope. This allows the doctor to see the back of the eye. Certain retinopathies have classic signs (for example, vascular "sea fans" in sickle cell, dot and blot hemorrhages in diabetes, flame-shaped hemorrhages in high blood pressure). Patients then may be referred for other tests to confirm the underlying cause of the retinopathy. These tests include blood tests and measurement of blood pressure.

Fluorescein **angiography**, where a dye is injected into the patient and the back of the eyes are viewed and photographed, helps to locate leaky vessels. Sometimes patients may become nauseated from the dye.

A newer diagnostic method called digital retinal photography can be used to screen those at high risk for retinopathies, in particular, diabetics. Some researchers say the technique could lead to more cost-effective screening for people with diabetic retinopathy.

Treatment

Retinal specialists are ophthalmologists who specialize in retinal disorders. Retinopathy is a disorder of the retina that can result from different underlying systemic causes, so general physicians should be consulted as well. For drug-related retinopathies, the treatment generally is discontinuation of the drug (only under the care of a physician).

Surgery with lasers can help to prevent blindness or lessen any losses in vision. The high-energy light from a laser is aimed at the weakened blood vessels in the eye, destroying them. **Scars** will remain where the laser treatment was performed. For that reason, laser treatment cannot be performed everywhere. For example, laser photocoagulation at the fovea would destroy the area for sharp vision. Panretinal photocoagulation may be performed. This is a larger area of treatment in the periphery of the retina; hopefully it will decrease neovascularization. Prompt treatment of proliferative retinopathy may reduce the risk of severe vision loss by 50%.

Patients with retinal artery occlusion should be referred to a cardiologist. Patients with retinal vein occlusion need to be referred to a physician, as they may have an underlying systemic disorder, such as high blood pressure.

Prognosis

Nonproliferative retinopathy has a better prognosis than proliferative retinopathy. Prognosis depends on the extent of the retinopathy, the cause, and promptness of treatment.

Prevention

Complete eye examinations done regularly can help detect early signs of retinopathy. Patients on certain medications should have more frequent eye exams. They also should have a baseline eye exam

KEY TERMS

Exudate—Cells, protein, fluid, or other material that passes through blood vessel walls to accumulate in the surrounding tissue.

Neovascularization—New blood vessel formation–usually leaky vessels.

Nonproliferative retinopathy—Retinopathy without the growth of new blood vessels.

Proliferative retinopathy—Retinopathy with the growth of new blood vessels (neovascularization).

when starting the drug. People with diabetes must take extra care to have thorough, periodic eye exams, especially if early signs of **visual impairment** are noticed. A 2003 report recommended re-screening eye exams every two years for diabetics whose blood sugar had remained in control, and more frequent exams if visual symptoms appear. Anyone experiencing a sudden loss of vision, decrease in vision or visual field, flashes of light, or floating spots should contact their eye doctor right away.

Proper medical treatment for any of the systemic diseases known to cause retinal damage will help prevent retinopathy. For diabetics, maintaining proper blood sugar and blood pressure levels is important as well; however, some form of retinopathy usually will occur in diabetics, given enough time. A proper diet, particularly for those persons with diabetes, and stopping **smoking** also will help delay retinopathy.

Frequent, thorough eye exams and control of systemic disorders are the best prevention.

Resources

PERIODICALS

Selby, Joe, Lynn Ackerson, and Talmadge Cooper. "Three-year Incidence of Treatable Diabetic Eye Disease After Negative Funduscopic Examination." *Diabetes* June 2003: A60.

Usher, David, et al. "Automated Detection of Diabetic Retinopathy in Digital Retinal Images." *Diabetes* June 2003: A204.

ORGANIZATIONS

American Academy of Ophthalmology. 655 Beach Street, P.O. Box 7424, San Francisco, CA 94120-7424. < http://www.eyenet.org >.

American Diabetes Association. 1701 North Beauregard Street, Alexandria, VA 22311. (800) 342-2383. < http://www.diabetes.org >.

American Optometric Association. 243 North Lindbergh Blvd., St. Louis, MO 63141. (314) 991-4100. < http://www.aoanet.org >.

Foundation Fighting Blindness. Executive Plaza I, Suite 800, 11350 McCormick Road, Hunt Valley, MD 21031-1014. (888) 394-3937. < http://www.blindness.org >.

Prevent Blindness America. 500 East Remington Road, Schaumburg, IL 60173. (800) 331-2020. < http://www.preventblindness.org >.

Faye A. Fishman
Teresa G. Odle

Retrocaval ureter *see* **Congenital ureter anomalies**

Retrograde cystography

Definition

A retrograde cystogram provides x-ray visualization of the bladder with injection of sterile dye.

Purpose

A retrograde cystogram is performed to evaluate the structure of the bladder and identify bladder disorders, such as tumors, or recurrent urinary tract infections. The presence of urine reflux (backward flow) into the ureters may also be visualized with this x-ray study.

Precautions

The doctor should be made aware of any previous history of reactions to shellfish, iodine, or any iodine-containing foods or dyes. Allergic reactions during previous dye studies is not necessarily a contraindication, as dye is not infused into the bloodstream for this study. Other conditions to be considered by the physician prior to proceeding with the test include active urinary tract infection, **pregnancy**, recent bladder surgery, or presence of obstruction that interferes with passage of a urinary catheter.

Description

After administration of anesthesia, the doctor will insert a thin, tubelike instrument called a catheter through the patient's urethra and into the bladder. The contrast medium is then injected through the catheter into the bladder. X-ray pictures are taken at various stages of filling, from various angles, to visualize the bladder. Additional films are taken after

KEY TERMS

Bladder—A balloon-like organ located in the lower abdomen that stores urine.

Catheter—A thin tube used to inject or withdraw fluids from the body.

Stones—Also known as calculi, stones result from an excessive build-up of mineral crystals in the kidney. Symptoms of stones include intense pain in the lower back or abdomen, urinary tract infection, fever, burning sensation on urination, and/or blood in the urine.

Ureter—Tube that carries urine from the kidney to the bladder.

Urethra—Tube that empties urine from the bladder to outside the body.

drainage of the dye. The procedure takes approximately one to one and one-half hours and the patient may be asked to wait while films are developed.

Alternately, instead of a contrast dye and x-ray pictures, the test can be done with a radioactive tracer and a different camera. This is known as a "radionuclide" retrograde cystogram.

Preparation

The patient will be required to sign a consent form after the risks and benefits of the procedure have been explained. **Laxatives** or **enemas** may be necessary before the procedure, as the bowel must be relatively empty of stool and gas to provide visualization of the urinary tract. Immediately before the procedure, the patient should remove all clothing and jewelry, and put on a surgical gown.

Aftercare

Sometimes, pulse, blood pressure, breathing status, and temperature are checked at regular intervals after the procedure, until they are stable. The patient may have some burning on urination for a few hours after the test, due to the irritation of the urethra from the catheter. The discomfort can be reduced by liberal fluid intake, in order to dilute the urine. The appearance and amount of urine output should be noted, and the doctor should be notified if blood appears in the urine after three urinations. Also, patients should report any signs of urinary infection, including chills, **fever**, rapid pulse, and rapid breathing rate.

Normal results

A normal result would reveal no anatomical or functional abnormalities.

Abnormal results

Abnormal results may indicate:

- stones
- blood clots
- tumors
- reflex (urine passing backward from the bladder into the ureters)

Resources

ORGANIZATIONS

American Kidney Fund (AKF). Suite 1010, 6110 Executive Boulevard, Rockville, MD 20852. (800) 638-8299. < http://216.248.130.102/Default.htm >.

National Kidney Foundation. 30 East 33rd St., New York, NY 10016. (800) 622-9010. < http://www.kidney.org >.

Kathleen D. Wright, RN

Retrograde ureteropyelography

Definition

A retrograde ureteropyelogram provides x-ray visualization of the bladder, ureters, and the kidney (renal) pelvis by injection of sterile dye into the renal collecting system.

Purpose

A retrograde ureteropyelogram is performed to determine the exact location of a ureteral obstruction when it cannot be visualized on an intravenous pyelogram (a dye is injected and an x ray taken of the kidneys and the tubes that carry urine to the bladder). This may occur due to poor renal function and inadequate excretion of the contrast medium (dye).

Precautions

The doctor should be made aware of any previous history of reactions to shellfish, iodine, or any iodine-containing foods or dyes. Allergic reactions during previous dye studies is not necessarily a contraindication, as dye is not infused into the bloodstream for this study. Other conditions to be considered by the physician prior to proceeding with the test include **pregnancy** and active urinary tract infection.

Description

After administration of anesthesia, the doctor will insert a thin, tubelike instrument (catheter) through the patient's urethra and into the bladder. A catheter is then placed into the affected ureter to instill the contrast medium. X-ray pictures are taken to visualize the ureter. If complete obstruction is found, a ureteral catheter may be left in place and secured to an indwelling urethral catheter to facilitate drainage of urine. The procedure takes approximately one hour.

Preparation

Laxatives or **enemas** may be necessary before the procedure, as the bowel must be relatively empty to provide visualization of the urinary tract. When **general anesthesia** is used for insertion of the ureteral catheter, there should be no eating and drinking after midnight prior to the procedure.

Aftercare

Even if no catheters are left in place after the procedure, the patient may have some burning on urination for a few hours after the procedure due to the irritation of the urethra. The discomfort can be reduced by liberal fluid intake, in order to dilute the urine. The appearance and amount of urine output should be noted for 24 hours after the procedure. If a stone was found, all urine should be strained to allow chemical analysis of any stones passed spontaneously. This will allow the doctor to provide advise on measures to prevent recurrent stone formation. **Antibiotics** are usually given after the procedure to prevent urinary tract infection.

Normal results

A normal result would reveal no anatomical or functional abnormalities.

Abnormal results

Abnormal results may indicate:

- congenital abnormalities
- fistulas or false passages
- renal stones
- strictures
- tumors

Resources

ORGANIZATIONS

American Kidney Fund (AKF). Suite 1010, 6110 Executive Boulevard, Rockville, MD 20852. (800) 638-8299. < http://216.248.130.102/Default.htm >.

National Kidney Foundation. 30 East 33rd St., New York, NY 10016. (800) 622-9010. < http://www.kidney.org >.

Kathleen D. Wright, RN

Retrograde urethrography

Definition

Retrograde urethrography involves the use of x-ray pictures to provide visualization of structural problems or injuries to the urethra.

Purpose

Retrograde urethrography is used, in combination with a doctor's observation and other tests, to establish a diagnosis for individuals, almost exclusively men, who may have structural problems of the urethra.

Precautions

The doctor should be made aware of any previous history of reactions to shellfish, iodine, or any iodine-containing foods or dyes. An earlier allergic reaction during a dye study is not necessarily something that makes the test inadvisable (a contraindication) as no dye is injected into the bloodstream for this study. Other conditions that should be considered by the physician before the test is done include **pregnancy**, recent urethral surgery, or severe inflammation of the urethra, bladder, or prostate.

Description

The urethra is first visually examined by the doctor, and the opening is cleansed with an antiseptic solution. A flexible rubber or plastic catheter is then inserted into the urethra, and dye is injected into the catheter. A clamp is applied to hold the dye in place while x-ray pictures are taken of the urethral structure. The clamp and catheter are then removed. The

KEY TERMS

Bladder—The balloonlike organ in the lower abdomen that holds urine.

Catheter—Tube used to inject into or withdraw fluids from the bladder.

Renal—Relating to the kidneys, from the Latin word for kidneys, *renes.*

Urethra—Tube that carries the urine from the bladder out of the body.

Visualization—The process of making an internal organ visible. A radiopaque subtance is introduced into the body, then an x-ray picture of the desired organ is taken.

procedure takes approximately 15 minutes. However, the patient may be asked to wait while films are developed, which also permits the patient to be observed for any immediate side effects from the dye. The test may be performed in a hospital, doctor's office, outpatient center, or freestanding surgical facility. The time involved for reporting of test results to the doctor may vary from a few minutes to a few days.

Preparation

The patient will be asked to sign a consent form after the risks and benefits of the procedure have been explained. No diet or activity changes are necessary in preparation for the procedure. The patient will be asked to remove all clothing and put on a surgical gown before the test begins.

Normal results

The presence of no anatomical or functional abnormalities is considered a normal result.

Abnormal results

Abnormal findings may indicate:

- congenital abormalities
- fistulas or false passages
- lacerations
- strictures
- valves, known as "posterior urethral valves"
- tumors

Resources

ORGANIZATIONS

American Kidney Fund (AKF). Suite 1010, 6110 Executive Boulevard, Rockville, MD 20852. (800) 638-8299. < http://216.248.130.102/Default.htm >.

National Kidney Foundation. 30 East 33rd St., New York, NY 10016. (800) 622-9010. < http://www.kidney.org >.

Kathleen D. Wright, RN

Retrograde urography *see* **Retrograde urethrography**

Retropharyngeal abscess *see* **Abscess**

Reye's syndrome

Definition

Reye's syndrome is a disorder principally affecting the liver and brain, marked by rapid development of life-threatening neurological symptoms.

Description

Reye's syndrome is an emergency illness chiefly affecting children and teenagers. It almost always follows a viral illness such as a cold, the flu, or chicken pox. Reye's syndrome may affect all the organs of the body, but most seriously affects the brain and liver. Rapid development of severe neurological symptoms, including lethargy, confusion, seizures, and **coma**, make Reye's syndrome a life-threatening emergency.

Reye's syndrome is a rare illness, even rarer now than when first described in the early 1970s. The incidence of the disorder peaked in 1980, with 555 cases reported. The number of cases declined rapidly thereafter due to decreased use of **aspirin** compounds for childhood **fever**, an important risk factor for Reye's syndrome development. Because of its rarity, it is often misdiagnosed as **encephalitis**, **meningitis**, diabetes, or **poisoning**, and the true incidence may be higher than the number of reported cases indicates.

Causes and symptoms

Reye's syndrome causes fatty accumulation in the organs of the body, especially the liver. In the brain, it causes fluid accumulation (**edema**), which leads to a rise in intracranial pressure. This pressure squeezes blood vessels, preventing blood from entering the

3228

brain. Untreated, this pressure increase leads to brain damage and **death**.

Although the cause remains unknown, Reye's syndrome appears to be linked to an abnormality in the energy-converting structures (mitochondria) within the body's cells.

Reye's syndrome usually occurs after a viral, fever-causing illness, most often an upper respiratory tract infection. Its cause is unknown. It is most often associated with use of aspirin during the fever, and for this reason aspirin and aspirin-containing products are not recommended for people under the age of 19 during fever. Reye's syndrome may occur without aspirin use, and in adults, although very rarely.

After the beginning of recovery from the viral illness, the affected person suddenly becomes worse, with the development of persistent **vomiting**. This may be followed rapidly by quietness, lethargy, agitation or combativeness, seizures, and coma. In infants, **diarrhea** may be more common than vomiting. Fever is usually absent at this point.

Diagnosis

Reye's syndrome may be suspected in a child who begins vomiting three to six days after a viral illness, followed by an alteration in consciousness. Diagnosis involves blood tests to determine the levels of certain liver enzymes, which are highly elevated in Reye's syndrome. Other blood changes may occur as well, including an increase in the level of ammonia and amino acids, a drop in blood sugar, and an increase in clotting time. A **liver biopsy** may also be done after clotting abnormalities are corrected with vitamin K or blood products. A lumbar puncture (spinal tap) may be needed to rule out other possible causes, including meningitis or encephalitis.

Treatment

Reye's syndrome is a life-threatening emergency that requires intensive management. The likelihood of recovery is greatest if it is recognized early and treated promptly. Children with Reye's syndrome should be managed in an intensive-care unit.

Treatment in the early stages includes intravenous sugar to return levels to normal and plasma **transfusion** to restore normal clotting time. Intracranial pressure is monitored, and if elevated, is treated with intravenous mannitol and hyperventilation to constrict the blood vessels in the brain.

KEY TERMS

Acetylsalicylic acid—Aspirin; an analgesic, antipyretic, and antirheumatic drug prescribed to reduce fever and for relief of pain and inflammation.

Edema—The abnormal accumulation of fluid in interstitial spaces of tissue.

Mitochondria—Small rodlike, threadlike, or granular organelle witin the cytoplasm that function in metabolism and respiration.

If the pressure remains high, **barbiturates** may be used.

Prognosis

The mortality rate for Reye's syndrome is between 30–50%. The likelihood of recovery is increased to 90% by early diagnosis and treatment. Almost all children who survive Reye's syndrome recover fully, although recovery may be slow. In some patients, permanent neurologic damage may remain, requiring physical or educational special services and equipment.

Prevention

Because Reye's syndrome is so highly correlated with use of aspirin for fever in young people, avoidance of aspirin use by children is strongly recommended. Aspirin is in many over-the-counter and prescription drugs, including drugs for **headache**, fever, menstrual cramps, muscle **pain**, **nausea**, upset stomach, and arthritis. It may be used in drugs taken orally or by suppository.

Any of the following ingredients indicates that aspirin is present:

- aspirin
- acetylsalicylate
- acetylsalicylic acid
- salicylic acid
- salicylate

Teenagers who take their own medications without parental consultation should be warned not to take aspirin-containing drugs.

Resources

ORGANIZATIONS

National Reye's Syndrome Foundation. P.O. Box 829, Bryan, OH 43506-0829. (800) 233-7393. < http://www.bright.net/~reyessyn >.

Richard Robinson

Rh disease *see* **Erythroblastosis fetalis**

Rh incompatibility *see* **Erythroblastosis fetalis**

Rh typing *see* **Blood typing and crossmatching**

Rheumatic fever

Definition

Rheumatic **fever** (RF) is an illness which arises as a complication of untreated or inadequately treated **strep throat** infection. Rheumatic fever can seriously damage the valves of the heart.

Description

Throat infection with a member of the Group A streptococcus (strep) bacteria is a common problem among school-aged children. It is easily treated with a ten-day course of **antibiotics** by mouth. However, when such a throat infection occurs without symptoms, or when a course of medication is not taken for the full ten days, there is a 3% chance of that person developing rheumatic fever. Other types of strep infections (such as of the skin) do not put the patient at risk for RF.

Children between the ages of five and fifteen are most susceptible to strep throat, and therefore most susceptible to rheumatic fever. Other risk factors include poverty, overcrowding (as in military camps), and lack of access to good medical care. Just as strep throat occurs most frequently in fall, winter, and early spring, so does rheumatic fever.

Causes and symptoms

Two different theories exist as to how a bacterial throat infection can develop into the disease called rheumatic fever. One theory, less supported by research evidence, suggests that the bacteria produce some kind of poisonous chemical (toxin). This toxin is sent into circulation throughout the bloodstream, thus affecting other systems of the body.

Research seems to point to a different theory, however. This theory suggests that the disease is caused by the body's immune system acting inappropriately. The body produces immune cells (called antibodies), which are specifically designed to recognize and destroy invading agents; in this case, streptococcal bacteria. The antibodies are able to recognize the bacteria because the bacteria contain special markers called antigens. Due to a resemblance between Group A streptococcus bacteria's antigens and antigens present on the body's own cells, the antibodies mistakenly attack the body itself.

It is interesting to note that members of certain families seem to have a greater tendency to develop rheumatic fever than do others. This could be related to the above theory, in that these families may have cell antigens which more closely resemble streptococcal antigens than do members of other families.

In addition to fever, in about 75% of all cases of RF one of the first symptoms is arthritis. The joints (especially those of the ankles, knees, elbows, and wrists) become red, hot, swollen, shiny, and extraordinarily painful. Unlike many other forms of arthritis, the arthritis may not occur symmetrically (affecting a particular joint on both the right and left sides, simultaneously). The arthritis of RF rarely strikes the fingers, toes, or spine. The joints become so tender that even the touch of bedsheets or clothing is terribly painful.

A peculiar type of involuntary movement, coupled with emotional instability, occurs in about 10% of all RF patients (the figure used to be about 50%). The patient begins experiencing a change in coordination, often first noted by changes in handwriting. The arms or legs may flail or jerk uncontrollably. The patient seems to develop a low threshold for anger and sadness. This feature of RF is called **Sydenham's chorea** or St. Vitus' Dance.

A number of skin changes are common to RF. A rash called erythema marginatum develops (especially in those patients who will develop heart problems from their illness), composed of pink splotches, which may eventually spread into each other. It does not itch. Bumps the size of peas may occur under the skin. These are called subcutaneous nodules; they are hard to the touch, but not painful. These nodules most commonly occur over the knee and elbow joint, as well as over the spine.

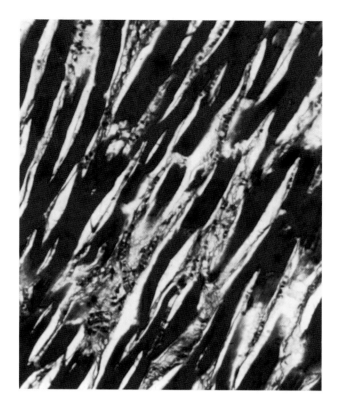

A magnified image of cardiac muscle damaged by chronic myocarditis caused by rheumatic fever. *(Science Photo Library. Custom Medical Stock Photo. Reproduced by permission.)*

The most serious problem occurring in RF is called pancarditis ("pan" means total; "carditis" refers to inflammation of the heart). Pancarditis is an inflammation that affects all aspects of the heart, including the lining of the heart (endocardium), the sac containing the heart (pericardium), and the heart muscle itself (myocardium). About 40-80% of all RF patients develop pancarditis. This RF complication has the most serious, long-term effects. The valves within the heart (structures which allow the blood to flow only in the correct direction, and only at the correct time in the heart's pumping cycle) are frequently damaged during the course of pancarditis. This may result in blood which either leaks back in the wrong direction, or has a difficult time passing a stiff, poorly moving valve. Either way, damage to a valve can result in the heart having to work very hard in order to move the blood properly. The heart may not be able to "work around" the damaged valve, which may result in a consistently inadequate amount of blood entering the circulation.

Diagnosis

Diagnosis of RF is done by carefully examining the patient. A list of diagnostic criteria has been created. These "Jones Criteria" are divided into major and minor criteria. A patient can be diagnosed with RF if he or she has either two major criteria (conditions), or one major and two minor criteria. In either case, it must also be proved that the individual has had a previous infection with streptococcus.

The major criteria include:

- carditis
- arthritis
- chorea
- subcutaneous nodules
- erythema marginatum

The minor criteria include:

- fever
- joint **pain** (without actual arthritis)
- evidence of electrical changes in the heart (determined by measuring electrical characteristics of the heart's functioning during a test called an electrocardiogram, or EKG)
- evidence (through a blood test) of the presence in the blood of certain proteins, which are produced early in an inflammatory/infectious disease.

Tests are also performed to provide evidence of recent infection with group A streptococcal bacteria. A swab of the throat can be taken, and smeared on a substance in a petri dish, to see if bacteria will multiply and grow over 24-72 hours. These bacteria can then be specially processed, and examined under a microscope, to identify streptococcal bacteria. Other tests can be performed to see if the patient is producing specific antibodies; that are only made in response to a recent strep infection.

Treatment

A 10-day course of penicillin by mouth, or a single injection of penicillin G-is the first line of treatment for RF. Patients will need to remain on some regular dose of penicillin to prevent recurrence of RF. This can mean a small daily dose of penicillin by mouth, or an injection every three weeks. Some practitioners keep patients on this regimen for five years, or until they reach 18 years of age (whichever comes first). Other practitioners prefer to continue treating those patients who will be regularly exposed to streptococcal bacteria (teachers, medical workers), as well as those patients with known RF heart disease.

Arthritis quickly improves when the patient is given a preparation containing **aspirin**, or some other anti-inflammatory agent (ibuprofen). Mild carditis will also improve with such anti-inflammatory agents, although more severe cases of carditis will require steroid medications. A number of medications are available to treat the involuntary movements of chorea, including diazepam for mild cases, and haloperidol for more severe cases.

Prognosis

The long-term prognosis of an RF patient depends primarily on whether he or she develops carditis. This is the only manifestation of RF which can have permanent effects. Those patients with no or mild carditis have an excellent prognosis. Those with more severe carditis have a risk of **heart failure**, as well as a risk of future heart problems, which may lead to the need for valve replacement surgery.

Prevention

Prevention of the development of RF involves proper diagnosis of initial strep throat infections, and adequate treatment within 10 days with an appropriate antibiotic. Prevention of RF recurrence requires continued antibiotic treatment, perhaps for life. Prevention of complications of already-existing RF heart disease requires that the patient always take a special course of antibiotics when he or she undergoes any kind of procedure (even dental cleanings) that might allow bacteria to gain access to the bloodstream.

Resources

ORGANIZATIONS

Centers for Disease Control and Prevention. 1600 Clifton Rd., NE, Atlanta, GA 30333. (800) 311-3435, (404) 639-3311. <http://www.cdc.gov>.

Rosalyn Carson-DeWitt, MD

Rheumatoid arthritis

Definition

Rheumatoid arthritis (RA) is a chronic autoimmune disease that causes inflammation and deformity of the joints. Other problems throughout the body (systemic problems) may also develop, including inflammation of blood vessels (**vasculitis**), the development of bumps (called rheumatoid nodules) in various parts of the body, lung disease, blood disorders, and weakening of the bones (**osteoporosis**).

Description

The skeletal system of the body is made up of different types of strong, fibrous tissue called connective tissue. Bone, cartilage, ligaments, and tendons are all forms of connective tissue that have different compositions and different characteristics.

The joints are structures that hold two or more bones together. Some joints (synovial joints) allow for movement between the bones being joined (articulating bones). The simplest synovial joint involves two bones, separated by a slight gap called the joint cavity. The ends of each articular bone are covered by a layer of cartilage. Both articular bones and the joint cavity are surrounded by a tough tissue called the articular capsule. The articular capsule has two components, the fibrous membrane on the outside and the synovial membrane (or synovium) on the inside. The fibrous membrane may include tough bands of tissue called ligaments, which are responsible for providing support to the joints. The synovial membrane has special cells and many tiny blood vessels (capillaries). This membrane produces a supply of synovial fluid that fills the joint cavity, lubricates it, and helps the articular bones move smoothly about the joint.

In rheumatoid arthritis (RA), the synovial membrane becomes severely inflamed. Usually thin and delicate, the synovium becomes thick and stiff, with numerous infoldings on its surface. The membrane is invaded by white blood cells, which produce a variety of destructive chemicals. The cartilage along the articular surfaces of the bones may be attacked and destroyed, and the bone, articular capsule, and ligaments may begin to wear away (erode). These processes severely interfere with movement in the joint.

RA exists all over the world and affects men and women of all races. In the United States alone, about two million people suffer from the disease. Women are three times more likely than men to have RA. About 80% of people with RA are diagnosed between the ages of 35-50. RA appears to run in families, although certain factors in the environment may also influence the development of the disease.

Causes and symptoms

The underlying event that promotes RA in a person is unknown. Given the known genetic factors involved in RA, some researchers have suggested that an outside event occurs that triggers the disease cycle in a person with a particular genetic makeup.

Many researchers are examining the possibility that exposure to an organism (like a bacteria or virus) may be the first event in the development of RA. The body's normal response to such an organism is to produce cells that can attack and kill the organism, protecting the body from the foreign invader. In an autoimmune disease like RA, this immune cycle spins out of control. The body produces misdirected immune cells, which accidentally identify parts of the person's body as foreign. These immune cells then produce a variety of chemicals that injure and destroy parts of the body.

RA can begin very gradually, or it can strike quickly. The first symptoms are **pain**, swelling, and stiffness in the joints. The most commonly involved joints include hands, feet, wrists, elbows, and ankles, although other joints may also be involved. The joints are affected in a symmetrical fashion. This means that if the right wrist is involved, the left wrist is also involved. Patients frequently experience painful joint stiffness when they first get up in the morning, lasting

for perhaps an hour. Over time, the joints become deformed. The joints may be difficult to straighten, and affected fingers and toes may be permanently bent (flexed). The hands and feet may curve outward in an abnormal way.

Many patients also notice increased **fatigue**, loss of appetite, weight loss, and sometimes **fever**. Rheumatoid nodules are bumps that appear under the skin around the joints and on the top of the arms and legs. These nodules can also occur in the tissue covering the outside of the lungs and lining the chest cavity (pleura), and in the tissue covering the brain and spinal cord (meninges). Lung involvement may cause **shortness of breath** and is seen more in men. Vasculitis (inflammation of the blood vessels) may interfere with blood circulation. This can result in irritated pits (ulcers) in the skin, tissue death (**gangrene**), and interference with nerve functioning that causes **numbness and tingling**.

Juvenile RA is a chronic inflammatory disease that affects the joints of children less than 16 years old. It is estimated to affect as many as 250,000 children in the United States alone. Most children with juvenile RA have arthritis when the illness starts, which affects multiple joints in 50% of these children, and only one joint in 30%. In all, 20% of the children affected by juvenile RA have the acute systemic form of the disease, which is characterized by fever, joint inflammation, rash, **liver disease**, and gastrointestinal disease.

Two periods of childhood are associated with an increased incidence of onset of juvenile RA. The first is from one to three years of age, and the second, from eight to 12 years. When more than four joints are affected, the disease is described as being polyarticular. If less than four joints are affected, the disease is known as pauciarticular. juvenile RA and this particular manifestation falls into two categories. The first occurs in girls aged one to four years old, and the onset of joint involvement is in the knees, ankles, or elbows. The second form occurs in boys aged eight years and older, and involves the larger joints, such as those of the hips and legs.

Diagnosis

There are no tests available that can absolutely diagnose RA. Instead, a number of tests exist that can suggest the diagnosis of RA. Blood tests include a special test of red blood cells (called **erythrocyte sedimentation rate**), which is positive in nearly 100% of patients with RA. However, this test is also positive in a variety of other diseases. Tests for anemia are usually positive in patients with RA, but can also be positive in many other unrelated diseases. Rheumatoid factor is another diagnostic test that measures the presence and amounts of rheumatoid factor in the blood. Rheumatoid factor is an autoantibody found in about 80% of patients with RA. It is often not very specific however, because it is found in about 5% of all healthy people and in 10-20% of healthy people over the age of 65. In addition, rheumatoid factor is also positive in a large number of other autoimmune diseases and other infectious diseases, including **systemic lupus erythematosus**, bacterial **endocarditis**, **malaria**, and **syphilis**. In addition, young people who have a process called juvenile rheumatoid arthritis often have no rheumatoid factor present in their blood.

Finally, the clinician may examine the synovial fluid, by inserting a thin needle into a synovial joint. In RA, this fluid has certain characteristics that indicate active inflammation. The fluid is cloudy, with increased protein and decreased or normal glucose. It also contains a higher than normal number of white blood cells. While these findings suggest inflammatory arthritis, they are not specific to RA.

Treatment

There is no cure available for RA. However, treatment is available to combat the inflammation in order to prevent destruction of the joints, and to prevent other complications of the disease. Efforts are also made to maintain flexibility and mobility of the joints.

The "first line" agents for the treatment of RA include nonsteroidal anti- inflammatory agents (NSAIDs) and **aspirin**, which are used to decrease inflammation and to treat pain. The NSAIDs include naproxen (Naprosyn), ibuprofen (Advil, Medipren, Motrin), and etodolac (Lodine). While these medications can be helpful, they do not interrupt the progress of the disease. Low-dose steroid medications can be helpful at both managing symptoms and slowing the progress of RA. Disease-modifying **antirheumatic drugs**, including gold compounds, D-penicillamine, certain antimalarial-like drugs, and sulfasalazine (Azulfadine) are also often the first agents clinicians use to treat RA, but in patients with the aggressive destructive type of RA, more slow-acting medications are needed. Methotrexate, azathioprine, and cyclophosphamide are all drugs that suppress the immune system and can decrease inflammation. All of the drugs listed have significant toxic side effects, which require healthcare professionals to carefully compare the risks associated with these medications versus the benefits.

Recently, several categories of drugs have been explored and developed for the treatment of RA. The first is a category of agents known as biological response modifiers. These work to reduce joint inflammation by blocking a substance called tumor necrosis factor (TNF). TNF is a protein that triggers inflammation during the body's normal immune responses. When TNF production is not regulated, the excess TNF can cause inflammation. Three agents in this class have become "second line" drugs for the treatment of RA. These are etanercept (Enbrel), leflunamide (Arava), and infliximab (Remicade), and they are recommended for patients in whom other medications have not been effective. Etanercept is approved by the FDA but is not recommended for patients with active infection. It is given twice weekly via subcutaneous injections by either the patient or a health care professional. Because this agent is so new, long-term side effects have not been fully studied. Infliximab is given intravenously once every eight weeks, and is approved for combined use with methotrexate to combat RA.

The cyclo-oxygenase-2 (COX-2) inhibitors are another category of drugs used to treat RA. Like the traditional NSAIDs, the **COX-2 inhibitors** work to block COX-2, which is an enzyme that stimulates inflammatory responses in the body. Unlike the NSAIDs, the COX-2 inhibitors do not carry a high risk of gastrointestinal ulcers and bleeding, because they do not inhibit COX-1, which is the enzyme that protects the stomach lining. These new agents include celecoxib (Celebrex) and rofecoxib (Vioxx). Celecoxib has been approved by the FDA for the treatment of RA and **osteoarthritis**, and is taken once or twice daily by mouth. Rofecoxib is approved for RA and osteoarthritis, and for acute pain caused by primary **dysmenorrhea** and surgery.

Total bed rest is sometimes prescribed during the very active, painful phases of RA. Splints may be used to support and rest painful joints. Later, after inflammation has somewhat subsided, physical therapists may provide a careful **exercise** regimen in an attempt to maintain the maximum degree of flexibility and mobility. **Joint replacement** surgery, particularly for the knee and the hip joints, is sometimes recommended when these joints have been severely damaged.

Alternative treatment

A variety of alternative therapies has been recommended for patients with RA. **Meditation**, hypnosis, **guided imagery**, and relaxation techniques have been used effectively to control pain. **Acupressure** and **acupuncture** have also been used for pain. Bodywork can be soothing, decreasing **stress** and tension, and is thought to improve/restore chemical balance within the body.

A multitude of **nutritional supplements** can be useful for RA. Fish oils, the enzymes bromelain and pancreatin, and the antioxidants (**vitamins** A, C, and E, selenium, and zinc) are the primary supplements to consider.

Many herbs also are useful in the treatment of RA. Anti-inflammatory herbs may be very helpful, including tumeric (*Curcuma longa*), ginger (*Zingiber officinale*), feverfew (*Chrysanthemum parthenium*), devil's claw (*Harpagophytum procumbens*), Chinese thoroughwax (*Bupleuri falcatum*), and licorice (*Glycyrrhiza glabra*). Lobelia (*Lobelia inflata*) and cramp bark (*Vibernum opulus*) can be applied topically to the affected joints.

Homeopathic practitioners recommended *Rhus toxicondendron* and *Bryonia* (*Bryonia alba*) for acute prescriptions, but constitutional treatment, generally used for chronic problems like RA, is more often recommended. **Yoga** has been used for RA patients to promote relaxation, relieve stress, and improve flexibility. Nutritionists suggest that a vegetarian diet low in animal products and sugar may help to decrease both inflammation and pain from RA. Beneficial foods for patients with RA include cold water fish (mackerel, herring, salmon, and sardines) and flavonoid-rich berries (cherries, blueberries, hawthorn berries, blackberries, etc.).

RA, considered an autoimmune disorder, is often connected with food allergies/intolerances. An elimination/challenge diet can help to decrease symptoms of RA as well as identify the foods that should be eliminated to prevent flare-ups and recurrences. **Hydrotherapy** can help to greatly reduce pain and inflammation. Moist heat is more effective than dry heat, and cold packs are useful during acute flare-ups.

Prognosis

About 15% of all RA patients will have symptoms for a short period of time and will ultimately get better, leaving them with no long-term problems. A number of factors are considered to suggest the likelihood of a worse prognosis. These include:

- race and gender (female and Caucasian).
- more than 20 joints involved.
- extremely high erythrocyte sedimentation rate.

KEY TERMS

Articular bones—Two or more bones connected to each other via a joint.

Joint—Structures holding two or more bones together.

Pauciarticular juvenile RA—Rheumatoid arthritis found in children that affects less than four joints.

Polyarticular juvenile RA—Rheumatoid arthritis found in children that affects more than four joints.

Synovial joint—A type of joint that allows articular bones to move.

Synovial membrane—The membrane that lines the inside of the articular capsule of a joint and produces a lubricating fluid called synovial fluid.

- extremely high levels of rheumatoid factor.
- consistent, lasting inflammation.
- evidence of erosion of bone, joint, or cartilage on x rays.
- poverty.
- older age at diagnosis.
- rheumatoid nodules.
- other coexisting diseases.
- certain genetic characteristics, diagnosable through testing.

Patients with RA have a shorter life span, averaging a decrease of three to seven years of life. Patients sometimes die when very severe disease, infection, and gastrointestinal bleeding occur. Complications due to the side effects of some of the more potent drugs used to treat RA are also factors in these deaths.

Prevention

There is no known way to prevent the development of RA. The most that can be hoped for is to prevent or slow its progress.

Resources

BOOKS

Arthritis Foundation. *The Good Living with Rheumatoid Arthritis*. New York: Longstreet Press Inc., 2000.

PERIODICALS

Case, J. P. "Old and New Drugs Used in Rheumatoid Arthritis: A Historical Perspective. Part 2: The Newer

Drugs and Drug Strategies." *American Journal of Therapeutics* May-June 2001: 163-79.

Goekoop, Y. P., et al. "Combination Therapy in Rheumatoid Arthritis." *Current Opinions in Rheumatology* May 2001: 177-83.

Koivuniemi, R., and M. Leirisalo-Repo. "Juvenile Chronic Arthritis in Adult Life: A Study of Long-term Outcome in Patients with Juvenile Chronic Arthritis or Adult Rhuematoid Arthritis." *Clinical Rheumatology* 1999: 220-6.

Liz Meszaros

Rheumatoid spondylit *see* **Ankylosing spondylitis**

Rhinitis

Definition

Rhinitis is inflammation of the mucous lining of the nose.

Description

Rhinitis is a nonspecific term that covers infections, **allergies**, and other disorders whose common feature is the location of their symptoms. In rhinitis, the mucous membranes become infected or irritated, producing a discharge, congestion, and swelling of the tissues. The most widespread form of infectious rhinitis is the **common cold**.

The common cold is the most frequent viral infection in the general population, causing more absenteeism from school or work than any other illness. Colds are self-limited, lasting about 3-10 days, although they are sometimes followed by a bacterial infection. Children are more susceptible than adults; teenage boys more susceptible than teenage girls; and adult women more susceptible than adult men. In the United States, colds are most frequent during the late fall and winter.

Causes and symptoms

Colds can be caused by as many as 200 different viruses. The viruses are transmitted by sneezing and coughing, by contact with soiled tissues or handkerchiefs, or by close contact with an infected person. Colds are easily spread in schools, offices, or any place where people live or work in groups. The incubation period ranges between 24 and 72 hours.

The onset of a cold is usually sudden. The virus causes the lining of the nose to become inflamed and produce large quantities of thin, watery mucus. Children sometimes run a **fever** with a cold. The inflammation spreads from the nasal passages to the throat and upper airway, producing a dry **cough**, **headache**, and watery eyes. Some people develop muscle or joint aches and feel generally tired or weak. After several days, the nose becomes less inflamed and the watery discharge is replaced by a thick, sticky mucus. This change in the appearance of the nasal discharge helps to distinguish rhinitis caused by a viral infection from rhinitis caused by an allergy.

Diagnosis

There is no specific test for viral rhinitis. The diagnosis is based on the symptoms. In children, the doctor will examine the child's throat and glands to rule out **measles** and other childhood illnesses that have similar early symptoms. Adults whose symptoms last longer than a week may require further testing to rule out a secondary bacterial infection, or an allergy. Bacterial infections can usually be identified from a laboratory culture of the patient's nasal discharge. Allergies can be evaluated by blood tests, skin testing for specific substances, or nasal smears.

Treatment

There is no cure for the common cold; treatment is given for symptom relief. Medications include **aspirin** or **nonsteroidal anti-inflammatory drugs** (NSAIDs) for headache and muscle **pain**, and **decongestants** to relieve stuffiness or runny nose. Patients should be warned against overusing decongestants, because they can cause a rebound effect. Over-the-counter (OTC) **antihistamines** are also available; however, most antihistamines carry warnings of drowsiness and the inability to do some tasks while medicated. Claritin is a prescription-strength OTC non-drowsy antihistamine that helps relieve symptoms of rhinitis. **Antibiotics** are not given for colds because they do not kill viruses.

Supportive care includes bed rest and drinking plenty of fluid.

Treatments under investigation include the use of ultraviolet light and injections of interferon.

Many prescription and over-the-counter drugs are available to help control the symptoms of **allergic rhinitis**. The most common class is antihistamines.

Alternative treatment

Homeopaths might prescribe any of 10 different remedies, depending on the appearance of the nasal discharge, the patient's emotional state, and the stage of infection. Naturopaths would recommend vitamin A and zinc supplements, together with botanical preparations made from goldenseal (*Hydrastis canadensis*), licorice (*Glycyrrhiza glabra*), or astragalus (*Astragalus membraneceus*) root.

At one time, the herb (*Echinacea* spp.) was touted as a remedy to relieve cold and rhinitis symptoms. However, a study published in 2004 reported that the herb failed to relieve cold symptoms in 400 children taking it and caused skin **rashes** in some children.

Prognosis

Most colds resolve completely in about a week. Complications are unusual but may include **sinusitis** (inflammation of the nasal sinuses), bacterial infections, or infections of the middle ear.

Prevention

There is no vaccine effective against colds, and infection does not confer immunity. Prevention depends on:

- washing hands often, especially before touching the face
- minimizing contact with people already infected
- not sharing hand towels, eating utensils, or water glasses.

Resources

PERIODICALS

"Study: Echinacea Is Ineffective." *Chain Drug Review* February 16, 2004: 25.

Rebecca J. Frey, PhD
Teresa G. Odle

Rhinoplasty

Definition

The term rhinoplasty means "nose molding" or "nose forming." It refers to a procedure in **plastic surgery** in which the structure of the nose is changed. The change can be made by adding or removing bone or cartilage, grafting tissue from another part of the body, or implanting synthetic material to alter the shape of the nose.

Rhinoplasty is the most frequently performed cosmetic surgical procedure in the United States as of the early 2000s. According to the American Society of Plastic Surgeons (ASPS), 356,554 rhinoplasties were performed in the United States in 2003, compared to 254,140 breast augmentations and 128,667 facelifts.

Purpose

Rhinoplasty is most often performed for cosmetic reasons. A nose that is too large, crooked, misshapen, malformed at birth, or deformed by an injury or **cancer** surgery can be given a more pleasing appearance. If breathing is impaired due to the form of the nose or to an injury, it can often be improved with rhinoplasty.

Precautions

The best candidates for rhinoplasty are those with relatively minor deformities. Nasal anatomy and proportions are quite varied and the final look of any rhinoplasty operation is the result of the patient's anatomy, as well as of the surgeon's skill.

The quality of the skin plays a major role in the outcome of rhinoplasty. Patients with extremely thick skin may not see a definite change in the underlying bone structure after surgery. On the other hand, thin skin provides almost no cushion to hide the most minor of bone irregularities or imperfections.

A cosmetic change in the shape of the nose will change a person's appearance, but it will not change self-image. A person who expects a different lifestyle after rhinoplasty is likely to be disappointed.

Rhinoplasty should not be performed until the pubertal growth spurt is complete, between ages 14-15 for girls and older for boys.

The cost of rhinoplasty depends on the difficulty of the work required and on the specialist chosen. Prices run from about $3,000 to over $6,000. If the problem was caused by an injury, insurance will usually cover the cost. A rhinoplasty done only to change a person's appearance is not usually covered by insurance.

Description

The external nose is composed of a series of inter-related parts which include the skin, the bony pyramid, cartilage, and the tip of the nose, which is both cartilage and skin. The strip of skin separating the nostrils is called the columella.

Surgical approaches to nasal reconstruction are varied. Internal rhinoplasty involves making all incisions inside the nasal cavity. The external or "open" technique involves a skin incision across the base of the nasal columella. An external incision allows the surgeon to expose the bone and cartilage more fully and is most often used for complicated procedures. During surgery, the surgeon will separate the skin from the bone and cartilage support. The framework of the nose is then reshaped in the desired form. Shape can be altered by removing bone, cartilage, or skin. The remaining skin is then replaced over the new framework. If the procedure requires adding to the structure of the nose, the donated bone, cartilage, or skin can come from the patient or from a synthetic source.

When the operation is over, the surgeon will apply a splint to help the bones maintain their new shape. The nose may also be packed, or stuffed with a dressing, to help stabilize the septum.

When a local anesthetic is used, light **sedation** is usually given first, after which the operative area is numbed. It will remain insensitive to **pain** for the length of the surgery. A general anesthetic is used for lengthy or complex procedures or if the doctor and patient agree that it is the best option.

Simple rhinoplasty is usually performed in an out-patient surgery center or in the surgeon's office. Most procedures take only an hour or two, and patients may return home right away. Complex procedures may be done in the hospital and require a short stay.

Preparation

During the initial consultation, the patient and surgeon will determine what changes can be made in the shape of the nose. Most doctors take photographs at the same time. The surgeon will also explain the techniques and anesthesia options available to the patient.

For legal reasons, many plastic surgeons now screen patients for psychological stability as well as general physical fitness for surgery. When a person consults a plastic surgeon about a rhinoplasty, the doctor will spend some time talking with the patient about his or her motives for facial surgery. The following are considered psychological warning signs:

- The patient is considering surgery to please someone else, most often a spouse or partner.

- The patient expects facial surgery to guarantee career advancement.

- The patient has a history of multiple cosmetic procedures and/or complaints about previous surgeons.

- The patient thinks that the surgery will solve all his or her life problems.

- The patient has an unrealistic notion of what he or she will look like after surgery.

- The patient seems otherwise emotionally unstable.

The patient and surgeon should also discuss guidelines for eating, drinking, **smoking**, taking or avoiding certain medications, and washing of the face.

Aftercare

Patients usually feel fine immediately after surgery; however, most surgery centers do not allow patients to drive themselves home after an operation.

The first day after surgery there will be some swelling of the face. Patients should stay in bed with their heads elevated for at least a day. The nose may hurt and a **headache** is not uncommon. The surgeon will prescribe medication to relieve these conditions. Swelling and bruising around the eyes will increase for a few days, but will begin to diminish after about the third day. Slight bleeding and stuffiness are normal, and vary according to the extensiveness of the surgery performed. Most people are up in two days, and back to school or work in a week. No strenuous activities are allowed for two to three weeks.

Patients are given a list of postoperative instructions, which include requirements for hygiene, **exercise**, eating, and follow-up visits to the doctor. Patients should not blow their noses for the first week to avoid disruption of healing. It is extremely important to keep the surgical dressing dry. Dressings, splints, and stitches are removed in one to two weeks. Patients should avoid **sunburn**.

Patients should remember that it may take as long as a year for the nose to assume its final shape; the tip of the nose in particular may be mildly swollen for several months.

KEY TERMS

Cartilage—Firm supporting tissue that does not contain blood vessels.

Columella—The strip of skin running from the tip of the nose to the upper lip, which separates the nostrils.

Septum—The dividing wall in the nose.

Risks

Any type of surgery carries a degree of risk. There is always the possibility of unexpected events, such as an infection or a reaction to the anesthesia. Some patients may have a so-called foreign body reaction to a nasal implant made from synthetic materials. In these cases the surgeon can replace the implant with a piece of cartilage from the patient's own body.

Some risks of rhinoplasty are social or psychological. The ASPS patient brochure about rhinoplasty mentions the possibility of criticism or rejection by friends or family if they feel threatened by the patient's new look. This type of reaction sometimes occurs with rhinoplasty if the friends or relatives consider the shape of the nose an important family or ethnic trait.

When the nose is reshaped or repaired from inside, the scars are not visible, but if the surgeon needs to make the incision on the outside of the nose, there will be some slight scarring. In addition, tiny blood vessels may burst, leaving small red spots on the skin. These spots are barely visible but may be permanent.

About 10% of patients require a second procedure; however, the corrections required are usually minor.

Resources

PERIODICALS

Chou, T. D., W. T. Lee, S. L. Chen, et al. "Split Calvarial Bone Graft for Chemical Burn-Associated Nasal Augmentation." *Burns* 30 (June 2004): 380–385.

Daniel, R. K., and J. W. Calvert. "Diced Cartilage Grafts in Rhinoplasty Surgery." *Plastic and Reconstructive Surgery* 113 (June 2004): 2156–2171.

Honigman, R. J., K. A. Phillips, and D. J. Castle. "A Review of Psychosocial Outcomes for Patients Seeking Cosmetic Surgery." *Plastic and Reconstructive Surgery* 113 (April 1, 2004): 1229–1237.

Raghavan, U., N. S. Jones, and T. Romo, 3rd. "Immediate Autogenous Cartilage Grafts in Rhinoplasty after Alloplastic Implant Rejection." *Archives of Facial and Plastic Surgery* 6 (May-June 2004): 192–196.

ORGANIZATIONS

American Academy of Facial Plastic and Reconstructive Surgery (AAFPRS). 310 South Henry Street, Alexandria, VA 22314. (703) 299-9291. < http://www.facemd.org >.

American Society of Plastic Surgeons (ASPS). 444 East Algonquin Road, Arlington Heights, IL 60005. (847) 228-9900. < http://www.plasticsurgery.org >.

OTHER

American Society of Plastic Surgeons. *Procedures: Rhinoplasty.* < http://www.plasticsurgery.org/public_education/procedures/Rhinoplasty.cfm >.

Dorothy Elinor Stonely
Rebecca J. Frey, PhD

Rhinovirus infection *see* **Common cold**

Rhytidoplasty *see* **Face lift**

Riboflavin deficiency

Definition

Riboflavin deficiency occurs when the chronic failure to eat sufficient amounts of foods that contain riboflavin produces lesions of the skin, lesions of smooth surfaces in the digestive tract, or nervous disorders.

Description

Riboflavin, also called vitamin B_2, is a water-soluble vitamin. The recommended dietary allowance (RDA) for riboflavin is 1.7 mg/day for an adult man and 1.3 mg/day for an adult woman. The best sources of this vitamin are meat, dairy products, and dark green vegetables, especially broccoli. Grains and legumes (beans and peas) also contribute riboflavin to the diet. Riboflavin is required for the processing of dietary fats, carbohydrates, and proteins to convert these nutrients to energy. Riboflavin is also used for the continual process of renewal and regeneration of all cells and tissues in the body.

Riboflavin is sensitive to light. For this reason, commercially available milk is sometimes supplied in cartons, rather than in clear bottles. Riboflavin is not rapidly destroyed by cooking. Milk contains about 1.7 mg riboflavin/kg. Cheese contains about 4.3 mg/kg, while beef has 2.4 mg/kg and broccoli has about 2.0

mg/kg. Apples, a food that is low in all nutrients, except water, contains only 0.1 mg riboflavin per kg.

Causes and symptoms

A deficiency only in riboflavin has never occurred in the natural environment. In contrast, diseases where people are deficient in one vitamin, such as thiamin, vitamin C, and vitamin D, for example, have been clearly documented. Poorer populations in the United States may be deficient in riboflavin, but when this happens, they are also deficient in a number of other nutrients as well. When riboflavin deficiency is actually detected, it is often associated with low consumption of milk, chronic **alcoholism**, or chronic **diarrhea**.

The symptoms of riboflavin deficiency include:

- swelling and fissuring of the lips (cheilosis)
- ulceration and cracking of the angles of the mouth (angular stomatitisis)
- oily, scaly skin **rashes** on the scrotum, vulva, or area between the nose and lips
- inflammation of the tongue
- red, itchy eyes that are sensitive to light

The nervous symptoms of riboflavin deficiency include:

- numbness of the hands
- decreased sensitivity to touch, temperature, and vibration

Diagnosis

Riboflavin status is diagnosed using a test conducted on red blood cells that measures the activity of an enzyme called glutathione reductase. An extract of the red blood cells is placed in two test tubes. One test tube contains no added riboflavin, while the second test tube contains a derivative of riboflavin, called flavin adenine dinucleotide. The added riboflavin derivative results in little or no stimulation of enzyme activity in patients with normal riboflavin levels. A stimulation of 20% or less is considered normal. A stimulation of over 20% means that the patient is deficient in riboflavin.

Treatment

Riboflavin deficiency can be treated with supplemental riboflavin (0.5 mg/kg body weight per day) until the symptoms disappear.

KEY TERMS

Recommended dietary allowance—The recommended daily allowances (RDAs) are quantities of nutrients of the diet that are required to maintain human health. RDAs are established by the Food and Nutrition Board of the National Academy of Sciences and may be revised every few years. A separate RDA value exists for each nutrient. The RDA values refer to the amount of nutrient needed to maintain health in a population of people. The actual amounts of each nutrient required to maintain health in any specific individual differs from person to person.

Water-soluble vitamin—Water-soluble vitamins can be dissolved in water or juice. Fat-soluble vitamins can be dissolved in oil or in melted fat.

Prognosis

The prognosis for correcting riboflavin deficiency is excellent.

Prevention

Riboflavin deficiency can be prevented by including milk, cheese, yogurt, meat, and/or certain vegetables in the daily diet. Of the vegetables, broccoli, asparagus, and spinach are highest in riboflavin. These vegetables have a riboflavin content that is similar to that of milk, yogurt, or meat.

Resources

BOOKS

Brody, Tom. *Nutritional Biochemistry*. San Diego: Academic Press, 1998.

Tom Brody, PhD

Rickets

Definition

Rickets is a childhood condition caused by serious **vitamin D deficiency**. This lacking in vitamin D results in weak, soft bones, along with slowed growth and skeletal development. Rickets is, by definition, a disorder which begins in childhood. If this problem occurs only later in life it is known as osteomalacia.

Description

Rickets occurs when the body has a severe lack of vitamin D during the developmental years. Vitamin D is essential to the development of strong, healthy bones. A child with rickets can experience stunted growth and will most likely be short in stature as an adult. This is because, without proper vitamin D levels, decreased mineralization of the bones at the growth plate level affects the strength, size and shape of the bones. A related condition called osteomalacia can occur in adults with the same sort of vitamin D deficiency, but osteomalacia occurs only in adulthood after the growth plates of the bones have closed.

Most vitamin D is produced by the body, although some can be directly supplied by diet. In order to accomplish production of vitamin D, the body requires both cholesterol and ultraviolet light. Most often, the cholesterol comes from digesting animal tissue, oils, fats, and egg yolks. The ultraviolet light is usually supplied by direct sunlight. Only when this light is available can the skin alter the cholesterol molecule to make vitamin D. Children who do not receive enough sunlight are at greater risk of developing rickets, as are children with darker skin, which can block the ultraviolet rays. Vitamin D is found naturally in the foods listed above, but more often children receive vitamin D supplements through foods which have had the vitamin added, as in milk or infant formula.

Vitamin D is necessary in the body, because it can be converted into a hormone which stimulates calcium intake by the intestines. This conversion begins in the liver, where vitamin D becomes a hormone called 25-OH-D, and is completed when the kidneys convert 25-OH-D into a hormone called 1,25-diOH-D. This is the hormone that causes the intestines to absorb calcium from the person's diet. Without proper levels of vitamin D, there is not enough 1,25-diOH-D produced, which results in lower levels of calcium in the body. Adequate calcium is needed by the bones for both development and maintenance.

Causes and symptoms

Rickets is directly caused by insufficient calcium for bone mineralization during growth and development. This is caused by vitamin D deficiency which can be a result of too little cholesterol, ultraviolet light, or vitamin D supplement. During the Industrial Revolution, rickets was quite common in cities because pollution in the air blocked much of the sunlight needed for vitamin D production in the body. There is also a hereditary type of rickets, called X-linked hypophosphatemia, that causes the kidneys bo be unable to retain phosphate.

The most commonly recognized symptoms of rickets occur in the arms and legs, where **stress** on the underdeveloped bones can cause bowing. Children with rickets may feel **pain** or tenderness in the bones of their arms, legs, spine, pelvis, and ribs. The skull may develop an odd or asymmetrical shape. Calcium levels in the blood will be low and overall growth is often impaired.

Diagnosis

The initial approach to diagnosing rickets involves a musculoskeletal examination followed by an x ray is often. Affected children may have obviously widened spaces between their joints or bowing of the bones in their arms and legs. Some children may not experience normal dental development as well. A doctor may also assess levels of serum calcium, alkaline phosphatase and other indicator chemicals by using a blood test. While calcium levels can be normal or slightly low, alkaline phosphatase levels in a child with rickets can be high even compared to a normal adult. While x rays can prove misleading, diagnosis by chemical analysis is highly accurate.

Treatment

The treatment for rickets primarily involves corrections of the conditions which led to the disorder. This can be as simple as a change in diet to include foods high in vitamin D such as milk, fish, or liver. Treatment might also mean a gradual increase in the amount sunlight received by the child. In more severe cases, bracing or surgery may be necessary to aid in the correction and repair of bones. Treatment is usually mild and bone deformities usually reduce over time.

Alternative Treatment

There is currently little known about any alternative method for treating rickets. Treatments which involve raising vitamin D levels and ultraviolet light exposure are usually simple and effective.

Prognosis

Children with rickets are likely to suffer from stunted growth, bone abnormalities and bone pain, however these symptoms often disappear with treatment. In women, deformation of the pelvic bone structure can prevent vaginal **childbirth** later in life. Most deformities correct with growth when proper levels of vitamin D are restored and normal bone calcification is maintained.

Prevention

Rickets caused by vitamin D deficiency is simple to prevent. Commercially available infant formula is usually fortified with more than enough vitamin D for infants. For parents who breastfeed their children, it is recommended by the U.S. Department of Health and Human Services that children also receive 400 international units (10 micrograms) of vitamin D supplement. This is because human breast milk contains little vitamin D. It is also important that children are allowed decent amounts of sunlight. As little as twenty minutes each day can be sufficient. For children living in cities, where pollution is likely to block ultraviolet light, and children with dark skin, which can block ultraviolet light, vitamin D supplement is especially important.

Resources

BOOKS

Hochber, Ze'ev, ed. *Vitamin D and Rickets* New York: Karger 2003.

PERIODICALS

Spence, Jean, T. and Janet R. Serwint."Secondary Prevention of Vitamin D-Deficiency Rickets." *Pediatrics.* 113, no 5: (Jan 2004),129.

Wharton, Brian and Nick Bishop. "Rickets." *The Lancet* 362 no9393: (Oct 2003). 1389.

OTHER

Finberg, Laurence. *Rickets.* E-Medicine December 18, 2003 [cited March 30, 2005]. < http://www.emedicine.com/ped/topic2014.htm >.

Tish Davidson, A.M.

Rickets *see* **Vitamin D deficiency**

Rickettsia rickettsii infection *see* **Rocky Mountain spotted fever**

Rickettsialpox

Definition

Rickettsialpox is a relatively mild disease caused by a member of the bacterial family called Rickettsia. Rickettsialpox causes rash, **fever**, chills, heavy sweating, **headache**, eye **pain** (especially when exposed to light), weakness, and achy muscles.

Description

Like other members of the family of Rickettsia, the bacteria causing rickettsialpox live in mice. Tiny mites feed on these infected mice, thus acquiring the organism. When these mites feed on humans, the bacteria can be transmitted.

Rickettsialpox occurs mostly within cities. In the United States, the disease has cropped up in such places as New York City, Boston, Philadelphia, Pittsburgh, and Cleveland. It has also been identified in Russia, Korea, and Africa.

Causes and symptoms

The specific bacteria responsible for rickettsialpox is called *Rickettsia akari*. A person contracts this bacteria through the bite of an infected mite. After a person has been bitten by an infected mite, there is a delay of about 10 days to three weeks prior to the onset of symptoms.

The first symptom is a bump which appears at the site of the original bite. The bump (papule) develops a tiny, fluid-filled head (vesicle). The vesicle sloughs

Resources

ORGANIZATIONS

Centers for Disease Control and Prevention. 1600 Clifton Rd., NE, Atlanta, GA 30333. (800) 311-3435, (404) 639-3311. < http://www.cdc.gov >.

Rosalyn Carson-DeWitt, MD

Rifampin *see* **Antituberculosis drugs**

Ringing ears *see* **Tinnitus**

away, leaving a crusty black scab in its place (eschar). In about a week, the patient develops a fever, chills, heavy sweating, headache, eye pain (especially when exposed to light), weakness, and achy muscles. The fever rises and falls over the course of about a weak. A bumpy rash spreads across the body. Each individual papule follows the same progression: papule, then vesicle, then eschar. The rash does not affect the palms of the hands or the soles of the feet.

Diagnosis

Most practitioners are able to diagnose rickettsialpox simply on the basis of its rising and falling fever, and its characteristic rash. Occasionally, blood will be drawn and tests performed to demonstrate the presence of antibodies (immune cells directed against specific bacterial agents) which would confirm a diagnosis of rickettsialpox.

Treatment

Because rickettsialpox is such a mild illness, some practitioners choose to simply treat the symptoms (giving **acetaminophen** for fever and achiness, pushing fluids to avoid **dehydration**). Others will give their patients a course of the antibiotic tetracycline, which will shorten the course of the illness to about one to two days.

Prognosis

Prognosis for full recovery from rickettsialpox is excellent. No deaths have ever been reported from this illness, and even the skin rash heals without scarring.

Prevention

As with all mite- or tick-borne illnesses, prevention includes avoidance of areas known to harbor the insects, and/or careful application of insect repellents. Furthermore, because mice pass the bacteria on to the mites, it is important to keep mice from nesting in or around residences.

Ringworm

Definition

Ringworm is a common fungal infection of the skin. The name is a misnomer since the disease is not caused by a worm.

Description

More common in males than in females, ringworm is characterized by patches of rough, reddened skin. Raised eruptions usually form the circular pattern that gives the condition its name. Ringworm may also be referred to as dermatophyte infection.

As lesions grow, the centers start to heal. The inflamed borders expand and spread the infection.

Types of ringworm

Ringworm is a term that is commonly used to encompass several types of fungal infection. Sometimes, however, only body ringworm is classified as true ringworm.

Body ringworm (tinea corporis) can affect any part of the body except the scalp, feet, and facial area where a man's beard grows. The well-defined, flaky sores can be dry and scaly or moist and crusty.

Scalp ringworm (tinea capitis) is most common in children. It causes scaly, swollen blisters or a rash that looks like black dots. Sometimes inflamed and filled with pus, scalp ringworm lesions can cause crusting, flaking, and round bald patches. Most common in black children, scalp ringworm can cause scarring and permanent hair loss.

Ringworm of the groin (tinea cruris or **jock itch**) produces raised red sores with well-marked edges. It can spread to the buttocks, inner thighs, and external genitals.

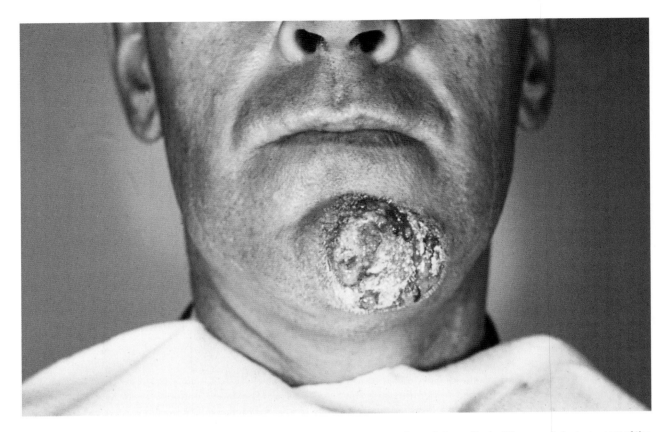

Ringworm on a man's chin. These infections are most common on the feet, scalp, or in toenails, but they can infect any part of the skin. *(Custom Medical Stock Photo. Reproduced by permission.)*

Ringworm of the nails (tinea unguium) generally starts at the tip of one or more toenails, which gradually thicken and discolor. The nail may deteriorate or pull away from the nail bed. Fingernail infection is far less common.

Causes and symptoms

Ringworm can be transmitted by infected people or pets or by towels, hairbrushes, or other objects contaminated by them. Symptoms include inflammation, scaling, and sometimes, **itching**.

Diabetes mellitus increases susceptibility to ringworm. So do dampness, humidity, and dirty, crowded living areas. Braiding hair tightly and using hair gel also raise the risk.

Diagnosis

Diagnosis is based on microscopic examination of scrapings taken from lesions. A dermatologist may also study the scalp of a patient with suspected tinea capitis under ultraviolet light.

Treatment

Some infections disappear without treatment. Others respond to such topical antifungal medications as naftifine (Caldesene Medicated Powder) or tinactin (Desenex) or to griseofulvin (Fulvicin), which is taken by mouth. Medications should be continued for two weeks after lesions disappear.

A person with body ringworm should wear loose clothing and check daily for raw, open sores. Wet dressings applied to moist sores two or three times a day can lessen inflammation and loosen scales. The doctor may suggest placing special pads between folds of infected skin, and anything the patient has touched or worn should be sterilized in boiling water.

Infected nails should be cut short and straight and carefully cleared of dead cells with an emery board.

Patients with jock itch should:

- wear cotton underwear and change it more than once a day
- keep the infected area dry
- apply antifungal ointment over a thin film of antifungal powder

Shampoo containing selenium sulfide can help prevent spread of scalp ringworm, but prescription shampoo or oral medication is usually needed to cure the infection.

Alternative treatment

The fungal infection ringworm can be treated with homeopathic remedies. Among the homeopathic remedies recommended are:

- *sepia* for brown, scaly patches
- *tellurium* for prominent, well-defined, reddish sores
- *graphites* for thick scales or heavy discharge
- *sulphur* for excessive itching.

Topical applications of antifungal herbs and essential oils also can help resolve ringworm. Tea tree oil (*Melaleuca* spp.), thuja (*Thuja occidentalis*), and lavender (*Lavandula officinalis*) are the most common. Two drops of essential oil in 1/4 oz of carrier oil is the dose recommended for topical application. Essential oils should not be applied to the skin undiluted. Botanical medicine can be taken internally to enhance the body's immune response. A person must be susceptible to exhibit this overgrowth of fungus on the skin. **Echinacea**(*Echinacea* spp.) and astragalus (*Astragalus membranaceus*) are the two most common immune-enhancing herbs. A well-balanced diet, including protein, complex carbohydrates, fresh fruits and vegetables, and good quality fats, is also important in maintaining optimal immune function.

Prognosis

Ringworm can usually be cured, but recurrence is common. Chronic infection develops in one patient in five.

It can take six to 12 months for new hair to cover bald patches, and three to 12 months to cure infected fingernails. Toenail infections do not always respond to treatment.

Prevention

Likelihood of infection can be lessened by avoiding contact with infected people or pets or contaminated objects and staying away from hot, damp places.

Resources

OTHER

"Ringworm." *YourHealth.com Page.* April 7, 1998. <http://www.yourhealth.com>.

Maureen Haggerty

Rinne test *see* **Hearing tests with a tuning fork**

Ritonavir *see* **Protease inhibitors**

River blindness *see* **Filariasis**

RMSF *see* **Rocky Mountain spotted fever**

Rocky Mountain spotted fever

Definition

Rocky Mountain spotted **fever** (RMSF) is a tick-borne illness caused by a bacteria, resulting in a high fever and a characteristic rash.

Description

The bacteria causing RMSF is passed to humans through the bite of an infected tick. The illness begins within about two weeks of such a bite. RMSF is the most widespread tick-borne illness in the United States, occurring in every state except Alaska and Hawaii. The states in the mid-Atlantic region, the Carolinas, and the Virginias have a great deal of tick activity during the spring and summer months, and the largest number of RMSF cases come from those states. About 5% of all ticks carry the causative bacteria. Children under the age of 15 years have the majority of RMSF infections.

Causes and symptoms

The bacterial culprit in RMSF is called *Rickettsia rickettsii*. It causes no illness in the tick carrying it, and can be passed on to the tick's offspring. When a tick attaches to a human, the bacteria is passed. The tick must be attached to the human for about six hours for this passage to occur. Although prompt tick removal will cut down on the chance of contracting RMSF, removal requires great care. If the tick's head and body are squashed during the course of removal, the bacteria can be inadvertently rubbed into the tiny bite wound.

Symptoms of RMSF begin within two weeks of the bite of the infected tick. Symptoms usually begin suddenly, with high fever, chills, **headache**, severe weakness, and muscle **pain**. Pain in the large muscle of the calf is very common, and may be particularly severe. The patient may be somewhat confused and delirious. Without treatment, these symptoms may last two weeks or more.

The rash of RMSF is quite characteristic. It usually begins on the fourth day of the illness, and occurs in at least 90% of all patients with RMSF. It starts around the wrists and ankles, as flat pink marks (called macules). The rash spreads up the arms and legs, toward the chest, abdomen, and back. Unlike **rashes** which accompany various viral infections, the rash of RMSF does spread to the palms of the hands and the soles of the feet. Over a couple of days, the macules turn a reddish-purple color. They are now called petechiae, which are tiny areas of bleeding under the skin (pinpoint hemorrhages). This signifies a new phase of the illness. Over the next several days, the individual petechiae may spread into each other, resulting in larger patches of hemorrhage.

The most severe effects of RMSF occur due to damage to the blood vessels, which become leaky. This accounts for the production of petechiae. As blood and fluid leak out of the injured blood vessels, other tissues and organs may swell and become damaged, and:

- breathing difficulties may arise as the lungs are affected.
- heart rhythms may become abnormal
- kidney failure occurs in very ill patients
- liver function drops
- the patient may experience **nausea**, **vomiting**, abdominal pain, and diarrhea
- the brain may swell (**encephalitis**) in about 25% of all RMSF patients (brain injury can result in seizures, changes in consciousness, actual **coma**, loss of coordination, imbalance on walking, **muscle spasms**, loss of bladder control, and various degrees of paralysis)
- the clotting system becomes impaired, and blood may be evident in the stools or vomit

Diagnosis

Diagnosis of RMSF is almost always made on the basis of the characteristic symptoms, coupled with either a known tick bite (noted by about 60–70% of patients) or exposure to an area known to harbor ticks. Complex tests exist to nail down a diagnosis of RMSF, but these are performed in only a few laboratories. Because the results of these tests take so long to obtain, they are seldom used. This is because delaying treatment is the main cause of **death** in patients with RMSF.

Treatment

It is essential to begin treatment absolutely as soon as RMSF is seriously suspected. Delaying treatment can result in death.

Antibiotics are used to treat RMSF. The first choice is a form of tetracycline; the second choice (used in young children and pregnant women) is chloramphenicol. If the patient is well enough, treatment by oral intake of medicine is perfectly effective. Sicker patients will need to be given the medication through a needle in the vein (intravenously). Penicillin and sulfa drugs are not suitable for treatment of RMSF, and their use may increase the death rate by delaying the use of truly effective medications.

Very ill patients will need to be hospitalized in an intensive care unit. Depending on the types of complications a particular patient experiences, a variety of treatments may be necessary, including intravenous fluids, blood transfusions, anti-seizure medications, **kidney dialysis**, and mechanical ventilation (a breathing machine).

Alternative treatment

Although alternative treatments should never be used in place of conventional treatment with antibiotics, they can be useful adjuncts to antibiotic therapy. The use of *Lactobacillus acidophilus* and *L. bifidus* supplementaion during and after antibiotic treatment can help rebalance the intestinal flora. **Acupuncture**, homeopathy, and botanical medicine can all be beneficial supportive therapies during recovery from this disease.

Prognosis

Prior to the regular use of antibiotics to treat RMSF, the death rate was about 25%. Although the death rate from RMSF has improved greatly with an understanding of the importance of early use of antibiotics, there is still a 5% death rate. This rate is believed to be due to delays in the administration of appropriate medications.

Certain risk factors suggest a worse outcome in RMSF. Death rates are higher in males and increase as people age. It is considered a bad prognostic sign to develop symptoms of RMSF within only two to five days of a tick bite.

Prevention

The mainstay of prevention involves avoiding areas known to harbor ticks. However, because

KEY TERMS

Encephalitis—Inflammation of the tissues of the brain.

Macule—A flat, discolored area on the skin.

Petechia—A small, round, reddish purple spot on the skin, representing a tiny area of bleeding under the skin.

many people enjoy recreational activities in just such areas, the following steps can be taken:

- Wear light colored clothing (so that attached ticks are more easily noticed).
- Wear long sleeved shirts and long pants; tuck the pants legs into socks.
- Spray clothing with appropriate tick repellents.
- Examine. Anybody who has been outside for any amount of time in an area known to have a population of ticks should examine his or her body carefully for ticks. Parents should examine their children at the end of the day.
- Remove any ticks using tweezers, so that infection doesn't occur due to handling the tick. Grasp the tick's head with the tweezers, and pull gently but firmly so that the head and body are entirely removed.
- Keep areas around homes clear of brush, which may serve to harbor ticks.

Resources

ORGANIZATIONS

Centers for Disease Control and Prevention. 1600 Clifton Rd., NE, Atlanta, GA 30333. (800) 311-3435, (404) 639-3311. < http://www.cdc.gov >.

Rosalyn Carson-DeWitt, MD

Rogaine *see* **Minoxidil**

Rolfing

Definition

Rolfing, also called Rolf therapy or structural integration, is a holistic system of bodywork that uses deep manipulation of the body's soft tissue to

IDA P. ROLF, PH.D. (1896–1979)

Born in New York City and raised in the Bronx, Ida P. Rolf attended school in the New York area, graduating from Barnard College in 1916. In 1920, she graduated from the Columbia University College of Physicians and Surgeons with a doctorate in biological chemistry. For the next 12 years, she worked in the departments of chemotherapy and organic chemistry at the Rockefeller Institute. During an extended leave of absence, she studied atomic physics and mathematics at the Swiss Technical University in Zurich and homeopathic medicine in Geneva. During the 1930s, she studied osteopathy, chiropractic medicine, tantric yoga, the Alexander Technique of tension reduction through body movement, and the philosophy of altered states of consciousness of Alfred H.S. Korzybski.

Her interest in body structure, movement, and manipulation began after being kicked by a horse shortly after graduating from Barnard. The accident left her with acute pneumonia. Dissatisfied with conventional medical treatment, she began her quest for more natural and effective ways of treating the body.

By 1940, Dr. Rolf had developed a technique of body movement she called structural integration, also known today as Rolfing. The therapy reshapes the body's muscular structure by applying pressure and energy, freeing the body from physical and emotional traumas. In 1977, she authored *Rolfing: The Integration of Human Structures*. She continued to teach and refine her therapy until her death in 1979. Dr. Rolf's desire to teach her work to others led to her establishing the Guild for Structural Engineering, now known as the Rolf Institute of Structural Integration, 205 Canyon Blvd., Boulder, CO 80302.

realign and balance the body's myofascial structure. Rolfing improves posture, relieves chronic **pain**, and reduces **stress**.

Purpose

Rolfing helps to improve posture and bring the body's natural structure into proper balance and alignment. This can bring relief from general aches and pains, improve breathing, increase energy, improve self-confidence, and relieve physical and mental stress. Rolfing has also been used to treat such specific physical problems as chronic back, neck, shoulder, and joint pain, and repetitive stress injuries, including **carpal tunnel syndrome**. Many amateur and professional athletes, including Olympic skaters and skiers, use Rolfing to keep in top condition, to prevent injuries, and to more quickly recover from injuries.

Description

Origins

Ida Pauline Rolf (1896–1979) was a biochemist from New York who developed structural integration over the course of many years after an accident as a young woman. She was kicked by a horse's hoof on a trip out West and developed symptoms resembling those of acute **pneumonia**. She made her way to a hospital in Montana, where she was treated by a physician who called in an osteopath to assist in her treatment. After the osteopath treated her, she was able to breathe normally. After her return to New York, her mother took her to a blind osteopath for further treatment. He taught her about the body's structure and function, after which Rolf became dissatisfied with conventional medical treatment. Following completion of a doctorate in biochemistry from Columbia University in 1920, Rolf studied atomic physics, mathematics, and **homeopathic medicine** in Europe. After 1928, when her father died and left her an inheritance that allowed her to pursue her own studies, she explored various forms of alternative treatment, including **osteopathy, chiropractic** medicine, tantric **yoga**, the **Alexander technique** of tension reduction through body movement, and Alfred Korzybski's philosophy of altered states of consciousness.

By 1940, Rolf had synthesized what she had learned from these various disciplines into her own technique of body movement that she called structural integration, which later became known as Rolfing. During the Second World War, Rolf continued to study with an osteopath in California named Amy Cochran. In the mid-1960s, Gestalt therapist Fritz Perls invited Rolf to Esalen, where she began to develop a following among people involved in the human potential movement. In 1977, she published *Rolfing: The Integration of Human Structures*, the definitive book on structural integration bodywork. She continued to refine the therapy until her death in 1979. Rolf's work is carried on through her Guild for Structural Integration, now known as the Rolf Institute of Structural Integration, which she founded in 1971 in Boulder, Colo.

Rolfing is more than just a massage of the body's surface. It is a system that reshapes the body's myofascial structure by applying pressure and energy, thereby freeing the body from the effects of physical and emotional traumas. Although Rolfing is used extensively to treat **sports injuries** and back pain, it is not designed as a therapy for any particular condition. Rather, it is a systematic approach to overall wellness. It works by counteracting the effects of gravity, which over time pulls the body out of alignment. This pull causes the body's connective tissue to become harder and stiffer, and the muscles to atrophy. Signs of this stiffening and contraction include slouching or an overly erect posture.

Rolfing identifies the vertical line as the ideal that the body should approximate. The mission statement of the Guild for Structural Integration describes Rolfing as "a method and a philosophy of personal growth and integrity.... The vertical line is our fundamental concept. The physical and psychological embodiment of the vertical line is a way of Being in the physical world [that] forms a basis for personal growth and integrity."

The basic ten

Basic Rolfing treatment consists of 10 sessions, each lasting 60–90 minutes and costing about $100 each. The sessions are spaced a week or longer apart. After a period of integration, specialized or advanced treatment sessions are available. A "tuneup" session is recommended every six months. In each session, the Rolfer uses his or her fingers, hands, knuckles, and elbows to rework the connective tissue over the entire body. The tissues are worked until they become pliable, allowing the muscles to lengthen and return to their normal alignment. The deep tissue manipulation improves posture and agility, and increases the body's range of movement. Rolfers also believe that the blocked energy accumulated in the tissue from emotional tension is released through Rolfing treatment, causing the patient to feel more energetic and have a more positive frame of mind.

Clients are asked to wait for a period of six to 12 months before scheduling advanced work, known as the PostTen/Advanced Series. This period allows the body to integrate the work done in the "Basic Ten."

Rolfing movement integration

Rolfing movement integration, or RMI, is intended to help clients develop better awareness of their vertical alignment and customary movement patterns. They learn to release tension and discover better ways to use body movement effectively.

Rolfing rhythms

Rolfing rhythms are a series of exercises intended to remind participants of the basic principles of Rolfing: ease, length, balance, and harmony with gravity. In addition, Rolfing rhythms improve the client's flexibility as well as muscle tone and coordination.

KEY TERMS

Atrophy—A progressive wasting and loss of function of any part of the body.

Carpal tunnel syndrome—A condition caused by compression of the median nerve in the carpal tunnel of the hand, characterized by pain.

Fascia—The sheet of connective tissue that covers the body under the skin and envelops every muscle, bone, nerve, gland, organ, and blood vessel. Fascia helps the body to retain its basic shape.

Osteopathy—A system of medical practice that believes that the human body can make its own remedies to heal infection. It originally used manipulative techniques but also added surgical, hygienic, and medicinal methods when needed.

Parasympathetic nervous system—A part of the autonomic nervous system that is concerned with conserving and restoring energy. It is the part of the nervous system that predominates in a state of relaxation.

Structural integration—The term used to describe the method and philosophy of life associated with Rolfing. Its fundamental concept is the vertical line.

Preparations

No pre-procedure preparations are needed to begin Rolfing treatment. The treatment is usually done on a massage table with the patient wearing only undergarments. Prior to the first session, however, the client is asked to complete a health questionnaire, and photographs are taken to assist with evaluation of his or her progress.

Precautions

Since Rolfing involves vigorous deep tissue manipulation, it is often described as uncomfortable and sometimes painful, especially during the first several sessions. In the past decade, however, Rolfers have developed newer techniques that cause less discomfort to participants. Since Rolfing is a bodywork treatment that requires the use of hands, it may be a problem for people who do not like or are afraid of being touched. It is not recommended as a treatment for any disease or a chronic inflammatory condition such as arthritis, and can worsen such a condition. Anyone with a serious medical condition, including heart disease, diabetes, or respiratory problems, should consult with a medical practitioner before undergoing Rolfing.

Side effects

There are no reported serious side effects associated with Rolfing when delivered by a certified practitioner to adults and juveniles.

Research and general acceptance

There is a growing amount of mainstream scientific research documenting the effectiveness of Rolf therapy. A 1988 study published in the *Journal of the American Physical Therapy Association* indicated that Rolfing stimulates the parasympathetic nervous system, which can help speed the recovery of damaged tissue. Other studies done in the 1980s concerned the effectiveness of Rolfing in treating figure skaters and children with **cerebral palsy**. In 1992 a presentation was made to the National Center of Medical **Rehabilitation** Research regarding Rolfing in the treatment of degenerative joint disease. A 1997 article in *The Journal of Orthopedic and Sports Physical Therapy* reported that Rolfing can provide effective and sustained pain relief from lower back problems.

Resources

BOOKS

Levine, Andrew S., and Valerie J. Levine. *The Bodywork and Massage Sourcebook*. Lincolnwood, IL: Lowell House. 1999.

ORGANIZATIONS

Rolf Institute of Structural Integration. 209 Canyon Blvd. P.O. Box 1868. Boulder, CO 80306-1868. (303) 449-5903. (800) 530-8875. < http://www.rolf.org >.

Ken R. Wells

Root canal treatment

Definition

Root canal treatment, also known as endodontic treatment, is a dental procedure in which the diseased or damaged pulp (core) of a tooth is removed and the inside areas (the pulp chamber and root canals) are filled and sealed.

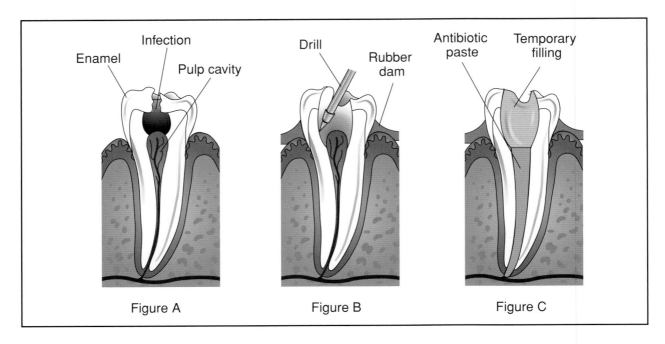

Root canal treatment is a dental procedure in which the diseased pulp of a tooth is removed and the inside areas are filled and sealed. In figure A, the infection can be seen above the pulp cavity. The dentist drills into the enamel and the pulp cavity is extracted (figure B). Finally, the dentist fills the pulp cavity with antibiotic paste and a temporary filling (figure C). *(Illustration by Electronic Illustrators Group.)*

Purpose

Inflamed or infected pulp (pulpitis) most often causes a **toothache**. To relieve the **pain** and prevent further complications, the tooth may be extracted (surgically removed) or saved by root canal treatment. Root canal treatment has become a common dental procedure; more than 14 million are performed every year, with a 95% success rate, according to the American Association of Endodontists.

Precautions

Once root canal treatment is performed, the patient must have a crown placed over the tooth to protect it. The cost of the treatment and the crown may be expensive. However, replacing an extracted tooth with a fixed bridge, a removable partial denture, or an implant to maintain the space and restore the chewing function is typically even more expensive.

Description

Root canal treatment may be performed by a general dentist or by an endodontist, a dentist who specializes in endodontic (literally "inside of the tooth") procedures. Inside the tooth, the pulp's soft tissue contains the blood supply, by which the tooth gets its nutrients, and the nerve, by which the tooth senses hot and cold. This tissue is vulnerable to damage from deep dental decay, accidental injury, tooth fracture, or trauma from repeated dental procedures (such as multiple fillings over time). If a tooth becomes diseased or injured, bacteria build up inside the pulp, spreading infection from the natural crown of the tooth to the root tips in the jawbone. Pus accumulates at the ends of the roots, forming a painful **abscess** which can damage the bone supporting the teeth. Such an infection may produce pain that is severe, constant, or throbbing, as well as prolonged sensitivity to heat or cold, swelling and tenderness in the surrounding gums, facial swelling, and discoloration of the tooth. However, in some cases, the pulp may die so gradually that there is little noticeable pain.

Root canal treatment is performed under **local anesthesia**. A thin sheet of rubber, called a rubber dam, is placed in the mouth to isolate the tooth. The dentist removes any **tooth decay** and makes an opening through the natural crown of the tooth into the pulp chamber. Creating this access also relieves the pressure inside the tooth and can dramatically ease pain.

The dentist determines the length of the root canals, usually with a series of x rays. Small wire-like files are then used to clean the entire canal space of diseased pulp tissue and bacteria. The debris is flushed out with large amounts of water (irrigation). The canals are also slightly enlarged and shaped to receive an inert (non-reactive) filling material called gutta percha. However, the tooth is not filled and permanently sealed until it is completely free of active infection. The dentist may place a temporary seal, or leave the tooth open to drain, and prescribe an antibiotic to counter any spread of infection from the tooth. This is why root canal treatment may require several visits to the dentist.

Once the canals are completely clean, they are filled with gutta percha and a sealer cement to prevent bacteria from entering the tooth in the future. A metal post may be placed in the pulp chamber for added structural support and better retention of the crown restoration. The tooth is protected by a temporary filling or crown until a permanent restoration may be made. This restoration is usually a gold or porcelain crown, although it may be a gold inlay, or an amalgam or composite filling (paste fillings that harden).

Preparation

There is no typical preparation for root canal treatment. Once the tooth is opened to drain, the dentist may prescribe an antibiotic, then the patient should take the full prescribed course. With the infection under control, local anesthetic is more effective, so that the root canal procedure may be performed without discomfort.

Aftercare

The tooth may be sore for several days after filling. Pain relievers, such as ibuprofen (Advil, Motrin) may be taken to ease the soreness. The tissues around the tooth may also be irritated. Rinsing the mouth with hot salt water several times a day will help. Chewing on that side of the mouth should be avoided for the first few days following treatment. A follow-up appointment should be scheduled with the dentist for six months after treatment to make sure the tooth and surrounding structures are healthy.

Risks

There is a possibility that the root canal treatment will not be successful the first time. If infection and inflammation recur and an x ray indicates retreatment is feasible, the old filling material is removed and the canals are thoroughly cleaned out. The dentist will try

---

KEY TERMS

Abscess—A hole in the tooth or gum tissue filled with pus as the result of infection. Its swelling exerts pressure on the surrounding tissues, causing pain.

Apicoectomy—Also called root resectioning. The root tip of a tooth is accessed in the bone and a small amount is shaved away. The diseased tissue is removed and a filling is placed to reseal the canal.

Crown—The natural crown of a tooth is that part of the tooth covered by enamel. Also, a restorative crown is a protective shell that fits over a tooth.

Endodontic—Pertaining to the inside structures of the tooth, including the dental pulp and tooth root, and the periapical tissue surrounding the root.

Endodontist—A dentist who specializes in the diagnosis and treatment of disorders affecting the inside structures of the tooth.

Extraction—The surgical removal of a tooth from its socket in the bone.

Gutta percha—An inert latex-like substance used for filling root canals.

Pulp—The soft innermost layer of a tooth, containing blood vessels and nerves.

Pulp chamber—The area within the natural crown of the tooth occupied by dental pulp.

Pulpitis—Inflammation of the pulp of a tooth involving the blood vessels and nerves.

Root canal—The space within a tooth that runs from the pulp chamber to the tip of the root.

Root canal treatment—The process of removing diseased or damaged pulp from a tooth, then filling and sealing the pulp chamber and root canals.

---

to identify and correct problems with the first root canal treatment before filling and sealing the tooth a second time.

In cases where an x ray indicates that retreatment cannot correct the problem, endodontic surgery may be performed. In a procedure called an apicoectomy, or root resectioning, the root end of the tooth is accessed in the bone, and a small amount is shaved away. The area is cleaned of diseased tissue and a filling is placed to reseal the canal.

In some cases, despite root canal treatment and endodontic surgery, the tooth dies anyway and must be extracted.

Normal results

With successful root canal treatment, the tooth will no longer cause pain. However, because it does not contain an internal nerve, it no longer has sensitivity to hot, cold, or sweets. These are signs of dental decay, so the patient must receive regular dental check-ups with periodic x rays to avoid further disease in the tooth. The restored tooth could last a lifetime; however, with routine wear, the filling or crown may eventually need to be replaced.

Resources

ORGANIZATIONS

American Association of Endodontists. 211 East Chicago Ave., Ste. 1100, Chicago, IL 60611-2691. (800) 872-3636. < http://www.aae.org >.

American Dental Association. 211 E. Chicago Ave., Chicago, IL 60611. (312) 440-2500. < http://www.ada.org >.

OTHER

"Endodontic (Root Canal) Therapy." *Tooth Talk and Your Health with Dr. Frank Gober.* < http://www.toothtalk.com >.

"Root Canal Treatment." *Annapolis Endodontics.* < http://users.erols.com/canals/index.html >.

"Root Canal Treatment." *Value Added Benefits.* < http://www.vab.com >.

Thivierge, Bethany. "What is the Value (and Cost) of a Root Canal?" *A Healthy Me Page.* < http://www.ahealthyme.com/topic/rootcanal >.

Bethany Thivierge

Rosacea

Definition

Rosacea is a skin disease typically appearing in people during their 30s and 40s. It is marked by redness (erythema) of the face, flushing of the skin, and the presence of hard pimples (papules) or pus-filled pimples (pustules), and small visible spider-like veins called telangiectasias. In later stages of the disease, the face may swell and the nose may take on a bulb-like appearance called rhinophyma.

Description

Rosacea produces redness and flushing of the skin, as well as pustules and papules. Areas of the face, including the nose, cheeks, forehead, and chin, are the primary sites, but some people experience symptoms on their necks, backs, scalp, arms, and legs.

The similarity in appearance of rosacea to **acne** led people in the past to erroneously call the disease acne rosacea or adult acne. Like acne, the skin can have pimples and papules. Unlike acne, however, people with rosacea do not have blackheads.

In early stages of rosacea, people typically experience repeated episodes of flushing. Later, areas of the face are persistently red, telangiectasia appear on the nose and cheeks, as well as inflamed papules and pustules. Over time, the skin may take on a roughened, orange peel texture. Very late in the disorder, a small group of patients with rosacea will develop rhinophyma, which can give the nose a bulb-like look.

Up to one half of patients with rosacea may experience symptoms related to their eyes. Ocular rosacea, as it is called, frequently precedes the other manifestations on the skin. Most of these eye symptoms do not threaten sight, however. Telangiectasia may appear around the borders of the eyelid, the eyelids may be chronically inflamed, and small lumps called chalazions may develop. The cornea of the eye, the transparent covering over the lens, can also be affected, and in some cases vision will be affected.

Causes and symptoms

There is no known specific cause of rosacea. A history of redness and flushing precedes the disease in most patients. The consensus among many experts is that multiple factors may lead to an overreaction of the facial blood vessels, which triggers flushing. Over time, persistent episodes of redness and flushing leave the face continually inflamed. Pimples and blood-vessel changes follow.

Certain genetic factors may also come into play, although these have not been fully described. The disease is more common in women and light-skinned, fair-haired people. It may be more common in people of Celtic background, although this is an area of disagreement among experts.

Certain **antibiotics** are useful in the treatment of rosacea, leading some researchers to suspect a bacterium or other infectious agent may be the cause. One of the newest suspects is a bacterium called *Helicobacter pylori*, which has been implicated in causing many cases of stomach ulcers but the evidence here is mixed.

Other investigators have observed that a particular parasite, the mite *Demodex folliculorum*, can be found in areas of the skin affected by rosacea. The mite can also be detected, however, in the skin of people who do not have the disease. It is likely that the mite does not cause rosacea, but merely aggravates it.

Diagnosis

Diagnosis of rosacea is made by the presence of clinical symptoms. There is no specific test for the disease. Episodes of persistent flushing, redness (erythema) of the nose, cheeks, chin, and forehead, accompanied by pustules and papules are hallmarks of the disease. A dermatologist will attempt to rule out a number of other diseases that have similar symptoms. Acne vulgaris is perhaps the disorder most commonly mistaken for rosacea, but redness and spider-like veins are not observed in patients with acne. Blackheads and cysts, however, are seen in acne patients, but not in those with rosacea.

Other diseases that produce some of the same symptoms as rosacea include perioral **dermatitis** and **systemic lupus erythematosus**.

Treatment

The mainstay of treatment for rosacea is oral antibiotics. These appear to work by reducing inflammation in the small blood vessels and structure of the skin, not by destroying bacteria that are present. Among the more widely used oral antibiotics is tetracycline. In many patients, antibiotics are effective against the papules and pustules that can appear on the face, but they appear less effective against the background redness, and they have no effect on telangiectasia. Patients frequently take a relatively high dose of antibiotics until their symptoms are controlled, and then they slowly reduce their daily dose to a level that just keeps their symptoms in check. Other oral antibiotics used include erythromycin and minocycline.

Some patients are concerned about long-term use of oral antibiotics. For them, a topical agent applied directly to the face may be tried in addition to an oral antibiotic, or in its place. **Topical antibiotics** are also useful for controlling the papules and pustules of rosacea, but do not control the redness, flushing, and telangiectasias. The newest of these topical agents is metronidazole gel, which can be applied twice daily. Like the oral antibiotics, topical preparations appear to work by reducing inflammation, not by killing bacteria.

Vitamin A derivatives, called retinoids, also appear useful in the treatment of rosacea. An oral retinoid, called isotretinoin, which is used in severe cases of acne also reduces the pustules and papules in severe cases of rosacea that do not respond to antibiotics. Isotretinoin must be taken with care, however,

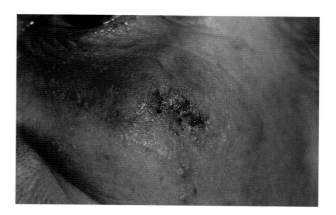

Rosacea on a woman's cheek. *(Custom Medical Stock Photo. Reproduced by permission.)*

particularly in women of childbearing age. They must agree to a reliable form of **contraception**, because the drug is known to cause **birth defects**.

Topical vitamin A derivatives that are used in the treatment of acne also may have a role in the treatment of rosacea. Accumulating evidence suggests that topical isotretinoin and topical azelaic acid can reduce the redness and pimples. Some patients who use these medications experience skin irritation that tends to resolve with time.

For later stages of the disorder, a surgical procedure may be needed to improve the appearance of the skin. To remove the telangiectasias, a dermatologist may use an electrocautery device to apply a current to the blood vessel in order to destroy it. Special lasers, called tunable dye lasers, can also be adjusted to selectively destroy these tiny blood vessels.

A variety of surgical techniques can be used to improve the shape and appearance of a bulbous nose in the later stages of the disease. Surgeons may use a scalpel or laser to remove excess tissue from the nose and restore a more natural appearance.

Alternative treatment

Alternative treatments have not been extensively studied in rosacea. Some reports advocate gentle circular massage for several minutes daily to the nose, cheeks, and forehead. Scientifically controlled studies are lacking, however.

Many people are able to avoid outbreaks by reducing things that trigger flushing. Alcoholic beverages, hot beverages, and spicy foods are among the more common factors in the diet that can provoke flushing. Reducing or eliminating these items in the diet can help limit rosacea outbreaks in many people. Exposure to heat, cold, and sunlight are also known triggers of flushing. The specific things that provoke flushing vary considerably from person to person, however. It usually takes some trial and error to figure these out.

A deficiency in hydrochloric acid (HCl) in the stomach may be a cause of rosacea, and supplementation with HCl capsules may bring relief in some cases.

Prognosis

The prognosis for controlling symptoms of rosacea and improving the appearance of the face is good. Many people require life-long treatment and achieve good results. There is no known cure for the disorder.

Prevention

Rosacea cannot be prevented, but once correctly diagnosed, outbreaks can be treated and repeated episodes can be limited.

Use mild soaps

Avoiding anything that irritates the skin is a good preventive measure for people with rosacea. Mild soaps and cleansers are recommended. Astringents and alcohol should be avoided.

Learn what triggers flushing

Reducing factors in the diet and environment that cause flushing of the face is another good preventive strategy. Alcoholic and hot beverages, and spicy foods are among the more common triggers.

Use sunscreen

Limiting exposure of the face to excesses of heat and cold can also help. A sunscreen with a skin protection factor (SPF) of 15 or greater used daily can limit the damage to the skin and small blood vessels caused by the sun, and reduce outbreaks.

Resources

ORGANIZATIONS

American Academy of Dermatology. 930 N. Meacham Road, P.O. Box 4014, Schaumburg, IL 60168-4014. (847) 330-0230. Fax: (847) 330-0050. < http://www.aad.org >.

National Rosacea Society. 800 S. Northwest Highway, Suite 200, Barrington, IL 60010. (888) 662-5874. < http://www.rosacea.org >.

Richard H. Camer

Rosary bead esophagus *see* **Diffuse esophageal spasm**

Roseola

Definition

Roseola is a common disease of babies or young children, in which several days of very high **fever** are followed by a rash.

Description

Roseola is an extraordinarily common infection, caused by a virus. About 90% of all children have been exposed to the virus, with about 33% actually demonstrating the syndrome of fever followed by rash.

The most common age for a child to contract roseola is between six and twelve months. Roseola infection strikes boys and girls equally. The infection may occur at any time of year, although late spring and early summer seem to be peak times for it.

Causes and symptoms

About 85% of the time, roseola is caused by a virus called Human Herpesvirus 6, or HHV-6. Although the virus is related to those herpesviruses known to cause sores on the lips or genitalia, HHV-6 causes a very different type of infection. HHV-6 is believed to be passed between people via infected saliva. A few other viruses (called enteroviruses) can

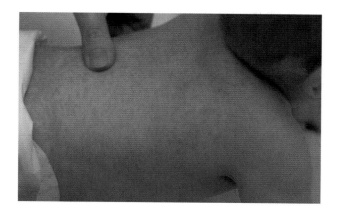

Roseola rash on infant's back and shoulders. *(Custom Medical Stock Photo. Reproduced by permission.)*

produce a similar fever-then-rash illness, which is usually also called roseola.

Researchers believe that it takes about 5-15 days to develop illness after having been infected by HHV-6. Roseola strikes suddenly, when a previously-well child spikes an impressively high fever. The temperature may reach 106°F. As is always the case with sudden fever spikes, the extreme change in temperature may cause certain children to have seizures. About 5-35% of all children with roseola will have these "febrile seizures."

The most notable thing about this early phase of roseola is the absence of symptoms, other than the high fever. Although some children have a slightly reddened throat, or a slightly runny nose, most children have no symptoms whatsoever, other than the sudden development of high fever. This fever lasts for between three and five days.

Somewhere around the fifth day, a rash begins on the body. The rash is usually composed of flat pink patches or spots, although there may be some raised patches as well. The rash usually starts on the chest, back, and abdomen, and then spreads out to the arms and neck. It may or may not reach the legs and face. The rash lasts for about three days, then fades.

Very rarely, roseola will cause more serious disease. Patients so afflicted will experience significant swelling of the lymph nodes, the liver, and the spleen. The liver may become sufficiently inflamed to interfere with its functioning, resulting in a yellowish color to the whites of the eyes and the skin (**jaundice**). This syndrome (called a mononucleosis-like syndrome, after the disease called mononucleosis that causes many of the same symptoms) has occurred in both infants and adults.

KEY TERMS

Jaundice—The development of a yellowish tone to the skin and the whites of the eyes, caused by poor liver function.

Mononuclosis—An infection which causes swelling of lymph nodes, spleen, and liver, usually accompanied by extremely sore throat, fever, headache, and intense long-lasting fatigue.

Diagnosis

The diagnosis of roseola is often made by carefully examining the feverish child to make sure that other illnesses are not causing the temperature spike. Once it is clear that no **pneumonia**, ear infection, **strep throat**, or other common childhood illness is present, the practitioner usually feels comfortable waiting to see if the characteristic rash of roseola begins.

Treatment

There are no treatments available to stop the course of roseola. **Acetaminophen** or ibuprofen is usually given to try to lower the fever. Children who are susceptible to seizures may be given a sedative medication when the fever first spikes, in an attempt to prevent such a seizure.

Prognosis

Children recover quickly and completely from roseola. The only complications are those associated with seizures, or the rare mononucleosis-like syndrome.

Prevention

Other than the usual good hygiene practices always recommended to decrease the spread of viral illness, no methods are available to specifically prevent roseola.

Resources

BOOKS

Kohl, Steve. "Human Herpesvirus 6." In *Nelson Textbook of Pediatrics*, edited by Richard E. Behrman. Philadelphia: W. B. Saunders Co., 1996.

Rosalyn Carson-DeWitt, MD

Roseola infantum *see* **Roseola**

Ross River Virus

Definition

Ross River Virus (RRV) is Australia's most common and widespread mosquito-borne pathogen. Also known as RRV disease, it can cause debilitating polyarthritis, rash, **fever**, and constitutional symptoms.

Description

Originally known as epidemic polyarthritis, RRV is a member of the *Togaviridae* family of arboviruses. RRV is transmitted in an animal host-vector-human cycle, where the vector is the mosquito. Serological investigations have indicated that native macropods are the main vertebrate hosts of RRV, although other animals can become infected as well. The RRV lives in the blood stream of an infected animal. When a mosquito feeds on the infected animal, the virus is transmitted to the insect where it rapidly multiplies. The virus is then passed onto the next animal or person the mosquito bites. It has been proposed that human-mosquito-human transmission can occur during RRV epidemics. One-third of all humans bitten by an infected mosquito will develop the RRV disease.

The RRV disease occurs throughout continental Australia. However, the majority of RRV infections occur in the northern states and along costal areas; in particular, the state of Queensland. Of the 4,800 cases reported annually in Australia, approximately 2,700 of these occur in Queensland. In addition to these cases, many more go unreported. Infection can occur year round, but outbreaks typically coincide with the increased mosquito activity of the wet season (between late November and the end of April). Also, areas with intensive irrigation and those near salt marches have higher mosquito populations, and, thus, tend to exhibit a higher number of RRV cases.

In addition to continental Australia, RRV is endemic to the Solomon Islands, East Timor, Papua New Guinea, and the adjacent islands of Indonesia. Epidemics have also been reported in the Cook Islands, Fiji, French Polynesia, New Caledonia, and Western Samoa.

Causes and symptoms

Many people that are infected with RRV will never develop symptoms. However, 25% to 45% of cases will develop symptoms within three days to three weeks (averaging nine days) of the infection. Symptoms will vary between patients, but typically include arthralgia, arthritis, myalgia, skin rash, fever, **fatigue**, **headache**, and swollen lymph nodes. **Tingling** and **pain** in the palms of the hands and soles of the feet can accompany these symptoms. Other, less frequent, symptoms can include general malaise, **nausea**, sore eyes, and **sore throat**.

Most patients with RRV disease (83% to 98%) experience symptoms of polyarthritis involving the wrists, knees, ankles, and small joints of the extremities. Less frequently affected joints include the elbows, toes, tarsal joints, vertebral joints, shoulders, and hips. Symptoms can range from restricted joint movement to prominent swell and severe pain. Although severe joint pain can last for only 2 to 6 weeks, over half of patients will continue to experience joint pain for 6 to 12 months after RRV infection. Symptoms typically diminish over time, but relapses are common and have been known to persist for several years. This persistent polyarthritis can lead to fatigue and myalgia, contributing to RRV diseases high morbidity.

Diagnosis

Diagnosis usually consists of serological tests to determine the presence and increase of RRV antibodies. Samples should be taken during the acute or convalescent stages of the illness. Testing will help clinicians differentiate between RRV disease and Barmah Forest virus disease, a very similar arbovirus. Virological tests can help distinguish between RRV disease and other causes of arthritis.

Treatment

No cure for RRV disease currently exists, so only its symptoms can be treated. In one of the few studies on RRV disease treatment, Cordon and Rouse (1995) found that roughly one-third of patients (36.4%) reported that **nonsteroidal anti-inflammatory drugs** (NSAIDS) provided them with the best symptomatic relief. In addition to NSAIDS, others patients found that rest (24.1%), **aspirin** and paracetamol (16.4%), or physical therapies (10.3%), such as **hydrotherapy**, massage, and physiotherapy, were their only source of symptom relief. Unfortunately, 20% of patients found none of these interventions effective. Health providers typically use one or a combination of these treatments for their patients. In particular, paracetamol has been found to be effective for treating the pain and fever associated with RRV disease.

Although some clinicians have found the use of oral corticosteroid useful and effective, this practice is considered unwise and unnecessary. The adverse

KEY TERMS

Arthralgia—Sharp, severe pain, extending along a nerve or group of nerves, experienced in a joint and/or joints.

Abrovirus viruses—Also known as arthropod-borne viruses, these viruses are maintained in nature through biological transmission between vertebrate hosts and blood-feeding arthropods. Infection occurs when an infected arthropod, such as a mosquito, feeds off a vertebrate, such as a human.

Macropods—Derived from the Greek, macropod literally means "large footed." Macropods are marsupials belonging to the family Macropodidae, which includes kangaroos, wallabies, tree kangaroos, pademelons, and several others.

Myalgia—Muscular pain or tenderness, typically of a diffuse and/or nonspecific nature.

Polyarthritis—A nonspecific term for arthritis involving two or more joints, typically associated with auto-immune forms of arthritis. Symptoms usually include pain, inflammation, and/or swelling in multiple joints.

effects associated with **corticosteroids** may outweigh their benefits, and may even worsen the RRV disease. More study is required on this and other treatment interventions of RRV disease.

Prognosis

Patients infected with RRV disease will fully recover within four to seven months. Although milder cases can recover within a few weeks, many cases have persisted for several years. Only the symptoms can be treated during this time, not the disease. Fortunately, RRV infection usually provides the patient with life-long immunity to future infection.

Prevention

Prevention techniques of RRV typically coincide with measures used to avoid mosquito bites; the primary source of the virus. These include the use of insect repellant (with 5% to 20% DEET) on exposed body parts, wearing loose-fitting clothes over the limbs and torso while outdoors, using mosquito coils and/or citronella candles outdoors, and limiting outdoor activities during peak biting periods and/or in areas with high mosquito density. While camping outdoors, knock-down spray or bed netting with pyrethrum is suggested.

Additional steps for reducing risk of being bitten include using screens in homes and removing mosquito-breeding areas near the home, such as uncovered water containers and old tires. Mosquito eradication programs can assist in reducing insect populations. An RRV vaccine is currently being developed.

Resources

BOOKS

Kay B.H., and J.G. Aaskov. "Ross River Virus (Epidemic Polyarthritis)". In *The Arboviruses: Epidemiology and Ecology (Vol. IV)*, edited by T.P. Monath. Boca Raton, FL: CRC Press, 1989, pp. 93-112.

PERIODICALS

Harley, D., A. Sleigh, S. Ritchie. "Ross River Virus Transmission, Infection, and Disease: A Cross-disciplinary Review." *Clinical Microbiology Reviews* 14 (October 2001): 909-932.

Harley, D., S. Ritchie, C. Bain, and A. Sleigh. "Risks for Ross River Virus Disease in Tropical Australia." *International Journal of Epidemiology* (January 26 2005): 1-8.

Flexman, J., D. Smith, J. Mackenzie, J. Fraser, S. Bass, L. Hueston, et al. "A Comparison of the Diseases Caused by Ross River Virus and Barmah Forest Virus." *Medical Journal of Australia* 169 (August 1998):159-163.

Hills, S. "Ross River Virus and Barmah Forest Virus Infection." *Australian Family Physician* 25 (December 1996):1822-1824.

OTHER

"Ross River Virus Infection- Fact Sheet" *Australian Government- Department of Health and Ageing* < http://www.health.gov.au/internet/wcms/Publishing.nsf/Content/health-arbovirus-pdf-fsrossriver.htm >.

Jason Fryer

Rotator cuff injury

Definition

A rotator cuff injury is a tear or inflammation of the rotator cuff tendons in the shoulder.

Description

Rotator cuff injury is known by several names, including pitcher's shoulder, swimmer's shoulder, and tennis shoulder. As these names imply, the injury occurs most frequently in athletes practicing sports that require the arm to be moved over the head repeatedly, such as pitching, swimming, tennis, and weight lifting. Rotator cuff tendonitis is an inflammation of the shoulder tendons while a rotator cuff tear is a ripping of one or more of the tendons.

The tendons of four muscles make up the rotator cuff. The muscles are the supraspinatus, infraspinatus, teres minor, and subscapularis. The tendons attach the muscles to four shoulder bones: the shoulder blade (scapula), the upper arm bone (humerus), and the collarbone (clavicle.) The rotator cuff tendons can also degenerate due to age, usually starting around age 40. Rotator cuff injury may also be caused by falling on the outstretched arm or joint of the elbow. Either of these may produce enough force to drive the humerus into the shoulder socket.

Causes and symptoms

Some areas of the rotator cuff tendons have poor blood supply. Thus, the tissue is very slow to heal and maintain itself during normal use. Tearing and inflammation in athletes is usually due to hard and repetitive use, especially in baseball pitchers. In non-athletes over age 40, the injuries usually occur as a result of lifting heavy objects. The two primary symptoms are **pain** and weakness in the shoulder or arm, especially with arm movement or at night. A partial tear may cause pain but still allow normal arm movement. A complete tear usually leaves the injured person unable to raise the arm away from the side.

Diagnosis

Diagnosis is usually made after a **physical examination**, often by a sports medicine physician. X rays are also sometimes used in diagnosis as well as an arthrogram. However, the arthrogram is an invasive procedure and may be painful afterwards. For this reason, **magnetic resonance imaging** (MRI) is preferred to determine tendon tears as it also show greater detail than the arthrogram.

Treatment

The primary treatment is resting the shoulder and, for minor tears and inflammation, applying ice packs. Anti-inflammatory medications may also be prescribed. As soon as pain decreases, physical therapy is usually started to help regain normal motion. If pain persists after several weeks, the physician may inject cortisone into the affected area.

Serious tears to the rotator cuff tendons usually require surgery to repair. An instrument called an arthroscope is used to view the shoulder joint and

---

KEY TERMS

Arthrogram—A test done by injecting dye into the shoulder joint and then taking x-rays. Areas where the dye leaks out indicate a tear in the tendons.

Arthroscope—An instrument for the visual examination of the interior of a joint.

Arthroscopy—Examination of a joint with an arthroscope or joint surgery using an arthroscope.

Cortisone—A hormone produced naturally by the adrenal glands or made synthetically.

Magnetic resonance imaging (MRI) scan—A special radiological test that uses magnetic waves to create pictures of an area, including bones, muscles, and tendons.

Spur—Any projection from a bone.

---

confirm the presence of a tear. The arthroscope can also be used to remove any bone spurs that may be present in the shoulder area. Current arthroscopic procedures usually involve a 2 in (5.1 cm) incision in the outer shoulder. Through this incision the torn rotator edge may be reattached to the humerus with stitches.

Alternative treatment

There are no effective alternative medicine treatments for rotator cuff injuries.

Prognosis

The prognosis for recovery from minor rotator cuff injuries is excellent. For serious injuries, the prognosis is usually good, some six weeks of physical therapy being required following surgery. Full recovery may take several more months. In some cases, the injury is so severe that it requires tendon grafts and muscle transfers. In rare cases, a severe injury is not repairable, usually because the tendon has been torn for too long a time.

Prevention

The best prevention is to avoid repetitive overhead arm movements and to develop shoulder strength.

Resources

PERIODICALS

Hersch, Jonathan C. "Arthroscopically Assisted Mini-Open Rotator Cuff Repairs." *The American Journal of Sports Medicine* May 2000: 301.

Huie, Gordon, and Peter D. McCann. "The Shoulder Exam and Diagnosing Rotator Cuff Injuries." *Physician Assistant* April 1999: 53.

Murrell, George A. C., and Judie R. Walton. "Diagnosis of Rotator Cuff Tears." *The Lancet* March 10, 2001: 769.

ORGANIZATIONS

American Academy of Orthopaedic Surgeons. 6300 N. River Road, Rosemont, IL 60018. (847) 823-7186. < http://www.aaos.org. >.

American Orthopaedic Society for Sports Medicine. 6300 N. River Road, Ste. 200, Rosemont, IL 60018. (847) 292-4900. < http://www.sportsmed.org. >.

OTHER

WebMD. < http://www.my.webmd.com >.

Ken R. Wells

Rotavirus infections

Definition

Rotavirus is the major cause of **diarrhea** and **vomiting** in young children worldwide. The infection is highly contagious and may lead to severe **dehydration** (loss of body fluids) and even **death**. In the United States, more than 50,000 children are hospitalized and up to 125 die each year as a result of rotavirus infection.

Description

Gastroenteritis, or inflammation of the stomach and the intestine, is the second most common illness in the United States, after the **common cold**. More than one-third of such cases are caused by viruses. Many different viruses can cause gastroenteritis, but the most common ones are the rotavirus and the Norwalk virus.

The name rotavirus comes from the Latin word "rota" for wheel and is given because the viruses have a distinct wheel-like shape. Rotavirus infection is also known as infantile diarrhea, or winter diarrhea, because it mainly targets infants and young children. The outbreaks are usually in the cooler months of winter.

The virus is classified into different groups (Group A through group G), depending on the type of protein marker (antigen) that is present on its surface. The diarrheal infection of children is caused by the Group A rotaviruses. Group B rotaviruses have caused major epidemics of adult diarrhea in China.

Group C rotavirus has been associated with rare cases of diarrheal outbreaks in Japan and England. Groups D through G have not been detected in humans.

Causes and symptoms

The main symptoms of the rotavirus infection are **fever**, stomach cramps, vomiting, and diarrhea (this could lead to severe dehydration). The symptoms last anywhere from four to six days. If a child has dry lips and tongue, dry skin, sunken eyes, and wets fewer than six diapers a day, it is a sign of dehydration and a physician needs to be notified. Because of the excellence of healthcare in this country, rotavirus is rarely fatal to American children. However, it causes deaths of up to a million children in the third world countries, every year.

The virus is usually spread by the "fecal-oral route." In other words, a child can catch a rotavirus infection if she puts her finger in her mouth after touching toys or things that have been contaminated by the stool of another infected child. This usually happens when children do not wash their hands after using the toilet, or before eating food.

The viruses can also spread by way of contaminated food and drinking water. Infected food handlers who prepare salads, sandwiches, and other foods that require no cooking can spread the disease. Generally, symptoms appear within 4–48 hours after exposure to the contaminated food or water.

Children between the ages of six months and two years, especially in a daycare setting, are the most susceptible to this infection. Breastfed babies may be less likely to become infected, because breast milk contains antibodies (proteins produced by the white blood cells of the immune system) that fight the illness. Nearly every child by the age of four has been infected by this virus, and has rotavirus antibodies in their body. The disease also targets the elderly and people who have weak immune systems.

Children who have been infected once can be infected again. However, second infections are less severe than the first infections. By the time a child has had two infections, the chances of subsequent severe infection is remote.

Diagnosis

The rotavirus infection is diagnosed by identifying the virus in the patient's stool. This is done using electron microscopy. Immunological tests such as ELISA (Enzyme-linked immunosorbent assay) are

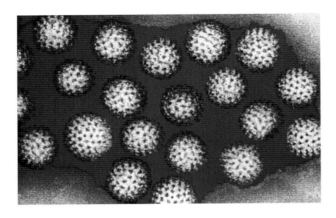

Rotaviruses are probably the most common viruses to infect humans and animals. These viruses are associated with gastroenteritis and diarrhea in humans and other animals. *(Photograph by Dr. Linda Stannard, Photo Researchers, Inc. Reproduced by permission.)*

also widely used for diagnosis, and several commercial kits are available.

Treatment

"Oral rehydration therapy," or drinking enough fluids to replace those lost through bowel movements and vomiting, is the primary aim of the treatment. Electrolyte and fluid replacement solutions are available over the counter in food and drug stores. Dehydration is one of the greatest dangers for infants and young children. If the diarrhea becomes severe, it may be necessary to hospitalize the patient so that fluids can be administered intravenously.

Anti-diarrheal medication should not be given to children unless directed to do so by the physician. Antibiotic therapy is not useful in viral illness. Specific drugs for the virus are not available.

Prognosis

Most of the infections resolve spontaneously. Dehydration due to severe diarrhea is one of the major complications.

Prevention

The best way to prevent the disease is by proper food handling and thorough hand washing, after using the toilet and whenever hands are soiled. In child care centers and hospital settings, the staff should be educated about personal and environmental hygiene. All dirty diapers should be regarded as infectious and disposed of in a sanitary manner.

Vaccines that prevent rotavirus in young children have been tested in nationwide trials. Researchers report that the vaccines appear to prevent the infection in 80% of the tested children. The vaccine is intended to be given orally (by mouth) at two, four, and six months of age. The only side effect of the vaccine is a low-grade fever in a small percentage of the children, three to four days after the **vaccination**. Within the next few years, a rotavirus vaccine may become part of every child's immunization schedule.

Resources

BOOKS

Fauci, Anthony S., et al., editors. *Harrison's Principles of Internal Medicine*. New York: McGraw-Hill, 1997.

Lata Cherath, PhD

Roundworm infections

Definition

Roundworm infections are diseases of the digestive tract and other organ systems caused by nematodes. Nematodes are parasitic worms with long, cylindrical bodies.

Description

Roundworm infections are widespread throughout the world, with some regional differences. Ascariasis and trichuriasis are more common in warm, moist climates where people use human or animal feces for fertilizer. Anisakiasis is most common in countries where raw or pickled fish or squid is a popular food item.

Causes and symptoms

The causes and symptoms of roundworm infection vary according to the species. Humans acquire most types of roundworm infection from contaminated food or by touching the mouth with unwashed hands.

Anisakiasis

Anisakiasis is caused by anisakid roundworms. Humans are not the primary host for these parasites. Anisakid roundworms infest whales, seals, and dolphins; crabs then ingest roundworm eggs from the feces of these animals. In the crabs, the eggs hatch into larvae that can infect fish. The larvae enter the muscles of marine animals further up the food chain, including squid, mackerel, herring, cod, salmon, tuna, and halibut. Humans become accidental hosts when they eat raw or undercooked fish containing anisakid larvae. The larvae attach themselves to the tissues lining the stomach and intestine, and eventually die inside the inflamed tissue.

In humans, anisakiasis can produce a severe syndrome that affects the stomach and intestines, or a mild chronic disease that may last for weeks or years. In acute anisakiasis, symptoms begin within one to seven hours after the patient eats infected seafood. Patients are often violently sick, with **nausea**, **vomiting**, **diarrhea**, and severe abdominal **pain** that may resemble **appendicitis**. In chronic anisakiasis, the patient has milder forms of stomach or intestinal irritation that resemble stomach ulcers or **irritable bowel syndrome**. In some cases, the acute form of the disease is followed by chronic infestation.

Ascariasis

Ascariasis, which is caused by *Ascaris lumbricoides*, is one of the most widespread parasitic infections in humans, affecting over 1.3 billion people worldwide. Ascarid roundworms cause a larger burden on the human host than any other parasite; adult worms can grow as long as 12 or 14 inches, and release 200,000 eggs per day. The eggs infect people who eat unwashed vegetables from contaminated soil or touch their mouths with unwashed hands. Once inside the digestive tract, the eggs release larvae that penetrate the intestinal wall and migrate to the lungs through the liver and the bloodstream. After about 10 days in the lungs, the larvae migrate further into the patient's upper lung passages and airway, where they are swallowed. When they return to the intestine, they mature into adults and reproduce. The time period from the beginning of the infection to egg production is 60–75 days.

The first symptoms of infection may occur when the larvae reach the lungs. The patient may develop chest pain, coughing, difficulty breathing, and inflammation of the lungs. In some cases, the patient's sputum is streaked with blood. This phase of the disease is sometimes called Loeffler's syndrome. It is marked by an accumulation of parasites in the lung tissue and by eosinophilia (an abnormal increase in the number of a specific type of white blood cell). The intestinal phase of ascariasis is marked by stomach pain, cramping, nausea, and intestinal blockage in severe cases.

Toxocariasis

Toxocariasis is sometimes called visceral larva migrans (VLM) because the larval form of the organism hatches inside the intestines and migrates throughout the body to other organs (viscera). The disease is caused by *Toxocara canis* and *T. cati*, which live within the intestines of dogs and cats. Most human patients are children between the ages of two and four years, who become infected after playing in sandboxes or soil contaminated by pet feces, although adults are also susceptible. The eggs can survive in soil for as long as seven years.

The organism's eggs hatch inside the human intestine and release larvae that are carried in the bloodstream to all parts of the body, including the eyes, liver, lungs, heart, and brain. The patient usually has a **fever**, with coughing or **wheezing** and a swollen liver. Some patients develop skin **rashes** and inflammation of the lungs. The larvae may survive inside the body for months, producing allergic reactions and small granulomas, which are tissue swellings or growths produced in response to inflammation. Infection of the eye can produce ocular larva migrans (OLM), which is the first symptom of toxocariasis in some patients.

Trichuriasis

Trichuriasis, caused by *Trichuris trichiura*, is sometimes called whipworm because the organism has a long, slender, whiplike front end. The adult worm is slightly less than an inch long. Trichuriasis is most common in warm, humid climates, including the southeastern United States. The number of people with trichuriasis may be as high as 800 million worldwide.

Whipworm larvae hatch from swallowed eggs in the small intestine and move on to the upper part of the large intestine, where they attach themselves to the lining. The adult worms produce eggs that are passed in the feces and mature in the soil. Patients with mild infections may have few or no symptoms. In cases of heavy infestation, the patient may have abdominal cramps and other symptoms resembling amebic **dysentery**. In children, severe trichuriasis may cause anemia and developmental retardation.

Diagnosis

Since the first symptoms of roundworm infection are common to a number of illnesses, a doctor is most likely to consider the possibility of a parasitic disease on the basis of the patient's history–especially in children.

The definite diagnosis is based on the results of stool or tissue tests. In trichuriasis, adult worms may also be visible in the lining of the patient's rectum. In ascariasis, adult worms may appear in the patient's feces or vomit; they can also be detected by x ray and ultrasound. In toxocariasis, larvae are sometimes found in tissue samples taken from a granuloma. If a patient with toxocariasis develops OLM, it is important to obtain a granuloma sample in order to distinguish between OLM and **retinoblastoma** (a type of eye tumor).

Anisakiasis is one of two roundworm infections that cannot be diagnosed from stool specimens. Instead, the diagnosis is made by x rays of the patient's stomach and small intestine. The larvae may appear as small threads when double contrast x rays are used. In acute cases, the doctor may use an endoscope (an instrument for examining the interior of a body cavity) to look for or remove larvae.

Blood tests cannot be used to differentiate among different types of roundworm infections, but the presence of eosinophilia can help to confirm the diagnosis.

Patients with trichuriasis or ascariasis should be examined for signs of infection by other roundworm species; many patients are infected by several parasites at the same time.

Treatment

Trichuriasis, ascariasis, and toxocariasis are treated with anthelminthic medications. These are drugs that destroy roundworms either by paralyzing them or by blocking them from feeding. Anthelminthic drugs include pyrantel pamoate, piperazine, albendazole, and mebendazole. Mebendazole cannot be given to pregnant women because it may harm the fetus. Treatment with anthelminthic drugs does not prevent reinfection.

There is no drug treatment for anisakiasis; however, symptoms usually resolve in one to two weeks when the larvae die. In some cases, the larvae are removed with an endoscope or by surgery.

Patients with an intestinal obstruction caused by ascariasis may be given **nasogastric suction**, followed by anthelminthic drugs, in order to avoid surgery. If suction fails, the worms must be removed surgically to prevent intestinal rupture or blockage.

Prognosis

The prognosis for recovery from roundworm infections is good for most patients. The severity of

---

KEY TERMS

Eosinophilia—An abnormal increase in the number of a specific type of white blood cell. Eosinophilia is a characteristic of all types of roundworm infections.

Granuloma—A tissue swelling produced in response to inflammation. Granulomas are important in diagnosing toxocariasis.

Loeffler's syndrome—The respiratory phase of ascariasis, marked by inflammation of the lungs and eosinophilia.

Nematode—A parasitic roundworm with a long, cylindrical body.

Ocular larva migrans (OLM)—A syndrome associated with toxocariasis, in which the eye is invaded by migrating larvae.

Visceral larva migrans (VLM)—Another name for toxocariasis. The name is derived from the life cycle of the organism.

Whipworm—Another name for trichuriasis. The name comes from the organism's long whiplike front end.

---

infection, however, varies considerably from person to person. Children are more likely to have heavy infestations and are also more likely to suffer from malabsorption and **malnutrition** than adults.

Ascariasis is the only roundworm infection with a significant mortality rate. *A. lumbricoides* grows large enough to perforate the bile or pancreatic ducts; in addition, a mass of worms in the digestive tract can cause rupture or blockage of the intestines. It is estimated that 20,000 children die every year from intestinal ascariasis.

Prevention

There are no effective vaccines against any of the soil-transmitted roundworms, nor does infection confer immunity. Prevention of infection or reinfection requires adequate hygiene and sanitation measures, including regular and careful handwashing before eating or touching the mouth with the hands.

With respect to specific infections, anisakiasis can be prevented by avoiding raw or improperly prepared fish or squid. Trichuriasis, ascariasis, and toxocariasis can be prevented by keeping children from playing in soil contaminated by human or animal feces; by teaching children to wash their hands before eating; and by having pets dewormed regularly by a veterinarian.

Resources

BOOKS

Goldsmith, Robert S. "Infectious Diseases: Protozoal & Helminthic." In *Current Medical Diagnosis and Treatment, 1998*, edited by Stephen McPhee, et al., 37th ed. Stamford: Appleton & Lange, 1997.

Rebecca J. Frey, PhD

Routine urinalysis *see* **Urinalysis**

RSV *see* **Respiratory syncytial virus infection**

RTA *see* **Renal tubular acidosis**

RU-486 *see* **Mifepristone**

Rubella

Definition

Rubella is a highly contagious viral disease, spread through contact with discharges from the nose and throat of an infected person. Although rubella causes only mild symptoms of low **fever**, swollen glands, joint **pain**, and a fine red rash in most children and adults, it can have severe complications for women in their first trimester of **pregnancy**. These complications include severe **birth defects** or **death** of the fetus.

Description

Rubella is also called German **measles** or three-day measles. This disease was once a common childhood illness, but its occurrence has been drastically reduced since vaccine against rubella became available in 1969. In the 20 years following the introduction of the vaccine, reported rubella cases dropped 99.6%. Only 229 cases of rubella were reported in the United States in 1996.

Rubella is spread through contact with fluid droplets expelled from the nose or throat of an infected person. A person infected with the rubella virus is contagious for about seven days before any symptoms appear and continues to be able to spread the disease for about four days after the appearance of symptoms. Rubella has an incubation period of 12–23 days.

Although rubella is generally considered a childhood illness, people of any age who have not been vaccinated or previously caught the disease can become infected. Having rubella once or being immunized against rubella normally gives lifetime immunity. This is why **vaccination** is so effective in reducing the number of rubella cases.

Women of childbearing age who do not have immunity against rubella should be the most concerned about getting the disease. Rubella infection during the first three months of pregnancy can cause a woman to miscarry or cause her baby to be born with birth defects. Although it has been practically eradicated in the United States, rubella is still common in less developed countries because of poor immunization penetration, creating a risk to susceptible travelers. Some countries have chosen to target rubella vaccination to females only and outbreaks in foreign-born males have occurred on cruise ships and at U.S. summer camps.

Causes and symptoms

Rubella is caused by the rubella virus (*Rubivirus*). Symptoms are generally mild, and complications are rare in anyone who is not pregnant.

The first visible sign of rubella is a fine red rash that begins on the face and rapidly moves downward to cover the whole body within 24 hours. The rash lasts about three days, which is why rubella is sometimes called the three-day measles. A low fever and swollen glands, especially in the head (around the ears) and neck, often accompany the rash. Joint pain and sometimes joint swelling can occur, more often in women. It is quite common to get rubella and not show any symptoms (subclinical infection).

Symptoms disappear within three to four days, except for joint pain, which may linger for a week or two. Most people recover fully with no complications. However, severe complications may arise in the unborn children of women who get rubella during the first three months of their pregnancy. These babies may be miscarried or stillborn. A high percentage are born with birth defects. Birth defects are reported to occur in 50% of women who contract the disease during the first month of pregnancy, 20% of those who contract it in the second month, and 10% of those who contract it in the third month.

The most common birth defects resulting from congenital rubella infection are eye defects such as **cataracts**, **glaucoma**, and blindness; deafness; congenital heart defects; and **mental retardation**. Taken together, these conditions are called congenital rubella

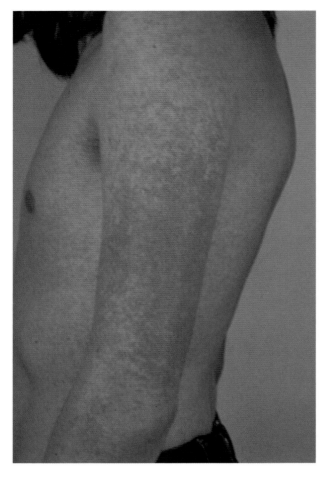

A red rash is one characteristic of rubella, or German measles, as seen on this man's arm. *(Custom Medical Stock Photo. Reproduced by permission.)*

syndrome (CRS). The risk of birth defects drops after the first trimester, and by the 20th week, there are rarely any complications.

Diagnosis

The rash caused by the rubella virus and the accompanying symptoms are so similar to other viral infections that it is impossible for a physician to make a confirmed diagnosis on visual examination alone. The only sure way to confirm a case of rubella is by isolating the virus with a blood test or in a laboratory culture.

A blood test is done to check for rubella antibodies. When the body is infected with the rubella virus, it produces both immunoglobulin G (IgG) and immunoglobulin M (IgM) antibodies to fight the infection. Once IgG exists, it persists for a lifetime, but the special IgM antibody usually wanes over six months. A blood test can be used either to confirm a recent infection (IgG

and IgM) or determine whether a person has immunity to rubella (IgG only). The lack of antibodies indicates that a person is susceptible to rubella.

All pregnant women should be tested for rubella early in pregnancy, whether or not they have a history of vaccination. If the woman lacks immunity, she is counseled to avoid anyone with the disease and to be vaccinated after giving birth.

Treatment

There is no drug treatment for rubella. Bed rest, fluids, and **acetaminophen** for pain and temperatures over 102°F (38.9°C) are usually all that is necessary.

Babies born with suspected CRS are isolated and cared for only by people who are sure they are immune to rubella. Congenital heart defects are treated with surgery.

Alternative treatment

Rather than vaccinating a healthy child against rubella, many alternative practitioners recommend allowing the child to contract the disease naturally at the age of five or six years, since the immunity conferred by contracting the disease naturally lasts a lifetime. It is, however, difficult for a child to contract rubella naturally when everyone around him or her has been vaccinated.

Ayurvedic practitioners recommend making the patient comfortable and giving the patient ginger or clove tea to hasten the progress of the disease. **Traditional Chinese medicine** uses a similar approach. Believing that inducing the skin rash associated with rubella hastens the progress of the disease, traditional Chinese practitioners prescribe herbs such as peppermint (*Mentha piperita*) and *chai-hu* (*Bupleurum chinense*). Cicada is often prescribed as well. Western herbal remedies may be used to alleviate rubella symptoms. Distilled witch hazel (*Hamamelis virginiana*) helps calm the **itching** associated with the skin rash and an eyewash made from a filtered diffusion of eyebright (*Euphrasia officinalis*) can relieve eye discomfort. Antiviral western herbal or Chinese remedies can be used to assist the immune system in establishing equilibrium during the healing process. Depending on the patient's symptoms, among the remedies a homeopath may prescribe are *Belladonna,Pulsatilla,* or *Phytolacca.*

Prognosis

Complications from rubella infection are rare in children, pregnant women past the 20th week of

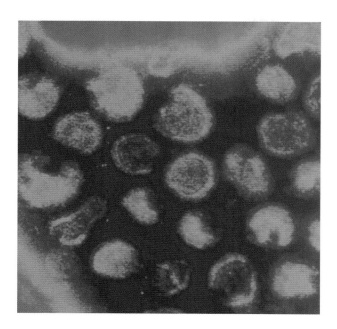

A digitized image of rubella virus particles. *(Custom Medical Stock Photo. Reproduced by permission.)*

date, however, accidental rubella vaccinations during pregnancy have not clearly been associated with the same risk as the natural infection itself. Women may be vaccinated while they are breastfeeding. People whose immune systems are compromised, either by the use of drugs such as steroids or by disease, should discuss possible complications with their doctor before being vaccinated.

Resources

ORGANIZATIONS

March of Dimes Birth Defects Foundation. 1275 Mamaroneck Ave., White Plains, NY 10605. (914) 428-7100. resourcecenter@modimes.org. < http://www.modimes.org >.

National Organization for Rare Disorders. P.O. Box 8923, New Fairfield, CT 06812-8923. (800) 999-6673. < http://www.rarediseases.org >.

Tish Davidson, A.M.

KEY TERMS

Incubation period—The time it takes for a person to become sick after being exposed to a disease.

Trimester—The first third or 13 weeks of pregnancy.

---

pregnancy, and other adults. For women in the first trimester of pregnancy, there is a high likelihood of the child being born with one or more birth defect. Unborn children exposed to rubella early in pregnancy are also more likely to be miscarried, stillborn, or have a low birthweight. Although the symptoms of rubella pass quickly for the mother, the consequences to the unborn child can last a lifetime.

Prevention

Vaccination is the best way to prevent rubella and is normally required by law for children entering school. Rubella vaccine is usually given in conjunction with measles and **mumps** vaccines in a shot referred to as MMR (mumps, measles, and rubella). Children receive one dose of MMR vaccine at 12-15 months and another dose at four to six years.

Pregnant women should not be vaccinated, and women who are not pregnant should avoid conceiving for at least three months following vaccination. To

Rubella test

Definition

The **rubella** test is a routine blood test performed as part of prenatal care of pregnant women. It is sometimes also used to screen women of childbearing age before the first **pregnancy**.

Purpose

The test is given to evaluate whether a woman is immune to rubella (German **measles**) as a result of childhood exposure or immunization, or whether she may be presently infected with the disease. The question of a current infection is particularly urgent for pregnant women. Although the disease itself is not serious in adults, it can cause **miscarriage**, **stillbirth**, or damage to the fetus during the first trimester (three months) of pregnancy. The rubella test is regarded as a more reliable indication of the patient's immune status than her history, because reinfection with rubella is possible even after immunization. The results of the test may influence decisions to terminate a pregnancy.

Description

The rubella test belongs to a category of blood tests called hemagglutination inhibition (HI) tests. Hemagglutination refers to the clumping or clustering of red blood cells caused by a disease antibody, virus, or certain other substances. Inhibition refers to interference with the clumping process. The presence of rubella antibodies inhibits the cell clumping caused by the rubella virus. Thus, the addition of the virus to a sample of the patient's blood allows a doctor to determine the presence and concentration of rubella antibodies and the patient's immunity to the disease.

When a person is infected with the rubella virus, the body produces both immunoglobulin G (IgG) and immunoglobulin M (IgM) antibodies to fight the infection. Once IgG exists, it persists for a lifetime, but the special IgM antibody usually wanes over six months. The rubella test can either confirm that a recent infection has occurred (both IgG and IgM are present) or that a patient has immunity to rubella (IgG only is present).

When the test is performed to confirm the diagnosis of rubella in a woman already pregnant, two blood samples are drawn. One is drawn during the acute phase of the illness about three days after the rash breaks out, and the second is drawn during the convalescent phase about three weeks later. The specimens are then tested simultaneously by a single laboratory. Alternatively, a pregnant woman with a rash suspected to be rubella can be tested for IgM antibody. If the test shows that IgM antibody is present, then a recent rubella infection has occurred.

Because there have been cases of children born with rubella syndrome even though the mother's blood test indicated that she was sufficiently immune to rubella, some researchers are presently recommending a second test, known as a synthetic peptide enzyme-linked immunosorbent assay (ELISA). This test screens for the presence of rubella virus neutralizing (RVN) antibodies in the mother's blood.

Normal results

If the patient has been successfully immunized against rubella or has had the disease, the HI antibody titer (concentration) will be greater than 1:10–1:20. The red blood cells will fail to clump when the rubella virus is added to the blood serum.

In the case of paired testing for pregnant women, a fourfold rise in antibody titer between the first and second blood samples indicates the suspicious rash was caused by rubella. The alternative test for IgM antibody confirms recent rubella infection if IgM is found in the patient's blood.

Abnormal results

If the patient has little or no immunity to rubella, her HI antibody titer will be 1:8 or less. Women

without immunity should receive immunization against rubella provided that they avoid pregnancy for a period of three months following immunization. Women with disease of the immune system or who are taking corticosteroid medications should receive immune serum globulin rather than rubella vaccine to prevent infection.

Resources

BOOKS

Beers, Mark H., MD, and Robert Berkow, MD., editors. "Childhood Infections: Viral Infections." In *The Merck Manual of Diagnosis and Therapy*. Whitehouse Station, NJ: Merck Research Laboratories, 2004.

PERIODICALS

Andrews, J. I. "Diagnosis of Fetal Infections" *Current Opinion in Obstetrics and Gynecology* 16 (April 2004): 163–166.

Giessauf, A., T. Letschka, G. Walder, et al. "A Synthetic Peptide ELISA for the Screening of Rubella Virus Neutralizing Antibodies in Order to Ascertain Immunity." *Journal of Immunological Methods* 287 (April 2004): 1–11.

ORGANIZATIONS

American Academy of Family Physicians (AAFP). 11400 Tomahawk Creek Parkway, Leawood, KS 66211-2672. (800) 274-2237 or (913) 906-6000. < http://www.aafp.org >.

Rebecca J. Frey, PhD

Rubeola *see* **Measles**

Ruptured disk *see* **Herniated disk**

RVT *see* **Renal vein thrombosis**

S

Sacroiliac disease

Definition

Sacroiliac disease is high-impact trauma to the sacroiliac joint that can cause **death**, or bone, and nerve damage.

Description

The sacroiliac joint is a strong, weight bearing synovial joint between the ilium and sacrum bones of the pelvis. The bones are held in place and allowed limited movements by a system of sacroiliac ligaments. Relaxation of this and other joints and ligaments is important during **pregnancy** and is accomplished by a special hormone called relaxin. Usually the sacroiliac is damaged by high-impact injuries. These injuries may be life threatening and mortality is approximately 20% if neighboring structures are also damaged. Injuries to this area often includes neurological deficits. Dislocation and nerve damage are frequently missed in the diagnosis.

Causes and symptoms

The primary cause of **dislocations, fractures**, and accompanying damage is usually a traumatic accident. Patients receiving such injuries require emergency medical attention. There may be severe blood loss due to breakage of large bones and resuscitative measures may be required for stabilization.

Diagnosis

The diagnosis can be difficult since nerve damage can mimic other conditions with similar symptoms (i.e., **low back pain** in persons with **sciatica**). Additionally imaging studies and **physical examination** maneuvers will miss the diagnosis. The definitive method for diagnosing sacroiliac pathology would be injection of local anesthetic in the correct area of the affected sacroiliac joint. This procedure is usually performed using advance guidance systems (CT or fluoroscopic assisted guidance). If the **pain** is relieved by anesthetic injection, then the diagnosis is confirmed. There are three typical patterns of pain: pain directly over the joint, pain in the groin extending down the affected leg that can mimic the signs associated with a herniated lumbar disc, and pain widely dispersed in the affected leg.

Treatment

Treatment initially can include emergency interventions, but usually is conservative. Treatment includes physical therapy, manipulation, and medications for pain control. In some cases a sacroiliac belt can help with symptoms. In sacroiliac joint disease that has already progressed and is chronic and severe, corrective joint fusion may be indicated.

Prognosis

Outcome is variable and takes into account the extent of injuries, early diagnosis, and responsiveness to conservative treatment.

Prevention

There is no known prevention since the disease is secondary to an accident.

Resources

BOOKS

Goetz, Christopher G., et al, editors. *Textbook of Clinical Neurology*. 1st ed. W. B. Saunders Company, 1999.

Ruddy, Shaun, et al, editors. *Kelly's Textbook of Rheumatology*. 6th ed. W. B. Saunders Company, 2001.

KEY TERMS

Herniated disk—A protrusion in a disk located in the spinal column.

Ligament—Fibrous tissue which connect bones.

Synovial joint—A joint that allows for bone movement.

OTHER

American Academy of Orthopaedic Surgeons. < http://www.aaos.org >.

Laith Farid Gulli, M.D.

SAD *see* **Seasonal affective disorder**

St. Anthony's fire *see* **Erysipelas**

▌St. John's wort

Definition

Hypericum perforatum is the most medicinally important species of the Hypericum genus, commonly known as St. John's wort. There are as many as 400 species in the genus, which is part of the Guttiferae family. Native to Europe, St. John's wort is found throughout the world. It thrives in sunny fields, open woods, and gravelly roadsides. Early colonists brought this valuable medicinal to North America, and the plant has become naturalized in the eastern United States and California, as well as in Australia, New Zealand, eastern Asia, and South America.

The entire plant, particularly the round, black seed, exudes a slight, turpentine-like odor. The woody, branched root spreads from the base with runners that produce numerous stalks. The simple, dark green leaves are veined and grow in opposite, oblong-obvate pairs on round, branching stalks that reach 3 ft (91.4 cm) high. Tiny holes, visible when the leaf is held to the light, are actually transparent oil glands containing the chemical photo sensitizer known as hypericin. These characteristic holes inspired the species name, *perforatum*, Latin for perforated. The bright yellow, star-shaped flowers, often clustered in a trio, have five petals. Each blossom has many showy stamens. Black dots along the margins of the blossom contain more of the red-pigmented chemical hypericin. The herb is also useful as a dye. The flowers bloom in branching, flat-topped clusters atop the stalks in mid-summer, around the time of the summer solstice. St. John's wort, sometimes called devil's flight or grace of God, was believed to have magical properties to ward off evil spirits. It's generic name hypericum is derived from a Greek word meaning "over an apparition." The herb was traditionally gathered on mid-summer's eve, June 23. This date was later christianized as the eve of the feast day of St. John the Baptist. This folk custom gave the plant its popular name. The Anglo-Saxon word wort means medicinal herb.

Purpose

St. John's wort has been known for its numerous medicinal properties as far back as Roman times. It was a valued remedy on the Roman battlefields where it was used to promote healing from trauma and inflammation. The herb is vulnerary and can speed the healing of **wounds**, **bruises**, ulcers, and **burns**. It is popularly used as a nervine for its calming effect, easing tension and **anxiety**, relieving mild depression, and soothing emotions during **menopause**. The bittersweet herb is licensed in Germany for use in cases of mild depression, anxiety, and sleeplessness. It is useful in circumstances of nerve injury and trauma, and has been used to speed healing after brain surgery. Its antispasmodic properties can ease uterine cramping and menstrual difficulties. St. John's wort acts medicinally as an astringent, and may also be used as an expectorant. The hypericin in St. John's wort possesses anti-viral properties that may be active in combating certain cancers, including many brain cancers. An infusion of the plant, taken as a tea, has been helpful in treating night-time incontinence in children. The oil, taken internally, has been used to treat **colic**, intestinal worms, and abdominal **pain**. The medicinal parts of St. John's wort are the fresh leaves and flowers. This valuable remedy has been extensively tested in West Germany, and is dispensed throughout Germany as a popular medicine called, *Johnniskraut*. Commercially prepared extracts are commonly standardized to 0.3% hypericin.

Clinical studies

A 1988 study at New York University found the antiviral properties in hypericin, a chemical component of Hypericum, to be useful in combating the virus that causes **AIDS**. Additional studies are under way through the Federal Drug Administration (FDA) to determine the effectiveness of the herb as a treatment for AIDS. Hypericin extract has also been reported to inhibit a form of leukemia that sometimes occurs after **radiation therapy**. Numerous clinical studies have found hypericum preparations to have an antidepressive effect when used in standardized extracts for treatment of mild depression. Clinical trials continue with this important herbal anti-depressant, particularly in view of its relative lack of undesirable side effects in humans.

Preparations

An oil extract can be purchased commercially or prepared by combining fresh flowers and leaves of St. John's wort in a glass jar and sunflower or olive oil. Seal the container with an airtight lid and leave on a sunny windowsill for four to six weeks, shaking daily. The oil will absorb the red pigment. Strain through muslin or cheesecloth, and store in a dark container. The medicinal oil will maintain its potency for two years or more. The oil of St. John's wort has been known in folk culture as "Oil of Jesus." This oil makes a good rub for painful joints, **varicose veins**, muscle strain, arthritis, and rheumatism. Used in a compress it can help to heal wounds and inflammation, and relieve the pain of deep bruising.

An infusion is made by pouring one pint of boiling water over 1 oz (28 g) of dried herb, or 2 oz (57 g) of fresh, minced flower and leaf. Steep in a glass or enamel pot for five to 10 minutes. Strain and cover. Drink the tea warm. A general dose is one cupful, up to three times daily.

Capsule: Dry the leaves and flowers and grind with mortar and pestle into a fine powder. Place in gelatin capsules. The potency of the herb varies with the soil, climate and harvesting conditions of the plant. A standardized extract of 0.3% hypericin extract, commercially prepared from a reputable source, is more likely to yield reliable results. Standard dosage is up to three 300 mg capsules of 0.3% standardized extract daily.

A tincture is prepared by combining one part fresh herb to three parts alcohol (50% alcohol/water solution) in glass container. Set aside in dark place, shaking the mixture daily for two weeks. Strain through muslin or cheesecloth, and store in dark bottle. The tincture should maintain potency for two years. Standard dosage, unless otherwise prescribed, is 0.24–1 tsp added to 8 oz (237 ml) of water, up to three times daily.

A salve is made by warming 2 oz (59 ml) of prepared oil extract in double boiler. Once warmed, 1 oz (28 g) of grated beeswax is added and mixed until melted. Pour into a glass jar and cool. The salve can be stored for up to one year. The remedy keeps best if refrigerated after preparation. The salve is useful in

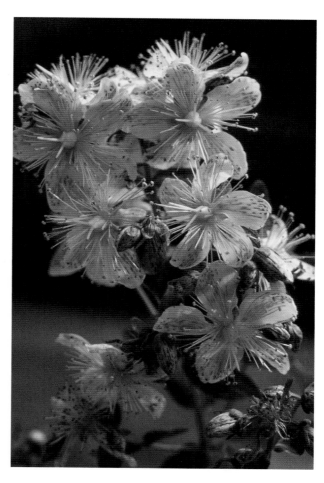

St. John's wort flowers. (Photo Researchers, Inc. Reproduced by permission.)

treating burns, wounds, and soothing painful muscles. It is also a good skin softener. St. John's wort salve may be prepared in combination with calendula extract (*Calendula officinalis*) for application on bruises.

Precautions

Consult a physician prior to use. Pregnant or lactating women should not use the herb. Individuals taking prescribed psychotropic medications classified as **selective serotonin reuptake inhibitors**, or **SSRI**, such as Prozac, should not simultaneously use St. John's wort. Many herbalists also discourage use of St. John's wort by individuals taking any other anti-depressant medication.

Cattlemen dislike the shrub because there have been some reports of toxicity to livestock that overgraze in fields abundant with the wild herb. Toxic

KEY TERMS

Antispasmodic—Relieves mild cramping or muscle spasm.

Expectorant—Promotes the discharge of mucus from respiratory system.

Nervine—Soothes and calms the nervous system.

Vulnerary—Heals wounds, bruises, sprains, and ulcers.

effects in livestock include reports of **edema** of the ears, eyelids, and the face due to photosensitization after ingestion of the herb. Exposure to sunlight activates the hypercin in the plant. Adverse effects have been reported in horses, sheep, and swine and include staggering, and blistering and peeling of the skin. Toxicity is greater in smaller mammals, such as rabbits.

Side effects

When used either internally or externally, the herb may cause photo-dermatitis in humans with fair or sensitive skin when exposed to sun light or other ultra-violet light source. There have been some reports of changes in **lactation** in some nursing women taking the hypericum extract. Changes in the nutritional quality and flavor of the milk, and reduction or cessation of lactation have also been reported. It can also cause headaches, stiff neck, **nausea and vomiting**, and high blood pressure.

Interactions

St. John's wort can interact with amphetamines, **asthma** inhalants, **decongestants**, diet pills, **narcotics**, and amino acid tryptophan and tyrosine, as well as certain foods. Reactions range from **nausea** to increased high blood pressure. Consult a practitioner prior to using St. John's wort.

Resources

ORGANIZATIONS

American Botanical Council. PO Box 201660, Austin, TX 78720-1660.

OTHER

Herb Research Foundation. < http://www.herbs.org >.

Clare Hanrahan

St. Vitus' dance *see* **Sydenham's chorea**

Salivary gland scan

Definition

A salivary gland scan is a nuclear medicine test that examines the uptake and secretion in the salivary glands of a radioactively labeled marker substance. The pattern of uptake and secretion shows if these glands are functioning normally.

Purpose

A salivary gland scan is done to help diagnose the cause of **dry mouth**. It is a test that is done when Sjogren's syndrome, salivary duct obstruction, asymmetric hypertrophy, or growths such as Warthin's tumors are suspected.

Precautions

Salivary gland scans are a safe and effective way to diagnose problems associated with dry mouth. The level of radioactivity in the marker substance is low and poses no threat to health. The only people who should not undergo this test are pregnant women.

Other recent nuclear medicine tests may affect the results of this scan. It may be necessary to wait until earlier radiopharmaceuticals have been cleared from the body before undergoing this scan.

Description

A salivary gland scan, also called a parotid gland scan, is a noninvasive test. The patient is positioned under a gamma scintillation camera that detects radiation. The patient then is injected with a low-level radioactive marker, usually technetium-99m or technetium pertechnetate.

Immediately after the injection, imaging begins. For accurate results, the patient must stay still during imaging. After several images, the patient is given lemon drop candies to suck on, which stimulate the salivary glands. Another set of images is made for comparison purposes. The entire process takes about ten minutes for the injection and 30–45 minutes for the scan.

Preparation

No special preparations are needed for this test. It is not necessary to fast or to restrict medications before testing. Any blood that needs to be drawn for other tests should be taken before the radiopharmaceutical is injected.

PERIODICALS

Baur, D. A., T. F. Heston, and J. I. Helman. "Nuclear Medicine in Oral and Maxillofacial Diagnosis: A Review for the Practicing Dental Professional." *Journal of Contemporary Dental Practice* 5 (February 15, 2004): 94–104.

Chae, S. W., J. H. Sohn, H. S. Shin, et al. "Unilateral, Multicentric Warthin's Tumor Mimicking a Tumor Metastatic to a Lymph Node. A Case Report." *Acta Cytologica* 48 (March-April 2004): 229–233.

ORGANIZATIONS

Society of Nuclear Medicine (SNM). 1850 Samuel Morse Drive, Reston, VA 20190-5316. (703) 708-9000. Fax: (703) 708-9015. < http://www.snm.org >.

OTHER

"Salivary Gland Scan." *HealthGate Page.* < http://www3.healthgate.com >.

Tish Davidson, AM
Rebecca J. Frey, PhD

> ## KEY TERMS
>
> **Hypertrophy**—Overgrowth of tissue not due to a tumor.
>
> **Parotid gland**—The salivary gland that lies below and in front of each ear.
>
> **Radiopharmaceutical**—A radioactive pharmaceutical or chemical (usually radioactive iodine or cobalt) used for diagnostic or therapeutic purposes.
>
> **Sjögren's syndrome**—A disease often associated with rheumatoid arthritis, that causes dry mouth, lesions on the skin, and enlargement of the parotid glands. It is often seen in menopausal women.
>
> **Technetium**—A synthetic element used in nuclear medicine; it is obtained from the fission of uranium.
>
> **Warthin's tumor**—A benign tumor of the parotid gland.

Aftercare

Patients can return to normal activities immediately.

Risks

A salivary gland scan is a safe test. The only risk is to the fetus of a pregnant woman. Women who are pregnant should discuss the risks and benefits of this procedure with their doctor.

Normal results

Normally functioning salivary glands take up the radiopharmaceutical then secrete it when stimulated by the lemon drops.

Abnormal results

Abnormally functioning salivary glands fail to exhibit a normal uptake and secretion pattern. This test does not differentiate between benign and malignant lesions.

Resources

BOOKS

Beers, Mark H., MD, and Robert Berkow, MD., editors. "Disorders of the Oral Region: Neoplasms." Section 9, Chapter 105 In *The Merck Manual of Diagnosis and Therapy*. Whitehouse Station, NJ: Merck Research Laboratories, 2004.

Salivary gland tumors

Definition

A salivary gland tumor is an uncontrolled growth of cells that originates in one of the many saliva-producing glands in the mouth.

Description

The tongue, cheeks, and palate (the hard and soft areas at the roof of the mouth) contain many glands that produce saliva. In saliva there are enzymes, or catalysts, that begin the breakdown (digestion) of food while it is still in the mouth. The glands are called salivary glands because of their function.

There are three big pairs of salivary glands in addition to many smaller ones. The parotid glands, submandibular glands and sublingual glands are the large, paired salivary glands. The parotids are located inside the cheeks, one below each ear. The submandibular glands are located on the floor of the mouth, with one on the inner side of each part of the lower jaw, or mandible. The sublingual glands are also in the floor of the mouth, but they are under the tongue.

The parotids are the salivary glands most often affected by tumors. Yet most of the tumors that grow in the parotid glands are benign, or not cancerous. Approximately 8 out of 10 salivary tumors diagnosed are in a parotid gland. One in 10 diagnosed is in a

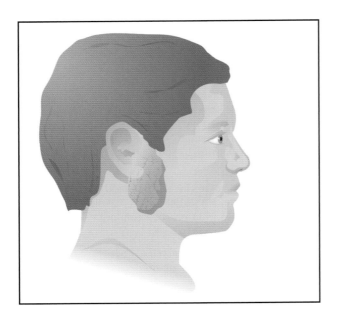

A salivary gland with a tumor. (Illustration by Argosy Inc.)

submandibular gland. The remaining 10% are diagnosed in other salivary glands.

In general, glands more likely to show tumor growth are also glands least likely to show malignant tumor growth. Thus, although tumors of the sublingual glands are rare, almost all of them are malignant. In contrast, about one in four tumors of the parotid glands is malignant.

Cancers of the salivary glands begin to grow in epithelial cells, or the flat cells that cover body surfaces. Thus, they are called carcinomas, cancers that by definition begin in epithelial cells.

Demographics

Cancers in the mouth account for fewer than 2% of all cases of **cancer** and about 1.5% of cancer deaths. About 7% of all cancers diagnosed in the head and neck region are diagnosed in a salivary gland. Men and women are at equal risk.

Mortality from salivary gland tumors in the United States is higher among male African Americans below the age of 50 than among older workers of any race or either sex. The reasons for these findings are not clear as of early 2004.

Causes and symptoms

When survivors of the 1945 atomic bombings of Nagasaki and Hiroshima began to develop salivary gland tumors at a high rate, radiation was suspected as a cause. Ionizing radiation, particularly gamma radiation, is a factor that contributes to tumor development. So is **radiation therapy**. Adults who received radiation therapy for enlarged adenoids or tonsils when they were children are at greater risk for salivary gland tumors.

Another reported risk factor is an association between wood dust inhalation and adenocarcinoma of the minor salivary glands of the nose and paranasal sinuses. There is also evidence that people infected with herpes viruses may be at greater risk for salivary gland tumors. And individuals infected with human **immunodeficiency** virus (HIV) have more salivary gland disease in general, and may be at greater risk for salivary gland tumors.

Although there has been speculation that the electromagnetic fields generated by cell phones increase the risk of salivary gland tumors, a recent study done in Denmark has concluded that the use of cell phones, pagers, and similar devices is not a risk factor.

There seems to be some link between **breast cancer** and salivary gland tumors. Women with breast cancer are more likely to be diagnosed with salivary gland tumors. Also linked to salivary gland tumors is alcohol use, exposure to sunlight (ultraviolet radiation) and hair dye use. There is evidence that people infected with herpes viruses may be at greater risk for salivary gland tumors. Individuals infected with human immunodeficiency virus (HIV) have more salivary gland disease in general, and may be at greater risk for salivary gland tumors.

Symptoms are often absent until the tumor is large or has metastasized (spread to other sites). In many cases, the tumor is first discovered by the patient's dentist. During regular dental examinations, the dentist looks for masses on the palate or under the tongue or in the cheeks, and such checkups are a good way to detect tumors early. Some symptoms are:

- a lump or mass in the mouth
- swelling in the face
- pain in the jaw or the side of the face
- difficulty swallowing
- difficulty breathing
- difficulty speaking

Diagnosis

A tissue sample will be taken for study via a biopsy. Usually an incision is necessary to take the tissue sample. Sometimes it is possible to take a tissue sample with a needle.

3272

Magnetic resonance imaging (MRI) and computed tomography (CT) scans are also used to evaluate the tumor. They help determine whether the cancer has spread to sites adjacent to the salivary gland where it is found. MRI offers a good way to examine the tonsils and the back of the tongue, which are soft tissues. CT is tapped as a way of studying the jaw, which is bone.

Treatment

To assess the stage of growth of a salivary gland tumor, many features are examined, including how big it is and the type of abnormal cell growth. Analysis of the types of abnormal cell growth in tissue is so specific that many salivary gland tumors are given unique names.

In stage I cancer the tumor is less than one inch in size and it has not spread. Stage II salivary gland cancers are larger than one inch and smaller than two and one-half inches, but they have not spread. Stage III cancers are smaller than one inch, but they have spread to a lymph node. Stage IV cancers have spread to adjacent sites in the head, which may include the base of the skull and nearby nerves, or they are larger than two and one-half inches and have invaded a lymph node.

Surgical removal (excision) of the tumor is the most common treatment. **Chemotherapy** and radiation therapy may be part of the treatment, particularly if the cancer has metastasized, or spread to other sites; chemotherapy of salivary gland cancers, however, does not appear to extend survival or improve the patient's quality of life. Because there are many nerves and blood vessels near the three major pairs of salivary glands, particularly the parotids, the surgery can be quite complicated. A complex surgery is especially true if the tumor has spread.

A promising form of treatment for patients at high risk of tumor recurrence in the salivary glands near the base of the skull is gamma knife surgery. Used as a booster treatment following standard neutron radiotherapy, gamma knife surgery appears to be well tolerated by the patients and to have minimal side effects.

Alternative treatment

Any technique, such as **yoga**, **meditation** or **biofeedback**, that helps a patient cope with **anxiety** over the condition and discomfort from treatment is useful and should be explored as an option.

KEY TERMS

Adenoids—Common name for the pharyngeal tonsils, which are lymph masses in the wall of the air passageway (pharynx) just behind the nose.

Biopsy—Tissue sample is taken from the body for examination.

Computed tomography (CT)—X rays are aimed at slices of the body (by rotating equipment) and results are assembled with a computer to give a three-dimensional picture of a structure.

Lymph—Tissue that is part of the lymphatic system, the system that collects and returns fluid to the blood vessels and produces substances that fight infection.

Magnetic resonance imaging (MRI)—Magnetic fields and radio frequency waves are used to take pictures of the inside of the body.

Tonsils—Common name for the palatine tonsils, which are lymph masses in the back of the mouth, on either side of the tongue.

Prognosis

Tumors in small salivary glands that are localized can usually be removed without much difficulty. The outlook for survival once the tumor is removed is very good if it has not metastasized.

For parotid cancers, the five-year survival rate is more than 85% whether or not a lymph node is involved at diagnosis. Ten-year survival rate is just under 50%.

Most early stage salivary gland tumors are removed, and they do not return. Those that do return, or recur, are the most troublesome and reduce the chance an individual will remain cancer-free.

Prevention

Minimizing intake of beverages containing alcohol may be important. Avoiding unnecessary exposure of the head to radiation and to sunlight may also be considered preventative. Anything that reduces the risk of contracting a sexually transmitted disease, such as the use of condoms, also may lower the risk of salivary gland cancer.

A salivary gland with a tumor.

Resources

BOOKS

Beers, Mark H., MD, and Robert Berkow, MD., editors. "Disorders of the Oral Region: Neoplasms." Section 9,

Chapter 105 In *The Merck Manual of Diagnosis and Therapy*. Whitehouse Station, NJ: Merck Research Laboratories, 2004.

PERIODICALS

Day, T. A., J. Deveikis, M. B. Gillespie, et al. "Salivary Gland Neoplasms." *Current Treatment Options in Oncology* 5 (February 2004): 11–26.

Douglas, J. G., D. L. Silbergeld, and G. E. Laramore. "Gamma Knife Stereotactic Radiosurgical Boost for Patients Treated Primarily with Neutron Radiotherapy for Salivary Gland Neoplasms." *Stereotactic and Functional Neurosurgery* 82 (March 2004): 84–89.

Johansen, C. "Electromagnetic Fields and Health Effects—Epidemiologic Studies of Cancer, Diseases of the Central Nervous System and Arrhythmia-Related Heart Disease." *Scandinavian Journal of Work and Environmental Health* 30, Supplement 1 (2004): 1–30.

Lawler, B., A. Pierce, P. J. Sambrook, et al. "The Diagnosis and Surgical Management of Major Salivary Gland Pathology." *Australian Dental Journal* 49 (March 2004): 9–15.

Wilson, R. T., L. E. Moore, and M. Dosemeci. "Occupational Exposures and Salivary Gland Cancer Mortality among African American and White Workers in the United States." *Journal of Occupational and Environmental Medicine* 46 (March 2004): 287–297.

Zheng, R., L. E. Wang, M. L. Bondy, et al. "Gamma Radiation Sensitivity and Risk of Malignant and Benign Salivary Gland Tumors: A Pilot Case-Control Analysis." *Cancer* 100 (February 1, 2004): 561–567.

ORGANIZATIONS

SPOHNC, Support for People with Oral and Head and Neck Cancer. P.O. Box 53, Locust Valley, NY 11560-0053. 800-377-0928. <http://www.spohnc.org>.

OTHER

"Oral Cavity and Pharyngeal Cancer." American Cancer Society. Revised May 22, 2000. <http://www3.cancer.org/cancerinfo>.

Diane M. Calabrese
Rebecca J. Frey, PhD

▌Salmonella food poisoning

Definition

Salmonella **food poisoning** is a bacterial food **poisoning** caused by the *Salmonella* bacterium. It results in the swelling of the lining of the stomach and intestines (**gastroenteritis**). While domestic and wild animals, including poultry, pigs, cattle, and pets such as turtles, iguanas, chicks, dogs, and cats can transmit this illness, most people become infected by ingesting foods contaminated with significant amounts of *Salmonella*.

Description

Salmonella food poisoning occurs worldwide, however it is most frequently reported in North America and Europe. Only a small proportion of infected people are tested and diagnosed, and as few as 1% of cases are actually reported. While the infection rate may seem relatively low, even an attack rate of less than 0.5% in such a large number of exposures results in many infected individuals. The poisoning typically occurs in small, localized outbreaks in the general population or in large outbreaks in hospitals, restaurants, or institutions for children or the elderly. In the United States, *Salmonella* is responsible for about 15% of all cases of food poisoning.

Improperly handled or undercooked poultry and eggs are the foods which most frequently cause Salmonella food poisoning. Chickens are a major carrier of *Salmonella* bacteria, which accounts for its prominence in poultry products. However, identifying foods which may be contaminated with *Salmonella* is particularly difficult because infected chickens typically show no signs or symptoms. Since infected chickens have no identifying characteristics, these chickens go on to lay eggs or to be used as meat.

At one time, it was thought that *Salmonella* bacteria were only found in eggs which had cracked, thus allowing the bacteria to enter. Ultimately, it was learned that, because the egg shell has tiny pores, even uncracked eggs which sat for a time on a surface (nest) contaminated with *Salmonella* could themselves become contaminated. It is known also that the bacteria can be passed from the infected female chicken directly into the substance of the egg before the shell has formed around it.

Anyone may contract Salmonella food poisoning, but the disease is most serious in infants, the elderly, and individuals with weakened immune systems. In these individuals, the infection may spread from the intestines to the blood stream, and then to other body sites, causing **death** unless the person is treated promptly with **antibiotics**. In addition, people who have had part or all of their stomach or their spleens removed, or who have sickle cell anemia, **cirrhosis** of the liver, leukemia, lymphoma, **malaria**, louse-borne **relapsing fever**, or Acquired Immunodeficiency Syndrome (**AIDS**) are particularly susceptible to Salmonella food poisoning.

Causes and symptoms

Salmonella food poisoning can occur when someone drinks unpasteurized milk or eats undercooked chicken or eggs, or salad dressings or desserts which contain raw eggs. Even if *Salmonella*-containing foods such as chicken are thoroughly cooked, any food can become contaminated during preparation if conditions and equipment for food preparation are unsanitary.

Other foods can then be accidentally contaminated if they come into contact with infected surfaces. In addition, children have become ill after playing with turtles or iguanas, and then eating without washing their hands. Because the bacteria are shed in the feces for weeks after infection with *Salmonella*, poor hygiene can allow such a carrier to spread the infection to others.

Symptoms appear about one-two days after infection, and include **fever** (in 50% of patients), **nausea** and vomiting, **diarrhea**, and abdominal cramps and pain. The diarrhea is usually very liquid, and rarely contains mucus or blood. Diarrhea usually lasts for about four days. The illness usually ends in about five-seven days.

Serious complications are rare, occurring most often in individuals with other medical illnesses. Complications occur when the *Salmonella* bacteria make their way into the bloodstream (**bacteremia**). Once in the bloodstream, the bacteria can enter any organ system throughout the body, causing disease. Other infections which can be caused by *Salmonella* include:

- bone infections (**osteomyelitis**)
- joint infections (arthritis)
- infection of the sac containing the heart (pericarditis)
- infection of the tissues which cover the brain and spinal cord (**meningitis**)
- infection of the liver (hepatitis)
- lung infections (**pneumonia**)
- infection of aneurysms (aneurysms are abnormal outpouchings which occur in weak areas of the walls of blood vessels)
- infections in the center of already-existing tumors or cysts.

Diagnosis

Under appropriate laboratory conditions, *Salmonella* can be grown and then viewed under a microscope for identification. Early in the infection, the blood is far more likely to positively show a

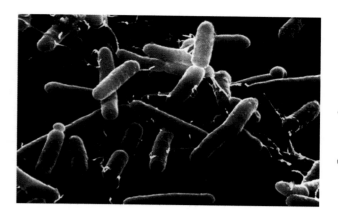

***Salmonella enteritidis.* Exposure to this bacterium usually occurs by contact with contaminated food.** *(Photograph by Oliver Meckes, Photo Researchers, Inc. Reproduced by permission.)*

presence of the *Salmonella* bacterium when a sample is grown on a nutrient substance (culture) for identification purposes. Eventually, however, positive cultures can be obtained from the stool and in some cases from a urine culture.

Treatment

Even though Salmonella food poisoning is a bacterial infection, most practitioners do not treat simple cases with antibiotics. Studies have shown that using antibiotics does not usually reduce the length of time that the patient is ill. Paradoxically, it appears that antibiotics do, however, cause the patient to shed bacteria in their feces for a *longer* period of time. In order to decrease the length of time that a particular individual is a carrier who can spread the disease, antibiotics are generally not given.

In situations where an individual has a more severe type of infection with *Salmonella* bacteria, a number of antibiotics may be used. Chloramphenicol was the first antibiotic successfully used to treat Salmonella food poisoning. It is still a drug of choice in developing countries because it is so inexpensive, although some resistance has developed to it. Ampicillin and trimethoprim-sulfonamide have been used successfully in the treatment of infections caused by chloramphenicol-resistant strains. Newer types of anibiotics, such as cephalosporin or quinolone, are also effective. These drugs can be given by mouth or through a needle in the vein (intravenously) for very ill patients. With effective antibiotic therapy, patients feel better in 24–48 hours, the temperature returns to normal in three-five days, and the patient is generally recovered by 10–14 days.

KEY TERMS

Carrier—Someone who has an organism (bacteria, virus, fungi) in his or her body, without signs of illness. The individual may therefore pass the organism on to others.

Gastroenteritis—Inflammation of the stomach and intestines. Usually causes nausea, vomiting, diarrhea, abdominal pain and cramps.

Alternative treatment

A number of alternative treatments have been recommended for food poisoning. One very effective treatment that is stongly recommended is supplementation with *Lactobacillus acidophilus*, *L. bulgaricus*, and/or *Bifidobacterium* to restore essential bacteria in the digestive tract. These preparations are available as powders, tablets, or capsules from health food stores; yogurt with live *L. acidophilus* cultures can also be eaten. Fasting or a liquid-only diet is often used for food poisoning. Homeopathic treatment can work very effectively in the treatment of Salmonella food poisoning. The appropriate remedy for the individual and his/her symptoms must be used to get the desired results. Some examples of remedies commonly used are *Chamomilla*, *Nux vomica*, *Ipecac*, and *Colchicum*. Juice therapy, including carrot, beet, and garlic juices, is sometimes recommended, although it can cause discomfort for some people. Charcoal tablets can help absorb toxins and remove them from the digestive tract through bowel elimination. A variety of herbs with antibiotic action, including citrus seed extract, goldenseal (*Hydrastis canadensis*), and Oregon grape (*Mahonia aquifolium*), may also be effective in helping to resolve cases of food poisoning.

Prognosis

The prognosis for uncomplicated cases of Salmonella food poisoning is excellent. Most people recover completely within a week's time. In cases where other medical problems complicate the illness, prognosis depends on the severity of the other medical conditions, as well as the specific organ system infected with *Salmonella*.

Prevention

Prevention of Salmonella food poisoning involves the proper handling and cooking of foods likely to carry the bacteria. This means that recipes utilizing uncooked eggs (Caesar salad dressing, meringue toppings, mousses) need to be modified to eliminate the raw eggs. Not only should chicken be cooked thoroughly, until no pink juices flow, but all surfaces and utensils used on raw chicken must be carefully cleaned to prevent *Salmonella* from contaminating other foods. Careful handwashing is a must before, during, and after all food preparation involving eggs and poultry. Handwashing is also important after handling and playing with pets such as turtles, iguanas, chicks, dogs and cats.

Resources

ORGANIZATIONS

Centers for Disease Control and Prevention. 1600 Clifton Rd., NE, Atlanta, GA 30333. (800) 311-3435, (404) 639-3311. < http://www.cdc.gov >.

Rosalyn Carson-DeWitt, MD

Salmonella paratyphi infection *see* **Paratyphoid fever**

Salmonella typhi infection *see* **Typhoid fever**

Salpingectomy

Definition

Salpingectomy is the removal of one or both of a woman's fallopian tubes, the tubes through which an egg travels from the ovary to the uterus.

Purpose

A salpingectomy may be performed for several different reasons. Removal of one tube (unilateral salpingectomy) is usually performed if the tube has become infected (a condition known as salpingitis).

Salpingectomy is also used to treat an **ectopic pregnancy**, a condition in which a fertilized egg has implanted in the tube instead of inside the uterus. In most cases, the tube is removed only after drug treatments designed to save the structure have failed. (Women with one remaining fallopian tube are still able to get pregnant and carry a **pregnancy** to term.) The other alternative to salpingectomy is surgery to remove the fetus from the fallopian tube, followed by surgery to repair the tube.

A bilateral salpingectomy (removal of both the tubes) is usually done if the ovaries and uterus are also going to be removed. If the fallopian tubes and the

KEY TERMS

Ectopic pregnancy—The development of a fetus at a site other than the inside of the uterus; most commonly, the egg implants itself in the fallopian tube.

Laparoscope—A surgical instrument with a light attached that is inserted through the abdominal wall to allow the surgeon to see the organs in the abdomen.

ovaries are both removed at the same time, this is called a **salpingo-oophorectomy**. A salpingo-oophorectomy is necessary when treating ovarian and endometrial cancer because the fallopian tubes and ovaries are the most common sites to which cancer may spread.

Description

Regional or **general anesthesia** may be used. Often a laparoscope (a hollow tube with a light on one end) is used in this type of operation, which means that the incision can be much smaller and the recovery time much shorter.

In this procedure, the surgeon makes a small incision just beneath the navel. The surgeon inserts a short hollow tube into the abdomen and, if necessary, pumps in carbon dioxide gas in order to move intestines out of the way and better view the organs. After a wider double tube is inserted on one side for the laparoscope, another small incision is made on the other side through which other instruments can be inserted. After the operation is completed, the tubes and instruments are withdrawn. The tiny incisions are sutured and there is very little scarring.

In the case of a pelvic infection, the surgeon makes a horizontal (bikini) incision 4-6 in (10-15 cm) long in the abdomen right above the pubic hairline. This allows the doctor to remove the scar tissue. (Alternatively, a surgeon may use a vertical incision from the pubic bone toward the navel, although this is less common.)

Preparation

The patient is given an injection an hour before surgery to encourage drowsiness.

Aftercare

Aftercare varies depending on whether the tube was removed by **laparoscopy** or through an abdominal incision. Even when major surgery is performed, most women are out of bed and walking around within three days. Within a month or two, a woman can slowly return to normal activities such as driving, exercising, and working.

Risks

All surgery, especially under general anesthesia, carries certain risks, such as the risk of scarring, hemorrhaging, infection, and reactions to the anesthesia. Pelvic surgery can also cause internal scarring which can lead to discomfort years afterward.

Resources

ORGANIZATIONS

National Women's Health Resource Center. 120 Albany St., Suite 820, New Brunswick, NJ 08901. (877) 986-9472. < http://www.healthywomen.org >.

Carol A. Turkington

Salpingitis *see* **Pelvic inflammatory disease**

Salpingo-oophorectomy

Definition

The surgical removal of a fallopian tube and an ovary.

Purpose

This surgery is performed to treat ovarian or other gynecological cancers, or infections as a result of **pelvic inflammatory disease**. Occasionally, removal of one or both ovaries may be done to treat **endometriosis**. If only one tube and ovary are removed, the woman may still be able to conceive and carry a **pregnancy** to term.

Description

If the procedure is performed through a laparoscope, the surgeon can avoid a large abdominal incision and can shorten recovery. With this technique, the surgeon makes a small cut through the abdominal wall just below the navel. When the laparoscope is used, the patient can be given either regional or **general anesthesia**; if there are no complications, the patient can leave the hospital in a day or two.

If a laparoscope is not used, the surgery involves an incision 4–6 in (10–long into the abdomen either extending vertically up from the pubic bone toward the navel, or horizontally (the "bikini incision") across the pubic hairline. The scar from a bikini incision is less noticeable, but some surgeons prefer the vertical incision because it provides greater visibility while operating.

Preparation

A spinal block or general anesthesia may be given before surgery.

Aftercare

If performed through an abdominal incision, salpingo-oophorectomy is major surgery that requires three to six weeks for full recovery. However, if performed laparascopically, the recovery time can be much shorter. There may be some discomfort around the incision for the first few days after surgery, but most women are walking around by the third day. Within a month or so, patients can gradually resume normal activities such as driving, exercising, and working.

Immediately following the operation, the patient should avoid sharply flexing the thighs or the knees. Persistent back **pain** or bloody or scanty urine indicates that a ureter may have been injured during surgery.

If both ovaries are removed in a premenopausal woman as part of the operation, the sudden loss of estrogen will trigger an abrupt **premature menopause** that may involve severe symptoms of hot flashes, vaginal dryness, painful intercourse, and loss of sex drive. (This is also called "surgical menopause.") In addition to these symptoms, women who lose both ovaries also lose the protection these hormones provide against heart disease and **osteoporosis** many years earlier than if they had experienced natural menopause. Women who have had their ovaries removed are seven times more likely to develop coronary heart disease and much more likely to develop bone problems at an early age than are premenopausal women whose ovaries are intact.

For these reasons, some form of estrogen replacement therapy (ERT) may be prescribed to relieve the symptoms of surgical **menopause** and to help prevent heart and bone disease.

In addition, to help offset the higher risks of heart and bone disease after loss of the ovaries, women

KEY TERMS

Androgens—Hormones (specifically testosterone) responsible for male sex characteristics.

Endometriosis—A painful disease in which cells from the lining of the uterus (endometrium) aren't shed during menstruation, but instead attach themselves to other organs in the pelvic cavity. The condition is hard to diagnose and often causes severe pain as well as infertility.

Fallopian tubes—Tubes that extend from either end of the uterus that convey the egg from the ovary to the uterus during each monthly cycle.

Ureter—The tube that carries urine from the bladder to the kidneys.

should get plenty of **exercise**, maintain a low-fat diet, and ensure intake of calcium is adequate.

Reaction to the removal of fallopian tubes and ovaries depends on a wide variety of factors, including the woman's age, the condition that required the surgery, her reproductive history, how much social support she has, and any previous history of depression. Women who have had many gynecological surgeries or chronic pelvic pain seem to have a higher tendency to develop psychological problems after the surgery.

Risks

Major surgery always involves some risk, including infection, reactions to the anesthesia, hemorrhage, and **scars** at the incision site. Almost all pelvic surgery causes some internal scars, which, in some cases, can cause discomfort years after surgery.

Resources

ORGANIZATIONS

Midlife Women's Network. 5129 Logan Ave. S., Minneapolis, MN 55419.(800) 886-4354.

Carol A. Turkington

San Joaquin fever *see* **Coccidioidomycosis**

Sanfilippo's syndrome *see* **Mucopolysaccharidoses**

Saquinavir *see* **Protease inhibitors**

Sarcoidosis

Definition

Sarcoidosis is a disease which can affect many organs within the body. It causes the development of granulomas. Granulomas are masses resembling little tumors. They are made up of clumps of cells from the immune system.

Description

Sarcoidosis is a very puzzling disorder. In addition to having no clear-cut understanding of the cause of sarcoidosis, researchers are also puzzled by its distribution in the world population. In the United States, for example, 10-17 times as many African-Americans are affected as white Americans. In Europe, whites are primarily affected.

Prevalence is a way of measuring the number of people affected per 100,000 people in a given population. The prevalence figures for sarcoidosis are very unusual. In the United States, prevalence figures range from five (5/100,000 in the United States) for whites to 40 for blacks. In Europe, prevalence ranges from three in Poland, to 10 in France, to 64 in Sweden, to 200 for Irish women living in London. Furthermore, a person from a group with very low prevalence who leaves his or her native land for a second location with a higher prevalence will then have the same risk as anyone living in that second location.

Sarcoidosis affects both men and women, although women are more likely to have the disorder. The average age for diagnosis is around 20-40 years.

Causes and symptoms

The cause of sarcoidosis is not known. Because the granulomas are primarily made up of cells from the immune system (macrophages and lymphocytes), an immune connection is strongly suspected. One of the theories which has been put forth suggests that exposure to some toxic or infectious material starts up an immune response. For some reason, the body is unable to stop the response, and it spreads from the original organ to other organs.

Because sarcoidosis has been noted to occur in family groups, a genetic cause has also been suggested. Research shows that identical twins are more likely to both have sarcoidosis than are nonidentical twins or other siblings.

Some cases of sarcoidosis occur without the patient even noting any symptoms. These cases are often discovered by chance during routine chest x rays. Most cases of sarcoidosis, however, begin with very nonspecific symptoms, such as decreased energy, weakness, and a dry **cough**. Occasionally, the cough is accompanied by some mild **pain** in the breastbone (sternum). Some patients note that they are having unusual **shortness of breath** while exercising. Some patients develop **fever**, decreased appetite, and weight loss.

Virtually every system of the body has the potential to suffer the effects of sarcoidosis:

- tender reddish bumps (nodules) or patches often appear on the skin
- the eyes may become red and teary, and the vision blurry
- the joints may become swollen and painful (arthritis)
- lymph nodes in the neck, armpits, and groin become enlarged and tender, lymph nodes within the chest, around the lungs, also become enlarged
- fluid may accumulate around the lungs (pleural effusion), making breathing increasingly difficult
- nasal stuffiness is common, as well as a hoarse sound to the voice
- cysts in the bone may cause pain in the hands and feet, or in other bony areas
- the bone marrow may decrease the production of all blood cells; decreased number of red blood cells causes anemia, fewer white blood cells increases the chance of infections, fewer platelets can increase the chance of bleeding
- the body's ability to process calcium often becomes abnormal, so that excess calcium passes through the kidneys and into the urine; this may cause kidney stones to form
- the liver may become enlarged
- the heart may suffer a variety of complications, including abnormal or missed beats (arrhythmias), inflammation of the covering of the heart (**pericarditis**), and an increasing tendency toward weak, ineffective pumping of the blood (heart failure)
- the nervous system may display the effects of sarcoidosis by hearing loss, chronic inflammation of the coverings of the brain and spinal cord (**meningitis**), abnormalities of the nerve that is involved in vision (optic nerve dysfunction), seizures, and the development of psychiatric disorders

Any, all, or even none of the above symptoms may be present in sarcoidosis.

Diagnosis

Diagnosis depends on information from a number of sources, including the patient's symptoms, the **physical examination**, x-ray pictures of the chest, and a number of other laboratory examinations of blood or other tissue. None of these categories of information are sufficient to make the diagnosis of sarcoidosis. There is no one test or sign or symptom which clearly points to sarcoidosis, excluding all other types of diseases. This is because nearly all of the symptoms and laboratory results in sarcoidosis also occur in other diseases. Diagnosis, then, requires careful consideration of many facts.

The physical examination in sarcoidosis may reveal the characteristic **skin lesions**. Wheezes may be heard throughout the lungs. The liver may be enlarged. Examination of the eyes using a special light called a slit-lamp may reveal changes indicative of sarcoidosis.

The **chest x ray** will show some pattern of abnormalities, which may include enlargement of the lymph nodes which drain the lung, scarring and abnormalities to the tissue of the lungs, and fluid accumulation around the lungs.

Lung function tests measure such things as the amount of air an individual can breathe in and breathe out, the speed at which the air flows in and out, and the amount of air left in the lung after blowing out as much as possible in one second. A variety of lung function tests may show abnormal results in sarcoidosis.

Other types of tests may be abnormal in sarcoidosis. The abnormal test results may also indicate other diseases. They include an elevation of a substance called angiotensin-converting enzyme in the blood, and an increased amount of calcium present in 24 hours worth of urine.

Bronchoscopy is a very helpful diagnostic test. This involves passing a tiny tube (bronchoscope) through the nose or mouth, down the trachea, and into the airways (bronchial tubes). The bronchial tubes can be inspected through the bronchoscope. The bronchoscope is also designed in such a way as to allow biopsies to be obtained. Bronchoalveolar lavage involves washing the surfaces with a sterile saltwater (saline) solution. The saline is then retrieved and examined in a laboratory. Cells and debris from within the bronchial tubes and the tiny sacs of the lung (the alveoli) will be obtained in this way, and can be studied for the presence of an abnormally large number of white blood cells. A tiny piece of the lung tissue can also be obtained through the bronchosocope. This can be studied under a microscope to look for the characteristic granulomas and inflammation of sarcoidosis.

KEY TERMS

Granuloma—Masses made up of a variety of immune cells, as well as fibroblasts (cells which make up connective tissue).

Immune system—The system of specialized organs, lymph nodes, and blood cells throughout the body which work together to prevent foreign invaders (bacteria, viruses, fungi, etc.) from taking hold and growing.

A gallium 67 scan involves the injection of a radioactive material called gallium 67. In sarcoidosis, areas of the body which are inflamed will retain the gallium 67. These areas will then show up on the scan.

Treatment

Many cases of sarcoidosis resolve without treatment. If treatment is needed, the most effective one for sarcoidosis is the administration of steroid medications. These medications work to decrease inflammation throughout the body. The long-term use of steroid medications has serious potential side-effects. Patients are only treated with steroids when the problems caused by sarcoidosis are particularly serious. Many cases of sarcoidosis resolve without treatment.

Prognosis

The prognosis for sarcoidosis is quite good. About 60-70% of the time, sarcoidosis cures itself within a year or two. In about 20-30% of patients, permanent damage occurs to the lungs. About 15-20% of all patients go on to develop a chronic, relapsing form of sarcoidosis. Death can be blamed on sarcoidosis in about 10% of all sarcoidosis cases.

Prevention

Until researchers are able to pinpoint the cause of sarcoidosis, there will be no available recommendations for how to prevent it.

Resources

PERIODICALS

Zitkus, Bruce S. "Sarcoidosis: Varied Symptoms Often Impede Diagnosis of this Multisystem Disorder." *American Journal of Nursing* 97, no. 10 (October 1997): 40 + .

Rosalyn Carson-DeWitt, MD

Sarcomas

Definition

A sarcoma is a bone tumor that contains **cancer** (malignant) cells. A benign bone tumor is an abnormal growth of noncancerous cells.

Description

A primary bone tumor originates in or near a bone. Most primary bone tumors are benign, and the cells that compose them do not spread (metastasize) to nearby tissue or to other parts of the body.

Malignant primary bone tumors account for fewer than 1% of all cancers diagnosed in the United States. They can infiltrate nearby tissues, enter the bloodstream, and metastasize to bones, tissues, and organs far from the original malignancy. Malignant primary bone tumors are characterized as either:

- bone cancers which originate in the hard material of the bone.
- soft-tissue sarcomas which begin in blood vessels, nerves, or tissues containing muscles, fat, or fiber.

Types of bone tumors

Osteogenic sarcoma, or osteosarcoma, is the most common form of bone cancer, accounts for 6% of all instances of the disease, and for about 5% of all cancers that occur in children. Nine hundred new cases of osteosarcoma are diagnosed in the United States every year. The disease usually affects teenagers, and is almost twice as common in boys as in girls.

Osteosarcomas, which grow very rapidly, can develop in any bone but most often occur along the edge or on the end of one of the fast-growing long bones that support the arms and legs. About 80% of all osteosarcomas develop in the parts of the upper and lower leg nearest the knee (the distal femur or in the proximal tibia). The next likely location for an osteosarcoma is the bone of the upper arm closest to the shoulder (the proximal humerus).

Ewing's sarcoma is the second most common form of childhood bone cancer. Accounting for fewer than 5% of bone tumors in children, Ewing's sarcoma usually begins in the soft tissue (the marrow) inside bones of the leg, hips, ribs, and arms. It rapidly infiltrates the lungs, and may metastasize to bones in other parts of the body.

More than 80% of patients who have Ewing's sarcoma are white, and the disease most frequently affects children between ages 5-9, and young adults between ages 20-30. About 27% of all cases of Ewing's sarcoma occur in children under age 10, and 64% occur in adolescents between ages 10-20.

Chondrosarcomas are cancerous bone tumors that most often appear in middle age. Usually originating in strong connective tissue (cartilage) in ribs or leg or hip bones, chondrosarcomas grow slowly. They rarely spread to the lungs. It takes years for a chondrosarcoma to metastasize to other parts of the body, and some of these tumors never spread.

Parosteal osteogenic sarcomas, fibrosarcomas, and chordomas are rare. Parosteal osteosarcomas generally involve both the bone and the membrane that covers it. Fibrosarcomas originate in the ends of the bones in the arm or leg, and then spread to soft tissue. Chordomas develop on the skull or spinal cord.

Osteochondromas, which usually develop between age 10-20, are the most common noncancerous primary bone tumors. Giant cell tumors generally develop in a section of the thigh bone near the knee. Giant cell tumors are originally benign but sometimes become malignant.

Causes and symptoms

The cause of bone cancer is unknown, but the tendency to develop it may be inherited. Children who have bone tumors are often tall for their age, and the disease seems to be associated with growth spurts that occur during childhood and adolescence. Injuries can make the presence of tumors more apparent but do not cause them.

A bone that has been broken or exposed to high doses of radiation used to treat other cancers is more likely than other bones to develop osteosarcoma. A history of noncancerous bone disease also increases bone-cancer risk.

The amount of radiation in diagnostic x rays poses little or no danger of bone-cancer development, but children who have a family history of the most common childhood cancer of the eye (**retinoblastoma**), or who have inherited rare cancer syndromes have a greater-than-average risk of developing bone cancer. Exposure to chemicals found in some paints and dyes can slightly raise the risk.

Both benign and malignant bone tumors can distort and weaken bone and cause **pain**, but benign tumors are generally painless and asymptomatic.

It is sometimes possible to feel a lump or mass, but pain in the affected area is the most common early symptom of bone cancer. Pain is not constant in the initial stages of the disease, but it is aggravated by activity and may be worse at night. If the tumor is located on a leg bone, the patient may limp. Swelling and weakness of the limb may not be noticed until weeks after the pain began.

Other symptoms of bone cancer include:

- a bone that breaks for no apparent reason
- difficulty moving the affected part of the body
- fatigue
- fever
- a lump on the trunk, an arm or leg, or another bone
- persistent, unexplained back pain
- weight loss

Diagnosis

Physical examination and routine x rays may yield enough evidence to diagnose benign bone tumors, but removal of tumor tissue for microscopic analysis (biopsy) is the only sure way to rule out malignancy.

A needle biopsy involves using a fine, thin needle to remove small bits of tumor, or a thick needle to extract tissue samples from the innermost part (the core) of the growth. An excisional biopsy is the surgical removal of a small, accessible tumor. An incisional biopsy is performed on tumors too large or inaccessible to be completely removed. The surgeon performing an incisional biopsy cuts into the patient's skin and removes a portion of the exposed tumor. Performed under local or general anesthetic, biopsy reveals whether a tumor is benign or malignant and identifies the type of cancer cells the malignant tumor contains.

Bone cancer is usually diagnosed about three months after symptoms first appear, and 20% of malignant tumors have metastasized to the lungs or other parts of the body by that time.

Imaging techniques

The following procedures are used, in conjunction with biopsy, to diagnose bone cancer:

- Bone x rays. These x rays usually provide a clear image of osteosarcomas.
- Computerized axial tomography (CAT scan) is a specialized x ray that uses a rotating beam to obtain detailed information about an abnormality and its physical relationship to other parts of the body. A CAT scan can differentiate between osteosarcomas and other types of bone tumors, illustrate how tumor

cells have infiltrated other tissues, and help surgeons decide which portion of a growth would be best to biopsy. Because more than four of every five malignant bone tumors metastasize to the lungs, a CAT scan of the chest is performed to see if these organs have been affected. Chest and abdominal CAT scans are used to determine whether Ewing's sarcoma has spread to the lungs, liver, or lymph nodes.

- Magnetic resonance imaging (MRI) is a specialized scan that relies on radio waves and powerful magnets to reflect energy patterns created by tissue abnormalities and specific diseases. An MRI provides more detailed information than does a CAT scan about tumors and marrow cavities of the bone, and can sometimes detect clusters of cancerous cells that have separated from the original tumor. This valuable information helps surgeons select the most appropriate approach for treatment.
- Radionuclide bone scans. These scans involve injecting a small amount of radioactive material into a vein. Primary tumors or cells that have metastasized absorb the radioactive material and show up as dark spots on the scan.

Cytogenic and molecular genetic studies, which assess the structure and composition of chromosomes and genes, may also be used to diagnose osteosarcoma. These tests can sometimes indicate what form of treatment is most appropriate.

Laboratory studies

A complete **blood count** (CBC) reveals abnormalities in the blood, and may indicate whether bone marrow has been affected. A blood test that measures levels of the enzyme lactate dehydrogenase (LDH) can predict the likelihood of a specific patient's survival.

Immunohistochemistry involves adding special antibodies and chemicals, or stains, to tumor samples. This technique is effective in identifying cells that are found in Ewing's sarcoma but are not present in other malignant tumors.

Reverse transcription polymerase chain reaction (RTPCR) relies on chemical analysis of the substance in the body that transmits genetic information (RNA) to:

- evaluate the effectiveness of cancer therapies
- identify mutations consistent with the presence of Ewing's sarcoma
- reveal cancer that recurs after treatment has been completed

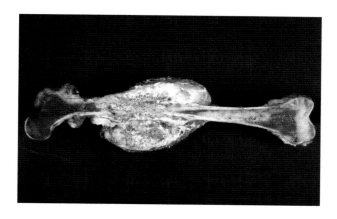

A specimen of a femur bone indicating the cancerous growth around the knee. Osteosarcoma is the most common primary cancer of the bone. *(Photo Researchers, Inc. Reproduced by permission.)*

Staging

Once bone cancer has been diagnosed, the tumor is staged. This process indicates how far the tumor has spread from its original location. The stage of a tumor suggests which form of treatment is most appropriate, and predicts how the condition will probably respond to therapy.

An osteosarcoma may be localized or metastatic. A localized osteosarcoma has not spread beyond the bone where it arose or beyond nearby muscles, tendons, and other tissues. A metastatic osteosarcoma has spread to the lungs, to bones not directly connected to the bone in which the tumor originated, or to other tissues or organs.

Treatment

Since the 1960s, when **amputation** was the only treatment for bone cancer, new **chemotherapy** drugs and innovative surgical techniques have improved survival with intact limbs. Because osteosarcoma is so rare, patients should consider undergoing treatment at a major cancer center staffed by specialists familiar with the disease.

A treatment plan for bone cancer, developed after the tumor has been diagnosed and staged, may include:

• Amputation. Amputation may be the only therapeutic option for large tumors involving nerves or blood vessels that have not responded to chemotherapy. MRI scans indicate how much of the diseased limb must be removed, and surgery is planned to create a cuff, formed of muscles and skin, around the amputated bone. Following surgery, an artificial (prosthetic) leg is fitted over the cuff. A patient who actively participates in the **rehabilitation** process may be walking independently as soon as three months after the amputation.

• Chemotherapy. Chemotherapy is usually administered in addition to surgery, to kill cancer cells that have separated from the original tumor and spread to other parts of the body. Although chemotherapy can increase the likelihood of later development of another form of cancer, the American Cancer Society maintains that the need for chemotherapeutic bone-cancer treatment is much greater than the potential risk.

• Surgery. Surgery, coordinated with diagnostic biopsy, enhances the probability that limb-salvage surgery can be used to remove the cancer while preserving nearby blood vessels and bones. A metal rod or bone graft is used to replace the area of bone removed, and subsequent surgery may be needed to repair or replace rods that have loosened or broken. Patients who have undergone limb-salvage surgery need intensive rehabilitation. It may take as long as a year for a patient to regain full use of a leg following limb-salvage surgery, and patients who have this operation may eventually have to undergo amputation.

• **Radiation therapy**. Radiation therapy is used often to treat Ewing's sarcoma.

• Rotationoplasty. Rotationoplasty, sometimes performed after a leg amputation, involves attaching the lower leg and foot to the thigh bone, so that the ankle replaces the knee. A prosthetic is later added to make the leg as long as it should be. Prosthetic devices are not used to lengthen limbs that remain functional after amputation to remove osteosarcomas located on the upper arm. When an osteosarcoma develops in the jaw bone, the entire lower jaw is removed. Bones from other parts of the body are later grafted on remaining bone to create a new jaw.

Follow-up treatments

After a patient completes the final course of chemotherapy, CAT scans, bone scans, x rays, and other diagnostic tests may be repeated to determine if any traces of tumor remain. If none are found, treatment is discontinued, but patients are advised to see their oncologist and orthopedic surgeon every two or three months for the next year. X rays of the chest and affected bone are taken every four months. An annual echocardiogram is recommended to evaluate any adverse effect chemotherapy may have had on the heart, and CT scans are performed every six months.

Patients who have received treatment for Ewing's sarcoma are examined often - at gradually lengthening intervals - after completing therapy. Accurate growth measurements are taken during each visit and blood is drawn to be tested for side effects of treatment. X rays, CT scans, bone scans, and other imaging studies are generally performed every three months during the first year. If no evidence of tumor growth or recurrence is indicated, these tests are performed less frequently in the following years.

Some benign bone tumors shrink or disappear without treatment. However, regular examinations are recommended to determine whether these tumors have changed in any way.

Alternative treatment

Alternative treatments should never be substituted for conventional bone-cancer treatments or used without the approval of a physician. However, some alternative treatments can be used as adjunctive and supportive therapies during and following conventional treatments.

Dietary adjustments can be very helpful for patients with cancer. Whole foods, including grains, beans, fresh fruits and vegetables, and high quality fats, should be emphasized in the diet, while processed foods should be avoided. Increased consumption of fish, especially cold water fish like salmon, mackerel, halibut, and tuna, provides a good source of **omega-3 fatty acids**. **Nutritional supplements** can build strength and help maintain it during and following chemotherapy, radiation, or surgery. These supplements should be individually prescribed by an alternative practitioner who has experience working with cancer patients.

Many cancer patients claim that **acupuncture** alleviates pain, **nausea**, and **vomiting**. It can also be effective in helping to maintain energy and relative wellness during surgery, chemotherapy, and radiation. Massage, **reflexology**, and relaxation techniques are said to relieve pain, tension, **anxiety**, and depression. **Exercise** can be an effective means of reducing mental and emotional **stress**, while increasing physical strength. **Guided imagery**, **biofeedback**, hypnosis, body work, and progressive relaxation can also enhance quality of life.

Claims of effectiveness in fighting cancer have been made for a variety of herbal medicines. These botanical remedies work on an individual basis and should only be used when prescribed by a practitioner familiar with cancer treatment.

Treating cancer is a complex and individual task. It should be undertaken by a team of support practitioners with varying specialities who can work together for healing the person with cancer.

Prognosis

Benign brain tumors rarely recur, but sarcomas can reappear after treatment was believed to have eliminated every cell.

Likelihood of long-term survival depends on:

- the type and location of the tumor
- how much the tumor has metastasized, and on what organs, bones, or tissues have been affected

More than 85% of patients survive for more than five years after complete surgical removal of low-grade osteosarcomas (tumors that arise in mature tissue and contain a small number of cancerous cells). About 25-30% of patients diagnosed with high-grade osteosarcomas (tumors that develop in immature tissue and contain a large number of cancer cells) will die of the disease.

Two-thirds of all children diagnosed with Ewing's sarcoma will live for more than five years after the disease is detected. The outlook is most favorable for children under age 10, and least favorable in patients whose cancer is not diagnosed until after it has metastasized: fewer than three of every 10 of these patients remain alive five years later. More than 80% of patients whose Ewing's sarcoma is confined to a small area and surgically removed live, for at least five years. Postsurgical radiation and chemotherapy add years to their lives. More than 70% of patients live five years or more with a small Ewing's sarcoma that cannot be removed, but only three out of five patients with large, unremovable tumors survive that long.

Prevention

There is no known way to prevent bone cancer.

Resources

ORGANIZATIONS

American Cancer Society. 1599 Clifton Rd., NE, Atlanta, GA 30329-4251. (800) 227-2345. < http://www.cancer.org >.

CancerCare, Inc. 1180 Avenue of the Americas, New York, NY 10036. (800) 813-4673. < http://www.cancercare.org >.

National Cancer Institute. Building 31, Room 10A31, 31 Center Drive, MSC 2580, Bethesda, MD 20892-2580. (800) 422-6237. < http://www.nci.nih.gov >.

Maureen Haggerty

Saw palmetto

Definition

Saw palmetto is an extract derived from the deep purple berries of the saw palmetto fan palm (*Serenoa repens*), a plant indigenous to the coastal regions of the southern United States and southern California. There is an estimated one million acres of wild saw palmetto palms in Florida, where the bulk of commercial saw palmetto is grown.

Purpose

Saw palmetto is used by natural health practitioners to treat a variety of ailments in men and women, such as testicular inflammation, urinary tract inflammation, coughs, and respiratory congestion. It is also used to strengthen the thyroid gland, balance the metabolism, stimulate appetite, and aid digestion. According to the American Dietetic Association, saw palmetto is one of the most commonly used dietary supplements among Americans between the ages of 50 and 76.

Most of the evidence supporting these uses is anecdotal and has not been proven by controlled clinical trials. However, there is much scientific documentation outlining the effectiveness of the herb in treating irritable bladder and urinary problems in men with benign prostate hyperplasia (BPH), an enlargement of the prostate gland. BPH results in a swelling of the prostate gland that obstructs the urethra. This causes painful urination, reduced urine flow, difficulty starting or stopping the flow, dribbling after urination, and more frequent nighttime urination. Saw palmetto does not reduce prostate enlargement. Instead, it is thought to work in a variety of ways. First, it inhibits the conversion of testosterone into dihydrotestosterone (DHT). BPH is thought to be caused by an increase in testosterone to DHT. Secondly, saw palmetto is believed to interfere with the production of estrogen and progesterone, hormones associated with DHT production.

In addition to causing **pain** and embarrassment, BPH can lead to serious kidney problems if undiagnosed and left untreated. It is a common problem in men over the age of 40. Estimates are that 50–60% of all men will develop BPH in their lifetimes. It is estimated that there are six million men between the ages of 50–79 who have BPH serious enough to require some type of therapy. Yet only half of them seek treatment from physicians. Health practitioners in both the allopathic and natural medicine communities recommend annual prostate examinations for men over the age of 50, and an annual blood test that measures prostate specific antigen, a marker for **prostate cancer**.

Recently, a number of clinical trials have confirmed the effectiveness of saw palmetto in treating BPH. Many of these trials have shown saw palmetto works better than the most commonly used prescription drug, Proscar. Saw palmetto is effective in nearly 90% of patients after six weeks of use, while Proscar is effective in less than 50% of patients. In addition, Proscar may take up to six months to achieve its full effect. Since Proscar blocks the production of testosterone, it can cause **impotence** and breast enlargement. Also, saw palmetto is significantly less expensive than Proscar. A one-month supply of saw palmetto costs $12–25, while a one month supply of Proscar costs $65–75. Other prescription drugs used to treat BPH are Cardura (doxazosin), Hytrin (terazosin), and Flomax (tamsulosin hydrochloride). Originally prescribed to treat **hypertension**, Cardura and Hytrin can drop blood pressure, causing lightheadedness and **fainting**. Presently, saw palmetto is being evaluated by the U.S. Food and Drug Administration (FDA) for treatment of BPH. If approved, it would become the first herbal product to be licensed by the agency as a treatment for a specific condition. Saw palmetto is also used as a treatment for prostate complaints and irritable bladder.

Since the 1960s, extensive clinical studies of saw palmetto have been done in Europe. A 1998 review of 24 European trials involved nearly 3,000 men, some taking saw palmetto, others taking Proscar, and a third group taking a placebo. The men taking saw palmetto had a 28% improvement in urinary tract symptoms, a 24% improvement in peak urine flow, and 43% improvement in overall urine flow. The results were nearly comparable to the group taking Proscar and superior to the men taking a placebo.

On the other hand, saw palmetto does not appear to be useful in treating **prostatitis** or chronic pelvic pain syndrome (CPPS) in men. A group of researchers at Columbia University reported in early 2004 that men given saw palmetto for CP/CPPS showed no appreciable improvement at the end of a year-long trial.

Uses in women

There is very little documentation or scientific research into saw palmetto use in women. However, several studies in the 1990s show that the BPH drug Proscar can be effective in stopping unwanted facial and body hair growth, and in treating thinning hair in

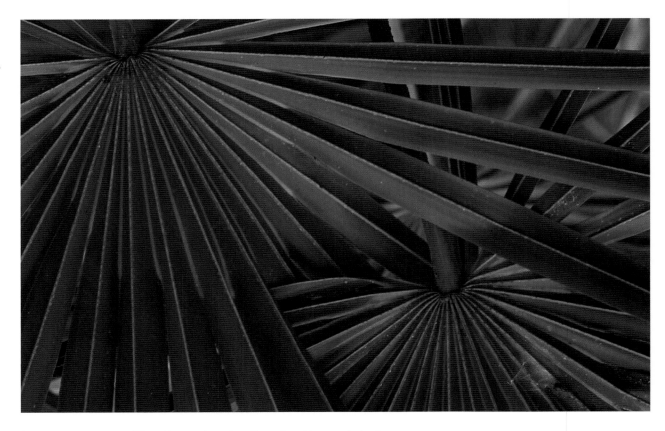

Saw palmetto leaves. *(Photo Researchers, Inc. Reproduced by permission.)*

women. It works by blocking the action of an enzyme called 5-alpha reductase. Anecdotal reports suggest that saw palmetto may be as effective as Proscar in treating unwanted hair growth and thinning hair, and in preventing some types of **acne**. It has also been used to treat urinary tract inflammation and help relieve the symptoms of menstruation. There are claims it can be used to enlarge breasts, but these claims have not been scientifically tested.

History

Saw palmetto berries have been used in American folk medicine for several hundred years as an aphrodisiac and for treating prostate problems. Native Americans in the southeast United States have used saw palmetto since the 1700s to treat male urinary problems. In the 1800s, medical botanist John Lloyd noted that animals that ate saw palmetto appeared healthier and fatter than other livestock. Early American settlers noticed the same effects and used the juice from saw palmetto berries to gain weight, to improve general disposition, as a sedative, and to promote reproductive health.

In the United States, the medicinal uses of saw palmetto were first documented in 1879 by Dr. J. B. Read, a physician in Savannah, Georgia, who published a paper on the medicinal benefits of the herb in the April 1879 issue of *American Journal of Pharmacy*. He found the herb useful in treating a wide range of conditions. "By its peculiar soothing power on the mucous membrane it induces sleep, relieves the most troublesome coughs, promotes expectoration, improves digestion, and increases fat, flesh and strength. Its sedative and diuretic properties are remarkable," Read wrote. "Considering the great and diversified power of the saw palmetto as a therapeutic agent, it seems strange that it should have so long escaped the notice of the medical profession."

A pungent tea made from saw palmetto berries was commonly used in the early 1900s to treat prostate enlargement and urinary tract infections. It was also used in men to increase sperm production and sex drive, although these uses are discounted today. One of the first published medical recommendations that saw palmetto was effective in treating prostate problems appeared in the 1926 edition of *United States Dispensatory*. In the late 1920s, the use of medicinal plants, including saw palmetto, began to decline in the United States, while at the same time, it was on the rise in Europe.

Preparations

The National Institute on Aging recommends that people taking saw palmetto should obtain it only from reputable sources. In addition, people should use only standardized extracts that contain 85–95% fatty acids and sterols. Dosages vary depending on the type of saw palmetto used. A typical dose is 320 mg per day of standardized extract (1–2 g) per day of ground dried whole berries. It may take up to four weeks of use before beneficial effects are seen. In late 1999, the web-based independent consumer organization ConsumerLab.com tested 27 leading brands of saw palmetto for fatty acid and sterol content. Ten of the brands contained less than the minimum recommended level of 85% fatty acids and sterols.

Precautions

There are no special precautions associated with taking saw palmetto, even in high doses. However, BPH can become a serious problem if left untreated. Men who are experiencing symptoms should be examined by a physician, since the symptoms of BPH are similar to those of prostate **cancer**. Men over the age of 50 should have a yearly prostate exam. Saw palmetto should only be used under a doctor's supervision by people with prostate cancer, **breast cancer**, or any sex hormone related diseases. Although the effects of saw palmetto on a fetus is unknown, pregnant women are advised not to take saw palmetto. Saw palmetto can alter hormonal activity that could have an adverse effect on the fetus. Women taking birth control pills or estrogen replacement products should consult a physician before taking saw palmetto. Persons taking testosterone or other anabolic steroids should not take saw palmetto without first consulting their doctor.

In rare cases, allergic reactions to saw palmetto have been reported. Symptoms include difficulty breathing, constricting of the throat, **hives**, and swelling of the lips, tongue, or face. Persons experiencing any of these symptoms should stop taking saw palmetto and seek immediate medical attention.

Side effects

The only reported minor side effects are rare and include cramps, **nausea**, **diarrhea**, and **headache**.

KEY TERMS

Anabolic steroids—A group of mostly synthetic hormones sometimes taken by athletes to temporarily increase muscle size.

Aphrodisiac—Any substance that excites sexual desire.

Estrogen—A hormone that stimulates development of female secondary sex characteristics.

Placebo—An inert or innocuous substance used in controlled experiments testing the efficacy of another substance.

Progesterone—A steroid hormone that is a biological precursor to corticoid (another steroid hormone) and androgen (a male sex hormone).

Testosterone—A male hormone produced in the testes or made synthetically that is responsible for male secondary sex characteristics.

Urethra—The canal that carries urine from the bladder.

Interactions

Saw palmetto may interfere with such hormone-related drugs as testosterone and estrogen replacements, including Premarin, Cenestin, Vivelle, Fempatch, and Climara. It may also interact with such birth control pills as Triphasil, Ovral, Lo-Ovral, Nordette, Alesse, Demulen, and Ortho-Novum. Anyone on these types of medications should consult their doctor before taking saw palmetto. There are no known restrictions on food, beverages, or physical activity while taking saw palmetto.

Several herbs and **minerals** have been used in conjunction with saw palmetto in treating BPH. A 1996 European study showed positive results in treating patients with a daily dose of 320 mg of saw palmetto extract and 240 mg of nettle root extract. Many alternative health practitioners also recommend saw palmetto be used in combination with the herb pygeum africanum, pumpkin seeds, zinc, flaxseed oil, certain amino acids, antioxidants, and **diets** high in protein and soy products. Some factors that can impair the effectiveness of saw palmetto include beer, cigarette smoke, and some chemical pesticides used on fruit and vegetables. Some physicians recommend using saw palmetto in addition to a prescription medicine, such as Proscar, Hytrin, or Cardura.

Resources

BOOKS

Foster, Steven W. *Guide to Herbal Dosages.* Loveland, CO: Interweave Press, 2000.

PERIODICALS

D'Epiro, Nancy Walsh. "Saw Palmetto and the Prostate." *Patient Care* April 15, 1999: 29.

Gong, E. M., and G. S. Gerber. "Saw Palmetto and Benign Prostatic Hyperplasia." *American Journal of Chinese Medicine* 32 (March 2004): 331–338.

Gunther, S., R. E. Patterson, A. R. Kristal, et al. "Demographic and Health-Related Correlates of Herbal and Specialty Supplement Use." *Journal of the American Dietetic Association* 104 (January 2004): 27–34.

Kaplan, S. A., M. A. Volpe, and A. E. Te. "A Prospective, 1-Year Trial Using Saw Palmetto Versus Finasteride in the Treatment of Category III Prostatitis/Chronic Pelvic Pain Syndrome." *Journal of Urology* 171 (January 2004): 284–288.

Peng, C. C., P. A. Glassman, L. E. Trilli, et al. "Incidence and Severity of Potential Drug-Dietary Supplement Interactions in Primary Care Patients: An Exploratory Study of 2 Outpatient Practices." *Archives of Internal Medicine* 164 (March 22, 2004): 630–636.

ORGANIZATIONS

National Institute on Aging (NIA) Information Center. P. O. Box 8057, Gaithersburg, MD 20892-8057. (800) 222-2225. < http://www.nih.gov/nia >.

Ken R. Wells
Rebecca J. Frey, PhD

Scabies

Definition

Scabies is a relatively contagious infection caused by a tiny mite(*Sarcoptes scabiei*).

Description

Scabies is caused by a tiny insect about 0.3 mm long called a mite. When a human comes in contact with the female mite, the mite burrows under the skin, laying eggs along the line of its burrow. These eggs hatch, and the resulting offspring rise to the surface of the skin, mate, and repeat the cycle either within the skin of the original host, or within the skin of its next victim.

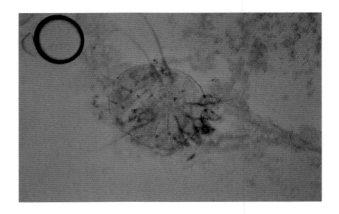

An enhanced image of a scab mite. *(Custom Medical Stock Photo. Reproduced by permission.)*

The intense **itching** almost always caused by scabies is due to a reaction within the skin to the feces of the mite. The first time someone is infected with scabies, he or she may not notice any itching for a number of weeks (four to six weeks). With subsequent infections, the itchiness will begin within hours of picking up the first mite.

Causes and symptoms

Scabies is most common among people who live in overcrowded conditions, and whose ability to practice good hygiene is limited. Scabies can be passed between people by close skin contact. Although the mites can only live away from human skin for about three days, sharing clothing or bedclothes can pass scabies among family members or close contacts. In May 2002, the Centers for Disease Control (CDC) included scabies in its updated guidelines for the treatment of **sexually transmitted diseases**.

The itching, or pruritus, from scabies is worse after a hot shower and at night. Burrows are seen as winding, slightly raised gray lines along the skin. The female mite may be seen at one end of the burrow, as a tiny pearl-like bump underneath the skin. Because of the intense itching, burrows may be obscured by scratch marks left by the patient. The most common locations for burrows include the sides of the fingers, between the fingers, the top of the wrists, around the elbows and armpits, around the nipples of the breasts in women, in the genitalia of men, around the waist (beltline), and on the lower part of the buttocks. Babies may have burrows on the soles of their feet, palms of their hands, and faces.

Scratching seems to serve some purpose in scabies, as the mites are apparently often inadvertently

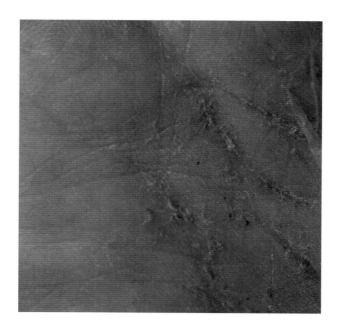

Scab mites have penetrated under the skin of this person' hand. *(Custom Medical Stock Photo. Reproduced by permission.)*

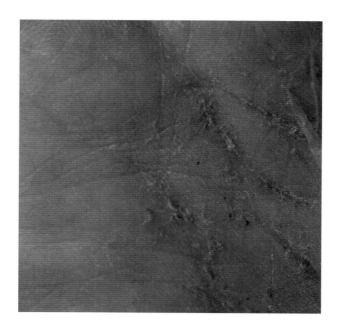

removed. Most infestations with scabies are caused by no more than 15 mites altogether.

Infestation with huge numbers of mites (on the order of thousands to millions) occurs when an individual does not scratch, or when an individual has a weakened immune system. These patients include those who live in institutions; are mentally retarded, or physically infirm; have other diseases which affect the amount of sensation they have in their skin (**leprosy** or syringomyelia); have leukemia or diabetes; are taking medications which lower their immune response (**cancerchemotherapy**, drugs given after organ transplantation); or have other diseases which lower their immune response (such as acquired **immunodeficiency** syndrome or **AIDS**). This form of scabies, with its major infestation, is referred to as crusted scabies or Norwegian scabies. Infected patients have thickened, crusty areas all over their bodies, including over the scalp. Their skin is scaly. Their fingernails may be thickened and horny.

Diagnosis

Diagnosis can be made simply by observing the characteristic burrows of the mites causing scabies. A sterilized needle can be used to explore the pearly bump at the end of a burrow, remove its contents, and place it on a slide to be examined. The mite itself may then be identified under a microscope.

Occasionally, a type of mite carried on dogs (*Sarcoptes scabiei var. canis*) may infect humans. These mites cannot survive for very long on humans, and so the infection is very light.

Treatment

Several types of lotions (usually containing 5% permethrin) can be applied to the body, and left on for 12–24 hours. One topical application is usually sufficient, although the scabicide may be reapplied after a week if mites remain. Preparations containing lindane are no longer recommended for treating scabies as of 2003 because of the potential for damage to the nervous system. Itching can be lessened by the use of calamine lotion or antihistamine medications.

In addition to topical medications, the doctor may prescribe oral ivermectin. Ivermectin is a drug that was originally developed for veterinary practice as a broad-spectrum antiparasite agent. Studies done in humans, however, have found that ivermectin is as safe and effective as topical medications for treating scabies. A study published in 2003 reported that ivermectin is safe for people in high-risk categories, including those with compromised immune systems.

Prognosis

The prognosis for complete recovery from scabies infestation is excellent. In patients with weak immune systems, the biggest danger is that the areas of skin involved with scabies will become secondarily infected with bacteria.

Prevention

Good hygiene is essential in the prevention of scabies. When a member of a household is diagnosed with scabies, all that person's recently-worn clothing and bedding should be washed in very hot water.

Resources

BOOKS

Beers, Mark H., MD, and Robert Berkow, MD., editors. "Scabies (The Itch)." Section 10, Chapter 114 In *The Merck Manual of Diagnosis and Therapy*. Whitehouse Station, NJ: Merck Research Laboratories, 2004.

PERIODICALS

Burroughs, R. F., and D. M. Elston. "What's Eating You? Canine Scabies." *Cutis* 72 (August 2003): 107–109.

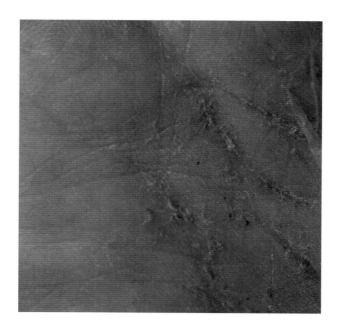

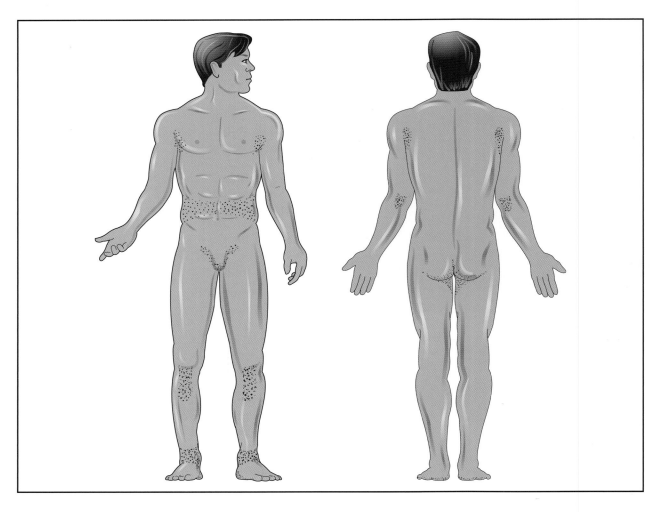

Scabies is a contagious skin infection common among people who live in overcrowded, less than ideal hygienic environments. It is caused by the infestation of female scab mites that, upon contact, burrows under the victim's skin and lays eggs along the lines of passage. Once the eggs hatch, the new mites rise to the skin's surface, mate, and repeats the infestation. Scabies can occur anywhere on the body, including the armpit, groin, buttocks, genital area, and ankles, as shown in the illustration above. *(Illustration by Electronic Illustrators Group.)*

KEY TERMS

Mite—An insect parasite belonging to the order Acarina. The organism that causes scabies is a mite.

Pruritus—An unpleasant itching sensation. Scabies is characterized by intense pruritus.

Topical—A type of medication applied to the skin or body surface.

Burstein, G. R., and K. A. Workowski. "Sexually Transmitted Diseases Treatment Guidelines." *Current Opinion in Pediatrics* 15 (August 2003): 391–397.

Fawcett, R. S. "Ivermectin Use in Scabies." *American Family Physician* 68 (September 15, 2003): 1089–1092.

Santoro, A. F., M. A. Rezac, and J. B. Lee. "Current Trend in Ivermectin Usage for Scabies." *Journal of Drugs in Dermatology* 2 (August 2003): 397–401.

ORGANIZATIONS

American Academy of Dermatology (AAD). 930 East Woodfield Road, Schaumburg, IL 60173. (847) 330-0230. < http://www.aad.org >.

Rosalyn Carson-DeWitt, MD
Rebecca J. Frey, PhD

Scarlatina *see* **Scarlet fever**

Scarlet fever

Definition

Scarlet **fever** is an infection that is caused by a bacteria called streptococcus. The disease is characterized by a sore throat, fever, and a sandpaper-like rash on reddened skin. It is primarily a childhood disease. If scarlet fever is untreated, serious complications such as **rheumatic fever** (a heart disease) or kidney inflammation (**glomerulonephritis**) can develop.

Description

Scarlet fever, also known as scarlatina, gets its name from the fact that the patient's skin, especially on the cheeks, is flushed. A **sore throat** and raised rash over much of the body are accompanied by fever and sluggishness (lethargy). The fever usually subsides within a few days and recovery is complete by two weeks. After the fever is gone, the skin on the face and body flakes; the skin on the palms of the hands and soles of the feet peels more dramatically.

This disease primarily affects children ages two to ten. It is highly contagious and is spread by sneezing, coughing, or direct contact. The incubation period is three to five days, with symptoms usually beginning on the second day of the disease, and lasting from four to ten days.

Early in the twentieth century, severe scarlet fever epidemics were common. Today, the disease is rare. Although this decline is due in part to the availability of **antibiotics**, that is not the entire reason since the decline began before the widespread use of antibiotics. One theory is that the strain of bacteria that causes scarlet fever has become weaker with time.

Causes and symptoms

Scarlet fever is caused by Group A streptococcal bacteria (*S. pyogenes*). Group A streptococci can be highly toxic microbes that can cause strep throat, wound or skin infections, **pneumonia**, and serious kidney infections, as well as scarlet fever. The Group A streptococci are; hemolytic bacteria, which means that the bacteria have the ability to lyse or break red blood cells. The strain of streptococcus that causes scarlet fever is slightly different from the strain that causes most strep throats. The scarlet fever strain of bacteria produces a toxin, called an erythrogenic toxin. This toxin is what causes the skin to flush.

The main symptoms and signs of scarlet fever are fever, lethargy, sore throat, and a bumpy rash that blanches under pressure. The rash appears first on the upper chest and spreads to the neck, abdomen, legs, arms, and in folds of skin such as under the arm or groin. In scarlet fever, the skin around the mouth tends to be pale, while the cheeks are flushed. The patient usually has a "strawberry tongue," in which inflamed bumps on the tongue rise above a bright red coating. Finally, dark red lines (called Pastia's lines) may appear in the creases of skin folds.

Diagnosis

Cases of scarlet fever are usually diagnosed and treated by pediatricians or family medicine practitioners. The chief diagnostic signs of scarlet fever are the characteristic rash, which spares the palms and soles of the feet, and the presence of a strawberry tongue in children. Strawberry tongue is rarely seen in adults.

The doctor will take note of the signs and symptoms to eliminate the possibility of other diseases. Scarlet fever can be distinguished from **measles**, a viral infection that is also associated with a fever and rash, by the quality of the rash, the presence of a sore throat in scarlet fever, and the absence of the severe eye inflammation and severe runny nose that usually accompany measles.

The doctor will also distinguish between a **strep throat**, a viral infection of the throat, and scarlet fever. With a strep infection, the throat is sore and appears beefy and red. White spots appear on the tonsils. Lymph nodes under the jawline may swell and become tender. However, none of these symptoms are specific for strep throat and may also occur with a viral infection. Other signs are more characteristic of bacterial infections. For example, inflammation of the lymph nodes in the neck is typical in strep infections, but not viral infections. On the other hand, cough, **laryngitis**, and stuffy nose tend to be associated with viral infections rather than strep infections. The main feature that distinguishes scarlet fever from a mere strep throat is the presence of the sandpaper-red rash.

Laboratory tests are needed to make a definitive diagnosis of a strep infection and to distinguish a strep throat from a viral sore throat. One test that can be performed is a blood cell count. Bacterial infections are associated with an elevated white blood cell count. In viral infections, the white blood cell count is generally below normal.

A throat culture can distinguish between a strep infection and a viral infection. A throat swab from the infected person is brushed over a nutrient gel (a sheep blood agar plate) and incubated overnight to detect the presence of hemolytic bacteria. In a positive culture, a clear zone will appear in the gel surrounding the bacterium, indicating that a strep infection is present.

Treatment

Although scarlet fever will often clear up spontaneously within a few days, antibiotic treatment with either oral or injectable penicillin is usually recommended to reduce the severity of symptoms, prevent complications, and prevent spread to others. Antibiotic treatment will shorten the course of the illness in small children but may not do so in adolescents or adults. Nevertheless, treatment with antibiotics is important to prevent complications.

Since penicillin injections are painful, oral penicillin may be preferable. If the patient is unable to tolerate penicillin, alternative antibiotics such as

KEY TERMS

Clindamycin—An antibiotic that can be used instead of penicillin.

Erythrogenic toxin—A toxin or agent produced by the scarlet fever-causing bacteria that causes the skin to turn red.

Erythromycin—An antibiotic that can be used instead of penicillin.

Glomerulonephritis—A serious inflammation of the kidneys that can be caused by streptococcal bacteria; a potential complication of untreated scarlet fever.

Hemolytic bacteria—Bacteria that are able to burst red blood cells.

Lethargy—The state of being sluggish.

Pastia's lines—Red lines in the folds of the skin, especially in the armpit and groin, that are characteristic of scarlet fever.

Penicillin—An antibiotic that is used to treat bacterial infections.

Procaine penicillin—An injectable form of penicillin that contains an anesthetic to reduce the pain of the injection.

Rheumatic fever—A heart disease that is a complication of a strep infection.

Sheep blood agar plate—A petri dish filled with a nutrient gel containing red blood cells that is used to detect the presence of streptococcal bacteria in a throat culture. Streptococcal bacteria will lyse or break the red blood cells, leaving a clear spot around the bacterial colony.

Strawberry tongue—A sign of scarlet fever in which the tongue appears to have a red coating with large raised bumps.

erythromycin or clindamycin may be used. However, the entire course of antibiotics, usually 10 days, will need to be followed for the therapy to be effective. Because symptoms subside quickly, there is a temptation to stop therapy prematurely. It is important to take all of the pills in order to kill the bacteria. Not completing the course of therapy increases the risk of developing rheumatic fever and kidney inflammation.

If the patient is considered too unreliable to take all of the pills or is unable to take oral medication, daily injections of procaine penicillin can be given in the hip or thigh muscle. Procaine is an anesthetic that makes the injections less painful.

Bed rest is not necessary, nor is **isolation** of the patient. Aspirin or Tylenol (acetaminophen) may be given for fever or relief of **pain**.

Prognosis

If treated promptly with antibiotics, full recovery is expected. Once a patient has had scarlet fever, they develop immunity and cannot develop it again.

Prevention

Avoiding exposure to children who have the disease will help prevent the spread of scarlet fever.

Resources

BOOKS

Bennett, J. Claude, and Fred Plum, editors. *Cecil Textbook of Medicine*. Philadelphia: W. B. Saunders Co., 1996.

Sally J. Jacobs, EdD

Scars

Definition

Scars are marks created during the healing of damage to the skin or tissues.

Description

A scar is a manifestation of the skin's healing process. After skin or tissue is wounded, the body releases collagen to mend the damage. Collagen, a protein, reattaches the damaged skin. As the wound heals, a temporary crust forms and covers it. The crust is a scab that protects the damaged area.

Causes of scars include cuts, sores, surgery, and **burns**. Severe **acne** and chicken pox may also scar skin. The degree that skin scars depends on more than the size and depth of the wound. Age also affects the process. The healing process is stronger in younger skin. That results in scars that are thicker than those of older people. Other factors affecting the type of scar are ethnicity, heredity, and the location of the injury.

Children are active and susceptible to cuts and injuries. They and people with fair complexions tend to get hypertophic scars. While Asians and blacks are likely to have keloid scars, people from other ethnic groups also experience this form of scarring.

Keloid and hypertophic scars have similar appearances. However, the keloid scar expands beyond the original wound.

The location of the wound also has an effect on its size. If the scar is located on places like the knee or shoulder, it will eventually widen because these areas are in motion.

Treatment could minimize a scar but will not erase the mark.

Causes and symptoms

Scarring is the natural process of repairing an open wound, injury, surgical incision, or other conditions like acne. Initially, a scar is red because blood vessels are created while the body forms scar tissue. The damaged area is covered by a protective scab that eventually falls off. The scar may become brown or pink. It generally fades over time and becomes less visible.

The healing process takes from one year to 18 months. Some scars heal naturally. Other scars require additional treatment.

Hypertophic scars and keloids

Hypertophic scars and **keloids** are caused by an over-active healing process. This produces an excessive amount of collagen at the wound site. Both types of scars are red, thick, and raised above the wound.

Hypertophic scars do not extend beyond the wound site. The scar may itch and usually heals without professional treatment in about a year.

Keloids are large scars that could form after surgery, an injury, burn, or body piercing. This scarring often occurs on the ear lobe or chest. Sometimes keloids develop spontaneously.

The keloid is raised, rigid, and grows beyond the wound. The keloid can continue to grow. Scars are generally harmless, but may itch or feel tender. In addition, a person may feel self-conscious about the scar's appearance.

Contracture scars

Contracture scars are caused by the loss of a large section of skin due to burns or other injury. The scar contracts or tightens around the wound. This contraction could impact a person's mobility. If the scar deepens, it could affect muscles and nerves.

Acne scars

Acne scars may appear after the severe stage of acne, a skin condition usually caused by hormonal changes. The inflammatory condition is seen in adolescence, but acne can occur later in life.

Severe acne is triggered by clogged pores that cause bacteria to multiply. It occurs more frequently in adolescent boys than girls. If the acne is not treated, there could be scarring. The types of scars include pit-like pockmarks.

Diagnosis

Since visible scars could make people self-conscious, they will probably seek treatment rather than a diagnosis. Medical professionals who treat scars include dermatologists and plastic surgeons. Dermatologists are physicians who care for the skin. Their expertise includes three or more years of medical and surgical training.

Scar treatment is usually not covered by insurance. Cosmetic procedures, those done to improve a person's appearance, are considered elective surgery and are paid for by the patient. However, if scars cause a physical impairment, coverage may be issued. Examples of impairments include burn scars and keloids that restrict motion. For coverage to be approved, it is helpful for the primary care doctor to document the patient's case in writing.

Treatment

A scar is permanent and cannot be completely removed. However, treatment can alter a scar's appearance. These procedures range from the application of over-the-counter ointment to surgery. Scar treatment should start after an injury because wound care affects scarring. The wound should be cleaned and covered. Picking at the scab breaks the collagen and allows germs to enter the wound. Time also helps with healing. Scars become smaller, and the color fades.

However, additional treatment is required for some scars. While some procedures are more effective for keloids and hypertrophic scars, the procedure for acne scars is based on the type of scarring. Treatment for burn scars may include skin grafts surgery.

Surgery

The surgical procedure for scars is referred to as scar revision because the procedure modifies the scar's appearance. The cost of scar revision averaged $1,129 in 2003, according to a membership survey of the American Academy of Facial Plastic and **Reconstructive Surgery** (AAFPRS).

This procedure works well on scars that are wide or long. Other treatments may be recommended for keloids because a surgical incision could cause a new scar and create another keloid. To reduce the risk of another scar, surgery may be followed by the injection of cortisone steroids.

Steroid Injections

Steroid injection is a singular form of treatment for scars, particularly keloid and hypertophic scars. **Corticosteroids** are an anti-inflammatory drug that helps to lessen the scar's red color and thickness. The treatment flattens the scar and helps with **itching**. Injection costs vary and could cost $150 per scar, according to a member of the American Academy of Dermatologists (AAD).

Cyrosurgery

Cryosurgery involves the freezing of freezes tissue with a probe containing nitrous oxide. It is used to modify scars, especially keloid and hypertrophic scars. Treatment vary could cost $175 per lesion, according to the AAD member.

Dermabrasion

Dermabrasion is the removal of a layer of the skin's surface. Scars including those caused by acne are smoothed or sanded by an instrument. The procedure costs approximately $150 per treatment.

Silicone gel sheets

Silicone gel sheets can be purchased over-the-counter. The sheets are worn over the scar area to seal moisture. The treatment helps with itching and to reduce scar thickness and color. Cost of sheets for small **wounds** ranges from $30 to $50.

Alternative treatment

Alternate methods of treating scars range from applying Vitamin E to massaging the skin. People should consult with a doctor or other health care professional before starting treatment involving contact with the scarred area.

These procedures include applying obtained Vitamin E, aloe vera, or cocoa butter to the scar. Vitamin E is sold as an oil or obtained by opening a vitamin capsule. Aloe is an African plant and is sold I capsule form and as a skin care product. Cocoa butter is a fat made from cacao seeds.

Those items are thought to help with healing so that a scar is less visible. However, time also helps to lessen the scar's appearance. Those substances should be applied only after a scar is well-healed.

Massaging mild scars is done to relax rigid scar tissue. The scar is massaged for about two minutes. Afterwards, Vitamin E oil is applied to the skin. The process should be discontinued if the area becomes sore or red.

Prognosis

The prognosis for scar treatment depends on factors including the type and severity of the scar. Keloids may return, and all scars are permanent. If treatment does not completely minimize a scar to the patient's satisfaction, the person can apply make-up to the scarred area.

Prevention

The primary way to prevent scarring is to avoid injuries. People should wear protective gear when participating in sports. Furthermore, acne should be treated before the condition reaches the severe stage.

If injured, a person should immediately treat the wound because this reduces the risk of scarring. The wound should be cleaned and covered. If stitches aren't needed, a butterfly bandage is effective at keeping the wound closed. Moreover, a balanced diet also helps with the healing process.

Picking at the scab should be avoided because this interferes with the healing process and raises the risk of scarring.

Resources

BOOKS

Turkington, Carol. *Skin Deep: An A-Z of Skin Disorders, Treatments, and Health.* Facts on File, Inc., 1998.

PERIODICALS

ORGANIZATIONS

American Academy of Dermatology. 1350 I Street NW, Suite 870, Washington, DC 20005-4355. 202-842-3555. < http://www.aad.org >.

American Academy of Facial Plastic and Reconstructive Surgery. 310 South Henry Street, Alexandria, VA 22314. 703) 299-9291. < http://www.aafprs.org >.

American Society of Plastic Surgeons, Plastic Surgery Educational Foundation. 444 East Algonquin Road, Arlington Heights, IL 60005. 847-228-9900. < http://www.plasticsurgery.org >.

OTHER

Treatment of Scars WebMD Medical Reference in collaboration with the Cleveland Clinic, Department of Plastic Surgery. September 2003 [cited March 28, 2005]. < http://my.webmd.com/content/article/76/90236.htm >.

What is a Scar? Academy of Dermatology pamphlet, 2004 [cited March 28, 2005]. < http://www.aad.org/public/Publications/pamphlets/WhatisaScar.htm >.

AAFPRS 2003 Statistics on Trends in Facial Plastic Surgery American Academy of Facial Plastic and Reconstructive Surgery. 2004 [cited March 28, 2005}. < http://www.aafprs.org/media/stats_polls/AAFPRS%20MEDIA%202004%20-%20Final.pd >.

Liz Swain

Schatzki's ring *see* **Lower esophageal ring**

Schistosomiasis

Definition

Schistosomiasis, also known as bilharziasis or snail **fever**, is a primarily tropical parasitic disease caused by the larvae of one or more of five types of flatworms or blood flukes known as schistosomes. The name bilharziasis comes from Theodor Bilharz, a German pathologist, who identified the worms in 1851.

Description

Infections associated with worms present some of the most universal health problems in the world. In fact, only **malaria** accounts for more diseases than schistosomiasis. The World Health Organization (WHO) estimates that 200 million people are infected and 120 million display symptoms. Another 600 million people are at risk of infection. Schistosomes are prevalent in rural and outlying city areas of 74 countries in Africa, Asia, and Latin America. In Central China and Egypt, the disease poses a major health risk.

There are five species of schistosomes that are prevalent in different areas of the world and produce somewhat different symptoms:

- *Schistosoma mansoni* is widespread in Africa, the Eastern-Mediterranean, the Caribbean, and South America and can only infect humans and rodents.

- *S. mekongi* is prevalent only in the Mekong river basin in Asia.

- *S. japonicum* is limited to China and the Philippines and can infect other mammals, in addition to humans, such as pigs, dogs, and water buffalos. As a result, it can be harder to control disease caused by this species.
- *S. intercalatum* is found in central Africa.
- *S. haematobium* occurs predominantly in Africa and the Eastern Mediterranean.

Intestinal schistosomiasis, caused by *Schistosoma japonicum, S. mekongi, S. mansoni,* and *S. intercalatum,* can lead to serious complications of the liver and spleen. Urinary schistosomiasis is caused by *S. haematobium.*

It is difficult to know how many individuals die of schistomiasis each year because death certificates and patient records seldom identify schistosomiasis as the primary cause of death. Mortality estimates vary related to the type of schistosome infection but is generally low, for example, 2.4 of 100,000 die each year from infection with *S. mansoni.*

Causes and symptoms

All five species are contracted in the same way, through direct contact with fresh water infested with the free-living form of the parasite known as cercariae. The building of dams, irrigation systems, and reservoirs, and the movements of refugee groups introduce and spread schistosomiasis.

Eggs are excreted in human urine and feces and, in areas with poor sanitation, contaminate freshwater sources. The eggs break open to release a form of the parasite called miracidium. Freshwater snails become infested with the miracidium, which multiply inside the snail and mature into multiple cercariae that the snail ejects into the water. The cercariae, which survive outside a host for 48 hours, quickly penetrate unbroken skin, the lining of the mouth, or the gastrointestinal tract. Once inside the human body, the worms penetrate the wall of the nearest vein and travel to the liver where they grow and sexually mature. Mature male and female worms pair and migrate either to the intestines or the bladder where egg production occurs. One female worm may lay an average of 200 to 2,000 eggs per day for up to twenty years. Most eggs leave the blood stream and body through the intestines. Some of the eggs are not excreted, however, and can lodge in the tissues. It is the presence of these eggs, rather than the worms themselves, that causes the disease.

Early symptoms of infection

Many individuals do not experience symptoms. If present, it usually takes four to six weeks for symptoms to appear. The first symptom of the disease may be a general ill feeling. Within twelve hours of infection, an individual may complain of a **tingling** sensation or light rash, commonly referred to as "swimmer's itch," due to irritation at the point of entrance. The rash that may develop can mimic **scabies** and other types of **rashes**. Other symptoms can occur two to ten weeks later and can include fever, aching, **cough**, **diarrhea**, or gland enlargement. These symptoms can also be related to avian schistosomiasis, which does not cause any further symptoms in humans.

Katayama fever

Another primary condition, called Katayama fever, may also develop from infection with these worms, and it can be very difficult to recognize. Symptoms include fever, lethargy, the eruption of pale temporary bumps associated with severe **itching** (urticarial) rash, liver and spleen enlargement, and bronchospasm.

Intestinal schistosomiasis

In intestinal schistosomiasis, eggs become lodged in the intestinal wall and cause an immune system reaction called a granulomatous reaction. This immune response can lead to obstruction of the colon and blood loss. The infected individual may have what appears to be a potbelly. Eggs can also become lodged in the liver, leading to high blood pressure through the liver, enlarged spleen, the build-up of fluid in the abdomen (**ascites**), and potentially life-threatening dilations or swollen areas in the esophagus or gastrointestinal tract that can tear and bleed profusely (esophageal varices). Rarely, the central nervous system may be affected. Individuals with chronic active schistosomiasis may not complain of typical symptoms.

Urinary tract schistosomiasis

Urinary tract schistosomiasis is characterized by blood in the urine, **pain** or difficulty urinating, and frequent urination and are associated with *S. haematobium.* The loss of blood can lead to **iron deficiency anemia**. A large percentage of persons, especially children, who are moderately to heavily infected experience urinary tract damage that can lead to blocking of the urinary tract and **bladder cancer**.

Diagnosis

Proper diagnosis and treatment may require a tropical disease specialist because the disease can be

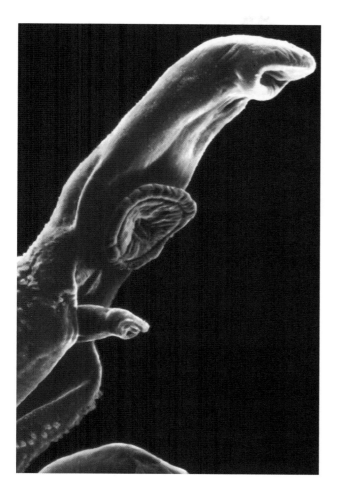

A scanning electron microscopy (SEM) of the head region of the male and female adult flukes of *Schistosoma sp.* These worms cause schistosomiasis (bilharziasis) in humans. Flukes live in human blood vessels and their eggs contaminate freshwater. *(Photo Researchers, Inc. Reproduced by permission.)*

confused with malaria or typhoid in the early stages. The healthcare provider should do a thorough history of travel in endemic areas. The rash, if present, can mimic scabies or other rashes, and the gastrointestinal symptoms may be confused with those caused by bacterial illnesses or other intestinal parasites. These other conditions will need to be excluded before an accurate diagnosis can be made. As a result, clinical evidence of exposure to infected water along with physical findings, a negative test for malaria, and an increased number of one type of immune cell, called an eosinophil, are necessary to diagnose acute schistosomiasis.

Eggs may be detected in the feces or urine. Repeated stool tests may be required to concentrate and identify the eggs. Blood tests may be used to detect a particular antigen or particle associated with the schistosome that induces an immune response. Persons infected with schistosomiasis may not test positive for six months, and as a result, tests may need to be repeated to obtain an accurate diagnosis. Blood can be detected visually in the urine or with chemical strips that react to small amounts of blood.

Sophisticated imaging techniques, such as ultrasound, computed tomography scan (CT scan), and **magnetic resonance imaging** (MRI), can detect damage to the blood vessels in the liver and visualize polyps and ulcers of the urinary tract, for example, that occur in the more advanced stages. *S. haematobium* is difficult to diagnose with ultrasound in pregnant women.

Treatment

The use of medications against schistosomiasis, such as praziquantel (Biltricide), oxamniquine, and metrifonate, have been shown to be safe and effective. Praziquantel is effective against all forms of schistososmiasis and has few side effects. This drug is given in either two or three doses over the course of a single day. Oxamniquine is typically used in Africa and South America to treat intestinal schistosomiasis. Metrifonate has been found to be safe and effective in the treatment of urinary schistosomiasis. Patients are typically checked for the presence of living eggs at three and six months after treatment. If the number of eggs excreted has not significantly decreased, the patient may require another course of medication.

Prognosis

If treated early, prognosis is very good and complete recovery is expected. The illness is treatable, but people can die from the effects of untreated schistosomiasis. The severity of the disease depends on the number of worms, or worm load, in addition to how long the person has been infected. With treatment, the number of worms can be substantially reduced, and the secondary conditions can be treated. The goal of the World Health Organization is to reduce the severity of the disease rather than to completely stop transmission of the disease. There is, however, little natural immunity to reinfection. Treated individuals do not usually require retreatment for two to five years in areas of low transmission. The World Health Organization has made research to develop a vaccine against the disease one of its priorities.

Prevention

Prevention of the disease involves several targets and requires long term community commitment. Infected patients require diagnosis, treatment, and education about how to avoid reinfecting themselves and others. Adequate healthcare facilities need to be available, water systems must be treated to kill the worms and control snail populations, and sanitation must be improved to prevent the spread of the disease.

To avoid schistosomiasis in endemic areas:

- contact the CDC for current health information on travel destinations.

- upon arrival, ask an informed local authority about the infestation of schistosomiasis before being exposed to freshwater in countries that are likely to have the disease.

- do not swim, stand, wade, or take baths in untreated water.

- treat all water used for drinking or bathing. Water can be treated by letting it stand for three days, heating it for five minutes to around 122°F (around 50°C), or filtering or treating water chemically, with chlorine or iodine, as with drinking water.

- Should accidental exposure occur, infection can be prevented by hastily drying off or applying rubbing alcohol to the exposed area.

Resources

ORGANIZATIONS

Centers for Disease Control and Prevention. 1600 Clifton Rd., NE, Atlanta, GA 30333. (800) 311-3435, (404) 639-3311. < http://www.cdc.gov >.

Ruth E. Mawyer, RN

Schizencephaly *see* **Congenital brain defects**

▌Schizoaffective disorder

Definition

Schizoaffective disorder is a mental illness that shares the psychotic symptoms of schizophrenia and the mood disturbances of depression or bipolar disorder.

Description

The term schizoaffective disorder was first used in the 1930s to describe patients with acute psychotic symptoms such as **hallucinations** and **delusions** along with disturbed mood. These patients tended to function well before becoming psychotic; their psychotic symptoms lasted relatively briefly; and they tended to do well afterward. Over the years, however, the term schizoaffective disorder has been applied to a variety of patient groups. The current definition contained in the American Psychiatric Association's *Diagnostic and Statistical Manual of Mental Disorders IV* (*DSM-IV*) recognizes patients with schizoaffective disorder as those whose mood symptoms are sufficiently severe to warrant a diagnosis of depression or other full-blown mood disorder and whose mood symptoms overlap at some period with psychotic symptoms that satisfy the diagnosis of **schizophrenia** (e.g. hallucinations, delusions, or thought process disorder).

Causes and symptoms

The cause of schizoaffective disorder remains unknown and subject to continuing speculation. Some investigators believe schizoaffective disorder is associated with schizophrenia and may be caused by a similar biological predisposition. Others disagree, stressing the disorder's similarities to **mood disorders** such as depression and bipolar disorder (manic depression). They believe its more favorable course and less intense psychotic episodes are evidence that schizoaffective disorder and mood disorders share a similar cause.

Many researchers, however, believe schizoaffective disorder may owe its existence to both disorders. These researchers believe that some people have a biologic predisposition to symptoms of schizophrenia that varies along a continuum of severity. On one end of the continuum are people who are predisposed to psychotic symptoms but never display them. On the other end of the continuum are people who are destined to develop outright schizophrenia. In the middle are those who may at some time show symptoms of schizophrenia, but require some other major trauma to set the progression of the disease into motion. It may be an early brain injury–either through a complicated delivery, prenatal exposure to the flu virus or illicit drugs; or it may be emotional, nutritional or other deprivation in early childhood. In this view, major life stresses, or a mood disorder like depression or **bipolar disorder**, may be sufficient to trigger the psychotic symptoms. In fact, patients with schizoaffective disorder frequently experience depressed mood or **mania** within days of the appearance of psychotic symptoms. Some clinicians believe that "schizomanic" patients are fundamentally different from "schizodepressed" types; the former are similar to bipolar patients, while the latter are a very heterogeneous group.

Symptoms of schizoaffective disorder vary considerably from patient to patient. Delusions, hallucinations, and evidence of disturbances in thinking–as observed in full-blown schizophrenia–may be seen. Similarly, mood fluctuations such as those observed in major depression or bipolar disorder may also be seen. These symptoms tend to appear in distinct episodes that impair the individual's ability to function well in daily life. But between episodes, some patients with schizoaffective disorder remain chronically impaired while some may do quite well in day-to-day living.

Diagnosis

There are no accepted tissue or brain imaging tests or techniques to diagnose schizophrenia, mood disorders, or schizoaffective disorder. Instead, physicians look for the hallmark signs and symptoms of schizoaffective disorder described above, and they attempt to rule out other illnesses or conditions that may produce similar symptoms. These include:

- Mania. True manic patients can experience episodes of hallucinations and delusions similar to those seen in schizoaffective disorder; but these do not persist for long periods after the mania recedes, as they do in schizoaffective disorder.

- Psychotic depression. Patients with psychotic depression experience hallucinations and delusions similar to those seen in schizoaffective disorder; but these symptoms do not persist after the depressive symptoms recede, as they do in schizoaffective disorder.

- Schizophrenia. Depressed mood, mania, or other symptoms may be present in patients with schizophrenia, but patients with schizoaffective disorder will meet all the criteria set out for a full-blown mood disorder.

- Medical and neurological disorders that mimic psychotic/affective disorders.

Treatment

Antipsychotic medications used to treat schizophrenia and the **antidepressant drugs** and mood stabilizers used in depression and bipolar disorder are the primary treatments for schizoaffective disorder.

Unfortunately these treatments have not been well studied in controlled investigations. Studies suggest that traditional antipsychotics such as haloperidol are effective in treating psychotic symptoms. Newer generation antipsychotics, such as clozaril and risperidone, have not been as well studied, but also appear effective. For patients with symptoms of bipolar disorder, lithium is often the mood stabilizer of choice; and it is often augmented with an anticonvulsant such as valproate. For those with depressive symptoms, the evidence supporting the use of antidepressant medications in addition to antipsychotic medications is more mixed. **Electroconvulsive therapy** (electric shock) is frequently tried in patients who otherwise do not respond to antidepressant or mood stabilizing drugs.

While the mainstay of treatment for schizoaffective disorder is antipsychotic medications and mood stabilizers, certain forms of psychotherapy for both patients and family members can be useful. Therapy designed to provide structure and help augment patients' ability to solve problems may aid in improving patients' ability to function in the day-to-day world, reducing **stress** and the risk of recurrence. Vocational and other rehabilitative training can help patients to work on skills they need to develop. Whereas hospitalization may be necessary for acute psychotic episodes, half-way houses and day hospitals can provide needed treatment while serving as a bridge for patients to reenter the community.

Alternative treatment

While alternative therapies should never be considered a replacement for medication, these treatments can help support people with schizoaffectve disorder and other mental illnesses. Dietary modifications that eliminate processed foods and emphasize whole foods, along with nutritional supplementation, may be helpful. Acupuncture, homeopathy, and botanical medicine can support many aspects of the person's life and may help decrease the side effects of any medications prescribed.

Prognosis

In general, patients with schizoaffective disorder have a more favorable prognosis than do those with schizophrenia, but a less favorable course than those with a pure mood disorder. Medication and other

KEY TERMS

Bipolar disorder—Also referred to as manic depression, it is a mood disorder marked by alternating episodes of extremely low mood (depression) and exuberant highs (mania).

Mood disorder—A collection of disorders that includes major depression and bipolar disorder. They are all characterized by major disruptions in patients' moods and emotions.

Schizophrenia—A major mental illness marked by psychotic symptoms, including hallucinations, delusions, and severe disruptions in thinking.

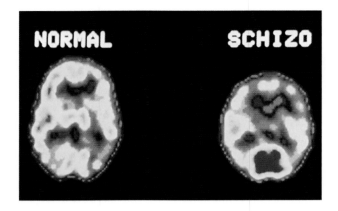

(Photo Researchers Inc. Reproduced by permission.)

interventions can help quell psychotic symptoms and stabilize mood in many patients, but there is great variability in outcome from patient to patient.

Prevention

There is no known way to prevent schizoaffective disorder. Treatment with antipsychotic and mood stabilizing drugs may prevent recurrences. Some researchers believe prompt treatment can prevent the development of full-blown schizophrenia, but this remains the subject of some disagreement.

Resources

ORGANIZATIONS

American Psychiatric Association. 1400 K Street NW, Washington DC 20005. (888) 357-7924. < http://www.psych.org >.

National Alliance for Research on Schizophrenia and Depression. 60 Cutter Mill Road, Suite 200, Great Neck, NY 11021. (516) 829-0091. < http://www.mhsource.com >.

Richard H. Camer

Schizophrenia

Definition

Schizophrenia is a psychotic disorder (or a group of disorders) marked by severely impaired thinking, emotions, and behaviors. Schizophrenic patients are typically unable to filter sensory stimuli and may have enhanced perceptions of sounds, colors, and other features of their environment. Most schizophrenics, if untreated, gradually withdraw from interactions with other people, and lose their ability to take care of personal needs and grooming.

The prevalence of schizophrenia is thought to be about 1% of the population around the world; it is thus more common than diabetes, **Alzheimer's disease**, or **multiple sclerosis**. In the United States and Canada, patients with schizophrenia fill about 25% of all hospital beds. The disorder is considered to be one of the top ten causes of long-term disability worldwide.

Description

The course of schizophrenia in adults can be divided into three phases or stages. In the acute phase, the patient has an overt loss of contact with reality (psychotic episode) that requires intervention and treatment. In the second or stabilization phase, the initial psychotic symptoms have been brought under control but the patient is at risk for relapse if treatment is interrupted. In the third or maintenance phase, the patient is relatively stable and can be kept indefinitely on antipsychotic medications. Even in the maintenance phase, however, relapses are not unusual and patients do not always return to full functioning.

The English term schizophrenia comes from two Greek words that mean "split mind." It was observed around 1908, by a Swiss doctor named Eugen Bleuler, to describe the splitting apart of mental functions that he regarded as the central characteristic of schizophrenia.

Recently, some psychotherapists have begun to use a classification of schizophrenia based on two main types. People with Type I, or positive schizophrenia, have a rapid (acute) onset of symptoms and tend to respond well to drugs. They also tend to suffer more from the "positive" symptoms, such as **delusions** and **hallucinations**. People with Type II, or negative schizophrenia, are usually described as poorly adjusted before their schizophrenia slowly overtakes them. They have predominantly "negative" symptoms, such as withdrawal from others and a slowing of mental and physical reactions (psychomotor retardation).

There are five subtypes of schizophrenia:

Paranoid

The key feature of this subtype of schizophrenia is the combination of false beliefs (delusions) and hearing voices (auditory hallucinations), with more nearly normal emotions and cognitive functioning (cognitive functions include reasoning, judgment, and memory). The delusions of paranoid schizophrenics usually involve thoughts of being persecuted or harmed by others or exaggerated opinions of their own importance, but may also reflect feelings of jealousy or excessive religiosity. The delusions are typically organized into a coherent framework. Paranoid schizophrenics function at a higher level than other subtypes, but are at risk for suicidal or violent behavior under the influence of their delusions.

Disorganized

Disorganized schizophrenia (formerly called hebephrenic schizophrenia) is marked by disorganized speech, thinking, and behavior on the patient's part, coupled with flat or inappropriate emotional responses to a situation (affect). The patient may act silly or withdraw socially to an extreme extent. Most patients in this category have weak personality structures prior to their initial acute psychotic episode.

Catatonic

Catatonic schizophrenia is characterized by disturbances of movement that may include rigidity, stupor, agitation, bizarre posturing, and repetitive imitations of the movements or speech of other people. These patients are at risk for **malnutrition**, exhaustion, or self-injury. This subtype is presently uncommon in Europe and the United States. **Catatonia** as a symptom is most commonly associated with **mood disorders**.

Undifferentiated

Patients in this category have the characteristic positive and negative symptoms of schizophrenia but do not meet the specific criteria for the paranoid, disorganized, or catatonic subtypes.

Residual

This category is used for patients who have had at least one acute schizophrenic episode but do not presently have strong positive psychotic symptoms, such as delusions and hallucinations. They may have negative symptoms, such as withdrawal from others, or mild forms of positive symptoms, which indicate that the disorder has not completely resolved.

The risk of schizophrenia among first-degree biological relatives is ten times greater than that observed in the general population. Furthermore the presence of the same disorder is higher in monozygotic twins (identical twins) than in dizygotic twins (nonidentical twins). The research concerning adoption studies and identical twins also supports the notion that environmental factors are important, because not all relatives who have the disorder express it. There are several chromosomes and loci (specific areas on chromosomes which contain mutated genes), which have been identified. Research is actively ongoing to elucidate the causes, types and variations of these mutations.

Most patients are diagnosed in their late teens or early twenties, but the symptoms of schizophrenia can emerge at any age in the life cycle. The male/female ratio in adults is about 1.2:1. Male patients typically have their first acute episode in their early twenties, while female patients are usually closer to age 30 when they are recognized with active symptoms.

Schizophrenia is rarely diagnosed in preadolescent children, although patients as young as five or six have been reported. Childhood schizophrenia is at the upper end of the spectrum of severity and shows a greater gender disparity. It affects one or two children in every 10,000; the male/female ratio is 2:1.

Causes and symptoms

Theories of causality

One of the reasons for the ongoing difficulty in classifying schizophrenic disorders is incomplete understanding of their causes. It is thought that these disorders are the end result of a combination of genetic, neurobiological, and environmental causes. A leading neurobiological hypothesis looks at the connection between the disease and excessive levels of dopamine, a chemical that transmits signals in the brain (neurotransmitter). The genetic factor in schizophrenia has been underscored by recent findings that first-degree biological relatives of schizophrenics are ten times as likely to develop the disorder as are members of the general population.

Prior to recent findings of abnormalities in the brain structure of schizophrenic patients, several generations of psychotherapists advanced a number of psychoanalytic and sociological theories about the origins of schizophrenia. These theories ranged from hypotheses about the patient's problems with **anxiety** or aggression to theories about **stress** reactions or interactions with disturbed parents. Psychosocial factors are now thought to influence the expression or severity of schizophrenia rather than cause it directly.

As of 2004, migration is a social factor that is known to influence people's susceptibility to **psychosis**. Psychiatrists in Europe have noted the increasing rate of schizophrenia and other psychotic disorders among immigrants to almost all Western European countries. Black immigrants from Africa or the Caribbean appear to be especially vulnerable. The stresses involved in migration include family breakup, the need to adjust to living in large urban areas, and social inequalities in the new country.

Another hypothesis suggests that schizophrenia may be caused by a virus that attacks the hippocampus, a part of the brain that processes sense perceptions. Damage to the hippocampus would account for schizophrenic patients' vulnerability to sensory overload. As of 2004, researchers are focusing on the possible role of the herpes simplex virus (HSV) in schizophrenia, as well as human endogenous retroviruses (HERVs). The possibility that HERVs may be associated with schizophrenia has to do with the fact that antibodies to these retroviruses are found more frequently in the blood serum of patients with schizophrenia than in serum from control subjects.

Symptoms of schizophrenia

Patients with a possible diagnosis of schizophrenia are evaluated on the basis of a set or constellation of symptoms; there is no single symptom that is unique to schizophrenia. In 1959, the German psychiatrist Kurt Schneider proposed a list of so-called first-rank symptoms, which he regarded as diagnostic of the disorder.

These symptoms include:

- delusions
- somatic
- hallucinations
- hearing voices commenting on the patient's behavior
- thought insertion or thought withdrawal

Somatic hallucinations refer to sensations or perceptions concerning body organs that have no known medical cause or reason, such as the notion that one's brain is radioactive. Thought insertion and/or withdrawal refer to delusions that an outside force (for example, the FBI, the CIA, Martians, etc.) has the power to put thoughts into one's mind or remove them.

POSITIVE SYMPTOMS. The positive symptoms of schizophrenia are those that represent an excessive or distorted version of normal functions. Positive symptoms include Schneider's first-rank symptoms as well as disorganized thought processes (reflected mainly in speech) and disorganized or catatonic behavior. Disorganized thought processes are marked by such characteristics as looseness of associations, in which the patient rambles from topic to topic in a disconnected way; tangentially, which means that the patient gives unrelated answers to questions; and "word salad," in which the patient's speech is so incoherent that it makes no grammatical or linguistic sense. Disorganized behavior means that the patient has difficulty with any type of purposeful or goal-oriented behavior, including personal self-care or preparing meals. Other forms of disorganized behavior may include dressing in odd or inappropriate ways, sexual self-stimulation in public, or agitated shouting or cursing.

NEGATIVE SYMPTOMS. Schizophrenia includes three so-called negative symptoms. They are called negative because they represent the lack or absence of behaviors. The negative symptoms that are considered diagnostic of schizophrenia are a lack of emotional response (affective flattening), poverty of speech, and absence of volition or will. In general, the negative symptoms are more difficult for doctors to evaluate than the positive symptoms.

Diagnosis

A doctor must make a diagnosis of schizophrenia on the basis of a standardized list of outwardly observable symptoms, not on the basis of internal psychological processes. There are no specific laboratory tests that can be used to diagnose schizophrenia. Researchers have, however, discovered that patients with schizophrenia have certain abnormalities in the structure and functioning of the brain compared to normal test subjects. These discoveries have been made with the help of imaging techniques such as **computed tomography scans** (CT scans).

When a psychiatrist assesses a patient for schizophrenia, he or she will begin by excluding physical conditions that can cause abnormal thinking and some other behaviors associated with schizophrenia. These conditions include organic brain disorders (including traumatic injuries of the brain), temporal lobe epilepsy, Wilson's disease, prion diseases, Huntington's chorea, and **encephalitis**. The doctor will also need to rule out **heavy metal poisoning** and **substance abuse** disorders, especially amphetamine use.

After ruling out organic disorders, the clinician will consider other psychiatric conditions that may include psychotic symptoms or symptoms resembling psychosis. These disorders include mood disorders with psychotic features; delusional disorder; dissociative disorder not otherwise specified (DDNOS) or **multiple personality disorder**; schizotypal, schizoid, or paranoid **personality disorders**; and atypical reactive disorders. In the past, many individuals were incorrectly diagnosed as schizophrenic. Some patients who were diagnosed prior to the changes in categorization should have their diagnoses, and treatment, reevaluated. In children, the doctor must distinguish between psychotic symptoms and a vivid fantasy life, and also identify learning problems or disorders. After other conditions have been ruled out, the patient must meet a set of criteria specified:

- the patient must have two (or more) of the following symptoms during a one-month period: delusions; hallucinations; disorganized speech; disorganized or catatonic behavior; negative symptoms

- decline in social, interpersonal, or occupational functioning, including self-care

- the disturbed behavior must last for at least six months

- mood disorders, substance **abuse** disorders, medical conditions, and developmental disorders have been ruled out

Treatment

The treatment of schizophrenia depends in part on the patient's stage or phase. Psychotic symptoms and behaviors are considered psychiatric emergencies, and persons showing signs of psychosis are frequently taken by family, friends, or the police to a hospital emergency room. A person diagnosed as psychotic can be legally hospitalized against his or her will, particularly if he or she is violent, threatening to commit **suicide**, or threatening to harm another person. A psychotic person may also be hospitalized if he or she has become malnourished or ill as a result of failure to feed, dress appropriately for the climate, or otherwise take care of him- or herself.

A patient having a first psychotic episode should be given a CT or MRI (**magnetic resonance imaging**) scan to rule out structural brain disease.

Antipsychotic medications

The primary form of treatment of schizophrenia is antipsychotic medication. **Antipsychotic drugs** help to control almost all the positive symptoms of the disorder. They have minimal effects on disorganized behavior and negative symptoms. Between 60–70% of schizophrenics will respond to antipsychotics. In the acute phase of the illness, patients are usually given medications by mouth or by intramuscular injection. After the patient has been stabilized, the antipsychotic drug may be given in a long-acting form called a depot dose. Depot medications last for two to four weeks; they have the advantage of protecting the patient against the consequences of forgetting or skipping daily doses. In addition, some patients who do not respond to oral neuroleptics have better results with depot form. Patients whose long-term treatment includes depot medications are introduced to the depot form gradually during their stabilization period. Most people with schizophrenia are kept indefinitely on antipsychotic medications during the maintenance phase of their disorder to minimize the possibility of relapse.

As of the early 2000s, the most frequently used antipsychotics fall into two classes: the older dopamine receptor antagonists, or DAs, and the newer serotonin dopamine antagonists, or SDAs. (Antagonists block the action of some other substance; for example, dopamine antagonists counteract the action of dopamine.) The exact mechanisms of action of these medications are not known, but it is thought that they lower the patient's sensitivity to sensory stimuli and so indirectly improve the patient's ability to interact with others.

DOPAMINE RECEPTOR ANTAGONIST. The dopamine antagonists include the older antipsychotic (also called neuroleptic) drugs, such as haloperidol (Haldol), chlorpromazine (Thorazine), and fluphenazine (Prolixin). These drugs have two major drawbacks: it is often difficult to find the best dosage level for the individual patient, and a dosage level high enough to control psychotic symptoms frequently produces extrapyramidal side effects, or EPS. EPSs include parkinsonism, in which the patient cannot walk normally and usually develops a tremor; dystonia, or painful **muscle spasms** of the head, tongue, or neck; and akathisia, or restlessness. A type of long-term EPS is called **tardive dyskinesia**, which features slow, rhythmic, automatic movements.

Schizophrenics with **AIDS** are especially vulnerable to developing EPS.

SEROTONIN DOPANINE ANTAGONISTS. The serotonin dopamine antagonists, also called atypical antipsychotics, are newer medications that include clozapine (Clozaril), risperidone (Risperdal), and olanzapine (Zyprexa). The SDAs have a better effect on the negative symptoms of schizophrenia than do the older drugs and are less likely to produce EPS than the older compounds. The newer drugs are significantly more expensive in the short term, although the SDAs may reduce long-term costs by reducing the need for hospitalization. They are also presently unavailable in injectable forms. The SDAs are commonly used to treat patients who respond poorly to the DAs. However, many psychotherapists now regard the use of these atypical antipsychotics as the treatment of first choice; in particular, clozapine appears to be more effective than other antipsychotics in controlling persistent aggression in some patients.

NEWER DRUGS. Some newer antipsychotic drugs have been approved by the Food and Drug administration (FDA) in the early 2000s. These drugs are sometimes called second-generation antipsychotics or SGAs. Aripiprazole (Abilify), which is classified as a partial dopaminergic agonist, received FDA approval in August 2003. Two drugs that are still under investigation, a neurokinin antagonist and a serotonin 2A/2C antagonist respectively, show promise in the treatment of schizophrenia and **schizoaffective disorder**.

Psychotherapy

Most schizophrenics can benefit from psychotherapy once their acute symptoms have been brought under control by antipsychotic medication. Psychoanalytic approaches are not recommended. Behavior therapy, however, is often helpful in assisting patients to acquire skills for daily living and social interaction. It can be combined with occupational therapy to prepare the patient for eventual employment.

Family therapy

Family therapy is often recommended for the families of schizophrenic patients, to relieve the feelings of guilt that they often have as well as to help them understand the patient's disorder. The family's attitude and behaviors toward the patient are key factors in minimizing relapses (for example, by reducing stress in the patient's life), and family therapy can often strengthen the family's ability to cope with the stresses caused by the schizophrenic's illness. Family therapy focused on communication skills and problem-solving strategies is particularly helpful. In addition to formal treatment, many families benefit from support groups and similar mutual help organizations for relatives of schizophrenics.

Prognosis

One important prognostic sign is the patient's age at onset of psychotic symptoms. Patients with early onset of schizophrenia are more often male, have a lower level of functioning prior to onset, a higher rate of brain abnormalities, more noticeable negative symptoms, and worse outcomes. Patients with later onset are more likely to be female, with fewer brain abnormalities and thought impairment, and more hopeful prognoses.

The average course and outcome for schizophrenics are less favorable than those for most other mental disorders, although as many as 30% of patients diagnosed with schizophrenia recover completely and the majority experience some improvement. Two factors that influence outcomes are stressful life events and a hostile or emotionally intense family environment. Schizophrenics with a high number of stressful changes in their lives, or who have frequent contacts with critical or emotionally over-involved family members, are more likely to relapse. Overall, the most important component of long-term care of schizophrenic patients is complying with their regimen of antipsychotic medications.

Resources

BOOKS

American Psychiatric Association. *Diagnostic and Statistical Manual of Mental Disorders.* 4th ed., revised. Washington, D.C.: American Psychiatric Association, 2000.

Beers, Mark H., MD, and Robert Berkow, MD., editors. "Psychiatric Emergencies." Section 15, Chapter 194 In *The Merck Manual of Diagnosis and Therapy.* Whitehouse Station, NJ: Merck Research Laboratories, 2004.

Beers, Mark H., MD, and Robert Berkow, MD., editors. "Schizophrenia and Related Disorders." Section 15, Chapter 193 In *The Merck Manual of Diagnosis and Therapy.* Whitehouse Station, NJ: Merck Research Laboratories, 2004.

Wilson, Billie Ann, Margaret T. Shannon, and Carolyn L. Stang. *Nurse's Drug Guide 2003.* Upper Saddle River, NJ: Prentice Hall, 2003.

PERIODICALS

DeLeon, A., N. C. Patel, and M. L. Crismon. "Aripiprazole: A Comprehensive Review of Its Pharmacology, Clinical Efficacy, and Tolerability." *Clinical Therapeutics* 26 (May 2004): 649–666.

KEY TERMS

Affective flattening—A loss or lack of emotional expressiveness. It is sometimes called blunted or restricted affect.

Akathisia—Agitated or restless movement, usually affecting the legs and accompanied by a sense of discomfort. It is a common side effect of neuroleptic medications.

Catatonic behavior—Behavior characterized by muscular tightness or rigidity and lack of response to the environment. In some patients rigidity alternates with excited or hyperactive behavior.

Delusion—A fixed, false belief that is resistant to reason or factual disproof.

Depot dosage—A form of medication that can be stored in the patient's body tissues for several days or weeks, thus minimizing the risk of the patient forgetting daily doses. Haloperidol and fluphenazine can be given in depot form.

Dopamine receptor antagonists (DAs)—The older class of antipsychotic medications, also called neuroleptics. These primarily block the site on nerve cells that normally receive the brain chemical dopamine.

Dystonia—Painful involuntary muscle cramps or spasms.

Extrapyramidal symptoms (EPS)—A group of side effects associated with antipsychotic medications. EPS include parkinsonism, akathisia, dystonia, and tardive dyskinesia.

First-rank symptoms—A set of symptoms designated by Kurt Schneider in 1959 as the most important diagnostic indicators of schizophrenia. These symptoms include delusions, hallucinations, thought insertion or removal, and thought broadcasting. First-rank symptoms are sometimes referred to as Schneiderian symptoms.

Hallucination—A sensory experience of something that does not exist outside the mind. A person can experience a hallucination in any of the five senses. Auditory hallucinations are a common symptom of schizophrenia.

Huntington's chorea—A hereditary disease that typically appears in midlife, marked by gradual loss of brain function and voluntary movement. Some of its symptoms resemble those of schizophrenia.

Negative symptoms—Symptoms of schizophrenia characterized by the absence or elimination of certain behaviors. DSM-IV specifies three negative symptoms: affective flattening, poverty of speech, and loss of will or initiative.

Neuroleptic—Another name for the older type of antipsychotic medications given to schizophrenic patients.

Parkinsonism—A set of symptoms originally associated with Parkinson disease that can occur as side effects of neuroleptic medications. The symptoms include trembling of the fingers or hands, a shuffling gait, and tight or rigid muscles.

Positive symptoms—Symptoms of schizophrenia that are characterized by the production or presence of behaviors that are grossly abnormal or excessive, including hallucinations and thought-process disorder. DSM-IV subdivides positive symptoms into psychotic and disorganized.

Poverty of speech—A negative symptom of schizophrenia, characterized by brief and empty replies to questions. It should not be confused with shyness or reluctance to talk.

Psychotic disorder—A mental disorder characterized by delusions, hallucinations, or other symptoms of lack of contact with reality. The schizophrenias are psychotic disorders.

Serotonin dopamine antagonist (SDA)—The newer second-generation antipsychotic drugs, also called atypical antipsychotics. SDAs include clozapine (Clozaril), risperidone (Risperdal), and olanzapine (Zyprexa).

Wilson disease—A rare hereditary disease marked by high levels of copper deposits in the brain and liver. It can cause psychiatric symptoms resembling schizophrenia.

Word salad—Speech that is so disorganized that it makes no linguistic or grammatical sense.

Frankenburg, Frances R., MD. "Schizophrenia." *eMedicine* June 17, 2004. < http://www.emedicine.com/med/topic2072.htm >.

Hutchinson, G., and C. Haasen. "Migration and Schizophrenia: The Challenges for European Psychiatry and Implications for the Future." *Social Psychiatry and Psychiatric Epidemiology* 39 (May 2004): 350–357.

Meltzer, H. Y., L. Arvanitis, D. Bauer, et al. "Placebo-Controlled Evaluation of Four Novel Compounds for the Treatment of Schizophrenia and Schizoaffective Disorder." *American Journal of Psychiatry* 161 (June 2004): 975–984.

Mueser, K. T., and S. R. McGurk. "Schizophrenia." *Lancet* 363 (June 19, 2004): 2063–2072.

Volavka, J., P. Czobor, K. Nolan, et al. "Overt Aggression and Psychotic Symptoms in Patients with Schizophrenia Treated with Clozapine, Olanzapine, Risperidone, or Haloperidol." *Journal of Clinical Psychopharmacology* 24 (April 2004): 225–228.

Yolken, R. "Viruses and Schizophrenia: A Focus on Herpes Simplex Virus." *Herpes* 11, Supplement 2 (June 2004): 83A–88A.

ORGANIZATIONS

American Psychiatric Association. 1400 K Street NW, Washington DC 20005. (888) 357-7924. < http://www.psych.org >.

National Alliance for the Mentally Ill (NAMI). Colonial Place Three, 2107 Wilson Blvd., Suite 300 Arlington, VA 22201. (703) 524-7600 HelpLine: (800) 950-NAMI. < http://www.nami.org/ >.

National Institute of Mental Health (NIMH). 6001 Executive Boulevard, Room 8184, MSC 9663, Bethesda, MD 20892-9663. (301) 443-4513. < http://www.nimh.nih.gov >.

Schizophrenics Anonymous. 15920 W. Twelve Mile, Southfield, MI 48076. (248) 477-1983.

United States Food and Drug Administration (FDA). 5600 Fishers Lane, Rockville, MD 20857-0001. (888) INFO-FDA. < http://www.fda.gov >.

OTHER

"Schizophrenia." *Internet Mental Health.* < http://www.mentalhealth.com/dis/p20-ps01.html >.

Laith Farid Gulli, M.D.
Rebecca Frey, PhD

Schwannoma *see* **Brain tumor**

Sciatic nerve pain *see* **Sciatica**

Sciatica

Definition

Sciatica refers to **pain** or discomfort associated with the sciatic nerve. This nerve runs from the lower part of the spinal cord, down the back of the leg, to the foot. Injury to or pressure on the sciatic nerve can cause the characteristic pain of sciatica: a sharp or burning pain that radiates from the lower back or hip, possibly following the path of the sciatic nerve to the foot.

Description

The sciatic nerve is the largest and longest nerve in the body. About the thickness of a person's thumb, it spans from the lower back to the foot. The nerve originates in the lower part of the spinal cord, the so-called lumbar region. As it branches off from the spinal cord, it passes between the bony vertebrae (the component bones of the spine) and runs through the pelvic girdle, or hip bones. The nerve passes through the hip joint and continues down the back of the leg to the foot.

Sciatica is a fairly common disorder and approximately 40% of the population experiences it at some point in their lives. However, only about 1% have coexisting sensory or motor deficits. Sciatic pain has several root causes and treatment may hinge upon the underlying problem.

Of the identifiable causes of sciatic pain, lumbosacral radiculopathy and back strain are the most frequently suspected. The term lumbosacral refers to the lower part of the spine, and radiculopathy describes a problem with the spinal nerve roots that pass between the vertebrae and give rise to the sciatic nerve. This area between the vertebrae is cushioned with a disk of shock- absorbing tissue. If this disk shifts or is damaged through injury or disease, the spinal nerve root may be compressed by the shifted tissue or the vertebrae.

This compression of the nerve roots sends a pain signal to the brain. Although the actual injury is to the nerve roots, the pain may be perceived as coming from anywhere along the sciatic nerve.

The sciatic nerve can be compressed in other ways. Back strain may cause **muscle spasms** in the lower back, placing pressure on the sciatic nerve. In rare cases, infection, **cancer**, bone inflammation, or other diseases may be causing the pressure. More likely, but often overlooked, is the piriformis syndrome. As the sciatic nerve passes through the hip joint, it shares the space with several muscles. One of these muscles, the piriformis muscle, is closely associated with the sciatic nerve. In some people, the nerve actually runs through the muscle. If this muscle is injured or has a spasm, it places pressure on the sciatic nerve, in effect, compressing it.

In many sciatica cases, the specific cause is never identified. About half of affected individuals recover from an episode within a month. Some cases can linger a few weeks longer and may require aggressive treatment. In some cases, the pain may return or potentially become chronic.

Causes and symptoms

Individuals with sciatica may experience some lower back pain, but the most common symptom is pain that radiates through one buttock and down the back of that leg. The most identified cause of the pain is compression or pressure on the sciatic nerve. The extent of the pain varies between individuals. Some people describe pain that centers in the area of the hip, and others perceive discomfort all the way to the foot. The quality of the pain also varies; it may be described as **tingling**, burning, prickly, aching, or stabbing.

Onset of sciatica can be sudden, but it can also develop gradually. The pain may be intermittent or continuous, and certain activities, such as bending, coughing, sneezing, or sitting, may make the pain worse.

Chronic pain may arise from more than just compression on the nerve. According to some pain researchers, physical damage to a nerve is only half of the equation. A developing theory proposes that some nerve injuries result in a release of neurotransmitters and immune system chemicals that enhance and sustain a pain message. Even after the injury has healed, or the damage has been repaired, the pain continues. Control of this abnormal type of pain is difficult.

Diagnosis

Before treating sciatic pain, as much information as possible is collected. The individual is asked to recount the location and nature of the pain, how long it has continued, and any accidents or unusual activities prior to its onset. This information provides clues that may point to back strain or injury to a specific location. Back pain from disk disease, piriformis syndrome, and back strain must be differentiated from more serious conditions such as cancer or infection. Lumbar stenosis, an overgrowth of the covering layers of the vertebrae that narrows the spinal canal, must also be considered. The possibility that a difference in leg lengths is causing the pain should be evaluated; the problem can be easily be treated with a foot orthotic or built-up shoe.

Often, a straight-leg-raising test is done, in which the person lies face upward and the health-care provider raises the affected leg to various heights. This test pinpoints the location of the pain and may reveal whether it is caused by a disk problem. Other tests, such as having the individual rotate the hip joint, assess the hip muscles. Any pain caused by these movements may provide information about involvement of the piriformis muscle, and piriformis weakness is tested with additional leg-strength maneuvers.

Further tests may be done depending on the results of the **physical examination** and initial pain treatment. Such tests might include **magnetic resonance imaging** (MRI) and **computed tomography scans** (CT scans). Other tests examine the conduction of electricity through nerve tissues, and include studies of the electrical activity generated as muscles contract (**electromyography**), nerve conduction velocity, and evoked potential testing. A more invasive test involves injecting a contrast substance into the space between the vertebrae and making x-ray images of the spinal cord (**myelography**), but this procedure is usually done only if surgery is being considered. All of these tests can reveal problems with the vertebrae, the disk, or the nerve itself.

Treatment

Initial treatment for sciatica focuses on pain relief. For acute or very painful flare-ups, bed rest is advised for up to a week in conjunction with medication for the pain. Pain medication includes **acetaminophen**, **nonsteroidal anti-inflammatory drugs** (NSAIDs), such as **aspirin**, or **muscle relaxants**. If the pain is unremitting, opioids may be prescribed for short-term use or a local anesthetic will be injected directly into the lower back. Massage and heat application may be suggested as adjuncts.

If the pain is chronic, different pain relief medications are used to avoid long-term dosing of NSAIDs, muscle relaxants, and opioids. **Antidepressant drugs**, which have been shown to be effective in treating pain, may be prescribed alongside short-term use of muscle relaxants or NSAIDs. Local anesthetic injections or epidural steroids are used in selected cases.

As the pain allows, physical therapy is introduced into the treatment regime. Stretching exercises that focus on the lower back, buttock, and hamstring muscles are suggested. The exercises also include finding comfortable, pain-reducing positions. Corsets and braces may be useful in some cases, but evidence for their general effectiveness is lacking. However, they may be helpful to prevent exacerbations related to certain activities.

With less pain and the success of early therapy, the individual is encouraged to follow a long-term program to maintain a healthy back and prevent re-injury. A physical therapist may suggest exercises and regular activity, such as water **exercise** or walking. Patients are instructed in proper body mechanics to minimize symptoms during light lifting or other activities.

If the pain is chronic and conservative treatment fails, surgery to repair a **herniated disk** or cut out part or all of the piriformis muscle may be suggested, particularly if there is neurologic evidence of nerve or nerve-root damage.

KEY TERMS

Disk—Dense tissue between the vertebrae that acts as a shock absorber and prevents damage to nerves and blood vessels along the spine.

Electromyography—A medical test in which a nerve's ability to conduct an impulse is measured.

Lumbosacral—Referring to the lower part of the backbone or spine.

Myelography—A medical test in which a special dye is injected into a nerve to make it visible on an x ray.

Piriformis—A muscle in the pelvic girdle that is closely associated with the sciatic nerve.

Radiculopathy—A condition in which the spinal nerve root of a nerve has been injured or damaged.

Spasm—Involuntary contraction of a muscle.

Vertebrae—The component bones of the spine.

Alternative treatment

Massage is a recommended form of therapy, especially if the sciatic pain arises from muscle spasm. Symptoms may also be relieved by icing the painful area as soon as the pain occurs. Ice should be left on the area for 30-60 minutes several times a day. After 2-3 days, a hot water bottle or heating pad can replace the ice. **Chiropractic** or **osteopathy** may offer possible solutions for relieving pressure on the sciatic nerve and the accompanying pain. **Acupuncture** and **biofeedback** may also be useful as pain control methods. Body work, such as the **Alexander technique**, can assist an individual in improving posture and preventing further episodes of sciatic pain.

Prognosis

Most cases of sciatica are treatable with pain medication and physical therapy. After 4-6 weeks of treatment, an individual should be able to resume normal activities.

Prevention

Some sources of sciatica are not preventable, such as disk degeneration, back strain due to **pregnancy**, or accidental falls. Other sources of back strain, such as poor posture, overexertion, being overweight, or wearing high heels, can be corrected or avoided. Cigarette **smoking** may also predispose people to pain, and should be discontinued.

General suggestions for avoiding sciatica, or preventing a repeat episode, include sleeping on a firm mattress, using chairs with firm back support, and sitting with both feet flat on the floor. Habitually crossing the legs while sitting can place excess pressure on the sciatic nerve. Sitting a lot can also place pressure on the sciatic nerves, so it's a good idea to take short breaks and move around during the work day, long trips, or any other situation that requires sitting for an extended length of time. If lifting is required, the back should be kept straight and the legs should provide the lift. Regular exercise, such as swimming and walking, can strengthen back muscles and improve posture. Exercise can also help maintain a healthy weight and lessen the likelihood of back strain.

Resources

PERIODICALS

Douglas, Sara. "Sciatic Pain and Piriformis Syndrome." *The Nurse Practitioner* 22 (May 1997): 166.

Julia Barrett

SCID *see* **Severe combined immunodeficiency**

Scleral buckling *see* **Retinal detachment**

Scleroderma

Definition

Scleroderma is a progressive disease that affects the skin and connective tissue (including cartilage, bone, fat, and the tissue that supports the nerves and blood vessels throughout the body). There are two major forms of the disorder. The type known as localized scleroderma mainly affects the skin. Systemic scleroderma, which is also called systemic sclerosis, affects the smaller blood vessels and internal organs of the body.

Description

Scleroderma is an autoimmune disorder, which means that the body's immune system turns against itself. In scleroderma, there is an overproduction of abnormal collagen (a type of protein fiber present in connective tissue). This collagen accumulates throughout the body, causing hardening (sclerosis), scarring (fibrosis), and other damage. The damage may affect the appearance of the skin, or it may involve only the internal organs. The symptoms and severity of scleroderma vary from person to person.

Scleroderma occurs in all races of people all over the world, but it affects about four females for every male. Among children, localized scleroderma is more common, and systemic sclerosis is comparatively rare. Most patients with systemic sclerosis are diagnosed between ages 30 and 50. In the United States, about 300,000 people have scleroderma. Young African-American women and Native Americans of the Choctaw tribe have especially high rates of the disease. In 2003, researchers reported that they had identified 12 different genetic markers associated with scleroderma in the Choctaw population.

Causes and symptoms

The cause of scleroderma is still a puzzle. Although the accumulation of collagen appears to be a hallmark of the disease, researchers do not know why it occurs. Some theories suggest that damage to blood vessels may cause the tissues of the body to receive an inadequate amount of oxygen—a condition called **ischemia**. Some researchers believe that the resulting damage causes the immune system to overreact, producing an autoimmune disorder. According to this theory of scleroderma, the immune system gears up to fight an invader, but no invader is actually present. Cells in the immune system called antibodies react to the body's own tissues as if they were foreign. The antibodies turn against the already damaged blood vessels and the vessels' supporting tissues. These immune cells are designed to deliver potent chemicals in order to kill foreign invaders. Some of these cells dump these chemicals on the body's own tissues instead, causing inflammation, swelling, damage, and scarring.

Most cases of scleroderma have no recognizable triggering event. Some cases, however, have been traced to exposure to toxic (poisonous) substances. For example, coal miners and gold miners, who are exposed to high levels of silica dust, have above-average rates of scleroderma. Other chemicals associated with the disease include polyvinyl chloride, benzine, toluene, and epoxy resins. In 1981, 20,000 people in Spain were stricken with a syndrome similar to scleroderma when their cooking oil was accidentally contaminated. Certain medications, especially a drug used in **cancer** treatment called bleomycin (Blenoxane), may lead to scleroderma. Some claims of a scleroderma-like illness have been made by women with silicone **breast implants**, but a link has not been proven in numerous studies.

Symptoms of systemic scleroderma

A condition called Raynaud's phenomenon is the first symptom in about 95% of all patients with systemic scleroderma. In Raynaud's phenomenon, the blood vessels of the fingers and/or toes (the digits) react to cold in an abnormal way. The vessels clamp down, preventing blood flow to the tip of the digit. Eventually, the flow is cut off to the entire finger or toe. Over time, oxygen deprivation may result in open ulcers on the skin surface. These ulcers can lead to tissue death (**gangrene**) and loss of the digit. When Raynaud's phenomenon is the first sign of scleroderma, the next symptoms usually appear within two years.

SKIN AND EXTREMITIES. Involvement of the skin leads to swelling underneath the skin of the hands, feet, legs, arms, and face. Swelling is followed by thickening and tightening of the skin, which becomes taut and shiny. Severe tightening may lead to abnormalities. For example, tightening of the skin on the hands may cause the fingers to become permanently curled (flexed). Structures within the skin are damaged (including those producing hair, oil, and sweat), and the skin becomes dry and scaly. Ulcers may form, with the danger of infection. Calcium deposits often appear under the skin.

In systemic scleroderma, the mouth and nose may become smaller as the skin on the face tightens. The small mouth may interfere with eating and dental hygiene. Blood vessels under the skin may become enlarged and show through the skin, appearing as purplish marks or red spots. This chronic dilation of the small blood vessels is called telangiectasis.

Muscle weakness, joint **pain** and stiffness, and **carpal tunnel syndrome** are common in scleroderma. Carpal tunnel syndrome involves scarring in the wrist, which puts pressure on the median nerve running through that area. Pressure on the nerve causes **numbness**, **tingling**, and weakness in some of the fingers.

DIGESTIVE TRACT. The tube leading from the mouth to the stomach (the esophagus) becomes stiff and scarred. Patients may have trouble swallowing food. The acid contents of the stomach may start to flow backward into the esophagus (esophageal reflux), causing a very uncomfortable condition known as **heartburn**. The esophagus may also become inflamed.

The intestine becomes sluggish in processing food, causing bloating and pain. Foods are not digested properly, resulting in **diarrhea**, weight loss, and anemia. Telangiectasis in the stomach or intestine may cause rupture and bleeding.

RESPIRATORY AND CIRCULATORY SYSTEMS. The lungs are affected in about 66% of all people with systemic scleroderma. Complications include **shortness of breath**, coughing, difficulty breathing due to tightening of the tissue around the chest, inflammation of the air sacs in the lungs (alveolitis), increased risk of

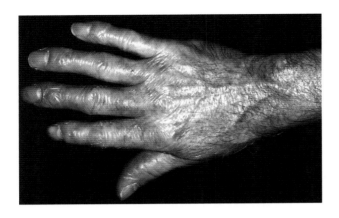

Scleroderma is a serious, progressive disease caused by the overproduction and accumulation of collagen throughout the body, resulting in hardening (sclerosis) and scarring (fibrosis) of the skin and connective tissue. *(Photo Researchers, Inc. Reproduced by permission.)*

pneumonia, and an increased risk of cancer. For these reasons, lung disease is the most likely cause of **death** associated with scleroderma.

The lining around the heart (pericardium) may become inflamed. The heart may have greater difficulty pumping blood effectively (heart failure). Irregular heart rhythms and enlargement of the heart also occur in scleroderma.

Kidney disease is another common complication. Damage to blood vessels in the kidneys often causes a major rise in the person's blood pressure. The blood pressure may be so high that there is swelling of the brain, causing severe headaches, damage to the retinas of the eyes, seizures, and failure of the heart to pump blood into the body's circulatory system. The kidneys may also stop filtering blood and go into failure. Treatments for high blood pressure have greatly improved these kidney complications. Before these treatments were available, kidney problems were the most common cause of death for people with scleroderma.

Other problems associated with scleroderma include painful dryness of the eyes and mouth, enlargement and destruction of the liver, and a low-functioning thyroid gland.

Diagnosis

Diagnosis of scleroderma is complicated by the fact that some of its symptoms can accompany other connective-tissue diseases. The most important symptom is thickened or hardened skin on the fingers, hands, forearms, or face. This symptom is found in 98% of people with scleroderma. It can be detected in the course of a physical examination. The person's medical history may also contain important clues, such as exposure to toxic substances on the job. There are a number of nonspecific laboratory tests on blood samples that may indicate the presence of an inflammatory disorder (but not specifically scleroderma). The antinuclear antibody (ANA) test is positive in more than 95% of people with scleroderma.

Other tests can be performed to evaluate the extent of the disease. These include a test of the electrical system of the heart (an electrocardiogram), lung-function tests, and x-ray studies of the gastrointestinal tract. Various blood tests can be given to study kidney function.

Treatment

Mainstream treatments

As of early 2004 there is no cure for scleroderma. A drug called D-penicillamine has been used to interfere with the abnormal collagen. It is believed to help decrease the degree of skin thickening and tightening, and to slow the progress of the disease in other organs. Taking vitamin D and using ultraviolet light may be helpful for localized scleroderma. One group of British researchers reported in 2003 that long-wavelength ultraviolet A light is particularly effective in treating localized scleroderma. **Corticosteroids** have been used to treat joint pain, **muscle cramps**, and other symptoms of inflammation. Other drugs have been studied that reduce the activity of the immune system (immunosuppressants). Because these medications can have serious side effects, they are used in only the most severe cases of scleroderma.

The various complications of scleroderma are treated individually. Raynaud's phenomenon requires that people try to keep their hands and feet warm constantly. Nifedipine is a medication that is sometimes given to help control Raynaud's. Thick ointments and creams are used to treat dry skin. **Exercise** and massage may help joint involvement; they may also help people retain more movement despite skin tightening. An exercise regimen for stretching the mouth opening has been reported to be a helpful alternative to surgery in managing this condition. Skin ulcers need prompt attention and may require **antibiotics**. People with esophageal reflux will be advised to eat small amounts more often, rather than several large meals a day. They should also avoid spicy foods and items containing **caffeine**. Some patients with esophageal reflux have been successfully treated with surgery. Acid-reducing medications may be given for heartburn. People must be monitored for the development of high blood pressure. If found, they should be promptly treated with appropriate medications, usually ACE inhibitors or other **vasodilators**. When fluid accumulates due to heart failure, diuretics can be given to get rid of the excess fluid.

Patients with scleroderma may also benefit from some form of counseling or psychotherapy, as they are at increased risk of depression. One study found that 46% of the patients in its sample met the criteria for a depressive disorder.

Alternative treatments

One alternative therapy that some naturopaths have used in treating patients with scleroderma is superoxide dismutase (SOD), an antioxidant enzyme used in its injectable form. More research, however, needs to be done on the benefits of this treatment.

Prognosis

The prognosis for people with scleroderma varies. Some have a very limited form of the disease called morphea, which affects only the skin. These individuals have a very good prognosis. Other people have a subtype of systemic scleroderma called limited scleroderma. For them, the prognosis is relatively good. Limited scleroderma is characterized by limited involvement of the patient's skin and a cluster of five symptoms called the CREST syndrome. CREST stands for:

- C = Calcinosis
- R = Raynaud's disease (phenomenon)
- E = Esophageal dysmotility (stiffness and malfunctioning of the esophagus)
- S = Sclerodactyly (thick, hard, rigid skin over the fingers)
- T = Telangiectasias

In general, people with very widespread skin involvement have the worst prognosis. This level of disease is usually accompanied by involvement of other organs and the most severe complications. Although women are more commonly stricken with scleroderma, men more often die of the disease. The two factors that negatively affect survival are male sex and older age at diagnosis. The most common causes of death include heart, kidney, and lung diseases. About 65% of all patients survive 11 years or more following a diagnosis of scleroderma.

As of early 2004 there are no known ways to prevent scleroderma. People can try to decrease occupational exposure to high-risk substances.

KEY TERMS

Autoimmune disorder—A disorder in which the body's immune cells mistake the body's own tissues as foreign invaders; the immune cells then work to destroy tissues in the body.

Collagen—The main supportive protein of cartilage, connective tissue, tendon, skin, and bone.

Connective tissue—A group of tissues responsible for support throughout the body; includes cartilage, bone, fat, tissue underlying skin, and tissues that support organs, blood vessels, and nerves throughout the body.

Fibrosis—The abnormal development of fibrous tissue; scarring.

Limited scleroderma—A subtype of systemic scleroderma with limited skin involvement. It is sometimes called the CREST form of scleroderma, after the initials of its five major symptoms.

Localized scleroderma—Thickening of the skin from overproduction of collagen.

Morphea—The most common form of localized scleroderma.

Raynaud phenomenon/Raynaud disease—A condition in which blood flow to the body's tissues is reduced by a malfunction of the nerves that regulate the constriction of blood vessels. When attacks of Raynaud's occur in the absence of other medical conditions, it is called Raynaud disease. When attacks occur as part of a disease (as in scleroderma), it is called Raynaud phenomenon.

Sclerosis—Hardening.

Systemic sclerosis—A rare disorder that causes thickening and scarring of multiple organ systems.

Telangiectasias—Very small arteriovenous malformations, or connections between the arteries and veins. The result is small red spots on the skin known as "spider veins."

Resources

BOOKS

Beers, Mark H., MD, and Robert Berkow, MD., editors. "Systemic Sclerosis." *The Merck Manual of Diagnosis and Therapy*. Whitehouse Station, NJ: Merck Research Laboratories, 2004.

Pelletier, Dr. Kenneth R. *The Best Alternative Medicine, Part II: CAM Therapies for Specific Conditions: Scleroderma*. New York: Simon and Schuster, 2002.

PERIODICALS

Dawe, R. S. "Ultraviolet A1 Phototherapy." *British Journal of Dermatology* 148 (April 2003): 626–637.

Hill, C. L., A. M. Nguyen, D. Roder, and P. Roberts-Thomson. "Risk of Cancer in Patients with Scleroderma: A Population Based Cohort Study." *Annals of the Rheumatic Diseases* 62 (August 2003): 728–731.

Matsuura, E., A. Ohta, F. Kanegae, et al. "Frequency and Analysis of Factors Closely Associated with the Development of Depressive Symptoms in Patients with Scleroderma." *Journal of Rheumatology* 30 (August 2003): 1782–1787.

Mayes, M. D., J. V. Lacey, Jr., J. Beebe-Dimmer, et al. "Prevalence, Incidence, Survival, and Disease Characteristics of Systemic Sclerosis in a Large US Population." *Arthritis and Rheumatism* 48 (August 2003): 2246–2255.

Pizzo, G., G. A. Scardina, and P. Messina. "Effects of a Nonsurgical Exercise Program on the Decreased Mouth Opening in Patients with Systemic Scleroderma." *Clinical Oral Investigations* 7 (September 2003): 175–178.

Zhou, X., F. K. Tan, N. Wang, et al. "Genome-Wide Association Study for Regions of Systemic Sclerosis Susceptibility in a Choctaw Indian Population with High Disease Prevalence." *Arthritis and Rheumatism* 48 (September 2003): 2585–2592.

ORGANIZATIONS

American College of Rheumatology. 60 Executive Park South, Suite 150, Atlanta, GA 30329. (404) 633-3777. < http://www.rheumatology.org >.

National Organization for Rare Disorders, Inc. (NORD). 55 Kenosia Avenue, P. O. Box 1968, Danbury, CT 06813. (800) 999-6673 or (203) 744-0100. < http://www.rarediseases.org >.

Scleroderma Foundation. 12 Kent Way, Suite 101, Byfield, MA 01922. (978) 463-5843 or (800) 722-HOPE. Fax: (978) 463-5809. < http://www.scleroderma.org. >.

Rebecca J. Frey, PhD

Sclerotherapy for esophageal varices

Definition

Sclerotherapy for esophageal varices (also called endoscopic sclerotherapy) is a treatment for esophageal bleeding that involves the use of an endoscope and the injection of a sclerosing solution into veins.

Purpose

In most hospitals, sclerotherapy for esophageal varices is the treatment of choice to stop esophageal bleeding during acute episodes, and to prevent further incidences of bleeding. Emergency sclerotherapy is often followed by preventive treatments to eradicate distended esophageal veins.

Precautions

Sclerotherapy for esophageal varices cannot be performed on an uncooperative patient, since movement during the procedure could cause the vein to tear or the esophagus to perforate and bleed. It should not be performed on a patient with a perforated gastrointestinal tract.

Description

Esophageal varices are enlarged or swollen veins on the lining of the esophagus which are prone to bleeding. They are life-threatening, and can be fatal in up to 50% of patients. They usually appear in patients with severe **liver disease**. Sclerotherapy for esophageal varices involves injecting a strong and irritating solution (a sclerosant) into the veins and/or the area beside the distended vein. The sclerosant injected into the vein causes **blood clots** to form and stops the bleeding. The sclerosant injected into the area beside the distended vein stops the bleeding by thickening and swelling the vein to compress the blood vessel. Most physicians inject the sclerosant directly into the vein, although injections into the vein and the surrounding area are both effective. Once bleeding has been stopped, the treatment can be used to significantly reduce or destroy the varices.

Sclerotherapy for esophageal varices is performed by a physician in a hospital, with the patient awake but sedated. Hyoscine butylbromide (Buscopan) may be administered to freeze the esophagus, making injection of the sclerosant easier. During the procedure, an endoscope is passed through the patient's mouth to the esophagus to view the inside. The branches of the blood vessels at or just above where the stomach and esophagus come together, the usual site of variceal bleeding, are located. After the bleeding vein is identified, a long, flexible sclerotherapy needle is passed through the endoscope. When the tip of the needle's sheath is in place, the needle is advanced, and the sclerosant is injected into the vein or the surrounding area. The most commonly used sclerosants are ethanolamine and sodium tetradecyl sulfate. The needle is withdrawn. The procedure is repeated as many times as necessary to eradicate all distended veins.

Sclerotherapy for esophageal varices controls acute bleeding in about 90% of patients, but it may have to be repeated within the first 48 hours to achieve this success rate. During the initial hospitalization, sclerotherapy is usually performed two or three times. Preventive treatments are scheduled every few weeks or so, depending on the patient's risk level and healing rate. Several studies have shown that the risk of recurrent bleeding is much lower in patients treated with sclerotherapy: 30-50%, as opposed to 70-80% for patients not treated with sclerotherapy.

Preparation

Before sclerotherapy for esophageal varices, the patient's vital signs and other pertinent data are recorded, an intravenous line is inserted to administer fluid or blood, and a sedative is prescribed.

Aftercare

After sclerotherapy for esophageal varices, the patient will be observed for signs of blood loss, lung complications, **fever**, a perforated esophagus, or other complications. Vital signs are monitored, and the intravenous line maintained. **Pain** medication is usually prescribed. After leaving the hospital, the patient follows a diet prescribed by the physician, and, if appropriate, can take mild pain relievers.

Risks

Sclerotherapy for esophageal varices has a 20-40% incidence of complications, and a 1–2% percent mortality rate. Complications can arise from the sclerosant or the endoscopic procedure. Minor complications, which are uncomfortable but do not require active treatment or prolonged hospitalization, include transient chest pain, difficulty swallowing, and fever, which usually go away after a few days. Some people have allergic reactions to the solution. Infection occurs in up to 50% of cases. In 2-10% of patients, the esophagus tightens, but this can usually be treated with dilatation. More serious complications may occur in 10-15% of patients treated with sclerotherapy. These include perforation or bleeding of the esophagus and lung problems, such as aspiration **pneumonia**. Long-term sclerotherapy can damage the esophagus, and increase the patient's risk of developing **cancer**.

Patients with advanced liver disease complicated by bleeding are very poor risks for this procedure. The surgery, premedications, and anesthesia may be sufficient to tip the patient into protein intoxication and

hepatic **coma**. The blood in the bowels acts like a high protein meal; therefore, protein intoxication may be induced.

Resources

PERIODICALS

Cello, J. P. "Endoscopic Management of Esophageal VaricealHemorrhage: Injection, Banding, Glue, Octreotide, or a Combination?" *Seminars in Gastrointestinal Diseases* 8 (October 1997): 179-187.

Lori De Milto

KEY TERMS

Endoscope—An instrument used to examine the inside of a canal or hollow organ. Endoscopic surgery is less invasive than traditional surgery.

Esophagus—The part of the digestive canal located between the pharynx (part of the digestive tube) and the stomach.

Sclerosant—An irritating solution that stops bleeding by hardening the blood or vein it is injected into.

Varices—Swollen or enlarged veins, in this case on the lining of the esophagus.

▌Scoliosis

Definition

Scoliosis is a side-to-side curvature of the spine.

Description

When viewed from the rear, the spine usually appears perfectly straight. Scoliosis is a lateral (side-to-side) curve in the spine, usually combined with a rotation of the vertebrae. (The lateral curvature of scoliosis should not be confused with the normal set of front-to-back spinal curves visible from the side.) While a small degree of lateral curvature does not cause any medical problems, larger curves can cause postural imbalance and lead to muscle **fatigue** and **pain**. More severe scoliosis can interfere with breathing and lead to arthritis of the spine (spondylosis).

Approximately 10% of all adolescents have some degree of scoliosis, though fewer than 1% have curves which require medical attention beyond monitoring. Scoliosis is found in both boys and girls, but a girl's spinal curve is much more likely to progress than a boy's. Girls require scoliosis treatment about five times as often. The reason for these differences is not known.

Causes and symptoms

Four out of five cases of scoliosis are *idiopathic*, meaning the cause is unknown. While idiopathic scoliosis tends to run in families, no responsible genes had been identified as of 1997. Children with idiopathic scoliosis appear to be otherwise entirely healthy, and have not had any bone or joint disease early in life. Scoliosis is not caused by poor posture, diet, or carrying a heavy bookbag exclusively on one shoulder.

Idiopathic scoliosis is further classified according to age of onset:

- Infantile. Curvature appears before age three. This type is quite rare in the United States, but is more common in Europe.

- Juvenile. Curvature appears between ages 3 and 10. This type may be equivalent to the adolescent type, except for the age of onset.

- Adolescent. Curvature appears between ages of 10 and 13, near the beginning of **puberty**. This is the most common type of idiopathic scoliosis.

- Adult. Curvature begins after physical maturation is completed.

Causes are known for three other types of scoliosis:

- Congenital scoliosis is due to congenital abnormal formation of the bones of the spine, and is often associated with other organ defects.

- Neuromuscular scoliosis is due to loss of control of the nerves or muscles which support the spine. The most common causes of this type of scoliosis are **cerebral palsy** and **muscular dystrophy**.

- Degenerative scoliosis may be caused by degeneration of the discs which separate the vertebrae or arthritis in the joints that link them.

Scoliosis causes a noticeable asymmetry in the torso when viewed from the front or back. The first sign of scoliosis is often seen when a child is wearing a bathing suit or underwear. A child may appear to be standing with one shoulder higher than the other, or to have a tilt in the waistline. One shoulder blade may appear more prominent than the other due to rotation. In girls, one breast may appear higher than the other, or larger if rotation pushes that side forward.

Curve progression is greatest near the adolescent growth spurt. Scoliosis that begins early on is more likely to progress significantly than scoliosis that begins later in puberty.

More than 30 states have screening programs in schools for adolescent scoliosis, usually conducted by trained school nurses or gym teachers.

Diagnosis

Diagnosis for scoliosis is done by an orthopedist. A complete medical history is taken, including questions about family history of scoliosis. The **physical examination** includes determination of pubertal development in adolescents, a neurological exam (which may reveal a neuromuscular cause), and measurements of trunk asymmetry. Examination of the trunk is done while the patient is standing, bending over, and lying down, and involves both visual inspection and use of a simple mechanical device called a scoliometer.

If a curve is detected, one or more x rays will usually be taken to define the curve or curves more precisely. An x ray is used to document spinal maturity, any pelvic tilt or hip asymmetry, and the location, extent, and degree of curvature. The curve is defined in terms of where it begins and ends, in which direction it bends, and by an angle measure known as the Cobb angle. The Cobb angle is found by projecting lines parallel to the vertebrae tops at the extremes of the curve; projecting perpendiculars from these lines; and measuring the angle of intersection. To properly track the progress of scoliosis, it is important to project from the same points of the spine each time.

Occasionally, **magnetic resonance imaging** (MRI) is used, primarily to look more closely at the condition of the spinal cord and nerve roots extending from it if neurological problems are suspected.

Treatment

Treatment decisions for scoliosis are based on the degree of curvature, the likelihood of significant progression, and the presence of pain, if any.

Curves less than 20 degrees are not usually treated, except by regular follow-up for children who are still growing. Watchful waiting is usually all that is required in adolescents with curves of 20–30 degrees, or adults with curves up to 40 degrees or slightly more, as long as there is no pain.

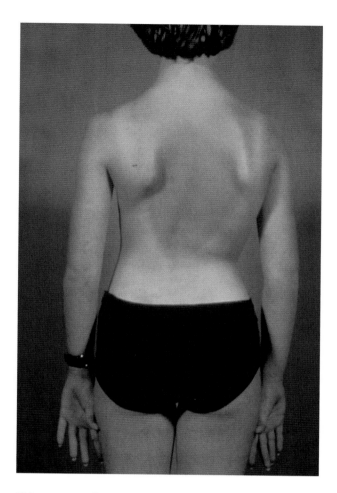

This woman suffers from scoliosis, or curvature of the spine. *(Custom Medical Stock Photo. Reproduced by permission.)*

For children or adolescents whose curves progress to 30 degrees, and who have a year or more of growth left, bracing may be required. Bracing cannot correct curvature, but may be effective in halting or slowing progression. Bracing is rarely used in adults, except where pain is significant and surgery is not an option, as in some elderly patients.

Two general styles of braces are used for daytime wear. The Milwaukee brace consists of metal uprights attached to pads at the hips, rib cage, and neck. The underarm brace uses rigid plastic to encircle the lower rib cage, abdomen, and hips. Both these brace types hold the spine in a vertical position. Because it can be worn out of sight beneath clothing, the underarm brace is better tolerated and often leads to better compliance. A third style, the Charleston bending brace, is used at night to bend the spine in the opposite direction. Braces are often prescribed to be worn for 22–23 hours per day, though some clinicians allow or encourage removal of the brace for **exercise**.

Bracing may be appropriate for scoliosis due to some types of neuromuscular disease, including spinal muscular atrophy, before growth is finished. Duchenne muscular dystrophy is not treated by bracing, since surgery is likely to be required, and since later surgery is complicated by loss of respiratory capacity.

Surgery for idiopathic scoliosis is usually recommended if:

- the curve has progressed despite bracing
- the curve is greater than 40–50 degrees before growth has stopped in an adolescent
- the curve is greater than 50 degrees and continues to increase in an adult
- there is significant pain

Orthopedic surgery for neuromuscular scoliosis is often done earlier. The goals of surgery are to correct the deformity as much as possible, to prevent further deformity, and to eliminate pain as much as possible. Surgery can usually correct 40–50% of the curve, and sometimes as much as 80%. Surgery cannot always completely remove pain.

The surgical procedure for scoliosis is called *spinal fusion*, because the goal is to straighten the spine as much as possible, and then to fuse the vertebrae together to prevent further curvature. To achieve fusion, the involved vertebra are first exposed, and then scraped to promote regrowth. Bone chips are usually used to splint together the vertebrae to increase the likelihood of fusion. To maintain the proper spinal posture before fusion occurs, metal rods are inserted alongside the spine, and are attached to the vertebrae by hooks, screws, or wires. Fusion of the spine makes it rigid and resistant to further curvature. The metal rods are no longer needed once fusion is complete, but are rarely removed unless their presence leads to complications.

Spinal fusion leaves the involved portion of the spine permanently stiff and inflexible. While this leads to some loss of normal motion, most functional activities are not strongly affected, unless the very lowest portion of the spine (the lumbar region) is fused. Normal mobility, exercise, and even contact sports are usually all possible after spinal fusion. Full recovery takes approximately six months.

Alternative treatment

Numerous alternative therapies have been touted to provide relief and help for individuals with scoliosis, but none have been proven beneficial in clinical trials. These include massage, physical therapy, and electrical stimulation. In addition, alternatives such as

KEY TERMS

Cobb angle —A measure of the curvature of scoliosis, determined by measurements made on x rays.

Rolfing —A system of soft tissue manipulation and movement education to realign and reorient the body.

Scoliometer —A tool for measuring trunk asymmetry; it includes a bubble level and angle measure.

Spondylosis —Arthritis of the spine.

physical therapy, **rolfing**, or chiropractice manipulation may provide improved flexibility, stronger muscles, and pain relief, but cannot prevent or correct the curvature of the spine or its natural progression.

Although important for general health and strength, exercise has not been shown to prevent or slow the development of scoliosis. It may help relieve pain from scoliosis by helping to maintain range of motion. Aquatic exercise, in particular, can increase flexibility and improve posture, balance, coordination, and range of motion. Because it decreases joint compression, it can lessen the pain caused by scoliosis or surgery.

Good **nutrition** is also important for general health, but no specific dietary regimen has been shown to control scoliosis development. In particular, dietary calcium levels do not influence scoliosis progression.

Chiropractic treatment may relieve pain, but it cannot halt scoliosis development, and should not be a substitute for conventional treatment of progressing scoliosis. **Acupuncture** and **acupressure** may also help reduce pain and discomfort, but they cannot halt scoliosis development either.

Prognosis

The prognosis for a person with scoliosis depends on many factors, including the age at which scoliosis begins and the treatment received. More importantly, mostly unknown individual factors affect the likelihood of progression and the severity of the curve. Most cases of mild adolescent idiopathic scoliosis need no treatment and do not progress. Untreated severe scoliosis often leads to spondylosis, and may impair breathing. Degenerative arthritis of the spine, **sciatica**, and severe physical deformities can also result if severe scoliosis is left untreated. Finally, scoliosis can also poorly affect the individual's self-esteem and cause serious emotional problems.

Prevention

There is no known way to prevent the development of scoliosis. Progression of scoliosis may be prevented through bracing or surgery.

Exercise and physical fitness are of paramount importance for all individuals affected with scoliosis. They not only work to maintain flexibility and health, but decrease the likelihood of **osteoporosis**, which in these individuals, can be extremely debilitating.

Resources

BOOKS

Lyons, Brooke, et al. *Scoliosis: Ascending the Curve*. New York: M. Evans & Co., 1999.

PERIODICALS

Bridwell, KH, et al., editors. "Parents' and Patients' Preferences and Concerns in Idiopathic Adolescent Scoliosis: A Cross-Sectional Preoperative Analysis." *Spine* 25, no. 18 (September 2000): 2392-9.

ORGANIZATIONS

American Physical Therapy Assocation. Scoliosis, P.O. Box 37257, Washington, DC 20013.

Center for Spinal Disorders, PC. 8515 Pearl Street, Suite 350, Thornton, CO 80229. (303) 287-2800; fax: (303) 287-7357. < http://www.cntrforspinaldisorders.com > .

National Scoliosis Foundation. 72 Mount Auburn St., Watertown, MA 02172. (617) 926-0397.

The Scoliosis Association. PO Box 811705, Boca Raton, FL 33481-0669. (407) 368-8518.

OTHER

"Chiropractic Treatment of Scoliosis." Scoliosis World.

Liz Meszaros

▌Scrotal nuclear medicine scan

Definition

Scrotal nuclear medicine scan is a study of the blood circulation in the scrotum using radioactive contrast agent to highlight obstruction.

Purpose

This test is used almost exclusively to differentiate infection in the testis (testicle) from twisting and infarction. Infection is called **epididymitis** because it mostly involves a collection of tubules on top of the testicle called the epididymis. Twisting of the testis shuts off its blood supply and is called testicular

KEY TERMS

Radioisotope—An unstable form of an element that gives off radiation to become stable.

Scrotum—The bag of skin below the penis that contains the testes.

torsion. Both conditions cause a very painful, swollen testis on one side. Both occur most often in young men, although infection usually occurs at a slightly greater age. The infection increases the blood supply, and the torsion cuts off the blood supply. This is an ideal situation for a blood flow study.

The distinction is critically important, because **testicular torsion** must be untwisted immediately or the testis will die. On the other hand, epididymitis responds to **antibiotics**, and surgery might further injure it.

Description

A radioisotope, technetium-99, combined in a chemical (pertechnate) is injected intravenously while the patient is under a special machine that detects radiation. This radiation detector, called a gamma camera, scans the scrotum at one minute intervals for about five minutes, then less often for another 10 or 15 minutes. It then creates pictures (either x ray or polaroid) that reveal where the isotope went in the scrotum. Since both sides are scanned, even greater accuracy is obtained by comparison.

Preparation

This procedure is usually done as an emergency to determine the need for immediate surgery.

Risks

The amount of radiation is so slight that even the sensitive testicular tissue is at minimum risk.

Normal results

Blood flow appears unobstructed.

Abnormal results

Three possible possible images appear. They are:

- Increased blood flow indicating infection
- No blood flow indicating testicular torsion

- Blood flow illuminated in a "donut" shaped pattern that indicates torsion that has resolved itself within the last few days.

Resources

BOOKS

Rajfer, Jacob. "Congenital Anomalies of the Testes and Scrotum." In *Campbell's Urology*, edited by Patrick C. Walsh, et al. Philadelphia: W. B. SaundersCo., 1998.

J. Ricker Polsdorfer, MD

Scrotal sonogram *see* **Scrotal ultrasound**

Scrotal ultrasound

Definition

Scrotal ultrasound is an imaging technique used for the diagnosis of suspected abnormalities of the scrotum. It uses harmless, high-frequency sound waves to form an image. The sound waves are reflected by scrotal tissue to form a picture of internal structures. It is not invasive and involves no radiation.

Purpose

Ultrasound of the scrotum is the primary imaging method used to evaluate disorders of the testicles and surrounding tissues. It is used when a patient has acute **pain** in the scrotum. Some of the problems for which the use of scrotal ultrasound is valuable include an absent or undescended testicle, an inflammation problem, testicular torsion, a fluid collection, abnormal blood vessels, or a mass (lump or tumor).

A sudden onset of pain in the scrotum is considered a serious problem, as delay in diagnosis and treatment can lead to loss of function. **Epididymitis** is the most common cause of this type of pain. Epididymitis is an inflammation of the epididymis, a tubular structure that transports sperm from the testes. It is most often caused by bacterial infection, but may occur after injury, or arise from an unknown cause. Epididymitis is treatable with antibiotics, which usually resolves pain quickly. Left untreated, this condition can lead to **abscess** formation or loss of blood supply to the testicle.

Testicular torsion is the twisting of the spermatic cord that contains the blood vessels which supply the testicles. It is caused by abnormally loose attachments of tissues that are formed during fetal development.

Torsion can be complete, incomplete, or intermittent. Spontaneous detorsion, or untwisting, can occur, making diagnosis difficult. Testicular torsion arises most commonly during adolescence, and is acutely painful. Scrotal ultrasound is used to distinguish this condition from inflammatory problems, such as epididymitis. Testicular torsion is a surgical emergency; it should be operated on as soon as possible to avoid permanent damage to the testes.

A scrotal sac with an absent testicle may be the result of a congenital anomaly (an abnormality present at birth), where a testicle fails to develop. More often, it is due to an undescended testicle. In the fetus, the testicles normally develop just outside the abdomen and descend into the scrotum during the seventh month. Approximately 3% of full-term baby boys have undescended testicles. It is important to distinguish between an undescended testicle and an absent testicle, as an undescended testicle has a very high probability of developing **cancer**.

Ultrasound can be used to locate and evaluate masses in the scrotum. Most masses within the testicle are malignant or cancerous, and most outside the testicle are benign. Primary cancer of the testicles is the most common malignancy in men between the ages of 15-35. Fluid collections and abnormalities of the blood vessels in the scrotum may appear to the physician as masses and need evaluation by ultrasound. A hydrocele, the most common cause of painless scrotal swelling, is a collection of fluid between two layers of tissue surrounding the testicle. An abnormal enlargement of the veins which drain the testicles is called a varicocele. It can cause discomfort and swelling, which can be examined by touch (palpated). Varicocele is a common cause of male infertility.

Precautions

Clear scrotal ultrasound images are difficult to obtain if a patient is unable to remain still.

Description

The patient lies on his back on an examining table. The technologist will usually take a history of the problem, then gently palpate the scrotum. A rolled towel is placed between the patient's legs to support the scrotum. The penis is lifted up onto the abdomen and covered. A gel that enhances sound transmission is put directly on the scrotum. The technologist then gently places a transducer (an electronic imaging device) against the skin. It is moved over the area creating images from reflected sound waves, which

<hr>

KEY TERMS

Hydrocele— A collection of fluid between two layers of tissue surrounding the testicle; the most common cause of painless scrotal swelling.

Varicocele— An abnormal enlargement of the veins which drain the testicles.

<hr>

appear on a monitor screen. There is no discomfort from the study itself. However, if the scrotum is very tender, even the slight pressure involved may be painful.

Normal results

A normal study would reveal testicles of normal size and shape, with no masses.

Abnormal results

An abnormal result of an ultrasound of the scrotum may reveal an absent or undescended testicle, an inflammation problem, testicular torsion, a fluid collection, abnormal blood vessels, or a mass.

Resources

BOOKS

Leonhardt, Wayne C. "Scrotum." In *Abdomen and Superficial Structures*, edited by Diane M. Kawamura, 2nd ed. Philadelphia: Lippincott, 1997.

Ellen S. Weber, MSN

<hr>

Scrub typhus

Definition

Scrub **typhus** is an infectious disease that is transmitted to humans from field mice and rats through the bite of mites that live on the animals. The main symptoms of the disease are **fever**, a wound at the site of the bite, a spotted rash on the trunk, and swelling of the lymph glands.

Description

Scrub typhus is caused by *Rickettsia tsutsugamushi*, a tiny parasite about the size of bacteria that belongs to the family Rickettsiaceae. Under the microscope, rickettsiae are either rod-like (bacilli) or spherical (cocci) in shape. Because they are intracellular parasites, they can live only within the cells of other animals.

R. tsutsugamushi lives primarily in mites that belong to the species *Leptotrombidium (Trombicula) akamushi* and *Leptotrombidium deliense*. In Japan, some cases of scrub typhus have been reportedly transmitted by mites of the species *Leptotrombidium scutellare* and *Leptotrombidium pallidum*. The mites have four-stage life cycles: egg, larva, nymph, and adult. The larva is the only stage that can transmit the disease to humans and other vertebrates.

The tiny chiggers (mite larvae) attach themselves to the skin. During the process of obtaining a meal, they may either acquire the infection from the host or transmit the rickettsiae to other mammals or humans. In regions where scrub typhus is a constant threat, a natural cycle of *R. tsutsugamushi* transmission occurs between mite larvae and small mammals (e.g., field mice and rats). Humans enter a cycle of rickettsial infection only accidentally.

Scrub typhus is also known as *tsutsugamushi disease*. The name tsutsugamushi is derived from two Japanese words: tsutsuga, meaning something small and dangerous, and mushi, meaning creature. The infection is called scrub typhus because it generally occurs after exposure to areas with secondary (scrub) vegetation. It has recently been found, however, that the disease can also be prevalent in such areas as sandy beaches, mountain deserts, and equatorial rain forests. Therefore, it has been suggested that the names mite-borne typhus, or chigger-borne typhus, are more appropriate. Since the disease is limited to eastern and southeastern Asia, India, northern Australia and the adjacent islands, it is also commonly referred to as tropical typhus.

The seasonal occurrence of scrub typhus varies with the climate in different countries. It occurs more frequently during the rainy season. Certain areas such as forest clearings, riverbanks, and grassy regions provide optimal conditions for the infected mites to thrive. These small geographic regions are high-risk areas for humans and have been called scrub-typhus islands.

Causes and symptoms

The incubation period of scrub typhus is about 10 to 12 days after the initial bite. The illness begins rather suddenly with shaking chills, fever, severe headache, infection of the mucous membrane lining the eyes (the conjunctiva), and swelling of the lymph nodes (lymphadenopathy). A wound (lesion) is often seen at the site of the chigger bite. Bite **wounds** are common in whites but rare in Asians.

The initial lesion, which is about 1 cm (0.4 in) in diameter and flat, eventually becomes elevated and filled with fluid. After it ruptures, it becomes covered with a black scab (eschar). The patient's fever rises during the first week, generally reaching 40–40.5°C (104–105°F). About the fifth day of fever, a red spotted rash develops on the trunk, often extending to the arms and legs. It may either fade away in a few days or may become spotted and elevated (maculopapular) and brightly colored. **Cough** is present during the first week of the fever. An infection of the lung (pneumonitis) may develop during the second week.

In severe cases, the patient's pulse rate increases and blood pressure drops. The patient may become delirious and lose consciousness. Muscular twitching may develop. Enlargement of the spleen is observed. Inflammation of the heart muscle (interstitial **myocarditis**) is more common in scrub typhus than in other rickettsial diseases. In untreated patients, high fever may last for more than two weeks. With specific therapy, however, the fever breaks within 36 hours. The patient's recovery is prompt and uneventful.

Diagnosis

Patient history and physical examination

Differentiating scrub typhus from other forms of typhus as well as from fever, typhoid and meningococcal infections is often difficult during the first several days before the initial rash appears. The geographical location of scrub typhus, the initial sore caused by the chigger bite, and the occurrence of specific proteins capable of destroying the organism (antibodies) in the blood, provide helpful clues and are useful in establishing the diagnosis.

Laboratory tests

Diagnostic procedures involving the actual isolation of rickettsiae from the blood or other body tissues are usually expensive, time-consuming, and hazardous to laboratory workers. As a result, several types of tests known as serological (immunological) tests are used widely to confirm the clinical diagnosis in the laboratory.

Specific antibodies develop in the body in response to an infection. The development of antibodies during the recovery period indicates that an immune response is present. The formation of antibodies is the basic principle of a serological test. Three different tests are available to diagnose rickettsial infections. The most widely used is the Weil-Felix test. This test is based on the fact that some of the antibodies that are formed in the body during a rickettsial infection can react with certain strains (OX-2 and OX-19) of *Proteus* bacteria and cause them to clump (agglutinate). The clumping is easily seen under the microscope. The Weil-Felix test is easy and inexpensive to perform, with the result that it is widely used. The Weil-Felix test, however, is not very specific. In addition, the clumping is not detectable until the second week of the illness, which limits the test's usefulness in early diagnosis.

A second test known as a complement fixation (CF) test is based on the principle that if antibodies are formed in the body in response to the illness, then the antigen and the antibody will form complexes. These antigen-antibody complexes have the ability to inactivate, or fix, a protein that is found in blood serum (serum complement). The serum complement fixation can be measured using standardized biochemical tests and confirms the presence of antibodies. A third test known as the fluorescent antibody test uses fluorescent tags that are attached to antibodies for easy detection. This test has been developed using three strains of *Rickettsia tsutsugamushi* and has proven to be the most specific for diagnosis.

Treatment

Scrub typhus is treated with **antibiotics**. Chloramphenicol (Chloromycetin, Fenicol) and tetracycline (Achromycin, Tetracyn) are the drugs of choice. They bring about prompt disappearance of the fever and dramatic clinical improvement. If the antibiotic treatment is discontinued too quickly, especially in patients treated within the first few days of the fever, relapses may occur. In patients treated in the second week of illness, the antibiotics may be stopped one to two days after the fever disappears.

Antibiotics are given intravenously to patients too sick to take them by mouth. Patients who are severely ill and whose treatment was delayed may be given **corticosteroids** in combination with antibiotics for three days.

Prognosis

Before the use of antibiotics, the mortality rate for scrub typhus varied from 1–60%, depending on the geographic area and the rickettsial strain. Recovery

---

---

also took a long time. With modern treatment methods, however, deaths are rare and the recovery period is short.

Prevention

General precautions

As of early 2004 there are no effective vaccines for scrub typhus. In endemic areas, precautions include wearing protective clothing. Insect repellents containing dibutyl phthalate, benzyl benzoate, diethyl toluamide, and other substances can be applied to the skin and clothing to prevent chigger bites. Clearing of vegetation and chemical treatment of the soil may help to break up the cycle of transmission from chiggers to humans to other chiggers.

Prophylactic antibiotic dosage

It has been shown that a single oral dose of chloramphenicol or tetracycline given every 5 days for a total of 35 days, with 5-day nontreatment intervals, actually produces active immunity to scrub typhus. This procedure is recommended under special circumstances in certain areas where the disease is endemic.

Resources

BOOKS

Beers, Mark H., MD, and Robert Berkow, MD., editors. "Scrub Typhus." Section 13, Chapter 159 In *The Merck Manual of Diagnosis and Therapy*. Whitehouse Station, NJ: Merck Research Laboratories, 2004.

PERIODICALS

Cheng, V. C., A. K. Wu, I. F. Hung, et al. "Clinical Deterioration in Community Acquired Infections Associated with Lymphocyte Upsurge in Immunocompetent Hosts." *Scandinavian Journal of Infectious Diseases* 36, no. 10 (2004): 743–751.

Ralph, A., M. Raines, P. Whelan, and B. J. Currie. "Scrub Typhus in the Northern Territory: Exceeding the Boundaries of Litchfield National Park." *Communicable Diseases Intelligence* 28 (February 2004): 267–269.

Takahashi, M., H. Misumi, H. Urakami, et al. "Mite Vectors (Acari: Trombiculidae) of Scrub Typhus in a New Endemic Area in Northern Kyoto, Japan." *Journal of Medical Entomology* 41 (January 2004): 107–114.

ORGANIZATIONS

Centers for Disease Control and Prevention. 1600 Clifton Rd., NE, Atlanta, GA 30333. (800) 311-3435, (404) 639-3311. <http://www.cdc.gov>.

Lata Cherath, PhD
Rebecca J. Frey, PhD

Scurvy

Definition

Scurvy is a condition caused by a lack of vitamin C (ascorbic acid) in the diet. Signs of scurvy include tiredness, muscle weakness, joint and muscle aches, a rash on the legs, and bleeding gums. In the past, scurvy was common among sailors and other people deprived of fresh fruits and vegetables for long periods of time.

Description

Scurvy is very rare in countries where fresh fruits and vegetables are readily available and where processed foods have vitamin C added. Vitamin C is an important antioxidant vitamin involved in the development of connective tissues, lipid and vitamin metabolism, biosynthesis of neurotransmitters, immune function, and wound healing. It is found in fruits, especially citrus fruits like oranges, lemons, and grapefruit, and in green leafy vegetables like broccoli and spinach. In adults, it may take several months of vitamin C deficiency before symptoms of scurvy develop.

Currently, the recommended dietary allowance (RDA) for vitamin C is 50–60 mg/day for adults; 35 mg/day for infants; 40–45 mg/day for children 1–14; 70 mg/day during **pregnancy**; and 90–95 mg/day during **lactation**. The body's need for vitamin C increases when a person is under **stress, smoking,** or taking certain medications.

Causes and symptoms

A lack of vitamin C in the diet is the primary cause of scurvy. This can occur in people on very restricted **diets,** who are under extreme physiological stress (for example, during an infection or after an injury), and in chronic alcoholics. Infants can develop scurvy if they are weaned from breast milk and switched to cow's milk without an additional supplement of vitamin C. Babies of mothers who took extremely high doses of vitamin C during pregnancy can develop infantile scurvy. In children, the deficiency can cause painful swelling of the legs along with **fever, diarrhea,** and **vomiting.** In adults, early signs of scurvy include feeling weak, tired, and achy. The appearance of tiny red blood-blisters to larger purplish blotches on the skin of the legs is a common symptom. Wound healing may be delayed and **scars** that had healed may start to break down. The gums swell and bleed easily, eventually leading to loosened teeth. Muscle and joint **pain** may also occur.

Diagnosis

Scurvy is often diagnosed based on the symptoms present. A dietary history showing little or no fresh fruits or vegetables are eaten may help to diagnose vitamin C deficiency. A blood test can also be used to check the level of ascorbic acid in the body.

Treatment

Adult treatment is usually 300–1,000 mg of ascorbic acid per day. Infants should be treated with 50 mg of ascorbic acid up to four times per day.

Prognosis

Treatment with vitamin C is usually successful, if the deficiency is recognized early enough. Left untreated, the condition can cause **death.**

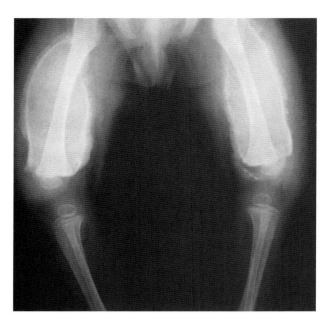

An x-ray image of an infant suffering from scurvy. *(Photograph by Lester V. Bergman, Corbis Images. Reproduced by permission.)*

KEY TERMS

Ascorbic acid—Another term for vitamin C, a nutrient found in fresh fruits and vegetables. Good sources of vitamin C in the diet are citrus fruits like oranges, lemons, limes, and grapefruits, berries, tomatoes, green peppers, cabbage, broccoli, and spinach.

Recommended dietary allowance (RDA)—The daily amount of a vitamin the average person needs to maintain good health.

Prevention

Eating foods rich in vitamin C every day prevents scurvy. A supplement containing the RDA of vitamin C will also prevent a deficiency. Infants who are being weaned from breast milk to cow's milk need a supplement containing vitamin C.

Resources

BOOKS

Stein, Jay H., editor. "Ascorbic Acid (Vitamin C) Deficiency." In *Internal Medicine*. St. Louis: Mosby, 1998.

Altha Roberts Edgren

Seafood poisoning *see* **Fish and shellfish poisoning**

Seasonal affective disorder

Definition

Seasonal affective disorder (SAD) is a form of depression most often associated with the lack of daylight in extreme northern and southern latitudes from the late fall to the early spring.

Description

Although researchers are not certain what causes seasonal affective disorder, they suspect that it has something to do with the hormone melatonin. Melatonin is thought to play an active role in regulating the "internal body clock," which dictates when humans feel like going to bed at night and getting up in the morning. Although seasonal affective disorder is most common when light is low, it may occur in the spring, and it is then often called reverse SAD.

Causes and symptoms

The body produces more melatonin at night than during the day, and scientists believe it helps people feel sleepy at nighttime. There is also more melatonin in the body during winter, when the days are shorter. Some researchers believe that excessive melatonin release during winter in people with SAD may account for their feelings of drowsiness or depression. One variation on this idea is that, during winter, people's internal clocks may become out of sync with the light-dark cycle, leading to a long-term disruption in melatonin release.

Seasonal affective disorder, while not an official category of mental illness listed by the American Psychiatric Association, is estimated to affect 10 million Americans, most of whom are women. Another 25 million Americans may have a mild form of SAD, sometimes called the "winter blues" or "winter blahs." The risk of SAD increases the further from the equator a person lives.

The symptoms of SAD are similar to those of other forms of depression. People with SAD may feel sad, irritable, or tired, and may find themselves sleeping too much. They may also lose interest in normal or pleasurable activities (including sex), become withdrawn, crave carbohydrates, and gain weight.

Diagnosis

Doctors usually diagnose seasonal affective disorder based on the patient's description of symptoms, including the time of year they occur.

Treatment

The first-line treatment for seasonal affective disorder is light therapy, exposing the patient to bright artificial light to compensate for the gloominess of winter. Light therapy uses a device called a light box, which contains a set of fluorescent or incandescent lights in front of a reflector. Typically, the patient sits for 30 minutes next to a 10,000-lux box (which is about 50 times as bright as ordinary indoor light). Light therapy appears to be safe for most people. However, it may be harmful for those with eye diseases. The most common side effects are vision problems such as eye strain, headaches, irritability, and **insomnia**. In addition, hypomania (elevated or expansive mood, characterized by hyperactivity and inflated self esteem) may occasionally occur.

Recently, researchers have begun testing whether people who do not completely respond to light therapy can benefit from tiny doses of the hormone melatonin to reset the body's internal clock. Early results look promising, but the potential benefits must be confirmed in larger studies before this type of treatment becomes widely accepted.

Like other types of **mood disorders**, seasonal affective disorder may also respond to medication and psychotherapy. The four different classes of drugs used for mood disorders are:

- heterocyclic antidepressants (HCAs), such as amitriptyline (Elavil)
- selective serotonin reuptake inhibitors (SSRIs), such as fluoxetine (Prozac), paroxetine (Paxil), and sertraline (Zoloft)
- monoamine oxidase inhibitors (MAO inhibitors), such as phenelzine sulfate (Nardil) and tranylcypromine sulfate (Parnate)
- Lithium salts, such as lithium carbonate (Eskalith), often used in people with bipolar mood disorders, are often useful with SAD patients; many SAD patients also suffer from **bipolar disorder** (excessive mood swings; formerly known as manic depression)

A number of psychotherapy approaches are useful as well. Interpersonal psychotherapy helps patients recognize how their mood disorder and their interpersonal relationships interact. Cognitive-behavioral therapy explores how the patient's view of the world may be affecting mood and outlook.

Prognosis

Most patients with seasonal affective disorder respond to light therapy and/or **antidepressant drugs**.

KEY TERMS

Cognitive behavioral therapy—Psychotherapy aimed at helping people change their attitudes, perceptions, and patterns of thinking.

Melatonin—A naturally occurring hormone involved in regulating the body's "internal clock."

Serotonin—A chemical messenger in the brain thought to play a role in regulating mood.

Resources

ORGANIZATIONS

American Psychiatric Association. 1400 K Street NW, Washington DC 20005. (888) 357-7924. <http://www.psych.org>.

National Depressive and Manic Depressive Association (NDMDA). 730 N. Franklin St., Ste. 501, Chicago, IL 60610. (800) 826-3632. <http://www.ndmda.org>.

National Institute of Mental Health. Mental Health Public Inquiries, 5600 Fishers Lane, Room 15C-05, Rockville, MD 20857. (888) 826-9438. <http://www.nimh.nih.gov>.

Robert Scott Dinsmoor

Seasonal depression *see* **Seasonal affective disorder**

Seatworm infection *see* **Enterobiasis**

Seborrheic dermatitis

Definition

Seborrheic **dermatitis** is a common inflammatory disease of the skin characterized by scaly lesions usually on the scalp, hairline, and face.

Description

Seborrheic dermatitis appears as red, inflamed skin covered by greasy or dry scales that may be white, yellowish, or gray. It can effect the scalp, eyebrows, forehead, face, folds around the nose and ears, the chest, armpits (axilla), and groin. Dandruff and cradle cap are mild forms of seborrheic dermatitis, and appear as fine white scales without inflammation.

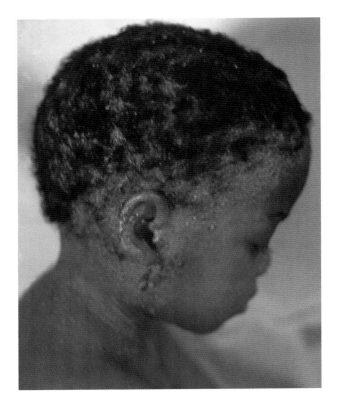

This young boy is afflicted with seborrheic dermatitis. *(Custom Medical Stock Photo. Reproduced by permission.)*

Causes and symptoms

The cause of seborrheic dermatitis is unclear, though it is has been linked to genetic or environmental factors. *Pityrosporum ovale*, a species of yeast normally found in hair follicles, has been proposed as one possible causative factor. A high fat diet and alcohol ingestion are thought to play some role. Other possible risk factors include:

- stress and **fatigue**
- weather extremes (e. g. hot, humid weather or cold, dry weather)
- oily skin
- infrequent shampoos
- obesity
- Parkinson's disease
- AIDS
- use of drying lotions that contain alcohol
- other skin disorders (for example **acne**, **rosacea**, or psoriasis)

Mild forms of the disorder may be asymptomatic. Symptoms also disappear and reappear, and vary in intensity over time. When scaling is present, it may be accompanied by **itching** that can lead to secondary infection.

Diagnosis

The diagnosis of seborrheic dermatitis is based on assessment of symptoms, accompanied by consideration of medical history.

Treatment

Treatment consists of vigorous shampoos with preparations that assist with softening and removing the scaly accumulations. For mild cases, a non-prescription shampoo with selenium sulfide or zinc pyrithione may be used. For more severe problems, the doctor may prescribe shampoos containing coal tar or scalp creams containing cortisone. The antiseborrheic shampoo should be left on the scalp for approximately five minutes before rinsing out. Hydrocortisone cream may also be ordered for application to the affected areas on the face and body. Application of the hydrocortisone should be discontinued when the condition clears and restarted with recurrence.

Prognosis

This chronic condition may be characterized by long periods of inactivity. Symptoms in the acute phase can be controlled with appropriate treatment.

Prevention

The condition cannot be prevented. The severity and frequency of flare-ups may be minimized with frequent shampoos, thorough drying of skin folds after bathing, and wearing of loose, ventilating clothing. Foods that appear to worsen the condition should be avoided.

Resources

BOOKS

Monahan, Frances, and Marianne Neighbors. *Medical Surgical Nursing: Foundations for Clinical Practice.* Philadelphia: W. B. Saunders,1998.

Kathleen D. Wright, RN

Secobarbital *see* **Barbiturates**

Secondary erythrocytosis *see* **Secondary polycythemia**

Secondary polycythemia

Definition

Secondary polycythemia is an acquired form of a rare disorder characterized by an abnormal increase in the number of mature red cells in the blood.

Secondary polycythemia is also called secondary erythrocytosis.

Description

Polycythemia means too many red blood cells. The resulting excess of red cells thickens the blood and impedes its passage through small blood vessels.

Secondary polycythemia usually affects people between the ages of 40 and 60.

Types of secondary polycythemia

Known as spurious polycythemia, **stress** polycythemia, or Gaisbock's syndrome, relative polycythemia is characterized by normal numbers of red blood cells but decreased levels of plasma (the fluid part of the blood). Overweight, middle-aged white men who smoke, have high blood pressure, and are on diuretic medicines to remove excess water from their bodies may develop Gaisbock's syndrome.

In smoker's polycythemia, the number of red blood cells is elevated. Plasma levels are abnormally low.

Causes and symptoms

Smoking, which impairs red blood cells' ability to deliver oxygen to body tissues, can cause secondary polycythemia. So can the following conditions:

- carbon monoxide **poisoning**
- chronic heart or lung disease
- hormonal (endocrine) disorders
- exposure to high altitudes
- kidney cysts
- tumors of the brain, liver, or uterus.

Causes of spurious polycythemia include:

- burns
- diarrhea
- hemoconcentration (higher-than-normal concentration of cells and solids in the blood, usually due to becoming dehydrated or taking **diuretics**)
- stress

Weakness, headaches, and **fatigue** are usually the first symptoms of secondary polycythemia. Patients may feel lightheaded or experience **shortness of breath**.

Visual disturbances associated with this disorder include distorted vision, blind spots, and flashes of light. The gums and small cuts are likely to bleed, and the hands and feet may burn. Extensive **itching** often occurs after taking a bath or shower.

Pain in the chest or leg muscles is common. The face often becomes ruddy, then turns blue after **exercise** or other exertion. Confusion and ringing in the ears (**tinnitus**) may also occur.

Diagnosis

A very important part of diagnosing secondary polycythemia is differentiating it from primary polycythemia (also called polycythemia rubra vera or Vaquez' disease). Unlike secondary polycythemia, primary polycythemia cannot be traced to an underlying condition such as smoking, high altitude, or chronic lung disease.

Doctors diagnose polycythemia by measuring oxygen levels in blood drawn from an artery. A patient whose oxygen level is abnormally low probably has secondary polycythemia. Erythropoietin may also be measured. Levels of this hormone, which stimulates the bone marrow to produce red blood cells, may be normal or elevated in a patient with secondary polycythemia. Red blood cell mass is also frequently measured in diagnosing the disorder.

Imaging studies are sometimes performed to determine whether the spleen and liver are enlarged and to detect erythropoietin-producing kidney lesions. Other diagnostic procedures include chest x rays and an electrocardiogram (EKG).

Treatment

Secondary polycythemia is treated primarily by treating the underlying condition causing the disorder. For example, patients with Gaisbock's syndrome are often taken off diuretics and encouraged to lose weight. Lung disorders, such as chronic obstructive pulmonary disease (COPD), may cause secondary polycythemia; treating the lung disorder generally improves the polycythemia.

Some medications may also be taken to treat symptoms caused by polycythemia. For example, **antihistamines** can alleviate itching, and **aspirin** can soothe burning sensations and bone pain.

Until the underlying condition is controlled, doctors use bloodletting (**phlebotomy**) to reduce the number of red blood cells in the patient's body. In most instances, a pint of blood is drained from the patient as needed and tolerated, until the hematocrit (the proportion of red cells in the blood) reaches an acceptable level. **Chemotherapy** is not used to treat secondary polycythemia; however, it may be used to treat the primary form.

Prognosis

Curing or removing the underlying cause of this disorder generally eliminates the symptoms.

Resources

OTHER

"Secondary Erythrocytosis." *The Merck Page.* June 3, 1998. < http://www.merck.com >.

Maureen Haggerty

SED rate *see* **Erythrocyte sedimentation rate**

Sedation

Definition

Sedation is the act of calming by administration of a sedative. A sedative is a medication that commonly induces the nervous system to calm.

Purpose

The process of sedation has two primary intentions. First, sedation is recommended to allow patients the ability to tolerate unpleasant diagnostic or surgical procedures and to relieve **anxiety** and discomfort. Second, sedation for uncooperative patients may expedite and simplify special procedures that require little or no movement. Additionally, sedation is often desirable to diminish fear associated with operative procedures. Sedation is typically used for common diagnostic tests that require prolonged **immobilization** such as **magnetic resonance imaging** (MRI) and computed axial tomography (CAT) scanning. Some cases that require sedation may also necessitate the use of **analgesics** to decrease **pain** associated with a procedure or test.

Precautions

Benzodiazepines (common sedative medication) have a cumulative effect. This means that if the patient has not had time to metabolize the previous dose and ingests more, then the sedative effect may increase. Because of these additive effects, these medications taken with other sedatives or alcohol (also a sedative hypnotic drug) may increase chances for accidental **death**. In general, most of the medications that induce sedation may alter breathing and cardiac stability. In patients with preexisting lung and/or heart disease, these medications should be monitored closely or not prescribed.

Description

The future of anesthetic care involves the simultaneous administration of several drugs including IV medications and inhaled anesthetics. An extensive survey of death in 100,000 cases published in 1988 revealed that death within seven days was 2.9 times greater when one or two anesthetic drugs were used than when using three or more medications. As of 2000 this study is accepted as standard practice and multiple IV anesthetics is the preferable recommendation for optimal patient care.

The procedure for sedation is usually explained to the patient by an attending clinician. An IV access line is set in place for fluid replacement and injection of medications. A history is usually taken to assess risk and choice of medication. The patient typically signs consent forms and the possible side effects are explained. The day before the test, the patient may be required to maintain specified dietary restriction.

For outpatient surgery there are two types of sedation, conscious and unconscious sedation. Patients receiving conscious sedation are capable of rational responses, and they are able to maintain their airway for ventilation. The hallmark of conscious sedation is that it does not alter respiratory, cardiac, or reflex functions (nerve reflexes from the brain) to the level that requires external support for these vital functions. Patients receiving conscious sedation are cooperative, have stable vital signs (pulse, respiratory rate, and temperature), shorter recovery room convalescence, and lower risk of developing drug-induced complications. Unconscious sedation is a controlled state of anesthesia, characterized by partial or complete loss of protective nerve reflexes, including the ability to independently breathe and respond to commands. The patient is unable to cooperate, has labile (fluctuating) vital signs, prolonged recovery room convalescence, and higher risk of anesthetic complications.

Preparation

Usually procedures for conscious sedation do not require preoperative or pre-testing orders. Clinical situations for unconscious sedation typically involve eating and drinking protocols starting the day before the procedure.

The age and physical status of the patient is useful in determining sensitivity. A detailed past history, especially prior experiences with sedatives and other anesthetics is an important part of preparatory assessment. It is important to determine if there were any untoward side effects associated with a previous medication. Patient positioning is important to prevent blood pressure changes or nerve damage associated with abnormal position.

Patients are also monitored for pulse rate, respiration, blood pressure, and temperature. Additionally, the heart is monitored using **electrocardiography** (ECG). Ventilation is assessed using a pulse oximeter. This machine is clipped with a special probe on one finger and can measure the levels of oxygen and carbon dioxide, which are reliable indicators of respiratory status.

Aftercare

The major goal for recovery room monitoring is assessment of residual drug effects. Recovery room monitoring primarily focuses on heart stability, respiratory adequacy and return to previous brain functioning.

KEY TERMS

Baseline— A return to an original state.

Diazepam— One of the most commonly used sedative-hypnotic medications.

Risks

The original forms of diazepam (Valium, a very common sedative) caused irritation of veins and phlebitis. Newer forms of diazepam (Dizac) are chemically improved to lower the possibility of vein irritation. Age and physical health are important risk factors. Preexisting medical conditions such as high blood pressure and heart and lung disease may increase the chance of developing undesirable side effects.

Normal results

Normal or uncomplicated results for sedation include alleviation of anxiety and discomfort. Coupled with analgesic, patients are usually pain-free. The normal progression post procedure or post operatively would be to return to baseline brain functioning, unassisted breathing, and normal heart rate and rhythm.

Abnormal results

Patients may have excessive **nausea and vomiting** associated with narcotic analgesia (if this is indicated). Excessive drowsiness can occur secondary to benzodiazepine-induced sedation. The patient can also develop hypoventilation (a decrease in ventilation), airway obstruction, high or low blood pressure, abnormal heart rhythms, **nausea**, **vomiting**, and shivering.

Resources

BOOKS

Fleisher, Gary R., et al. *Textbook of Pediatric Emergency Medicine.* 4th ed. Lippincott Wlliams &Wilkins, 2000.
Miller, Ronald D., et al, editors. *Anesthesia.* 5th ed. Churchill Livingstone, Inc., 2000.

Laith Farid Gulli, M.D.
Bilal Nasser, M.Sc.

Sedative-hypnotic drugs *see* **Anti-insomnia drugs**

Sedimentation rate *see* **Erythrocyte sedimentation rate**

Seizure disorder

Definition

A seizure is a sudden disruption of the brain's normal electrical activity accompanied by altered consciousness and/or other neurological and behavioral manifestations. Epilepsy is a condition characterized by recurrent seizures that may include repetitive muscle jerking called convulsions.

Description

There are more than 20 different seizure disorders. One in ten Americans will have a seizure at some time, and at least 200,000 have at least one seizure a month.

Epilepsy affects 1–2% of the population of the United States. Although epilepsy is as common in adults over 60 as in children under 10, 25% of all cases develop before the age of five. One in every two cases develops before the age of 25. About 125,000 new cases of epilepsy are diagnosed each year, and a significant number of children and adults that have not been diagnosed or treated have epilepsy.

Most seizures are benign, but a seizure that lasts a long time can lead to status epilepticus, a life-threatening condition characterized by continuous seizures, sustained loss of consciousness, and respiratory distress. Non-convulsive epilepsy can impair physical coordination, vision, and other senses. Undiagnosed seizures can lead to conditions that are more serious and more difficult to manage.

Types of seizures

Generalized epileptic seizures occur when electrical abnormalities exist throughout the brain. A partial seizure does not involve the entire brain. A partial seizure begins in an area called an epileptic focus, but may spread to other parts of the brain and cause a generalized seizure. Some people who have epilepsy have more than one type of seizure.

Motor attacks cause parts of the body to jerk repeatedly. A motor attack usually lasts less than an hour and may last only a few minutes. Sensory seizures begin with **numbness** or **tingling** in one area. The sensation may move along one side of the body or the back before subsiding.

Visual seizures, which affect the area of the brain that controls sight, cause people to see things that are not there. Auditory seizures affect the part of the brain that controls hearing and cause the patient to imagine voices, music, and other sounds. Other types of seizures can cause confusion, upset stomach, or emotional distress.

GENERALIZED SEIZURES. A generalized tonic-clonic (grand-mal) seizure begins with a loud cry before the person having the seizure loses consciousness and falls to the ground. The muscles become rigid for about 30 seconds during the tonic phase of the seizure and alternately contract and relax during the clonic phase, which lasts 30–60 seconds. The skin sometimes acquires a bluish tint and the person may bite his tongue, lose bowel or bladder control, or have trouble breathing.

A grand mal seizure lasts between two and five minutes, and the person may be confused or have trouble talking when he regains consciousness (post-ictal state). He may complain of head or muscle aches, or weakness in his arms or legs before falling into a deep sleep.

PRIMARY GENERALIZED SEIZURES. A primary generalized seizure occurs when electrical discharges begin in both halves (hemispheres) of the brain at the same time. Primary generalized seizures are more likely to be major motor attacks than to be absence seizures.

ABSENCE SEIZURES. Absence (petit mal) seizures generally begin at about the age of four and stop by the time the child becomes an adolescent.

Absence seizures usually begin with a brief loss of consciousness and last between one and 10 seconds. A person having a petit mal seizure becomes very quiet and may blink, stare blankly, roll his eyes, or move his lips. A petit mal seizure lasts 15-20 seconds. When it ends, the person who had the seizure resumes whatever he was doing before the seizure began. He will not remember the seizure and may not realize that anything unusual has happened. Untreated, petit mal seizures can recur as many as 100 times a day and may progress to grand mal seizures.

MYOCLONIC SEIZURES. Myoclonic seizures are characterized by brief, involuntary spasms of the tongue or muscles of the face, arms, or legs. Myoclonic seizures are most apt to occur when waking after a night's sleep.

A jacksonian seizure is a partial seizure characterized by tingling, stiffening, or jerking of an arm or leg. Loss of consciousness is rare. The seizure may progress in characteristic fashion along the limb.

Limp posture and a brief period of unconsciousness are features of akinetic seizures, which occur in young children. Akinetic seizures, which cause the child to fall, also are called drop attacks.

PARTIAL SEIZURES. Simple partial seizures do not spread from the focal area where they arise. Symptoms are determined by the part of the brain affected. The patient usually remains conscious during the seizure and can later describe it in detail. In 2003, it was reported that people who experience partial seizures are twice as likely to have sleep disturbances as people their same age and gender.

COMPLEX PARTIAL SEIZURES. A distinctive smell, taste, or other unusual sensation (aura) may signal the start of a complex partial seizure.

Complex partial seizures start as simple partial seizures, but move beyond the focal area and cause loss of consciousness. Complex partial seizures can become major motor seizures. Although a person having a complex partial seizure may not seem to be unconscious, he does not know what is happening and may behave inappropriately. He will not remember the seizure, but may seem confused or intoxicated for a few minutes after it ends.

Causes and symptoms

The origin of 50-70% of all cases of epilepsy is unknown. Epilepsy sometimes is the result of trauma at birth. Such causes include insufficient oxygen to the brain; **head injury**; heavy bleeding or incompatibility between a woman's blood and the blood of her newborn baby; and infection immediately before, after, or at the time of birth.

Other causes of epilepsy include:

- head trauma resulting from a car accident, gunshot wound, or other injury.
- alcoholism
- brain **abscess** or inflammation of membranes covering the brain or spinal cord
- phenylketonuria (PKU, a disease that is present at birth, often is characterized by seizures, and can result in **mental retardation**) and other inherited disorders
- infectious diseases like **measles**, **mumps**, and diphtheria
- degenerative disease
- lead **poisoning**, mercury poisoning, **carbon monoxide poisoning**, or ingestion of some other poisonous substance
- genetic factors

Status epilepticus, a condition in which a person suffers from continuous seizures and may have trouble breathing, can be caused by:

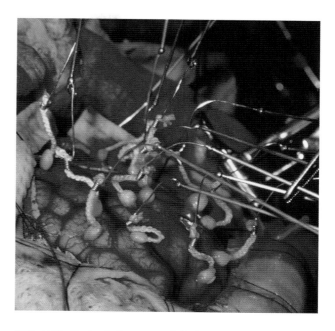

This patient's brain is exposed during surgery in order for surgeons to remove the mass responsible for his epilepsy. *(Custom Medical Stock Photo. Reproduced by permission.)*

- suddenly discontinuing anti-seizure medication
- hypoxic or metabolic encephalopathy (brain disease resulting from lack of oxygen or malfunctioning of other physical or chemical processes)
- acute head injury
- blood infection caused by inflammation of the brain or the membranes that cover it

Diagnosis

Personal and family medical history, description of seizure activity, and physical and neurological examinations help primary care physicians, neurologists, and epileptologists diagnose this disorder. Doctors rule out conditions that cause symptoms that resemble epilepsy, including small strokes (transient ischemic attacks, or TIAs), **fainting**, (syncope), pseudoseizures, and sleep attacks (narcolepsy.)

Neuropsychological testing uncovers learning or memory problems. Neuroimaging provides views of brain areas involved in seizure activity.

The electroencephalogram (EEG) is the main test used to diagnose epilepsy. EEGs use electrodes placed on or within the skull to record the brain's electrical activity and pinpoint the exact location of abnormal discharges.

The patient may be asked to remain motionless during a short-term EEG or to go about his normal activities during extended monitoring. Some patients are deprived of sleep or exposed to seizure triggers, such as rapid, deep breathing (hyperventilation) or flashing lights (photic stimulation). In some cases, people may be hospitalized for EEG monitorings that can last as long as two weeks. Video EEGs also document what the patient was doing when the seizure occurred and how the seizure changed his behavior.

Other techniques used to diagnose epilepsy include:

• Magnetic resonance imaging (MRI), which provides clear, detailed images of the brain. Functional MRI (fMRI), performed while the patient does various tasks, can measure shifts in electrical intensity and blood flow and indicate which brain region each activity affects.

• Positron emission tomography (**PET**) and single photon emission tomography (SPECT) monitor blood flow and chemical activity in the brain area being tested. PET and SPECT are very effective in locating the brain region where metabolic changes take place between seizures.

Treatment

The goal of epilepsy treatment is to eliminate seizures or make the symptoms less frequent and less severe. Long-term anticonvulsant drug therapy is the most common form of epilepsy treatment.

Medication

A combination of drugs may be needed to control some symptoms, but most patients who have epilepsy take one of the following medications:

• Dilantin (phenytoin)

• Tegretol (carbamazepine)

• Barbita (phenobarbital)

• Mysoline (primidone)

• Depakene (valproic acid, sodium valproate)

• Klonopin (clonazepam)

• Zarontin (ethosuximide).

Dilantin, Tegretol, Barbita, and Mysoline are used to manage or control generalized tonic-clonic and complex partial seizures. Depakene, Klonopin, and Zarontin are prescribed for patients who have absence seizures.

Neurontin (gabapentin), Lamictal (lamotrigine), and topiramate (Topamax) are among the medications more recently approved in the United States to treat adults who have partial seizures or partial and grand mal seizures. Another new medication called Levetiracetam (Keppra) has been approved and shows particularly good results in reducing partial seizures among elderly patients with few side effects. This is important, because elderly patients often have other conditions and must take other medications that might interact with seizure medications. In 2003, Keppra's manufacturer was working on a new antiepilectic drug from the same chemical family as Keppra that should be more potent and effective. Available medications frequently change, and it the physician will determine the best treatment for an individual patient. A 2003 report found that monotherapy, or using just one medication rather than a combination, works better for most patients. The less complicated the treatment, the more likely the patient will comply and better manager the seizure disorder.

Even a patient whose seizures are well controlled should have regular blood tests to measure levels of anti-seizure medication in his system and to check to see if the medication is causing any changes in his blood or liver. A doctor should be notified if any signs of drug toxicity appear, including uncontrolled eye movements; sluggishness, **dizziness**, or hyperactivity; inability to see clearly or speak distinctly; **nausea** or **vomiting**; or sleep problems.

Status epilepticus requires emergency treatment, usually with Valium (Ativan), Dilantin, or Barbita. An intravenous dextrose (sugar) solution is given to patients whose condition is due to low blood sugar, and a vitamin B_1 preparation is administered intravenously when status epilepticus results from chronic alcohol withdrawal. Because dextrose and thiamine are essentially harmless and because delay in treatment can be disastrous, these medications are given routinely, as it is usually difficult to obtain an adequate history from a patient suffering from status epilepticus.

Intractable seizures are seizures that cannot be controlled with medication or without **sedation** or other unacceptable side effects. Surgery may be used to eliminate or control intractable seizures.

Surgery

Surgery can be used to treat patients whose intractable seizures stem from small focal lesions that can be removed without endangering the patient, changing the patient's personality, dulling the

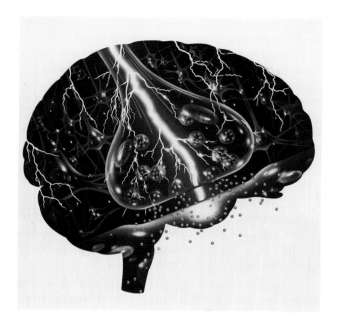

This abstract artwork is based on a patient's description of what an epileptic seizure feels like. Epileptic seizures are caused by chaotic electrical activity in the brain. They can be triggered by a variety of factors, such as illness or stress, although the underlying causes is not completely understood. *(Illustration by John Bavosi, Photo Researchers, Inc. Reproduced by permission.)*

patient's senses, or reducing the patient's ability to function.

Each year, as many as 5,000 new patients may become suitable candidates for surgery, which most often is performed at a comprehensive epilepsy center. Potential surgical candidates include patients with:

- partial seizures and secondarily generalized seizures (attacks that begin in one area and spread to both sides of the brain)

- seizures and childhood **paralysis** on one side of the body (hemiplegia)

- complex partial seizures originating in the temporal lobe (the part of the brain associated with speech, hearing, and smell) or other focal seizures. (However, the risk of surgery involving the speech centers is that the patient will lose speech function.)

- Generalized myoclonic seizures or generalized seizures featuring temporary paralysis (akinetic) or loss of muscle tone (atonal)

A **physical examination** is conducted to verify that a patient's seizures are caused by epilepsy, and surgery is not used to treat patients with severe psychiatric disturbances or medical problems that raise risk factors to unacceptable levels.

Surgery is never indicated unless:

- the best available anti-seizure medications have failed to control the patient's symptoms satisfactorily

- the origin of the patient's seizures has been precisely located

- there is good reason to believe that surgery will significantly improve the patient's health and quality of life.

Every patient considering epilepsy surgery is carefully evaluated by one or more neurologists, neurosurgeons, neuropsychologists, and/or social workers. A psychiatrist, chaplain, or other spiritual advisor may help the patient and his family cope with the **stress** that occurs during and after the selection process.

TYPES OF SURGERY. Surgical techniques used to treat intractable epilepsy include:

- Lesionectomy. Removing the lesion (diseased brain tissue) and some surrounding brain tissue is very effective in controlling seizures. Lesionectomy is generally more successful than surgery performed on patients whose seizures are not caused by clearly defined lesions, but removing only part of the lesion lessens the effectiveness of the procedure.

- Temporal resections. Removing part of the temporal lobe and the part of the brain associated with feelings, memory, and emotions (the hippocampus) provides good or excellent seizure control in 75-80% of properly selected patients with appropriate types of temporal lobe epilepsy. Some patients experience post-operative speech and memory problems.

- Extra-temporal resection. This procedure involves removing some or all of the frontal lobe, the part of the brain directly behind the forehead. The frontal lobe helps regulate movement, planning, judgment, and personality, and special care must be taken to prevent post-operative problems with movement and speech. Extra-temporal resection is most successful in patients whose seizures are not widespread.

- Hemispherectomy. This method of removing brain tissue is restricted to patients with severe epilepsy and abnormal discharges that often extend from one side of the brain to the other. Hemispherectomies most often are performed on infants or young children who have had an extensive brain disease or disorder since birth or from a very young age.

- Corpus callosotomy. This procedure, an alternative to hemispherectomy in patients with congenital hemiplegia, removes some or all of the white matter that separates the two halves of the brain. Corpus callosotomy is performed almost exclusively on children who are frequently injured during falls caused by seizures. If removing two-thirds of the corpus callosum doesn't produce lasting improvement in the patient's condition, the remaining one-third will be removed during another operation.

- Multiple subpial transection. This procedure is used to control the spread of seizures that originate in or affect the "eloquent" cortex, the area of the brain responsible for complex thought and reasoning.

Other forms of treatment

KETOGENIC DIET. A special high-fat, low-protein, low-carbohydrate diet sometimes is used to treat patients whose severe seizures have not responded to other treatment. Calculated according to age, height, and weight, the ketogenic diet induces mild **starvation** and **dehydration**. This forces the body to create an excessive supply of ketones, natural chemicals with seizure-suppressing properties.

The goal of this controversial approach is to maintain or improve seizure control while reducing medication. The ketogenic diet works best with children between the ages of one and 10. It is introduced over a period of several days, and most children are hospitalized during the early stages of treatment.

If a child following this diet remains seizure-free for at least six months, increased amounts of carbohydrates and protein gradually are added. If the child shows no improvement after three months, the diet is gradually discontinued. A 2003 study of the diet and its effect on growth noted that If used, clinicians should recommend adequate intake of energy and protein and a higher proportion of unsaturated to saturated dietary fats. The report also recommended use of vitamin and mineral supplements with the diet.

Introduced in the 1920s, the ketogenic diet has had limited, short-term success in controlling seizure activity. Its use exposes patients to such potentially harmful side effects as:

- staphylococcal infections
- atunted or delayed growth
- low blood sugar (**hypoglycemia**)
- excess fat in the blood (hyperlipidemia)
- disease resulting from calcium deposits in the urinary tract (urolithiasis)
- disease of the optic nerve (optic neuropathy)

VAGUS NERVE STIMULATION. The United States Food and Drug Administration (FDA) has approved the use of vagus nerve stimulation (VNS) in patients over the age of 16 who have intractable partial seizures.

This non-surgical procedure uses a pacemaker-like device implanted under the skin in the upper left chest, to provide intermittent stimulation to the vagus nerve. Stretching from the side of the neck into the brain, the vagus nerve affects swallowing, speech, breathing, and many other functions, and VNS may prevent or shorten some seizures. A 2003 report said that this treatment has reduced partial seizures by 50% or more in about one-third of patient with no adverse effects.

First aid for seizures

A person having a seizure should not be restrained, but sharp or dangerous objects should be moved out of reach. Anyone having a complex partial seizure can be warned away from danger by someone calling his/her name in a clear, calm voice.

A person having a grand mal seizure should be helped to lie down. Tight clothing should be loosened. A soft, flat object like a towel or the palm of a hand should be placed under the person's head. Forcing a hard object into the mouth of someone having a grand mal seizure could cause injuries or breathing problems. If the person's mouth is open, placing a folded cloth or other soft object between his teeth will protect his tongue. Turning his head to the side will help him breathe. After a grand mal seizure has ended, the person who had the seizure should be told what has happened and reminded of where he is.

Alternative treatment

Stress increases seizure activity in 30% of people who have epilepsy. Relaxation techniques can provide some sense of control over the disorder, but they should never be used instead of anti-seizure medication or used without the approval of the patient's doctor. **Yoga**, **meditation**, and favorite pastimes help some people relax and manage stress more successfully. **Biofeedback** can teach adults and older adolescents how to recognize an aura and what to do to stop its spread. Children under 14 are not usually able to understand and apply principles of biofeedback. **Acupuncture** treatments (acupuncture needles inserted for a few minutes or left in place for as long as 30 minutes) make some people feel pleasantly relaxed. **Acupressure** can have the same effect on children or on adults who dislike needles.

Aromatherapy involves mixing aromatic plant oils into water or other oils and massaging them into the skin or using a special burner to waft their fragrance throughout the room. Aromatherapy oils affect the body and the brain, and undiluted oils should never be applied directly to the skin. Ylang ylang, chamomile,

---

KEY TERMS

Acupressure—Needleless acupuncture.

Acupuncture—An ancient Chinese method of relieving pain or treating illness by piercing specific areas of the body with fine needles.

Biofeedback—A learning technique that helps individuals influence automatic body functions.

Epileptologist—A physician who specializes in the treatment of epilepsy.

---

or lavender can create a soothing mood. People who have epilepsy should not use rosemary, hyssop, sage or sweet fennel, which seem to make the brain more alert.

Dietary changes that emphasize whole foods and eliminate processed foods may be helpful. Homeopathic therapy also can work for people with seizures, especially constitutional homeopathic treatment that acts at the deepest levels to address the needs of the individual person.

Prognosis

People who have epilepsy have a higher-than-average rate of **suicide**; sudden, unexplained **death**; and drowning and other accidental fatalities.

Benign focal epilepsy of childhood and some absence seizures may disappear in time, but remission is unlikely if seizures occur several times a day, several times in a 48-hour period, or more frequently than in the past.

Seizures that occur repeatedly over time and always involve the same symptoms are called stereotypic seizures. The probability that stereotypic seizures will abate is poor.

About 85% of all seizure disorders can be partially or completely controlled if the patient takes antiseizure medication according to directions; avoids seizure-inducing sights, sounds, and other triggers; gets enough sleep; and eats regular, balanced meals.

Anyone who has epilepsy should wear a bracelet or necklace identifying his seizure disorder and listing the medication he takes.

Prevention

Eating properly, getting enough sleep, and controlling stress and fevers can help prevent seizures. A person who has epilepsy should be careful not to hyperventilate. A person who experiences an aura should find a safe place to lie down and stay there until the seizure passes. Anticonvulsant medications should not be stopped suddenly and, if other medications are prescribed or discontinued, the doctor treating the seizures should be notified. In some conditions, such as severe head injury, brain surgery, or **subarachnoid hemorrhage**, anticonvulsant medications may be given to the patient to prevent seizures.

Resources

PERIODICALS

Dilorio, Colleen, et al. "The Epilelpsy Medication and Treatment Complexity Index: Reliability and Validity Testing." *Journal of Neuroscience Nursing* June 2003: 155–158.

"Epilepsy Surgery and Vagus Nerve Stimulation Are Effective When Drugs Fail." *Medical Devices & Surgical Technology Week* May 4, 2003: 33.

Finn, Robert. "Partial Seizures Double Risk of Sleep Disturbances (Consider in Diagnosis, Management)." *Clinical Psychiatry News* June 2003: 36–41.

Liu, Yeou-Mei Christiana, et al. "A Prospetive Study: Growth and Nutritional Status of Children Treated With the Ketogenic Diet." *Journal of the American Dietetic Association* June 2003: 707.

"New Drug Candidate Shows Promise." *Clinical Trials Week* April 7, 2003: 26.

ORGANIZATIONS

American Epilepsy Society. 342 North Main Street, West Hartford, CT 06117-2507. (860) 586-7505. < http://www.aesnet.org >.

Epilepsy Concern International Service Group. 1282 Wynnewood Drive, West Palm Beach, FL 33417. (407) 683-0044.

Epilepsy Foundation of America. 4351 Garden City Drive, Landover, MD 20785. (800) 332-1000. < http://www.efa.org >.

Epilepsy Information Service. (800) 642-0500.

Maureen Haggerty
Teresa G. Odle

Selective abortion *see* **Abortion, selective**

Selective mutism *see* **Mutism**

Selective serotonin reuptake inhibitors

Definition

Selective serotonin reuptake inhibitors are medicines that relieve symptoms of depression.

Purpose

Selective serotonin reuptake inhibitors are used to treat serious, continuing depression that interferes with a person's ability to function. Like other **antidepressant drugs**, they help reduce the extreme sadness, hopelessness, and lack of interest in life that are typical in people with depression. Selective serotonin reuptake inhibitors also are used to treat **panic disorder**, obsessive compulsive disorder (OCD), and have shown promise for treating a variety of other conditions, such as **premenstrual syndrome**, eating disorders, **obesity**, **self-mutilation**, and **migraine headache**.

As of late 2003, SSRIs have been found to have other off-label applications, including treatment of **premature ejaculation** and **diabetic neuropathy**.

Description

Selective serotonin reuptake inhibitors, also known as SSRIs or serotonin boosters, are thought to work by correcting chemical imbalances in the brain. Normally, chemicals called neurotransmitters carry signals from one nerve cell to another. These chemicals are constantly being released and taken back up at the ends of nerve cells. Selective serotonin reuptake inhibitors act on one particular neurotransmitter, serotonin, reducing its re-entry into nerve cells and thus allowing serotonin to build up. Although scientists are not exactly sure how it works, serotonin is involved in the control of moods, as well as other functions such as sleep, body temperature, and appetite for sweets and other carbohydrates. Somehow, drugs that prevent the uptake of serotonin improve the moods of people with serious depression, OCD, and some types of **anxiety disorders**.

Selective serotonin reuptake inhibitors are available only with a doctor's prescription and are sold in tablet, capsule, and liquid forms. Commonly used selective serotonin reuptake inhibitors are fluoxetine (Prozac), paroxetine (Paxil), sertraline (Zoloft), and fluvoxamine (Luvox).

Recommended dosage

The recommended dosage depends on the type of **SSRI** and the type and severity of depression for which it is being taken. Dosages may be different for different people. It is important for people taking SSRIs to take the drug exactly as prescribed. Taking larger or more frequent doses or taking the drug for longer than directed, for example, can cause unwanted effects.

SSRIs are about as effective as other antidepressants. About 60–80% of people taking the drugs as directed will find that their conditions improve. However, it may take four weeks or more for the effects of this medicine to be felt. Therefore, when people begin SSRI therapy, it is important to continue taking the medication, even if an improvement in mood doesn't begin immediately.

People who take SSRIs should ask their doctors about how to stop taking the medication. Usually, doctors advise patients to taper down gradually to reduce the chance of withdrawal symptoms or SSRI discontinuation syndrome.

SSRIs may be taken with food to prevent stomach upset.

Precautions

There have been reports that some patients taking SSRIs have an increase in thoughts about **suicide**. It is not clear whether the medicine causes this effect because suicidal thoughts are very often a part of depression itself. While some patients may experience worsening of such thoughts early in the treatment of their depression, there is no credible evidence that SSRIs alone cause people to become suicidal or violent.

Serious and possibly life-threatening reactions may occur when SSRIs are used in combination with **monoamine oxidase inhibitors** (MAO inhibitors), such as Nardil and Parnate, which also are used to treat depression. These reactions also are possible when a person stops taking an SSRI and immediately begins taking an MAOI. SSRIs and MAO inhibitors should never be taken at the same time. When switching from an SSRI to an MAOI or vice versa, it may be necessary to allow two to five weeks or more between stopping one and starting the other. The physician prescribing the medications should tell the patient exactly how much time to allow before beginning the other medication.

People with a history of manic disorders should use any antidepressant, including an SSRI, with caution.

It is important to see a doctor regularly while taking SSRIs. The doctor will check to make sure the medicine is working as it should and will watch for unwanted side effects. The doctor may also need to adjust the dosage during this period.

Some people feel drowsy, dizzy, or lightheaded when using SSRIs. The drugs may also cause blurred vision in some people. Since SSRIs can sometimes cause drowsiness, driving or operating heavy machinery should be undertaken cautiously, particularly when the person first begins taking the medication.

These medicines make some people feel lightheaded, dizzy, or faint when they get up after sitting or lying down, a condition known as **orthostatic hypotension**. People may try to lessen the problem by getting up gradually and holding onto something for support if possible. If the problem is severe or doesn't improve, the patient should discuss it with his or her doctor.

Because SSRIs work on the central nervous system, they may add to the effects of alcohol and other drugs that slow down the central nervous system, such as **antihistamines**, cold medicine, allergy medicine, sleep aids, medicine for seizures, tranquilizers, some **pain** relievers, and **muscle relaxants**. They may also add to the effects of anesthetics, including those used for dental procedures. Anyone taking SSRIs should check with his or her doctor before taking any of the drugs mentioned above.

SSRIs may occasionally cause **dry mouth**, although this side effect is much more common with an older class of antidepressants known as tricyclics. To temporarily relieve the discomfort, doctors sometimes suggest chewing sugarless gum, sucking on sugarless candy or ice chips, or using saliva substitutes, which come in liquid and tablet forms and are available without a prescription. If the problem continues for more than two weeks, check with a doctor or dentist. Mouth dryness that continues over a long time may contribute to **tooth decay** and other dental problems.

Changes in sexual functioning are among the more common side effects with SSRIs. Depending on the particular SSRI prescribed, 8–15% of patients may report these side effects. The most common problem for men is delayed ejaculation. Women may be unable to have orgasms. A doctor should be contacted if any changes in sexual functioning occur.

Special conditions

People with certain medical conditions or who are taking certain other medicines can have problems if they take SSRIs. Before taking these drugs, a patient should let the doctor know about any of these conditions:

ALLERGIES. Anyone who has had unusual reactions to SSRIs in the past should let his or her doctor know before taking the drugs again. The doctor should also be told about any **allergies** to foods, dyes, preservatives, or other substances.

PREGNANCY. In studies of laboratory animals, some SSRIs have caused **miscarriage** and other problems in pregnant females and their offspring. However, at least two studies in humans (by Pastuszak in 1993 and Kuhlin in 1998) have shown SSRIs to be safe during **pregnancy**, and newer studies done in 2003 have reported that SSRIs do not appear to increase the risks of **birth defects** in the offspring. Still, women who are pregnant or who may become pregnant should check with their doctors before using SSRIs.

BREASTFEEDING. SSRIs pass into breast milk and some may occasionally cause unwanted side effects in nursing babies whose mothers take the drugs. These effects include **vomiting**, watery stools, crying, and sleep problems. Women who are breastfeeding should talk to their doctors about the use of SSRIs. They may need to switch to a different medicine while breastfeeding. If SSRIs must be taken, it may be necessary to stop breastfeeding while being treated with these drugs. However, several studies in people (for example, Yoshida in 1998) have indicated that SSRIs in breast milk have no effect on infant development.

DIABETES. SSRIs may affect blood sugar levels. People with diabetes who notice changes in their blood or urine tests while taking this medicine should check with their doctors.

OTHER MEDICAL CONDITIONS. Before using SSRIs, people with any of these medical problems should make sure their doctors are aware of their conditions: diabetes, **kidney disease**, **liver disease**, seizure disorders, current or past drug **abuse** or dependence, or diseases or conditions that affect the metabolism or blood circulation.

Side effects

The most common side effects are **anxiety** and nervousness (reported by 5–13% of people taking various SSRIs), tremor (5–14%), trouble sleeping (2–8%), tiredness or weakness (4–15%), **nausea** (11–26%), **diarrhea** (11–26%), **constipation** (1–8%), loss of appetite (3–18%), weight loss (1–13%), dry mouth (10–22%), **headache** (1–5%), sweating (5–9%), trouble urinating (1–2%), and decreased sexual ability (8–15%). Many of these problems diminish or disappear as the body adjusts to the drug and do not require medical treatment unless they interfere with normal activities. Persistent problems, such as **sexual dysfunction**, should be discussed with the doctor.

More serious side effects are possible, but extremely rare. People taking SSRIs who notice unusual joint or muscle pain; breathing problems; chills or **fever**; excessive excitement, fast talking, or actions that are out of control; or mood swings should contact their doctors. People who develop skin **rashes** or **hives** after taking an SSRI should stop taking the medication and contact their doctors as soon as possible. Other rare side effects may occur. Anyone who has unusual symptoms after taking an SSRI should get in touch with his or her doctor.

Side effects may continue for some time after treatment with this medicine ends. How long the effects continue depends on how long the drug was taken and how much of it was used. In most cases, doctors recommend that patients taper off SSRIs rather than abruptly stopping them, because of the risk of developing a condition known as SSRI discontinuation syndrome. This syndrome can mimic serious illness. People who experience agitation, confusion, or restlessness; **dizziness** or lightheadedness; vision problems; tremor; sleep problems; unusual tiredness or weakness; **nausea and vomiting** or diarrhea; headache; excessive sweating; runny nose; or muscle pain for more than a few days after stopping or tapering an SSRI should consult their doctors.

Interactions

SSRIs may interact with other medicines. When this happens, the effects of one or both of the drugs may change or the risk of side effects may be greater. Anyone who takes SSRIs should let the doctor know about all other medicines he or she is taking. Among the drugs that may interact with SSRIs are:

- such central nervous system (CNS) depressants as medicine for allergies, colds, hay fever, and **asthma**; sedatives; tranquilizers; prescription pain medicine; muscle relaxants; medicine for seizures; sleep aids; **barbiturates**; and anesthetics.

- blood thinners (anticoagullants)

- such monoamine oxidase inhibitors (MAOIs) as Nardil or Parnate, used to treat conditions including depression and Parkinson's disease

- the antiseizure drug phenytoin (Dilantin)

- the food supplement (and sleep aid) tryptophan, which has been withdrawn from the United States market, but may be found in some herbal preparations

- digitalis and other heart medicines

- **St. John's wort** (*Hypericum perforatum*). St. John's wort is a herb used in Europe and the United States to relieve mild-to-moderate symptoms of depression. Research indicates that it acts as an SSRI and not as an MAO inhibitor, as previously believed. People

KEY TERMS

Anesthetic—Medicine that causes a loss of feeling, especially of pain. Some anesthetics also cause a loss of consciousness.

Anxiety—Worry or tension in response to real or imagined stress, danger, or dreaded situations. Physical reactions, such as fast pulse, sweating, trembling, fatigue, and weakness may accompany anxiety.

Central nervous system—The brain and spinal cord.

Depression—A mental condition in which people feel extremely sad and lose interest in life. People with depression may also have sleep problems and loss of appetite and may have trouble concentrating and carrying out everyday activities.

Metabolism—All the physical and chemical changes that occur in cells to allow growth and maintain body functions. These include processes that break down substances to yield energy and processes that build up other substances necessary for life.

Obsessive-compulsive disorder—An anxiety disorder in which people cannot prevent themselves from dwelling on unwanted thoughts, acting on urges, or performing repetitious rituals, such as washing their hands or checking to make sure they turned off the lights.

Off-label application—The use of a prescription medication to treat conditions outside the indications approved by the Food and Drug Administration (FDA).

Premenstrual syndrome—(PMS) A set of symptoms that occur in some women 2–14 days before they begin menstruating each month. Symptoms include headache, fatigue, irritability, depression, abdominal bloating, and breast tenderness.

who are using St. John's wort to relieve depression should not take a prescription SSRI at the same time.

The list above does not include every drug that may interact with SSRIs. Patients should be sure to check with a doctor or pharmacist before combining SSRIs with any other prescription or nonprescription (over-the-counter) medicine, including herbal preparations.

Resources

BOOKS

Beers, Mark H., MD, and Robert Berkow, MD., editors. "Depression (Unipolar Disorder)." Section 15, Chapter

189 In *The Merck Manual of Diagnosis and Therapy.* Whitehouse Station, NJ: Merck Research Laboratories, 2002.

Pelletier, Dr. Kenneth R. *The Best Alternative Medicine, Part I: Western Herbal Medicine.* New York: Simon and Schuster, 2002.

Pies, Ronald W. *Handbook of Essential Psychopharmacology.* Washington, DC: American Psychiatric Press, Inc.

PERIODICALS

Aronson, Sarah A., MD. "Depression." *eMedicine* December 31, 2003. < http://www.emedicine.com/ med/topic532.htm > .

Ditto, K. E. "SSRI Discontinuation Syndrome. Awareness as an Approach to Prevention." *Postgraduate Medicine* 114 (August 2003): 79–84.

Nonacs, R., and L. S. Cohen. "Assessment and Treatment of Depression During Pregnancy: An Update." *Psychiatric Clinics of North America* 26 (September 2003): 547–562.

Roose, S. P. "Treatment of Depression in Patients with Heart Disease." *Biological Psychiatry* 54 (August 1, 2003): 262–268.

Stone, K. J., A. J. Viera, and C. L. Parman. "Off-Label Applications for SSRIs." *American Family Physician* 68 (August 1, 2003): 425–427.

ORGANIZATIONS

American Psychiatric Association (APA). 1400 K Street, NW, Washington, DC 20005. (888) 357-7924. < http://www.psych.org >.

National Center for Complementary and Alternative Medicine (NCCAM) Clearinghouse. P.O. Box 7923, Gaithersburg, MD 20898-7923. (888) 644-6226. < http://nccam.nih.gov >.

National Institute of Mental Health (NIMH). 6001 Executive Boulevard, Room 8184, MSC 9663, Bethesda, MD 20892-9663. (301) 443-4513. < www.nimh.nih.gov. >.

U. S. Food and Drug Administration (FDA). 5600 Fishers Lane, Rockville, MD 20857. (888) 463-6332. < http://www.fda.gov >.

Nancy Ross-Flanigan
Rebecca J. Frey, PhD

Self-mutilation

Definition

Self-mutilation is a general term for a variety of forms of intentional self-harm without the wish to die. Cutting one's skin with razors or knives is the most common pattern of self-mutilation. Others include biting, hitting, or bruising oneself; picking or pulling at skin or hair; burning oneself with lighted cigarettes, or amputating parts of the body.

Description

Self-mutilation has become a major public health concern as its incidence appears to have risen since the early 1990s. One source estimates that 0.75% of the general American population practices self-mutilation. The incidence of self-mutilation is highest among teenage females, patients diagnosed with borderline personality disorder, and patients diagnosed with one of the dissociative disorders. Over half of self-mutilators were sexually abused as children, and many also suffer from eating disorders.

Self-mutilation should not be confused with current fads for **tattoos** and body **piercing**. In some cases, however, it may be difficult to distinguish between an interest in these fads and the first indications of a disorder.

The relationship of self-mutilation to **suicide** is still debated even though statistics show that nearly 50% of individuals who injure themselves also attempt suicide at some point in their lives. Many researchers think that suicide attempts reflect feelings of rejection or hopelessness, while self-mutilation results from feelings of shame or a need to relieve tension.

Causes and symptoms

Several different theories have been proposed to explain self-mutilation:

- self-mutilation is an outlet for strong negative emotions, especially anger or shame, that the person is afraid to express in words or discuss with others.

- self-mutilation represents anger at someone else directed against the self.

- self-mutilation relieves unbearable tension or **anxiety** Many self-mutilators do report feeling relief after an episode of self-cutting or other injury.

- self-mutilation is a technique for triggering the body's biochemical responses to **pain**. **Stress** and trauma release endorphins, which are the body's natural pain-killing substances

- self-mutilation is a way of stopping a dissociative episode. Dissociation is a process in which the mind splits off, or dissociates, certain memories and thoughts that are too painful to keep in conscious awareness. Some people report that they feel "numb" or "dead" when they dissociate, and self-injury allows them to feel "alive."

- self-mutilation is a symbolic acting-out of the larger culture's mistreatment of women. This theory is sometimes offered to explain why the great majority (about 75%) of self-mutilators are girls and women

The symptoms of self-mutilation typically include wearing long-sleeved or baggy clothing, even in hot weather; and an unusual need for privacy. Self-mutilators are often hesitant to change their clothes or undress around others. In most cases the person has also shown signs of depression.

Diagnosis

Self-mutilation is usually diagnosed by a psychiatrist or psychotherapist. A family practitioner or nurse who notices **scars**, **bruises**, or other physical evidence of self-injury may refer the person to a specialist for evaluation.

Treatment

Persons who mutilate themselves should seek treatment from a therapist with some specialized training and experience with this behavior. Most self-mutilators are treated as outpatients, although there are some inpatient programs, such as S.A.F.E., for adolescent females. A number of different treatment approaches are used with self-mutilators, including psychodynamic psychotherapy, **group therapy**, journaling, and behavioral therapy.

Although there are no medications specifically for self-mutilation, antidepressants are often given, particularly if the patient meets the diagnostic criteria for a depressive disorder.

Alternative treatment

Mindfulness training, which is a form of **meditation**, has been used to teach self-mutilators to observe and identify their feelings in order to have some control over them.

Prognosis

The prognosis depends on the presence and severity of other emotional disorders, and a history of sexual **abuse** and/or suicide attempts. In general, teenagers without a history of abuse or other disorders have a good prognosis. Patients diagnosed with borderline personality disorder and/or a history of

---

KEY TERMS

Borderline personality disorder (BPD)—A pattern of behavior characterized by impulsive acts, intense but chaotic relationships with others, identity problems, and emotional instability.

Dissociation—The splitting off of certain mental processes from conscious awareness.

Dissociative disorders—A group of mental disorders in which dissociation is a prominent symptom. Patients with dissociative disorders have a high rate of self-mutilation.

Endorphins—Pain-killing substances produced in the human body and released by stress or trauma. Some researchers think that people who mutilate themselves are trying to trigger the release of endorphins.

---

attempted suicide are considered to have the worst prognosis.

Prevention

Some society-wide factors that influence self-mutilation, such as the high rate of sexual abuse of children and media stereotypes of women, are difficult to change. In general, however, young people who have learned to express themselves in words or through art and other creative activities are less likely to deal with painful feelings by injuring their bodies.

Resources

BOOKS

Eisendrath, Stuart J., M.D., and Jonathan E. Lichtmacher, M.D. "Psychiatric Disorders." In *Current Medical Diagnosis & Treatment 2001*, edited by L. M. Tierney, Jr., MD, et al., 40th ed. N. New York: Lange Medical Books/McGraw-Hill, 2001.

ORGANIZATIONS

American Psychiatric Association. 1400 K Street, NW. Washington, DC 20005. (202) 682-6220. < http:// www.psych.org >.

Focus Adolescent Services. (877) 362-8727. < http// www.focusas.com >.

National Institute of Mental Health. 5600 Fishers Lane, Rockville, MD 20857. (301) 443-4513. Fax: (301) 443-4513. < http://www.nimh.nih.gov >.

Rebecca J. Frey, PhD

Semen analysis

Definition

Semen analysis evaluates a man's sperm and semen. It is done to discover cause for infertility and to confirm success of **vasectomy**.

Purpose

Semen analysis is an initial step in investigating why a couple has been unable to conceive a child. Abnormalities of sperm and semen can cause male **infertility**. Semen is the thick yellow-white male ejaculate containing sperm. Sperm are the male sex cells that fertilize the female egg (ovum). They contain the genetic information that the male will pass on to a child.

Vasectomy is an operation done to sterilize a man by stopping the release of sperm into semen. Success of vasectomy is confirmed by the absence of sperm in semen.

Description

The semen analysis test is usually done manually, though computerized test systems are available. Many laboratories base their procedures on standards published by the World Health Organization (WHO).

The volume of semen in the entire ejaculate is measured. The appearance, color, thickness, and pH is noted. A pH test looks at the range from a very acid solution to a very alkaline solution. Semen, like many other body fluids, has a standard pH range that would be considered optimal for fertilization of the egg to take place. The thick semen is then allowed to liquify; this usually takes 20-60 minutes.

Drops of semen are placed on a microscope slide and examined under the microscope. Motility, or movement, of 100 sperm are observed and graded in categories, such as rapid progressive or immotile.

The structure of sperm (sperm morphology) is assessed by carefully examining sperm for abnormalities in the size and shape in the head, tail, and neck regions. WHO standards define normal as a specimen with less than 30% abnormal forms. An alternative classification system (Kruger's) measures the dimensions of sperm parts. Normal specimens are allowed 14% or less abnormalities.

Sperm are counted by placing semen in a special counting chamber. The sperm within the chamber are counted under a microscope. White blood cells are recorded; these may indicate a reproductive tract infection. Laboratories may test for other biochemicals such as fructose, zinc, and citric acid. These are believed to contribute to sperm health and fertility.

Results of semen analysis for infertility must be confirmed by a second analysis seven days to three months after the first. Sperm counts may vary from day to day.

Semen analysis to confirm success of vasectomy is concerned only with discovering if sperm are still present. Semen is collected six weeks after surgery. If sperm are seen, another specimen is collected 2 to 4 weeks later. The test is repeated until two consecutive specimens are free of sperm.

Preparation

A man should collect an entire ejaculate, by masturbation, into a container provided by his physician. To examine the best quality sperm, the specimen must be collected after two to three days of sexual abstinence, but not more than five to seven days. The specimen must not come into contact with any spermicidal agents used by a female partner for birth control purposes. The man should not have alcohol before the test.

A semen specimen to investigate infertility must be brought to the testing laboratory within one hour of obtaining it. Timing is not as critical for the postvasectomy test but the semen must be kept at body temperature. The most satisfactory sample is one obtained in the lab rather than at home.

Normal results

WHO standards have established these normal values:

- volume less than or equal to 2.0 mL
- sperm count greater than or equal to 20 million per mL
- motility (movement of the sperm) value is greater than or equal to 50% with forward progression, or greater than or equal to 25% with rapid progression within 60 minutes of ejaculation
- morphology greater than or equal to 30% with normal forms
- white blood cell count less than 1 million per mL.

If infertility continues, despite normal semen analysis and female studies, further tests are done to evaluate sperm function.

Abnormal results

Abnormalities of semen volume and liquidity, and sperm number and morphology decrease fertility. These abnormalities may be inherited or caused by a hormone imbalance, medications, or a recent infection. Further tests may be done to determine the cause of abnormalities.

Resources

PERIODICALS

Kamada, M., et al. "Semen Analysis and Antisperm Antibody." *Archives of Andrology* March-April 1998): 117-128.

Nancy J. Nordenson

Senile tremor *see* **Tremors**

Seniors' health

Definition

Seniors' health refers to the physical and mental conditions of senior citizens, those who are in their 60s and older. The proportion of people age 65 years and older in the United States is on the rise and will continue to increase through 2030.

Purpose

For a senior, the **aging** process and a person's lifestyle will affect health. People who maintain a healthy weight, exercise regularly, eat nutritionally, and don't smoke reduce the risk for many health conditions. This wellness allows people to live longer and to remain independent for more years. **Smoking, obesity** (excess weight), and lack of exercise shorten life and increase the risk for many health conditions. According to a 2003 report, about 80% of people in the United States age 65 and older have at least one chronic (long-lasting) condition and 50% have two.

Diet and exercise

Proper diet and regular **exercise** form the foundation of senior health. A nutritional diet and physical activity can help prevent diseases such as **cancer**, **stroke**, heart disease, and diabetes. A healthy diet also can help manage diabetes, high blood pressure, and heart disease.

As people age, there is more of a need to exercise on a regular basis. According to the American Heart Association, the inactive person loses from 3–5% of muscle fiber each decade after age 30. That loss would total 30% of lost muscle fiber at age 60. Exercise helps to boost muscle strength. It can help improve balance and coordination, and therefore help to prevent falls.

Organizations including the heart association advise that regular physical activity helps prevent bone loss (**osteoporosis**) and the risk of conditions such as heart disease, Type II diabetes, **colon cancer**, **stress**, and depression. In addition, exercise can help extend the lives of people with conditions such as diabetes, high blood pressure, and high cholesterol. Good health later in life helps to prevent serious illness or **death** from common infections as well. If a senior catches the flu, for instance, it can have more detrimental effects than in a healthier, younger person. When the **SARS** outbreak occurred in 2002 and 2003, clinicians expressed concern about the elderly Americans and again expressed the importance of diet and exercise. As people age, their immune system response weakens. Seniors need to be proactive in keeping their systems strong.

Osteoporosis

Osteoporosis is a condition in which bones become less dense (solid). Bones become brittle, thinner, and break easily. Although osteoporosis is associated with aging, it is only the risk of osteoporosis that increases as a person ages. It is linked to approximately 70% of bone fractures in people age 46 and older. According to the National Institutes of Health (NIH), one out of two women over age 50 will experience an osteoporosis-related fracture. So will one out of eight men over 50.

Osteoporosis is associated primarily with the changes that occur to women during menopause. During **menopause**, there is a decrease in the level of estrogen, the hormone that helps maintain bone mass. Other causes of osteoporosis include lack of exercise and a diet deficient in vitamin D.

Osteoporosis is largely preventable, however, research released in 2003said that evidence is increasing to suggest that the condition starts as far back as in the womb. If this is true, it still is preventable, but by the behavior of the mother carrying a child. More research needs to be done, but it is clear that childhood growth rates are linked to hip **fractures** that occur decades later.

Osteoarthritis

Osteoarthritis is a joint disease in which cartilage wears out and bones rub against each other. This condition can occur gradually over time as activities performed throughout the years cause wear on joints. In addition, bones thin as a person ages.

Excess weight and injuries can aggravate this condition. About 16 million Americans experience some form of osteoarthritis. It generally affects the neck, fingers, lower back, knees, and toes. Symptoms include **pain**, stiffness, swelling, and creaking. The pain may disrupt sleep, and joint stiffness may make it difficult for a person to dress.

Falls

More than two million Americans each year fall and experience serious injuries, according to the American Academy of Otolaryngology-Head and Neck Surgery. For seniors, fall-related injuries can reduce mobility and hinder independence.

As people age, their reflexes slow down so it may be more difficult to prevent a fall. Deteriorating vision and hearing can affect balance, which can cause an accidental fall. Furthermore, conditions such as arthritis, **dizziness**, and sleeping disorders can increase the likelihood of a fall. In addition, a person may fall at the start of a condition such as a stroke or **heart attack**.

Falls can result in broken bones or fractures because bones are weakened by osteoporosis. In addition, healing takes longer. Head injuries could affect sight and hearing. Injuries sustained during falls could reduce an active person's mobility and independence.

Vision

Eyesight changes as people age. Generally, people are in their 40s when they experience presbyopia, a form of farsightedness. This is a progressive condition involving a decrease in the eye's ability to focus on close objects (near vision). By age 65, little near focusing ability remains.

Glaucoma is a condition caused by pressure from the build-up of a large amount of fluid in the eye. This progressive condition is often seen in people in their 50s. It starts with the gradual loss of peripheral vision. If not treated, it can lead to some vision loss.

People in their 60s may experience the first signs of age-related macular degeneration (AMD). It is a progressive condition affecting the retina. The macula in the retina distinguishes detail. Degeneration in the macula could cause scarring and a gradual reduction in vision. The person experiences a circle of blindness, an area of sightlessness that grows as the condition progress.

More than half of people age 65 or older will be diagnosed with **cataracts**. Cataract refers to the loss of the transparency in the lens of the eye. As the loss progresses, the person is able to see less detail. This condition generally affects both eyes.

Hearing

Presbycusis, age-related **hearing loss**, is a progressive condition. It usually starts with a difficulty in hearing high-frequency sound such as people talking. A senior has less trouble with low-frequency tones. Background noise will make it even more difficult to hear. Presbycusis affects approximately 25% of people between the ages of 65 and 75 and half of those over 75. Many people diagnosed with this condition say they have lost hearing in both ears. They also report feelings of dizziness and that they experience a ringing in their ears.

Sleep disorders

Sleep patterns change when a person ages. Many people in their 60s and 70s experience less time in the stages of deep sleep known as delta sleep. Despite this change, many healthy older people don't experience **sleep disorders**. Overall health plays a role in whether a senior experiences trouble sleeping.

Obesity is linked to **snoring** and sleep apnea. Snoring can turn into apnea. A person with apnea stops breathing for up to one minute until the brain restarts the breathing process. This action could be repeated several hundred times each night.

Furthermore, a senior's sleep can be disrupted by conditions such as arthritis, osteoporosis, and **Alzheimer's disease**. Insomnia, or the inability to stay asleep, is a symptom of conditions including depression, **anxiety**, chronic pain, and restless leg syndrome (RLS).

RLS involves movement of legs when a person is at rest. The person moves legs in response to a **tingling** sensation in the upper leg, calf, or foot. In other cases, legs move involuntarily. Sensations that trigger movement can re-occur within seconds.

A person with RLS is likely to have PLMD (periodic limb movement disorder). A sleeping person with this condition will kick legs or move arms repeatedly. These involuntary movements can last from 20 seconds to an hour. Approximately 45% of the elderly have a mild form of PLMD, according to the National Sleep Foundation.

The cause of these disorders is not known. They are thought to be caused by a chemical reaction in the brain. In addition, the conditions may be hereditary.

Mental health

While age has little effect on the mind, social and emotional factors affect an older person's health. After a lifetime of work or raising a family, retirement brings several challenges. A person who has been identified for years by a profession may experience a sense of lost identity.

A senior may find that the thinking process has changed. Learning something new may take longer. However, older people have excellent recall of new information.

Memory loss may be a concern, particularly since this is a symptom of Alzheimer's disease.

Dementia

Alzheimer's disease is a form of **dementia**, a condition in which mental abilities decline. Symptoms of dementia include memory loss that goes beyond forgetting a word or where an item was placed. The person with dementia may never recognize family members or remember how to perform functions such as preparing a meal. Sometimes they experience a change in personality, with some uncharacteristic aggression or **paranoia**.

Alzheimer's disease is the most prevalent form of dementia. Although the cause of this condition is not known, the risk of Alzheimer's increases as a person ages. In 2000, the condition affected one in 15 people over the age of 65. The ratio rises to one in three people age 85 and older.

Alzheimer's is a progressive condition. In most cases, after five to eight years, a patient with this condition is unable to perform basic functions. There is no known cure for Alzheimer s. However, as of 2003, the U.S. Food and Drug Administration had approved four medications that could help delay the degenerative process.

Leading causes of death in persons 65 and older

Cause of death	Number of deaths	Death rate (per 100,000 population)	Percentage of all deaths in those >65 years old
All causes	1,542,493	4,963.2	100.0
Heart disease	594,858	1,914.0	38.6
Malignant neoplasms, including neoplasms of lymphatic and hematopoietic tissues	345,387	1,111.3	22.4
Cerebrovascular diseases	125,409	403.5	8.1
Chronic obstructive pulmonary disease and associated conditions	72,755	234.1	4.7
Pneumonia and influenza	70,485	226.8	4.6
Diabetes mellitus	35,523	114.3	2.3
Accidents and adverse effects	26,213	84.3	1.7
	7,210	23.2	0.5
Motor vehicle accidents	19,003	61.1	1.2
All other accidents and adverse effects			
Nephritis, nephrotic syndrome, and nephrosis	17,306	55.7	1.1
Atherosclerosis	17,158	55.2	1.1
Septicemia	15,351	49.4	1.0
All other causes, residual	222,048	2,045.9	14.4

Precautions

A health condition may result in a doctor recommending against some forms of exercise. However, even if a person can't jog, other forms of exercise include those designed for people in wheelchairs and those who are bedridden.

Treatments for menopause and osteoporosis include Raloxifene, a medication that may cause **blood clots**.

Description

The cost of treatment varies. Cost of medical treatment will be determined by the type of procedure and whether a person has medical insurance. Health plan and Medicare coverage and copayments impact an individual's cost for various preventions and treatments.

Nutrition

Nutrition plays an important role in senior health. Not only does a well-balanced diet keep a person from becoming obese, that same diet is a safeguard against health conditions that seniors face. Proper diet can help prevent a condition like diabetes or keep it from worsening.

The senior diet should consist of foods that are low in fat, particularly saturated fat and cholesterol. A person should choose foods that provide nutrients such as iron and calcium. Other healthy menu choices include:

- fish, skinless poultry, and lean meat.
- proteins such as dry beans (red beans, navy beans, and soybeans), lentils, chickpeas, and peanuts.
- low-fat dairy products
- vegetables, especially those that are dark green and leafy
- citrus fruits or juices, melons, and berries
- whole grains like wheat, rice, oats, corn, and barley
- whole grain breads and cereals

Exercise

Physical activity should be rhythmic, repetitive, and should challenge the circulatory system. It also should be enjoyable so that a senior gets in the habit of exercising regularly for 30 minutes each day. It may be necessary to check with a doctor to determine the type of exercise that can be done.

Walking is recommended for weight loss, stress release, and many other conditions. Brisk walking is said to produce the same benefits as jogging. Other forms of exercise can include gardening, bicycling, hiking, swimming, dancing, skating or ice-skating. If weather prohibits outdoor activities, a person can work out indoors with an exercise video.

Exercise also offers a chance to socialize. In some cities, groups of seniors meet for regular walks at shopping malls. Senior centers offer exercise classes ranging from line dancing to belly dancing.

Costs for exercise range from the price of walking shoes to the fees for joining a gym.

Osteoporosis

Prevention is the best method of treating osteoporosis. Methods of preventing osteoporosis include regular weight-bearing exercise such as walking, jogging, weight lifting, **yoga**, and stair climbing.

People should not smoke since smoking makes the body produce less estrogen. Care should be taken to avoid falling.

Diet should include from 1,000–1,300 mg. of calcium each day. Sources of calcium include:

- leafy, dark-green vegetables such as spinach, kale, mustard greens, and turnip greens
- low-fat dairy products such as milk, yogurt, and cheeses such as cheddar, Swiss, mozzarella, and parmesan; also helpful are foods made with milk such as pudding and soup
- canned fish such as salmon, sardine, and anchovies
- tortillas made from lime-processed corn
- tofu processed with calcium-sulfate
- calcium and vitamin D tablets

MEDICAL TREATMENT. An x ray will indicate bone loss when much of the density has decreased. A more effective way of detecting osteoporosis is the DEXA-scan (dual-energy x-ray absorbtiometry). This whole-body scan will indicate whether a person is at risk for fractures. It could be useful for people at risk for osteoporosis as well as women near the age of menopause or older. People should ask their doctors about whether this test is needed.

During menopause, a woman loses estrogen. A pill or skin patch containing estrogen and progesterone eases symptoms of menopause has been used to treat osteoporosis. This treatment is known as **hormone replacement therapy** (HRT). In 2002, the Women's Health Initiative found that HRT produced harmful effects in postmenopausal women, including increased incidence of **breast cancer**, heart disease and dementia. The effects were bad enough to stop the study. In 2003, researchers were looking for alternatives to HRT for women who had been using the hormones for osteoporosis. Until an alternative is identified, women and physicians have been advised to closely weigh the risks and benefits of hormone therapy. Several drugs are available to help reduce the risk of fractures in seniors with osteoporosis. In 2003, the FDA approved a new treatment option called Teriparatide. Some alternative treatments show promise in studies, including SAMe, (S-adenosylmethionine). However, long-term safety and effectiveness of SAMe have yet to be established.

Osteoarthritis

Treatments for osteoarthritis range from preventative measures such as walking to joint replacement surgery. Treatment costs vary from no cost for soaking a joint in cold water, the price of over-the-counter remedies to fees for surgery.

Preventive and maintenance remedies include low-impact exercise such as swimming and walking, along with maintaining proper posture. Nutritional aids include foods rich in vitamin C such as citrus fruits and broccoli. Also recommended is daily consumption of 400 international units of Vitamin E. Cutting back on fats, sugar, salt, cholesterol, and alcohol helps relieve the symptoms of osteoarthritis.

HOME REMEDIES AND PHYSICAL THERAPY. The Arthritis Foundation recommends several remedies for easing pain. To treat inflammation, a person should use a cold treatment. Methods include soaking the affected area in cold water or applying an ice pack. To soothe aches and stimulate circulation, a person applies heat to the affected area for 20 minutes. This should be done three times a day.

Over-the-counter (OTC) remedies such as **aspirin** and ibuprofen and salves containing capsaicin can be helpful. Furthermore, a doctor may recommend anti-inflammatory medications.

SURGICAL TREATMENT. If osteoarthritis is suspected, a doctor's diagnosis will include an assessment of whether joint pain is part of a patient's medical history. The doctor may take an x ray to determine the presence of cartilage loss and how much degeneration occurred.

Acupuncture may be helpful in treating mild osteoarthritis. Generally, a person should have one to two treatments a week for several weeks. Afterward, one treatment is recommended. An assessment of results should be made after 10 treatments.

In cases of severe osteoarthritis, **joint replacement** surgery or joint **immobilization** may be required. Joints are replaced with metal, plastic, or ceramic material.

Fall prevention

Fall prevention starts with regular exercise such as walking. This improves balance and muscles. The walk route should be on level ground. Other methods for preventing falls include:

- when rising from a chair or bed, a senior should move slowly to avoid dizziness
- people who smoke should quit
- shoes with low heels and rubber soles are recommended
- medications should be monitored because of side effects that increase the probability of a fall
- vision and hearing should be checked periodically
- fall-proofing the home, including the installation of lighting, especially on stairways, clearing clutter and electrical cords that can cause falls, and installing handrails and strips in bathtubs and rails on stairs.

MEDICAL TREATMENT FOR FALLS. After a fall, a senior may need first aid treatment for cuts or fractures. The doctor may evaluate whether medications cause balance problems. If indicated, the doctor may examine the patient's central nervous system function, balance, and muscle/joint function. A hearing or vision test may be ordered.

Corrective measures could include adjusting prescriptions, vision surgery or having the patient use a cane or walker.

Vision

A person diagnosed with **presbyopia** may need bifocals or reading glasses to read print that appears too small. These lenses may need to be changed as vision changes over the years. Eventually, a person relies on glasses to focus on items that are near. Other seniors who never needed corrective lenses may need to wear eyeglasses. Publishers aware of this condition produce books with large print.

A senior should schedule periodic vision exams because early treatment helps prevent or lessen a risk of cataracts or glaucoma. Diet also plays a role in vision care. Dark green vegetables like broccoli are said to help prevent cataracts from progressing. Physical exercise is thought to reduce the pressure associated with glaucoma.

Glaucoma can be treated with eyedrops. Surgery can remove cataracts. The affected lens is removed and replaced with a permanent synthetic lens called an intraocular lens. There was no successful treatment for age-related **macular degeneration** as of 2001.

Hearing

An audiologist can administer tests to determine the amount of hearing loss. Although there is no cure for presbycusis, **hearing aids** can help a senior affected by age-related hearing loss. If this treatment is not effective, the person might need to learn to read lips.

Sleep disorders

Losing weight can help with conditions such as snoring and **sleep apnea**. A doctor may advise the senior to quit smoking, reduce alcohol consumption, or to sleep on his or her side. In some cases, a doctor may refer the senior to a sleep disorder clinic. The senior may be prescribed a continuous positive airway pressure device. Known as a CPAP, the device is placed over the nose. It sends air into the nose.

PLMD and restless leg syndrome may be treated with the prescription drug Dopar. These disorders could be signs of kidney or circulation conditions. Treatment of those conditions should end these sleeping disorders.

Insomnia treatments include exercising and treating depression, stress, and other causes of sleeplessness.

Mental health

After retirement, a senior must find activities and interests to provide a sense of fulfillment. Otherwise, feelings of loneliness and isolation can lead to depression and susceptibility to poor health.

Activities that stimulate a person physically and intellectually contribute to good health. A senior can start an exercise program, take up hobbies, take classes, or volunteer. Senior centers offer numerous activities. Lunch programs provide nutritional meals and companionship. This is important because a senior living alone may not feel motivated to prepare healthy meals.

Dementia

Diagnosis of Alzheimer's disease starts with a thorough medical examination. The doctor should administer memory tests. Blood tests may be required, as well as a CT scan or MRI scan of the brain. If Alzheimer's is diagnosed, the doctor may prescribe medication to slow down progression of this form of dementia.

As of 2003, the FDA had approved four prescription medications for treatment of Alzheimer's. Tacrine, donepezil, riviastigmine, and galantamine are cholinesterase inhibitors that enhance memory. Modest improvement was reported in clinical trials on donepezil, riviastigmine, and galantamine. Tacrine's possible side effects include liver damage, so it is seldom prescribed.

Preparation

Before beginning a weight loss or exercise program, seniors should check with their doctors. The doctor will determine whether a patient is at a healthy weight, or needs to gain or lose weight. The medical professional should be informed about a health condition or a family history of a condition like heart disease. The doctor may order a physical exam or recommend a specific exercise program.

Exercise preparation

A senior should select a form of exercise enjoyable enough to become a regular routine. Suitable clothing or equipment such as walking shoes or a bicycle helmet should be purchased. If a person is active for more than a half-hour, the American Heart Association recommends drinking water every 15 minutes.

In addition to packing a water bottle, a person should pick an exercise buddy. Exercising with a friend or a group makes the activity more enjoyable. In addition, a person is more apt to stick with a routine if a buddy is involved.

Before exercising, a warmup with slow stretching exercises is recommended. This could take longer for a senior because muscular elasticity slows down as a person ages. The exercise session should end with a cool-down that includes slow stretches.

Aftercare

Some recovery time may be needed after surgery. However, a healthy person will heal more quickly. A senior needs to maintain a schedule of regular exercise in order to remain mobile. Otherwise, a minor illness could make them dependent on others for daily care, according to the American Heart Association.

If mobility becomes limited due to a condition such as osteoarthritis, equipment like a walker and devices that make it easier to open bottles and grip cutlery can be helpful.

Risks

Exercising too long or too strenuously can be physically harmful. The over-exertion could cause the person to lose interest in exercise and put off establishing a regular routine. Experts recommend starting out slowly and building up to more intense or longer sessions. This is particularly important for a sedentary person.

Osteoporosis

The long-term effects of hormone replacement therapy have ruled this treatment out for some women.

Normal results

Seniors who stay active and eat nutritionally will be at less risk for conditions such as diabetes. A senior also should seek mental stimulation and social interaction. These provide enjoyment, boost self-esteem, and help reduce feelings of isolation and depression.

Although eyesight and hearing will weaken, glasses and hearing aids help seniors keep the senses of sight and hearing.

When surgery is required for osteoarthritis, hip replacement surgery is extremely successful. In about 98% of surgeries, flexibility returns and pain is eased. Knee replacement surgery also is effective.

If a person maintains a healthy lifestyle, the ability to avoid falls and recover from them is increased.

After a fall, seniors needs to build up physical strength and the confidence needed so they don't fear falling again. Care should be taken so that seniors don't feel isolated by their injuries. Isolation could lead to decreased mobility and loss of independence.

There is no cure for Alzheimer's disease. However, several medications have proved moderately effective in stopping memory loss. Since Alzheimer's is progressive, a person diagnosed with this condition should make arrangements for the future. Finances should be taken care of and plans should be made for future care. Family should be brought into the discussion.

After diagnosis, a person should stay active for as long as possible. Not only does this help with enjoying this stage of life, activities can help to fight depression. Alzheimer and other support groups can be helpful. In addition, modifications to environment can be effective.

Resources

BOOKS

Gillick, Muriel R. *Lifelines: Living Longer, Growing Frail, Taking Heart.* New York: W.W. Norton and Co., 2001.

Honn Qualls, Sara, and Norman Abeles, editors. *Psychology and the Aging Revolution: How We Adapt to Longer Life.* Washington, DC: American Psychological Association, 2000.

Powell, Douglas H. *The Nine Myths of Aging: Maximizing the Quality of Later Life.* Thorndike, ME: Thorndike Press,1998.

Wei, Jeanne Y., and Sue Levkoff. *Aging Well: The Complete Guide to Physical and Emotional Health.* New York: Wiley, 2000.

PERIODICALS

"Aging Americans Face Growing Health Threats." *Health & Medicine Week* June 23, 2003: 3.

Evans, Jeff. "Aging U.S. Population Will Force Changes in Health Care Services." *Family Practice News* April 1, 2003: 54-61.

"Increasing Evidence That Osteoporosis Begins in the Womb." *Womenós Health Weekly* June 19, 2003: 30.

"Update on the Treatment of Osteoporosis Released." *Drug Week* June 27, 2003: 344.

Vernarec, Emil. "An Emerging Alternative to NSAIDs for Osteoarthritis?" *RN* May 2003: 24-31.

ORGANIZATIONS

Alzheimer's Association. 919 N. Michigan Ave., Suite 1100, Chicago, IL 60611-1676. (800) 272-3900. < http://www.alz.org >.

American Academy of Otolaryngology-Head and Neck Surgery. One Prince St., Alexandria, VA 22314-3357. (703) 836-4444. < http://www.ent.org >.

American Dietetic Association. 216 W. Jackson Blvd., Chicago, IL 60606-6995. (312) 899-0040. < http://www.eatright.org >.

American Heart Association. 7272 Greenville Ave., Dallas, TX75231. (800) AHA-USA1. < http://www.americanheart.org >.

National Institute on Aging. P.O. Box 8057, Gaithersburg, MD20898-8057. (800) 222-2225. < http://www.nih.gov >.

National Osteoporosis Foundation. 1232 22nd St., NW,Washington, DC 20037. (800) 624-BONE. < http://www.osteo.org >.

National Sleep Foundation. 1522 K St., NW, Suite 500Washington, DC 20005. Fax: (202) 347-3472. < http://www.sleepfoundation.org >.

Liz Swain
Teresa G. Odle

Sensory hearing loss *see* **Hearing loss**

Sensory integration disorder

Definition

Sensory integration disorder or dysfunction (SID) is a neurological disorder that results from the brain's inability to integrate certain information received from the body's five basic sensory systems. These sensory systems are responsible for detecting sights, sounds, smell, tastes, temperatures, **pain**, and the position and movements of the body. The brain then forms a combined picture of this information in order for the body to make sense of its surroundings and react to them appropriately. The ongoing relationship between behavior and brain functioning is called sensory integration (SI), a theory that was first pioneered by A. Jean Ayres, Ph.D., OTR in the 1960s.

Description

Sensory experiences include touch, movement, body awareness, sight, sound, smell, taste, and the pull of gravity. Distinguishing between these is the process of sensory integration (SI). While the process of SI occurs automatically and without effort for most, for some the process is inefficient. Extensive effort and attention are required in these individuals for SI to occur, without a guarantee of it being accomplished. When this happens, goals are not easily completed, resulting in sensory integration disorder (SID).

The normal process of SI begins before birth and continues throughout life, with the majority of SI development occurring before the early teenage years. The ability for SI to become more refined and effective coincides with the **aging** process as it determines how well motor and speech skills, and emotional stability develop. The beginnings of the SI theory by Ayres instigated ongoing research that looks at the crucial foundation it provides for complex learning and behavior throughout life.

Causes and symptoms

The presence of a sensory integration disorder is typically detected in young children. While most children develop SI during the course of ordinary childhood activities, which helps establish such things as the ability for motor planning and adapting to incoming sensations, others' SI ability does not develop as efficiently. When their process is disordered, a variety of problems in learning, development, or behavior become obvious.

Those who have sensory integration dysfunction may be unable to respond to certain sensory information by planning and organizing what needs to be done in an appropriate and automatic manner. This may cause a primitive survival technique called "fright, flight, and fight," or withdrawal response, which originates from the "primitive" brain. This response often appears extreme and inappropriate for the particular situation.

The neurological disorganization resulting in SID occurs in three different ways: the brain does not receive messages due to a disconnection in the neuron cells; sensory messages are received inconsistently; or sensory messages are received consistently, but do not connect properly with other sensory messages. When the brain poorly processes sensory messages, inefficient motor, language, or emotional output is the result.

According to Sensory Integration International (SII), a non-profit corporation concerned with the impact of sensory integrative problems on people's lives, the following are some signs of sensory integration disorder (SID):

- oversensitivity to touch, movement, sights, or sounds
- underreactivity to touch, movement, sights, or sounds
- tendency to be easily distracted
- social and/or emotional problems
- activity level that is unusually high or unusually low
- physical clumsiness or apparent carelessness
- impulsive, lacking in self-control
- difficulty in making transitions from one situation to another
- inability to unwind or calm self
- poor self concept
- delays in speech, language, or motor skills
- delays in academic achievement

While research indicates that sensory integrative problems are found in up to 70% of children who are considered learning disabled by schools, the problems of sensory integration are not confined to children with learning disabilities. SID transfers through all age groups, as well as intellectual levels and socioeconomic groups. Factors that contribute to SID include: premature birth; **autism** and other developmental disorders; learning disabilities; delinquency and **substance abuse** due to learning disabilities; stress-related disorders; and brain injury. Two of the biggest contributing conditions are autism and attention-deficit hyperactivity disorder (**ADHD**).

Diagnosis

In order to determine the presence of SID, an evaluation may be conducted by a qualified occupational or physical therapist. An evaluation normally consists of both standardized testing and structured observations of responses to sensory stimulation, posture, balance, coordination, and eye movements. These test results and assessment data, along with information from other professionals and parents, are carefully analyzed by the therapist who then makes recommendations about appropriate treatment.

Treatment

Occupational therapists play a key role in the conventional treatment of SID. By providing sensory integration therapy, occupational therapists are able to supply the vital sensory input and experiences that children with SID need to grow and learn. Also referred to as a "sensory diet," this type of therapy involves a planned and scheduled activity program implemented by an occupational therapist, with each "diet" being designed and developed to meet the needs of the child's nervous system. A sensory diet stimulates the "near" senses (tactile, vestibular, and proprioceptive) with a combination of alerting, organizing, and calming techniques.

Motor skills training methods that normally consist of adaptive physical education, movement education, and gymnastics are often used by occupational and physical therapists. While these are important skills to work on, the sensory integrative approach is vital to treating SID.

The sensory integrative approach is guided by one important aspect—the child's motivation in selection of the activities. By allowing them to be actively involved, and explore activities that provide sensory experiences most beneficial to them, children become more mature and efficient at organizing sensory information.

Alternative treatment

Sensory integration disorder (SID) is treatable with occupational therapy, but some alternative methods are emerging to complement the conventional methods used for SID.

Therapeutic body brushing is often used on children (not infants) who overreact to tactile stimulation. A specific non-scratching surgical brush is used to make firm, brisk movements over most of the body, especially the arms, legs, hands, back and soles of the feet. A technique of deep joint compression follows the brushing. Usually begun by an occupational therapist, the technique is taught to parents who need to complete the process for three to five minutes, six to eight times a day. The time needed for brushing is reduced as the child begins to respond more normally to touch. In order for this therapy to be effective, the correct brush and technique must be used.

A report in 1998 indicated the use of cerebral electrical stimulation (CES) as being helpful to children with conditions such as moderate to severe autistic spectrum disorders, learning disabilities, and sensory integration dysfunction. CES is a modification of Transcutaneous Electrical Nerve Stimulation (TENS) technology that has been used to treat adults with various pain problems, including arthritis and carpal tunnel syndrome. TENS therapy uses a low voltage signal applied to the body through the skin with the goal of replacing painful impressions with a massage-like sensation. A much lower

signal is used for CES than that used for traditional TENS, and the electrodes are placed on the scalp or ears. Occupational therapists who have studied the use of CES suggest that CES for children with SID can result in improved brain activity. The device is worn by children at home for 10 minutes at a time, twice per day.

Music therapy helps promote active listening. Hypnosis and biofeedback are sometimes used, along with psychotherapy, to help those with SID, particularly older patients.

Prognosis

By providing treatment at an early age, sensory integration disorder may be managed successfully. The ultimate goal is for the individual to be better able to interact with his or her environment in a more successful and adaptive way.

Resources

ORGANIZATIONS

Sensory Integration International/The Ayres Clinic. 1514 Cabrillo Avenue, Torrance, CA 90501-2817.

OTHER

Sensory Integration Dysfunction. < http://home.ptd.net/blnelson/SIDEWEBPAGE2.htm >.

Sensory Integration International. < http://www.sensoryint.com >.

KEY TERMS

Axon—A process of a neuron that conducts impulses away from the cell body. Axons are usually long and straight.

Cortical—Regarding the cortex, or the outer layer of the brain, as distinguished from the inner portion.

Neurotransmission—When a neurotransmitter, or chemical agent released by a particular brain cell, travels across the synapse to act on the target cell to either inhibit or excite it.

Proprioceptive—Pertaining to proprioception, or the awareness of posture, movement, and changes in equilibrium and the knowledge of position, weight, and resistance of objects as they relate to the body.

Tactile—The perception of touch.

Vestibular—Pertaining to the vestibule; regarding the vestibular nerve of the ear which is linked to the ability to hear sounds.

Sensory Integration Network. <http://
www.sinetwork.org>.
Southpaw Enterprises, Inc. <http://
www.southpawenterprises.com>.

Beth A. Kapes

Sepsis

Definition

Sepsis refers to a bacterial infection in the bloodstream or body tissues. This is a very broad term covering the presence of many types of microscopic disease-causing organisms.

Description

Sepsis is also called **bacteremia**. Closely related terms include septicemia and septic syndrome. In the general population, the incidence of sepsis is two people in 10,000. The number of deaths from sepsis each year has almost doubled in the United States since 1980 because more patients are developing the condition. There are three major factors responsible for this increase: a rise in the number of organ transplants and other surgical procedures that require suppressing the patient's immune system; the greater number of elderly people in the population; and the overuse of **antibiotics** to treat infectious illnesses, resulting in the development of drug-resistant bacteria.

Causes and symptoms

Sepsis can originate anywhere bacteria can gain entry to the body; common sites include the genitourinary tract, the liver and its bile ducts, the gastrointestinal tract, and the lungs. Broken or ulcerated skin can also provide access to bacteria commonly present in the environment. Invasive medical procedures, including dental work, can introduce bacteria or permit them to accumulate in the body. Entry points and equipment left in place for any length of time present a particular risk. **Heart valve replacement**, catheters, ostomy sites, intravenous (IV) or arterial lines, surgical **wounds**, or surgical drains are examples. IV drug users are at high risk as well.

People with inefficient immune systems, HIV infection, spinal cord injuries, or blood disorders are at particular risk for sepsis and have a higher **death** rate (up to 60%); in people who have no underlying chronic disease, the death rate is far lower (about 5%). The growing problem of antibiotic resistance has increased the incidence of sepsis, partly because ordinary preventive measures (such as prophylactic antibiotics) are less effective.

Cancer patients are at an increased risk of developing sepsis because **chemotherapy** and other forms of treatment for cancer weaken their immune systems.

The most common symptom of sepsis is **fever**, often accompanied by chills or shaking, or other flu-like symptoms. A history of any recent invasive procedure or dental work should raise the suspicion of sepsis and medical help should be sought.

Diagnosis

The presence of sepsis is indicated by blood tests showing particularly high or low white blood cell counts. The causative agent is determined by blood culture.

In some cases the doctor may order imaging studies to rule out **pneumonia**, or to determine whether the sepsis has developed from a ruptured appendix or other leakage from the digestive tract into the abdomen.

Treatment

Identifying the specific causative agent ultimately determines how sepsis is treated. However, time is of the essence, so a broad-spectrum antibiotic or multiple antibiotics will be administered until blood cultures reveal the culprit and treatment can be made specific to the organism. Intravenous antibiotic therapy is usually necessary and is administered in the hospital. The patient's chances of survival are increased by rapid admission to an intensive care unit followed by aggressive treatment with antibiotics.

Resources

BOOKS

Beers, Mark H., MD, and Robert Berkow, MD., editors. "Bacteremia and Septic Shock." Section 13, Chapter 156 In *The Merck Manual of Diagnosis and Therapy*. Whitehouse Station, NJ: Merck Research Laboratories, 2004.

PERIODICALS

Cunha, Burke A., MD. "Sepsis, Bacterial." *eMedicine* September 29, 2004. < http://www.emedicine.com/med/topic3163.htm >.

Koranyi, K. I., and M. A. Ranalli. "*Mycobacterium aurum* Bacteremia in an Immunocompromised Child." *Pediatric Infectious Diseases Journal* 22 (December 2003): 1108–1109.

Larche, J., E. Azoulay, F. Fieux, et al. "Improved Survival of Critically Ill Cancer Patients with Septic Shock." *Intensive Care Medicine* 29 (October 2003): 1688–1695.

Paphitou, N. I., and K. V. Rolston. "Catheter-Related Bacteremia Caused by *Agrobacterium radiobacter* in a Cancer Patient: Case Report and Literature Review." *Infection* 31 (December 2003): 421–424.

Petrosillo, N., L. Pagani, G. Ippolito, et al. "Nosocomial Infections in HIV-Positive Patients: An Overview." *Infection* 31, Supplement 2 (December 2003): 28–34.

Wall, B. M., T. Mangold, K. M. Huch, et al. "Bacteremia in the Chronic Spinal Cord Injury Population: Risk Factors for Mortality." *Journal of Spinal Cord Medicine* 26 (Fall 2003): 248–253.

ORGANIZATIONS

American College of Epidemiology. 1500 Sunday Drive, Suite 102, Raleigh, NC 27607. (919) 861-5573. < http://www.acepidemiology.org >.

American Public Health Association (APHA). 800 I Street NW, Washington, DC 20001-3710. (202) 777-APHA. < http://www.apha.org >.

Centers for Disease Control and Prevention. 1600 Clifton Rd., NE, Atlanta, GA 30333. (800) 311-3435, (404) 639-3311. < http://www.cdc.gov >.

OTHER

"Supportive Care for Patients—Fever, Chills, and Sweats." *National Cancer Institute CancerNet* 16 April 16, 2001. < http://cancernet.nci.nih.gov/coping.html >.

Jill S. Lasker
Rebecca J. Frey, PhD

Sepsis syndrome *see* **Septic shock**

Septal deviation *see* **Deviated septum**

Septic arthritis *see* **Infectious arthritis**

Septic shock

Definition

Septic **shock** is a potentially lethal drop in blood pressure due to the presence of bacteria in the blood.

Description

Septic shock is a possible consequence of **bacteremia**, or bacteria in the bloodstream. Bacterial toxins, and the immune system response to them, cause a dramatic drop in blood pressure, preventing the delivery of blood to the organs. Septic shock can lead to multiple organ failure including **respiratory failure**, and may cause rapid **death**. Toxic shock syndrome is one type of septic shock.

Causes and symptoms

During an infection, certain types of bacteria can produce and release complex molecules, called endotoxins, that may provoke a dramatic response by the body's immune system. Released in the bloodstream, endotoxins are particularly dangerous, because they become widely dispersed and affect the blood vessels themselves. Arteries and the smaller arterioles open wider, increasing the total volume of the circulatory system. At the same time, the walls of the blood vessels become leaky, allowing fluid to seep out into the tissues, lowering the amount of fluid left in circulation. This combination of increased system volume and decreased fluid causes a dramatic decrease in blood pressure and reduces the blood flow to the organs. Other changes brought on by immune response may cause coagulation of the blood in the extremities, which can further decrease circulation through the organs.

Septic shock is seen most often in patients with suppressed immune systems, and is usually due to bacteria acquired during treatment at the hospital. The immune system is suppressed by drugs used to treat **cancer**, autoimmune disorders, organ transplants, and diseases of immune deficiency such as **AIDS**. **Malnutrition**, chronic drug **abuse**, and long-term illness increase the likelihood of succumbing to bacterial infection. Bacteremia is more likely with preexisting infections such as urinary or gastrointestinal tract infections, or skin ulcers. Bacteria may be introduced to the blood stream by surgical procedures, catheters, or intravenous equipment.

Toxic shock syndrome most often occurs in menstruating women using highly absorbent tampons. Left in place longer than other types, these tampons provide the breeding ground for *Staphylococcus* bacteria, which may then enter the bloodstream through small tears in the vaginal lining. The incidence of toxic shock syndrome has declined markedly since this type of tampon was withdrawn from the market.

Symptoms

Septic shock is usually preceded by bacteremia, which is marked by **fever**, malaise, chills, and **nausea**. The first sign of shock is often confusion and decreased consciousness. In this beginning stage, the extremities are usually warm. Later, they become cool, pale, and bluish. Fever may give way to lower than normal temperatures later on in sepsis.

Other symptoms include:

- rapid heartbeat
- shallow, rapid breathing
- decreased urination.
- reddish patches in the skin

Septic shock may progress to cause "adult respiratory distress syndrome," in which fluid collects in the lungs, and breathing becomes very shallow and labored. This condition may lead to ventilatory collapse, in which the patient can no longer breathe adequately without assistance.

Diagnosis

Diagnosis of septic shock is made by measuring blood pressure, heart rate, and respiration rate, as well as by a consideration of possible sources of infection. Blood pressure may be monitored with a catheter device inserted into the pulmonary artery supplying the lungs (Swan-Ganz catheter). Blood cultures are done to determine the type of bacteria responsible. The levels of oxygen, carbon dioxide, and acidity in the blood are also monitored to assess changes in respiratory function.

Treatment

Septic shock is treated initially with a combination of **antibiotics** and fluid replacement. The antibiotic is chosen based on the bacteria present, although two or more types of antibiotics may be used initially until the organism is identified. Intravenous fluids, either blood or protein solutions, replace the fluid lost by leakage. Coagulation and hemorrhage may be treated with transfusions of plasma or platelets. Dopamine may be given to increase blood pressure further if necessary.

Respiratory distress is treated with mechanical ventilation and supplemental oxygen, either using a nosepiece or a tube into the trachea through the throat.

Identification and treatment of the primary infection site is important to prevent ongoing proliferation of bacteria.

KEY TERMS

Bacteremia—Invasion of the bloodstream by bacteria.

Prognosis

Septic shock is most likely to develop in the hospital, since it follows infections which are likely to be the objects of treatment. Because of this, careful monitoring and early, aggressive therapy can minimize the likelihood of progression. Nonetheless, death occurs in at least 25% of all cases.

The likelihood of recovery from septic shock depends on may factors, including the degree of immunosuppression of the patient, underlying disease, promptness of treatment, and type of bacteria responsible. Mortality is highest in the very young and the elderly, those with persistent or recurrent infection, and those with compromised immune systems.

Prevention

The risk of developing septic shock can be minimized through treatment of underlying bacterial infections, and prompt attention to signs of bacteremia. In the hospital, scrupulous aseptic technique on the part of medical professionals lowers the risk of introducing bacteria into the bloodstream.

Resources

OTHER

The Merck Page. April 13, 1998. < http://www.merck.com >.

Richard Robinson

Septoplasty

Definition

Septoplasty is a surgical procedure to correct the shape of the septum of the nose. The nasal septum is the separation between the two nostrils. In adults, the septum is composed partly of cartilage and partly of bone.

Purpose

Septoplasty is performed to correct a crooked (deviated) or dislocated septum, often as part of **plastic surgery** of the nose (**rhinoplasty**). The nasal septum has three functions: to support the nose, regulate air flow, and support the mucous membranes (mucosa) of the nose. Septoplasty is done to correct the shape of the nose caused by a deformed septum or correct deregulated air flow caused by a **deviated septum**. Septoplasty is often needed when the patient is having an operation to reduce the size of the nose (reductive rhinoplasty), because this operation usually reduces the amount of breathing space in the nose.

Septoplasty may also be done as a follow-up procedure following facial trauma, as the nose is frequently broken or dislocated by blows to the face resulting from automobile accidents, criminal assaults, or **sports injuries**.

Precautions

Septoplasty is ordinarily not performed within six months of a traumatic injury to the nose.

Description

Septoplasties are performed in the hospital with a combination of local and intravenous anesthesia. In some cases, hypnosis has been successfully used as anesthesia. After the patient is anesthetized, the surgeon makes a cut (incision) in the mucous tissue that covers the part of the septum that is made of cartilage. The tissue is lifted, exposing the cartilage and bony part of the septum. Usually, one side of the mucous tissue is left intact to provide support during healing. Cartilage is cut away as needed.

As the surgeon cuts away the cartilage, deformities tend to straighten themselves out, reducing the amount of cartilage that must be cut. Once the cartilage is cut, bony deformities can be corrected. For most patients, this is the extent of the surgery required to improve breathing through the nose and correct deformities. Some patients have bony obstructions at the base of the nasal chamber and require further surgery. These obstructions include bony spurs and ridges that contribute to drying, ulceration, or bleeding of the mucous tissue that covers the inside of the nasal passages. In these cases, the extent of the surgery depends on the nature of the deformities that need correcting.

During surgery, the patient's own cartilage that has been removed can be reused to provide support for

the nose if needed. External septum supports are not usually needed. Splints may be needed occasionally to support cartilage when extensive cutting has been done. External splints can be used to support the cartilage for the first few days of healing. Tefla gauze is inserted in the nostril to support the flaps and cartilage and to absorb any bleeding or mucus.

A newer option for closing perforations in the septum is a button made of Silastic, a compound of silicone and rubber.

Preparation

Before performing a septoplasty, the surgeon will evaluate the difference in airflow between the two nostrils. In children, this assessment can be done very simply by asking the child to breathe out slowly on a small mirror held in front of the nose.

As with any other operation under **general anesthesia**, patients are evaluated for any physical conditions that might complicate surgery and for any medications that might affect blood clotting time.

Aftercare

Patients with septoplasties are usually sent home from the hospital later the same day or the morning after the surgery. All dressings inside the nose are removed before the patient leaves. Aftercare includes a list of detailed instructions for the patient that focus on preventing trauma to the nose.

Risks

The risks from a septoplasty are similar to those from other operations on the face: postoperative **pain** with some bleeding, swelling, bruising, or discoloration. A few patients may have allergic reactions to the anesthetics. The operation in itself, however, is relatively low-risk in that it does not involve major blood vessels or vital organs. Infection is unlikely if proper surgical technique is observed.

Normal results

Normal results include improved breathing and airflow through the nostrils, and an acceptable outward shape of the nose.

Resources

BOOKS

Beers, Mark H., MD, and Robert Berkow, MD., editors. "Septal Deviation and Perforation." Section 7, Chapter 86 In *The Merck Manual of Diagnosis and Therapy.* Whitehouse Station, NJ: Merck Research Laboratories, 2004.

PERIODICALS

Piatti, G., A. Scotti, and U. Ambrosetti. "Nasal Ciliary Beat after Insertion of Septo-Valvular Splints." *Otolaryngology and Head and Neck Surgery* 130 (May 2004): 558–562.

Wain, H. J. "Reflections on Hypnotizability and Its Impact on Successful Surgical Hypnosis: A Sole Anesthetic for Septoplasty." *American Journal of Clinical Hypnosis* 46 (April 2004): 313–321.

ORGANIZATIONS

American Academy of Facial Plastic and Reconstructive Surgery (AAFPRS). 310 South Henry Street, Alexandria, VA 22314. (703) 299-9291. < http://www.facemd.org >.

American Society of Plastic Surgeons (ASPS). 444 East Algonquin Road, Arlington Heights, IL 60005. (847) 228-9900. < http://www.plasticsurgery.org >.

John T. Lohr, PhD
Rebecca J. Frey, PhD

Septum perforation *see* **Perforated septum**

Serenoa repens see **Saw palmetto**

Serotonin boosters *see* **Selective serotonin reuptake inhibitors**

Serum albumin test *see* **Protein components test**

Serum globulin test *see* **Protein components test**

Serum hepatitis *see* **Hepatitis B**

Serum protein electrophoresis *see* **Protein electrophoresis**

Serum sickness

Definition

Serum sickness is a type of delayed allergic response, appearing four to 10 days after exposure to some **antibiotics** or antiserum, the portion of serum that contains antibodies, such as gamma globulin, which may be given to provide immunization against some diseases.

Description

Serum sickness is very similar to an allergic reaction. The patient's immune system recognizes the proteins in the drug or antiserum as foreign proteins, and produces its own antibodies to protect against the foreign proteins. The newly formed antibodies bind with the foreign protein to form immune complexes. These immune complexes may enter the walls of blood vessels where they set off an inflammatory reaction.

While other types of allergic reactions may produce a rapid response, the serum sickness reaction is delayed because it takes time for the body to produce antibodies to the new protein.

Causes and symptoms

The usual symptoms are severe skin reactions, often on the palms of the hands and soles of the feet. **Fever**, sometimes as high as 104o F, is always present and usually appears before the skin rash.

Joint **pain** may be reported in up to 50% of cases. This is usually seen in the larger joints, but occasionally the finger and toe joints may also be involved.

Swelling of lymph nodes, particularly around the site of the injection, is seen in 10–20% of cases. There may also be swelling of the head and neck.

Urine analysis may show traces of blood and protein in the urine.

Other symptoms may involve the heart and central nervous system. These may include changes in vision, and difficulty in movement. Breathing difficulty may occur.

Traditionally, antitoxins were the most common cause of serum sickness, but those reports date from a time when most antitoxins were made from horse serum. As many as 16% of the people who received antirabies serum derived from horses developed serum sickness. The risk of a reaction to antitoxins has dropped dramatically since manufacturers have started using human serum instead of horse serum to make their products.

Although antitoxins are the most common cause of serum sickness, a number of drugs have been reported to cause a serum sickness reaction. The following list is not complete, but indicates some of the drugs that have been associated with this type of reaction:

- allopurinol (Zyloprim)
- barbiturates
- captopril (Capoten)
- cephalosporin antibiotics
- griseofulvin (Fulvicin, Grifulvin)
- penicillins
- pehnytoin (Dilantin)
- procainamide (Procan SR, Procanbid, Pronestyl-SR)
- quinidine (Quinaglute, Quinidex, Quinora)
- streptokinase (Streptase, Kabikinase)
- sulfonamide antibacterial drugs

Of cases of serum sickness reported to the United States Food and Drug Administration, the drugs most commonly associated with the reaction have been the cephalosporin antibiotics, including cefaclor (Ceclor) and cefalexin (Keflex) and the sulfonamide combination trimethoprim-sulfamethoxazole (Bactrim, Septra.) This does not mean that these are high-risk drugs, since these drugs are very widely used, so that there are many people exposed to them.

In addition to these substances, allergenic extracts used for testing and immunization, hormones, and vaccines have been known to cause serum sickness.

Diagnosis

Diagnosis is made by observing the symptoms and reviewing the patient's medical and medication history. Although the symptoms of serum sickness may be similar to other conditions, patients who present with symptoms of serum sickness and who have a recent history of exposure to a drug or other product which may cause this type of reaction should be suspected of having serum sickness.

Treatment

The first step in treatment of serum sickness is always to discontinue the drug or other substance which is suspected of causing the reaction. After that, all treatment is symptomatic. Antihistamines, pain

relievers, and **corticosteroids** may be given to relieve the symptoms. The choice of treatment depends on the severity of the reaction.

Prognosis

Most serum sickness reactions are mild, and disappear on their own after one or two weeks as long as the cause is removed. Sometimes, symptoms of pain and discomfort may continue for several weeks, even after all the observable reactions such as skin rash and protein in the urine have disappeared. In very rare cases, however, there can be severe reactions and permanent damage. In very rare but extreme cases, serum sickness can lead to **shock**, permanent kidney damage, and even **death**.

Prevention

The most effective method of prevention is simple avoidance of antitoxins that may cause serum sickness. If patients have had a reaction in the past, particularly if the reaction was to a commonly used drug, they should be made aware of it, and be advised to alert physicians and hospitals in the future. Patients who have had particularly severe reactions may be advised to wear identification bracelets, or use other means to alert health care providers.

When it is necessary to administer an antitoxin, skin tests may be used to identify people who are at risk of a reaction. If the situation does not allow enough time for skin testing, the antitoxin should be given along with an intravenous antihistamine. Other drugs, such as epinephrine, which may be needed for an emergency, should be available.

Resources

BOOKS

1999 Year Book: Allergy and Clinical Immunology. Saint Louis: Mosby, Inc., 1999.

PERIODICALS

"Children at Rrisk from Medication Mistakes." *Houston Chronicle* May 18, 2001.
"Drug allergies." *Pediatrics for Parents* 18 (2000):1.
Fielding, Jonathan. "Our Health; Drug Reactions Differ From Side Effects." *The Los Angeles Times* February 7, 2000.
"VA Hospitals Test Smart Cards for Patient Information." *Computerworld* May 14, 2001.

ORGANIZATIONS

Action Against Allergy (AAA). PO Box 278, Twickenham Middlesex, Greater London TW1 4QQ, England.
American Allergy Association (AAA). 3104 E Camelback, Ste. 459 Phoenix, AZ 85016.

Samuel D. Uretsky, PharmD

Serum therapy *see* **Gammaglobulin**

Severe acute respiratory syndrome (SARS)

Definition

Severe acute respiratory syndrome (SARS) is the first emergent and highly transmissible viral disease to appear during the twenty-first century.

Description

Patients with SARS develop flu-like **fever, headache**, malaise, dry **cough** and other breathing difficulties. Many patients develop **pneumonia**, and in 5–10% of cases, the pneumonia and other complications are severe enough to cause **death**. SARS is caused by a virus that is transmitted usually from person to person—predominantly by the aerosolized droplets of virus infected material.

The first known case of SARS was traced to a November 2002 case in Guangdong province, China. By mid-February 2003, Chinese health officials tracked more than 300 cases, including five deaths in Guangdong province from what was at the time described as an acute respiratory syndrome. Many flu-causing viruses have previously originated from Guangdong province because of cultural and exotic cuisine practices that bring animals, animal parts, and humans into close proximity. In such an environment, pathogens can more easily genetically mutate and make the leap from animal hosts to humans. The first cases of SARS showed high rates among Guangdong food handlers and chefs.

Chinese health officials initially remained silent about the outbreak, and no special precautions were taken to limit travel or prevent the spread of the disease. The world health community, therefore, had no chance to institute testing, **isolation**, and quarantine measures that might have prevented the subsequent global spread of the disease.

On February 21, Liu Jianlun, a 64-year-old Chinese physician from Zhongshan hospital (later determined to have been "super-spreader," a person capable of infecting unusually high numbers of contacts) traveled to Hong Kong to attend a family wedding despite the fact that he had a fever. Epidemiologists subsequently determined that, Jianlun passed on the SARS virus to other guests at the Metropole Hotel where he stayed—including an American businessman en route to Hanoi, three women from Singapore, two Canadians, and a Hong Kong resident. Jianlun's travel to Hong Kong and the subsequent travel of those he infected allowed SARS to spread from China to the infected travelers' destinations.

Johnny Chen, the American businessman, grew ill in Hanoi, Vietnam, and was admitted to a local hospital. Chen infected 20 health care workers at the hospital including noted Italian epidemiologist Carlo Urbani who worked at the Hanoi World Health Organization (WHO) office. Urbani provided medical care for Chen and first formally identified SARS as a unique disease on February 28, 2003. By early March, 22 hospital workers in Hanoi were ill with SARS.

Unaware of the problems in China, Urbani's report drew increased attention among epidemiologists when coupled with news reports in mid-March that Hong Kong health officials had also discovered an outbreak of an acute respiratory syndrome among health care workers. Unsuspecting hospital workers admitted the Hong Kong man infected by Jianlun to a general ward at the Prince of Wales Hospital because it was assumed he had a typical severe pneumonia—a fairly routine admission. The first notice that clinicians were dealing with an unusual illness came—not from health notices from China of increasing illnesses and deaths due to SARS—but from the observation that hospital staff, along with those subsequently determined to have been in close proximity to the infected persons, began to show signs of illness. Eventually, 138 people, including 34 nurses, 20 doctors, 16 medical students, and 15 other health care workers, contracted pneumonia.

One of the most intriguing aspects of the early Hong Kong cases was a cluster of more than 250 SARS cases that occurred in a cluster of high-rise apartment buildings—many housing health care workers—that provided evidence of a high rate of secondary transmission. Epidemiologists conducted extensive investigations to rule out the hypothesis that the illnesses were related to some form of local contamination (e.g., sewage, bacteria on the ventilation system, etc.). Rumors began that the illness was due to cockroaches or rodents, but no scientific evidence supported the hypothesis that the disease pathogen was carried by insects or animals.

Hong Kong authorities then decided that those suffering the flu-like symptoms would be given the option of self-isolation, with family members allowed to remain confined at home or in special camps. Compliance checks were conducted by police.

One of the Canadians infected in Hong Kong, Kwan Sui-Chu, return to Toronto, Ontario, and died in a Toronto hospital on March 5. As in Hong Kong, because there were no alert from China about the SARS outbreak, Canadian officials did not initially suspect that Sui-Chu had been infected with a highly contagious virus, until Sui-Chu's son and five health care workers showed similar symptoms. By mid-April, Canada reported more than 130 SARS cases and 15 fatalities.

Increasingly faced with reports that provided evidence of global dissemination, on March 15, 2003, the World Health Organization (WHO) took the unusual step of issuing a travel warning that described SARS is a "worldwide health threat." WHO officials announced that SARS cases, and potential cases, had been tracked from China to Singapore, Thailand, Vietnam, Indonesia, Philippines, and Canada.

Although the exact cause of the "acute respiratory syndrome" had not, at that time, been determined, WHO officials issuance of the precautionary warning to travelers bound for Southeast Asia about the potential SARS risk served as notice to public health officials about the potential dangers of SARS.

Within days of the first WHO warning, SARS cases were reported in United Kingdom, Spain, Slovenia, Germany, and in the United States.

WHO officials were initially encouraged that isolation procedures and alerts were working to stem the spread of SARS, as some countries reporting small numbers of cases experienced no further dissemination to hospital staff or others in contact with SARS victims. However, in some countries, including Canada, where SARS cases occurred before WHO alerts, SARS continued to spread beyond the bounds of isolated patients.

WHO officials responded by recommending increased screening and quarantine measures that included mandatory screening of persons returning from visits to the most severely affected areas in China, Southeast Asia, and Hong Kong.

In early April 2003, WHO took the controversial additional step of recommending against non-essential travel to Hong Kong and the Guangdong province of China. The recommendation, sought by infectious disease specialists, was not controversial within the medical community, but caused immediate concern regarding the potentially widespread economic impacts.

Mounting reports of SARS showed a increasing global dissemination of the virus. By April 9, the first confirmed reports of SARS cases in Africa reached WHO headquarters, and eight days later, a confirmed case was discovered in India.

Causes and symptoms

In mid-April 2003, Canadian scientists at the British Columbia **Cancer** Agency in Vancouver announced that they that sequenced the genome of the coronavirus most likely to be the cause of SARS. Within days, scientists at the Centers for Disease Control (CDC) in Atlanta, Georgia, offered a genomic map that confirmed more than 99% of the Canadian findings.

Both genetic maps were generated from studies of viruses isolated from SARS cases. The particular coronavirus mapped had a genomic sequence of 29,727 nucleotides—average for the family of coronavirus that typically contain between 29,000-31,000 nucleotides.

Proof that the coronavirus mapped was the specific virus responsible for SARS would eventually come from animal testing. Rhesus monkeys were exposed to the virus via injection and inhalation and then monitored to determine whether SARS like symptoms developed, and then if sick animals exhibited a histological pathology (i.e., an examination of the tissue and cellular level pathology) similar to findings in human patients. Other tests, including polymerase chain reaction (PCR) testing helped positively match the specific coronavirus present in the lung tissue, blood, and feces of infected animals to the exposure virus.

Identification of a specific pathogen can be a complex process, and positive identification requires thousands of tests. All testing is conducted with regard to testing Koch's postulates—the four conditions that must be met for an organism to be determined to the cause of a disease. First, the organism must be present in every case of the disease. Second, the organism must be able to be isolated from the host and grown in laboratory conditions. Third, the disease must be reproduced when the isolated organism is introduced into another, healthy host. The fourth postulate stipulates that the same organism must be able to be recovered and purified from the host that was experimentally infected.

Early data indicates that SARS has an incubation period range of two to 10 days, with an average incubation of about four days. Much of the inoculation period allows the virus to be both transported and spread by an asymptomatic carrier. With air travel, asymptotic carriers can travel to anywhere in the world. The initial symptoms are non-specific and common to the flu. Infected cases then typically spike a high fever 100.4°F (38°C) as they develop a cough, **shortness of breath**, and difficulty breathing. SARS often fulminates (reaches it maximum progression) in a severe pneumonia that can cause **respiratory failure** and death in about 10% of its victims.

Diagnosis

Currently, initial tests include blood cultures, Gram stain, chest radiograph, and tests for other viral respiratory pathogens such as **influenza** A and B. Other serologic techniques are used, and if SARS is suspected, samples are forwarded to state/local public health departments and/or the CDC for coronavirus antibody testing.

Treatment

As of May 1, 2003, no therapy was demonstrated to have clinical effectiveness against the virus that causes SARS, and physicians could offer only supportive therapy (e.g. administration of fluids, oxygen, ventilation, etc.).

Prognosis

By late April/early May 2003, WHO officials had confirmed reports of more than 3,000 cases of SARS from 18 different countries with 111 deaths attributed to the disease (about a 5–10% death rate). United States health officials reported 193 cases with no deaths. Significantly, all but 20 of the U.S. cases were linked to travel to infected areas, and the other 20 cases were accounted for by secondary transmission from infected patients to family members and health care workers.

Information on countries reporting SARS and the cumulative total of cases and deaths is updated each day on the WHO SARS web site at <http://www.who.int/csr/sarscountry/en/>.

Prevention

Until a vaccine is developed, isolation and quarantine remain potent tools in the modern public health arsenal. Both procedures seek to control exposure to infected individuals or materials. Isolation procedures are used with patients with a confirmed illness. Quarantine rules and procedures apply to individuals who are not currently ill, but are known to have been exposed to the illness (e.g., been in the company of a infected person or come in contact with infected materials).

Isolation and quarantine both act to restrict movement and to slow or stop the spread of disease within a community. Depending on the illness, patients placed in isolation may be cared for in hospitals, specialized health care facilities, or in less severe cases, at home. Isolation is a standard procedure for TB patients. In most cases, isolation is voluntary; however, isolation can be compelled by federal, state, and some local law.

States governments within the United States have a general authority to set and enforce quarantine conditions. At the federal level, the Centers for Disease Control and Prevention's (CDC) Division of Global Migration and Quarantine is empowered to detain, examine, or conditionally release (release with restrictions on movement or with a required treatment protocol) individuals suspected of carrying certain listed communicable diseases.

As of April 27, 2003, the CDC in Atlanta recommended SARS patients be voluntarily isolated, but had not recommended enforced isolation or quarantine. Regardless, CDC and other public heath officials, including the Surgeon General, sought and secured increased powers to deal with SARS. On April 4, 2003, U.S. President George W. Bush signed Presidential Executive Order 13295 that added SARS to a list of quarantinable communicable diseases. The order provided health officials with the broader powers to seek "...apprehension, detention, or conditional release of individuals to prevent the introduction, transmission, or spread of suspected communicable diseases..."

Travel advisories issued by WHO should be reviewed and people who must travel to areas with SARS outbreaks should follow such preventative measures as frequent hand washing and avoidance of large crowds. Likewise, family members caring for suspected and/or confirmed SARS patients should wash hands frequently, avoid direct contact with the patient's bodily fluids, and monitor their own possible development of symptoms closely.

Brenda Wilmoth Lerner
K. Lee Lerner

Severe combined immunodeficiency

Definition

Severe combined **immunodeficiency** (SCID) is the most serious human immunodeficiency disorder(s). It is a group of congenital disorders in which both the humoral part of the patient's immune system and the cells involved in immune responses fail to work properly. Children with SCID are vulnerable to recurrent severe infections, retarded growth, and early **death**.

Description

SCID is thought to affect between one in every 100,000 persons, and one in every 500,000 infants. Several different immune system disorders are currently grouped under SCID:

- Swiss-type agammaglobulinemia. This was the first type of SCID discovered, in Switzerland in the 1950s.
- Adenosine deaminase deficiency (ADA). About 50% of SCID cases are of this type. ADA deficiency

leads to low levels of B and T cells in the child's immune system.

- Autosomal recessive. About 40% of SCID cases are inherited from the parents in an autosomal recessive pattern.
- Bare lymphocyte syndrome. In this form of SCID, the white blood cells (lymphocytes) in the baby's blood are missing certain proteins. Without these proteins, the lymphocytes cannot activate the T cells in the immune system.
- SCID with leukopenia. Children with this form of SCID are lacking a type of white blood cell called a granulocyte.

In order to understand why SCID is considered the most severe immunodeficiency disorder, it is helpful to have an outline of the parts of the human immune system. It has three parts: cellular, humoral, and nonspecific. The cellular and humoral parts of the system are both needed to fight infections–they recognize disease agents and attack them. The cellular system is composed of many classes of T-lymphocytes (white blood cells that detect foreign invaders called antigens). The humoral system is made up of B cells, which are the only cells in the body that make antibodies. In SCID, neither the cellular nor the humoral part of the immune system is working properly.

Causes and symptoms

SCID is an inherited disorder. There are two ways in which a developing fetus' immune system can fail to develop normally. In the first type of genetic problem, both B and T cells are defective. In the second type, only the T cells are abnormal, but their defect affects the functioning of the B cells.

For the first few months of life, a child with SCID is protected by antibodies in the mother's blood. As early as three months of age, however, the SCID child begins to suffer from mouth infections (thrush), chronic **diarrhea**, otitis media and pulmonary infections, including pneumocystis pneumonia. The child loses weight, becomes very weak, and eventually dies from an opportunistic infection.

Diagnosis

SCID is diagnosed by the typing of T and B cells in the child's blood. B cells can be detected by immuno-fluorescence tests for surface markers (unique proteins)on the cells. T cells can be identified in tissue sections (samples) using enzyme-labeled antibodies.

KEY TERMS

Adenosine deaminase (ADA)—An enzyme that is lacking in a specific type of SCID. Children with an ADA deficiency have low levels of both B and T cells.

Antigens—A substance that usually causes the formation of an antibody. A foreign invaders in the body.

Autosomal recessive inheritance—A pattern of inheritance of a recessive gene where, among other things, both parents may not show symptoms.

B cell—A type of lymphocyte or white blood cell that is derived from precursor cells in the bone marrow.

Congenital—Present at the time of birth. Most forms of SCID are hereditary as well as congenital.

Gene therapy—An experimental treatment for SCID that consists of implanting a gene for ADA into an activated virus and merging it with some of the patient's own T cells. The corrected T cells are infused back into the patient every few months.

Humoral—Pertaining to or derived from a body fluid. The humoral part of the immune system includes antibodies and immunoglobulins in blood serum.

Lymphocyte—A type of white blood cell that is important in the formation of antibodies.

Orphan drug—A drug that is known to be useful in treatment but lacks sufficient funding for further research and development.

PEG-ADA—An orphan drug that is useful in treating SCID related to ADA deficiency.

T cells—Lymphocytes that originate in the thymus gland. T cells regulate the immune system's response to infections. The thymus gland is small or underdeveloped in children with SCID.

Thrush—A disease of the mouth caused by a yeast, *Candida albicans*.

Treatment

Patients with SCID can be treated with **antibiotics** and immune serum to protect them from infections, but these treatments cannot cure the disorder. Bone marrow transplants are currently regarded as one of the few effective standard treatments for SCID.

Investigational treatments

In 1990, the Food and Drug Administration (FDA) approved PEG-ADA, an orphan drug (not available in US but available elsewhere), for the treatment of SCID. PEG-ADA, which is also called pegademase bovine, works by replacing the ADA deficiency in children with this form of SCID. Children who receive weekly injections of PEG-ADA appear to have normal immune functions restored. Another treatment that is still in the experimental stage is **gene therapy**. In gene therapy, the children receive periodic infusions of their own T cells corrected with a gene for ADA that has been implanted in an activated virus.

Prognosis

Currently, there is no cure for SCID. Most untreated patients die before age two.

Prevention

Genetic counseling is recommended for parents of a child with SCID.

Resources

ORGANIZATIONS

Immune Deficiency Foundation. 25 W. Chesapeake Ave., Suite 206, Towson, MD 21204. (800) 296-4433. < http://www.primaryimmune.org >.

National Organization for Rare Disorders. P.O. Box 8923, New Fairfield, CT 06812-8923. (800) 999-6673. < http://www.rarediseases.org >.

Rebecca J. Frey, PhD

Sex hormones tests

Definition

Sex hormones tests measure levels of the sex hormones, including estrogen, progesterone, and testosterone.

Purpose

The sex hormone tests are ordered to determine if secretion of these hormones is normal. Estrogen fraction test is done to evaluate sexual maturity, menstrual problems, and fertility problems in females. This test may also be used to test for tumors that excrete estrogen. In pregnant women it aids in determining fetal-placental health. Estrogen fraction is also used to evaluate males who have enlargement of one or both breasts (gynecomastia), or who have feminization syndromes, where they display female sex characteristics.

Progesterone assay test is ordered to evaluate women who are having difficulty becoming pregnant or maintaining a **pregnancy**, and to monitor high-risk pregnancies.

Testosterone levels are ordered to evaluate:

- ambiguous sex characteristics
- **precocious puberty**
- virilizing syndromes in the female
- infertility in the male
- rare tumors of the ovary and testicle

Description

The sex hormones control the development of primary and secondary sexual characteristics. They regulate the sex-related functions of the body, such as the menstrual cycle or the production of eggs or sperm. There are three main types of sex hormones:

- the female sex hormones (called the estrogen hormones)
- the progesterone hormones (which help the body prepare for and maintain pregnancy)
- the male sex hormones, or the androgen hormones

Female sex hormones are responsible for normal menstruation and the development of secondary female characteristics. Testosterone is a hormone that induces **puberty** in the male and maintains male secondary sex characteristics. In females, the adrenal glands and the ovaries secrete small amounts of testosterone.

Estrogen

Estrogen is tested to evaluate menstrual status, sexual maturity, and **gynecomastia** (or feminization syndromes). It is a tumor marker for patients with certain ovarian tumors. E1, a type of estrogen, is the most active estrogen in the nonpregnant female.

E3 (estriol) is the major estrogen in the pregnant female. It is produced in the placenta. Excretion of estriol increases around the eighth week of gestation and continues to rise until shortly before delivery. Serial urine and blood studies of this hormone are used to assess placental function and fetal normality in high-risk pregnancies. Falling values during

pregnancy suggest fetoplacental deterioration and require prompt reassessment of the pregnancy, including the possibility of early delivery.

Progesterone

Progesterone is essential for the healthy functioning of the female reproductive system. Produced in the ovaries during the second half of the menstrual cycle, and by the placenta during pregnancy, small amounts of progesterone are also produced in the adrenal glands and testes.

After ovulation, an increase of progesterone causes the uterine lining to thicken in preparation for the implantation of a fertilized egg. If this event does not take place, progesterone and estrogen levels fall, resulting in shedding of the uterine lining.

Progesterone is essential during pregnancy, not only ensuring normal functioning of the placenta, but passing into the developing baby's circulation, where it is converted in the adrenal glands to corticosteroid hormones.

Testosterone

Testosterone is the most important of the male sex hormones. It is responsible for stimulating bone and muscle growth, and sexual development. It is produced by the testes and in very small amounts by the ovaries. Most testosterone tests measure total testosterone.

Testosterone stimulates sperm production (spermatogenesis), and influences the development of male secondary sex characteristics. Overproduction of testosterone caused by testicular, adrenal, or **pituitary tumors** in the young male may result in precocious puberty.

Overproduction of testosterone in females, caused by ovarian and adrenal tumors, can result in masculinization, the symptoms of which include cessation of the menstrual cycle (amenorrhea) and excessive growth of body hair (**hirsutism**).

When reduced levels of testosterone in the male indicate underactivity of the testes (hypogonadism), testosterone stimulation tests may be ordered.

Preparation

The progesterone and testosterone tests require a blood sample; it is not necessary for the patient to restrict food or fluids before the test. Testosterone specimens should be drawn in the morning, as testosterone levels are highest in the early morning hours.

The estrogen fraction test can be performed on blood and/or urine. It is not necessary for the patient to restrict food or fluids for either test. If a 24-hour urine test has been requested, the patient should call the laboratory for instructions.

Risks

Risks for these blood tests are minimal, but may include slight bleeding from the puncture site, **fainting** or feeling lightheaded after having blood drawn, or blood accumulating under the puncture site (hematoma).

Normal results

Estrogen levels vary in women, ranging from 24–149 picograms per ml of blood. In men, the normal range is between 12–34 picograms per ml of blood.

Progesterone levels vary from less than 150 nanograms per deciliter (ng/dL) of blood to 2,000 nanograms in menstruating women. During pregnancy, progesterone levels range from 1,500–20,000 ng/dL of blood.

Testosterone values vary from laboratory to laboratory, but can generally be found within the following levels:

• Men. 300–1,200 ng/dL

• Women. 30–95 ng/dL

• Prepubertal children. Less than 100 ng/dL (boys), less than 40 ng/dL (girls).

Abnormal results

Increased levels of estrogen are seen in feminization syndromes:

• when a male begins to develop female secondary sex characteristics

• during precocious puberty

• when children develop secondary sexual characteristics at an abnormally early age

• because of ovarian, testicular, or adrenal tumor

• During normal pregnancy, **cirrhosis**, and increased thyroid levels (hyperthyroidism)

Decreased levels of estrogen are found in the following conditions:

• a failing pregnancy

• during **menopause**

• anorexia nervosa

• primary and secondary hypogonadism

• turner's syndrome, seen in females with one missing X chromosome

Increased levels of progesterone are seen:

• during ovulation and pregnancy

• with certain types of ovarian cysts

• with a tumor of the ovary known as a choriocarcinoma

Decreased levels of progesterone are seen:

• in toxemia of pregnancy

• with a threatened abortion

• during placental failure

• after fetal **death**

• with amenorrhea

• due to ovarian dysfunction

Increased levels (male) of testosterone are found in:

• sexual precocity

• the viral infection of encephalitis

• tumors involving the adrenal glands

• testicular tumors

• excessive thyroid production (hyperthyroidism)

• testosterone resistance syndromes.

Decreased levels (male) of testosterone are seen in:

• Klinefelter syndrome

• a chromosomal deficiency

• primary and secondary hypogonadism

• down syndrome

• surgical removal of the testicles

• cirrhosis.

Increased levels (females) of testosterone are found in ovarian and adrenal tumors and in the presence of excessive hair growth of unknown cause (hirsutism).

Resources

BOOKS

Pagana, Kathleen Deska. *Mosby's Manual of Diagnostic and Laboratory Tests*. St. Louis: Mosby, Inc., 1998.

Janis O. Flores

Sex reassignment surgery *see* **Gender reassignment surgery**

Sex therapy

Definition

Sex therapy is the treatment of **sexual dysfunction**.

Purpose

Sex therapy utilizes various techniques in order to relieve sexual dysfunction commonly caused by **premature ejaculation** or sexual **anxiety** and to improve the sexual health of the patient.

Precautions

Sexual dysfunction conjures up feelings of guilt, anger, insecurity, frustration, and rejection. Therapy is slow and requires open communication and understanding between sexual partners. Therapy may inadvertently address interpersonal communication problems.

Description

Sex therapy is conducted by a trained therapist, doctor, or psychologist. The initial sessions should cover a complete history not only of the sexual problem but of the entire relationship and each individual's background and personality. The sexual relationship should be discussed in the context of the entire relationship. In fact, sexual counseling may de-emphasize sex until other aspects of the relationship are better understood and communicated.

There are several techniques that combat sexual dysfunction and are used in sex therapy. They include:

- Semans' technique:which is used to help combat premature ejaculation with a "start-stop" approach to penis stimulation. By stimulating the man up to the point of ejaculation and then stopping, the man will become more aware of his response. More awareness leads to greater control, and open stimulation of both partners leads to greater communication and less anxiety. The start-stop technique is conducted four times until the man is allowed to ejaculate.

- Sensate focus therapy, the practice of nongenital and genital touching between partners in order to decrease sexual anxiety and build communication. First, partners explore each other's bodies without touching the genitals or breasts. Once the couple is comfortable with nongenital touching, they can expand to genital stimulation. Intercourse is prohibited in order to allow the partners to expand their intimacy and communication.

- Squeeze technique, which is used to treat premature ejaculation. When the man feels the urge to ejaculate, his partner squeezes his penis just below the head. This stops ejaculation and gives the man more control over his response.

Aftercare

Habits change slowly. All the techniques must be practiced faithfully for long periods of time to relearn behaviors. Communication is imperative.

Resources

BOOKS

Masters, William H., Virginia E. Johnson, and Robert C. Kolodny. *Heterosexuality*. New York: Harper Collins Publishers, Inc., 1994.

J. Ricker Polsdorfer, MD

Sexual abuse *see* **Rape and sexual assault**

Sexual arousal disorders *see* **Sexual dysfunction**

Sexual desire disorders *see* **Sexual dysfunction**

Sexual dysfunction

Definition

Sexual dysfunction is broadly defined as the inability to fully enjoy sexual intercourse. Specifically, sexual dysfunctions are disorders that interfere with a full sexual response cycle. These disorders make it difficult for a person to enjoy or to have sexual intercourse. While sexual dysfunction rarely threatens physical health, it can take a heavy psychological toll, bringing on depression, **anxiety**, and debilitating feelings of inadequacy.

Description

Sexual dysfunction takes different forms in men and women. A dysfunction can be life-long and always present, acquired, situational, or generalized, occurring despite the situation. A man may have a sexual problem if he:

- ejaculates before he or his partner desires

- does not ejaculate, or experiences delayed ejaculation

is unable to have an erection sufficient for pleasurable intercourse

- feels **pain** during intercourse
- lacks or loses sexual desire

A woman may have a sexual problem if she:

- lacks or loses sexual desire
- has difficulty achieving orgasm
- feels anxiety during intercourse
- feels pain during intercourse
- feels vaginal or other muscles contract involuntarily before or during sex
- has inadequate lubrication

The most common sexual dysfunctions in men include:

- **Erectile dysfunction**: an impairment of the erectile reflex. The man is unable to have or maintain an erection that is firm enough for coitus or intercourse.
- **Premature ejaculation**: rapid ejaculation with minimal sexual stimulation before, on, or shortly after penetration and before the person wishes it.
- Ejaculatory incompetence: the inability to ejaculate within the vagina despite a firm erection and relatively high levels of sexual arousal.
- Retarded ejaculation: a condition in which the bladder neck does not close off properly during orgasm so that the semen spurts backward into the bladder.

Until recently, it was presumed that women were less sexual than men. In the past two decades, traditional views of female sexuality were all but demolished, and women's sexual needs became accepted as legitimate in their own right.

Female sexual dysfunctions include:

- Sexual arousal disorder: the inhibition of the general arousal aspect of sexual response. A woman with this disorder does not lubricate, her vagina does not swell, and the muscle that surrounds the outer third of the vagina does not tighten—a series of changes that normally prepare the body for orgasm ("the orgasmic platform"). Also, in this disorder, the woman typically does not feel erotic sensations.
- Orgasmic disorder: the impairment of the orgasmic component of the female sexual response. The woman may be sexually aroused but never reach orgasm. Orgasmic capacity is less than would be reasonable for her age, sexual experience, and the adequacy of sexual stimulation she receives.

- Vaginismus: a condition in which the muscles around the outer third of the vagina have involuntary spasms in response to attempts at vaginal penetration.
- Painful intercourse: a condition that can occur at any age. Pain can appear at the start of intercourse, midway through coital activities, at the time of orgasm, or after intercourse is completed. The pain can be felt as burning, sharp searing, or cramping; it can be external, within the vagina, or deep in the pelvic region or abdomen.

Causes and symptoms

Many factors, of both physical and psychological natures, can affect sexual response and performance. Injuries, ailments, and drugs are among the physical influences; in addition, there is increasing evidence that chemicals and other environmental pollutants depress sexual function. As for psychological factors, sexual dysfunction may have roots in traumatic events such as **rape** or incest, guilt feelings, a poor self-image, depression, chronic **fatigue**, certain religious beliefs, or marital problems. Dysfunction is often associated with anxiety. If a man operates under the misconception that all sexual activity must lead to intercourse and to orgasm by his partner, and if the expectation is not met, he may consider the act a failure.

Men

With premature ejaculation, physical causes are rare, although the problem is sometimes linked to a neurological disorder, prostate infection, or **urethritis**. Possible psychological causes include anxiety (mainly performance anxiety), guilt feelings about sex, and ambivalence toward women. However, research has failed to show a direct link between premature ejaculation and anxiety. Rather, premature ejaculation seems more related to sexual inexperience in learning to modulate arousal.

When men experience painful intercourse, the cause is usually physical; an infection of the prostate, urethra, or testes, or an allergic reaction to spermicide or condoms. Painful erections may be caused by **Peyronie's disease**, fibrous plaques on the upper side of the penis that often produce a bend during erection. **Cancer** of the penis or testes and arthritis of the lower back can also cause pain.

Retrograde ejaculation occurs in men who have had prostate or urethral surgery, take medication that keeps the bladder open, or suffer from diabetes, a disease that can injure the nerves that normally close the bladder during ejaculation.

Erectile dysfunction is more likely than other dysfunctions to have a physical cause. Drugs, diabetes (the most common physical cause), Parkinson's disease, **multiple sclerosis**, and spinal cord lesions can all be causes of erectile dysfunction. When physical causes are ruled out, anxiety is the most likely psychological cause of erectile dysfunction.

Women

Dysfunctions of arousal and orgasm in women also may be physical or psychological in origin. Among the most common causes are day-to-day discord with one's partner and inadequate stimulation by the partner. Finally, sexual desire can wane as one ages, although this varies greatly from person to person.

Pain during intercourse can occur for any number of reasons, and location is sometimes a clue to the cause. Pain in the vaginal area may be due to infection, such as urethritis; also, vaginal tissues may become thinner and more sensitive during breast-feeding and after **menopause**. Deeper pain may have a pelvic source, such as **endometriosis**, pelvic **adhesions**, or uterine abnormalities. Pain can also have a psychological cause, such as fear of injury, guilt feelings about sex, fear of **pregnancy** or injury to the fetus during pregnancy, or recollection of a previous painful experience.

Vaginismus may be provoked by these psychological causes as well, or it may begin as a response to pain, and continue after the pain is gone. Both partners should understand that the vaginal contraction is an involuntary response, outside the woman's control.

Similarly, insufficient lubrication is involuntary, and may be part of a complex cycle. Low sexual response may lead to inadequate lubrication, which may lead to discomfort, and so on.

Diagnosis

In deciding when a sexual dysfunction is present, it is necessary to remember that while some people may be interested in sex at almost any time, others have low or seemingly nonexistent levels of sexual interest. Only when it is a source of personal or relationship distress, instead of voluntary choice, is it classified as a sexual dysfunction.

The first step in diagnosing a sexual dysfunction is usually discussing the problem with a doctor, who will need to ask further questions in an attempt to differentiate among the types of sexual dysfunction. The physician may also perform a physical exam of the genitals, and may order further medical tests, including measurement of hormone levels in the blood. Men may be referred to a specialist in diseases of the urinary and genital organs (urologist), and primary care physicians may refer women to a gynecologist.

Treatment

Treatments break down into two main kinds: behavioral psychotherapy and physical. **Sex therapy**, which is ideally provided by a member of the American Association of Sexual Educators, Counselors, and Therapists (AASECT), universally emphasizes correcting sexual misinformation, the importance of improved partner communication and honesty, anxiety reduction, sensual experience and pleasure, and interpersonal tolerance and acceptance. Sex therapists believe that many sexual disorders are rooted in learned patterns and values. These are termed psychogenic. An underlying assumption of sex therapy is that relatively short-term outpatient therapy can alleviate learned patterns, restrict symptoms, and allow a greater satisfaction with sexual experiences.

In some cases, a specific technique may be used during intercourse to correct a dysfunction. One of the most common is the "squeeze technique" to prevent premature ejaculation. When a man feels that an orgasm is imminent, he withdraws from his partner. Then, the man or his partner gently squeezes the head of the penis to halt the orgasm. After 20–30 seconds, the couple may resume intercourse. The couple may do this several times before the man proceeds to ejaculation.

In cases where significant sexual dysfunction is linked to a broader emotional problem, such as depression or **substance abuse**, intensive psychotherapy and/or pharmaceutical intervention may be appropriate.

In many cases, doctors may prescribe medications to treat an underlying physical cause or sexual dysfunction. Possible medical treatments include:

- clomipramine and fluoxetine for premature ejaculation
- papaverine and prostaglandin for erectile difficulties
- hormone replacement therapy for female dysfunctions
- Viagra, a pill approved in 1998 as a treatment for impotence

Alternative treatment

A variety of alternative therapies can be useful in the treatment of sexual dysfunction. Counseling or

KEY TERMS

Ejaculatory incompetence—The inability to ejaculate within the vagina.

Erectile dysfunction—Difficulty achieving or maintaining an erect penis.

Orgasmic disorder—The impairment of the ability to reach sexual climax.

Painful intercourse (dyspareunia)—Generally thought of as a female dysfunction but also affects males. Pain can occur anywhere.

Premature ejaculation—Rapid ejaculation before the person wishes it, usually in less than one to two minutes after beginning intercourse.

Retrograde ejaculation—A condition in which the semen spurts backward into the bladder.

Sexual arousal disorder—The inhibition of the general arousal aspect of sexual response.

Vaginismus—Muscles around the outer third of the vagina have involuntary spasms in response to attempts at vaginal penetration, not allowing for penetration.

psychotherapy is highly recommended to address any emotional or mental components of the disorder. Botanical medicine, either western, Chinese, or ayurvedic, as well as nutritional supplementation, can help resolve biochemical causes of sexual dysfunction. **Acupuncture** and homeopathic treatment can be helpful by focusing on the energetic aspects of the disorder.

Some problems with sexual function are normal. For example, women starting a new or first relationship may feel sore or bruised after intercourse and find that an over-the-counter lubricant makes sex more pleasurable. Simple techniques, such as soaking in a warm bath, may relax a person before intercourse and improve the experience. **Yoga** and **meditation** provide needed mental and physical relaxation for several conditions, such as vaginismus. Relaxation therapy eases and relieves anxiety about dysfunction. Massage is extremely effective at reducing **stress**, especially if performed by the partner.

Prognosis

There is no single cure for sexual dysfunctions, but almost all can be controlled. Most people who have a sexual dysfunction fare well once they get into a treatment program. For example, a high percentage of men

with premature ejaculation can be successfully treated in two to three months. Furthermore, the gains made in sex therapy tend to be long-lasting rather than short-lived.

Resources

ORGANIZATIONS

American Academy of Clinical Sexologists. 1929 18th St. NW, Suite 1166, Washington, DC 20009. (202) 462-2122.

American Association for Marriage and Family Therapy. 1133 15th St., NW Suite 300, Washington, DC 20005-2710. (202) 452-0109. < http://www.aamft.org >.

David James Doermann

Sexual perversions

Definition

Sexual perversions are conditions in which sexual excitement or orgasm is associated with acts or imagery that are considered unusual within the culture. To avoid problems associated with the stigmatization of labels, the neutral term paraphilia, derived from Greek roots meaning "alongside of" and "love," is used to describe what used to be called sexual perversions. A paraphilia is a condition in which a person's sexual arousal and gratification depend on a fantasy theme of an unusual situation or object that becomes the principal focus of sexual behavior.

Description

Paraphilias can revolve around a particular sexual object or a particular act. They are defined by *DSM-IV* as "sexual impulse disorders characterized by intensely arousing, recurrent sexual fantasies, urges and behaviors considered deviant with respect to cultural norms and that produce clinically significant distress or impairment in social, occupational or other important areas of psychosocial functioning." The nature of a paraphilia is generally specific and unchanging, and most of the paraphilias are far more common in men than in women.

Paraphilias differ from what some people might consider "normal" sexual activity in that these behaviors cause significant distress or impairment in areas of life functioning. They do not refer to the normal use of sexual fantasy, activity, or objects to heighten sexual excitement where there is no distress or impairment. The most common signs of sexual activity that can be classified as paraphilia include: the inability to resist an impulse for the sexual act, the requirement of participation by non-consenting or under-aged individuals, legal consequences, resulting sexual dysfunction, and interference with normal social relationships.

Paraphilias include fantasies, behaviors, and/or urges which:

- involve nonhuman sexual objects, such as shoes or undergarments
- require the suffering or humiliation of oneself or partner
- involve children or other non-consenting partners

The most common paraphilias are:

- exhibitionism, or exposure of the genitals
- fetishism, or the use of nonliving objects
- frotteurism, or touching and rubbing against a non-consenting person
- pedophilia, or the focus on prepubescent children
- sexual masochism, or the receiving of humiliation or suffering
- sexual sadism, or the inflicting of humiliation or suffering
- transvestic fetishism, or cross-dressing
- voyeurism, or watching others engage in undressing or sexual activity

A paraphiliac often has more than one paraphilia. Paraphilias often result in a variety of associated problems, such as guilt, depression, shame, isolation, and impairment in the capacity for normal social and sexual relationships. A paraphilia can, and often does, become highly idiosyncratic and ritualized.

Causes and symptoms

There is very little certainty about what causes a paraphilia. Psychoanalysts generally theorize that these conditions represent a regression to or a fixation at an earlier level of psychosexual development resulting in a repetitive pattern of sexual behavior that is not mature in its application and expression. In other words, an individual repeats or reverts to a sexual habit arising early in life. Another psychoanalytic theory holds that these conditions are all expressions of hostility in which sexual fantasies or unusual sexual acts become a means of obtaining revenge for a childhood trauma. The persistent, repetitive nature of the paraphilia is caused by an inability to erase the underlying trauma completely. Indeed, a history of childhood sexual **abuse** is sometimes seen in individuals with paraphilias.

However, behaviorists suggest, instead, that the paraphilia begins via a process of conditioning. Nonsexual objects can become sexually arousing if they are frequently and repeatedly associated with a pleasurable sexual activity. The development of a paraphilia is not usually a matter of conditioning alone; there must usually be some predisposing factor, such as difficulty forming person-to-person sexual relationships or poor self-esteem.

The following are situations or causes that might lead someone in a paraphiliac direction:

- parents who humiliate and punish a small boy for strutting around with an erect penis
- a young boy who is sexually abused
- an individual who is dressed in a woman's clothes as a form of parental punishment
- fear of sexual performance or intimacy
- inadequate counseling
- excessive alcohol intake
- physiological problems
- sociocultural factors
- psychosexual trauma

Diagnosis

Whatever the cause, paraphiliacs apparently rarely seek treatment unless they are induced into it by an arrest or discovery by a family member. This makes diagnosis before a confrontation very difficult.

Paraphiliacs may select an occupation, or develop a hobby or volunteer work, that puts them in contact with the desired erotic stimuli, for example, selling women's shoes or lingerie in fetishism, or working with children in pedophilia. Other coexistent problems may be alcohol or drug abuse, intimacy problems, and personality disturbances, especially emotional immaturity. Additionally, there may be sexual dysfunctions. **Erectile dysfunction** and an inability to ejaculate may be common in attempts at sexual activity without the paraphiliac theme.

Paraphilias may be mild, moderate, or severe. An individual with mild paraphilia is markedly distressed by the recurrent paraphiliac urges but has never acted on them. The moderate has occasionally acted on the paraphilic urge. A severe paraphiliac has repeatedly acted on the urge.

Treatment

The literature describing treatment is fragmentary and incomplete. Traditional **psychoanalysis** has not been particularly effective with paraphilia and generally requires several years of treatment. Therapy with hypnosis has also had poor results. Current interests focus primarily on several behavioral techniques that include the following:

- Aversion imagery involves the pairing of a sexually arousing paraphilic stimulus with an unpleasant image, such as being arrested or having one's name appear in the newspaper.

- Desensitization procedures neutralize the anxiety-provoking aspects of nonparaphilic sexual situations and behavior by a process of gradual exposure. For example, a man afraid of having sexual contact with women his own age might be led through a series of relaxation procedures aimed at reducing his **anxiety**.

- Social skills training is used with either of the other approaches and is aimed at improving a person's ability to form interpersonal relationships.

- Orgasmic reconditioning may instruct a person to masturbate using his paraphilia fantasy and to switch to a more appropriate fantasy just at the moment of orgasm.

In addition to these therapies, drugs are sometimes prescribed to treat paraphilic behaviors. Drugs that drastically lower testosterone temporarily (anti-androgens) have been used for the control of repetitive deviant sexual behaviors and have been prescribed for paraphilia-related disorders as well. Cyproterone acetate inhibits testosterone directly at androgen receptor sites. In its oral form, the usual prescribed dosage range is 50–200 mg per day.

Serotonergics (drugs that boost levels of the brain chemical serotonin) are prescribed for anxious and depressive symptoms. Of the serotonergic agents reported, fluoxetine has received the most attention, although lithium, clomipramine, buspirone, and sertraline are reported as effective in case reports and open clinical trials with outpatients. Other alternative augmentation strategies that may be effective include adding a low dose of a secondary amine tricyclic antidepressant to the primary serotonergics, but these reports are only anecdotal.

Prognosis

Despite more than a decade of experience with psychotherapeutic treatment programs, most workers in the field are not convinced that they have a high degree of success. Furthermore, because some cases involve severe abuse, many in the general public would prefer to "lock up" the sex offender than to have him out in the community in a treatment program or on parole after the treatment program has been completed.

Paraphilia and paraphilia-related disorders are more prevalent than most clinicians suspect. Since these disorders are cloaked in shame and guilt, the presence of these conditions may not be adequately revealed until a therapeutic alliance is firmly established. Once a diagnosis is established, appropriate education about possible behavioral therapies and appropriate use of psychopharmacological agents can improve the prognosis for these conditions.

Resources

ORGANIZATIONS

American Academy of Clinical Sexologists. 1929 18th St., N.W., Suite 1166, Washington, DC 20009. (202) 462-2122.

American Association for Marriage and Family Therapy. 1133 15th St., NW Suite 300, Washington, DC 20005-2710. (202) 452-0109. < http://www.aamft.org >.

David James Doermann

KEY TERMS

Exhibitionism—Obtaining sexual arousal by exposing genitals to an unsuspecting stranger.

Fetishism—Obtaining sexual arousal using or thinking about an inanimate object or part of the body.

Frotteurism—Obtaining sexual arousal and gratification by rubbing one's genitals against others in public places.

Masochism—Sexual arousal by having pain and/or humiliation inflicted upon oneself.

Pedophilia—Sex or sexual activity with children who have not reached puberty.

Sadism—Sexual arousal through inflicting pain on another person.

Transvestitism—Sexual arousal from dressing in the clothes of the opposite sex.

Voyeurism—Sexual arousal by observing nude individuals without their knowledge.

Sexually transmitted diseases

Definition

Sexually transmitted disease (STD) is a term used to describe more than 20 different infections that are transmitted through exchange of semen, blood, and other body fluids; or by direct contact with the affected body areas of people with STDs. Sexually transmitted diseases are also called venereal diseases.

Description

The Centers for Disease Control and Prevention (CDC) has reported that 85% of the most prevalent infectious diseases in the United States are sexually transmitted. The rate of STDs in this country is 50 to 100 times higher than that of any other industrialized nation. One in four sexually active Americans will be affected by an STD at some time in his or her life.

About 12 million new STD infections occur in the United States each year. One in four occurs in someone between the ages of 16 and 19. Almost 65% of all STD infections affect people under the age of 25.

Types of STDs

STDs can have very painful long-term consequences as well as immediate health problems. They can cause:

- birth defects
- blindness
- bone deformities
- brain damage
- cancer
- heart disease
- infertility and other abnormalities of the reproductive system
- mental retardation
- **death**

Some of the most common and potentially serious STDs in the United States include:

- Chlamydia. This STD is caused by the bacterium *Chlamydia trachomatis*, a microscopic organism that lives as a parasite inside human cells. Although over 526,000 cases of chlamydia were reported in the United States in 1997, the CDC estimates that nearly three million cases occur annually because 75% of women and 50% of men show no symptoms of the disease after infection. Approximately 40% of women will develop **pelvic inflammatory disease** (PID) as a result of chlamydia infection, a leading cause of infertility.

- Human papillomavirus (HPV). HPV causes **genital warts** and is the single most important risk factor for **cervical cancer** in women. Over 100 types of HPV exist, but only about 30 of them can cause genital **warts** and are spread through sexual contact. In some instances, warts are passed from mother to child during **childbirth**, leading to a potentially life-threatening condition for newborns in which warts develop in the throat (laryngeal papillomatosis).

- **Genital herpes**. Herpes is an incurable viral infection thought to be one of the most common STDs in this country. It is caused by one of two types of herpes simplex viruses: HSV-1 (commonly causing oral herpes) or HSV-2 (usually causing genital herpes). The CDC estimates that 45 million Americans (one out of every five individuals 12 years of age or older) are infected with HSV-2; this number has increased 30% since the 1970s. HSV-2 infection is more common in women (one out of every four women) than men (one out of every five men) and in African Americans (45.9%) than Caucasians (17.6%).

- **Gonorrhea**. The bacterium *Neisseria gonorrhoeae* is the causative agent of gonorrhea and can be spread by vaginal, oral, or anal contact. The CDC reports that approximately 650,000 individuals are infected with gonorrhea each year in the United States, with 132.2 infections per 100,000 individuals occurring in 1999. Approximately 75% of American gonorrhea infections occur in persons aged 15 to 29 years old. In 1999, 75% of reported gonorrhea cases occurred among African Americans.

- **Syphilis**. Syphilis is a potentially life-threatening infection that increases the likelihood of acquiring or transmitting HIV. In 1998, the CDC reported approximately 38,000 cases of syphilis in the United States; this included 800 cases of congenital syphilis. Congenital syphilis causes irreversible health problems or death in as many as 40% of all live babies born to women with untreated syphilis.

- Human immunodeficiencyvirus (HIV) infection. In 2000, the CDC reported that 120,223 people in the United States are HIV-positive and 426,350 are living with **AIDS**. In addition, approximately 1,000-2,000 children are born each year with HIV infection. It is also estimated that 33 million adults and 1.3 million children worldwide were living with HIV/AIDS as of 1999 with 5.4 million being newly infected that year. There is no cure for this STD.

Drugs Used To Treat STDS	
Brand Name (Generic Name)	**Possible Common Side Effects Include:**
Achromycin V (tetracyline hydrochloride)	Blurred vision, headache, dizziness, rash, hives, appetite loss, nausea and vomiting
Amoxil (amoxicillin)	Behaviorial changes, diarrhea, hives, nausea and vomiting
Ceftin (cerfuroxime axetil)	Nausea and vomiting, diarrhea, irritated skin
Doryx (doxycycline hyclate)	Itching (genital and/or rectal), nausea and vomiting, appetite loss, diarrhea, swelling
E.E.S., E-Mycin, ERYC, Ery-Tab, Erythrocin, Ilosone (erthromycin)	Diarrhea, nausea and vomiting, appetite loss, abdominal pain
Flagyl (metronidazole)	Numbness, tingling sensation in extremities, seizures
Floxin (ofloxacin)	Genital itching, nausea and vomiting, headache, diarrhea, dizziness
Minocin (minocycline hydrochloride)	Blurred vision, anemia, hives, rash, throat irritation
Noroxin (norfloxacin)	Headache, nausea, dizziness
Omnipen (ampicillin)	Itching, rash, hives, peeling skin, nausea and vomiting
Penetrex (enoxacin)	Nausea and vomiting
Zithromax (azithromycin)	Nausea and vomiting, diarrhea, abdominal pain
Zovirax (acyclovir)	Fluid retention, headache, rash, tingling sensation

Social groups and STDs

STDs affect certain population groups more severely than others. Women, young people, and members of minority groups are particularly affected. Women in any age bracket are more likely than men to develop medical complications related to STDs. With respect to racial and ethnic categories, the incidence of syphilis is 60 times higher among African Americans than among Caucasians, and four times higher in Hispanics than in Anglos. According to the CDC, in 1999 African Americans accounted for 77% of the total number of gonorrhea cases and nearly 46% of all genital herpes cases.

Causes and symptoms

The symptoms of STDs vary somewhat according to the disease agent (virus or bacterium), the sex of the patient, and the body systems affected. The symptoms of some STDs are easy to identify; others produce infections that may either go unnoticed for some time or are easy to confuse with other diseases.

Syphilis in particular can be confused with disorders ranging from **infectious mononucleosis** to allergic reactions to prescription medications. In addition, the incubation period of STDs varies. Some produce symptoms close enough to the time of sexual contact—often less than 48 hours later%mdash;for the patient to recognize the connection between the behavior and the symptoms. Others have a longer incubation period, so that the patient may not recognize the early symptoms as those of a sexually transmitted infection.

Some symptoms of STDs affect the genitals and reproductive organs:

- A woman who has an STD may bleed when she is not menstruating or has abnormal vaginal discharge. Vaginal burning, **itching**, and odor are common, and she may experience **pain** in her pelvic area while having sex

- A discharge from the tip of the penis may be a sign that a man has an STD. Males may also have painful or burning sensations when they urinate.

- There may be swelling of the lymph nodes near the groin area.

- Both men and women may develop skin **rashes**, sores, bumps, or blisters near the mouth or genitals. Homosexual men frequently develop these symptoms in the area around the anus.

Other symptoms of STDs are systemic, which means that they affect the body as a whole. These symptoms may include:

- fever, chills, and similar flu-like symptoms
- skin rashes over large parts of the body
- arthritis-like pains or aching in the joints
- throat swelling and redness that lasts for three weeks or longer

Diagnosis

A sexually active person who has symptoms of an STD or who has had an STD or symptoms of infection should be examined without delay by one of the following health care professionals:

- a specialist in **women's health** (gynecologist)
- a specialist in disorders of the urinary tract and the male sexual organs (urologist)
- a family physician
- a nurse practitioner
- a specialist in skin disorders (dermatologist).

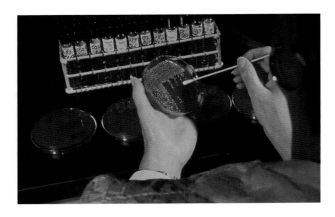

Cultures on agar plates. *(Photograph by T. McCarthy, Custom Medical Stock Photo. Reproduced by permission.)*

The diagnostic process begins with a thorough **physical examination** and a detailed medical history that documents the patient's sexual history and assesses the risk of infection.

The doctor or other healthcare professional will:

- Describe the testing process. This includes all blood tests and other tests that may be relevant to the specific infection.

- Explain the meaning of the test results.

- Provide the patient with information regarding high-risk behaviors and any necessary treatments or procedures.

The doctor may suggest that a patient diagnosed with one STD be tested for others, as its possible to have more than one STD at a time. One infection may hide the symptoms of another or create a climate that fosters its growth. At present, it is particularly important that persons who are HIV-positive be tested for syphilis as well.

Notification

The law in most parts of the United States requires public health officials to trace and contact the partners of persons with STDs. Minors, however, can get treatment without their parents' permission. Public health departments in most states can provide information about STD clinic locations; Planned Parenthood facilities provide testing and counseling. These agencies can also help with or assume the responsibility of notifying sexual partners who must be tested and may require treatment.

Treatment

Although self-care can relieve some of the pain of genital herpes or genital warts that has recurred after

being diagnosed and treated by a physician, other STD symptoms require immediate medical attention.

Antibiotics are prescribed to treat gonorrhea, chlamydia, syphilis, and other STDs caused by bacteria. Although prompt diagnosis and early treatment almost always cures these STDs, new infections can develop if exposure continues or is renewed. Viral infections can be treated symptomatically with antiviral medications.

Prognosis

The prognosis for recovery from STDs varies among the different diseases. The prognosis for recovery from gonorrhea, syphilis, and other STDs caused by bacteria is generally good, provided that the disease is diagnosed early and treated promptly. Untreated syphilis in particular can lead to long-term complications and disability. Viral STDs (genital herpes, genital warts, HIV) cannot be cured but must be treated on a long-term basis to relieve symptoms and prevent life-threatening complications.

Prevention

Vaccines

Vaccines for the prevention of **hepatitis A** and **hepatitis B** are currently recommended for gay and bisexual men, users of illegal drugs, health care workers, and others at risk of contracting these diseases. Vaccines to prevent other STDs are being tested and may be available within several years.

Lifestyle choices

The risk of becoming infected with an STD can be reduced or eliminated by changing certain personal behaviors. Abstaining from sexual relations or maintaining a mutually monogamous relationship with a partner are legitimate options. It is also wise to avoid sexual contact with partners who are known to be infected with an STD, whose health status is unknown, who **abuse** drugs, or who are involved in prostitution.

Use of condoms and other contraceptives

Men or women who have sex with a partner of known (or unsure) infection should make sure a new **condom** is used every time they have genital, oral, or anal contact. Used correctly and consistently, male condoms provide good protection against HIV and other STDs such as gonorrhea, chlamydia, and syphilis. Female condoms (lubricated sheaths inserted into

Chlamydia—A microorganism that resembles certain types of bacteria and causes several sexually transmitted diseases in humans.

Condom—A thin sheath worn over the penis during sexual intercourse to prevent pregnancy or the transmission of STDs. There are also female condoms.

Diaphragm—A dome-shaped device used to cover the back of a woman's vagina during intercourse in order to prevent pregnancy.

Pelvic inflammatory disease (PID)—An inflammation of the tubes leading from a woman's ovaries to the uterus (the Fallopian tubes), caused by a bacterial infection. PID is a leading cause of fertility problems in women.

Venereal disease—Another term for sexually transmitted disease.

the vagina) have also been shown to be effective in preventing HIV and other STDs. Condoms provide a measure of protection against genital herpes, genital warts, and hepatitis B.

Spermicides and diaphragms can decrease the risk of transmission of some STDs. They do not protect women from contracting HIV. Birth-control pills, patches, or injections do not prevent STDs. Neither do surgical sterilization or **hysterectomy**.

Hygienic measures

Urinating and washing the genital area with soap and water immediately after having sex may eliminate some germs before they cause infection. Douching, however, can spread infection deeper into the womb. It may also increase a woman's risk of developing pelvic inflammatory disease (PID).

Resources

ORGANIZATIONS

National STD Hotline. (800)227-8922.
Planned Parenthood Federation of America. (800)230-7526. < http://www.planned parenthood.org >.

OTHER

Sexually Transmitted Diseases. March 24, 2001. < http://www.cdc.gov/nchstp/dstd/dstdp.html >.

Maureen Haggerty

Sexually transmitted diseases cultures

Definition

Sexually transmitted diseases are infections spread from person to person through sexual contact. A culture is a test in which a laboratory attempts to grow and identify the microorganism causing an infection.

Purpose

Sexually transmitted diseases (STDs) produce symptoms such as genital discharge, **pain** during urination, bleeding, pelvic pain, skin ulcers, or **urethritis**. Often, however, they produce no immediate symptoms. Therefore, the decision to test for these diseases must be based not only the presence of symptoms, but on whether or not a person is at risk of having one or more of the diseases. Activities, such as drug use and sex with more than one partner, put a person at high risk for these diseases.

STD cultures are necessary to diagnose certain types of STDs. Only after the infection is diagnosed can it be treated and further spread of the infection prevented. Left untreated, consequences of these diseases range from discomfort to **infertility** to **death**. In addition, these diseases, if present in a pregnant woman, can be passed from mother to fetus.

Description

Gonorrhea, **syphilis**, chlamydia, **chancroid**, herpes, human papillomavirus, human **immunodeficiency** virus (HIV), and mycoplasma are common sexually transmitted diseases. Not all are diagnosed with a culture. For those that are, a sample of material is taken from the infection site, placed in a sterile container, and sent to the laboratory.

Bacterial cultures

In the laboratory, a portion of material from the infection site is spread over the surface of several different types of culture plates and placed in an incubator at body temperature for one to two days. Bacteria present in the sample will multiply and appear on the plates as visible colonies. They are identified by the appearance of their colonies and by the results of biochemical tests and a gram stain. The Gram stain is done by smearing part of a colony onto a microscope slide. After it dries, the slide is stained with purple and red stains, then examined under a microscope. The color of stain picked up by the bacteria (purple or red), the shape (such as round or rectangle), and the size provide valuable clues as to the identity and which **antibiotics** might work best. Bacteria that stain purple are called Gram-positive; those that stain red are called gram-negative.

The result of the gram stain is available the same day or in less than an hour if requested by the physician. An early report, known as a preliminary report, is usually available after one day. This report will tell if any microorganisms have been found yet, and if so, their Gram stain appearance—for example, a Gram-negative rod or a gram-positive cocci. The final report, usually available in one to seven days, includes complete identification and an estimate of the quantity of the microorganisms isolated.

A sensitivity test, also called antibiotic susceptibility test, commonly done on bacteria isolated from an infection site, is not always done on bacteria isolated from a sexually transmitted disease. These bacteria often are treated using antibiotics that are part of a standard treatment protocol.

GONORRHEA. *Neisseria gonorrhoeae*, also called gonococcus or GC, causes gonorrhea. It infects the surfaces of the genitourinary tract, primarily the urethra in males and the cervix in females. On a gram stain done on material taken from an infection site, the bacteria appear as small gram-negative diplococci (pairs of round bacteria) inside white blood cells. *Neisseria gonorrhoeae* grows on a special culture plate called Thayer-Martin (TM) media in an environment with low levels of oxygen and high levels of carbon dioxide.

The best specimen from which to culture *Neisseria gonorrhoeae* is a swab of the urethra in a male or the cervix in a female. Other possible specimens include vagina, body fluid discharge, swab of genital lesion, or the first urine of the day. Final results usually are available after two days. Rapid nonculture tests are available to test for GC and provide results on the same or following day.

CHANCROID. Chancroid is caused by *Haemophilus ducreyi*. It is characterized by genital ulcers with nearby swollen lymph nodes. The specimen is collected by swabbing one of these pus-filled ulcers. The gram stain may not be helpful as this bacteria looks just like other Haemophilus bacteria. This bacteria only grows on special culture plates, so the physician must request a specific culture for a person who has symptoms of chancroid. Even using special culture plates, *Haemophilus ducreyi* is isolated from less than 80% of the ulcers it infects. If a culture is negative, the physician must diagnose chancroid based on the person's symptoms and by ruling out other possible causes of these symptoms, such as syphilis.

MYCOPLASMA. Three types of mycoplasma organisms cause sexually transmitted urethritis in males and **pelvic inflammatory disease** and **cervicitis** in females: *Mycoplasma hominis*, *Mycoplasma gentialium*, and *Ureaplasma urealyticum*. These organisms require special culture plates and may take up to six days to grow. Samples are collected from the cervix in a female, the urethra or semen in a male, or urine.

SYPHILIS. Syphilis is caused by *Treponema pallidum*, one in a group of bacteria called spirochetes. It causes ulcers or chancres at the site of infection. The organism does not grow in culture. Using special techniques and stains, it is identified by looking at a sample of the ulcer or chancre under the microscope. Various blood tests also may be done to detect the treponema organism.

CHLAMYDIA. Chlamydia is caused by the gram-negative baterium *Chlamydia trachomatis*. It is one of the most common STDs in the United States and generally appears in sexually active adolescents and young adults. While chlamydia often does not have any initial symptoms, it can, if left untreated, lead to pelvic inflammatory disease and sterility. Samples are collected from one or more of these infection sites: cervix in a female, urethra in a male, or the rectum. A portion of specimen is combined with a specific type of cell and allowed to incubate. Special stains are performed on the cultured cells, looking for evidence of the chlamydia organism within the cells. A swab can also be taken from the woman's vulva. Men and women can now be screened for Chlamydia with a urine sample. Urine-based screening has increased screening significantly, especially among men.

Viral cultures

To culture or grow a virus in the laboratory, a portion of specimen is mixed with commercially prepared animal cells in a test tube. Characteristic changes to the cells caused by the growing virus help identify the virus. The time to complete a viral culture varies with the type of virus. It may take several days or up to several weeks.

HERPES VIRUS. Herpes simplex virus type 2 is the cause of **genital herpes**. Diagnosis is usually made based on the person's symptoms. If a diagnosis needs confirmation, a viral culture is performed using material taken from an ulcer. A Tzanck smear is a microscope test that can rapidly detect signs of herpes infection in cells taken from an ulcer. The culture takes up to 14 days. In 2004, the FDA approved a blood test to detect the antibodies to herpes virus.

HUMAN PAPILLOMAVIRUS. Human papilloma-virus causes **genital warts**. This virus will not grow in culture; the diagnosis is based on the appearance of the **warts** and the person's symptoms. In late 2003, the U.S. Food and Drug Administration (FDA) approved a human papillomavirus (HPV) DNA test with a Pap smear for screening women age 30 and older. The combined test would help physicians determine which women were at extremely low risk for **cervical cancer** and which should be more closely monitored.

HIV. Human immunodeficiency virus (HIV) is usually diagnosed with a blood test. Cultures for HIV are possible, but rarely needed for diagnosis. However, newer rapid tests were developed in 2003 and approved by the FDA in 2004. These tests are cheaper and can deliver results in as little as three minutes. The FDA also approved an HIV test in 2004 that can detect HIV in saliva.

Preparation

Generally, the type of specimen depends on the type of infection. Cultures always should be collected before the person begins taking antibiotics. After collection of these specimens, each is placed into a sterile tube containing a liquid in which the organism can survive while in route to the laboratory. The new rapid HIV tests rely on blood samples collected from a finger stick or vein or on saliva collected from the mouth. Initial results are not sent to a lab but are processed onsite.

Urethral specimen

Men should not urinate one hour before collection of a urethral specimen. The physician inserts a sterile, cotton-tipped swab into the urethra.

Cervical specimen

Women should not douche or take a bath within 24 hours of collection of a cervical or vaginal culture. The physician inserts a moistened, nonlubricated vaginal speculum. After the cervix is exposed, the physician removes the cervical mucus using a cotton ball. Next, he or she inserts a sterile cotton-tipped swab into the endocervical canal and rotates the swab with firm pressure for about 30 seconds.

Vaginal specimen

Women should not douche or take a bath within 24 hours of collection of a cervical or vaginal culture.

KEY TERMS

Culture—A laboratory test done to grow and identify microorganisms causing infection.

Gram stain—Microsopic examination of a portion of a bacterial colony or sample from an infection site after it has been stained by special stains. Certain bacteria pick up the purple stain; these bacteria are called gram positive. Other bacteria pick up the red stain; these bacteria are called gram negative. The color of the bacteria, in addition to their size and shape, provide clues as to the identity of the bacteria.

Sensitivity test—A test that determines which antibiotics will kill the bacteria isolated from a culture.

Vulva—The external part of the woman's genital organs, including the vaginal vestibule.

The physician inserts a sterile, cotton-tipped swab into the vagina.

Anal specimen

The physician inserts a sterile, cotton-tipped swab about 1 inch into the anus and rotates the swab for 30 seconds. Stool must not contaminate the swab.

Oropharynx (throat) specimen

The person's tongue is held down with a tongue depressor, as a healthcare worker moves a sterile, cotton-tipped swab across the back of the throat and tonsil region.

Urine specimen

To collect a "clean-catch" urine, the person first washes the perineum, and the penis or labia and vulva. He or she begins urinating, letting the first portion pass into the toilet, then collecting the remainder into a sterile container.

Normal results

These microorganisms are not found in a normal culture. Many types of microorganisms, normally found on a person's skin and in the genitourinary tract, may contaminate the culture. If a mixture of these microorganisms grow in the culture, they are reported as normal flora.

Abnormal results

If a person has a positive culture for one or more of these microorganisms, treatment is started and his or her sexual partners should be notified and tested. Certain laws govern reporting and partner notification of various STDs. After treatment is completed, the person's physician may want a follow-up culture to confirm the infection is gone.

Resources

PERIODICALS

"Answer Back: Is there a Vulval Swwab Test for Chlamydia?" *Pulse* September 13, 2004: 100.

"Approval Sought for HIV-1 Test that Detects Antibodies in Oral Fluid or Plasma." *AIDS Weekly* October 27, 2003: 23.

Boschert, Sherry. "Chlaymdia Urine Test: Males Still Underscreened: Noninvasive Screening Test." *Pediatric News* August 2004: 10–12.

"FDA Approves DNAwithPap for Screening Women (Greater than or Equal to) Age 30)." *Contemporary OB/Gyn* October 2003: 105.

"FDA Approves OraQuick HIV-1/2 Test to Detect HIV-2 in Oral Fluid." *Biotech Week* July 21, 2004: 401.

Kaye, Donald. "FDA Approves Herpes Antibody Test." *Clinical Infectious Diseases* September 15, 2004: 1.

"New HIV Rapid Test Is 100 Percent Accurate." *Health & Medicine Week* September 15, 2003: 194.

"New Three-minute Rapid HIV Test Launched in the United States." *Medical Devices & Surgical Technology Week* September 12, 2004: 102.

"One-step HIV Test May Be Cheaper, Faster, Less Wasteful." *Medical Letter on the CDC & FDA* October 5, 2003: 5.

St. Lawrence, Janet S., et al. "STD Screening, Testing, Case Reporting, and Clinical and Partner Notification Practices: A National Survey of U.S. Physicians." *The American Journal of Public Health* November 2002: 1784.

ORGANIZATIONS

American Social Health Association. PO Box 13827, Research Triangle Park, NC 27709. (800) 227-8922. < http://sunsite.unc.edu/ASHA >.

Centers for Disease Control and Prevention. National Center for HIV, STD, and TB Prevention. 1600 Clifton Road NE, Atlanta, GA 30333. (404) 639-8000. < http://www.cdc.gov/nchstp/od/nchstp.html >.

Nancy J. Nordenson
Teresa G. Odle

SGOT *see* **Aspartate aminotransferase test**

Shaken baby syndrome

Definition

Shaken baby syndrome (SBS) is a collective term for the internal head injuries a baby or young child sustains from being violently shaken.

Description

Shaken baby syndrome was first described in medical literature in 1972. Physicians earlier labeled these injuries as accidental, but as more about child abuse became known, more cases of this syndrome were properly diagnosed.

Every year, nearly 50,000 children in the United States are forcefully shaken by their caretakers. More than 60% of these children are boys. The victims are on average six to eight months old, but may be as old as five years or as young as a few days.

Men are more likely than women to shake a child; typically, these men are in their early 20s and are the baby's father or the mother's boyfriend. Women who inflict SBS are more likely to be baby-sitters or child care providers than the baby's mother. The shaking may occur as a response of frustration to the baby's inconsolable crying or as an action of routine **abuse**.

Causes and symptoms

Infants and small children are especially vulnerable to SBS because their neck muscles are still too weak to adequately support their disproportionately large heads, and their young brain tissue and blood vessels are extremely fragile. When an infant is vigorously shaken by the arms, legs, shoulders, or chest, the **whiplash** motion repeatedly jars the baby's brain with tremendous force, causing internal damage and bleeding. While there may be no obvious external signs of injury following shaking, the child may suffer internally from brain bleeding and bruising (called subdural hemorrhage and hematoma); brain swelling and damage (called cerebral **edema**); mental retardation; blindness, **hearing loss**, **paralysis**, speech impairment, and learning disabilities; and **death**. Nearly 2,000 children die every year as a result of being shaken.

Physicians may have difficulty initially diagnosing SBS because there are usually few witnesses to give a reliable account of the events leading to the trauma, few if any external injuries, and, upon close examination, the physical findings may not agree with the account given. A shaken baby may present one or

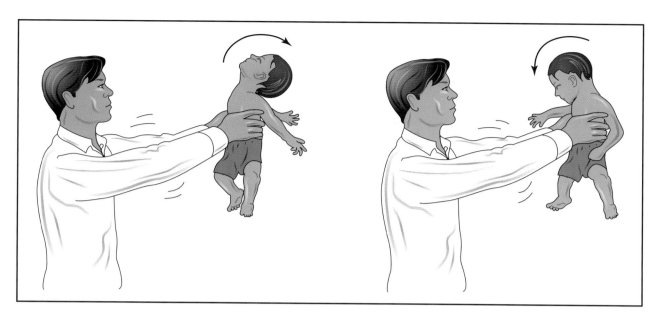

Shaken baby syndrome is a collective term for the internal head injuries a baby or young child sustains from being violently shaken. Because of the fragile state of an infant's brain tissue and blood vessels, when a baby is vigorously shaken by the chest, as shown in the illustration above, the whiplash motion repeatedly jars the baby's brain with extreme force, causing serious internal damage and bleeding. Nearly 2,000 American children die annually from this condition. *(Illustration by Electronic Illustrators Group.)*

more signs, including **vomiting**; difficulty breathing, sucking, swallowing, or making sounds; seizures; and altered consciousness.

Diagnosis

To diagnose SBS, physicians look for at least one of three classic conditions: bleeding at the back of one or both eyes (**retinal hemorrhage**), subdural hematoma, and cerebral edema. The diagnosis is confirmed by the results of either a computed tomography scan (CT scan) or magnetic resonance imaging (MRI).

Treatment

Appropriate treatment is determined by the type and severity of the trauma. Physicians may medically manage both internal and external injuries. Behavioral and educational impairments as a result of the injuries require the attention of additional specialists. Children with SBS may need physical therapy, speech therapy, vision therapy, and special education services.

Alternative treatment

There is no alternative to prompt medical treatment. An unresponsive child should never be put

---

KEY TERMS

Cerebral edema—Fluid collecting in the brain, causing tissue to swell.

Hematoma—A localized accumulation of blood in tissues as a result of hemorrhaging.

Hemorrhage—A condition of bleeding, usually severe.

Retinal hemorrhage—Bleeding of the retina, a key structure in vision located at the back of the eye.

Subdural hematoma—A localized accumulation of blood, sometimes mixed with spinal fluid, in the space of the brain beneath the membrane covering called the dura mater.

---

to bed, but must be taken to a hospital for immediate care.

Prognosis

Sadly, children who receive violent shaking have a poor prognosis for complete recovery. Those who do not die may experience permanent blindness, **mental retardation**, seizure disorders, or loss of motor control.

Prevention

Shaken baby syndrome is preventable with public education. Adults must be actively taught that shaking a child is never acceptable and can cause severe injury or death.

When the frustration from an incessantly crying baby becomes too much, caregivers should have a strategy for coping that does not harm the baby. The first step is to place the baby in a crib or playpen and leave the room in order to calm down. Counting to 10 and taking deep breaths may help. A friend or relative may be called to come over and assist. A calm adult may then resume trying to comfort the baby. A warm bottle, a dry diaper, soft music, a bath, or a ride in a swing, stroller, or car may be offered to soothe a crying child. Crying may also indicate **pain** or illness, such as from abdominal cramps or an earache. If the crying persists, the child should be seen by a physician.

Resources

ORGANIZATIONS

American Humane Association, Children's Division. 63 Inverness Drive East, Englewood, CO 80112-5117. (800) 227-4645. < www.americanhumane.org >.

Child Abuse Prevention Center of Utah. 2955 Harrison Boulevard, #102, Ogden, UT 84403. (888) 273-0071.

National Center on Shaken Baby Syndrome. 2955 Harrison Blvd., #102, Ogden, UT 84403. (801) 627-3399. < http://www.dontshake.com >.

Bethany Thivierge

Shiatsu

Definition

Shiatsu is a manipulative therapy developed in Japan and incorporating techniques of *anma* (Japanese traditional massage), **acupressure**, stretching, and Western massage. Shiatsu involves applying pressure to special points or areas on the body in order to maintain physical and mental well being, treat disease, or alleviate discomfort. This therapy is considered holistic because it attempts to treat the whole person instead of a specific medical complaint. All types of acupressure generally focus on the same pressure points and so-called energy pathways, but may differ in terms of massage technique. Shiatsu, which can be translated as finger pressure, has been described as needle-free **acupuncture**.

Purpose

Shiatsu has a strong reputation for reducing **stress** and relieving **nausea and vomiting**. Shiatsu is also believed to improve circulation and boost the immune system. Some people use it to treat **diarrhea**, **indigestion**, **constipation**, and other disorders of the gastrointestinal tract; menstrual and menopausal problems; chronic **pain**; migraine; arthritis; **toothache**; **anxiety**; and depression. Shiatsu can be used to relieve muscular pain or tension, especially neck and back pain. It also appears to have sedative effects and may alleviate **insomnia**. In a broader sense, shiatsu is believed to enhance physical vitality and emotional well being.

Description

Origins

Shiatsu is an offshoot of anma that developed during the period after the Meiji Restoration in 1868. Traditional massage (anma) used during the age of shoguns was being criticized, and practitioners of *koho anma* (ancient way) displeased with it introduced new practices and new names for their therapies.

During the twentieth century, shiatsu distinguished itself from anma through the merging of Western knowledge of anatomy, koho anma, *ampuku* (abdominal massage), acupressure, *Do-In* (breathing practices), and Buddhism. Based on the work of Tamai Tempaku, shiatsu established itself in Japan and worldwide. The Shiatsu Therapists Association was founded in 1925 and clinics and schools followed. Students of Tempaku began teaching their own brand of shiatsu, creating branch disciplines. By 1955, the Japanese Ministry of Health and Welfare acknowledged shiatsu as a beneficial treatment, and licensing was established for practitioners.

Shiatsu and other forms of Japanese acupressure are based on the concept of *ki*, the Japanese term for the all-pervading energy that flows through everything in the universe. (This notion is borrowed from the Chinese, who refer to the omnipresent energy as qi or chi.) Ki tends to flow through the body along special energy pathways called meridians, each of which is associated with a vital organ. In Asian systems of traditional medicine, diseases are often believed to occur due to disruptions in the flow this energy through the body. These disruptions may stem from emotional factors, climate, or a host of other causes including stress, the presence of impurities in the body, and physical trauma.

The aim of shiatsu is to restore the proper flow of bodily energy by massaging the surface of the skin along the meridian lines. Pressure may also be applied to any of the 600 or so acupoints. Acupoints, which are supposedly located just under the skin along the meridians, are tiny energy structures that affect the flow of ki through the body. When ki either stagnates and becomes deflected or accumulates in excess along one of these channels, stimulation to the acupoints, which are sensitive to pressure, can unblock and regulate the ki flow through toning or sedating treatment.

Western medicine has not proven the existence of meridians and acupoints. However, in one study, two French medical doctors conducted an experiment at Necher Hospital in Paris to test validity of the theory that energy is being transported along acupuncture meridians. They injected and traced isotpes with gamma-camera imaging. The meridians may actually correspond to nerve transmission lines. In this view, shiatsu and other forms of healing massage may trigger the emission of naturally occurring chemicals called neurotransmitters. Release of these chemical messengers may be responsible for some of the therapeutic effects associated with shiatsu, such as pain relief.

Preparations

People usually receive shiatsu therapy while lying on a floor mat or massage table or sitting up. The massage is performed through the clothing—preferably a thin garment made from natural fibers—and disrobing is not required. Pressure is often applied using the thumbs, though various other parts of the body may be employed, including fingertips, palms, knuckles, elbows, and knees—some therapists even use their feet. Shiatsu typically consists of sustained pressure (lasting up to 10 seconds at a time), squeezing, and stretching exercises. It may also involve gentle holding as well as rocking motions. A treatment session lasts anywhere from 30 to 90 minutes.

Before shiatsu treatment begins, the therapist usually performs a general health assessment. This involves taking a family medical history and discussing the physical and emotional health of the person seeking therapy. Typically, the practitioner also conducts a diagnostic examination by palpating the abdomen or back for any energy imbalances present in other parts of the body.

Precautions

While shiatsu is generally considered safe, there are a few precautions to consider. Because it may increase blood flow, this type of therapy is not recommended in people with bleeding problems, heart disease, or **cancer**.

KEY TERMS

Acupressure—An ancient form of Asian healing massage that involves applying pressure to special points or areas on the body in order to maintain good health, cure disease, and restore vitality.

Analgesic—Pain reliever.

Osteoporosis—A disease of the bones due to deficiency of bone matrix, occurring most frequently in postmenopausal women.

Palpate—Feel.

Massage therapy should always be used with caution in those with **osteoporosis**, fresh **wounds** or scar tissue, bone fractures, or inflammation.

Applying pressure to areas of the head is not recommended in people with epilepsy or high blood pressure, according to some practitioners of shiatsu.

Shiatsu is not considered effective in the treatment of fever, burns, and infectious diseases.

Shiatsu should not be performed right after a meal.

Side effects

When performed properly, shiatsu is not associated with any significant side effects. Some people may experience mild discomfort, which usually disappears during the course of the treatment session.

Research and general acceptance

Like many forms of massage, shiatsu is widely believed to have a relaxing effect on the body. There is also a significant amount of research suggesting that acupressure techniques can relieve **nausea** and **vomiting** associated with a variety of causes, including **pregnancy** and anesthetics and other drugs. In one study, acupressure was shown to significantly reduce the effects of nausea in 12 of 16 women suffering from morning sickness. Five days of this therapy also appeared to reduce anxiety and improve mood. Another investigation, published in 1999, studied the effects of acupressure on nausea resulting from the use of anesthetics. Pressure applied to an acupoint on the inside of the wrist appeared to alleviate nausea in patients who received anesthetics during the course of laparoscopic surgery.

Shiatsu may also produce sedative and analgesic effects. The sedative powers of acupressure were investigated in a study published in the *Journals of Gerontology* 1999, which involved over 80 elderly people who suffered from sleeping difficulties. Compared to the people in the control groups, the 28 participants who received acupressure were able to sleep better. They slept for longer periods of time and were less likely to wake up during the night. The researchers concluded that acupressure may improve the quality of sleep in older adults. The use of acupressure in postoperative pain was investigated in a study published in 1996. In this study, which involved 40 knee surgery patients, one group received acupressure (15 acupoints were stimulated) while the control group received sham acupressure. Within an hour of treatment, members of the acupressure group reported less pain than those in the control group. The pain-relieving effects associated with acupressure lasted for 24 hours.

Shiatsu may benefit **stroke** victims. The results of at least one study (which did not include a control group) suggest that shiatsu may be useful during stroke rehabilitation when combined with other treatments.

Resources

BOOKS

Cook, Allan R. *Alternative Medicine Source book*. Detroit: Omnigraphics, 1999.

PERIODICALS

Chen, M.L., L.C. Lin, S.C. Wu, et al. "The effectiveness of Acupressure in Improving the Quality of Sleep of Institutionalized Residents." *J Gerontol A Biol Sci Med Sci* 1999: M389-94.

Harmon, D., J. Gardiner, R. Harrison, et al. "Acupressure and the Prevention of nausea and vomiting after laparoscopy." *Br J Anaesth* 1999: 387-390

ORGANIZATIONS

Acupressure Institute. 1533 Shattuck Avenue, Berkeley, CA 94709.

American Massage Therapy Association. 820 Davis Street, Suite 100, Evanston, IL. <http://www.amtamassage.org>.

American Oriental Bodywork Therapy Association. 50 Maple Place, Manhasset, NY 11030.

International School of Shiatsu. 10 South Clinton Street, Doylestown, PA 18901.

National Certification Board for Therapeutic Massage and Bodywork. 8201 Greensboro Drive, Suite 300, McLean, VA 22102.

OTHER

International School of Shiatsu. <http://www.shiatsubo.com>.

MEDLINE. <http://igm.nlm.nih.gov>.

Greg Annussek

Shigellosis

Definition

Shigellosis is an infection of the intestinal tract by a group of bacteria called *Shigella*. The bacteria is named in honor of Shiga, a Japanese researcher, who discovered the organism in 1897. The major symptoms are **diarrhea**, abdominal cramps, **fever**, and severe fluid loss (**dehydration**). Four different groups of *Shigella* can affect humans; of these, *S. dysenteriae* generally produces the most severe attacks, and *S. sonnei* the mildest.

Description

Shigellosis is a well-known cause of **traveler's diarrhea** and illness throughout the world. *Shigella* are extremely infectious bacteria, and ingestion of just 10 organisms is enough to cause severe diarrhea and dehydration. *Shigella* accounts for 10-20% of all cases of diarrhea worldwide, and in any given year infects over 140 million persons and kills 600,000, mostly children and the elderly. The most serious form of the disease is called **dysentery**, which is characterized by severe watery (and often blood- and mucous-streaked) diarrhea, abdominal cramping, rectal **pain**, and fever. *Shigella* is only one of several organisms that can cause dysentery, but the term bacillary dysentery is usually another name for shigellosis.

Most deaths are in less-developed or developing countries, but even in the United States, shigellosis can be a dangerous and potentially deadly disease. Poor hygiene, overcrowding, and improper storage of food are leading causes of infection. The following statistics show the marked difference in the frequency of cases between developed and less-developed countries; in the United States, about 30,000 individuals are hit by the disease each year or about 10 cases/100,000 population. On the other hand, infection in some areas of South America is 1,000 times more frequent. Shigellosis is most common in children below age five, and occurs less often in adults over 20.

Causes and symptoms

Shigella share several of the characteristics of a group of bacteria that inhabit the intestinal tract. *E coli,* another cause of food-borne illness, can be mistaken for *Shigella* both by physicians and the laboratory. Careful testing is needed to assure proper diagnosis and treatment.

Shigella are very resistant to the acid produced by the stomach, and this allows them to easily pass through the gastrointestinal tract and infect the colon (large intestine). The result is a colitis that produces multiple ulcers, which can bleed. *Shigella* also produce a number of toxins (Shiga toxin and others) that increase the amount of fluid secretion by the intestinal tract. This fluid secretion is a major cause of the diarrhea symptoms.

Shigella infection spreads through food or water contaminated by human waste. Sources of transmission are:

- contaminated milk, ice cream, vegetables and other foods which often cause epidemics
- household contacts (40% of adults and 20% of children will develop infection from such a source)
- poor hygiene and overcrowded living conditions
- day care centers
- sexual practices which lead to oral-anal contact, directly or indirectly

Symptoms can be limited to only mild diarrhea or go on to full-blown dysentery. Dehydration results from the large fluid losses due to diarrhea, **vomiting**, and fever. Inability to eat or drink worsens the situation.

In developed countries, most infections are of the less severe type, and are often due to *S. sonnei*. The period between infection and symptoms (incubation period) varies from one to seven days. Shigellosis can last from a few days to several weeks, with an average of seven days.

Complications

Areas outside the intestine can be involved, including:

- nervous system (irritation of the meninges or meningitis, encephalitis, and seizures)
- kidneys (producing hemolytic uremic syndrome or HUS which leads to kidney failure)
- joints (leading to an unusual form of arthritis called Reiter's syndrome)
- skin (rash)

One of the most serious complications of this disease is HUS, which involves the kidney. The main findings are kidney failure and damage to red blood cells. As many as 15% of patients die from this complication, and half the survivors develop chronic kidney failure, requiring dialysis.

Another life-threatening condition is toxic megacolon. Severe inflammation causes the colon to dilate or stretch, and the thin colon wall may eventually tear. Certain medications (particularly those that diminish intestinal contractions) may increase this risk, but this

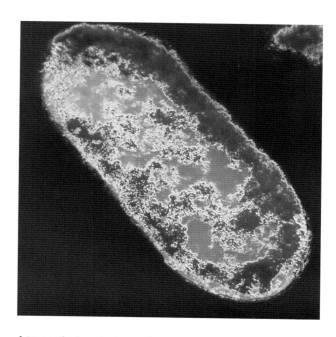

A transmission electron microscopy (TEM) scan of *Shigella*, a genus of aerobic bacteria that causes dysentery in humans and animals. *(Custom Medical Stock Photo. Reproduced by permission.)*

interaction is unclear. Clues to this diagnosis include sudden decrease in diarrhea, swelling of the abdomen, and worsening abdominal pain.

Diagnosis

Shigellosis is one of the many causes of acute diarrhea. Culture (growing the bacteria in the laboratory) of freshly obtained diarrhea fluid is the only way to be certain of the diagnosis. But even this is not always positive, especially if the patient is already on **antibiotics**. *Shigella* are identified by a combination of their appearance under the microscope and various chemical tests. These studies take several days, so quicker means to recognize the bacteria and its toxins are being developed.

Treatment

The first aim of treatment is to keep up **nutrition** and avoid dehydration. Ideally, a physician should be consulted before starting any treatment. Antibiotics may not be necessary, except for the more severe infections. Many cases resolve before the diagnosis is established by culture. Medications that control diarrhea by slowing intestinal contractions can cause problems and should be avoided by patients with bloody diarrhea or fever, especially if antibiotics have not been started.

KEY TERMS

Dysentery—A disease marked by frequent watery bowel movements, often with blood and mucus, and characterized by pain, urgency to have a bowel movement, fever, and dehydration.

Traveler's diarrhea—An illness due to infection from a bacteria or parasite that occurs in persons traveling to areas where there is a high frequency of the illness. The disease is usually spread by contaminated food or water.

Oral Rehydration Solution(ORS)—A liquid preparation developed by the World Health Organization that can decrease fluid loss in persons with diarrhea. Originally developed to be prepared with materials available in the home, commercial preparations have recently come into use.

Antibiotic—A medication that is designed to kill or weaken bacteria.

Anti-motility medications—Medications such as loperamide (Imodium), dephenoxylate (Lomotil), or medications containing codeine or narcotics which decrease the ability of the intestine to contract. These may worsen the condition of a patient with dysentery or colitis.

Food-borne illness—A disease that is transmitted by eating or handling contaminated food.

Fluoroquinolones—A relatively new group of antibiotics that have had good success in treating infections with many gram-negative bacteria, such as *Shigella*. One drawback is that they should not be used in children under 17 years of age, because of possible effect on bone or cartilage growth.

Dialysis—A form of treatment for patients with kidneys that do not function properly. The treatment removes toxic wastes from the body that are normally removed by the kidneys.

Colitis—Inflammation of the colon or large bowel which has several causes. The lining of the colon becomes swollen, and ulcers often develop. The ability of the colon to absorb fluids is also affected, and diarrhea often results.

Carrier state—The continued presence of an organism (bacteria, virus, or parasite) in the body that does not cause symptoms, but is able to be transmitted and infect other persons.

Stool—Passage of fecal material; a bowel movement.

Meninges—Outer covering of the spinal cord and brain. Infection is called meningitis, which can lead to damage to the brain or spinal cord and lead to death.

Rehydration

The World Health Organization (WHO) has developed guidelines for a standard solution taken by mouth, and prepared from ingredients readily available at home. This Oral Rehydration Solution (ORS) includes salt, baking powder, sugar, orange juice, and water. Commercial preparations, such as Pedialyte, are also available. In many patients with mild symptoms, this is the only treatment needed. Severe dehydration usually requires intravenous fluid replacement.

Antibiotics

In the early and mid-1990s, researchers began to realize that not all cases of bacterial dysentery needed antibiotic treatment. Many patients improve without such therapy, and therefore these drugs are indicated only for treatment of moderate or severe disease, as found in the tropics. Choice of antibiotic is based on the type of bacteria found in the geographical area and on laboratory results. Recommendations as

of 1997 include ampicillin, sulfa derivatives such as Trimethoprim-Sulfamethoxazole (TMP-SMX) sold as Bactrim, or **fluoroquinolones** (such as Ciprofloxacin which is not FDA approved for use in children).

Prognosis

Many patients with mild infections need no specific treatment and recover completely. In those with severe infections, antibiotics will decrease the length of symptoms and the number of days bacteria appear in the feces. In rare cases, an individual may fail to clear the bacteria from the intestinal tract; the result is a persistent carrier state. This may be more frequent in **AIDS** (Acquired Immune Deficiency Syndrome) patients. Antibiotics are about 90% effective in eliminating these chronic infections.

In patients who have suffered particularly severe attacks, some degree of cramping and diarrhea can last for several weeks. This is usually due to damage to the intestinal tract, which requires some time to heal. Since antibiotics can also produce a form of colitis, this must be considered as a possible cause of persistent or recurrent symptoms.

Prevention

Shigellosis is an extremely contagious disease; good hand washing techniques and proper precautions in food handling will help in avoiding spread of infection. Children in day care centers need to be reminded about hand washing during an outbreak to minimize spread. *Shigellosis* in schools or day care settings almost always disappears when holiday breaks occur, which sever the chain of transmission.

Traveler's diarrhea (TD)

Shigella accounts for about 10% of diarrhea illness in travelers to Mexico, South America, and the tropics. Most cases of TD are more of a nuisance than a life-threatening disease. However, bloody diarrhea is an indication that *Shigella* may be responsible.

In some cases though, aside from ruining a well deserved vacation, these infections can interrupt business conference schedules and, in the worst instances, lead to a life-threatening illness. Therefore, researchers have tried to find a safe, yet effective, way of preventing TD. Of course the best prevention is to follow closely the rules outlined by the WHO and other groups regarding eating fresh fruits, vegetables, and other foods.

One safe and effective method of preventing TD is the use of large doses of Pepto Bismol. Tablets are now available which are easier for travel; usage must start a few days before departure. Patients should be aware that Bismuth will turn bowel movements black.

Antibiotics have also proven to be highly effective in preventing TD. They can also produce significant side effects, and therefore a physician should be consulted before use. Like Pepto Bismol, antibiotics need to be started before beginning travel.

Resources

ORGANIZATIONS

Centers for Disease Control and Prevention. 1600 Clifton Rd., NE, Atlanta, GA 30333. (800) 311-3435, (404) 639-3311. <http://www.cdc.gov>.

David Kaminstein, MD

Shin splints

Definition

Shin splints refer to the sharp pains that occur down the front of the lower leg. They are a common complaint, particularly among runners and other athletes.

Description

Shin splints may refer to a number of lower leg complaints and injuries. In most cases, shin splints refer to the **pain** that results from overload on the tissues that connect muscles to the shin bone (tibia). They also may come from the small bone of the lower leg and ankle, called the fibula. The medical term for shin splints is medial tibial **stress** syndrome.

Next to ankle **sprains**, shin splints are probably the most common complaint of injury to the lower body. Most shin splints occur in the front (anterior) portion of the tibia; some also occur in the inside of the leg along the tibia. Runners probably suffer shin splints more than other people, but they also occur in people who play basketball and tennis and those who walk long distances, particularly on treadmills.

Causes and symptoms

The most common cause of shin splints is overdoing activities that constantly pound on the legs and feet. This may include sports with many stops and starts, running down hills or other tilted surfaces, or repeated walking. Simply training too long or too hard, especially without proper stretching and warm-up, can cause shin splints. People with flat feet, high arches, or feet that turn outward may be more prone to shin splints. Shoes that are worn or don't provide proper foot support also add to the problem.

Diagnosis

The physician will check the leg for tenderness. If the pain is in a single area of the tibia and hurts to the touch, the cause may by a stress fracture. The physician may order an x ray to rule out a stress fracture, but shin splints often can be diagnosed without x rays.

Treatment

Physicians usually recommend a period of rest for people with shin splints to let the area heal.

KEY TERMS

Podiatrist—A physician who specializes in the medical care and treatment of the human foot.

Stress fracture—A hairline fracture (narrow crack along the surface of a bone) that is caused by repeated stress to the bone, such as from jogging, rather than from a single heavy blow.

Usually, about three to four weeks is recommended, though the time varies depending on the patient and injury severity. Shin splints may be treated in phases, beginning with absolute rest and gradual return to activity. Ice and elevation of the foot may be used to help relieve pain and swelling in the first phase. If the person needs to keep in shape, stretching and water exercises that keep the foot from bearing weight may be allowed after initial treatment. As the patient returns to normal function, orthotic footwear and braces may be added to prevent re-injury.

Alternative treatment

Various massage techniques may help speed up recovery. Homeopathic physicians may recommend Rhus tox. Those using alternative remedies should ensure they are certified practitioners and should coordinate care with allopathic providers.

Prognosis

With proper rest, management, and prevention, people with shin splints can return to normal activity in a few weeks or more. However, continuing to perform the activity that caused the shin splints can lead to stress **fractures** of the tibia.

Prevention

Re-injury is most common in the first month after return to normal activity, and patients who have had shin splints should return to previous activities cautiously. The following can help prevent shin splints from occurring in people who run and perform stop and start physical activities:

- Warming up and stretching calf muscles before running or jogging. A podiatrist specializing in sports medicine or other sports medicine specialist may recommend specific stretching exercises.

- Strengthening muscles in the front lower leg (anterior tibialis) with resistance exercises or by walking on the heels three times daily for about 30 yards.

- Wearing quality shoes with arch supports. Runners should purchase new shoes about every 400 miles. A podiatrist can design special arch supports or orthotics for people with flat feet.

- Runs should be started at a slow pace and gradually increased.

- Athletes can cross-train in a sport that does not impact the feet and lower legs as much, such as swimming or riding a bicycle.

Resources

PERIODICALS

Metzi, Jordan D., Joshua A. Metzi. " Shin Pain in an Adolescent Soccer Player: A Case-based Look at 'Shin Splints': Do you Care for Children Who Regularly Run or Play Sports? Then You Should Have a Basic Understanding of the Different Entities that Can Cause Shin Pain. That List Includes Tibial Stress Injuries and Exertional Compartment Syndrome." *Contemporary Pediatrics* (Sept. 2004):36–39.

"Shunning Shin Splints." *Muscle & Fitness* (Aug. 2003):38.

Smith, Ian. "World of Hurt." *Men's Health* (June 2003):40.

ORGANIZATIONS

American Academy of Podiatric Sports Medicine. P.O. Box 723, Rockville, MD 20853. 888-854-3338. http://www.aapsm.org.

OTHER

Shin Splints.Foot.com Web site, 2005. http://www.foot.com/info/cond_cond_shin_splints.jsp.

Teresa G. Odle

Shingles

Definition

Shingles, also called herpes zoster or zona, gets its name from both the Latin and French words for belt or girdle and refers to girdle-like skin eruptions that may occur on the trunk of the body. The virus that causes **chickenpox**, the varicella zoster virus (VSV), can become dormant in nerve cells after an episode of chickenpox and later reemerge as shingles. Initially, red patches of rash develop into blisters. Because the virus travels along the nerve to the skin, it can damage the nerve and cause it to become inflamed. This condition can be very painful. If the **pain** persists long after the rash disappears, it is known as postherpetic **neuralgia**.

Description

Any person who has had chickenpox can develop shingles. Approximately 500,000 cases of shingles occur every year in the United States, according to the National Institute of Allergy and Infectious Diseases (NIAID). Overall, approximately 20% of those who had chickenpox as children develop shingles at some time in their lives. People of all ages, even children, can be affected, but the incidence increases with age. Newborn infants, bone marrow and other transplant recipients, as well as indivduals with immune systems weakened by disease or drugs are also at increased risk. However, most individuals who develop shingles do not have any underlying malignancy or other immunosuppressive condition.

Causes and symptoms

Shingles erupts along the course of the affected nerve, producing lesions anywhere on the body and may cause severe nerve pain. The most common areas to be affected are the face and trunk, which correspond to the areas where the chickenpox rash is most concentrated. The disease is caused by a reactivation of the chickenpox virus that has lain dormant in certain nerves following an episode of chickenpox. Exactly how or why this reactivation occurs is not clear; however, it is believed that the reactivation is triggered when the immune system becomes weakened, either as a result of **stress**, **fatigue**, certain medications, **chemotherapy**, or diseases, such as **cancer** or HIV. Further, it can be an early sign in persons with HIV that the immune system has deteriorated.

In some cases, the virus appears to be reactivated by mechanical irritation or minor surgical procedures. In one instance, the patient had an attack of shingles following **liposuction**.

Early signs of shingles are often vague and can easily be mistaken for other illnesses. The condition may begin with **fever** and malaise (a vague feeling of weakness or discomfort). Within two to four days, severe pain, **itching**, and numbness/tingling (paresthesia) or extreme sensitivity to touch (hyperesthesia) can develop, usually on the trunk and occasionally on the arms and legs. Pain may be continuous or intermittent, usually lasting from one to four weeks. It may occur at the time of the eruption, but can precede the eruption by days, occasionally making the diagnosis difficult. Signs and symptoms may include the following:

- itching, **tingling**, or severe burning pain
- red patches that develop into blisters
- grouped, dense, deep, small blisters that ooze and crust
- swollen lymph nodes

Diagnosis

Diagnosis is usually not possible until the skin lesions develop. Once they develop, however, the pattern and location of the blisters and the type of cell damage displayed are characteristic of the disease, allowing an accurate diagnosis primarily based upon the **physical examination**.

Although tests are rarely necessary, they may include the following:

- viral culture of skin lesion
- microscopic examination using a **Tzanck preparation**. This involves staining a smear obtained from a blister. Cells infected with the herpes virus will appear very large and contain many dark cell centers or nuclei.
- complete **blood count** (CBC) may show an elevated white blood cell count (WBC), a nonspecific sign of infection
- Rise in antibody to the virus
- Polymerase chain reaction (PCR) analysis. PCR testing has been found to be much faster and significantly more accurate than culturing the virus.

Treatment

Shingles almost always resolves spontaneously and may not require any treatment except for the relief of symptoms. In most people, the condition clears on its own in one or two weeks and seldom recurs.

Cool, wet compresses may help reduce pain. If there are blisters or crusting, applying compresses made with diluted vinegar will make the patient more comfortable. Mix one-quarter cup of white vinegar in two quarts of lukewarm water. Use the compress twice each day for 10 minutes. Stop using the compresses when the blisters have dried up.

Soothing baths and lotions such as colloidal oatmeal baths, starch baths or lotions, and calamine lotion may help to relieve itching and discomfort. Keep the skin clean, and do not re-use contaminated items. While the lesions continue to ooze, the person should be isolated to prevent infecting other susceptible individuals.

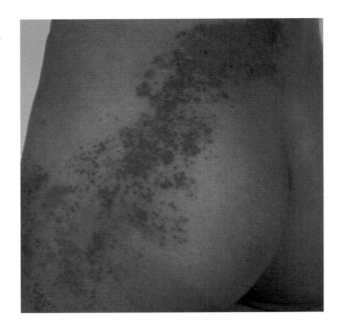

Shingles, or herpes zoster, on patient's buttocks and thigh.
(Custom Medical Stock Photo. Reproduced by permission.)

Later, when the crusts and scabs are separating, the skin may become dry, tight, and cracked. If that happens, rub on a small amount of plain petroleum jelly three or four times a day.

The **antiviral drugs** acyclovir, valacyclovir, and famciclovir can be used to treat shingles. These drugs may shorten the course of the illness. Their use results in more rapid healing of the blisters when drug therapy is started within 72 hours of the onset of the rash. In fact, the earlier the drugs are administered, the better, because early cases can sometimes be stopped. If taken later, these drugs are less effective but may still lessen the pain. Antiviral drug treatment does not seem to reduce the incidence of postherpetic neuralgia, but recent studies suggest famciclovir may cut the duration of postherpetic neuralgia in half. Side effects of typical oral doses of these antiviral drugs are minor with **headache** and nausea reported by 8–20 % of patients. Severely immunocompromised individuals, such as those with **AIDS**, may require intravenous administration of antiviral drugs.

Corticosteroids, such as prednisone, may be used to reduce inflammation but they do interfere with the functioning of the immune system. Corticosteroids, in combination with antiviral therapy, also are used to treat severe infections, such as those affecting the eyes, and to reduce severe pain.

Once the blisters are healed, some people continue to experience pain for months or even years (postherpetic neuralgia). This pain can be excruciating. Consequently, the doctor may prescribe tranquilizers, sedatives, or antidepressants to be taken at night. As noted above attempts to treat postherpetic neuralgia with the antiviral drug famciclovir have shown some promising results. When all else fails, severe pain may require a permanent nerve block.

A newer medication to treat postherpectic neuralgia is pregabalin, to be marketed in the United States under the trade name Lyrica. Pregabalin was approved by the Food and Drug Administration in September 2004 for the treatment of **diabetic neuropathy** as well as postherpetic neuralgia. The drug has been shown to improve patients' sleep and overall quality of life as well as relieve pain. Its most common side effects are drowsiness, headache, **dry mouth**, and **dizziness**.

Alternative treatment

There are nonmedical methods of prevention and treatment that may speed recovery. For example, getting lots of rest, eating a healthy diet, exercising regularly, and minimizing stress are always helpful in preventing disease. Supplementation with vitamin B_{12} during the first one to two days and continued supplementation with vitamin B complex, high levels of vitamin C with bioflavenoids, and calcium, are recommended to boost the immune system. Herbal antivirals such as **echinacea** can be effective in fighting infection and boosting the immune system.

Although no single alternative approach, technique, or remedy has yet been proven to reduce the pain, there are a few options which may be helpful. For example, topical applications of lemon balm (*Melissa officinalis*) or licorice (*Glycyrrhiza glabra*) and peppermint (*Mentha piperita*) may reduce pain and blistering. Homeopathic remedies include *Rhus toxicodendron* for blisters, *Mezereum* and *Arsenicum album* for pain, and *Ranunculus* for itching. Practitioners of Eastern medicine recommend self-hypnosis, **acupressure**, and **acupuncture** to alleviate pain.

Prognosis

Shingles usually clears up in two to three weeks and rarely recurs. Involvement of the nerves that cause movement may cause a temporary or permanent nerve **paralysis** and/or **tremors**. The elderly or debilitated patient may have a prolonged and difficult course. For them, the eruption is typically more extensive and inflammatory, occasionally resulting in blisters that bleed, areas where the skin actually dies,

KEY TERMS

Acyclovir—An antiviral drug that is available under the trade name Zovirax, in oral, intravenous, and topical forms. The drug blocks the replication of the varicella zoster virus.

Antibody—A specific protein produced by the immune system in response to a specific foreign protein or particle called an antigen.

Corticosteroid—A steroid that has similar properties to the steroid hormone produced by the adrenal cortex. It is used to alter immune responses to shingles.

Famciclovir—An oral antiviral drug that is available under the trade name Famvir. The drug blocks the replication of the varicella zoster virus.

Immunocompromised—A state in which the immune system is suppressed or not functioning properly.

Postherpetic neuralgia (PHN)—The term used to describe the pain after the rash associated with herpes zoster is gone.

Tzanck preparation—Procedure in which skin cells from a blister are stained and examined under the microscope. Visualization of large skin cells with many cell centers or nuclei indicates a positive diagnosis of herpes zoster when combined with results from a physical examination.

Valacyclovir—An oral antiviral drug that is available under the trade name Valtrex. The drug blocks the replication of the varicella zoster virus.

secondary bacterial infection, or extensive and permanent scarring.

Similarly, an immunocompromised patient usually has a more severe course that is frequently prolonged for weeks to months. They develop shingles frequently and the infection can spread to the skin, lungs, liver, gastrointestinal tract, brain, or other vital organs. Cases of chronic shingles have been reported in patients infected with AIDS, especially when they have a decreased number of one particular kind of immune cell, called CD4 lymphocytes. Depletion of CD4 lymphocytes is associated with more severe, chronic, and recurrent varicella-zoster virus infections. These lesions are typical at the onset but may turn into ulcers that do not heal.

Potentially serious complications can result from herpes zoster. Many individuals continue to experience persistent pain long after the blisters heal. This pain, called postherpetic neuralgia or PHN, can be severe and debilitating. Postherpetic neuralgia can persist for months or years after the lesions have disappeared. The incidence of postherpetic neuralgia increases with age, and episodes in older individuals tend to be of longer duration. Most patients under 30 years of age experience no persistent pain. By age 40, the risk of prolonged pain lasting longer than one month increases to 33%. By age 70, the risk increases to 74%. The pain can adversely affect quality of life, but it does usually diminish over time. Another risk factor for PHN is female sex.

Other complications include a secondary bacterial infection, and rarely, potentially fatal inflammation of the brain (**encephalitis**) and the spread of an infection throughout the body. These rare, but extremely serious, complications are more likely to occur in those individuals who have weakened immune systems (immunocompromised).

Prevention

Strengthening the immune system by making lifestyle changes is thought to help prevent the development of shingles. A lifestyle designed to strengthen the immune system and maintain good overall health includes eating a well-balanced diet rich in essential **vitamins** and **minerals**, getting enough sleep, exercising regularly, and reducing stress.

Resources

BOOKS

Beers, Mark H., MD, and Robert Berkow, MD., editors. "Herpesvirus Infections." Section 13, Chapter 162 In *The Merck Manual of Diagnosis and Therapy*. Whitehouse Station, NJ: Merck Research Laboratories, 2004.

PERIODICALS

Andrews, T. R., G. Perdikis, and R. B. Shack. "Herpes Zoster as a Rare Complication of Liposuction." *Plastic and Reconstructive Surgery* 113 (May 2004): 1838–1840.

Feder, H. M. Jr., and D. M. Hoss. "Herpes Zoster in Otherwise Healthy Children." *Pediatric Infectious Disease Journal* 451–457.

Jung, B. F., R. W. Johnson, D. R. Griffin, and R. H. Dworkin. "Risk Factors for Postherpetic Neuralgia in Patients with Herpes Zoster." *Neurology* 62 (May 11, 2004): 1545–1551.

Sabatowski, R., R. Galvez, D. Cherry, et al. "Pregabalin Reduces Pain and Improves Sleep and Mood Disturbances in Patients with Postherpetic Neuralgia: Results of a Randomised, Placebo-Controlled Clinical Trial." *Pain* 109 (May 2004): 26–35.

Stranska, R., R. Schuurman, M. de Vos, and A. M. van Loon. "Routine Use of a Highly Automated and Internally Controlled Real-Time PCR Assay for the Diagnosis of Herpes Simplex and Varicella-Zoster Virus Infections." *Journal of Clinical Virology* 30 (May 2004): 39–44.

ORGANIZATIONS

American Academy of Dermatology. 930 N. Meacham Road, P.O. Box 4014, Schaumburg, IL 60168-4014. (847) 330-0230. Fax: (847) 330-0050. < http://www.aad.org >.

National Institute of Allergy and Infectious Diseases (NIAID). Office of Communications and Public Liaison, 6610 Rockledge Drive, MSC 6612, Bethesda, MD 20892-6612. < http://www.niaid.nih.gov >.

David James Doermann
Rebecca J. Frey, PhD

Shock

Definition

Shock is a medical emergency in which the organs and tissues of the body are not receiving an adequate flow of blood. This deprives the organs and tissues of oxygen (carried in the blood) and allows the buildup of waste products. Shock can result in serious damage or even **death**.

Description

There are three stages of shock: Stage I (also called compensated, or nonprogressive), Stage II (also called decompensated or progressive), and Stage III (also called irreversible).

In Stage I of shock, when low blood flow (perfusion) is first detected, a number of systems are activated in order to maintain/restore perfusion. The result is that the heart beats faster, the blood vessels throughout the body become slightly smaller in diameter, and the kidney works to retain fluid in the circulatory system. All this serves to maximize blood flow to the most important organs and systems in the body. The patient in this stage of shock has very few symptoms, and treatment can completely halt any progression.

In Stage II of shock, these methods of compensation begin to fail. The systems of the body are unable to improve perfusion any longer, and the patient's symptoms reflect that fact. Oxygen deprivation in the brain causes the patient to become confused and disoriented, while oxygen deprivation in the heart may cause chest **pain**. With quick and appropriate treatment, this stage of shock can be reversed.

In Stage III of shock, the length of time that poor perfusion has existed begins to take a permanent toll on the body's organs and tissues. The heart's functioning continues to spiral downward, and the kidneys usually shut down completely. Cells in organs and tissues throughout the body are injured and dying. The endpoint of Stage III shock is the patient's death.

Causes and symptoms

Shock is caused by three major categories of problems: cardiogenic (meaning problems associated with the heart's functioning); hypovolemic (meaning that the total volume of blood available to circulate is low); and **septic shock** (caused by overwhelming infection, usually by bacteria).

Cardiogenic shock can be caused by any disease, or event, which prevents the heart muscle from pumping strongly and consistently enough to circulate the blood normally. **Heart attack**, conditions which cause inflammation of the heart muscle (myocarditis), disturbances of the electrical rhythm of the heart, any kind of mass or fluid accumulation and/or blood clot which interferes with flow out of the heart can all significantly affect the heart's ability to adequately pump a normal quantity of blood.

Hypovolemic shock occurs when the total volume of blood in the body falls well below normal. This can occur when there is excess fluid loss, as in **dehydration** due to severe **vomiting** or diarrhea, diseases which cause excess urination (diabetes insipidus, diabetes mellitus, and kidney failure), extensive **burns**, blockage in the intestine, inflammation of the pancreas (**pancreatitis**), or severe bleeding of any kind.

Septic shock can occur when an untreated or inadequately treated infection (usually bacterial) is allowed to progress. Bacteria often produce poisonous chemicals (toxins) which can cause injury throughout the body. When large quantities of these bacteria, and their toxins, begin circulating in the bloodstream, every organ and tissue in the body is at risk of their damaging effects. The most damaging consequences of these bacteria and toxins include poor functioning of the heart muscle; widening of the diameter of the blood vessels; a drop in blood pressure; activation of the blood clotting system, causing **blood clots**, followed by a risk of uncontrollable bleeding; damage to the lungs, causing acute respiratory distress syndrome; liver failure; kidney failure; and **coma**.

Initial symptoms of shock include cold, clammy hands and feet; pale or blue-tinged skin tone; weak, fast pulse rate; fast rate of breathing; low blood pressure. A variety of other symptoms may be present, but they are dependent on the underlying cause of shock.

Diagnosis

Diagnosis of shock is based on the patient's symptoms, as well as criteria including a significant drop in blood pressure, extremely low urine output, and blood tests that reveal overly acidic blood with a low circulating concentration of carbon dioxide. Other tests are performed, as appropriate, to try to determine the underlying condition responsible for the patient's state of shock.

Treatment

The most important goals in the treatment of shock include: quickly diagnosing the patient's state of shock; quickly intervening to halt the underlying condition (stopping bleeding, re-starting the heart, giving **antibiotics** to combat an infection, etc.); treating the effects of shock (low oxygen, increased acid in the blood, activation of the blood clotting system); and supporting vital functions (blood pressure, urine flow, heart function).

Treatment includes keeping the patient warm, with legs raised and head down to improve blood flow to the brain, putting a needle in a vein in order to give fluids or blood transfusions, as necessary; giving the patient extra oxygen to breathe and medications to improve the heart's functioning; and treating the underlying condition which led to shock.

Prognosis

The prognosis of an individual patient in shock depends on the stage of shock when treatment was begun, the underlying condition causing shock, and the general medical state of the patient.

Prevention

The most preventable type of shock is caused by dehydration during illnesses with severe vomiting or **diarrhea**. Shock can be avoided by recognizing that a patient who is unable to drink in order to replace lost fluids needs to be given fluids intravenously (through a needle in a vein). Other types of shock are only preventable insofar as one can prevent their underlying conditions, or can monitor and manage those conditions well enough so that they never progress to the point of shock.

Resources

PERIODICALS

Kerasote, Ted. "After Shock: Recognizing and Treating Shock." *Sports Afield* 217 (May 1997): 60+.

Rosalyn Carson-DeWitt, MD

Shock I *see* **Adult respiratory distress syndrome**

Shock therapy *see* **Electroconvulsive therapy**

Shortness of breath

Definition

Shortness of breath, or dyspnea, is a feeling of difficult or labored breathing that is out of proportion to the patient's level of physical activity. It is a symptom of a variety of different diseases or disorders and may be either acute or chronic.

Description

The experience of dyspnea depends on its severity and underlying causes. The feeling itself results from a combination of impulses relayed to the brain from nerve endings in the lungs, rib cage, chest muscles, or diaphragm, combined with the patient's perception and interpretation of the sensation. In some cases, the patient's sensation of breathlessness is intensified by **anxiety** about its cause. Patients describe dyspnea variously as unpleasant shortness of breath, a feeling of increased effort or tiredness in moving the chest muscles, a panicky feeling of being smothered, or a sense of tightness or cramping in the chest wall.

Causes and symptoms

ACUTE DYSPNEA. Acute dyspnea with sudden onset is a frequent cause of emergency room visits. Most cases of acute dyspnea involve pulmonary (lung and breathing) disorders, cardiovascular disease, or chest trauma.

PULMONARY DISORDERS. Pulmonary disorders that can cause dyspnea include airway obstruction by a foreign object, swelling due to infection, or anaphylactic **shock**; acute **pneumonia**; hemorrhage from the lungs; or severe bronchospasms associated with **asthma**.

CARDIOVASCULAR DISEASE. Acute dyspnea can be caused by disturbances of the heart rhythm, failure of the left ventricle, mitral valve (a heart valve) dysfunction, or an embolus (a clump of tissue, fat, or gas) that is blocking the pulmonary circulation. Most pulmonary emboli (**blood clots**) originate in the deep veins of the lower legs and eventually migrate to the pulmonary artery.

TRAUMA. Chest injuries, both closed injuries and penetrating **wounds**, can cause **pneumothorax** (the presence of air inside the chest cavity), **bruises**, or fractured ribs. **Pain** from these injuries results in dyspnea. The impact of the driver's chest against the steering wheel in auto accidents is a frequent cause of closed chest injuries.

OTHER CAUSES. Anxiety attacks sometimes cause acute dyspnea; they may or may not be associated with chest pain. Anxiety attacks are often accompanied by hyperventilation, which is a breathing pattern characterized by abnormally rapid and deep breaths. Hyperventilation raises the oxygen level in the blood, causing chest pain and **dizziness**.

Chronic dyspnea

PULMONARY DISORDERS. Chronic dyspnea can be caused by asthma, chronic obstructive pulmonary disease (COPD), **bronchitis**, **emphysema**, inflammation of the lungs, **pulmonary hypertension**, tumors, or disorders of the vocal cords.

HEART DISEASE. Disorders of the left side of the heart or inadequate supply of blood to the heart muscle can cause dyspnea. In some cases a tumor in the heart or inflammation of the membrane surrounding the heart may cause dyspnea.

NEUROMUSCULAR DISORDERS. Neuromuscular disorders cause dyspnea from progressive deterioration of the patient's chest muscles. They include muscular dystrophy, myasthenia gravis, and amyotrophic lateral sclerosis.

OTHER CAUSES. Patients who are severely anemic may develop dyspnea if they **exercise** vigorously. **Hyperthyroidism** or **hypothyroidism** may cause shortness of breath, and so may gastroesophageal reflux disease (GERD). Both chronic **anxiety disorders** z of physical fitness can also cause episodes of dyspnea. Deformities of the chest or **obesity** can cause dyspnea by limiting the movement of the chest wall and the ability of the lungs to fill completely.

Diagnosis

Patient history

The patient's history provides the doctor with such necessary information as a history of gastroesophageal reflux disease (GERD), asthma, or other allergic conditions; the presence of chest pain as well as difficulty breathing; recent accidents or recent surgery; information about **smoking** habits; the patient's baseline level of physical activity and exercise habits; and a psychiatric history of panic attacks or anxiety disorders.

ASSESSMENT OF BODY POSITION. How a person's body position affects his/her dyspnea symptoms sometimes gives hints as to the underlying cause of the disorder. Dyspnea that is worse when the patient is sitting up is called platypnea and indicates the possibility of **liver disease**. Dyspnea that is worse when the patient is lying down is called orthopnea, and is associated with heart disease or **paralysis** of the diaphragm. Paroxysmal nocturnal dyspnea (PND) refers to dyspnea that occurs during sleep and forces the patient to awake gasping for breath. It is usually relieved if the patient sits up or stands. PND may point to dysfunction of the left ventricle of the heart, **hypertension**, or narrowing of the mitral valve.

Physical examination

The doctor will examine the patient's chest in order to determine the rate and depth of breathing, the effort required, the condition of the patient's breathing muscles, and any evidence of chest deformities or trauma. He or she will listen for **wheezing**, **stridor**, or signs of fluid in the lungs. If the patient has a **fever**, the doctor will look for other signs of pneumonia. The doctor will check the patient's heart functions, including blood pressure, pulse rate, and the presence of **heart murmurs** or other abnormal heart sounds. If the doctor suspects a blood clot in one of the large veins leading to the heart, he or she will examine the patient's legs for signs of swelling.

Diagnostic tests

BASIC DIAGNOSTIC TESTS. Patients who are seen in emergency rooms are given a **chest x ray** and electro-cardiogram (ECG) to assist the doctor in evaluating abnormalities of the chest wall, also to determine the position of the diaphragm, possible rib **fractures** or pneumothorax, irregular heartbeat, or the adequacy of the supply of blood to the heart muscle. Also, the patient may be given a breathing test on an instrument called a spirometer to screen for airway disorders.

The doctor may order blood tests and arterial blood gas tests to rule out anemia, hyperventilation–from an anxiety attack –, or thyroid dysfunction. A **sputum culture** can be used to test for pneumonia.

SPECIALIZED TESTS. Specialized tests may be ordered for patients with normal results from basic diagnostic tests for dyspnea. High-resolution CT scans can be used for suspected airway obstruction or mild emphysema. Tissue biopsy performed with a bronchoscope can be used for patients with suspected lung disease.

If the doctor suspects a **pulmonary embolism**, he or she may order ventilation-perfusion scanning to inspect lung function, an angiogram of blood vessels, or ultrasound studies of the leg veins. **Echocardiography** can be used to test for pulmonary hypertension and heart disease.

Pulmonary function studies or **electromyography** (EMG) are used to assess neuromuscular diseases. Exercise testing is used to assess dyspnea related to COPD, anxiety attacks, poor physical fitness, and the severity of lung or heart disease. The level of acidity in the patient's esophagus may be monitored to rule out GERD.

Treatment

Treatment of dyspnea depends on its underlying cause.

Acute dyspnea

Patients with acute dyspnea are given oxygen in the emergency room, with the following treatments for specific conditions:

- Asthma. Treatment with Alupent, epinephrine, or aminophylline.

- Anaphylactic shock. Treatment with Benadryl, ster-oids, or aminophylline, with hydrocortisone if necessary.

- Congestive **heart failure**. Treatment with oxygen, **diuretics**, and placing patient in upright position.

- Pneumonia. Treatment with **antibiotics** and removal of lung secretions.

- Anxiety attacks. Immediate treatment includes anti-depressant medications. If the patient is hyperventi-lating, he or she may be asked to breathe into a paper bag to normalize breathing rhythm and the oxygen level of the blood.

- Pneumothorax. Surgical placement of a chest tube.

Chronic dyspnea

The treatment of chronic dyspnea depends on the underlying disorder. Asthma can often be managed with a combination of medications to reduce airway spasms and removal of allergens from the patient's environment. COPD requires both medication, life-style changes, and long-term physical **rehabilitation**. Anxiety disorders are usually treated with a combina-tion of medication and psychotherapy. GERD can usually be managed with **antacids**, other medications, and dietary changes. There are no permanent cures for myasthenia gravis or muscular dystrophy.

Tumors and certain types of chest deformities can be treated surgically.

Alternative treatment

The appropriate alternative therapy for shortness of breath depends on the underlying cause of the con-dition. When dyspnea is acute and severe, **oxygen therapy** is used either in the doctor's office or in the emergency room. For shortness of breath with an underlying physical cause like asthma, anaphylactic shock, or pneumonia, the physical condition should be treated. Botanical and homeopathic remedies can be used for acute dyspnea, if the proper remedies and formulas are prescribed. If the dyspnea has a psycho-logical basis (especially if it is caused by anxiety), **acupuncture**, botanical medicine, and homeopathy can help the patient heal at a deep level.

Prognosis

The prognosis for recovery depends on the under-lying cause of the dyspnea, its severity, and the type of treatment required.

Prevention

Dyspnea caused by asthma can be minimized or prevented by removing dust and other triggers from the patient's environment. Long-term prevention of chronic dyspnea includes such lifestyle choices as reg-ular aerobic exercise and avoidance of smoking.

KEY TERMS

Anaphylactic shock—A severe systemic reaction to an allergen that occurs in hypersensitive individuals. It can cause spasms of the larynx that block the patient's airway and cause dyspnea.

Dyspnea—A sensation of difficult or labored breathing.

Electromyography—A technique for recording electric currents in an active muscle in order to measure its level of function.

Orthopnea—Difficulty in breathing that occurs while the patient is lying down.

Paroxysmal nocturnal dyspnea (PND)—A form of dyspnea characterized by the patient's waking from sleep unable to breathe.

Platypnea—Dyspnea that occurs when the patient is sitting up.

Pneumothorax—The presence of air or gas inside the chest cavity.

Spirometer—An instrument that is used to test lung capacity. It is used to screen patients with dyspnea.

Stridor—A harsh or crowing breath sound caused by partial blockage of the patient's upper airway.

Wheezing—A whistling or musical sound caused by tightening of the air passages inside the patient's chest. Wheezing is most commonly associated with asthma.

Resources

BOOKS

Gillespie, D. J., and E. J. Olson. "Dyspnea." In *Current Diagnosis*. Vol. 9. Edited by Rex B. Conn, et al. Philadelphia: W. B. Saunders Co., 1997.

Rebecca J. Frey, PhD

Shy-Drager syndrome

Definition

Shy-Drager syndrome (SDS) is a rare condition that causes progressive damage to the autonomic nervous system. The autonomic nervous system controls vital involuntary body functions such as heart rate, breathing, and intestinal, urinary, and sexual functions. The autonomic nervous system also controls skin and body temperature, and how the body responds to **stress**. Shy-Drager syndrome leads to dizziness or **fainting** when standing up, urinary incontinence, **impotence**, and muscle **tremors**.

Description

SDS was named for neurologists Milton Shy, M.D., from the National Institutes of Health, and Glenn Drager, M.D., from the Baylor College of Medicine, who first described the condition in 1960. It typically affects those between ages 50–70. It affects more men than women. In severe cases, the person cannot even stand up. Symptoms can be mild as well. Sometimes, people with mild cases are misdiagnosed as having **anxiety** or **hypertension**.

Many nonprescription drugs, such as cold medicines and diet capsules, can trigger extremely high blood pressure spikes in patients with SDS, even in very low doses. Therefore, these patients are at risk for strokes and excessive bleeding (hemorrhage) if they take even the recommended dosage of these drugs.

Causes and symptoms

The cause of SDS is unknown. Symptoms develop because of degeneration of certain groups of nerve cells in the spinal cord.

Patients with SDS usually have problems with the function of the autonomic nervous system. Progressive degeneration may occur in other areas of the nervous system as well. The hallmark of the syndrome is **dizziness** and fainting when arising or after standing still for a long time (postural **hypotension**). This is caused by low blood pressure and inadequate blood flow to the brain. When this problem becomes severe (for example, a blood pressure below 70/40 mmHg), it can lead to a momentary loss of consciousness. When the person faints, the blood pressure returns to normal and the person wakes up.

Many patients also notice impotence, **urinary incontinence**, dry mouth and skin, and trouble regulating body temperature because of abnormal sweating. Since the autonomic nervous system also controls the narrowing and widening of the iris, some patients with SDS have vision problems, such as trouble focusing.

In later stages, problems in the autonomic nervous system lead to breathing difficulties such as **sleep apnea**, loud breathing, and **snoring**. In advanced stages of the disease, patients can die from irregular heartbeat.

Other symptoms of SDS do not involve the autonomic nervous system. These include parkinsonism (muscle tremor, rigidity, and slow movements), double vision, problems controlling emotions, and wasting of muscles in the hands and feet. Eventually, patients may have problems chewing, swallowing, speaking, and breathing. There may be a loss of color pigment in the iris.

Diagnosis

While no blood test can reveal the disorder, a careful assessment of symptoms should alert a neurologist to suspect SDS. A combination of parkinsonism and certain autonomic problems (especially impotence, incontinence, and postural hypotension) are clear indications of the syndrome.

Tests of the autonomic nervous system may help diagnose the condition. In normal patients, blood levels of norepinephrine rise when they stand up. This doesn't happen in people with SDS. Norepinephrine is a hormone that helps maintain blood pressure by triggering certain blood vessels to constrict when blood pressure falls below normal. Another test for the condition is the Valsalva maneuver. In this test, the patient holds his or her breath and strains down as if having a bowel movement while the doctor monitors blood pressure and heart rate for 10 seconds. Patients with SDS will not have the normal increase in blood pressure and heart rate.

A variety of other tests can identify a broad range of autonomic problems in patients with SDS. Brain scans, however, don't usually reveal any problems.

Treatment

Medication can relieve many of the symptoms, especially the parkinsonism and low blood pressure. However, typical antiparkinsonism drugs such as carbidopa-levodopa (Sinemet) should be used with caution, since they often worsen the postural low blood pressure and may cause fainting.

Because postural hypotension is the most troublesome of the symptoms in the early years, treatments center on relieving this problem. Patients are encouraged to eat a liberal salt diet and drink plenty of fluids. They are advised to wear waist-high elastic hosiery and to sleep with the head elevated at least 5 in (13 cm). Other drug treatment includes fludrocortisone, indomethacin, nonsteroidal anti-inflammatory drugs, beta blockers, central stimulants, and other medications.

Occasionally, a pacemaker, **gastrostomy**, or tracheostomy may be needed. A pacemaker is a device

---

KEY TERMS

Autonomic nervous system—The part of the nervous system that controls the involuntary (apparently automatic) activities of organs, blood vessels, glands, and many other body tissues.

Degenerative—Degenerative disorders involve progressive impairment of both the structure and function of part of the body.

Gastrostomy—An artificial opening into the stomach through the abdomen to enable a patient to be fed via a feeding tube. The procedure is given to patients with SDS who are unable to chew or swallow.

Norepinephrine—A hormone that helps maintain blood pressure by triggering certain blood vessels to constrict when blood pressure falls below normal.

Sleep apnea—A sleep disorder characterized by periods of breathing cessation lasting for 10 seconds or more.

Tracheostomy—An opening through the neck into the trachea through which a tube may be inserted to maintain an effective airway and help a patient breathe.

---

that delivers electrical impulses to the heart to keep it beating regularly. A gastrostomy creates an opening in the stomach to connect a feeding tube from outside the body. In a tracheostomy an opening is made in the windpipe and a tube is inserted to maintain breathing.

Prognosis

While the course of the disease varies, and some patients live for up to 20 years after the symptoms first appear, most patients become severely disabled within seven or eight years. It is unusual for someone to survive more than 15 years after diagnosis.

Symptoms (especially tremor) often get worse if the patient smokes, because of the nicotine.

Many patients develop swallowing problems which may lead to recurrent episodes of pneumonia, a frequent cause of **death**. Others experience Cheyne-Stokes (periodic breathing). One of the most common causes of death is pulmonary embolus. This is caused by a blood clot in the main artery in the lung.

Prevention

Since scientists don't know the cause of Shy-Drager syndrome, there is no way to prevent the condition.

Resources

ORGANIZATIONS

American Academy of Neurology. 1080 Montreal Ave., St. Paul, MN 55116. (612) 695-1940. < http://www.aan.com >.

Association for Neuro-Metabolic Disorders. 5223 Brookfield Lane, Sylvania, OH 43560-1809. (419) 885-1497.

National Institute of Neurological Disorders and Stroke. P.O. Box 5801, Bethesda, MD 20824. (800) 352-9424. < http://www.ninds.nih.gov/index.htm >.

National Organization for Rare Disorders. P.O. Box 8923, New Fairfield, CT 06812-8923. (800) 999-6673. < http://www.rarediseases.org >.

Shy-Drager Syndrome Support Group. 2004 Howard Lane, Austin, TX 78728. (800) 288-5582. < http://www.shy-drager.com >.

Carol A. Turkington

Shyness

Definition

Shyness is a personality trait that produces behaviors ranging from feeling uncomfortable at a party to an extreme fear of being watched by others while talking on the telephone.

Description

Shyness affects people of all ages. A toddler might run from strangers and cling to her parents. While kindergarten is frightening for many children; some students are anxious about the first day of school until they graduate from college. Job interviews are stressful for people uncomfortable talking about themselves. For some people, feelings of self-worth are related to their careers. Retirement may bring feelings of lower self-esteem.

Shyness is linked to brain activity, how a person was raised and other experiences, and the person's reaction to those experiences.

Social phobia

Extreme shyness is sometimes referred to as a social phobia. Also known as social **anxiety** disorder, a social phobia is a psychiatric condition defined as a "marked and persistent fear" of some situations. The shy person continues to go on job interviews. Social phobia may cause a person to remain unemployed,

according to the National Mental Health Association (NMHA). True social phobia affects about 3% of people.

Introversion

The introvert enjoy being alone and intentionally avoids situations like a party. The shy person wants to be around people. However, shyness is stronger than the desire to be sociable. The shy person is afraid to go to the party and stays home alone.

Causes and symptoms

Temperament is related to the amygdala, the part of the brain related to emotions and new situations. The amygdala evaluates new situations based on memories of past experiences. If the new situation appears threatening, the amygdala sends a warning signal. The amygdala in a shy person is extremely sensitive and much more active than that of an outgoing person. The increased activity causes the person to withdraw either physically or emotionally. This withdrawal is known as inhibition.

The baby runs from strangers; the job applicant laughs nervously when talking about his accomplishments. Brain activity is one component of shyness. Environment also plays a role. If the inhibited child has outgoing, nurturing parents, she will probably imitate their behavior. If parents and teachers are mocking and critical, a child may have a lifelong fear of the first day of school. A person with that background may compare himself with others and feel they are more capable than he is. The person embarrassed in a job interview could become anxious in future interviews.

At the root of shyness is a feeling of self-consciousness. This may cause the person to blush, tense up, or start sweating. Those are some reactions caused when the brain signals its warning. The person may avoid eye contact, look down, become very quiet, or fumble over words.

Symptoms vary because there are degrees of shyness. A person might be very quiet when meeting new people, but then become talkative when she feels comfortable with them. The jobseeker may not be afraid of social gatherings.

Social Phobia

Social phobia causes an extreme fear of being humiliated or embarrassed in front of people, according to the according to the NMHA. It may be connected to low self-esteem or feelings of inferiority. The phobic is not fearful in all situations and may feel comfortable around people in most of the time.

However, social **phobias** have caused people to drop out of school, avoid making friends, and keep away from other fear-provoking situations. Phobic fears range from speaking in pubic and dating to using public restrooms or writing when other people are present.

According to the NMHA, phobic may feel that everyone is looking at them, A trivial mistake is regarded as much more serious, and blushing is painfully embarrassing. Social phobia is frequently accompanied by depression or **substance abuse**.

Diagnosis

In many cases, adults realize they are shy. In a sense they have diagnosed themselves, and may take steps to overcome their shyness. Teen-agers may also try to remedy their situations.

Adults and youths may buy self-help books or take classes on subjects like overcoming shyness and assertiveness training. These classes may be taught by counselors, psychologists, or people with experience conquering shyness. Health-care providers often schedule these classes. They are also taught in settings ranging from adult schools to social service agencies. Costs will vary at these classes.

Children may not know there are treatment solutions for their shyness. Parents and educators should be alert for symptoms of shyness in younger children. Schools and family resource centers can provide referrals if it appears counseling want their child diagnosed.

Medical diagnosis

Based on the child's circumstances, parents may take the child to their health care provider. Some insurance plans require an appointment with a doctor before a referral to a counselor or a psychologist. The health professional conducts an assessment and then recommends treatment.

Children and adults may need medical treatment for social phobia. The adult's diagnosis also starts with a medical exam to determine if there is a physical cause for symptoms. If that has been ruled out, the patient undergoes a psychiatric evaluation.

Diagnostic fees and the time allocated for evaluation vary for both shy and phobic people. Diagnosis could span several hour-long sessions that cover an initial evaluation, personality tests, and a meeting to set therapy goals. Each session could cost around $90. Insurance may cover part of the costs.

Treatment

Shyness treatment concentrates on changing behavior so the person feels more at ease in shyness-provoking situations. The person may be guided by a self-help book or participate in individual or **group therapy**.

Books and therapy generally focus on behavioral therapy and **cognitive-behavioral therapy**. One method of behavioral therapy is to expose the person to the situation that triggers fear. This could start with rehearsing a job interview with a friend or making eye contact with a store clerk. Over time, the person goes on interviews to get experience rather than to be hired. Another person might move from eye contact to attending an enjoyable event like a concert to become more at ease around strangers.

Therapy also focuses on developing skills to cope in new situation. These include taking deep breaths to relax and practicing small talk. Cognitive-therapy helps the person learn how thinking patterns contribute to symptoms, according to NMHA. The person is taught techniques to change those thoughts or stop symptoms. This association maintains this therapy is very effective for people with social phobias.

Treatment costs very from the price of a self-help book to the fees for therapy. Therapy sessions may be led by a licensed marriage and family counselor, a psychologist or psychiatrist. The cost of group therapy is for is generally an hourly fee, with therapy planned for a set time. The therapist might charge $80 an hour for a social phobia group that meets three hours a week for 16 weeks.

Treatment may include medication. Prescription drugs like Paxil (paroxetine) are generally only prescribed to people with social **anxiety disorders**. Paxil is prescribed for depression and other **mood disorders**. The patient takes one tablet daily. Costs will vary, and a 30-day order could be priced at $74 to $84.

Insurance may cover part of the costs of therapy and medicine.

Alternative treatment

Alternative treatments for shyness focus on symptoms like tension and **stress**. Relaxation tapes and CDs guide the listener through a series of actions to relieve tension. The activity starts with deep breathing and then the person progressively focuses on the head and different parts of the body. The **exercise** may start with the head, neck, shoulders, moving down to the one foot and then the other. Some techniques involve tightly tensing and then releasing each part. Another method is to concentrate on relaxing each part or imagine that it becomes warm.

Another self-treatment is **aromatherapy**. Lavender is a relaxing scent and is available in liquid form as an essential oil. Stress can be relieved by adding oil to a bath. Some people carry the oil with them. If they become anxious, the people can dab the oil on a cotton pad. They breathe in the lavender and feel calmer.

Prognosis

Shyness may not be a permanent. Children often outgrow shyness. Behavioral changes and therapy can help people feel more at ease. Furthermore, some aspects of shyness are positive. Shy people are frequently good listeners and are empathetic, aware of others' feelings.

Prevention

Shyness is a personality trait related to a person's biology and experiences. The part of shyness related to the brain cannot be changed. However, parents can provide a nurturing environment that helps prevent shyness. This will provide the child with a healthy mental attitude that helps prevent shyness. When faced with situations that could cause self-defeating shyness, children will have coping skills.

According to the National Mental Health Association, the basics of good mental health for children include:

- A family that provides unconditional love not related on accomplishments.

- Nurturing self-confidence and high self-esteem by praising children. Methods include encouraging a child to learn a new game. The parents should set realistic goals, assure children, and smile frequently. Parents should avoid sarcastic remarks, set realistic goals and let children know that all people make mistakes.

- Playing with other children helps the young learn how to develop friendships and problem-solving skills.

- Emphasizing that school is fun. Parents can play school with their child to demonstrate that learning is enjoyable. Enrolling children in preschool or children's programs allows them to learn, be creative, and develop social skills.

- When disciplining, parents should criticize the behavior, rather than berating the child.

Shyness prevention and adults

For adults prone to shyness, the issue is related more to treatment than prevention. Shyness for these people has probably been an issue, one that surfaces at various times in their lives. A move, a **death** in the family, job loss, and other unsettling changes could cause emotions that include the fear associated with shyness.

In some circumstances, the person must go through the grieving process. In other situations, the person needs to do things that build self-confidence. Like the child, the adult needs a support system. A network of friends helps with encouragement and listens to the person's concerns.

To combat the avoidance symptom caused by shyness, the person should look into enjoyable pursuits. Recreational activities like walking groups combine physical exercise with the opportunity to socialize. Enrolling in a class at an adult school or community college provides the opportunity to learn and make new friends. Class topics range from upholstery to mystery book discussions. Classes like these can boost confidence as a person learns a hands-on skill or discovers that other mystery readers value her or his opinion.

Resources

PERIODICALS

Carducci, Bernardo. "Shyness: the New Solution." *Psychology Today* January/February 2000 [cited April 5, 2005]. < http://cms.psychologytoday.com/articles/index.php?term = PTO-20000101-000032 >.

ORGANIZATIONS

American Psychological Association.750 First Street, NE, Washington, DC 20002-4242. 800-374-2721. < http://www.apa.org >.

National Mental Health Association. 2001 N. Beauregard Street, 12th Floor, Alexandria, VA 22311. 703-684-7722. < http://www.nmha.org >.

Shyness Research Institute. 4201 Grant Line Road, New Albany, IN 47150. 812-941-2295. < http://homepages.ius.edu/Special/Shyness >.

OTHER

Jaret, Peter. "Is Shyness a Mental Disorder?" WebMD Feature. April 10, 2000 [cited April 5, 2005]. < http://my.webmd.com/content/article/13/1674_50379.htm >.

Painful Shyness in Children and Adults *American Psychological Association pamphlet*. [cited April 5, 2005]. < http://www.apa.org/topics/topicshyness.html >.

Shy Child, Shy Adult. WebMD: Science, June 20, 2003: News release, American Association for the Advancement of Science. [cited April 5, 2005]. < http://my.webmd.com/content/article/67/79975.htm >.

Putting Shyness in the Spotlight. Teens Health. April 2004 [cited April 1, 2005]. < http://www.kidshealth.org/teen/your_mind/emotions/shyness.html >.

Liz Swain

Sick sinus syndrome

Definition

Sick sinus syndrome is a disorder of the sinus node of the heart, which regulates heartbeat. With sick sinus syndrome, the sinus node fails to signal properly, resulting in changes in the heart rate.

Description

The sinus node in the heart functions as the heart's pacemaker, or beat regulator. In sick sinus syndrome, patients normally will experience bradycardia, or slowed heart rate. Also, it is not uncommon to see fluctuations between slow and rapid heart rate (tachycardia). This makes the diagnosis and treatment of sick sinus syndrome more complicated than most other cardiac arrhythmias (irregular heart beats). A sick sinus node may be responsible for starting beats too slowly, pausing too long between initiation of heartbeats, or not producing heartbeats at all.

Causes and symptoms

Sick sinus syndrome may be brought on by the use of certain drugs, but is most common in elderly patients. Cardiac **amyloidosis**, a condition in which amyloid, a kind of protein, builds up in heart tissue, may affect the sinus node. Other conditions, such as **sarcoidosis** (round bumps in the tissue surrounding the heart and other organs), **Chagas' disease** (resulting from the bite of a bloodsucking insect) or certain cardiac **myopathies** can cause fiber-like tissue to grow around the normal sinus node, causing the node to malfunction.

A patient may not show any symptoms of sick sinus syndrome. In general, however, the common symptoms are those associated with slow heart rate, such as light-headedness, or dizziness, **fatigue** and **fainting**. Patients may also experience confusion, heart **palpitations**, **angina** or heart failure.

Diagnosis

A slow pulse, especially one that is irregular, may be the first indication of sick sinus syndrome. **Electrocardiography** (ECGs) is a commonly used method of detecting sick sinus syndrome. ECG monitoring for 24 hours is most useful, since with this syndrome, heart rate may alternate between slow and fast, and the determination of this fact can help differentiate sick sinus syndrome from other **arrhythmias**.

Treatment

If drugs are causing the problem, their withdrawal may effectively eliminate the disorder. However, the treatment of sick sinus syndrome is normally delayed until a patient shows symptoms. Once treatment is indicated, most patients will receive a pacemaker. This is a permanent treatment involving implantation of a small device under the skin below the collarbone. Small electrodes run from the device to the heart; they deliver and regulate the electrical signals that cause the heart to beat. Patients with sick sinus syndrome should generally receive dual chamber pacing systems to prevent atrial fibrillation (involuntary contraction of the muscles of the atria). Some drugs are used to treat sick sinus syndrome, but digitalis should be used with caution. Often the use of drugs to regulate the heartbeat should be implemented only after the pacemaker has been placed, since these drugs may further worsen the slow heart rate.

Alternative treatment

The reduction or elimination of certain foods and substances, such as alcohol or **caffeine**, may be advised to control heart rate. Stress reduction may also assist with changes in rate. Homeopathic treatment can work on a deep healing level, while **acupuncture** and botanical medicine can offer supportive treatment for symptoms.

Prognosis

Patients with sick sinus syndrome face relatively normal lives if the disorder is controlled by a pacemaker. However, in some patients, the pacemaker does not adequately control the fluctuations in heart rate. Left untreated, or in severe cases, the heart could stop beating.

Prevention

Elimination of a drug therapy which aggravates sick sinus syndrome is the first line of treatment for some patients. Other causes of the syndrome are not preventable. However, proper treatment of those underlying conditions which affect the tissues of the heart may intervene to prevent sick sinus syndrome from becoming a significant problem.

Resources

ORGANIZATIONS

American Heart Association. 7320 Greenville Ave. Dallas, TX 75231. (214) 373-6300. < http://www.americanheart.org >.

National Heart, Lung and Blood Institute. P.O. Box 30105, Bethesda, MD 20824-0105. (301) 251-1222. < http://www.nhlbi.nih.gov >.

Teresa Odle

Sickle cell disease

Definition

Sickle cell disease describes a group of inherited blood disorders characterized by chronic anemia, painful events, and various complications due to associated tissue and organ damage.

Because sickle cell diseases are characterized by the rapid loss of red blood cells as they enter the circulation, they are classified as hemolytic disorders, "hemolytic" referring to the destruction of the cell membrane of red blood cells resulting in the release of hemoglobin.

Description

The most common and best-known type of sickle cell disease is sickle cell anemia, which is also called meniscocytosis, sicklemia, or SS disease. All types of sickle cell disease are caused by a genetic change in hemoglobin, the oxygen-carrying protein inside the red blood cells. The red blood cells of affected individuals contain a predominance of a structural variant of the usual adult hemoglobin. This variant hemoglobin, called sickle hemoglobin, has a tendency to polymerize into rod-like structures that alter the shape of the usually flexible red blood cells. The cells take on a shape that resembles the curved blade of the sickle, an agricultural tool. Sickle cells have a shorter life span than normally shaped red blood cells. This results in chronic anemia characterized by low levels of hemoglobin and decreased numbers of red blood cells. Sickle cells are also less flexible and stickier than normal red blood cells, and can become trapped in small blood vessels preventing blood flow. This compromises the delivery of oxygen, which can result in **pain** and damage to associated tissues and organs. Sickle cell disease presents with marked variability, even within families.

Carriers of the sickle cell gene are said to have sickle cell trait. Unlike sickle cell disease, sickle cell trait does not cause health problems. In fact, sickle cell trait is protective against **malaria**, a disease caused by blood-borne parasites transmitted through mosquito bites. According to a widely accepted theory, the genetic mutation associated with the sickle cell trait occurred thousands of years ago. Coincidentally, this mutation increased the likelihood that carriers would survive malaria infection. Survivors then passed the mutation on to their offspring, and the trait became established throughout areas where malaria was common. As populations migrated, so did the sickle cell trait. Today, approximately one in 12 African Americans has sickle cell trait.

Worldwide, it has been estimated that one in every 250,000 babies is born annually with sickle cell disease. Sickle cell disease primarily affects people of African, Mediterranean, Middle Eastern, and Asian Indian ancestry. In the United States, sickle cell disease is most often seen in African Americans, in whom the disease occurs in one out of every 400 births. The disease has been described in individuals from several different ethnic backgrounds and is also seen with increased frequency in Latino Americans—particularly those of Caribbean, Central American, and South American ancestry. Approximately one in every 1000-1400 Latino births are affected.

Causes and symptoms

Humans normally make several types of the oxygen-carrying protein hemoglobin. An individual's stage in development determines whether he or she makes primarily embryonic, fetal, or adult hemoglobins. All types of hemoglobin are made of three components: heme, alpha (or alpha-like) globin, and beta (or beta-like) globin. Sickle hemoglobin is the result of a genetic change in the beta globin component of normal adult hemoglobin. The beta globin gene is located on chromosome 11. The sickle cell form of the beta globin gene results from the substitution of a single DNA nucleotide, or genetic building-block. The change from adenine to thymine at codon (position) 6 of the beta globin gene leads to insertion of the amino acid valine–instead of glutamic acid–at this same position in the beta globin protein. As a result of this change, sickle hemoglobin has unique properties in comparison to the usual type of adult hemoglobin.

Most individuals have two normal copies of the beta globin gene, which make normal beta globin that is incorporated into adult hemoglobin. Individuals who have sickle cell trait (called sickle cell carriers) have one normal beta globin gene and one sickle cell gene. These individuals make both the usual adult hemoglobin and sickle hemoglobin in roughly equal proportions, so they do not experience any health problems as a result of having the trait. Although traces of blood in the urine and difficulty in concentrating the urine can occur, neither represents a significant health problem as a result of sickle cell trait. Of the millions of people with sickle cell trait worldwide, a small handful of individuals have experienced acute symptoms. In these very rare cases, individuals were subject to very severe physical strain.

When both members of a couple are carriers of sickle cell trait, there is a 25% chance in each **pregnancy** for the baby to inherit two sickle cell genes and have sickle cell anemia, or SS disease. Correspondingly, there is a 50% chance the baby will have sickle cell trait and a 25% chance that the baby will have the usual type of hemoglobin. Other types of sickle cell disease include SC disease, SD disease, and S/beta **thalassemia**. These conditions are caused by the co-inheritance of the sickle cell gene and another altered beta globin gene. For example, one parent may have sickle cell trait and the other parent may have hemoglobin C trait (another hemoglobin trait that does not cause health problems). For this couple, there would be a 25% chance of SC disease in each pregnancy.

Normal adult hemoglobin transports oxygen from the lungs to tissues throughout the body. Sickle hemoglobin can also transport oxygen. However, once the oxygen is released, sickle hemoglobin tends to polymerize (line-up) into rigid rods that alter the shape of the red blood cell. Sickling of the red blood cell can be triggered by low oxygen, such as occurs in organs with slow blood flow. It can also be triggered by cold temperatures and **dehydration**.

Sickle cells have a decreased life span in comparison to normal red blood cells. Normal red blood cells survive for approximately 120 days in the bloodstream; sickle cells last only 10–12 days. As a result, the bloodstream is chronically short of red blood cells and hemoglobin, and the affected individual develops anemia.

Sickle cells can create other complications. Due to their shape, they do not fit well through small blood vessels. As an aggravating factor, the outside surfaces of sickle cells may have altered chemical properties that increase the cells' 'stickiness'. These sticky sickle cells are more likely to adhere to the inside surfaces of small blood vessels, as well as to other blood cells. As a result of the sickle cells' shape and stickiness, blockages form in small blood vessels. Such blockages prevent oxygenated blood from reaching areas where it is needed, causing pain as well as organ and tissue damage.

The severity of symptoms cannot be predicted based solely on the genetic inheritance. Some individuals with sickle cell disease develop health- or life-threatening problems in infancy, but others may have only mild symptoms throughout their lives. Individuals may experience varying degrees of health at different stages in the life cycle. For the most part, this clinical variability is unpredictable, and the reasons for the observed variability can not usually be determined. However, certain types of sickle cell disease (i.e. SC disease) tend to result in fewer and less severe symptoms on average than other types of sickle cell disease (i.e. SS disease). Some additional modifying factors are known. For example, elevated levels of fetal hemoglobin in a child or adult can decrease the quantity and severity of some symptoms and complications. Fetal hemoglobin is a normally occurring hemoglobin that usually decreases from over 90% of the total hemoglobin to under 1% during the first year of life. This change is genetically determined, although some individuals may experience elevated levels of fetal hemoglobin due to variation in the genes that control fetal hemoglobin production. Such individuals often experience a reduction in their symptoms and complications due to the ability of fetal hemoglobin to prevent the polymerization of sickle hemoglobin, which leads to sickling of the red blood cell.

There are several symptoms that warrant immediate medical attention, including the following:

- signs of infection (**fever** greater than $>101°F$ or $38.3°C$, coughs frequently or breathing trouble, unusual crankiness, feeding difficulties)

- signs of severe anemia (pale skin or lips, yellowing of the skin or eyes, very tired, very weak)

- signs indicating possible dehydration (**vomiting**, **diarrhea**, fewer wet diapers)

- other signs (pain or swelling in the abdomen, swollen hands or feet, screams when touched)

These can be signs of various complications that occur in sickle cell disease.

Infections and effects on the spleen

Children with sickle cell disease who are under age three are particularly prone to life-threatening bacterial infections. *Streptococcus pneumoniae* is the most common offending bacteria, and invasive infection from this organism leads to **death** in 15% of cases. The spleen, an organ that helps to fight bacterial infections, is particularly vulnerable to the effects of sickling. Sickle cells can impede blood flow through the spleen, causing organ damage, which usually results in loss of spleen function by late childhood. The spleen can also become enlarged due to blockages and/or increased activity of the spleen. Rapid enlargement of the spleen may be a sign of another complication called *splenic sequestration*, which occurs mostly in young children and can be life-threatening. Widespread sickling in the spleen prevents adequate blood flow from the organ, removing increasing volumes of blood from the circulation and leading to accompanying signs of severe anemia.

Painful events

Painful events, also known as *vaso-occlusive events*, are a hallmark symptom of sickle cell disease. The frequency and duration of the pain can vary tremendously from person to person and over an individual's life cycle. Painful events are the most common cause of hospitalizations in sickle cell disease. However, only a small portion of individuals with sickle cell disease experience frequent and severe painful events. Most painful events can be managed at home. Pain results when small blood vessel blockages prevent oxygen from reaching tissues. Pain can affect any area of the body, although the extremities, chest, abdomen, and bones are frequently affected sites. There is some evidence that cold temperatures or infection can trigger a painful event, but most events occur for unknown reasons. The hand-foot syndrome, or *dactylitis* , is a particular type of painful event. Most common in toddlers, dactylitis results in pain and swelling in the hands and feet, sometimes accompanied by a fever.

Anemia

Sickle cells have a high turnover rate leading to a deficit of red blood cells in the bloodstream. Common symptoms of anemia include **fatigue**, paleness, and a **shortness of breath**. A particularly severe form of anemia—aplastic anemia—occurs following infection with parvovirus. Parvovirus causes extensive destruction of the bone marrow, bringing production of new red blood cells to a halt. Bone marrow production resumes after seven to 10 days; however, given the short lives of sickle cells, even a brief shut-down in red blood cell production can cause a rapid decline in hemoglobin concentrations.

Delayed growth

The energy demands of the bone marrow for red blood cell production compete with the demands of a growing body. Children with sickle cell anemia may have delayed growth and reach **puberty** at a later age than normal. By early adulthood, they catch up on growth and attain normal height; however, weight typically remains below average.

Stroke

Children with sickle cell disease have a significantly elevated risk of having a **stroke**, which can be one of the most concerning complications of sickle cell disease. Approximately 11% of individuals with sickle cell disease will have a recognizable stroke by the age of 20. **Magnetic resonance imaging** studies have found that 17% of children with sickle cell anemia have evidence of a previous stroke or clinically 'silent' stroke-like events called *transient ischemic events*. Stroke in sickle cell disease is usually caused by a blockage of a blood vessel, but about one fourth of the time may be caused by a hemorrhage (or rupture) of a blood vessel.

Strokes result in compromised delivery of oxygen to an area of the brain. The consequences of stroke can range from life-threatening, to severe physical or cognitive impairments, to apparent or subtle learning disabilities, to undetectable effects. Common stroke symptoms include weakness or **numbness** that affects one side of the body, sudden behavioral changes, loss of vision, confusion, loss of speech or the ability to understand spoken words, **dizziness**, **headache**, seizures, vomiting, or even **coma**.

Approximately two-thirds of the children who have a stroke will have at least one more. Transfusions have been shown to decrease the incidence of a second stroke. A recent study showed that children at highest risk to experience a first stroke were 10 times more likely to stroke if untreated when compared to high-risk children treated with chronic blood **transfusion** therapy. High-risk children were identified using transcranial doppler ultrasound technology to detect individuals with increased blood flow speeds due to constricted intracranial blood vessels.

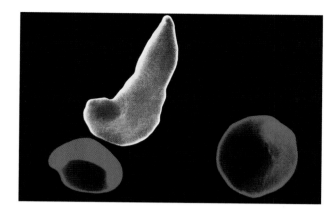

A scanning electron microscopy (SEM) scan of red blood cells taken from a person with sickle cell anemia. The blood cells at the bottom are normal; the diseased, sickle-shaped cells appear at the top. *(Photograph by Dr. Gopal Murti, Photo Researchers, Inc. Reproduced by permission.)*

As of 2003, researchers are investigating various techniques for helping children with memory loss related to strokes caused by sickle cell disease.

Acute chest syndrome

Acute chest syndrome (ACS) is a leading cause of death for individuals with sickle cell disease, and recurrent attacks can lead to permanent lung damage. Therefore rapid diagnosis and treatment is of great importance. ACS can occur at any age and is similar but distinct from **pneumonia**. Affected persons may experience fever, **cough**, chest pain, and shortness of breath. ACS seems to have multiple causes including infection, sickling in the small blood vessels of the lungs, fat embolisms to the lungs, or a combination of factors.

Priapism

Males with sickle cell anemia may experience **priapism**, a condition characterized by a persistent and painful erection of the penis. Due to blood vessel blockage by sickle cells, blood is trapped in the tissue of the penis. Priapism may be short in duration or it may be prolonged. Priapism can be triggered by low oxygen (hypoxemia), alcohol consumption, or sexual intercourse. Since priapism can be extremely painful and result in damage to this tissue causing **impotence**, rapid treatment is essential.

Kidney disease

The environment in the kidney is particularly prone to damage from sickle cells. Signs of kidney damage can include blood in the urine, incontinence, and enlarged kidneys. Adults with sickle cell disease often experience insufficient functioning of the kidneys, which can progress to kidney failure in a small percentage of adults with sickle cell disease.

Jaundice and gallstones

Jaundice is indicated by a yellow tone in the skin and eyes, and alone it is not a health concern. Jaundice may occur if bilirubin levels increase, which can occur with high levels of red blood cell destruction. Bilirubin is the final product of hemoglobin degradation, and is typically removed from the bloodstream by the liver. Therefore, jaundice can also be a sign of a poorly functioning liver, which may also be evidenced by an enlarged liver. Increased bilirubin also leads to increased chance for **gallstones** in children with sickle cell disease. Treatment, which may include removal of the gall bladder, may be selected if the gallstones start causing symptoms.

Retinopathy

The blood vessels that supply oxygen to the retina—the tissue at the back of the eye—may be blocked by sickle cells, leading to a condition called retinopathy. This is one of the only complications that is actually more common in SC disease as compared to SS disease. Retinopathy can be identified through regular ophthalmology evaluations and effectively treated in order to avoid damage to vision.

Joint problems

Avascular necrosis of the hip and shoulder joints, in which bone damage occurs due to compromised blood flow due to sickling, can occur later in childhood. This complication can affect an individual's physical abilities and result in substantial pain.

Diagnosis

Inheritance of sickle cell disease or trait cannot be prevented, but it may be predicted. Screening is recommended for individuals in high-risk populations. In the United States, African Americans and Latino Americans have the highest risk of having the disease or trait. Sickle cell is also common among individuals of Mediterranean, Middle Eastern, and Eastern Indian descent.

A complete **blood count** (CBC) will describe several aspects of an individual's blood cells. A person with sickle cell disease will have a lower than normal hemoglobin level, together with other characteristic red blood cell abnormalities. A *hemoglobin electrophoresis* is a test that can help identify the types and quantities of hemoglobin made by an individual. This test uses an electric field applied across a slab of gel-like material. Hemoglobins migrate through this gel at various rates and to specific locations, depending on their size, shape, and electrical charge. Although sickle hemoglobin (Hb S) and regular adult hemoglobin (called Hb A) differ by only one amino acid, they can be clearly separated using **hemoglobin electrophoresis**. *Isoelectric focusing* and *high-performance liquid chromatography (HPLC)* use similar principles to separate hemoglobins and can be used instead of or in various combinations with hemoglobin electrophoresis to determine the types of hemoglobin present.

Another test called the sickledex can help confirm the presence of sickle hemoglobin, although this test cannot provide accurate or reliable diagnosis when used alone. When Hb S is present, but there is an absence or only a trace of Hb A, sickle cell anemia is a likely diagnosis. Additional beta globin *DNA testing*, which looks directly at the beta globin gene, can be performed to help confirm the diagnosis and establish the exact genetic type of sickle cell disease. CBC and hemoglobin electrophoresis are also typically used to diagnose sickle cell trait and various other types of beta globin traits.

Diagnosis of sickle cell disease can occur under various circumstances. If an individual has symptoms that are suggestive of this diagnosis, the above-described screening tests can be performed followed by DNA testing, if indicated. Screening at birth using HPLC or a related technique offers the opportunity for early intervention. More than 40 states include sickle cell screening as part of the usual battery of blood tests done for newborns. This allows for early identification and treatment. Hemoglobin trait screening is recommended for any individual of a high-risk ethnic background who may be considering having children. When both members of a couple are found to have sickle cell trait, or other related hemoglobin traits, they can receive **genetic counseling** regarding the risk of sickle cell disease in their future children and various testing options.

Sickle cell disease can be identified before birth through the use of prenatal diagnosis. *Chorionic villus sampling (CVS)* can be offered as early as 10 weeks of pregnancy and involves removing a sample of the placenta made by the baby and testing the cells. CVS carries a risk of causing a **miscarriage** that is between one-half to one percent.

Amniocentesis is generally offered between 15 and 22 weeks of pregnancy, but can sometimes be offered earlier. Two to three tablespoons of the fluid surrounding the baby is removed. This fluid contains fetal cells that can be tested. This test carries a risk of causing a miscarriage, which is not greater than one percent. Pregnant woman and couples may choose prenatal testing in order to prepare for the birth of a baby that may have sickle cell disease. Alternately, knowing the diagnosis during pregnancy allows for the option of pregnancy termination.

Preimplantation genetic diagnosis (PGD) is a relatively new technique that involves in-vitro fertilization followed by **genetic testing** of one cell from each developing embryo. Only the embryos unaffected by sickle cell disease are transferred back into the uterus. PGD is currently available on a research basis only, and is relatively expensive.

Treatment

There are several practices intended to prevent some of the symptoms and complications of sickle cell disease. These include preventative **antibiotics**, good hydration, immunizations, and access to comprehensive care. Maintaining good health through adequate **nutrition**, avoiding stresses and infection, and getting proper rest is also important. Following these guidelines is intended to improve the health of individuals with sickle cell disease.

Penicillin

Infants are typically started on a course of penicillin that extends from infancy to age six. Use of this antibiotic is meant to ward off potentially fatal infections. Infections at any age are treated aggressively with antibiotics. Vaccines for common infections, such as *pneumococcal pneumonia*, are also recommended.

Pain management

Pain is one of the primary symptoms of sickle cell anemia, and controlling it is an important concern. The methods necessary for pain control are based on individual factors. Some people can gain adequate pain control through over-the-counter oral painkillers (**analgesics**). Other individuals, or painful events, may require stronger methods that can include administration of **narcotics**. Alternative therapies may be useful in avoiding or controlling pain, including relaxation, hydration, avoiding extremes of temperature, and the application of local warmth.

Blood transfusions

Blood transfusions are not usually given on a regular basis but are used to treat individuals with

Purpose

Sigmoidoscopy is used most often in screening for colorectal **cancer** or to determine the cause of rectal bleeding. It is also used for the diagnosis of inflammatory bowel disease and other benign diseases of the lower intestine.

Cancer of the rectum and colon is the second most common cancer in the United States, and claims the lives of approximately 56,000 people annually. As a result, The American Cancer Society recommends that people age 50 and over be screened for colorectal cancer every five years. The screening includes a flexible sigmoidoscopy. Screening at an earlier age should be done on patients who have a family history of colon or **rectal cancer**, or small growths in the colon (polyps).

Individuals with inflammatory bowel disease (Crohn's colitis or **ulcerative colitis**) are at increased risk for colorectal cancer and should begin their screenings at a younger age, and be screened more frequently. Many doctors screen such patients more often than every three to five years. Those with ulcerative colitis should be screened beginning 10 years after the onset of disease; those with Crohn's colitis beginning 15 years after the onset of disease.

Some doctors prefer to do this screening with a colonoscope, which allows them to see the entire colon (certain patients, such as those with Crohn's colitis or ulcerative colitis, must be screened with a colonoscope). However, compared with sigmoidoscopy, **colonoscopy** is a longer process, causes more discomfort, and is more costly.

Studies have indicated that about one-fourth of all precancerous or small cancerous growths in the colorectal region can be seen with a rigid sigmoidoscope. The longer, flexible version, which is the primary type of sigmoidoscope used in the screening process, can detect more than one-half of all growths in this region. This examination is usually performed in combination with a **fecal occult blood test**, in an effort to increase detection of polyps and cancers that lie beyond the scope's reach.

Precautions

Sigmoidoscopy can usually be conducted in a doctor's office or a health clinic. However, some individuals should have the procedure done in a hospital day surgery facility. These include patients with rectal bleeding, and patients whose blood does not clot well (possibly as a result of blood-thinning medications).

The exam is not always adequate. A 2004 study reported that among older patients and women, sigmoidoscopy is not always effective, particularly because insertion depth is not adequate. For unknown reasons, this is almost twice as true for women as for men.

Description

Most sigmoidoscopy is done with a flexible fiber-optic tube. The tube contains a light source and a camera lens. The doctor moves the sigmoidoscope up beyond the rectum (the first 1 ft/30 cm of the colon), examining the interior walls of the rectum. If a 2 ft/60 cm scope is used, the next portion of the colon can also be examined for any irregularities.

The procedure takes 20 to 30 minutes, during which time the patient will remain awake. Light **sedation** may be given to some patients. There is some discomfort (usually bloating and cramping) because air is injected into the bowel to widen the passage for the sigmoidoscope. **Pain** is rare except in individuals with active inflammatory bowel disease.

In a colorectal cancer screening, the doctor is looking for polyps or tumors. Studies have shown that over time, many polyps develop into cancerous lesions and tumors. Using instruments threaded through the fiber-optic tube, cancerous or precancerous polyps can either be removed or biopsied during the sigmoidoscopy. People who have cancerous polyps removed can be referred for full colonoscopy, or more frequent sigmoidoscopy, as necessary.

The doctor may also look for signs of ulcerative colitis, which include a loss of blood flow to the lining of the bowel, a thickening of the lining, and sometimes a discharge of blood and pus mixed with stool. The doctor can also look for **Crohn's disease**, which often appears as shallow or deep ulcerations, or erosions and fissures in the lining of the colon. In many cases, these signs appear in the first few centimeters of the colon above the rectum, and it is not necessary to do a full colonoscopic exam.

Private insurance plans often cover the cost of sigmoidoscopy for screening in healthy individuals over 50, or for diagnostic purposes. Medicare covers the cost for diagnostic exams, and may cover the costs for screening exams.

Preparation

The purpose of preparation for sigmoidoscopy is to clean the lower bowel of stool so that the doctor can see the lining. Many patients are required to consume only clear liquids on the day before the test, and to take two **enemas** on the morning of the procedure. The

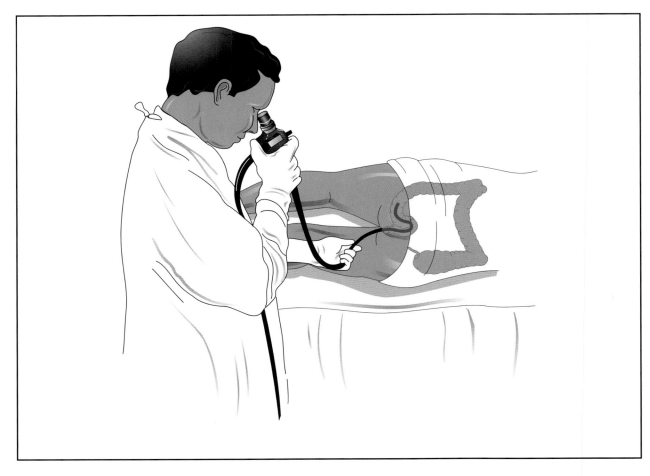

Sigmoidoscopy is a procedure most often used in screening for colorectal cancer and as a test in diagnosis of possible inflammatory bowel disease. As illustrated above, the physician can view the rectum and colon through a sigmoidoscope, a 12 inch (30 cm) or 24 inch (60 cm) flexible fiber-optic tube which contains a light source and a lens. *(Illustration by Electronic Illustrators Group.)*

bowel is cleaner, however, if patients also take an oral laxative preparation of 1.5 oz phospho-soda the evening before the sigmoidoscopy.

Certain medications should be avoided for a week before having a sigmoidoscopy. These include:

- aspirin, or products containing aspirin
- ibuprofen products (Nuprin, Advil, or Motrin)
- iron or **vitamins** containing iron

Although most prescription medication can be taken as usual, patients should check with their doctor in advance.

Aftercare

Patients may feel mild cramping after the procedure that will improve after passing gas. Patients can resume their normal activities almost immediately.

Risks

There is a slight risk of bleeding from the procedure. This risk is heightened in individuals whose blood does not clot well, either due to disease or medication, and in those with active inflammatory bowel disease. The most serious complication of sigmoidoscopy is bowel perforation (tear). This complication is very rare, however, occurring only about once in every 7,500 procedures.

Normal results

A normal exam shows a smooth bowel wall with no evidence of inflammation, polyps or tumors.

Abnormal results

For a cancer screening sigmoidoscopy, an abnormal result involves one or more noncancerous or

KEY TERMS

Biopsy—A procedure where a piece of tissue is removed from a patient for diagnostic testing.

Colorectal cancer—Cancer of the large intestine, or colon, including the rectum (the last 16 in of the large intestine before the anus).

Inflammatory bowel disease—Ulcerative colitis or Crohn's colitis; chronic conditions characterized by periods of diarrhea, bloating, abdominal cramps, and pain, sometimes accompanied by weight loss and malnutrition because of the inability to absorb nutrients.

Polyp—A small growth that can be precancerous when it appears in the colon.

precancerous polyps or tumors. Patients showing polyps have an increased risk of developing colorectal cancer in the future.

Small polyps can be completely removed. Larger polyps or tumors usually require the doctor to remove a portion of the growth for diagnostic testing. Depending on the test results, the patient is then scheduled to have the growth removed surgically, either as an urgent matter if it is cancerous, or as an elective surgery within a few months if it is noncancerous.

In a diagnostic sigmoidoscopy, an abnormal result shows signs of active inflammatory bowel disease, either a thickening of the intestinal lining consistent with ulcerative colitis, or ulcerations or fissures consistent with Crohn's disease.

Sigmoidoscopy is a procedure most often used in screening for colorectal cancer and as a test in diagnosis of possible inflammatory bowel disease. As illustrated above, the physician can view the rectum and colon through a sigmoidoscope, a 12 inch (30 cm) or 24 inch (60 cm) flexible fiber-optic tube which contains a light source and a lens.

Resources

PERIODICALS

Johnson, Brett Andrew. "Flexible Sigmoidoscopy: Screening for Colorectal Cancer." *American Family Physician* March 15, 1999: 1537–46.

Manoucheri, Manoucher, et al. "Bowel Preparations for Flexible Sigmoidoscopy: Which Method Yields the Best Results?" *The Journal of Family Practice* 48, no. 4 (April, 1999): 272–4.

"Women are Twice as Likely as Men to Have an Inadequate Signoidoscopy Examination." *Doctor* February 5, 2004: 13.

OTHER

"Diagnostic Tests." *The National Digestive Diseases Information Clearing house (National Institutes of Health)*. July 5, 2001. < http://www.niddk.nih.gov/health/digest/pubs/diagtest/index.htm >.

"Overview: Colon and Rectum Cancer." *The American Cancer Society*. Jan. 20, 2005. http://www.cancer.org/docroot/CRI/content/CRI_2_2_1X_How_Many_People_Get_Colorectal_Cancer.asp?sitearea = .

Jon H. Zonderman
Teresa G. Odle

Sildenafil citrate

Definition

Sildenafil citrate (Viagra) is a medication used to treat *erectile dysfunction* (ED), or **impotence**, in men.

Purpose

Labeled use

Viagra treats **erectile dysfunction**, the inability to achieve and/or maintain an erection of the penis that is adequate for sexual intercourse. Ten to fifteen million men in the United States suffer from ED, and by age 65, up to 25% of men have experienced impotence problems. Erectile dysfunction can be caused by a number of physical and psychological conditions, including diabetes, depression, **prostate cancer**, **spinal cord injury**, **multiple sclerosis**, artherosclerosis, and heart disease. Injuries to the penis that cause nerve, tissue, or vascular damage can trigger impotence. It is also a common side effect of some prescription medications, including **antihistamines**, antidepressants, antihypertensives, antipsychotics, **beta blockers**, **diuretics**, tranquilizers, appetite suppressants, cimetidine (Tagamet), and **finasteride** (Propecia).

A study of African American and Hispanic men published in 2002 reported that Viagra appears to be equally safe and equally effective across different racial and ethnic groups in the United States.

Investigational uses

Although not approved for use in women, clinical studies have shown that sildenafil citrate may be effective in relieving female **sexual dysfunction** for some women. In one study, both female and male study participants who suffered from sexual dysfunction related to their use of such psychotropic medications as **benzodiazepines** reported an increase in arousal and overall sexual satisfaction when they began taking Viagra. Several studies have also indicated the drug may be effective in improving libido and arousal in women taking selective serotonin uptake inhibitors (SSRIs).

Another possible use of sildenafil in women is the treatment of **infertility**. Women who have had repeated failures with **in vitro fertilization** (IVF) due to poor development of the tissue that lines the uterus may benefit from treatment with vaginal suppositories containing sildenafil. One study reported that 70% of patients had a significant thickening of the uterine lining, with 29% having a successful implantation of a new embryo, and 45% achieving ongoing pregnancies.

Another investigational study conducted by researchers at Johns Hopkins University School of Medicine in Baltimore, and published in the August 2000 issue of the *Journal of Clinical Investigation* found that Viagra may have additional clinical promise for people with diabetes beyond treating ED. In animal studies, Viagra was effective in relaxing the pyloric muscle of stomach, improving digestion and relieving the symptoms of gastroparesis. Up to 75% of people with diabetes suffer from gastroparesis, which causes bloating, **nausea**, loss of appetite, and **vomiting**. Further human studies are needed to evaluate Viagra's effectiveness in treating this common diabetic complication.

Because of its capacity to enhance nitric oxide production, sildenafil has been investigated as a possible treatment for other disorders that are caused by impaired nitric oxide production. One such disorder is esophageal motility dysfunction (**achalasia**), in which the smooth muscles of the esophagus and the cardiac sphincter remain constricted, causing difficulty in swallowing, regurgitation of food, and chest **pain** when eating. A study published in 2000 in the journal *Gastroenterology* found that sildenafil temporarily improved the condition in some patients by relaxing the lower esophageal muscles. An Italian study reported in 2002 that sildenafil shows genuine promise as a treatment for spastic **esophageal disorders**.

Precautions

Viagra is not labeled or approved for use by women or children, or by men without erectile dysfunction. The medication may also be contraindicated (not recommended for use) in patients with certain medical conditions.

Because sexual activity can **stress** the heart, men who have heart problems should check with their physician to see if sexual activity is recommended. Viagra may trigger temporary **hypotension** (low blood pressure) and is known to increase cardiovascular nerve activity, so it is prescribed with caution in men with a history of **heart attack**, artherosclerosis, **angina**, arrhythmia, and chronic low blood pressure problems. However, a study published in the March 15, 2001, *British Medical Journal* found no evidence that the drug causes a higher incidence of heart attack. A four-year update on the safety of Viagra published in September 2002 corroborated the findings of the British report, and stated that the only absolute contraindication for the use of sildenafil is the concurrent use of nitrates.

Anyone experiencing cardiovascular symptoms such as **dizziness**, chest or arm pain, and nausea when participating in sexual activity after taking Viagra should stop the encounter. They should also not take Viagra again until they have discussed the episode with their healthcare provider.

It is recommended that men with kidney or liver impairments, and men over age 65, start at the lowest possible dosage of Viagra (25 mg). Clinical studies have shown that the drug builds up in the plasma of these patients to a concentration that is three to eight times higher than normal. Caution is also recommended in prescribing the drug to individuals with *retinitis pigmentosa*, a rare genetic eye disorder. Viagra should not be taken more than once per day by anyone.

Viagra has not been studied for use on patients with stomach ulcers and bleeding disorders, and its safety in these individuals is unknown. Men who have either of these conditions should let their physician know before taking Viagra. It should also be used with caution in men with misshapen or deformed penises, such as those with Peyronie's disease, cavernosal fibrosis, or with angulation of the penis.

Men who take medications containing nitrates (e.g., nitroglycerin, isosorbide mononitrate, isosorbide dinitrate) should never take Viagra, as the interaction between the two drugs may cause a dramatic drop in blood pressure, and possibly trigger a heart attack or **stroke**. This includes illegal recreational drugs such as amyl nitrates (also known as poppers).

Viagra may also interact with other prescription and over-the-counter (OTC) medications, either magnifying or diluting the intended therapeutic effects of one or both drugs. Some drugs that have a known interaction with Viagra include the protease inhibitor ritonavir and the antibiotic erythromycin. For this reason, it is critical that men who are prescribed Viagra let their healthcare providers know all the medications they are taking.

Other medications and therapies for erectile dysfunction, including vacuum or pump devices, drug injections (Caverject), and urethral suppositories (MUSE), should never be used in conjunction with Viagra.

Description

Sildenafil citrate was originally developed in 1991 as a treatment for angina, or chest pain. The drug, marketed under the name Viagra, received FDA market clearance as a treatment for impotence in March 1998, and since that time it has been prescribed for over 10 million men worldwide. It was the first oral medication approved for ED treatment. A newer drug, tadalafil, has been developed to treat men who do not respond to sildenafil. Tadalafil has gained preliminary approval in the European Union (EU), and is in the final stages of regulatory approval in Canada as of November 2002.

Viagra is a vasodilator, a drug that has the effect of dilating the blood vessels. It works by improving blood circulation to the penis, and by enhancing the effects of *nitric oxide*, the agent that relaxes the smooth muscle of the penis and regulates blood vessels during sexual stimulation, allowing the penis to become engorged and achieve an erection.

The average recommended dose of Viagra is 50 mg. For men that do not respond adequately to this amount, the dosage may be increased up to 100 mg or decreased to 25 mg. The medication is taken approximately one hour before sexual activity is planned, and may remain effective for up to four hours.

Viagra does not increase sexual desire. Sexual stimulation and arousal are required for the medication to be effective. Despite its widespread use as a recreational drug, it is not an aphrodisiac and there is no clinical evidence that it improves sexual performance in men who are not suffering from ED.

Many insurance plans provide coverage or reimbursement for sildenafil citrate provided it is prescribed to treat erectile dysfunction. A 1999 report issued by a health insurance consulting group indicated that almost half of the men taking Viagra at least once weekly receive insurance reimbursement for the drug. The pills cost approximately $10 each,

and insurers may limit coverage to a specific number of pills each month.

Preparation

Viagra requires time to be absorbed by the body and become effective. The average recommended time frame for taking the drug is one hour before initiating sexual activity, although depending on an individual's response to the drug, this time can vary from four hours to 30 minutes.

Men should always consult with their physician before beginning treatment with sildenafil citrate. The medication is not for everyone, and a healthcare professional needs to evaluate medical history and perform a thorough medical examination before prescribing the drug. In addition, erectile dysfunction may be a symptom of an undiagnosed condition (i.e., diabetes) for which treatment is critical, and may actually reverse the impotence problem.

Risks

The most commonly reported side effects of Viagra are **headache**, flushing of the face, upset stomach, and nasal congestion.

Other less common side effects include, but are not limited to:

- vision problems, including sensitivity to light, blurred vision, and a color tinge to vision
- urinary tract infection
- diarrhea
- dizziness
- rash

Side effects may be reduced or eliminated through adjustments to dosage. Men who experience these symptoms should consult their physician.

Priapism, a painful and prolonged erection that lasts for two to six hours, is a rare but potentially serious side effect of Viagra. Because prolonged erection can permanently damage the tissues of the penis, anyone who experiences an erection lasting over four hours should call a healthcare professional immediately.

Men who are taking Viagra and inadvertently or intentionally take a medication containing nitrates may suffer from life-threatening hypotension—a severe drop in blood pressure.

The cardiovascular risks of sildenafil citrate are still under investigation. The drug is known to cause

KEY TERMS

Angina—Angina pectoris, or chest pain, caused by an insufficient supply of oxygen and decreased blood flow to the heart muscle. Angina is frequently the first sign of coronary artery disease.

Angulation of the penis—Abnormal bend or angle to the structure of the penis.

Antidepressants—Medications prescribed to relieve major depression. Classes of antidepressants include selective serotonin reuptake inhibitors (fluoxetine/Prozac, sertraline/Zoloft), tricyclics (amitriptyline/Elavil), MAOIs (phenelzine/Nardil), and heterocyclics (bupropion/Wellbutrin, trazodone/Desyrel).

Antihistamines—A drug used to treat allergic conditions that counteracts histamines — a substance in the body that causes itching, vascular changes, and mucus secretion when released by cells.

Antihypertensives—Medications used to treat high blood pressure.

Antipsychotics—A class of drugs used to control psychotic symptoms in patients with psychotic disorders such as schizophrenia and delusional disorder. Antipsychotics include risperidone (Risperdal), haloperidol (Haldol), and chlorpromazine (Thorazine).

Arrhythmia—Irregular heartbeat caused by erratic electrical signals or nerve impulses to the cardiac muscles.

Artherosclerosis—The cause of coronary artery disease, in which the walls of the coronary arteries thicken due to the accumulation of plaque in the blood vessels.

Beta blockers—Drugs that lower blood pressure and reduce stress to the heart by blocking the actions of beta receptors that control the speed and strength of heart muscle contractions and blood vessel dilation.

Cavernosal fibrosis—The formation of abnormal fibrous tissue in the erectile tissue of the penis.

Diuretics—Any substance that increases urine output.

Erectile dysfunction—Impotence; the inability of a man to achieve and/or maintain an erection of sufficient quality for sexual intercourse.

Gastroparesis—Nerve damage of the stomach that delays or stops stomach emptying, resulting in nausea, vomiting, bloating, discomfort, and weight loss.

Peyronie's disease—A disease which causes a hardening of the corpora cavernosa, the erectile tissue of the penis. The penis may become misshapen and/or curved as a result.

Placebo—An inactive substance with no pharmacological action that is administered to some patients in clinical trials to determine the relative effectiveness of another drug administered to a second group of patients.

Priapism—A painful, abnormally prolonged erection (i.e., four or more hours).

Protease inhibitor—A drug that inhibits the action of enzymes.

Retinitis pigmentosa—An inherited degenerative eye disease that impairs night vision and drastically narrows the field of vision.

Selective serotonin uptake inhibitors (SSRIs)—Drugs that regulate depression by blocking the reabsorption of serotonin in the brain consequently raising serotonin levels. SSRIs include fluoxetine (Prozac), sertraline (Zoloft), and paroxetine (Paxil).

Serotonin—One of three major neurotransmitters found in the brain that is linked to emotions.

---

dips in blood pressure and to boost cardiovascular nerve activity. Some cardiovascular-related deaths have been reported in men who use Viagra, but it is unclear whether the fatalities were due to the drug itself or to the underlying heart disease. Further complicating the picture is the fact that the stress of sexual activity may have triggered the fatal cardiac event with or without the use of Viagra. The *BMJ* study, and a report published in the April 18, 2001 issue of the *Journal of the American Medical Association* (*JAMA*) suggest that the drug does not increase the risk of heart attack. However, *JAMA* also notes

that further studies are necessary to confirm this finding.

Although it is a prescription drug, as of early 2001 there was still a thriving illicit market for Viagra via the Internet. Aside from the health risks recreational use of the drug poses to individuals with heart conditions and other contraindicated disorders, any adverse effects caused by Viagra cannot be tracked by regulatory authorities if it has been illegally obtained. In addition, the drug appears to be toxic in large doses. In November 2002, a group of French toxicologists reported the case of a 56-year-old male who took a fatal overdose of Viagra.

Normal results

When used as directed, Viagra allows men with erectile dysfunction to achieve and maintain a penile erection when aroused during sexual activity. Double-blind, randomized clinical trials of sildenafil citrate have shown that the drug has an 63–82% efficacy rate in improving erectile activity among men with ED, depending on the dose administered (between 25 and 100 mg), compared to a 24% improvement in men receiving a placebo.

Resources

BOOKS

Medical Economics Company. *The Physicians DeskReference (PDR)*. 55th ed. Montvale, NJ: Medical Economics Company, 2001.

Stolar, Mark. *Viagra & You*. New York:Berkley Books, 1999.

PERIODICALS

Bortolotti, M., N. Pandolfo, M. Giovannini, et al. " Effect of Sildenafil on Hypertensive Lower Oesophageal Sphincter" *European Journal of Clinical Investigation* 32 (September 2002): 682–685.

Boyce, E. G., and E. M. Umland. "Sildenafil Citrate: A Therapeutic Update." *Clinical Therapeutics* 1 (January 2001): 2–23.

Kuan, J., and G. Brock. " Selective Phosphodiesterase Type 5 Inhibition using Tadalafil for the Treatment of Erectile Dysfunction." *Expert Opinion on Investigational Drugs* 11 (November 11, 2002): 1605–1613.

Mitka, Mike. "Studies of Viagra Offer Some Reassurance to Men With Concerns About Cardiac Effects." *The Journal of the American Medical Association* 285, no.15 (April 18, 2001): 1950.

Padma-nathan, H., I. Eardley, R. A. Kloner, et al. " A 4-year Update on the Safety of Sildenafil Citrate (Viagra)." *Urology* 60, no.2, Supplement 2 (September 2002): 67–90.

Shakir, S. A., et al. "Cardiovascular Events in Users of Sildenafil: Results from First Phase of Prescription Event Monitoring in England." *British Medical Journal* 322, no.7287 (March 17, 2001): 651–2.

Sher, G., and J. D. Fisch. " Effect of Vaginal Sildenafil on the Outcome of in vitro Fertilization (IVF) After Multiple IVF Failures Attributed to Poor Endometrial Development." *Fertility and Sterility* 78 (November 2002): 1256–1257.

Tracqui, A., A. Miras, A. Tabib, et al. " Fatal Overdosage with Sildenafil Citrate (Viagra): First Report and Review of the Literature." *Human and Experimental Toxicology* 21 (November 2002): 623–629.

"Viagra Increases Nerve Activity Associated with Cardiovascular Function." *Drug Week* January 26, 2001: 11.

Young, J. M., C. Bennett, P. Gilhooly, et al. " Efficacy and Safety of Sildenafil Citrate (Viagra) in Black and Hispanic American Men." *Urology* 60, no. 2, Supplement 2 (September 2002): 39–48.

ORGANIZATIONS

American Heart Association. American Heart Association. 7320 Greenville Ave. Dallas, TX 75231. (214) 373-630 or (800) 242-8721. inquire@heart.org. < http://www.americanheart.org >.

U.S. Food and Drug Administration (FDA), Center for Drug Evaluation and Research. Viagra Information. < http://www.fda.gov/cder/consumerinfo/viagra/default.htm >.

OTHER

Pfizer, Inc. Viagra Information Site. < http://www.viagra.com/ >.

Paula Anne Ford-Martin
Rebecca J. Frey, PhD

Silent thyroiditis *see* **Thyroiditis**

Silicosis

Definition

Silicosis is a progressive disease that belongs to a group of lung disorders called pneumoconioses. Silicosis is marked by the formation of lumps (nodules) and fibrous scar tissue in the lungs. It is the oldest known occupational lung disease, and is caused by exposure to inhaled particles of silica, mostly from quartz in rocks, sand, and similar substances.

Description

It is estimated that there are TWO million workers in the United States employed in occupations at risk for the development of silicosis. These include miners, foundry workers, stonecutters, potters and ceramics workers, sandblasters, tunnel workers, and rock drillers. Silicosis is mostly found in adults over 40. It has four forms:

- Chronic. Chronic silicosis may take 15 or more years of exposure to develop. There is only mild impairment of lung functioning. Chronic silicosis may progress to more advanced forms.

- Complicated. Patients with complicated silicosis have noticeable **shortness of breath**, weight loss, and extensive formation of fibrous tissue (fibrosis) in the lungs. These patients are at risk for developing **tuberculosis** (TB).

- Accelerated. This form of silicosis appears after 5-10 years of intense exposure. The symptoms are similar to those of complicated silicosis. Patients in this group often develop rheumatoid arthritis and other autoimmune disorders.

- Acute. Acute silicosis develops within six months to two years of intense exposure to silica. The patient loses a great deal of weight and is constantly short of breath. These patients are at severe risk of TB.

Causes and symptoms

The precise mechanism that triggers the development of silicosis is still unclear. What is known is that particles of silica dust get trapped in the tiny sacs (alveoli) in the lungs where air exchange takes place. White blood cells called macrophages in the alveoli ingest the silica and die. The resulting inflammation attracts other macrophages to the region. The nodule forms when the immune system forms fibrous tissue to seal off the reactive area. The disease process may stop at this point, or speed up and destroy large areas of the lung. The fibrosis may continue even after the worker is no longer exposed to silica.

Early symptoms of silicosis include shortness of breath after exercising and a harsh, dry cough. Patients may have more trouble breathing and **cough** up blood as the disease progresses. Congestive **heart failure** can give their nails a bluish tint. Patients with advanced silicosis may have trouble sleeping and experience chest **pain**, hoarseness, and loss of appetite. Silicosis patients are at high risk for TB, and should be checked for the disease during the doctor's examination.

Diagnosis

Diagnosis of silicosis is based on:

- A detailed occupational history.

- Chest x rays will usually show small round opaque areas in chronic silicosis; the round areas are larger in complicated and accelerated silicosis.

- bronchoscopy

- lung function tests

It should be noted that the severity of the patient's symptoms does not always correlate with x-ray findings or lung function test results.

KEY TERMS

Fibrosis—The development of excess fibrous connective tissue in an organ. Fibrosis of the lungs is a symptom of silicosis.

Pneumoconiosis (plural, pneumoconioses)—Any chronic lung disease caused by inhaling particles of silica or similar substances that lead to loss of lung function.

Silica—A substance (silicon dioxide) occurring in quartz sand, flint, and agate. It is used in making glass, scouring and grinding powders, pottery, etc.

Treatment

Symptom management

There is no cure for silicosis. Therapy is intended to relieve symptoms, treat complications, and prevent respiratory infections. It includes careful monitoring for signs of TB. Respiratory symptoms may be treated with bronchodilators, increased fluid intake, steam inhalation, and physical therapy. Patients with severe breathing difficulties may be given **oxygen therapy** or placed on a mechanical ventilator. Acute silicosis may progress to complete **respiratory failure**. Heart-lung transplants are the only hope for some patients.

Patients with silicosis should call their doctor for any of the following symptoms:

- tiredness or mental confusion

- continued weight loss

- coughing up blood

- fever, chest pain, breathlessness, or new unexplained symptoms

Lifestyle changes

Patients with silicosis should be advised to quit smoking, prevent infections by avoiding crowds and persons with colds or similar infections, and receive vaccinations against **influenza** and **pneumonia**. They should be encouraged to increase their **exercise** capacity by keeping up regular activity, and to learn to pace themselves with their daily routine.

Prognosis

Silicosis is currently incurable. The prognosis for patients with chronic silicosis is generally good. Acute silicosis, however, may progress rapidly to respiratory failure and death.

Prevention

Silicosis is a preventable disease. Preventive occupational safety measures include:

- controls to minimize workplace exposure to silica dust
- substitution of substances–especially in sandblasting–that are less hazardous than silica
- clear identification of dangerous areas in the workplace
- Informing workers about the dangers of overexposure to silica dust, training them in safety techniques, and giving them appropriate protective clothing and equipment.

Coworkers of anyone diagnosed with silicosis should be examined for symptoms of the disease. The state health department and the Occupational Safety and Health Administration (OSHA) or the Mine Safety and Health Administration (MSHA) must be notified whenever a diagnosis of silicosis is confirmed.

Resources

ORGANIZATIONS

Centers for Disease Control and Prevention. 1600 Clifton Rd., NE, Atlanta, GA 30333. (800) 311-3435, (404) 639-3311. <http://www.cdc.gov>.

Maureen Haggerty

Silo-filler's disease *see* **Lung diseases due to gas or chemical exposure**

Simethicone *see* **Antigas agents**

Singer's nodules *see* **Vocal cord nodules and polyps**

Sinus endoscopy

Definition

An endoscope is a narrow flexible tube which contains an optical device like a telescope or magnifying lens with a bright light. In sinus endoscopy, the endoscope is inserted into the nose, and the interior of the nasal passages, sinuses, and throat is examined.

Purpose

Sinus endoscopy is used to help diagnose structural defects, infection or damage to the sinuses, or structures in the nose and throat. It may be used to view polyps and growths in the sinuses and to investigate causes of recurrent inflammation of the sinuses (**sinusitis**). During surgical procedures, an endoscope may be used to view the area to correct sinus-drainage problems or to remove polyps from the nose and throat.

Precautions

Insertion of the endoscope may cause a gag reflex and some discomfort, however, no special precautions are required to prepare for nasal endoscopy.

Description

This procedure can be done in a physician's office. The endoscope is inserted into a nostril and is threaded through the sinus passages to the throat. To make viewing of these areas easier, and to record the areas being examined, a camera, monitor, or other such viewing device is connected to the endoscope

Preparation

For the procedure, the patient is usually awake and seated upright in a chair. A local anesthetic spray or liquid may be applied to the throat to make insertion of the endoscope less uncomfortable.

Aftercare

After the endoscope is removed, the patient can return to most normal activities. If an anesthetic was used, the patient may have to wait until the **numbness** wears off to be able to eat or drink.

Risks

The insertion and removal of the endoscope may stimulate a gag reflex, and can cause some discomfort. The procedure may also irritate the tissues of the nose and throat, causing a **nosebleed** or coughing.

Normal results

Under normal conditions, no polyps, or growths are found in the sinuses. There should also be no evidence of infection, swelling, injury, or any structural defect that would prevent normal draining of the sinuses.

Abnormal results

Polyps, growths, infections, or structural defects of the nasal passages are considered abnormal.

Resources

ORGANIZATIONS

American Academy of Otolaryngology-Head and Neck Surgery, Inc. One Prince St., Alexandria VA 22314-3357. (703) 836-4444. < http://www.entnet.org >.

Ear Foundation. 1817 Patterson St., Nashville, TN 37203. (800) 545-4327. < http://www.earfoundation.org >.

OTHER

"Endoscopic Plastic Surgery." *Southern California Plastic Surgery Group' Page.* < http://www.face-doctor.com >.

Altha Roberts Edgren

Sinus x ray *see* **Skull x rays**

Sinusitis

Definition

Sinusitis refers to an inflammation of the sinuses, airspaces within the bones of the face. Sinusitis is most often due to an infection within these spaces.

Description

The sinuses are paired air pockets located within the bones of the face. They are:

- the frontal sinuses; located above the eyes, in the center region of each eyebrow
- the maxillary sinuses; located within the cheekbones, just to either side of the nose
- the ethmoid sinuses; located between the eyes, just behind the bridge of the nose.
- the sphenoid sinuses; Located just behind the ethmoid sinuses, and behind the eyes.

The sinuses are connected with the nose. They are lined with the same kind of skin found elsewhere within the respiratory tract. This skin has tiny little hairs projecting from it, called cilia. The cilia beat constantly, to help move the mucus produced in the sinuses into the respiratory tract. The beating cilia sweeping the mucus along the respiratory tract helps to clear the respiratory tract of any debris, or any organisms which may be present. When the lining of the sinuses is at all swollen, the swelling interferes with the normal flow of mucus. Trapped mucus can then fill the sinuses, causing an uncomfortable sensation of pressure and providing an excellent environment for the growth of infection-causing bacteria.

Causes and symptoms

Sinusitis is almost always due to an infection, although swelling from **allergies** can mimic the symptoms of pressure, **pain**, and congestion; and allergies can set the stage for a bacterial infection. Bacteria are the most common cause of sinus infection. *Streptococcus pneumoniae* causes about 33% of all cases, while *Haemophilus influenzae* causes about 25% of all cases. Sinusitis in children may be caused by *Moraxella catarrhalis* (20%). In people with weakened immune systems (including patients with diabetes; acquired **immunodeficiency** syndrome or **AIDS**; and patients who are taking medications which lower their immune resistance, such as **cancer** and transplant patients), sinusitis may be caused by fungi such as *Aspergillus*, *Candida*, or Mucorales.

Acute sinusitis usually follows some type of upper respiratory tract infection or cold. Instead of ending, the cold seems to linger on, with constant or even worsening congestion. Drainage from the nose often changes from a clear color to a thicker, yellowish-green. There may be **fever**. **Headache** and pain over the affected sinuses may occur, as well as a feeling of pressure which may worsen when the patient bends over. There may be pain in the jaw or teeth. Some children, in particular, get upset stomachs from the infected drainage going down the back of their throats, and being swallowed into their stomachs. Some patients develop a **cough**.

Chronic sinusitis occurs when the problem has existed for at least three months. There is rarely a fever with chronic sinusitis. Sinus pain and pressure is frequent, as is nasal congestion. Because of the nature of the swelling in the sinuses, they may not be able to drain out the nose. Drainage, therefore, drips constantly down the back of the throat, resulting in a continuously sore throat and **bad breath**.

Diagnosis

Diagnosis is sometimes tricky, because the symptoms so often resemble those of an uncomplicated cold. However, sinusitis should be strongly suspected when a cold lingers beyond about a week's time.

Medical practitioners have differing levels of trust of certain basic examinations commonly conducted in the office. For example, tapping over the sinuses may

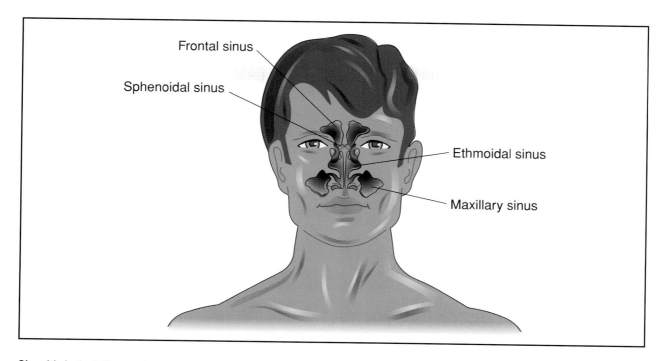

Frontal sinus

Sphenoidal sinus

Ethmoidal sinus

Maxillary sinus

Sinusitis is the inflammation of the sinuses caused by a bacterial infection. Sometimes diagnosis may be problematic because the symptoms often mimic those of the common cold. Sinusitis is usually treated with antibiotics. *(Illustration by Electronic Illustrators Group.)*

cause pain in patients with sinusitis, but it may not. A procedure called "sinus transillumination" may, or may not, also be helpful. Using a flashlight pressed up against the skin of the cheek, the practitioner will look in the patient's open mouth. When the sinuses are full of air (under normal conditions), the light will project through the sinus, and will be visible on the roof of the mouth as a lit-up, reddened area. When the sinuses are full of mucus, the light will be stopped. While this simple test can be helpful, it is certainly not a perfect way to diagnose or rule out the diagnosis of sinusitis.

X-ray pictures and CT scans of the sinuses are helpful for both acute and chronic sinusitis. People with chronic sinusitis should also be checked for allergies; and they may need a procedure with a scope to see if any kind of anatomic obstruction is causing their illness. For example, the septum (the cartilage which separates the two nasal cavities from each other) may be slightly displaced, called a **deviated septum**. This can result in chronic obstruction, setting the person up for the development of an infection.

Treatment

Antibiotic medications are used to treat acute sinusitis. Suitable **antibiotics** include sulfa drugs, amoxicillin, and a variety of **cephalosporins**. These medications are usually given for about two weeks, but may be given

for even longer periods of time. **Decongestants**, or the short-term use of decongestant nose sprays, can be useful. **Acetaminophen** and ibuprofen can decrease the pain and headache associated with sinusitis. Also, running a humidifier can prevent mucus within the nasal passages from drying out uncomfortably, and can help soothe any accompanying **sore throat** or cough.

Chronic sinusitis is often treated initially with antibiotics. Steroid nasal sprays may be used to decrease swelling in the nasal passages. If an anatomic reason is found for chronic sinusitis, it may need to be corrected with surgery. If a surgical procedure is necessary, samples are usually taken at the same time to allow identification of any organisms present which may be causing infection.

Fungal sinusitis will require surgery to clean out the sinuses. Then, a relatively long course of a very strong antifungal medication called amphotericin B is given through a needle in the vein (intravenously).

Alternative treatment

Chronic sinusitis is often associated with **food allergies**. An elimination/challenge diet is recommended to identify and eliminate allergenic foods. Irrigating the sinuses with a salt water solution is often recommended for sinusitis and allergies, in order to clear the nasal passages of mucus. Another solution for nasal lavage (washing) utilizes powdered goldenseal (*Hydrastis canadensis*). Other herbal treatments, taken internally, include a mixture made of eyebright (*Euphrasia officinalis*), goldenseal, yarrow (*Achillea millefolium*), horseradish, and ephedra (*Ephedra sinica*), or, when infection is present, a mixture made of echinacea (*Echinacea* spp.), wild indigo, and poke root (*Phytolacca decandra-Americana*).

Homeopathic practitioners find a number of remedies useful for treating sinusitis. Among those they recommend are: *Arsenicum album*, *Kalium bichromium*, *Nux vomica*, *Mercurius iodatus*, and *Silica*.

Acupuncture has been used to treat sinusitis, as have a variety of dietary supplements, including **vitamins** A, C, and E, and the mineral zinc. Contrast **hydrotherapy** (hot and cold compresses, alternating 3 minutes hot, 30 seconds cold, repeated 3 times always ending with cold) applied directly over the sinuses can relieve pressure and enhance healing. A direct inhalation of essential oils (2 drops of oil to 2 cups of water) using thyme, rosemary, and lavender can help open the sinuses and kill bacteria that cause infection.

Prognosis

Prognosis for sinus infections is usually excellent, although some individuals may find that they are particularly prone to contracting such infections after a cold. Fungal sinusitis, however, has a relatively high **death** rate.

Prevention

Prevention involves the usual standards of good hygiene to cut down on the number of colds an individual catches. Avoiding exposure to cigarette smoke, identifying and treating allergies, and avoiding deep dives in swimming pools may help prevent sinus infections. During the winter, it is a good idea to use a humidifier. Dry nasal passages may crack, allowing bacteria to enter. When allergies are diagnosed, a number of nasal sprays are available to try to prevent

inflammation within the nasal passageways, thus allowing the normal flow of mucus.

Resources

ORGANIZATIONS

American Academy of Otolaryngology-Head and Neck Surgery, Inc. One Prince St., Alexandria VA 22314-3357. (703) 836-4444. <http://www.entnet.org>.

Rosalyn Carson-DeWitt, MD

Situs inversus

Definition

Situs inversus is a condition in which the organs of the chest and abdomen are arranged in a perfect mirror image reversal of the normal positioning.

Description

Normal human development results in an asymmetrical arrangement of the organs within the chest and abdomen. Typically, the heart lies on the left side of the body (*levocardia*), the liver and spleen lie on the right, and the lung on the left has two lobes while the lung on the right has three lobes. This normal arrangement is known as *situs solitus*.

However, in about 1 in 8,500 people, the organs of the chest and abdomen are arranged in the exact opposite position: the heart is on the right (*dextrocardia*), as is the two-lobed lung, and the liver, spleen, and three-lobed lung are on the left. Yet because this arrangement, called *situs inversus*, is a perfect mirror image, the relationship between the organs is not changed, so functional problems rarely occur.

Causes and symptoms

Early in the normal development of an embryo, the tube-like structure that becomes the heart forms a loop toward the left, identifying the left/right axis along which the other organs should be positioned. Although the mechanism that causes the heart loop to go left is not fully understood, at least one gene has been identified to have a role in this process. However, it is thought that many factors may be involved in causing situs inversus. Rarely, situs inversus can run in families, but most often it is an isolated and accidental event occurring in an individual for the first time in the family.

Most people with situs inversus have no medical symptoms or complications resulting from the condition. Although only 3-5% of people with situs inversus have any type of functional heart defect, this is higher than the rate of heart defects in the general population, which is less than 1%.

It is estimated that about 25% of people with situs inversus have an underlying condition called primary ciliary dyskinesia (PCD). PCD, also known as Kartagener's syndrome, is characterized as situs inversus, chronic sinus infections, increased mucous secretions from the lungs, and increased susceptibility to respiratory infections. PCD is caused by a defect in the cilia that impairs their normal movements.

Diagnosis

Situs inversus should detected by a thorough **physical examination**. It is often picked up when a physician, using a stethoscope, hears otherwise normal heart sounds on the right side of the body instead of the left. To confirm the a suspected diagnosis of situs inversus, imaging studies such as MRI, CT, or ultrasound may be ordered, and a referral may be made to a cardiologist or internist for completeness. Imaging studies will also rule out the possibility of random arrangement of the organs, or heterotaxy, which has a much higher risk for serious medical complications.

Treatment

There is no treatment for situs inversus. In the unlikely case that a heart defect is present, it should be treated accordingly by a cardiologist.

Individuals who have situs inversus should be sure to inform all physicians involved in their medical care. In addition to preventing unnecessary confusion, this will reduce the risk of missing a crucial diagnosis that presents with location-specific symptoms (such as **appendicitis**).

Alternative treatment

Not applicable.

Prognosis

The prognosis for an individual with situs inversus is good, and in the absence of a heart defect or other underlying diagnosis, life expectancy is normal.

Prevention

There is no known method of preventing situs inversus.

KEY TERMS

Cilia—Tiny hairlike projections on certain cells within the body; cilia produce lashing or whipping movements to direct or cause motion of substances or fluids within the body.

Gene—A single unit of genetic information, providing the body with instruction for a specific biological task.

MRI—An imaging study that uses magnetic forces to produce an image of the body's internal structures.

CT—A special technique that uses a computer to create a cross-sectional image of the body from a series of x rays.

Ultrasound—An imaging study that uses high-frequency sound waves to form a visual image of the body's internal structures.

Resources

PERIODICALS

Ainsworth, Claire. "Left Right and Wrong." *New Scientist* 66, no. 2243 (June 17, 2000): 40-45.

Janchar, T., Milzman, D., and Clement, M. "Situs Inversus: Emergency Evaluations of Atypical Presentations." *American Journal of Emergency Medicine* 18, no. 3 (May 2000): 349-50.

Travis, John. "Twirl Those Organs into Place." *Science News* 156, no. 8 (21 August 1999): 124-125.

ORGANIZATIONS

American Heart Association. National Center. 7272 Greenville Avenue, Dallas, TX 75231-4596. (214) 373-6300. (800) 242-8721. inquire@heart.org.

NIH/National Heart, Lung and Blood Institute Information Center. P.O. Box 30105. Bethesda, MD 20824-0105. (301) 592-8573.

Stefanie B. N. Dugan, M.S.

Sitz bath

Definition

A sitz bath (also called a hip bath) is a type of bath in which only the hips and buttocks are soaked in water or saline solution. Its name comes from the German verb "sitzen," meaning "to sit."

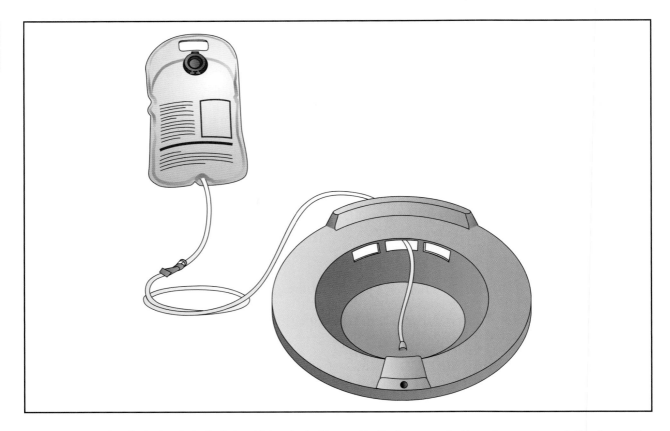

Equipment used for sitz baths. A sitz bath, in which only the hips and buttocks are soaked in water or saline solution, is used for patients who have had surgery in the rectal area or to ease discomfort from bladder, prostate, or vaginal infections. *(Illustration by Electronic Illustrators Group.)*

Purpose

A sitz bath is used for patients who have had surgery in the area of the rectum, or to ease the **pain** of **hemorrhoids**, uterine cramps, prostate infections, painful ovaries, and/or testicles. It is also used to ease discomfort from infections of the bladder, prostate, or vagina. Inflammatory bowel diseases are also treated with sitz baths.

Precautions

Some patients may become dizzy when standing up after sitting in hot water; it is best to have someone else present when doing a contrast sitz bath.

Description

The sitz bath is a European tradition in which only the pelvis and abdominal area are placed in water, with the upper body, arms, legs, and feet out of the water. The water can be warm or cool and one or two tubs may be used.

Warm sitz baths are one of the easiest and most effective ways to ease the pain of hemorrhoids. A warm bath is also effective in lessening the discomfort associated with **genital herpes**, uterine cramps, and other painful conditions in the pelvic area.

For prostate pain, patients should take two hot sitz baths a day, for about 15 minutes each.

To ease discomfort from a vaginal yeast infection, women should take a warm saline sitz bath. To prepare, fill the tub to hip height with warm water and add 1/2 c of salt (enough to make the water taste salty) and 1/2 vinegar. Sit in the bath for 20 minutes (or until the water gets cool). The vinegar will help bring the vaginal pH back to 4.5 (pH is a measurement of how acid or alkaline a fluid is).

A brief, cool sitz bath helps ease inflammation, **constipation**, and vaginal discharge. It can be used to tone the muscles in cases of bladder or bowel incontinence.

Other conditions respond to a "contrast bath" of both hot and cold. For this a patient should have a tub of hot water (about 110°F/43°C) and one tub of ice water. The patient should sit in the hot water for three to four minutes and in the cold for 30–60 seconds. This is repeated three to five times, always ending with the cold water.

If two tubs are not handy, the patient may sit in a hot bath (up to the navel). Then the patient stands up in the water and pulls a cold towel between the legs and over the pelvis in front and back. The cold towel is held in place for up to 60 seconds. Then the patient should sit back into the hot bath, and repeat the process 3–5 times, ending with the cold towel.

Preparation

The bath should be filled with 3–4 in (8–10cm) of water. For most conditions, nothing else should be added (no bubble bath or oil).

Aftercare

The area should be carefully patted dry and, if necessary, clean dressings should be applied.

Risks

Sitz baths pose almost no risk. On rare occasions, patients can feel dizzy or experience rapid heart beat because of blood vessel dilation.

Normal results

Swelling goes down; discomfort is eased; healing is promoted.

Carol A. Turkington

Sjögren's syndrome

Definition

Sjögren's syndrome (SS) is a disorder in which the mouth and eyes become extremely dry. Sjögren's syndrome is often associated with other autoimmune disorders. It is named for Henrik Sjögren, a Swedish ophthalmologist.

Description

Like other **autoimmune disorders**, Sjögren's syndrome occurs when the body's immune system mistakenly begins treating parts of the body as foreign invaders. While the immune cells should attack and kill invaders like bacteria, viruses, and fungi, these cells should not attack the body itself. In autoimmune disorders, however, cells called antibodies see tissues of the body as foreign, and help to start a chain of events that results in damage and destruction of those tissues.

There are three types of Sjögren's syndrome. Primary Sjögren's syndrome occurs by itself, with no other associated disorders. Secondary Sjögren's syndrome occurs along with other autoimmune disorders, like systemic lupus erythematosus, **rheumatoid arthritis**, **scleroderma**, **vasculitis**, or **polymyositis**. When the disorder is limited to involvement of the eyes, with no other organ or tissue involvement evident, it is called sicca complex.

Women are about nine times more likely to suffer from Sjögren's syndrome than are men. SS affects all age groups, although most patients are diagnosed when they are between 40 and 55 years old. Sjögren's syndrome is commonly associated with other autoimmune disorders. In fact, 30% of patients with certain autoimmune disorders will also have Sjögren's syndrome.

SS is found in all races and ethnic groups. It is thought to affect between 0.1% and 3% of the population in the United States; this range reflects the lack of a uniform set of diagnostic criteria. According to the American College of Rheumatology, between 1 million and 4 million Americans have Sjögren's syndrome.

Causes and symptoms

The cause of Sjögren's syndrome has not been clearly defined, but several causes are suspected. The syndrome sometimes runs in families. Other potential causes include hormonal factors (since there are more women than men with the disease) and viral factors. The viral theory suggests that the immune system is activated in response to a viral invader, but then fails to turn itself off. Some other immune malfunction then causes the overly active immune system to begin attacking the body's own tissues. In 2004 a group of Greek researchers presented evidence that a coxsackievirus may be the disease organism that triggers SS.

The main problem in Sjögren's syndrome is dryness. The salivary glands are often attacked and slowly destroyed, leaving the mouth extremely dry and sticky. Swallowing and talking become difficult. Normally, the saliva washes the teeth clean. Saliva cannot perform this function in Sjögren's syndrome, so the teeth develop many cavities and decay quickly. The parotid glands produce the majority of the mouth's saliva. They are located lying over the jaw bones behind the area of the cheeks and in front of the ears, and may become significantly enlarged in Sjögren's syndrome.

The eyes also become extremely dry as the tear glands (called glands of lacrimation) are slowly destroyed. Eye symptoms include **itching**, burning, redness, increased sensitivity to light, and thick secretions gathering at the eye corners closest to the nose. The cornea may have small irritated pits in its surface (ulcerations).

Destruction of glands in other areas of the body may cause a variety of symptoms. In the nose, dryness may result in nosebleeds. In the rest of the respiratory tract, the rates of ear infection, hoarseness, **bronchitis**, and **pneumonia** may increase. Vaginal dryness can be quite uncomfortable. Rarely, the pancreas may slow production of enzymes important for digestion. The kidney may malfunction. About 33% of all patients with Sjögren's syndrome have other symptoms unrelated to gland destruction. These symptoms include fatigue, decreased energy, fevers, muscle aches and pains, and joint **pain**.

Many patients with SS also develop a variety of skin problems that include dry patches, vasculitis, and cutaneous B-cell lymphoma. These and other dermatologic disorders are more common in SS than was previously thought.

Patients who also have other autoimmune diseases will suffer from the symptoms specific to those conditions.

In addition to physical symptoms, patients with SS appear to be at increased risk for depression and other **mood disorders**.

Diagnosis

Diagnosis of Sjögren's syndrome is based on the patient having at least three consecutive months of bothersome eye and/or mouth dryness. A variety of tests can then be done to determine the quantity of tears produced, the quantity of saliva produced, and the presence or absence of antibodies that could be involved in the destruction of glands.

KEY TERMS

Autoimmune disorder—A disorder in which the body's immune cells mistake the body's own tissues as foreign invaders; the immune cells then work to destroy tissues in the body.

Cornea—A transparent structure of the eye over the iris and pupil; light must pass through the cornea to make vision possible.

Coxsackievirus—Any of a group of enteroviruses that produce a disease in humans characterized by fever and rash. Coxsackieviruses are named for the town in upstate New York where they were first identified.

Immune system—The complex network of organs and blood cells that protect the body from foreign invaders, like bacteria, viruses, and fungi.

Treatment

There is no cure for Sjögren's syndrome. Instead, treatment usually attempts to reduce the discomfort and complications associated with dryness of the eyes and mouth (and other areas). Artificial tears are available, and may need to be used up to every 30 minutes. By using these types of products, the patient is more comfortable and avoids the complications associated with eyes that are overly dry. **Dry mouth** is treated by sipping fluids slowly but constantly throughout the day. Sugarless chewing gum can also be helpful. An artificial saliva is available for use as a mouthwash. Patients may also be given such drugs as pilocarpine (Salagen) or cevimeline (Evoxac) to increase saliva and tear secretions. Careful dental hygiene is important in order to avoid **tooth decay**, and it is wise for patients to decrease sugar intake. Vaginal dryness can be treated with certain gel preparations. Steroid medications may be required when other symptoms of autoimmune disorders complicate Sjögren's syndrome. However, these medications should be avoided when possible because they may make the cornea thin and even more susceptible to injury.

Prognosis

The prognosis for patients with primary Sjögren's syndrome is particularly good; these patients have a normal life expectancy. Although the condition is quite annoying, serious complications rarely occur. The prognosis for patients with secondary Sjögren's syndrome varies since it depends on the prognosis for the accompanying autoimmune disorder.

Prevention

Since the cause of Sjögren's syndrome is unknown as of 2004, there are no known ways to prevent this syndrome.

Resources

BOOKS

Beers, Mark H., MD, and Robert Berkow, MD., editors. "Diffuse Connective Tissue Disease." Section 5, Chapter 50 In *The Merck Manual of Diagnosis and Therapy*. Whitehouse Station, NJ: Merck Research Laboratories, 2004.

Moutsopoulos, Haralampos M. "Sjögren's Syndrome." In *Harrison's Principles of Internal Medicine*, edited by Anthony S. Fauci, et al. New York: McGraw-Hill, 1997.

PERIODICALS

Bell, Mary, et al. "Sjögren's Syndrome: A Critical Review of Clinical Management." *The Journal of Rheumatology* 26, no. 9 (2001): 2051–2059.

Francis, Mark L., MD. "Sjogren Syndrome." *eMedicine* July 1, 2004. < http://emedicine.com/med/topic2136.htm >.

Ono, M., E. Takamura, K. Shinozaki, et al. "Therapeutic Effect of Cevimeline on Dry Eye in Patients with Sjögren's Syndrome: A Randomized, Double-Blind Clinical Study." *American Journal of Ophthalmology* 138 (July 2004): 6–17.

Roguedas, A. M., L. Misery, B. Sassolas, et al. "Cutaneous Manifestations of Primary Sjögren's Syndrome Are Underestimated." *Clinical and Experimental Rheumatology* 22 (September-October 2004): 632–636.

Stevenson, H. A., M. E. Jones, J. L. Rostron, et al. "UK Patients with Primary Sjögren's Syndrome Are at Increased Risk from Clinical Depression." *Gerodontology* 21 (September 2004): 141–145.

Triantafyllopoulou, A., N. Tapinos, and H. M. Moutsopoulos. "Evidence for Coxsackievirus Infection in Primary Sjögren's Syndrome." *Arthritis and Rheumatism* 50 (September 2004): 2897–2902.

ORGANIZATIONS

American College of Rheumatology. 1800 Century Place, Suite 250, Atlanta, GA 30345-4300. (404) 633-3777. Fax: (404) 633-1870. < http://www.rheumatology.org >.

Sjögren's Syndrome Foundation, Inc. 8120 Woodmont Avenue, Bethesda, MD 20814. (800) 475-6473. Fax: (301) 718-0322. < http://www.sjogrens.org >.

OTHER

American College of Rheumatology Fact Sheet. "Sjögren's Syndrome." < http://www.rheumatology.org/public/factsheets/sjogrens_new.asp?aud = pat >.

Rosalyn Carson-DeWitt, MD
Rebecca J. Frey, PhD

Skeletal traction *see* **Traction; Immobilization**

Skin abrasion *see* **Skin resurfacing**

Skin allergy test *see* **Allergy tests**

Skin biopsy

Definition

A skin biopsy is a procedure in which a small piece of living skin is removed from the body for examination, usually under a microscope, to establish a precise diagnosis. Skin biopsies are usually brief, straightforward procedures performed by a skin specialist (dermatologist) or family physician.

Purpose

The word *biopsy* is taken from Greek words that mean "to view life." The term describes what a specialist in identifying diseases (pathologist) does with tissue obtained from a skin biopsy. The pathologist *visually* examines the tissue under a microscope.

A skin biopsy is used to make a diagnosis of many skin disorders. Information from the biopsy also helps the doctor choose the best treatment for the patient.

Doctors perform skin biopsies to:

- make a diagnosis
- confirm a diagnosis made from the patient's medical history and a **physical examination**
- check whether a treatment prescribed for a previously diagnosed condition is working
- check the edges of tissue removed with a tumor to make certain it contains all the diseased tissue

Skin biopsies also can serve a therapeutic purpose. Many skin abnormalities (lesions) can be removed completely during the biopsy procedure.

Precautions

A patient taking **aspirin** or another blood thinner (anticoagulant) may be asked to stop taking them a week or more before the skin biopsy. This adjustment in medication will prevent excessive bleeding during the procedure and allow for normal blood clotting.

Some patients are allergic to lidocaine, the numbing agent most frequently used during a skin biopsy. The doctor can usually substitute another anesthetic agent.

Description

The first part of the skin biopsy test is obtaining a sample of tissue that best represents the lesion being evaluated. Many biopsy techniques are available. The choice of technique and precise location from which to take the biopsy material are determined by factors such as the type and shape of the lesion. Biopsies can be classified as excisional or incisional. In excisional biopsy, the lesion is completely removed; in incisional biopsy, a portion of the lesion is removed.

The most common biopsy techniques are:

- Shave biopsy. A scalpel or razor blade is used to shave off a thin layer of the lesion parallel to the skin.
- Punch biopsy. A small cylindrical punch is screwed into the lesion through the full thickness of the skin and a plug of tissue is removed. A stitch or two may be needed to close the wound.
- Scalpel biopsy. A scalpel is used to make a standard surgical incision or excision to remove tissue. This technique is most often used for large or deep lesions. The wound is closed with stitches.
- Scissors biopsy. Scissors are used to snip off surface (superficial) skin growths and lesions that grow from a stem or column of tissue. Such growths are sometimes seen on the eyelids or neck.

After the biopsy tissue is removed, bleeding may be controlled by applying pressure or by burning with electricity or chemicals. **Antibiotics** often are applied to the wound to prevent infection. Stitches may be placed in the wound, or the wound may be bandaged and allowed to heal on its own.

The second part of the skin biopsy test is handling and examining the tissue sample. Drying and structural damage to the tissue sample must be prevented, so it should be placed immediately in an appropriate preservative, such as formaldehyde.

The pathologist can use a variety of laboratory techniques to process the biopsy tissue. Tissue stains and several different kinds of microscopes are used. Because there are many skin disorders (broadly called dermatosis and **dermatitis**), the pathologist has extensive training in their accurate identification. Cases of melanoma, the most malignant kind of skin **cancer**, have almost tripled in the past 30 years. Because melanoma grows very rapidly in the skin, quick and accurate diagnosis is important.

Preparation

The area of the biopsy is cleansed thoroughly with alcohol or a disinfectant containing iodine. Sterile

---

KEY TERMS

Benign—Noncancerous.

Dermatitis—A skin disorder that causes inflammation, that is, redness, swelling, heat, and pain.

Dermatologist—A doctor who specializes in skin care and treatment.

Dermatosis—A noninflammatory skin disorder.

Lesion—An area of abnormal or injured skin.

Malignant—Cancerous.

Pathologist—A person who specializes in studying diseases. In particular, this person examines the structural and functional changes in the tissues and organs of the body that are caused by disease or that cause disease themselves.

---

cloths (drapes) may be positioned, and a local anesthetic, usually lidocaine, is injected into the skin near the lesion. Sometimes the anesthetic contains epinephrine, a drug that helps reduce bleeding during the biopsy. Sterile gloves and surgical instruments are always used to reduce the risk of infection.

Aftercare

If stitches have been placed, they should be kept clean and dry until removed. Stitches are usually removed five to 10 days after the biopsy. Sometimes the patient is instructed to put protective ointment on the stitches before showering. **Wounds** that have not been stitched should be cleaned with soap and water daily until they heal. Adhesive strips should be left in place for two to three weeks. **Pain** medications usually are not necessary.

Risks

Infection and bleeding occur rarely after skin biopsy. If the skin biopsy may leave a scar, the patient usually is asked to give informed consent before the test.

Normal results

The biopsy reveals normal skin layers.

Abnormal results

The biopsy reveals a noncancerous (benign) or cancerous (malignant) lesion. Benign lesions may require treatment.

Resources

ORGANIZATIONS

American Academy of Dermatology. 930 N. Meacham Road, P.O. Box 4014, Schaumburg, IL 60168-4014. (847) 330-0230. Fax: (847) 330-0050. <http://www.aad.org>.

Collette L. Placek

Skin cancer *see* **Melanoma**

Skin cancer, non-melanoma

Definition

Non-melanoma skin **cancer** is a malignant growth of the external surface or epithelial layer of the skin.

Description

Skin cancer is the growth of abnormal cells capable of invading and destroying other associated skin cells. Skin cancer is often subdivided into either melanoma or non-melanoma. Melanoma is a dark-pigmented, usually malignant tumor arising from a skin cell capable of making the pigment melanin (a melanocyte). Non-melanoma skin cancer most often originates from the external skin surface as a squamous cell carcinoma or a basal cell carcinoma.

The cells of a cancerous growth originate from a single cell that reproduces uncontrollably, resulting in the formation of a tumor. Exposure to sunlight is documented as the main cause of almost 800,000 cases of non-melanoma skin cancer diagnosed each year in the United States. The incidence increases for those living where direct sunshine is plentiful, such as near the equator.

Basal cell carcinoma affects the skin's basal layer and has the potential to grow progressively larger in size, although it rarely spreads to distant areas (metastasizes). Basal cell carcinoma accounts for 80% of skin cancers (excluding melanoma), whereas squamous cell cancer makes up about 20%. Squamous cell carcinoma is a malignant growth of the external surface of the skin. Squamous cell cancers metastasize at a rate of 2–6%, with up to 10% of lesions affecting the ear and lip.

Causes and symptoms

Cumulative sun exposure is considered a significant risk factor for non-melanoma skin cancer. There is evidence suggesting that early, intense exposure causing blistering **sunburn** in childhood may also play an important role in the cause of non-melanoma skin cancer. Basal cell carcinoma most frequently affects the skin of the face, with the next most common sites being the ears, the backs of the hands, the shoulders, and the arms. It is prevalent in both sexes and most commonly occurs in people over 40.

About 1–2% of all skin cancers develop within burn **scars**; squamous cell carcinomas account for about 95% of these cancers, with 3% being basal cell carcinomas and the remainder malignant melanomas.

Basal cell carcinomas usually appear as small **skin lesions** that persist for at least three weeks. This form of non-melanomatous skin cancer looks flat and waxy, with the edges of the lesion translucent and rounded. The edges also contain small fresh blood vessels. An ulcer in the center of the lesion gives it a dimpled appearance. Basal cell carcinoma lesions vary from 4–6mm in size, but can slowly grow larger if untreated.

Squamous cell carcinoma also involves skin exposed to the sun, such as the face, ears, hands, or arms. This form of non-melanoma is also most common among people over 40. Squamous cell carcinoma presents itself as a small, scaling, raised bump on the skin with a crusting ulcer in the center, but without **pain** and **itching**.

Basal cell and squamous cell carcinomas can grow more easily when people have a suppressed immune system because they are taking immunosuppressive drugs or are exposed to radiation. Some people must take immunosuppressive drugs to prevent the rejection of a transplanted organ or because they have a disease in which the immune system attacks the body's own tissues (autoimmune illnesses); others may need **radiation therapy** to treat another form of cancer. Because of this, everyone taking these immunosuppressive drugs or receiving radiation treatments should undergo complete skin examination at regular intervals. If proper treatment is delayed and the tumor continues to grow, the tumor cells can spread (metastasize) to muscle, bone, nerves, and possibly the brain.

Diagnosis

To diagnose skin cancer, doctors must carefully examine the lesion and ask the patient about how long it has been there, whether it itches or bleeds, and other questions about the patient's medical history. If skin cancer cannot be ruled out, a sample of the tissue is removed and examined under a microscope (a biopsy). A definitive diagnosis of squamous or basal cell cancer can only be made with microscopic examination of the tumor cells. Once skin cancer has been diagnosed, the stage of the disease's development is determined. The information from the biopsy and staging allows the physician and patient to plan for treatment and possible surgical intervention.

Treatment

A variety of treatment options are available for those diagnosed with non-melanoma skin cancer. Some carcinomas can be removed by cryosurgery, the process of freezing with liquid nitrogen. Uncomplicated and previously untreated basal cell carcinoma of the trunk and arms is often treated with curettage and electrodesiccation, which is the scraping of the lesion and the destruction of any remaining malignant cells with an electrical current. Removal of a lesion layer-by-layer down to normal margins (Mohs' surgery) is an effective treatment for both basal and squamous cell carcinoma. Radiation therapy is best reserved for older, debilitated patients or when the tumor is considered inoperable. Laser therapy is sometimes useful in specific cases; however, this form of treatment is not widely used to treat skin cancer.

A newer type of radiation treatment for non-melanoma skin cancers consists of low-energy x rays delivered through the tip of a portable needle-like probe at a high dosage rate. This method allows the radiologist to treat the cancer while sparing the surrounding normal skin. The device was effective in treating 83% of skin lesions in a group of patients diagnosed with non-melanomatous skin cancers during a Phase I trial for the Food and Drug Administration (FDA). There were no cases of damage to surrounding tissues.

Some topical (applied onto the skin) creams and ointments may be used to treat certain types of non-melanoma skin cancers. For example, imiquimod cream, a topical immune stimulator, has been shown effective in treating superficial basal cell carcinoma. The company who marketed the drug was seeking FDA approval.

Alternative treatment

Alternative medicine aims to prevent rather than treat skin cancer. **Vitamins** have been shown to prevent sunburn and, possibly, skin cancer. Some dermatologists have suggested that taking vitamins E and C may help prevent sunburn. In one particular study, men and women took these vitamins for eight days prior to being exposed to ultraviolet light. The researchers found that those who consumed vitamins

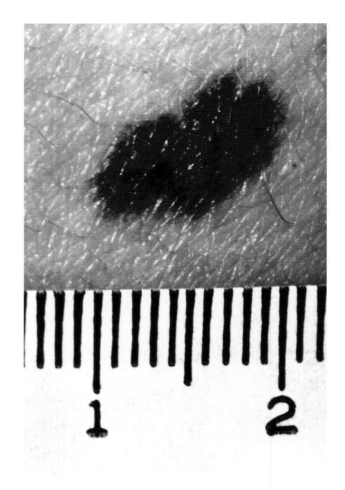

A close up image of a precancerous mole that could develop into a melanoma. Melanomas arise from pigment-producing cells, while non-melanoma skin cancer arises from squamous cells or basal cells. (*Custom Medical Stock Photo. Reproduced by permission.*)

required about 20% more ultraviolet light to induce sunburn than did people who didn't take vitamins. This is the first study that indicates the oral use of vitamins E and C increases resistance to sunburn. These antioxidants are thought to reduce the risk of skin cancer, and are expected to provide protection from the sun even in lower doses. Other anitoxidant nutrients, including beta carotene, selenium, zinc, and the bioflavonoid quercetin have been suggested as possibly preventing skin cancer. However, a 2003 study reported that selenium was not effective in preventing basal cell carcinoma and may even increase risk of squamous cell carcinoma and total non-melanoma skin cancer. Antioxidant herbs such as bilberry (*Vaccinium myrtillus*), hawthorn (*Crataegus laevigata*), tumeric (*Curcuma longa*), and ginkgo (*Ginkgo biloba*) also have been presented as helpful in preventing skin cancers.

KEY TERMS

Autoimmune—Pertaining to an immune response by the body against one of its own tissues or types of cells.

Curettage—The removal of tissue or growths by scraping with a curette.

Dermatologist—A physician specializing in the branch of medicine concerned with skin.

Electrodesiccation—To make dry, dull, or lifeless with the use of electrical current.

Lesion—A patch of skin that has been infected or diseased.

Topical—Referring to a medication or other preparation applied to the skin or the outside of the body.

A team of researchers at Duke University reported in 2003 that topical application of a combination of 15% vitamin C and 1% vitamin E over a four-day period offered significant protection against sunburn. The researchers suggest that this combination may protect skin against **aging** caused by sunlight as well.

Another antioxidant that appears to counter the effects of severe sun exposure is superoxide dismutase, or SOD. SOD must be given in injectable form, however, because it is destroyed in the digestive tract.

As of 2003, researchers were also looking at botanical compounds that could be added to skin care products applied externally to lower the risk of skin cancer. Several botanical compounds had been tested on animals and found to be effective in preventing skin cancer, but further research needs to be done in human subjects.

Prognosis

Both squamous and basal cell carcinoma are curable with appropriate treatment, although basal cell carcinomas have about a 5% rate of recurrence. Early detection remains critical for a positive prognosis. Although it is rare for basal cell carcinomas to metastasize, their metastases can rapidly lead to **death** if they invade the eyes, ears, mouth, or the membranes covering the brain.

Prevention

Avoiding exposure to the sun reduces the incidence of non-melanoma skin cancer. Sunscreen with a sun-protective factor of 15 or higher is helpful in prevention, along with a hat and clothing to shield the skin from sun damage. People should examine their skin monthly for unusual lesions, especially if previous skin cancers have been experienced.

Advances in photographic technique have now made it easier to track the development of **moles** with the help of whole-body photographs. A growing number of hospitals are offering these photographs as part of outpatient mole-monitoring services.

Resources

BOOKS

Beers, Mark H., MD, and Robert Berkow, MD., editors. "Dermatologic Disorders: Malignant Tumors." Section 10, Chapter 126 In *The Merck Manual of Diagnosis and Therapy*. Whitehouse Station, NJ: Merck Research Laboratories, 2004.

Beers, Mark H., MD, and Robert Berkow, MD., editors. "Dermatologic Disorders: Reactions to Sunlight." Section 10, Chapter 119 In *The Merck Manual of Diagnosis and Therapy*. Whitehouse Station, NJ: Merck Research Laboratories, 2004.

Pelletier, Kenneth R., MD. *The Best Alternative Medicine*, Part I: Food for Thought. New York: Simon & Schuster, 2002.

PERIODICALS

Bodner, W. R., B. S. Hilaris, M. Alagheband, et al. "Use of Low-Energy X-Rays in the Treatment of Superficial Nonmelanomatous Skin Cancers." *Cancer Investigation* 21 (June 2003): 355–362.

Bray, C. "The Development of an Improved Method of Photography for Mole-Monitoring at the University Hospital of North Durham." *Journal of Audiovisual Media in Medicine* 26 (June 2003): 60–66.

Brown, C. K., and J. M. Kirkwood. "Medical Management of Melanoma." *Surgical Clinics of North America* 83 (April 2003): 283–322.

Duffield-Lillico, Anna J., et al. "Selenium Supplementation and Secondary Prevention of Nonmelanoma Skin Cancer in A Randomized Trial." *Journal of the National Cancer Institute* 95 (October 1, 2003): 1477-1485.

F'guyer, S., F. Afaq, and H. Mukhtar. "Photochemoprevention of Skin Cancer by Botanical Agents." *Photodermatology, Photoimmunology and Photomedicine* 19 (April 2003): 56–72.

Jellouli-Elloumi, A., L. Kochbati, S. Dhraief, et al. "Cancers Arising from Burn Scars: 62 Cases." [in French] *Annales de dermatologie et de venereologie* 130 (April 2003): 413–416.

Lin, J. Y., M. A. Selim, C. R. Shea, et al. "UV Photoprotection by Combination Topical Antioxidants Vitamin C and Vitamin E." *Journal of the American Academy of Dermatology* 48 (June 2003): 866-874.

Spates, S. T., J. R. Mellette, Jr., and J. Fitzpatrick. "Metastatic Basal Cell Carcinoma." *Dermatologic Surgery* 29 (June 2003): 650–652.

Zoler, Mitchell L. "Imiquimod Up for FDA Approval to Treat BCC, AK; Phase III Trial Results." *Internal Medicine News* 36 (October 1, 2003): 52.

ORGANIZATIONS

American Academy of Dermatology. 930 N. Meacham Road, P.O. Box 4014, Schaumburg, IL 60168-4014. (847) 330-0230. Fax: (847) 330-0050. <http://www.aad.org>.

American Cancer Society. 1599 Clifton Rd., NE, Atlanta, GA 30329-4251. (800) 227-2345. <http://www.cancer.org>.

Centers for Disease Control and Prevention (CDC). Cancer Prevention and Control Program. 4770 Buford Highway, NE, MS K64, Atlanta, GA 30341. (888) 842-6355. <http://www.cdc.gov/cancer/comments.htm>.

National Cancer Institute (NCI). NCI Public Inquiries Office, Suite 3036A, 6116 Executive Boulevard, MSC8332, Bethesda, MD 20892-8322. (800) 4-CANCER or (800) 332-8615 (TTY). <http://www.nci.nih.gov>.

Jeffrey P. Larson, RPT
Rebecca J. Frey, PhD
Teresa G. Odle

Skin culture

Definition

A skin culture is a test that is done to identify the microorganism (bacteria, fungus, or virus) causing a skin infection and to determine the antibiotic or other treatment that will effectively treat the infection.

Purpose

Microorganisms can infect healthy skin, but more often they infect skin already damaged by an injury or abrasion. Skin infections are contagious and, if left untreated, can lead to serious complications. A culture enables a physician to diagnose and treat a skin infection.

Description

Several groups of microorganisms cause skin infections: bacteria, fungi (molds and yeast), and viruses. Based on the appearance of the infection, the physician determines what group of microorganisms is likely causing the infection, then he or she collects a specimen for one or more types of cultures. A sample of material–such as skin cells, pus, or fluid–is taken from the infection site, placed in a sterile container, and sent to the laboratory. In the laboratory, each type of culture is handled differently.

Bacterial infections are the most common. Bacteria cause lesions, ulcers, **cellulitis**, and **boils**. Pyoderma are pus-containing skin infections, such as **impetigo**, caused by *Staphylococcus* or group A *Streptococcus* bacteria. To culture bacteria, a portion of material from the infection site is spread over the surface of a culture plate and placed in an incubator at body temperature for one to two days. Bacteria in the skin sample multiply and appear on the plates as visible colonies. They are identified by noting the appearance of their colonies, and by performing biochemical tests and a Gram's stain.

The Gram's stain is done by smearing part of a colony onto a microscope slide. After it dries, the slide is colored with purple and red stains, then examined under a microscope. The color of stain picked up and retained by the bacteria (purple or red), their shape (such as round or rectangle), and their size provide valuable clues as to their identity.

A sensitivity test, also called antibiotic susceptibility test, is also done. The bacteria are tested against different **antibiotics** to determine which will effectively treat the infection by killing the bacteria.

Fungal cultures are done less frequently. A group of fungi called dermatophytes cause a skin infection called **ringworm**. Yeast causes an infection called thrush. These infections are usually diagnosed using a method other than culture, such as the KOH test. A culture is done only when specific identification of the mold or yeast is necessary. The specimen is spread on a culture plate designed to grow fungi, then incubated. Several different biochemical tests and stains are used to identify molds and yeasts.

Viruses, such as herpes, can also cause skin infections. Specimens for viral cultures are mixed with commercially-prepared animal cells in a test tube. Characteristic changes to the cells caused by the growing virus help identify the virus.

Results for bacterial cultures are usually available in one to three days. Cultures for fungi and viruses may take longer–up to three weeks. Cultures are covered by insurance.

Preparation

After cleaning the infected area with sterile saline and alcohol, the physician collects skin cells, pus, or

Pyoderma—A pus-containing skin infection, such as impetigo, caused by *Staphylococcus* or group A *Streptococcus* bacteria.

Sensitivity test—A test that determines which antibiotics will treat an infection by killing the bacteria.

fluid using a needle or swab. If necessary, the physician will open a lesion to collect the specimen. To collect a specimen for a fungal culture, the physician uses a scalpel to scrape skin cells into a sterile container.

Normal results

Many types of microorganisms are normally found on a person's skin. Presence of these microorganisms is noted on a skin culture report as "normal flora."

Abnormal results

A microorganism is considered to be a cause of the infection if it is either the only or predominant microorganism that grew, if it grew in large numbers, or if it is known to produce infection.

Resources

PERIODICALS

Carroll, John A. "Common Bacterial Pyodermas." *Postgraduate Medicine* September 1996: 311-322.

Nancy J. Nordenson

Skin grafting

Definition

Skin grafting is a surgical procedure by which skin or skin substitute is placed over a burn or non-healing wound to permanently replace damaged or missing skin or provide a temporary wound covering.

Purpose

Wounds such as third-degree **burns** must be covered as quickly as possible to prevent infection or loss of fluid. Wounds that are left to heal on their own can contract, often resulting in serious scarring; if the wound is large enough, the scar can actually prevent movement of limbs. Non-healing wounds, such as diabetic ulcers, venous ulcers, or pressure sores, can be treated with skin grafts to prevent infection and further progression of the wounded area.

Precautions

Skin grafting is generally not used for first- or second-degree burns, which generally heal with little or no scarring. Also, the tissue for grafting and the recipient site must be as sterile as possible to prevent later infection that could result in failure of the graft.

Description

The skin is the largest organ of the human body. It consists of two main layers: the epidermis is the outer layer, sitting on and nourished by the thicker dermis. These two layers are approximately 0.04–0.08 in (1–2 mm) thick. The epidermis consists of an outer layer of dead cells, which provides a tough, protective coating, and several layers of rapidly dividing cells called keratinocytes. The dermis contains the blood vessels, nerves, sweat glands, hair follicles, and oil glands. The dermis consists mainly of connective tissue, primarily the protein collagen, which gives the skin its flexibility and provides structural support. Fibroblasts, which make collagen, are the main cell type in the dermis.

Skin protects the body from fluid loss, aids in temperature regulation, and helps prevent disease-causing bacteria or viruses from entering the body. Skin that is damaged extensively by burns or non-healing wounds can compromise the health and well-being of the patient. More than 50,000 people are hospitalized for burn treatment each year in the United States, and 5,500 die. Approximately 4 million people suffer from non-healing wounds, including 1.5 million with venous ulcers and 800,000 with diabetic ulcers, which result in 55,000 amputations per year in the United States.

Skin for grafting can be obtained from another area of the patient's body, called an autograft, if there is enough undamaged skin available, and if the patient is healthy enough to undergo the additional surgery required. Alternatively, skin can be obtained from another person (donor skin from cadavers is frozen, stored, and available for use), called an allograft, or from an animal (usually a pig), called a xenograft. Allografts and xenografts provide only temporary covering–they are rejected by the patient's immune system within seven to 10 days and must be replaced with an autograft.

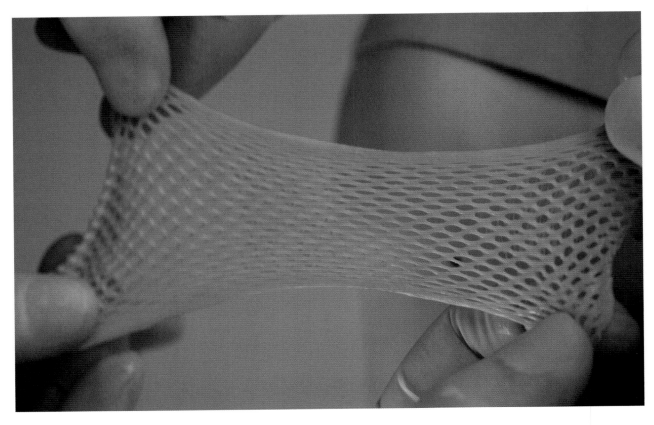

This skin graft is ready for application. *(Photograph by Ted Horowitz, The Stock Market. Reproduced by permission.)*

A split-thickness skin graft takes mainly the epidermis and a little of the dermis, and usually heals within several days. The wound must not be too deep if a split-thickness graft is going to be successful, since the blood vessels that will nourish the grafted tissue must come from the dermis of the wound itself.

A full-thickness graft involves both layers of the skin. Full-thickness autografts provide better contour, more natural color, and less contraction at the grafted site. The main disadvantage of full-thickness skin grafts is that the wound at the donor site is larger and requires more careful management; often a split-thickness graft must be used to cover the donor site.

A composite skin graft is sometime used, consisting of combinations of skin and fat, skin and cartilage, or dermis and fat. Composite grafts are used where three-dimensional reconstruction is necessary. For example, a wedge of ear containing skin and cartilage can be used to repair the nose.

Several artificial skin products are available for burns or non-healing wounds. Unlike allographs and xenographs, these products are not rejected by the patient's body and actually encourage the generation of new tissue. Artificial skin usually consists of a synthetic epidermis and a collagen-based dermis. This artificial dermis, the fibers of which are arranged in a lattice, acts as a template for the formation of new tissue. Fibroblasts, blood vessels, nerve fibers, and lymph vessels from surrounding healthy tissue cross into the collagen lattice, which eventually degrades as these cells and structures build a new dermis. The synthetic epidermis, which acts as a temporary barrier during this process, is eventually replaced with a split-thickness autograft or with an epidermis cultured in the laboratory from the patient's own epithelial cells. The cost for the synthetic products in about $1,000 for a 40-in (100-cm) square piece of artificial skin, in addition to the costs of the surgery. This procedure is covered by insurance.

Aftercare

Once a skin graft has been put in place, even after it has healed, it must be maintained carefully. Patients

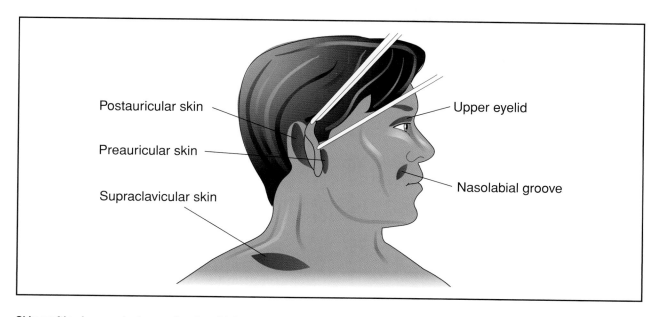

Skin grafting is a surgical procedure by which skin or a skin substitute is placed over a burn or non-healing wound to replace the damaged skin or provide a temporary wound covering. Skin for grafting can be obtained from another area of the patient's body, such as the face and neck, as shown in the illustration above. *(Illustration by Electronic Illustrators Group.)*

---

who have grafts on their legs should remain in bed for seven to 10 days, with their legs elevated. For several months, the patient should support the graft with an Ace bandage or Jobst stocking. Grafts in other areas of the body should be similarly supported after healing to decrease the amount of contracture.

Grafted skin does not contain sweat or oil glands, and should be lubricated daily for two to three months with a bland oil (e.g., mineral oil) to prevent drying and cracking.

Risks

The risks of skin grafting include those inherent in any surgical procedure that involves anesthesia. These include reactions to the medications, problems breathing, bleeding, and infection. In addition, the risks of an allograft procedure include transmission of infectious disease.

Normal results

A skin graft should provide significant improvement in the quality of the wound site, and may prevent the serious complications associated with burns or non-healing wounds.

Abnormal results

Failure of a graft can result from poor blood flow, swelling, or infection.

Resources

ORGANIZATIONS

American Burn Association. 625 N. Michigan Ave., Suite 1530, Chicago, IL 60611. (800) 548-2876. < http://www.ameriburn.org >.

American Diabetes Association. 1701 North Beauregard Street, Alexandria, VA 22311. (800) 342-2383. < http://www.diabetes.org >.

Lisa Christenson, PhD

Skin lesion removal

Definition

Skin lesion removal employs a variety of techniques, from relatively simple biopsies to more complex surgical excisions, to remove lesions that range from benign growths to **malignant melanoma**.

Purpose

Sometimes the purpose of skin lesion removal is to excise an unsightly mole or other cosmetically unattractive skin growth. Other times, physicians will remove a skin lesion to make certain it is not cancerous, and, if it proves cancerous, to prevent its spread to other parts of the body.

Precautions

Most skin lesion removal procedures require few precautions. The area to be treated is cleaned before the procedure with alcohol or another antibacterial preparation, but generally it is not necessary to use a sterile operating room. Most procedures are performed on an outpatient basis, using a local anesthetic. Some of the more complex procedures may require specialized equipment available only in an outpatient surgery center. Most of the procedures are not highly invasive and, frequently, can be well-tolerated by young and old patients, as well as those with other medical conditions.

Description

A variety of techniques are used to remove **skin lesions**. The particular technique selected will depend on such factors as the seriousness of the lesion, its location, and the patient's ability to tolerate the procedure. Some of the simpler techniques, such as a biopsy or cryosurgery, can be performed by a primary care physician. Some of the more complex techniques, such as excision with a scalpel, electrosurgery, or laser surgery, are typically performed by a dermatologic surgeon, plastic surgeon, or other surgical specialist. Often, the technique selected will depend on how familiar the physician is with the procedure and how comfortable he or she is with performing it.

Biopsy

In this procedure, the physician commonly injects a local anesthetic at the site of the skin lesion, then removes a sample of the lesion, so that a definite diagnosis can be made. The sample is sent to a pathology laboratory, where it is examined under a microscope. Certain characteristic skin cells, and their arrangement in the skin, offer clues to the type of skin lesion, and whether it is cancerous or otherwise poses danger. Depending on the results of the microscopic examination, additional surgery may be scheduled.

A variety of methods are used to obtain a **skin biopsy**. The physician may use a scalpel to cut a piece or remove all of the lesion for examination. Lesions that are confined to the surface may be sampled with a shave biopsy, where the physician holds a scalpel blade parallel to the surface of the skin and slides the blade across the base of the lesion, removing a sample. Some physicians use a single-edge razor blade for this, instead of a scalpel. A physician may also perform a punch biopsy, in which a small circular punch removes a plug of skin.

Excision

When excising a lesion, the physician attempts to remove it completely by using a scalpel to cut the shape of an ellipse around the lesion. Leaving an elliptical wound, rather than a circular wound, makes it easier to insert stitches. If a lesion is suspected to be cancerous, the physician will not cut directly around the lesion, but will attempt to also remove a healthy margin of tissue surrounding it. This is to ensure that no cancerous cells remain, which would allow the tumor to reappear. To prevent recurrence of basal and squamous cell skin cancers, experts recommend a margin of 0.08–0.16 in (2–4 mm) for malignant melanoma, the margin may be 1.2 in (3 cm) or more.

Destruction

Not all lesions need to be excised. A physician may simply seek to destroy the lesion using a number of destructive techniques. These techniques do not leave sufficient material to be examined by a pathologist, however, and are best used in cases where a visual diagnosis is certain.

- Cryosurgery. This technique employs an extremely cold liquid or instrument to freeze and destroy abnormal skin cells that require removal. Liquid nitrogen is the most commonly used cryogen. It is typically sprayed on the lesion in several freeze-thaw cycles to ensure adequate destruction of the lesion.

- Curettage. In this procedure, an instrument with a circular cutting loop at the end is drawn across the lesion, starting at the middle and moving outward. With successive strokes, the physician scrapes portions of the lesion away. Sometimes a physician will use the curet to reduce the size of the lesion before turning to another technique to finish removing it.

- Electrosurgery. This utilizes an alternating current to selectively destroy skin tissue. Depending on the type of current and device used, physicians may use electrosurgical equipment to dry up surface lesions (electrodessication), to burn off the lesion (electrocoagulation), or to cut the lesion (electrosection). One advantage of electrosurgery is that it minimizes bleeding.

Mohs' micrographic surgery

The real extent of some lesions may not be readily apparent to the eye, making it difficult for the surgeon to decide where to make incisions. If some cancer cells are left behind, for example, the **cancer** may reappear or spread. In a technique called Mohs' micrographic surgery, surgeons begin by removing a lesion and examining its margins under a microscope for evidence of cancer. If cancerous cells are found, the surgeon then removes another ring of tissue and examines the margins again. The process is repeated until the margins appear clear of cancerous cells. The technique is considered ideal for aggressive tumors in areas such as the nose or upper lip, where an excision with wide margins may be difficult to repair, and may leave a cosmetically poor appearance.

Lasers

Laser surgery is now applied to a variety of skin lesions, ranging from spider veins to more extensive blood vessel lesions called hemangiomas. Until recently, CO_2 lasers were among the more common laser devices used by physicians, primarily to destroy skin lesions. Other lasers, such as the Nd:YAG and flashlamp-pumped pulse dye laser have been developed to achieve more selective results when used to treat vascular lesions, such as hemangiomas, or pigmented lesions, such as café-au-lait spots.

Preparation

No extensive preparation is required for skin lesion removal. Most procedures can be performed on an outpatient basis with a local anesthetic. The lesion and surrounding area is cleaned with an antibacterial compound before the procedure. A sterile operating room is not required.

Aftercare

The amount of aftercare will vary, depending on the skin lesion removal technique. For biopsy, curettage, cryosurgery, and electrosurgery procedures, the patient is told to keep the wound clean and dry. Healing will take at least several weeks, and may take longer, depending on the size of the wound and other factors. Healing times will also vary with excisions and with Mohs' micrographic surgery, particularly if a skin graft or skin flap is needed to repair the resulting wound. Laser surgery may produce changes in skin coloration that often resolve in time. **Pain** is usually minimal following most outpatient procedures, so pain medicines are not routinely prescribed. Some areas of the body, such as the scalp and fingers, can be more painful than others, however, and a pain medicine may be required.

Risks

All surgical procedures present risk of infection. Keeping the wound clean and dry can minimize the risk. **Antibiotics** are not routinely given to prevent infection in skin surgery, but some doctors believe they have a role. Other potential complications include:

- bleeding below the skin, which may create a hematoma and sometimes requires the wound to be reopened and drained,

- temporary or permanent nerve damage resulting from excision in an area with extensive and shallow nerve branches,

- wounds that may reopen after they have been stitched closed, increasing the risk of infection and scarring.

Normal results

Depending on the complexity of the skin lesion removal procedure, patients can frequently resume

KEY TERMS

Curet—A surgical instrument with a circular cutting loop at one end. The curet is pulled over the skin lesion in repeated strokes to remove one portion of the lesion at a time.

Mohs' micrographic surgery—A surgical technique in which successive rings of skin tissue are removed and examined under a microscope to ensure that no cancer is left.

Shave biopsy—A method of removing a sample of skin lesion so it can be examined by a pathologist. A scalpel or razor blade is held parallel to the skin's surface and is used to slice the lesion at its base.

their normal routine the day of surgery. Healing frequently will take place within weeks. Some excisions will require later reconstructive procedures to improve the appearance left by the original procedure.

Abnormal results

In addition to the complications outlined above, it is always possible that the skin lesion will reappear, requiring further surgery.

Resources

ORGANIZATIONS

American Academy of Dermatology. 930 N. Meacham Road, P.O. Box 4014, Schaumburg, IL 60168-4014. (847) 330-0230. Fax: (847) 330-0050. < http://www.aad.org >.

American Society for Dermatologic Surgery. 930 N. Meacham Road, P.O. Box 4014, Schaumburg, IL 60168-4014. (847) 330-9830. < http://www.asds-net.org >.

American Society of Plastic and Reconstructive Surgeons. 44 E. Algonquin Rd., Arlington Heights, IL 60005. (847) 228-9900. < http://www.plasticsurgery.org >.

Richard H. Camer

Skin lesions

Definition

A skin lesion is a superficial growth or patch of the skin that does not resemble the area surrounding it.

Description

Skin lesions can be grouped into two categories: primary and secondary. Primary skin lesions are variations in color or texture that may be present at birth, such as **moles** or **birthmarks**, or that may be acquired during a person's lifetime, such as those associated with infectious diseases (e.g. **warts**, **acne**, or **psoriasis**), allergic reactions (e.g. **hives** or **contact dermatitis**), or environmental agents (e.g. **sunburn**, pressure, or temperature extremes). Secondary skin lesions are those changes in the skin that result from primary skin lesions, either as a natural progression or as a result of a person manipulating (e.g. scratching or picking at) a primary lesion.

The major types of primary lesions are:

- Macule. A small, circular, flat spot less than $^2/_5$ in (1 cm) in diameter. The color of a macule is not the same as that of nearby skin. Macules come in a variety of shapes and are usually brown, white, or red. Examples of macules include freckles and flat moles. A macule more than $^2/_5$ in (1 cm) in diameter is called a patch.

- Vesicle. A raised lesion less than $^1/_5$ in (5 mm) across and filled with a clear fluid. Vesicles that are more than $^1/_5$ in (5 mm) across are called bullae or blisters. These lesions may may be the result of sunburns, insect bites, chemical irritation, or certain viral infections, such as herpes.

- Pustule. A raised lesion filled with pus. A pustule is usually the result of an infection, such as acne, imptigeo, or **boils**.

- Papule. A solid, raised lesion less than $^2/_5$ in (1 cm) across. A patch of closely grouped papules more than $^2/_5$ in (1 cm) across is called a plaque. Papules and plaques can be rough in texture and red, pink, or brown in color. Papules are associated with such conditions as warts, **syphilis**, psoriasis, seborrheic and actinic keratoses, **lichen planus**, and skin **cancer**.

- Nodule. A solid lesion that has distinct edges and that is usually more deeply rooted than a papule. Doctors often describe a nodule as "palpable," meaning that, when examined by touch, it can be felt as a hard mass distinct from the tissue surrounding it. A nodule more than 2 cm in diameter is called a tumor. Nodules are associated with, among other conditions, keratinous cysts, lipomas, fibromas, and some types of lymphomas.

- Wheal. A skin elevation caused by swelling that can be itchy and usually disappears soon after erupting. Wheals are generally associated with an allergic reaction, such as to a drug or an insect bite.

• Telangiectasia. Small, dilated blood vessels that appear close to the surface of the skin. Telangiectasia is often a symptom of such diseases as **rosacea** or **scleroderma**.

The major types of secondary skin lesions are:

• Ulcer. Lesion that involves loss of the upper portion of the skin (epidermis) and part of the lower portion (dermis). Ulcers can result from acute conditions such as bacterial infection or trauma, or from more chronic conditions, such as scleroderma or disorders involving peripheral veins and arteries. An ulcer that appears as a deep crack that extends to the dermis is called a fissure.

• Scale. A dry, horny build-up of dead skin cells that often flakes off the surface of the skin. Diseases that promote scale include fungal infections, psoriasis, and **seborrheic dermatitis**.

• Crust. A dried collection of blood, serum, or pus. Also called a scab, a crust is often part of the normal healing process of many infectious lesions.

• Erosion. Lesion that involves loss of the epidermis.

• Excoriation. A hollow, crusted area caused by scratching or picking at a primary lesion.

• Scar. Discolored, fibrous tissue that permanently replaces normal skin after destruction of the dermis. A very thick and raised scar is called a keloid.

• Lichenification. Rough, thick epidermis with exaggerated skin lines. This is often a characteristic of scratch **dermatitis** and **atopic dermatitis**.

• Atrophy. An area of skin that has become very thin and wrinkled. Normally seen in older individuals and people who are using very strong topical corticosteroid medication.

Causes and symptoms

Skin lesions can be caused by a wide variety of conditions and diseases. A tendency toward developing moles, freckles, or birthmarks may be inherited. Infection of the skin itself by bacteria, viruses, fungi, or parasites is the most common cause of skin lesions. Acne, **athlete's foot** (tinea pedis), warts, and **scabies** are examples of skin infections that cause lesions. Allergic reactions and sensitivity to outside environmental factors can also lead to the formation of skin lesions. Underlying conditions can also precipitate the appearance of skin lesions. For example, the decreased sensitivity and poor circulation that accompanies **diabetes mellitus** can contribute to the formation of extensive ulcers on extremities such as the feet. Infections of body's entire system can cause the sudden onset of skin lesions. For example, skin lesions are a hallmark symptom of such diseases as chicken pox, herpes, and small pox. Cancers affecting the skin, including basal cell carcinoma, squamous cell carcinoma, **malignant melanoma**, and **Kaposi's sarcoma**, are recognized by their lesions.

Diagnosis

Diagnosis of the underlying cause of skin lesions is usually based on patient history, characteristics of the lesion, and where and how it appears on the patient's body (e.g. pustules confined to the face, neck and upper back can indicate acne, while scales appearing on the scalp and face may indicate seborrheic dermatitis). To determine the cause of an infection, doctors may also take scrapings or swab samples from lesions for examination under a microscope or for use in bacterial, fungal, or viral cultures. In cases where a fungal infection is suspected, a doctor may examine a patient's skin under ultraviolet light using a filter device called a Woods light–under these conditions, certain species will taken on specific fluorescent colors. Dermatologists may also use contrast lighting and subdued lighting to detect variations in the skin. When involvement of the immune system is suspected, doctors may order a immunofluorescence test, which detects antibodies to specific antigens using a fluorescent chemical. In cases of contact dermatitis, a condition in which a allergic reaction to something irritates the skin, doctors may use patch tests, in which samples of specific antigens are introduced into the skin via a scratch or a needle prick, to determine what substances are provoking the reaction.

The vast majority of skin lesions are noncancerous. However, doctors will determine whether or not a particular lesion or lesions are cancerous based on observation and the results of an excisional or punch biopsy, in which a tissue sample is excised for microscopic analysis. Since early detection is a key to successful treatment, individuals should examine their skin on a monthly basis for changes to existing moles, the presence of new moles, or a change in a certain area of skin. When examining moles, factors to look for include:

• Asymmetry. A normal mole is round, whereas a suspicious mole is uneven.

• Border. A normal mole has a clear-cut border with the surrounding skin, whereas the edges of a suspect mole may be irregular.

• Color. Normal moles are uniformly tan or brown, but cancerous moles may appear as mixtures of red, white, blue, brown, purple, or black.

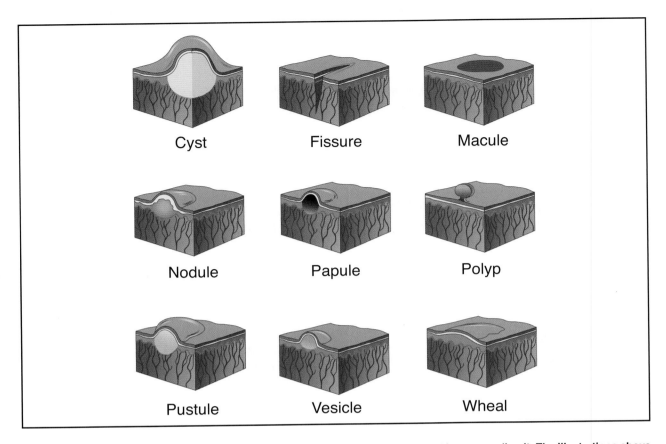

Cyst   Fissure   Macule

Nodule   Papule   Polyp

Pustule   Vesicle   Wheal

A skin lesion is an abnormal growth or an area of skin that does not resemble the skin surrounding it. The illustrations above feature some of the different types of skin lesions. *(Illustration by Electronic Illustrators Group.)*

- Diameter. Normal moles are usually less than $^1/_5$ in (5 mm) in diameter, a skin lesion greater than this may be suspected as cancerous.

Treatment

Treatment of skin lesions depends upon the underlying cause, what type of lesions they are, and the patient's overall health. If the cause of the lesions is an allergic reaction, removing the allergen from the patient's environment is the most effective treatment. Topical preparations can also be used to clean and protect irritated skin as well as to remove dead skin cells and scales. These may come in a variety of forms, including ointments, creams, lotions, and solutions. **Topical antibiotics**, fungicides, pediculicides (agents that kill lice), and scabicides (agents that kill the scabies parasite) can be applied to treat appropriate skin infections. Oral medications may be taken to address systemic infections or conditions. Deeply infected lesions may require minor surgery to lance and drain pus. Topical agents to sooth irritated skin and reduce inflammation may also be applied. **Corticosteroids** are particularly effective in reducing inflammation and **itching** (puritis). Oatmeal baths, baking soda mixtures, and calamine lotion are also recommended for the relief of these symptoms. A type of corticosteroid may be used to reduce the appearance of keloid **scars**. Absorbent powders may also be used to reduce moisture and prevent the spread of infection. In cases of ulcers that are slow to heal, pressure dressings may be used. At times, surgical removal of a lesion may be recommended–this is the usual course of therapy for skin cancer. Surgical removal usually involves a simple excision under local anesthetic, but it may also be accomplished through freezing (**cryotherapy**) or **laser surgery**.

Prognosis

Skin lesions such as moles, freckles, and birthmarks are a normal part of skin and will not disappear unless deliberately removed by a surgical procedure. Lesions due to an allergic reaction often subside soon after the offending agent is removed. Healing of lesions due to infections or disorders depends upon

KEY TERMS

Corticosteroid—A type of steroid medication that helps relieve itching (puritis) and reduce inflammation.

Fibroma—A usually benign tumor consisting of fiborous tissue.

Lesion—A possibly abnormal change or difference in a tissue or structure, such as the skin.

Lipoma—A usually benign tumor of fatty tissue.

Patch test—Test in which different antigens (substances that cause an allergic reaction) are introduced into a patient's skin via a needle prick or scratch and then observed for evidence of an allergic reaction to one or more of them. Also known as a scratch test.

Woods light—Device that allows only ultraviolet light to pass through it.

the type of infection or disorder and the overall health of the individual. Prognosis for skin cancer primarily depends upon whether or not the lesion is localized and whether or not it has spread to other areas of the body, such as the lymph nodes. In cases where the lesion is localized and has not spread to other parts of the body, the cure rate is 95-100%.

Prevention

Not all skin lesions are preventable; moles and freckles, for example, are benign growths that are common and unavoidable. However others can be avoided or minimized by taking certain precautions. Skin lesions caused by an allergic reaction can be avoided by determining what the offending agent is and removing it from the home or workplace, or, if this is impossible, developing strategies for safely handling it, such as with gloves and protective clothing. Keeping the skin, nails, and scalp clean and moisturized can help reduce or prevent the incidence of infectious skin diseases, as can not sharing personal care items such as combs and make-up with others. Skin lesions associated with **sexually transmitted diseases** can be prevented by the use of condoms. Scratching or picking at existing lesions should be avoided since this usually serves only to spread infection and may result in scarring. Individuals who have systemic conditions, such as diabetes mellitus or poor circulation, that could lead to serious skin lesions should inspect their bodies regularly for changes in their skin's condition. Regular visual inspection of

the skin is also a key to preventing or minimizing the occurrence of skin cancer, as is the regular use of sun screens with an SPF of 15 or more.

Resources

BOOKS

Rosen, Theodore, Marilyn B. Lanning, and Marcia J. Hill. *The Nurse's Atlas of Dermatology.* Boston: Little Brown & Co., 1983.

Bridget Travers

Skin pigmentation disorders

Definition

Skin pigmentation disorders are conditions that cause the skin to appear lighter or darker than normal, or blotchy and discolored.

Description

People of all races have skin pigmentation disorders. Some disorders, like **albinism** (which affects one out of every 17,000 people) are rare. Others, such as age spots, are very common.

Skin pigmentation disorders occur because the body produces either too much or too little melanin, a pigment that creates hair, skin, and eye color. Melanin protects the body by absorbing ultraviolet light.

In hypopigmentation means the body does not produces enough melanin. Albinism, for example, is an inherited condition that causes a lack of pigment. So people with albinism typically have light skin, white or pale yellow hair, and light blue or gray eyes. Another condition called vitilgo, creates smooth, depigmented white spots on the skin. Vitilgo affects nearly 2% of the population, but it strikes people between 10 and 30 years old more often, and is more evident in people with darker skin.

In **hyperpigmentation**, the body produces too much melanin, causing skin to become darker than usual. Lichen simplex chronicus is a skin disorder with severe **itching** that causes thick, dark patches of skin to develop. Lamellar **ichthyosis** (fish scale disease) is an inherited disease that also is characterized by darkened, scaly, dry patches of skin.

Hyperpigmentation also occurs in melasma, a dark mask-like discoloration that covers the cheeks and bridge of the nose. Melasma can occur during the end of **pregnancy**. People with the autoimmune disease (when immune cells, which attack invaders, become abnormally programed to kill self cells inside the body) systemic lupus also may develop a similar butterfly-shaped mask on their faces. In addition, many people have moles, freckles, age spots, and **birthmarks**, ranging from red or brown to bluish, black, covering various parts of their bodies.

Causes and symptoms

Scientists are still studying the reasons why skin pigmentation disorders occur. In some cases there are tangible causes, such as sun exposure, drug reactions or genetic inheritance. In other cases, it is not as clear.

Albinism is an inherited recessive trait. Albinism has many different forms, but most people who have this condition have pale skin, hair, and eyes. Melanin also creates eye color, and serves as a filter that prevents too much light from entering the eye. Since they lack melanin in their eyes, many people with albinism also have **visual impairment**. With little skin pigmentation, they also **sunburn** easily and are more prone to skin **cancer**.

The hypopigmentation spots associated with vitilgo sometimes form where a person has been cut or injured. Research has shown that the light patches associated with vitilgo do not contain melanocytes, the type of skin cells that create melanin. Some scientists believe vitilgo may be caused by an autoimmune disorder. It also has been linked to other conditions such as **hyperthyroidism** (too much thyroid hormone) and Addison's Disease, which affects the adrenal gland.

Hyperpigmentation can be caused by many factors, from too much sunbathing to drug reactions or poor **nutrition**. Wounds and **scars** also can develop darker patches of skin. A psychological syndrome gives people with lichen simplex chronicus to develop a compulsive need to scratch, which causes dark, leathery skin to form. This can lead to permanent scarring and infection if untreated. Scientists believe lamellar ichthyosis is caused by genetics.

The mask caused by melasma may be related to pregnancy hormones, and usually disappears after a woman gives birth. Birthmarks, **moles**, and **aging** spots usually are harmless. Some moles, however, can change in size, color, texture, or start bleeding, which could indicate possible skin cancer.

Diagnosis

Diagnostic tests vary for different types of skin pigmentation disorders. Physicians usually can

---

KEY TERMS

Melanin—A pigment that creates hair, skin and eye color. Melanin also protects the body by absorbing ultraviolet light.

Melanocytes— The type of skin cells that create melanin.

Albinism— An inherited condition that causes a lack of pigment. People with albinism typically have light skin, white or pale yellow hair and light blue or gray eyes

Hypopigmentation—A skin condition that occurs when the body has too little melanin, or pigment.

Hyperpigmentation— A skin condition that occurs when the body has too much melanin, or pigment.

Lichen simplex chronicus—A skin disorder with severe itching that causes thick, dark patches of skin to develop.

Vitilgo—A skin disorder that creates smooth, depigmented white spots on the skin.

Lamellar ichthyosis— Also called fish scale disease, this inherited condition is characterized by darkened, scaly, dry patches of skin.

Melasma—A dark mask-like discoloration that covers the cheeks and bridge of the nose. Also called "the mask of pregnancy."

---

diagnose albinism by looking carefully at a person's hair, skin, and eyes. They may order blood tests and eye exams as well. A visual exam also is enough to diagnose vitilgo.

For most hyperpigmentation disorders, doctors can make a diagnosis by looking at a person's appearance. To detect conditions like **lichen simplex chronicus** or lamellar ichthyosis, or skin cancer, they may also do a biopsy to remove some of the affected skin for further study under a microscope. Some physicians also use a wood's lamp, or black light test, to diagnose skin conditions. Affected areas would absorb the ultraviolet light and stand out with flourescent colors in the darkened room.

Treatment

For albinism, healthcare providers advise people to cover up, use sunscreen and avoid excess sunlight to prevent skin cancer. People with albinism also must wear protective sunglasses and, in some cases, prescription corrective lenses. Surgery may be necessary to correct visual impairments.

To treat vitilgo, physicians may prescribe a combination of photo-sensitive medications like trimethylpsoralen and ultraviolet light therapy to darken the spots. If the person has depigmented patches covering more than 50% of the body, doctors also may be able to use skin bleaching agents like monobenzone to give the skin a lighter, more uniform appearance. Other options include cosmetic concealers and **skin grafting**.

Skin-lightening creams are available for hyperpigmentation disorders. Doctors also advise staying out of the sun. Counseling with a dietitian may help in cases caused by poor nutrition. For lichen simplex chronicus, doctors could prescribe antihistamines and topical steroid creams to stop the itching. If a mole or birthmark appears suspicious, physicians often will surgically remove it to prevent skin cancer.

Prognosis

Most skin pigmentation disorders do not affect a person's health, only the outward appearance.

Prevention

In most cases, doctors will recommend using sunscreen and avoiding too much sun exposure.

Resources

PERIODICALS

Wilson, Tracy. "The Paler Side of Beauty." *Heart and Soul* 6, no. 1 (February 1999): 30-33.

ORGANIZATIONS

American Academy of Dermatology. 930 N. Meacham Road, P.O. Box 4014, Schaumburg, IL 60168-4014. (847) 330-0230. < http://www.aad.org > .

National Organization for Albinism and Hypopigmentation (NOAH), 1530 Locust St., #29, Philadelphia, PA, 19102-4415. (800) 473-2310. < http://www.albinism.org >.

OTHER

MelanomaNet. < http://www.skincarephysicians.com/melanomanet/index.html >.

National Weather Service. "Ultraviolet Light Index." < http://www.nws.noaa.gov/pa/secnews/uv/index.html >.

Melissa Knopper

Skin resurfacing

Definition

Skin resurfacing employs a variety of techniques to change the surface texture and appearance of the skin. Common skin resurfacing techniques include chemical peels, dermabrasion, and laser resurfacing.

Purpose

Skin resurfacing procedures may be performed for cosmetic reasons, such as diminishing the appearance of wrinkles around the mouth or eyes. They may also be used as a medical treatment, such as removing large numbers of certain precancerous lesions called actinic keratoses. Physicians sometimes combine techniques, using dermabrasion or laser resurfacing on some areas of the face, while performing a chemical peel on other areas.

Precautions

As the popularity of skin resurfacing techniques has increased, many unqualified or inexperienced providers have entered the field. Patients should choose their provider with the same degree of care they take for any other medical procedure. Complications of skin resurfacing techniques can be serious, including severe infection and scarring.

Patient's with active herpesvirus infections are not good candidates for resurfacing procedures. Persons who tend to scar easily may also experience poor results. Patients who have recently used the oral **acne** medication isotretinoin (Accutane) may be at higher risk of scarring following skin resurfacing.

Description

Chemical peel

Chemical peels employ a variety of caustic chemicals to selectively destroy several layers of skin. The peeling solutions are "painted on," area-by-area, to ensure that the entire face is treated. After the skin heals, discoloration, wrinkles, and other surface irregularities are often eliminated.

Chemical peels are divided into three types: superficial, medium-depth, and deep. The type of peel depends on the strength of the chemical used, and on how deeply it penetrates. Superficial peels are used for fine wrinkles, sun damage, acne, and **rosacea**. The medium-depth peel is used for more obvious wrinkles and sun damage, as well as for precancerous lesions like actinic keratoses. Deep peels are used for the most severe wrinkling and sun damage.

Dermabrasion

Dermabrasion uses an abrasive tool to selectively remove layers of skin. Some physicians use a hand-held motorized tool with a small wire brush or diamond-impregnated grinding wheel at the end. Other physicians prefer to abrade the skin by hand with an abrasive pad or other instrument. Acne scarring is one of the prime uses for dermabrasion. It also can be used to treat wrinkling, remove surgical **scars**, and obliterate **tattoos**.

Laser resurfacing

Laser resurfacing is the most recently developed technique for skin resurfacing. Specially designed, pulsed CO_2 lasers can vaporize skin layer-by-layer, causing minimal damage to other skin tissue. Special scanning devices move the laser light across the skin in predetermined patterns, ensuring proper exposure. Wrinkling around the eyes, mouth, and cheeks are the primary uses for laser resurfacing. Smile lines or those associated with other facial muscles tend to reappear after laser resurfacing. Laser resurfacing appears to achieve its best results as a spot treatment; patients expecting complete elimination of their wrinkles will not be satisfied.

Preparation

Chemical peel

Preparation for the chemical peel begins several weeks before the actual procedure. To promote turnover of skin cells, patients use a mild glycolic acid lotion or cream in the morning, and the acne cream tretinoin in the evening. They also use hydroquinone cream, a bleaching product that helps prevent later discoloration. To prevent reappearance of a herpes simplex virus infection, antiviral medicine is started a few days before the procedure and continues until the skin has healed.

Patients arrive for the procedure wearing no makeup. The physician "degreases" the patient's face using alcohol or another cleanser. Some degree of **pain** accompanies all types of peels. For a superficial peel, use of a hand held fan to cool the face during the procedure is often sufficient. For medium-depth peels, the patient may take a sedative or **aspirin**. During the procedure, cold compresses and a hand-held fan can also reduce pain. Deep peels can be extremely painful. Some physicians prefer **general**

anesthesia, but local anesthetics combined with intravenous sedatives are frequently sufficient to control pain.

Dermabrasion

Dermabrasion does not require much preparation. It is usually performed under **local anesthesia**, although some physicians use intravenous **sedation** or general anesthesia. The physician begins by marking the areas to be treated and then chilling them with ice packs. In order to stiffen the skin, a spray refrigerant is applied to the area, which also helps control pain. Some physicians prefer to inject the area with a solution of saline and local anesthetic, which also leaves the skin's surface more solid. Since dermabrasion can cause quite a bit of bleeding, physicians and their assistants will wear gloves, gowns, and masks to protect themselves from possible blood-transmitted infection.

Laser resurfacing

Antiviral medications should be started several days before the procedure. Laser resurfacing is performed under local anesthesia. An oral sedative may also be taken. The patient's eyes must be shielded, and the area surrounding the face should be shielded with wet drapes or crumpled foil to catch stray beams of laser light. The physician will mark the areas to be treated before beginning the procedure.

Aftercare

Chemical peel

Within a day or so following a superficial peel, the skin will turn faint pink or brown. Over the next few days, dead skin will peel away. Patients will be instructed to wash their skin frequently with a mild cleanser and cool water, then apply an ointment to the skin to keep it moist. After a medium-depth peel, the skin turns deep red or brown, and crusts may form. Care is similar to that following a superficial peel. Redness may persist for a week or more. Deep-peeled skin will turn brown and crusty. There may also be swelling and some oozing of fluid. Frequent washing and ointments are favored over dressings. The skin typically heals in about two weeks, but redness may persist.

Dermabrasion

Following the procedure, an ointment may be applied, and the wound will be covered with a dressing and mask. Patients with a history of herpesvirus

KEY TERMS

Actinic keratosis—A crusty, scaly skin lesion, caused by exposure to the sun, which can transform into skin cancer.

Herpesviruses—A family of viruses responsible for cold sores, chicken pox, and genital herpes.

Isotretinoin—A powerful vitamin A derivative used in the treatment of acne. It can promote scarring after skin resurfacing procedures.

infections will begin taking an antiviral medication to prevent a recurrence. After 24 hours, the dressing is removed, and ointment is reapplied to keep the wound moist. Patients are encouraged to wash their face with plain water and reapply ointment every few hours. This relieves **itching** and pain and helps remove oozing fluid and other matter. Patients may require a pain medication. A steroid medication may be taken during the first few days to reduce swelling. The skin will take a week or more to heal, but may remain very red.

Laser resurfacing

The skin should be kept moist following laser resurfacing. This promotes more rapid healing and reduces the risk of infection. Some physicians favor application of ointments only to the skin; others prefer the use of dressings. In either case, care of the skin is similar to that given following a chemical peel. The face is washed with plain water to remove ooze, and an ointment is reapplied. Healing will take approximately two weeks. Pain medications and a steroid to reduce swelling may also be taken.

Risks

All resurfacing procedures can lead to infection and scarring. It is also possible that skin coloration will be altered, or that redness of the skin will be prolonged for many months. Some of the peeling agents used in deep chemical peels can affect the function of the heart.

Normal results

Depending on the resurfacing techniques selected, it is possible to improve the appearance of skin damaged by sun, age, or disease in many people. Skin resurfacing techniques address only the surface of the skin; procedures such as face-lift surgery or **blepharoplasty** may be needed to repair other age-related skin changes. All resurfacing procedures are accompanied by some pain, redness, and skin color changes. These may persist for several months following the procedure, but they usually resolve over time.

Abnormal results

As noted above, resurfacing procedures can reactivate herpesvirus infections or lead to new, sometimes serious infections. All resurfacing techniques intentionally create skin **wounds**, creating the possibility for scarring. Abnormal results such as these can be minimized with use of antiviral medications prior to the procedure and good wound care afterward. Selection of an experienced, reputable provider also is key.

Resources

ORGANIZATIONS

American Society for Dermatologic Surgery. 930 N. Meacham Road, P.O. Box 4014, Schaumburg, IL 60168-4014. (847) 330-9830. < http://www.asds-net.org >.

American Society for Laser Medicine and Surgery. 2404 Stewart Square, Wausau, WI 54401.(715) 845-9283. < http://www.aslms.org >.

American Society of Plastic and Reconstructive Surgeons. 44 E. Algonquin Rd., Arlington Heights, IL 60005. (847) 228-9900. < http://www.plasticsurgery.org >.

Richard H. Camer

Skin traction *see* **Traction; Immobilization**

Skull x rays

Definition

Skull x rays are performed to examine the nose, sinuses, and facial bones. These studies may also be referred to as sinus x rays. X-ray studies produce films, also known as radiographs, by aiming x rays at soft bones and tissues of the body. X-ray beams are similar to light waves, except their shorter wavelength allows them to penetrate dense substances, producing images and shadows on film.

Purpose

Doctors may order skull x rays to aid in the diagnosis of a variety of diseases or injuries.

Sinusitis

Sinus x rays may be ordered to confirm a diagnosis of **sinusitis**, or sinus infection.

Fractures

A skull x ray may detect bone **fractures** resulting from injury or disease. The skull x ray should clearly show the skull cap, jaw bones, and facial bones.

Tumors

Skull radiographs may indicate tumors in facial bones, tissues, or the sinuses. Tumors may be benign (not cancerous) or malignant (cancerous).

Other

Birth defects (referred to as congenital anomalies) may be detected on a skull x ray by changes in bone structure. Abnormal tissues or glands resulting from various conditions or diseases may also be shown on a skull radiograph.

Precautions

As with any x-ray procedure, women who may be pregnant are advised against having a skull x ray if it is not absolutely necessary. However, a lead apron may be worn across the abdomen during the procedure to protect the fetus. Children are also more sensitive to x-ray exposure. Children of both sexes should wear a protective covering (a lead apron) in the genital/reproductive area. In general, skull x-ray exposure is minimal and x-ray equipment and procedures are monitored to ensure radiation safety.

Description

Skull or sinus x rays may be performed in a doctor's office that has x-ray equipment and a technologist available. The exam may also be performed in an outpatient radiology facility or a hospital radiology department.

In many instances, particularly for sinus views, the patient will sit upright in a chair, perhaps with the head held stable by a foam vise. A film cassette is located behind the patient. The x-ray tube is in front of the patient and may be moved to allow for different positions and views. A patient may also be asked to move his or her head at various angles and positions.

In some cases, technologists will ask the patient to lie on a table and will place the head and neck at various angles. In routine skull x rays, as many as

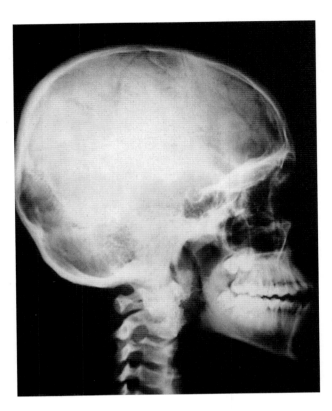

A skull x ray. *(Photo Researchers. Reproduced by permission.)*

five different views may be taken to allow a clear picture of various bones and tissues. The length of the test will vary depending on the number of views taken, but in general, it should last about 10 minutes. The technologist will usually ask a patient to wait while the films are being developed to ensure that they are clear before going to the radiologist.

Preparation

There is no preparation for the patient prior to arriving at the radiology facility. Patients will be asked to remove jewelry, dentures, or other metal objects that may produce artifacts on the film. The referring doctor or x-ray technologist can answer any questions regarding the procedure. Any woman who is, or may be, pregnant should tell the technologist.

Aftercare

There is no aftercare required following skull or sinus x-ray procedures.

Risks

There are no common side effects from skull or sinus x ray. The patient may feel some discomfort in

KEY TERMS

Radiograph—The actual picture or film produced by an x-ray study.

X ray—A form of electromagnetic radiation with shorter wavelengths than normal light. X rays can penetrate most structures.

the positioning of the head and neck, but will have no complications. Any x-ray procedure carries minimal radiation risk, and children and pregnant women should be protected from radiation exposure to the abdominal or genital areas.

Normal results

Normal results should indicate sinuses, bones, tissues, and other observed areas are of normal size, shape, and thickness for the patient's age and medical history. Results, whether normal or abnormal, will be provided to the referring doctor in a written report.

Abnormal results

Abnormal results may include:

Sinusitis

Air in sinuses will show up on a radiograph as black, but fluid will be cloudy or white (opaque). This helps the radiologist to identify trapped fluids in the sinuses. In chronic sinusitis, the radiologist may also note thickening or hardening of the bony wall of an infected sinus.

Fractures

Radiologists may recognize even tiny facial bone fractures as a line of defect.

Tumors

Tumors may be visible if the bony sinus wall is distorted or destroyed. Abnormal findings may result in follow-up imaging studies.

Other

Skull x rays may also detect disorders that show up as changes in bone structure, such as Paget's disease of the bone or acromegaly (a disorder associated with excess growth hormones from the pituitary gland). Areas of calcification, or gathering of calcium

deposits, may indicate a condition such as an infection of bone or bone marrow (**osteomyelitis**).

Resources

ORGANIZATIONS

National Cancer Institute. Building 31, Room 10A31, 31 Center Drive, MSC 2580, Bethesda, MD 20892-2580. (800) 422-6237. < http://www.nci.nih.gov >.

National Head Injury Foundation, Inc. (888) 222-5287. < http://www.nhif.org/home.html >.

Radiological Society of North America. 820 Jorie Boulevard, Oak Brook, IL 60523-2251. (630) 571-2670. < http://www.rsna.org >.

Teresa Odle

SLE *see* **Systemic lupus erythematosus**

Sleep apnea

Definition

Sleep apnea is a condition in which breathing stops for more than ten seconds during sleep. Sleep apnea is a major, though often unrecognized, cause of daytime sleepiness. It can have serious negative effects on a person's quality of life, and is thought to be considerably underdiagnosed in the United States.

Description

A sleeping person normally breathes continuuously and uninterruptedly throughout the night. A person with sleep apnea, however, has frequent episodes (up to 400–500 per night) in which he or she stops breathing. This interruption of breathing is called "apnea." Breathing usually stops for about 30 seconds; then the person usually startles awake with a loud snort and begins to breathe again, gradually falling back to sleep.

There are two forms of sleep apnea. In obstructive sleep apnea (OSA), breathing stops because tissue in the throat closes off the airway. In central sleep apnea, (CSA), the brain centers responsible for breathing fail to send messages to the breathing muscles. OSA is much more common than CSA. It is thought that about 1–10% of adults are affected by OSA; only about one tenth of that number have CSA. OSA can affect people of any age and of either sex, but it is most common in middle-aged, somewhat overweight men, especially those who use alcohol.

Causes and symptoms

Obstructive sleep apnea

Obstructive sleep apnea occurs when part of the airway is closed off (usually at the back of the throat) while a person is trying to inhale during sleep. People whose airways are slightly narrower than average are more likely to be affected by OSA. **Obesity**, especially obesity in the neck, can increase the risk of developing OSA, because the fat tissue tends to narrow the airway. In some people, the airway is blocked by enlarged tonsils, an enlarged tongue, jaw deformities, or growths in the neck that compress the airway. Blocked nasal passages may also play a part in some people.

When a person begins to inhale, the expansion of the lungs lowers the air pressure inside the airway. If the muscles that keep the airway open are not working hard enough, the airway narrows and may collapse, shutting off the supply of air to the lungs. OSA occurs during sleep because the neck muscles that keep the airway open are not as active then. Congestion in the nose can make collapse more likely, since the extra effort needed to inhale will lower the pressure in the airway even more. Drinking alcohol or taking tranquilizers in the evening worsens this situation, because these cause the neck muscles to relax. (These drugs also lower the "respiratory drive" in the nervous system, reducing breathing rate and strength.)

People with OSA almost always snore heavily, because the same narrowing of the airway that causes **snoring** can also cause OSA. Snoring may actually help cause OSA as well, because the vibration of the throat tissues can cause them to swell. However, most people who snore do not go on to develop OSA.

Other risk factors for developing OSA include male sex; **pregnancy**; a family history of the disorder; and **smoking**. With regard to gender, it has been found that male sex hormones sometimes cause changes in the size or structure of the upper airway. The weight gain that accompanies pregnancy can affect a woman's breathing patterns during sleep, particularly during the third trimester. With regard to family history, OSA is known to run in families even though no gene or genes associated with the disorder have been identified as of 2002. Smoking increases the risk of developing OSA because it causes inflammation, swelling, and narrowing of the upper airway.

Some patients being treated for **head and neck cancer** develop OSA as a result of physical changes in the muscles and other tissues of the neck and throat. Doctors recommend prompt treatment of the OSA to improve the patient's quality of life.

Central sleep apnea

In central sleep apnea, the airway remains open, but the nerve signals controlling the respiratory muscles are not regulated properly. This can cause wide fluctuations in the level of carbon dioxide (CO_2) in the blood. Normal activity in the body produces CO_2, which is brought by the blood to the lungs for exhalation. When the blood level of CO_2 rises, brain centers respond by increasing the rate of respiration, clearing the CO_2. As blood levels fall again, respiration slows down. Normally, this interaction of CO_2 and breathing rate maintains the CO_2 level within very narrow limits. CSA can occur when the regulation system becomes insensitive to CO_2 levels, allowing wide fluctuations in both CO_2 levels and breathing rates. High CO_2 levels cause very rapid breathing (hyperventilation), which then lowers CO_2 so much that breathing becomes very slow or even stops. CSA occurs during sleep because when a person is awake, breathing is usually stimulated by other signals, including conscious awareness of breathing rate.

A combination of the two forms is also possible, and is called mixed sleep apnea. Mixed sleep apnea episodes usually begin with a reduced central respiratory drive, followed by obstruction.

OSA and CSA cause similar symptoms. The most common symptoms are:

- daytime sleepiness
- morning headaches
- a feeling that sleep is not restful
- disorientation upon waking
- poor judgment
- personality changes

Sleepiness is caused not only by the frequent interruption of sleep, but by the inability to enter long periods of deep sleep, during which the body performs numerous restorative functions. OSA is one of the leading causes of daytime sleepiness, and is a major risk factor for motor vehicle accidents. Headaches and disorientation are caused by low oxygen levels during sleep, from the lack of regular breathing.

Other symptoms of sleep apnea may include **sexual dysfunction**, loss of concentration, memory loss, intellectual impairment, and behavioral changes including **anxiety** and depression.

Sleep apnea is also associated with night sweats and nocturia, or increased frequency of urination at night. Bedwetting in children is also linked to sleep apnea.

Sleep apnea can also cause serious changes in the cardiovascular system. Daytime **hypertension** (high blood pressure) is common. An increase in the number of red blood cells (polycythemia) is possible, as is an enlarged left ventricle of the heart (**cor pulmonale**), and left ventricular failure. In some people, sleep apnea causes life-threatening changes in the rhythm of the heart, including heartbeat slowing (bradycardia), racing (tachycardia), and other types of "arrhythmias." Sudden **death** may occur from such **arrhythmias**. Patients with the **Pickwickian syndrome** (named after a Charles Dickens character) are obese and sleepy, with right **heart failure**, **pulmonary hypertension**, and chronic daytime low blood oxygen (hypoxemia) and increased blood CO_2 (hypercapnia).

Diagnosis

Excessive daytime sleepiness is the complaint that usually brings a person to see the doctor. A careful medical history will include questions about alcohol or tranquilizer use, snoring (often reported by the person's partner), and morning headaches or disorientation. A physical exam will include examination of the throat to look for narrowing or obstruction. Blood pressure is also measured. Measuring heart rate or blood levels of oxygen and CO_2 during the daytime will not usually be done, since these are abnormal only at night in most patients.

In some cases the person's dentist may suggest the diagnosis of OSA on the basis of a dental checkup or evaluation of the patient for oral surgery.

Confirmation of the diagnosis usually requires making measurements while the person sleeps. These tests are called a **polysomnography** study, and are conducted during an overnight stay in a specialized sleep laboratory. Important parts of the polysomnography study include measurements of:

• heart rate

• airflow at the mouth and nose

• respiratory effort

• sleep stage (light sleep, deep sleep, dream sleep, etc.)

• oxygen level in the blood, using a noninvasive probe (ear oximetry)

Simplified studies done overnight at home are also possible, and may be appropriate for people whose profile strongly suggests the presence of obstructive sleep apnea; that is, middle-aged, somewhat overweight men, who snore and have high blood pressure. The home-based study usually includes ear oximetry and cardiac measurements. If these measurements support the diagnosis of OSA, initial treatment is usually suggested without polysomnography. Home-based measurements are not used to rule out OSA, however, and if the measurements do not support the OSA diagnosis, polysomnography may be needed to define the problem further.

Both types of studies are usually covered by insurance with the appropriate referral from a physician. Without insurance, lab-based polysomnography cost approximately $1,500 in 1997, while overnight home monitoring cost between $500 and $1,000.

Treatment

Behavioral changes

Treatment of obstructive sleep apnea begins with reducing the use of alcohol or tranquilizers in the evening, if these have been contributing to the problem. Weight loss is also effective, but if the weight returns, as it often does, so does the apnea. Changing sleeping position may be effective; snoring and sleep apnea are both most common when a person sleeps on his back. Turning to sleep on the side may be enough to clear up the symptoms. Raising the head of the bed may also help. Opening of the nasal passages can provide some relief. There are a variety of nasal devices such as clips, tapes, or holders which may help, though discomfort may limit their use. Nasal **decongestants** may be useful, but should not be taken for sleep apnea without the consent of the treating physician.

Oxygen and drug therapy

Supplemental nighttime oxygen can be useful for some people with either central and obstructive sleep apnea. Tricyclic **antidepressant drugs** such as protriptyline (Vivactil) may help by increasing the muscle tone of the upper airway muscles, but their side effects may severely limit their usefulness.

Mechanical ventilation

For moderate to severe sleep apnea, the most successful treatment is nighttime use of a ventilator, called a CPAP machine. CPAP (continuous positive airway pressure) blows air into the airway continuously, preventing its collapse. CPAP requires the use of a nasal mask. The appropriate pressure setting for the CPAP machine is determined by polysomnography in the sleep lab. Its effects are dramatic; daytime sleepiness usually disappears within one to two days after treatment begins. CPAP is used to treat both obstructive and central sleep apnea.

CPAP is tolerated well by about two-thirds of patients who try it. Bilevel positive airway pressure (BiPAP), is an alternative form of ventilation. With BiPAP, the ventilator reduces the air pressure when the person exhales. This is more comfortable for some.

Surgery

Surgery can be used to correct obstructions in the airways. The most common surgery is called UPPP, for uvulopalatopharngyoplasty. This surgery removes tissue from the rear of the mouth and top of the throat. The tissues removed include parts of the uvula (the flap of tissue that hangs down at the back of the mouth), the soft palate, and the pharynx. Tonsils and adenoids are usually removed in this operation. This operation significantly improves sleep apnea in slightly more than half of all cases.

Reconstructive surgery is possible for those whose OSA is due to constriction of the airway by lower jaw deformities. Genioplasty, which is a procedure that plastic surgeons usually perform to reshape a patient's chin to improve his or her appearance, is now being done to reshape the upper airway in patients with OSA.

When other forms of treatment are not successful, obstructive sleep apnea may be treated by a tracheostomy. In this procedure, an opening is made into the trachea (windpipe) below the obstruction, and a tube inserted to maintain an air passage. A tracheostomy requires a great deal of care to prevent infection of the tracheostomy site. In addition, since air is no longer being filtered and moistened by the nasal passages before entering the lungs, the lower airways can become dry and susceptible to infection as well. Tracheostomy is usually reserved for those whose apnea has led to life-threatening heart arrhythmias, and who have not been treated successfully with other treatments.

Oral appliances

Another approach to treating OSA involves the use of oral appliances intended to improve breathing either by holding the tongue in place or by pushing the lower jaw forward during sleep to increase the air volume in the upper airway. The first type of oral appliance is known as a tongue retaining device or TRD. The second type is variously called an oral protrusive device (OPD) or mandibular advancement splint (MAS), because it holds the mandible, or lower jaw, forward during sleep. These oral devices appear to work best for patients with mild-to-moderate OSA, and in some cases can postpone or prevent the need for surgery. Their rate of patient compliance is about

---

KEY TERMS

Continuous positive airway pressure (CPAP)—A ventilation system that blows a gentle stream of air into the nose to keep the airway open.

Genioplasty—An operation performed to reshape the chin. Genioplasties are often done to treat OSA because the procedure changes the structure of the patient's upper airway.

Mandible—The medical term for the lower jaw. One type of oral appliance used to treat OSA pushes the mandible forward in order to ease breathing during sleep.

Nocturia—Excessive need to urinate at night. Nocturia is a symptom of OSA and often increases the patient's daytime sleepiness.

Polysomnography—A group of tests administered to analyze heart, blood, and breathing patterns during sleep.

Tracheotomy—A surgical procedure in which a small hole is cut into the trachea, or windpipe, below the level of the vocal cords.

Uvulopalatopharyngoplasty (UPPP)—An operation to remove excess tissue at the back of the throat to prevent it from closing off the airway during sleep.

50%; most patients who stop using oral appliances do so because their teeth are in poor condition. TRDs and OPDs can be fitted by dentists; however, most dentists work together with the patient's physician following a polysomnogram rather than prescribing the device by themselves.

Prognosis

The combination of behavioral changes, ventilation assistance, drug therapy, and surgery allow most people with sleep apnea to be treated successfully, although it may take some time to determine the most effective and least intrusive treatment. Polysomnography testing is usually required after beginning a treatment to determine how effective it has been.

Prevention

For people who snore frequently, weight control, avoidance of evening alcohol or tranquilizers, and adjustment of sleeping position may help reduce the risk of developing obstructive sleep apnea.

Resources

BOOKS

Beers, Mark H., MD, and Robert Berkow, MD., editors. "Disorders of the Oral Region." Section 9, Chapter 105 In *The Merck Manual of Diagnosis and Therapy*. Whitehouse Station, NJ: Merck Research Laboratories, 2004.

Beers, Mark H., MD, and Robert Berkow, MD., editors. "Sleep Disorders." Section 14, Chapter 173 In *The Merck Manual of Diagnosis and Therapy*. Whitehouse Station, NJ: Merck Research Laboratories, 2004.

PERIODICALS

Chasens, E. R., and M. G. Umlauf. "Nocturia: A Problem That Disrupts Sleep and Predicts Obstructive Sleep Apnea" *Geriatric Nursing* 24 (March-April 2003): 76–81, 105.

Chung, S. A., S. Jairam, M. R. Hussain, and C. M. Shapiro. "How, What, and Why of Sleep Apnea. Perspectives for Primary Care Physicians." *Canadian Family Physician* 48 (June 2002): 1073–1080.

Edwards, N., P. G. Middleton, D. M. Blyton, and C. E. Sullivan. "Sleep Disordered Breathing and Pregnancy." *Thorax* 57 (June 2002): 555–558.

Hisanaga, A., T. Itoh, Y. Hasegawa, et al. "A Case of Sleep Choking Syndrome Improved by the Kampo Extract of Hange-Koboku-To." *Psychiatry and Clinical Neuroscience* 56 (June 2002): 325–327.

Kapur, V., K. P. Strohl, S. Redline, et al. "Underdiagnosis of Sleep Apnea Syndrome in U.S. Communities." *Sleep and Breathing* 6 (June 2002): 49–54.

Koliha, C. A. "Obstructive Sleep Apnea in Head and Neck Cancer Patients Post Treatment ... Something to Consider?" *ORL—Head and Neck Nursing* 21 (Winter 2003): 10–14.

Neill, A., R. Whyman, S. Bannan, et al. "Mandibular Advancement Splint Improves Indices of Obstructive Sleep Apnoea and Snoring but Side Effects Are Common." *New Zealand Medical Journal* 115 (June 21, 2002): 289–292.

Rose, E., R. Staats, J. Schulte-Monting, et al. "Long-Term Compliance with an Oral Protrusive Appliance in Patients with Obstructive Sleep Apnoea." [in German] *Deutsche medizinische Wochenschrift* 127 (June 7, 2002): 1245–1249.

Shiomi, T., A. T. Arita, R. Sasanabe, et al. "Falling Asleep While Driving and Automobile Accidents Among Patients with Obstructive Sleep Apnea-Hypopnea Syndrome." *Psychiatry and Clinical Neuroscience* 56 (June 2002): 333–334.

Stanton, D. C. "Genioplasty." *Facial Plastic Surgery* 19 (February 2003): 75–86.

Umlauf, M. G., and E. R. Chasens. "Bedwetting—Not Always What It Seems: A Sign of Sleep-Disordered Breathing in Children." *Journal for Specialists in Pediatric Nursing* 8 (January-March 2003): 22–30.

Veale, D., G. Poussin, F. Benes, et al. "Identification of Quality of Life Concerns of Patients with Obstructive Sleep Apnoea at the Time of Initiation of Continuous Positive Airway Pressure: A Discourse Analysis." *Quality of Life Research* 11 (June 2002): 389–399.

Viera, A. J., M. M. Bond, and S. J. Yates. "Diagnosing Night Sweats." *American Family Physician* 67 (March 1, 2003): 1019–1024.

ORGANIZATIONS

American Academy of Otolaryngology, Head and Neck Surgery, Inc. One Prince Street, Alexandria, VA 22314-3357. (703) 836-4444. < http://www.entnet.org >.

American Dental Association. 211 East Chicago Avenue, Chicago, IL 60611. (312) 440-2500. < www.ada.org >.

American Sleep Apnea Association. 1424 K Street NW, Suite 302, Washington, DC 20005. (202) 293-3650. Fax: (202) 293-3656. < www.sleepapnea.org >.

Canadian Coordinating Office for Health Technology Assessment. < www.ccohta.ca/pubs/english/sleep/ treatmnt >.

National Sleep Foundation. 1522 K Street, NW, Suite 500, Washington, DC 20005. < www.sleepfoundation.org >.

OTHER

American Sleep Apnea Association (ASAA). *Considering Surgery for Snoring?* < http://www.sleepapnea.org/ snoring.html >.

National Heart, Lung, and Blood Institute (NHLBI). *Facts About Sleep Apnea*. NIH Publication No. 95-3798. < http://www.nhlbi.nih.gov/health/public/ sleep/sleepapn.htm >.

Richard Robinson
Rebecca J. Frey, PhD

Sleep disorders

Definition

Sleep disorders are a group of syndromes characterized by disturbance in the patient's amount of sleep, quality or timing of sleep, or in behaviors or physiological conditions associated with sleep. There are about 70 different sleep disorders. To qualify for the diagnosis of sleep disorder, the condition must be a persistent problem, cause the patient significant emotional distress, and interfere with his or her social or occupational functioning.

Although sleep is a basic behavior in animals as well as humans, researchers still do not completely understand all of its functions in maintaining health. In the past 30 years, however, laboratory studies on human volunteers have yielded new information about the different types of sleep. Researchers have learned about the cyclical patterns of different types of sleep and their relationships to breathing, heart rate, brain waves, and other physical functions. These measurements are obtained by a technique called **polysomnography**.

There are five stages of human sleep. Four stages have non-rapid eye movement (NREM) sleep, with unique brain wave patterns and physical changes occurring. Dreaming occurs in the fifth stage, during rapid eye movement (REM) sleep.

- Stage 1 NREM sleep. This stage occurs while a person is falling asleep. It represents about 5% of a normal adult's sleep time.

- Stage 2 NREM sleep. In this stage, (the beginning of "true" sleep), the person's electroencephalogram (EEG) will show distinctive wave forms called sleep spindles and K complexes. About 50% of sleep time is stage 2 REM sleep.

- Stages 3 and 4 NREM sleep. Also called delta or slow wave sleep, these are the deepest levels of human sleep and represent 10–20% of sleep time. They usually occur during the first 30–50% of the sleeping period.

- REM sleep. REM sleep accounts for 20-25% of total sleep time. It usually begins about 90 minutes after the person falls asleep, an important measure called REM latency. It alternates with NREM sleep about every hour and a half throughout the night. REM periods increase in length over the course of the night.

Sleep cycles vary with a person's age. Children and adolescents have longer periods of stage 3 and stage 4 NREM sleep than do middle aged or elderly adults. Because of this difference, the doctor will need to take a patient's age into account when evaluating a sleep disorder. Total REM sleep also declines with age.

The average length of nighttime sleep varies among people. Most people sleep between seven and nine hours a night. This population average appears to be constant throughout the world. In temperate climates, however, people often notice that sleep time varies with the seasons. It is not unusual for people in North America and Europe to sleep about 40 minutes longer per night during the winter.

Description

Sleep disorders are classified based on what causes them. Primary sleep disorders are distinguished from those that are not caused by other mental disorders,

prescription medications, **substance abuse**, or medical conditions. The two major categories of primary sleep disorders are the dyssomnias and the parasomnias.

Dyssomnias

Dyssomnias are primary sleep disorders in which the patient suffers from changes in the amount, restfulness, and timing of sleep. The most important dyssomnia is primary **insomnia**, which is defined as difficulty in falling asleep or remaining asleep that lasts for at least one month. It is estimated that 35% of adults in the United States experience insomnia during any given year, but the number of these adults who are experiencing true primary insomnia is unknown. Primary insomnia can be caused by a traumatic event related to sleep or bedtime, and it is often associated with increased physical or psychological arousal at night. People who experience primary insomnia are often anxious about not being able to sleep. The person may then associate all sleep-related things (their bed, bedtime, etc.) with frustration, making the problem worse. The person then becomes more stressed about not sleeping. Primary insomnia usually begins when the person is a young adult or in middle age.

Hypersomnia is a condition marked by excessive sleepiness during normal waking hours. The patient has either lengthy episodes of daytime sleep or episodes of daytime sleep on a daily basis even though he or she is sleeping normally at night. In some cases, patients with primary hypersomnia have difficulty waking in the morning and may appear confused or angry. This condition is sometimes called sleep drunkenness and is more common in males. The number of people with primary hypersomnia is unknown, although 5–10% of patients in sleep disorder clinics have the disorder. Primary hypersomnia usually affects young adults between the ages of 15 and 30.

Nocturnal myoclonus and **restless legs syndrome** (RLS) can cause either insomnia or hypersomnia in adults. Patients with nocturnal myoclonus wake up because of cramps or twitches in the calves. These patients feel sleepy the next day. Nocturnal myoclonus is sometimes called periodic limb movement disorder (PLMD). RLS patients have a crawly or aching feeling in their calves that can be relieved by moving or rubbing the legs. RLS often prevents the patient from falling asleep until the early hours of the morning, when the condition is less intense.

Kleine-Levin syndrome is a recurrent form of hypersomnia that affects a person three or four times a year. Doctors do not know the cause of this syndrome. It is marked by two to three days of sleeping 18–20 hours per day, hypersexual behavior, compulsive eating, and irritability. Men are three times more likely than women to have the syndrome. Currently, there is no cure for this disorder.

Narcolepsy is a dyssomnia characterized by recurrent "sleep attacks" that the patient cannot fight. The sleep attacks are about 10–20 minutes long. The patient feels refreshed by the sleep, but typically feels sleepy again several hours later. Narcolepsy has three major symptoms in addition to sleep attacks: cataplexy, **hallucinations**, and sleep **paralysis**. Cataplexy is the sudden loss of muscle tone and stability ("drop attacks"). Hallucinations may occur just before falling asleep (hypnagogic) or right after waking up (hypnopompic) and are associated with an episode of REM sleep. Sleep paralysis occurs during the transition from being asleep to waking up. About 40% of patients with narcolepsy have or have had another mental disorder. Although narcolepsy is often regarded as an adult disorder, it has been reported in children as young as three years old. Almost 18% of patients with narcolepsy are 10 years old or younger. It is estimated that 0.02–0.16% of the general population suffer from narcolepsy. Men and women are equally affected.

Breathing-related sleep disorders are syndromes in which the patient's sleep is interrupted by problems with his or her breathing. There are three types of breathing-related sleep disorders:

- Obstructive **sleep apnea** syndrome. This is the most common form of breathing-related sleep disorder, marked by episodes of blockage in the upper airway during sleep. It is found primarily in obese people. Patients with this disorder typically alternate between periods of **snoring** or gasping (when their airway is partly open) and periods of silence (when their airway is blocked). Very loud snoring is a clue to this disorder.

- Central sleep apnea syndrome. This disorder is primarily found in elderly patients with heart or neurological conditions that affect their ability to breathe properly. It is not associated with airway blockage and may be related to brain disease.

- Central alveolar hypoventilation syndrome. This disorder is found most often in extremely obese people. The patient's airway is not blocked, but his or her blood oxygen level is too low.

- Mixed-type sleep apnea syndrome. This disorder combines symptoms of both obstructive and central sleep apnea.

Circadian rhythm sleep disorders are dyssomnias resulting from a discrepancy between the person's daily sleep/wake patterns and demands of social activities, shift work, or travel. The term circadian comes from a Latin word meaning daily. There are three circadian rhythm sleep disorders. Delayed sleep phase type is characterized by going to bed and arising later than most people. **Jet lag** type is caused by travel to a new time zone. Shift work type is caused by the schedule of a person's job. People who are ordinarily early risers appear to be more vulnerable to jet lag and shift work-related circadian rhythm disorders than people who are "night owls." There are some patients who do not fit the pattern of these three disorders and appear to be the opposite of the delayed sleep phase type. These patients have an advanced sleep phase pattern and cannot stay awake in the evening, but wake up on their own in the early morning.

PARASOMNIAS. Parasomnias are primary sleep disorders in which the patient's behavior is affected by specific sleep stages or transitions between sleeping and waking. They are sometimes described as disorders of physiological arousal during sleep.

Nightmare disorder is a parasomnia in which the patient is repeatedly awakened from sleep by frightening dreams and is fully alert on awakening. The actual rate of occurrence of nightmare disorder is unknown. Approximately 10–50% of children between three and five years old have nightmares. They occur during REM sleep, usually in the second half of the night. The child is usually able to remember the content of the nightmare and may be afraid to go back to sleep. More females than males have this disorder, but it is not known whether the sex difference reflects a difference in occurrence or a difference in reporting. Nightmare disorder is most likely to occur in children or adults under severe or traumatic **stress**.

Sleep terror disorder is a parasomnia in which the patient awakens screaming or crying. The patient also has physical signs of arousal, like sweating, shaking, etc. It is sometimes referred to as pavor nocturnus. Unlike nightmares, sleep terrors typically occur in stage 3 or stage 4 NREM sleep during the first third of the night. The patient may be confused or disoriented for several minutes and cannot recall the content of the dream. He or she may fall asleep again and not remember the episode the next morning. Sleep terror disorder is most common in children four to 12 years old and is outgrown in adolescence. It affects about 3% of children. Fewer than 1% of adults have the disorder. In adults, it usually begins between the ages of 20 and 30. In children, more males than females have the disorder. In adults, men and women are equally affected.

Sleepwalking disorder, which is sometimes called somnambulism, occurs when the patient is capable of complex movements during sleep, including walking. Like sleep terror disorder, sleepwalking occurs during stage 3 and stage 4 NREM sleep during the first part of the night. If the patient is awakened during a sleepwalking episode, he or she may be disoriented and have no memory of the behavior. In addition to walking around, patients with sleepwalking disorder have been reported to eat, use the bathroom, unlock doors, or talk to others. It is estimated that 10–30% of children have at least one episode of sleepwalking. However, only 1–5% meet the criteria for sleepwalking disorder. The disorder is most common in children eight to 12 years old. It is unusual for sleepwalking to occur for the first time in adults.

Unlike sleepwalking, REM sleep behavior disorder occurs later in the night and the patient can remember what they were dreaming. The physical activities of the patient are often violent.

Sleep disorders related to other conditions

In addition to the primary sleep disorders, there are three categories of sleep disorders that are caused by or related to substance use or other physical or mental disorders.

SLEEP DISORDERS RELATED TO MENTAL DISORDERS. Many mental disorders, especially depression or one of the **anxiety disorders**, can cause sleep disturbances. Psychiatric disorders are the most common cause of chronic insomnia.

SLEEP DISORDERS DUE TO MEDICAL CONDITIONS. Some patients with chronic neurological conditions like Parkinson's disease or Huntington's disease may develop sleep disorders. Sleep disorders have also been associated with viral **encephalitis**, brain disease, and hypo- or **hyperthyroidism**.

SUBSTANCE-INDUCED SLEEP DISORDERS. The use of drugs, alcohol, and **caffeine** frequently produces disturbances in sleep patterns. Alcohol **abuse** is associated with insomnia. The person may initially feel sleepy after drinking, but wakes up or sleeps fitfully during the second half of the night. Alcohol can also increase the severity of breathing-related sleep disorders. With amphetamines or **cocaine**, the patient typically suffers from insomnia during drug use and hypersomnia during drug withdrawal. Opioids usually make short-term users sleepy. However, long-term users develop tolerance and may suffer from insomnia.

In addition to alcohol and drugs that are abused, a variety of prescription medications can affect sleep patterns. These medications include **antihistamines**, **corticosteroids**, **asthma** medicines, and drugs that affect the central nervous system.

Sleep disorders in children and adolescents

Pediatricians estimate that 20–30% of children have difficulties with sleep that are serious enough to disturb their families. Although sleepwalking and night terror disorder occur more frequently in children than in adults, children can also suffer from narcolepsy and sleep apnea syndrome.

Causes and symptoms

The causes of sleep disorders have already been discussed with respect to the classification of these disorders.

The most important symptoms of sleep disorders are insomnia and sleepiness during waking hours. Insomnia is by far the more common of the two symptoms. It covers a number of different patterns of sleep disturbance. These patterns include inability to fall asleep at bedtime, repeated awakening during the night, and/or inability to go back to sleep once awakened.

Diagnosis

Diagnosis of sleep disorders usually requires a psychological history as well as a medical history. With the exception of sleep apnea syndromes, physical examinations are not usually revealing. The patient's sex and age are useful starting points in assessing the problem. The doctor may also talk to other family members in order to obtain information about the patient's symptoms. The family's observations are particularly important to evaluate sleepwalking, kicking in bed, snoring loudly, or other behaviors that the patient cannot remember.

Sleep logs

Many doctors ask patients to keep a sleep diary or sleep log for a minimum of one to two weeks in order to evaluate the severity and characteristics of the sleep disturbance. The patient records medications taken as well as the length of time spent in bed, the quality of the sleep, and similar information. Some sleep logs are designed to indicate circadian sleep patterns as well as simple duration or restfulness of sleep.

Psychological testing

The doctor may use **psychological tests** or inventories to evaluate insomnia because it is frequently

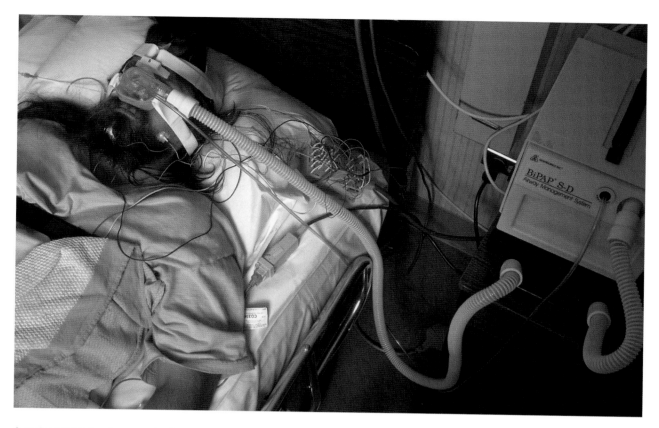

A patient suffering from acute sleep apnea is hooked up to monitors in preparation for a night's sleep at a Stanford University sleep lab. (Photograph by Russell D. Curtis, Photo Researchers, Inc. Reproduced by permission.)

associated with mood or affective disorders. The **Minnesota Multiphasic Personality Inventory** (MMPI), the Millon Clinical Multiaxial Inventory (MCMI), the Beck Depression Inventory, and the Zung Depression Scale are the tests most commonly used in evaluating this symptom.

SELF-REPORT TESTS. The Epworth Sleepiness Scale, a self-rating form recently developed in Australia, consists of eight questions used to assess daytime sleepiness. Scores range from 0–24, with scores higher than 16 indicating severe daytime sleepiness.

Laboratory studies

If the doctor is considering breathing-related sleep disorders, myoclonus, or narcolepsy as possible diagnoses, he or she may ask the patient to be tested in a sleep laboratory or at home with portable instruments.

POLYSOMNOGRAPHY. Polysomnography can be used to help diagnose sleep disorders as well as conduct research into sleep. In some cases the patient is tested in a special sleep laboratory. The advantage of this testing is the availability and expertise of trained technologists, but it is expensive. As of 2001, however, portable equipment is available for home recording of certain specific physiological functions.

MULTIPLE SLEEP LATENCY TEST (MSLT). The multiple sleep latency test (MSLT) is frequently used to measure the severity of the patient's daytime sleepiness. The test measures sleep latency (the speed with which the patient falls asleep) during a series of planned naps during the day. The test also measures the amount of REM sleep that occurs. Two or more episodes of REM sleep under these conditions indicates narcolepsy. This test can also be used to help diagnose primary hypersomnia.

REPEATED TEST OF SUSTAINED WAKEFULNESS (RTSW). The repeated test of sustained wakefulness (RTSW) is a test that measures sleep latency by challenging the patient's ability to stay awake. In the RTSW, the patient is placed in a quiet room with dim lighting and is asked to stay awake. As with the MSLT, the testing pattern is repeated at intervals during the day.

Treatment

Treatment for a sleep disorder depends on what is causing the disorder. For example, if major depression is the cause of insomnia, then treatment of the depression with antidepressants should resolve the insomnia.

Medications

Sedative or hypnotic medications are generally recommended only for insomnia related to a temporary stress (like surgery or grief) because of the potential for **addiction** or overdose. Trazodone, a sedating antidepressant, is often used for chronic insomnia that does not respond to other treatments. Sleep medications may also cause problems for elderly patients because of possible interactions with their other prescription medications. Among the safer hypnotic agents are lorazepam, temazepam, and zolpidem. Chloral hydrate is often preferred for short-term treatment in elderly patients because of its mildness. Short-term treatment is recommended because this drug may be habit forming.

Narcolepsy is treated with stimulants such as dextroamphetamine sulfate or methylphenidate. Nocturnal myoclonus has been successfully treated with clonazepam.

Children with sleep terror disorder or sleepwalking are usually treated with **benzodiazepines** because this type of medication suppresses stage 3 and stage 4 NREM sleep.

Psychotherapy

Psychotherapy is recommended for patients with sleep disorders associated with other mental disorders. In many cases the patient's scores on the Beck or Zung inventories will suggest the appropriate direction of treatment.

Sleep education

"Sleep hygiene" or sleep education for sleep disorders often includes instructing the patient in methods to enhance sleep. Patients are advised to:

- wait until he or she is sleepy before going to bed
- avoid using the bedroom for work, reading, or watching television
- get up at the same time every morning no matter how much or how little he or she slept
- avoid **smoking** and avoid drinking liquids with caffeine

- get some physical **exercise** early in the day every day
- limit fluid intake after dinner; in particular, avoid alcohol because it frequently causes interrupted sleep
- learn to meditate or practice relaxation techniques
- avoid tossing and turning in bed; instead, he or she should get up and listen to relaxing music or read

Lifestyle changes

Patients with sleep apnea or hypopnea are encouraged to stop smoking, avoid alcohol or drugs of abuse, and lose weight in order to improve the stability of the upper airway.

In some cases, patients with sleep disorders related to jet lag or shift work may need to change employment or travel patterns. Patients may need to avoid rapid changes in shifts at work.

Children with nightmare disorder may benefit from limits on television or movies. Violent scenes or frightening science fiction stories appear to influence the frequency and intensity of children's nightmares.

Surgery

Although making a surgical opening into the windpipe (a tracheostomy) for sleep apnea or hypopnea in adults is a treatment of last resort, it is occasionally performed if the patient's disorder is life threatening and cannot be treated by other methods. In children and adolescents, surgical removal of the tonsils and adenoids is a fairly common and successful treatment for sleep apnea. Most sleep apnea patients are treated with continuous positive airway pressure (CPAP). Sometimes an oral prosthesis is used for mild sleep apnea.

Alternative treatment

Some alternative approaches may be effective in treating insomnia caused by **anxiety** or emotional stress. **Meditation** practice, breathing exercises, and **yoga** can break the vicious cycle of sleeplessness, worry about inability to sleep, and further sleeplessness for some people. Yoga can help some people to relax muscular tension in a direct fashion. The breathing exercises and meditation can keep some patients from obsessing about sleep.

Homeopathic practitioners recommend that people with chronic insomnia see a professional homeopath. They do, however, prescribe specific remedies for at-home treatment of temporary insomnia: *Nux vomica* for alcohol or substance-related insomnia, *Ignatia* for insomnia caused by

KEY TERMS

Apnea—The temporary absence of breathing. Sleep apnea consists of repeated episodes of temporary suspension of breathing during sleep.

Cataplexy—Sudden loss of muscle tone (often causing a person to fall), usually triggered by intense emotion. It is regarded as a diagnostic sign of narcolepsy.

Circadian rhythm—Any body rhythm that recurs in 24-hour cycles. The sleep-wake cycle is an example of a circadian rhythm.

Dyssomnia—A primary sleep disorder in which the patient suffers from changes in the quantity, quality, or timing of sleep.

Electroencephalogram (EEG)—The record obtained by a device that measures electrical impulses in the brain.

Hypersomnia—An abnormal increase of 25% or more in time spent sleeping. Patients usually have excessive daytime sleepiness.

Hypnotic—A medication that makes a person sleep.

Hypopnea—Shallow or excessively slow breathing usually caused by partial closure of the upper airway during sleep, leading to disruption of sleep.

Insomnia—Difficulty in falling asleep or remaining asleep.

Jet lag—A temporary disruption of the body's sleep-wake rhythm following high-speed air travel across several time zones. Jet lag is most severe in people who have crossed eight or more time zones in 24 hours.

Kleine-Levin syndrome—A disorder that occurs primarily in young males, three or four times a year. The syndrome is marked by episodes of hypersomnia, hypersexual behavior, and excessive eating.

Narcolepsy—A life-long sleep disorder marked by four symptoms: sudden brief sleep attacks, cataplexy, temporary paralysis, and hallucinations. The hallucinations are associated with falling asleep or the transition from sleeping to waking.

Nocturnal myoclonus—A disorder in which the patient is awakened repeatedly during the night by cramps or twitches in the calf muscles. Nocturnal myoclonus is sometimes called periodic limb movement disorder (PLMD).

Non-rapid eye movement (NREM) sleep—A type of sleep that differs from rapid eye movement (REM) sleep. The four stages of NREM sleep account for 75–80% of total sleeping time.

Parasomnia—A primary sleep disorder in which the person's physiology or behaviors are affected by sleep, the sleep stage, or the transition from sleeping to waking.

Pavor nocturnus—Another term for sleep terror disorder.

Polysomnography—Laboratory measurement of a patient's basic physiological processes during sleep. Polysomnography usually measures eye movement, brain waves, and muscular tension.

Primary sleep disorder—A sleep disorder that cannot be attributed to a medical condition, another mental disorder, or prescription medications or other substances.

Rapid eye movement (REM) sleep—A phase of sleep during which the person's eyes move rapidly beneath the lids. It accounts for 20–25% of sleep time. Dreaming occurs during REM sleep.

REM latency—After a person falls asleep, the amount of time it takes for the first onset of REM sleep.

Restless legs syndrome (RLS)—A disorder in which the patient experiences crawling, aching, or other disagreeable sensations in the calves that can be relieved by movement. RLS is a frequent cause of difficulty falling asleep at night.

Sedative—A medication given to calm agitated patients; sometimes used as a synonym for hypnotic.

Sleep latency—The amount of time that it takes to fall asleep. Sleep latency is measured in minutes and is important in diagnosing depression.

Somnambulism—Another term for sleepwalking.

grief, *Arsenicum* for insomnia caused by fear or anxiety, and *Passiflora* for insomnia related to mental stress.

Melatonin has also been used as an alternative treatment for sleep disorders. Melatonin is produced in the body by the pineal gland at the base of the brain. This substance is thought to be related to the body's circadian rhythms.

Practitioners of Chinese medicine usually treat insomnia as a symptom of excess yang energy. Cinnabar is recommended for chronic nightmares. Either magnetic magnetite or "dragon bones" is recommended for insomnia associated with **hysteria** or fear. If the insomnia appears to be associated with excess yang energy arising from the liver, the practitioner will give the patient oyster shells. **Acupuncture** treatments can help bring about balance and facilitate sleep.

Dietary changes like eliminating stimulant foods (coffee, cola, chocolate) and late-night meals or snacks can be effective in treating some sleep disorders. Nutritional supplementation with magnesium, as well as botanical medicines that calm the nervous system, can also be helpful. Among the botanical remedies that may be effective for sleep disorders are valerian (*Valeriana officinalis*), passionflower (*Passiflora incarnata*), and skullcap (*Scutellaria lateriflora*).

Prognosis

The prognosis depends on the specific disorder. Children usually outgrow sleep disorders. Patients with Kleine-Levin syndrome usually get better around age 40. Narcolepsy is a life-long disorder. The prognosis for sleep disorders related to other conditions depends on successful treatment of the substance abuse, medical condition, or other mental disorder. The prognosis for primary sleep disorders is affected by many things, including the patient's age, sex, occupation, personality characteristics, family circumstances, neighborhood environment, and similar factors.

Resources

BOOKS

Moe, Paul G., and Alan R. Seay. "Neurologic & Muscular Disorders: Sleep Disorders." In *Current Pediatric Diagnosis & Treatment*, edited by William W. Hay Jr., et al. Stamford: Appleton & Lange, 1997.

Rebecca J. Frey, PhD

Sleep study *see* **Polysomnography**

Sleeping drugs *see* **Anti-insomnia drugs**

Sleeping sickness

Definition

Sleeping sickness (also called trypanosomiasis) is an infection caused by *Trypanosoma* protozoa; it is passed to humans through the bite of the tsetse fly. If left untreated, the infection progresses to **death** within months or years.

DAVID BRUCE (1855–1931)

David Bruce was born in Melbourne, Australia, on May 29,1855, to Scottish immigrants. Bruce's family moved back to Scotland when he was five years old. Bruce attended the University of Edinburgh where he studied natural history and medicine. Following his graduation, he accepted a position working with a doctor. In 1883, Bruce married Mary Elizabeth Steele who would help him with his work throughout his life.

In 1884, Bruce began to study the disease "Malta, Mediterranean" when he and Mary were stationed in Malta with the Army Medical Service. Using a microscope, Bruce discovered that the disease was caused by a "microccus" that grew in the individual's spleen. The organism responsible for this disease was ultimately isolated by Bernhard L. F. Bang. In 1905, Bruce led a scientific team that discovered that the soldiers who contracted the disease had ingested the milk of infected goats. The disease disappeared when the soldiers quit drinking goat's milk. Many physicians began calling the disease "brucellosis" in honor of Bruce's discoveries. Bruce also conducted research in Africa where he found that the tsetse fly could infect humans, as well as animals, with the "nagana" disease. Ultimately, his work would prove that sleeping sickness was caused by the tsetse fly.

In 1903, Bruce became the director of the Royal Society's Sleeping Sickness Commission and, in 1908, he was knighted. He served as commandant of the Royal Army Medical College after he and his wife returned to England. Bruce died on November 20, 1931.

Description

Protozoa are single-celled organisms considered to be the simplest life form in the animal kingdom. The protozoa responsible for sleeping sickness are a variety that bear numerous flagella (hair-like projections from the cell that help the cell to move). These protozoa exist only on the continent of Africa. The type of protozoa causing sleeping sickness in humans is referred to as the *Trypanasoma brucei* complex, which can be divided further into Rhodesian (Central and East African) and Gambian (Central and West African) subspecies.

The Rhodesian variety live within antelopes in savanna and woodland areas, and they cause no problems with the antelope's health. The protozoa are then acquired by tsetse flies when they bite and suck the blood of an infected antelope or cow.

Within the tsetse fly, the protozoa cycle through several different life forms; ultimately they migrate to the salivary glands of the tsetse fly. Once the protozoa are harbored in the salivary glands, they are ready to be deposited into the bloodstream of the fly's next source of a blood meal.

Humans most likely to become infected by Rhodesian trypanosomes are people such as game wardens and visitors to game parks in East Africa, who may be bitten by a tsetse fly that has fed on game (antelope) carrying the protozoa. The Rhodesian variety of sleeping sickness causes a much more severe illness, with even greater likelihood of eventual death than the Gambian form.

The Gambian variety of *Trypanosoma* thrives in tropical rain forests throughout Central and West Africa; it does not infect game or cattle, and is primarily a threat to people dwelling in such areas, rarely infecting visitors.

Causes and symptoms

The first sign of infection with the trypanosome may be a sore appearing at the site of the tsetse fly bite about two to tree days after having been bitten. Redness, **pain**, and swelling occur, but are often ignored by the patient.

Stage I illness

Two to three weeks later, Stage I disease develops as a result of the protozoa being carried through the blood and lymph circulation of the host. This systemic (meaning that symptoms affect the whole body) phase of the illness is characterized by a **fever** that rises quite high, then falls to normal, then respikes (rises rapidly). A rash with intense **itching** may be present, and **headache** and mental confusion may occur. The Gambian form, in particular, includes extreme swelling of lymph tissue, with enlargement of both the spleen and liver, and greatly swollen lymph nodes. "Winterbottom's sign" is classic of Gambian sleeping sickness, and consists of a visibly swollen area of lymph nodes located behind the ear and just above the base of the neck. During this stage, the heart may be affected by a severe inflammatory reaction, particularly when the infection is caused by the Rhodesian variety of trypanosomiasis.

Many of the symptoms of sleeping sickness are actually the result of attempts by the patient's immune system to get rid of the invading organism. The heightened activity of the cells of the immune system result in damage to the patient's own organs, anemia, and leaky blood vessels. These leaks in the blood vessels end up helping to further spread the protozoa throughout the afflicted person's body.

One reason for the intense reaction of the immune system to the presence of the trypanosomes is also the reason why the trypanosomes survive so well despite the efforts of the immune system to eradicate them. The protozoa causing sleeping sickness are able to rapidly change specific markers (unique proteins) on their outer coats. These kinds of markers usually serve to stimulate the host's immune system to produce immune cells that will specifically target the marker, allowing quick destruction of those cells bearing the markers. Trypanosomes, however, are able to express new markers at such a high rate of change that the host's immune system is constantly trying to catch up.

Stage II illness

Stage II sleeping sickness involves the nervous system. Gambian sleeping sickness, in particular, has a clearly delineated phase in which the predominant symptoms involve the brain. The patient's speech becomes slurred, mental processes slow, and the patient sits and stares for long periods of time, or sleeps. Other symptoms resemble Parkinson's disease, including imbalance when walking, slow and shuffling gait, trembling of the limbs, involuntary movements, muscle tightness, and increasing mental confusion. Untreated, these symptoms eventually lead to **coma** and then to death.

Diagnosis

Diagnosis of sleeping sickness can be made by microscopic examination of fluid from the original sore at the site of the tsetse fly bite. Trypanosomes will be present in the fluid for a short period of time following the bite. If the sore has already resolved, fluid can be obtained from swollen lymph nodes for examination. Other methods of trypanosome diagnosis involve culturing blood, lymph node fluid, bone marrow, or spinal fluid. These cultures are then injected into rats, which develop blood-borne protozoa infection that can be detected in blood smears within one to two weeks. However, this last method is effective only for the Rhodesian variety of sleeping sickness.

Treatment

Without treatment, sleeping sickness will lead to death. Unfortunately, however, those medications effective against the *Trypanosoma brucei* complex protozoa all have significant potential side effects for the patient. Suramin, eflornithine, pentamidine, and several drugs that contain arsenic (a chemical which in higher doses is highly poisonous to humans), are all effective anti-trypanosomal agents. Each of these drugs, however, requires careful monitoring to ensure that the drugs themselves do not cause serious complications such as fatal hypersensitivity (allergic) reaction, kidney or liver damage, or inflammation of the brain.

Prevention

Prevention of sleeping sickness requires avoiding contact with the tsetse fly. Insect repellents and clothing that covers the limbs to the wrists and ankles are advisable. Public health measures have included drug treatment of humans who are infected with one of the *Trypanosoma brucei* complex. There are currently no immunizations available to prevent the acquisition of sleeping sickness.

Resources

ORGANIZATIONS

Centers for Disease Control and Prevention. 1600 Clifton Rd., NE, Atlanta, GA 30333. (800) 311-3435, (404) 639-3311. < http://www.cdc.gov >.

Rosalyn Carson-DeWitt, MD

Sleepwalking *see* **Sleep disorders**

Slipped disk *see* **Herniated disk**

Slit lamp examination *see* **Eye examination**

Small-for-gestational-age infant *see* **Intrauterine growth retardation**

Small bowel follow-through (SBFT) *see* **Upper GI exam**

Small cell lung cancer *see* **Lung cancer, small cell**

Small intestine biopsy

Definition

A biopsy is a diagnostic procedure in which tissue or cells are removed from a part of the body and specially prepared for examination under a microscope. When the tissue involved is part of the small intestine, the procedure is called a small-intestine (or small-bowel) biopsy.

Purpose

The small-bowel biopsy is used to diagnose and confirm disease of the intestinal mucosa (the lining of the small intestine). The test is most commonly done to test for tumors of the small bowel or malabsorption syndromes.

Precautions

Due to the slight risk of bleeding during or after this procedure, **aspirin**, aspirin-containing medications, **nonsteroidal anti-inflammatory drugs**, and anticoagulants and **antiplatelet drugs** should be withheld for at least five days before the test.

Description

The small intestine is approximately 21 ft (6.4m). It has three sections: the duodenum (a short, curved segment fixed to the back wall of the abdomen), the jejunum, and the ileum (two larger, coiled, and mobile segments). Some digestion occurs in the stomach, but the small intestine is mainly responsible for digestion and absorption of foods.

Malabsorption syndromes occur when certain conditions result in impaired absorption of nutrients, **vitamins**, or **minerals** from the diet by the lining of the small intestine. For example, injury to the intestinal lining can interfere with absorption, as can infections, intestinal parasites, some drugs, blockage of the lymphatic vessels, poor blood supply to the intestine, or diseases like sprue.

Malabsorption is suspected when a patient not only loses weight, but has **diarrhea** and nutritional deficiencies despite eating well (weight loss alone can have other causes). Laboratory tests like fecal fat, a measurement of fat in stool samples collected over 72 hours, are the most reliable tests for diagnosing fat malabsorption, but abnormalities of the small intestine itself are diagnosed by small-intestine biopsy.

Several different methods are used to detect abnormalities of the small intestine. A tissue specimen can be obtained by using an endoscope (a flexible viewing tube), or by using a thin tube with a small cutting instrument at the end. This latter procedure is ordered when specimens larger than those provided by endoscopic biopsy are needed, because it allows removal of tissue from areas beyond the reach of an endoscope.

Several similar types of capsules are used for tissue collection. In each, a mercury-weighted bag is attached to one end of the capsule, while a thin polyethylene tube about 5 ft (1.5m) long is attached to the other end. Once the bag, capsule, and tube are in place in the small bowel, suction on the tube draws the tissue into the capsule and closes it, cutting off the piece of tissue within. This is an invasive procedure, but it causes little **pain** and complications are rare.

A newer method of obtaining diagnostic information about the small intestine was approved by the Food and Drug Administration (FDA) in 2001. Known as the M2A Imaging System, the device was developed by a company in Atlanta, Georgia. The M2A system consists of an imaging capsule, a portable belt-pack image receiver and recorder, and a specially modified computer. The patient swallows the capsule, which is the size of a large pill. A miniature lens in the capsule transmits images through an antenna/transmitter to the belt-pack receiver, which the patient wears under ordinary clothing as he or she goes about daily activities. The belt-pack recording device is returned after seven or eight hours to the doctor, who then examines the images recorded as a digital video. The capsule itself is simply allowed to pass through the digestive tract.

Preparation requires only **fasting** the night before the M2A examination and taking nothing but clear liquids for two hours after swallowing the capsule. After four hours the patient can eat food without interfering with the test. As of the early 2000s, the M2A system is used to evaluate gastrointestinal bleeding from unknown causes, inflammatory bowel disease, some malabsorption syndromes, and to monitor surgical patients following small-bowel transplantation. The system has shown good results in detecting **Crohn's disease** undiagnosed by conventional methods.

Small-intestine biopsy procedure

After application of a topical anesthetic to the back of the patient's throat, the capsule and the tube are introduced, and the patient is asked to swallow as the tube is advanced. The patient is then placed on the right side and the instrument tip is advanced another 20 in (51cm) or so. The tube's position is checked by fluoroscopy or by instilling air through the tube and listening with a stethoscope for air to enter the stomach.

The tube is advanced 2–4 in (5.1–10 cm)at a time to pass the capsule through the stomach outlet (pylorus). When fluoroscopy confirms that the capsule has passed the pylorus, small samples of small intestine tissue are obtained by the instrument's cutting edge, after which the instrument and tube are withdrawn. The entire procedure may be completed in minutes.

Preparation

This procedure requires tissue specimens from the small intestine through means of a tube inserted into the stomach through the mouth. The patient is to withhold food and fluids for at least eight hours before the test.

Aftercare

The patient should not have anything to eat or drink until the topical anesthetic wears off (usually about one to two hours). If intravenous sedatives were administered during the procedure, the patient should not drive for the remainder of the day. Complications from this procedure are uncommon, but can occur. The patient is to note any abdominal pain or bleeding and report either immediately to the doctor.

Risks

Complications from this procedure are rare, but can include bleeding (hemorrhage), bacterial infection with **fever** and pain, and bowel puncture (perforation). The patient should immediately report any abdominal pain or bleeding to the physician in charge. Biopsy is contraindicated in uncooperative patients, those taking aspirin or anticoagulants, and in those with uncontrolled bleeding disorders.

Normal results

Normal results are no abnormalities seen on gross examination of the specimen(s) or under the microscope after tissue preparation.

Abnormal results

Small-intestine tissue exhibiting abnormalities may indicate Whipple's disease, a malabsorption disease; lymphoma, a group of cancers; and parasitic infections like **giardiasis**, strongyloidiasis, and coccidiosis. When biopsy indicates celiac sprue (a malabsorption disorder), infectious **gastroenteritis**

KEY TERMS

Sprue—A disorder of impaired absorption of nutrients from the diet by the small intestine (malabsorption), resulting in malnutrition. Two forms of sprue exist: tropical sprue, which occurs mainly in tropical regions; and celiac sprue, which occurs more widely and is due to sensitivity to the wheat protein gluten.

Whipple's disease—A disorder of impaired absorption of nutrients by the small intestine. Symptoms include diarrhea, abdominal pain, progressive weight loss, joint pain, swollen lymph nodes, abnormal skin pigmentation, anemia, and fever. The precise cause is unknown, but it is probably due to an unidentified bacterial infection.

Wireless capsule endoscopy—A newer method of examining the small bowel by means of a capsule swallowed by the patient. The capsule contains a miniaturized lens and an antenna that transmits information to a belt-pack recorder worn by the patient during the day.

(inflammation of the gastrointestinal tract), folate and B_{12} deficiency, or **malnutrition**, confirmation studies are needed for conclusive diagnosis.

Resources

BOOKS

Beers, Mark H., MD, and Robert Berkow, MD., editors. "Malabsorption Syndromes." Section 3, Chapter 30 In *The Merck Manual of Diagnosis and Therapy.* Whitehouse Station, NJ: Merck Research Laboratories, 2004.

Beers, Mark H., MD, and Robert Berkow, MD., editors. "Small-Bowel Tumors." Section 3, Chapter 34 In *The Merck Manual of Diagnosis and Therapy*. Whitehouse Station, NJ: Merck Research Laboratories, 2004.

PERIODICALS

Adler, Douglas J., MD, and Christopher J. Gostout, MD. "Wireless Capsule Endoscopy." *Hospital Physician* May 2003: 17–22.

Ge, Z. Z., Y. B. Hu, and S. D. Xiao. "Capsule Endoscopy in Diagnosis of Small Bowel Crohn's Disease." *World Journal of Gastroenterology* 10 (May 1, 2004): 1349–1352.

Thompson, B. F., L. C. Fry, C. D. Wells, et al. "The Spectrum of GI Strongyloidiasis: An Endoscopic-Pathologic Study." *Gastrointestinal Endoscopy* 59 (June 2004): 906–910.

Janis O. Flores
Rebecca J. Frey, PhD

Smallpox

Definition

Smallpox is an infection caused by the variola virus, a member of the poxvirus family. Throughout history, smallpox has been a greatly feared disease because it was responsible for huge epidemics worldwide that resulted in large numbers of deaths. In 1980, the World Health Organization (WHO) announced that an extensive program of **vaccination** against the disease had resulted in the complete eradication of the virus, with the exception of samples of stored virus in two laboratories.

Description

Smallpox is strictly an infection of human beings. Animals and insects can neither be infected by smallpox, nor carry the virus in any form. Most infections are caused by contact with a person who has already developed the characteristic **skin lesions** (pox) of the disease, although a person who has a less severe infection (not symptomatic or diagnosable in the usual way) can unwittingly spread the virus.

Causes and symptoms

Smallpox is a relatively contagious disease, which accounts for its ability to cause massive epidemics. The variola virus is acquired from direct contact with individuals infected with the disease, from contaminated air droplets, and even from objects used by another smallpox victim (books, blankets, utensils, etc.). The respiratory tract is the usual entry point for the variola virus into a human being.

After the virus enters the body, there is a 12–14 day incubation period during which the virus multiplies, although no symptoms are recognizable. After the incubation period, symptoms appear abruptly and include **fever**, chills, and muscle aches. Two to three days later, a bumpy rash begins appearing first on the face and forearms. The rash progresses, ultimately reaching the chest, abdomen, and back. Seven to ten days after the rash appears, the patient is most infectious. The individual bumps (papules) fill with clear fluid and eventually become pus-filled over the course of 10–12 days. These pox eventually scab over, each leaving a permanently scarred pock or pit when the scab drops off.

Initially, the smallpox symptoms and rash appear similar to **chickenpox**. However, unlike chickenpox, smallpox lesions develop at the same rate so that they are all visible in the same stage. Another major difference is that smallpox occurs primarily on the face and entremities, whereas chickenpox tends to be concentrate on the face and trunk area.

Complications such as bacterial infection of the open skin lesions, **pneumonia**, or bone infections are the major causes of **death** from smallpox. A very severe and quickly fatal form called "sledgehammer smallpox," occurs in 5-10% of patients and results in massive, uncontrollable bleeding (hemorrhage) from the skin lesions, as well as from the mouth, nose, and other areas of the body. This form is very infectious and usually fatal five to seven days after onset.

Fear of smallpox comes from both the epidemic nature of the disease, as well as from the fact that no therapies have ever been discovered to either treat the symptoms of smallpox, or shorten the course of the disease.

Diagnosis

In modern times, a diagnosis of smallpox is made using an electron microscope to identify virus in fluid from the papules, urine, or in the patient's blood prior to the appearance of the papular rash.

Treatment

No treatments have been developed to halt the progression of the disease. Treatment for smallpox is only supportive, meaning that it is aimed at keeping a patient as comfortable as possible. **Antibiotics** are sometimes administered to prevent secondary bacterial infections.

Prognosis

Approximately one in three patients die from smallpox, with the more severe, hemorrhagic form nearly 100% fatal. Patients who survive smallpox infection nearly always have multiple areas of scarring where each pock has been.

Prevention

From about the tenth century in China, India, and the Americas, it is noted that individuals who had even a mild case of smallpox could not be infected again. Fascinating accounts appear in writings from all over the world of ways in which people tried to prevent smallpox. Material from people mildly ill with smallpox (fluid or pus from the papules, scabs over the pox) was scratched into the skin of people who had never had the illness, in an attempt to produce a mild

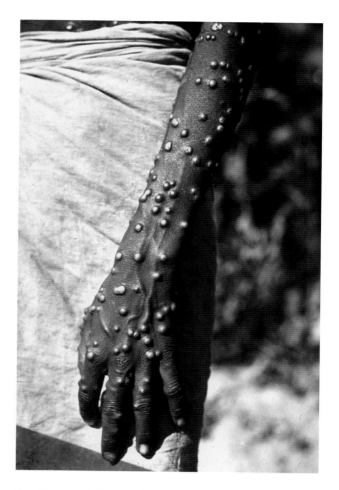

Smallpox pustules on the arm of an Asian Indian man. *(Photograph by C. James Webb, Phototake NYC. Reproduced by permission.)*

reaction and its accompanying protective effect. These efforts often resulted in full-fledged smallpox, and probably served only to help effectively spread the infection throughout a community. In fact, such crude smallpox "vaccinations" were against the law in Colonial America.

In 1798, Edward Jenner published a paper in which he discussed his important observation that milkmaids who contracted a mild infection of the hands (called cowpox, and caused by a relative of the variola virus) appeared to be immune to smallpox. Jenner created an immunization against smallpox using the pus found in the lesions of cowpox infection. Jenner's paper led to much work in the area of vaccinations, and ultimately resulted in the creation of a very effective vaccination against smallpox that utilized the vaccinia virus, another close relative of variola. Indeed, the term vaccination is derived from *vacce*, Latin for cow and related to the cowpox link. Later, the term was applied to other vaccinations.

In 1967, WHO began its attempt to eradicate the smallpox virus worldwide. The methods used in the program were simple:

- Careful surveillance for all smallpox infections worldwide, to allow for quick diagnosis and immediate quarantine of patients.

- Immediate vaccination of all contacts diagnosed with infection, in order to interrupt the virus' usual pattern of infection.

The WHO's program was extremely successful, and the virus was declared eradicated worldwide in May 1980.

Future concerns

Today, two laboratories (the Centers for Disease Control and Prevention in Atlanta, Georgia, and the Russian State Centre for Research on Virology and Biotechnology in Koltsovo, Novosibirsk Region) officially retain samples of the smallpox virus. These samples, as well as stockpiles of the smallpox vaccine, are stored because some level of concern exists that another poxvirus could undergo genetic changes (mutate) and cause human infection. There is also the remote chance that smallpox virus could somehow escape from the laboratories where it is stored. For these reasons, surveillance continues of various animal groups that continue to be infected with viruses related to the variola virus, and large quantities of vaccine are stored in different countries around the world, so that response to any future threat by the smallpox virus could be prompt.

Of greatest concern is the potential use of smallpox as a biological weapon. Since 1980, when the WHO announced smallpox had been eradicated, essentially no one has been vaccinated against the disease. Those individuals vaccinated prior to 1980 are believed to be susceptible as well because immunity only lasts 15-20 years. These circumstances coupled with the nature of smallpox to spread quickly from person to person could lead to devastating consequences.

The United States and Russia are the only two countries to officially house remaining samples of the virus. However, it is believed that other countries, such as Iraq, may have obtained samples of the smallpox virus during the Cold War through their association with Russia. It is also possible that scientists with access to the virus may have sold their services and knowledge to other governments.

On June 22-23, 2001, four U.S. organizations (CSIS—Center for Strategic and International Studies, Johns Hopkins Center for Civilian Biodefense Studies, ANSER—Analytic Services Inc., and MIPT—Memorial Institute for the Prevention of Terrorism) presented a fictitious scenario of the United States' response to a deliberate introduction of smallpox titled *Dark Winter*. This **exercise** demonstrated that if such an event were to occur, the United States would be ill prepared on several fronts. The primary concern is an inadequate supply of vaccine, which is essential to preventing disease development in exposed persons. Between 1997 and 2001, two companies were contracted to produce additional smallpox vaccines for both military and civilian use. Through these contracts, an additional 40 million doses would be made available for civilian use by 2005. In the meantime, studies are underway to determine if the existing vaccines can be diluted in order to increase the number of doses available for immediate use. Results from a very small group of volunteers tested in 2000 found that at one-tenth strength, the existing smallpox vaccines are approximately 70% effective. In late 2001, a new study began evaluating the effectiveness of the vaccine at one-fifth strength.

In the event that smallpox is reintroduced into the current population, it will be imperative that doctors immediately recognize the symptoms and isolate the individual to prevent further spread of the disease. Prompt vaccination of any persons who had contact with the patient is also necessary to prevent additional cases of smallpox from developing. Controlling and containing spread of this disease is critical for prevention of a world-wide epidemic that would have a devastating impact on current populations.

Resources

PERIODICALS

Broad, William J. "U.S. Acts to Make Vaccines and Drugs Against Smallpox." *The New York Times* October 9, 2001: D1-2.

Miller, Judith, and Sheryl Gay Stolberg. "Sept. 11 Attaks Led to Push for More Smallpox Vaccine." *The New York Times* October 22, 2001: A1.

OTHER

Hamre, John, Randy Larsen, Mark DeMier, General Dennis Reimer, and Tara O'Toole. "Dark Winter." ANSER Analytic Services Inc. [cited October 25, 2001]. < http://www.aha.org/Emergency/Readiness/FieldLessons.asp >.

Henderson, D. A. "Smallpox: Clinical and Epidemiologic Features." In: *Emerging Infectious Diseases* 15, no. 4 (July-August 1999) [Online Journal]. [cited October 25, 2001]. < http://www.cdc.gov/ncidod/EID/vol5no4/henderson.htm >.

Rotz, Lisa D., Debra A. Dotson, Inger K. Damon, and John A. Becher. "Vaccinia (Smallpox) Vaccine Recommendations of the Advisory Committee on Immunization Practices (ACIP), 2001." In: *Morbidity and Mortality Weekly Report* 50, rr 10 (June 22, 2001): 1-25. [cited October 25, 2001]. < http://www.cdc.gov/mmwr/preview/mmwrhtml/rr5010a1.htm >.

Rosalyn Carson-DeWitt, MD

Smelling disorders

Definition

Smelling disorders are disturbances of the olfactory sense, which is known as the sense of smell. These nasal dysfunctions range from the total loss of smell (**anosmia**) to dysosmia, a distorted sense of smell.

Description

An awareness of how the olfactory system works is helpful for understanding how smelling disorders affect the sense of smell. People detect odors because sensory receptors located in the nose carry smell sensations to the brain. The receptors, which are nerve cell endings, are found in the mucous membrane in the roof of the nose. This section of the nose called the olfactory area is located just below the brain's frontal lobes.

In the olfactory area are millions of tiny olfactory cells. Each cell contains about 12 cilia, tiny hairs that extend into a mucus layer. The mucus moistens the cilia. Mucus also catches odor molecules, while receptors in the cilia stimulate the molecules and send nerve impulses to the brain.

Olfactory nerve fibers carry the impulse to two olfactory bulbs located in the brain. Information is processed in the bulbs and then sent to the cerebral cortex. Once the transmission is inside the smell center of the brain, a person experiences the sense of smell.

A person with a normal sense of smell (normosmia) is able to distinguish 10,000 odors. The sense of smell stimulates salivary glands. As a result, smelling disorders often affect the sense of taste. The olfactory sense allows people to experience pleasurable odors like the scent of roses. And smell is thought to contribute to sexual attraction.

A smelling disorder that affects the sense of smell is generally not life-threatening. However, it can be dangerous. Without a sense of smell, a person might eat spoiled food. Lack of a sense of smell could pose a health risk if a person has little appetite and fails to eat enough. Furthermore, without a sense of smell, a person might not detect a gas leak or the smell of something burning. Loss of smell and the resulting loss of taste may lead to depression.

Types of smelling disorders

Smelling disorders differ in the way that the sense of smell is affected and how long a person has the disorder. For example, anosmia, the loss of the sense of smell, is often a temporary symptom of a cold or flu. However, a **head injury** could cause permanent anosmia. In addition, a head injury could produce dysosmia, the distorted sense of smell that could cause a person to hallucinate a foul odor.

Smelling disorders are categorized as:

- Anosmia, the loss of the sense of smell. It is the most common smelling disorder. This condition can be temporary or permanent.

- Dysosmia is a distorted sense of smell. A person senses non-existent unpleasant odors. It can be caused by medical and mental conditions.

- Hyperosmia is an increased sensitivity to smell. It can be a characteristic of someone with a neurotic or histrionic personality.

- Hyposmia is the diminished sense of smell. This is usually a temporary condition that a person may experience after a case of acute **influenza**. Sometimes this condition is referred to as partial anosmia.

- Presbyosmia refers to the lessening or loss of the olfactory sense that occurs when a person ages.

Smelling disorder demographics

Anosmia occurs in about 10% of head trauma injuries, and head trauma is a leading cause of anosmia in young adults. In older adults, the disorder is generally caused by viral infection. **Aging** may also bring a loss of the sense of smell. In rare cases, anosmia is inherited. It is a symptom of male **hypogonadism** (Kallmann's syndrome).

Olfactory **hallucinations** known as dysosmia are generally associated with psychological conditions. In some cases, people may believe they are the source of foul odors.

Causes and symptoms

Anosmia is the most common type of smelling disorder. Loss of the olfactory sense is generally caused by nasal congestion or obstruction. Temporary partial anosmia often occurs when a person has a cold, the flu, or some types of **rhinitis**, especially hay **fever** (**allergic rhinitis**). During these conditions, nasal mucus membranes become inflamed. Other causes for anosmia are:

- **Nasal polyps** and other disorders that prevent air from getting to the area in the nose where the smell receptors are found. Hay fever or an allergy may cause one or more polyps to show up.

- Viral upper respiratory infection.

- Atrophic rhinitis. This condition causes mucus membrane to waste away. The person may experience some level of permanent anosmia. One symptom of this condition is that a person expels a foul-smelling discharge.

- Hypertrophic rhinitis. Mucous membrane thickens, covering the olfactory nerve endings. If not treated, hypertrophic rhinitis can lead to permanent anosmia. This discharge could overpower other odors.

- Cigarettes. **Smoking** aggravates the nose's membrane and intensifys nasal polyp symptoms.

- A crooked nose or a deviated septum.

- When the olfactory bulbs, tracts, or central connections are destroyed. This can occur in situations such as head trauma, infections or nasal or sinus surgery.

- Head injury. If both olfactory nerves are torn during a head injury, permanent anosmia results.

- Medications such as **antihistamines** and **decongestants**, especially prolonged use of decongestants.

- Drugs like amphetamines, estrogen, naphazoline, phenothiazines, and resperine.

- The aging process may cause the sense to lessen. In most cases, there is no other obvious cause for the disorder.

- A tumor behind the nose or in the membranes surrounding the brain.

- Lead poisoning.

- Exposure to insecticides or other chemicals.

- Radiation therapy.

- Nervous disorders.

- Idiopathic loss, which means there is no diagnosable cause for the condition.

Anosmia symptoms

Most people with anosmia can distinguish salty, sweet, bitter, and sour tastes since the tongue senses these tastes. However, people with anosmia cannot sense other tastes. Since taste is largely based on the olfactory sense, people complain of losing the sense of taste (ageusia).

Dysosmia

Infected nasal sinuses and damage to the olfactory bulbs can cause dysosmia, the distorted sense of smell. Head trauma can cause this disorder. Poor **oral hygiene** can lead to dysosmia. In these cases, a person may also find that disagreeable odors are accompanied by the sensing of unpleasant tastes. In addition, brain-stem disease can cause smelling disorders. An epileptic seizure can include olfactory hallucinations.

Mental conditions such as depression and **schizophrenia** may be accompanied by dysosmia. In addition, when people who are person severely dependent on alcohol quit drinking, they may experience dysosmia.

Diagnosis

If a smelling disorder is a symptom of a mental condition such as schizophrenia, diagnosis should be part of treatment for that condition.

When the condition is caused by a medical condition such as **allergies** or a viral infection, a person may notice that the olfactory sense is impaired during that condition. If the smelling disorder continues after the person is well, an appointment should be made with a primarily health care provider.

Diagnosis of smelling disorders begins with a health assessment to determine the cause of the olfactory impairment. The patient's primary care doctor will ask if the patient has a cold, allergies, **sinusitis**, or an upper respiratory infection.

Treatment of a head injury or follow-up medical appointment should address smelling disorders. In all cases, discussion of the symptoms covers issues such as when the smelling disorder started, if this has been an ongoing problem, and whether the disorder is becoming more intense. The assessment will include questions about whether the patient can taste food and if the disorder affects all odors or specific smells. The patient will also be asked about medications taken.

Physical examinations

The **physical examination** will include a thorough inspection of the nose, nasopharynx, and the examination of the upper respiratory tract. The examination could include sinus transillumination, placement of a light on the face to help determine if sinuses are full. **Skull x rays** may be required to determine the presence of tumors in the nose or brain.

The patient may be referred to a neurologist;—an ear, nose, and throat specialist;—or to a center that specializes in treatment of smelling disorders.

Other diagnostic tests could be required. These include:

- A CT scan (**computed tomography scans**) of the head. Also known as a CAT scan, this process provides a more detailed image than the x ray.

- Olfactory nerve testing.

- Nasal cytology, which involves the study of mucus under a microscope.

- Testing to determine the scope of smelling disorder. A basic smell test involves the patient trying to identify each one of a group of different odors. A variation of this is a scratch-and-sniff test. The patient may be asked to differentiate among concentrations of one odor. The alcohol sniff test that involves use of a material soaked in isopropyl alcohol. Patients close their eyes and the doctor moves around. Patients tell the doctor when they smell the alcohol.

- The patient may also take a taste test.

Medical costs

The costs for diagnosis and treatment vary because of the different types of smelling disorders, the range of causes for olfactory dysfunction, and the different types of treatment.

There are also differences in what health plans require in terms of patient co-pay. A health plan could cover treatments ranging from the initial appointment with a primary care provider to the surgery to remove brain tumors.

In addition, some health plans cover costs of treatment at specialized facilities like the Center for Smell and Taste Disorders at the University of Colorado Health Sciences Center in Denver. A series of tests including a taste-and-smell test cost $250 in May of 2001.

Treatment

Treating a condition that causes a smelling disorder can sometimes restore the olfactory sense. Treatments for smelling disorders are as varied as the olfactory dysfunctions. Treatment for smelling disorders ranges from lifestyle changes to surgery. Treatment of mental conditions could affect the smelling disorder. In some cases, the disorder can't be treated, and the person must adjust to the loss of the sense of smell. Anosmia associated with aging is not treatable.

Basic treatments for anosmia

The sense of smell should return after a condition like a cold or the flu ends. Decongestants such as Sudafed help reduce congestion related to colds, allergies, and sinus conditions. Manufacturer's dosage recommendations should be followed. If anosmia is related to excessive use of nasal decongestants, a person should discontinue use of those medications.

Saline sprays can be used to clean the interior of the nose.

If smoking causes anosmia, a person should quit smoking.

The sense of smell may return after treatment of allergic or bacterial rhinitis and sinusitis. An over-the-counter antihistamine such as Actifed may provide relief.

If allergies cause anosmia, adjustments should be made to avoid allergens. If dust causes allergies, care should be taken to clean areas such as the bedroom.

Antibiotics may be prescribed for infections.

Other medications prescribed for smelling disorders include steroids such as Prednisone. It should only be used for a short time since longterm use could lessen resistance to infection.

Surgical treatment

Removal of nasal polyps and benign tumors may cause the sense of smell to return. Polyp removal is an uncomplicated surgery. Generally, only a local anesthetic is needed.

Septoplasty straightens the nasal passage. It is generally an outpatient surgery, with local or **general anesthesia** required. **Rhinoplasty** straightens the structure of the nose. This surgery could be combined with septoplasty.

Endoscopic sinus surgery opens sinus drainage channels. This outpatient surgery is an option after a person sees no improvement after trying treatments such as medications.

Surgical treatment may not be effective in conditions that result in the destruction of the olfactory nerve or its central passages. However, regeneration of those tissues may cause the sense to return.

Enhancing taste

Without a sense of smell, most people can still taste salt and flavors that are sweet, sour, and bitter. People with anosmia could distinguish other tastes by adding spices such as pepper to food. These spices stimulate facial nerves that also sense flavors.

Alternative treatment

Alternative treatments for smelling disorder center around the theory that zinc supplements help improve the sense of smell. The supplement is said to be effective when the olfactory sense is impaired by conditions such as a head injury or an upper respiratory infection. A person should take 50 mg of zinc picolinate each day after eating. This procedure might be effective in the case of head injury. However, it may be several months before results are seen. **Acupuncture** may also produce results.

If polyps cause a smelling disorder, a change in diet could be helpful. A person should avoid dairy products, take supplements such as garlic, and follow other recommendations from a health care practitioner. A daily dosage of 5,000–10,000 mg of vitamin C could cut back on the amount of polyps. **Vitamins** should not be taken all at once. A multi-vitamin and mineral complex could also help.

Prognosis

In cases where smelling disorders are treatable, the outcome is positive because the olfactory sense is restored. In those cases where the sense of smell is lost, the person must make adjustments to adapt to life without that sense. Those adjustments include using spices like pepper to stimulate tastebuds.

Since a person with anosmia can no longer smell food to determine whether it is safe to eat, care should be taken. The person who lives with other people can ask them if food smells fresh. People who live alone should discard food if there is a chance that it has spoiled. Other home safety measures include installing smoke alarms and gas detectors. Cooking on an electric stove is preferable to a gas stove.

Furthermore, people with smelling disorders can find support groups. These are often associated with smell and taste clinics. In addition, there are on-line bulletin board where people can share experiences. One site contains descriptions of how things smell. Those words provide a connection to a missing sense in the same way that sign language allows the hearing-impaired to understand the spoken word.

Prevention

Not all causes of smelling disorders can be prevented. However, people with a disorder should not smoke and should ask those around them not to smoke. Those with smelling disorders related to allergies should be taken to avoid allergens. Since head trauma injuries can lead to smelling disorders, people should wear protective helmets when bicycling or participating in sports like football.

Resources

BOOKS

Watson, Lyall. *Jacob's Organ and the Remarkable Sense of Smell.* New York: W. W. Norton &Company, 2000.

ORGANIZATIONS

American Academy of Otolaryngology-Head and Neck Surgery. One Prince St., Alexandria, VA 23314-3357. (703) 836-4444. < http://www.ent.org >.

Center for Taste and Smell Disorders. University of Colorado Health Sciences Center, 4200 E, Ninth Ave., Denver, CO 80262. (303) 315-5660. < http://www.hsc.colorado.edu >.

U.S. Department of Health and Human Services. 200 Independence Avenue, SW, Washington, DC 20201.(877) 696-6775. < http://www.hhs.gov >.

Liz Swain

Smoke inhalation

Definition

Smoke inhalation is breathing in the harmful gases, vapors, and particulate matter contained in smoke.

Description

Smoke inhalation typically occurs in victims or firefighters caught in structural fires. However, cigarette **smoking** also causes similar damage on a smaller scale over a longer period of time. People who are trapped in fires may suffer from smoke inhalation independent of receiving skin **burns**; however, the incidence of smoke inhalation increases with the percentage of total body surface area burned. Smoke inhalation contributes to the total number of fire-related deaths each year for several reasons: the damage is serious; its diagnosis is not always easy and there are no sensitive diagnostic tests; and patients may not show symptoms until 24–48 hours after the event. Children under age 11 and adults over age 70 are most vulnerable to the effects of smoke inhalation.

Causes and symptoms

The harmful materials given off by combustion injure the airways and lungs in three ways: heat damage, tissue irritation, and oxygen **starvation** of tissues (asphyxiation). Signs of heat damage are singed nasal hairs, burns around and inside the nose and mouth, and internal swelling of the throat. Tissue irritation of the throat and lungs may appear as noisy breathing, coughing, hoarseness, black or gray spittle, and fluid in the lungs. Asphyxiation is apparent from **shortness of breath** and blue-gray or cherry-red skin color. In some cases, the patient may not be conscious or breathing.

Diagnosis

In addition to looking for the signs of heat damage, tissue irritation, and asphyxiation, the physician will assess the patient's breathing by the respiratory rate (number of breaths per minute) and motion of the chest as the lungs inflate and deflate. The patient's circulation is also evaluated by the pulse rate (number of heartbeats per minute) and blood pressure. Blood tests will indicate the levels of oxygen and byproducts of poisonous gases. Chest x rays are too insensitive to show damage to delicate respiratory tissues, but can show fluid in the lungs (**pulmonary edema**).

The physician may perform a **bronchoscopy**, a visual examination in which the airways and lungs are seen through a fiber optic tube inserted down the patient's windpipe (trachea). Other pulmonary function tests may be performed to measure how efficiently the lungs are working.

Treatment

Treatment will vary with the severity of the damage caused by smoke inhalation. The primary focus of treatment is to maintain an open airway and provide an adequate level of oxygen. If the airway is open and stable, the patient may be given high-flow humidified 100% oxygen by mask. If swelling of the airway tissues is closing off the airway, the patient may require the insertion of an endotracheal tube to artificially maintain an open airway.

Oxygen is often the only medication necessary. However, patients who have a **cough** with **wheezing** (bronchospasm), indicating that the bronchial airways are narrowed or blocked, may be given a bronchodilator to relax the muscles and increase ventilation. There are also antidotes for specific poisonous gases in the blood; dosage is dependent upon the level indicated by blood tests. **Antibiotics** are not given until sputum and blood cultures confirm the presence of a bacterial infection.

In institutions where it is available, hyperbaric **oxygen therapy** may be used to treat smoke inhalation resulting in severe carbon monoxide or cyanide **poisoning**. This treatment requires a special chamber in which the patient receives pure oxygen at three times the normal atmospheric pressure, thus receiving more oxygen faster to overcome loss of consciousness, altered mental state, cardiovascular dysfunction, pulmonary **edema**, and severe neurological damage.

Alternative treatment

Botanical medicine can help to maintain open airways and heal damaged mucous membranes. It can also help support the entire respiratory system. **Acupuncture** and homeopathic treatment can provide support to the whole person who has suffered a traumatic injury such as smoke inhalation.

Prognosis

Although the outcome depends of the severity of the smoke inhalation and the severity of any accompanying burns or other injuries, with prompt medical treatment, the prognosis for recovery is good. However, some patients may experience chronic pulmonary problems following smoke inhalation, and those with **asthma** or other chronic respiratory conditions prior to smoke inhalation may find their original conditions have been aggravated by the inhalation injury.

Prevention

Smoke inhalation is best avoided by preventing structural fires. This includes inspection of wiring, safe use and storage of flammable liquids, and maintenance of clean, well-ventilated chimneys, wood stoves, and space heaters. Properly placed and working smoke detectors in combination with rapid evacuation plans will minimize a person's exposure to smoke in the event of a fire. When escaping a burning building, a person should move close to the floor where there is more cool, clear air to breathe because hot air rises, carrying gases and particulate matter upward. Finally, firefighters should wear proper protective gear.

Resources

OTHER

Johnson, Norma Jean. "Smoke Inhalation." *eMedicine World Medical Library.* < http://www.emedicine.com >.

Bethany Thivierge

Smoking-cessation drugs

Definition

Smoking cessation drugs are medicines that help people stop smoking cigarettes or using other forms of tobacco.

Purpose

People who smoke cigarettes or use other forms of tobacco often have a difficult time when they try to stop. The difficulty is partly psychological; they get in the habit of using tobacco at certain times of day or while they are doing certain things, such as having a cup of coffee or reading the newspaper. But the habit is also hard to break for physical reasons. Tobacco contains nicotine, a drug that is as addictive as **cocaine** or heroin. Of those who have ever tried even a single cigarette, about a third will become nicotine-dependent. A person who is addicted to nicotine has withdrawal symptoms, such as irritability, **anxiety**, difficulty concentrating, and craving for tobacco when he or she stops using tobacco.

Some people can stop smoking through will-power alone, but most do better if they have support from friends, family, a physician or pharmacist, or a formal stop-smoking program. Heavy tobacco users

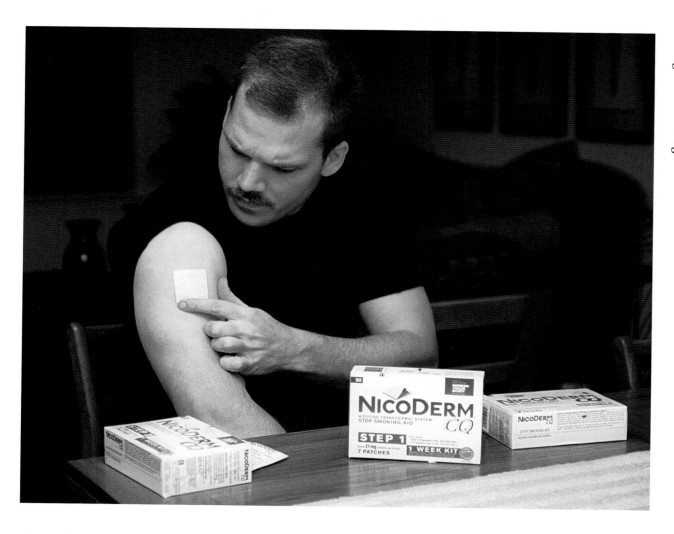

The nicotine patch brand Nicoderm. *(Fieldmark Publications. Reproduced by permission.)*

may find that smoking cessation products also help by easing their withdrawal symptoms. Most smoking cessation products contain nicotine, but the nicotine is delivered in small, steady doses spread out over many hours. In contrast, when a person inhales a cigarette, nicotine enters the lungs and then travels to the brain within seconds, delivering the "rush" that smokers come to crave. Another difference is that smoking cessation products do not contain the tar, carbon monoxide, and other toxins that make cigarettes so harmful to people's health. According to one Canadian study, tobacco smoke contains over 40 different chemicals known to cause **cancer**.

The importance of smoking cessation is reflected in legal penalties against the tobacco industry for its long-standing denial of the harm caused by tobacco products. Recent legal findings against the tobacco industry have led to legislation in three states concerning lawsuits against the industry. In Florida, state agencies can sue on behalf of Medicaid recipients for repayment of benefits. Maryland allows the use of statistical analysis in lawsuits against tobacco companies. In Vermont, the state can bring direct lawsuits against tobacco manufacturers to recover Medicaid benefits for tobacco-related illnesses paid after April 1998. Nineteen states (Alabama, Alaska, Connecticut, Florida, Hawaii, Louisiana, Maryland, Massachusetts, Minnesota, Mississippi, Montana, New Hampshire, New York, Rhode Island, Texas, Vermont, Virginia, Washington, and Wisconsin) have set aside as of 2001 a portion of their money from tobacco settlements to smoking prevention programs.

Description

Nicotine replacement products

Smoking cessation drugs that contain nicotine are also called nicotine substitution products or nicotine replacement therapy. There are four forms approved by the Food and Drug Administration (FDA) as of 2001–chewing gum, skin patch, nasal spray, and inhaler. The nasal spray and inhaler are available only with a prescription, but the gum and some brands of the patch can be bought over the counter (without a prescription). People who buy the nonprescription products should check with a physician before starting to use them. The patches are sold under the brand names Nicotrol, Nicoderm CQ, and Habitrol (prescription only). The gum is sold under the brand name Nicorette. The nasal spray and inhaler are marketed as Nicotrol NS and Nicotrol respectively. The costs of these products are about $30 for a box of 48 pieces of the gum and about $30 per week for the patches.

Other medications

Another type of smoking cessation drug, bupropion (Zyban), also reduces craving and withdrawal symptoms, although it is not a nicotine replacement product. Bupropion is an antidepressant medication that is thought to help people stop smoking by mimicking some of the effects of tobacco on brain tissue. Bupropion can be used together with nicotine replacement products; several studies indicate that the combination helps more smokers quit than either method by itself.

Buspirone (BuSpar) is a tranquilizer that appears to be effective in helping smokers deal with feelings of anxiety resulting from tobacco withdrawal.

Alternative approaches

Other approaches that have been used to help smokers quit include hypnosis and **acupuncture**. The evidence for the usefulness of hypnosis is largely anecdotal; it appears to be most helpful when used in combination with nicotine replacement products or bupropion. Although acupuncture has been used in Western countries since the 1970s to help people quit smoking, it does not appear to be particularly effective in this regard. A British study that was published in 1999 found that smokers who received acupuncture did not have a higher quit rate than those who received only sham acupuncture.

Recommended dosage

The recommended dosage of nicotine replacement products depends on the method of administration.

Each form of this medicine comes with detailed instructions for its use. Following directions exactly is very important. For example, nicotine gum should not be chewed like regular chewing gum. It must be chewed very slowly until it has a slight taste or causes a slight **tingling** sensation in the mouth; then "parked" between the cheek and gum until the taste and tingling goes away; then chewed and parked in the same way for about 30 minutes. Nicotine patches and other products also must be used correctly to be effective. Some patches are meant to be worn only during the day and removed at night; others are worn 24 hours a day.

Smokers who are heavily dependent on nicotine may want to ask their doctors about using a combination of nicotine replacement products. Studies done between 1995 and 2000 indicate that combining the transdermal patch with either the gum or the nasal spray helps more smokers quit than any of the three products by themselves. It is thought that the higher success rate is due to the different rates of speed at which these products deliver nicotine to the body. The nasal spray delivers nicotine very rapidly, and can be used to relieve intense cravings at times of the day when the smoker is accustomed to having a cigarette, while the patch delivers a smaller dosage of nicotine to the body at a steadier rate.

Precautions

Seeing a physician regularly while using smoking cessation drugs is important. The physician will check to make sure the medicine is working as it should and will watch for unwanted side effects.

Seeing a physician regularly while using smoking cessation drugs is important. The physician will check to make sure the medicine is working as it should and will watch for unwanted side effects.

- nausea
- vomiting
- severe **pain** in the stomach or abdomen
- severe diarrhea
- severe dizziness
- fainting
- convulsions (seizures)
- low blood pressure
- fast, weak, or irregular heartbeat
- hearing or vision problems
- severe breathing problems
- severe watering of the mouth or drooling

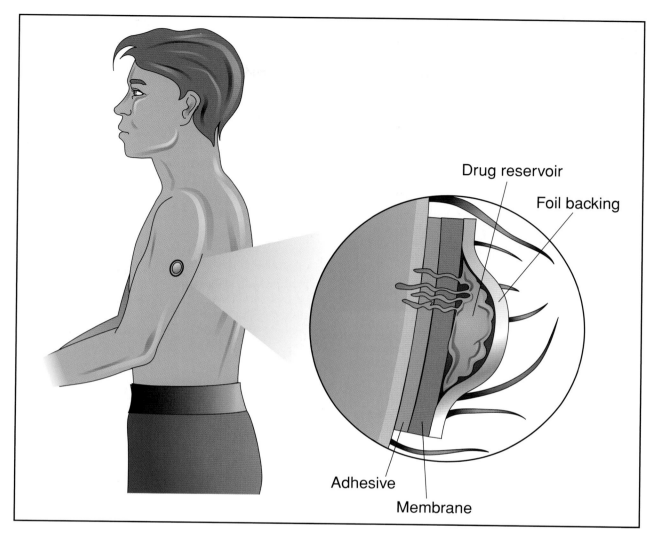

Drug reservoir

Foil backing

Adhesive

Membrane

The nicotine patch is a type of transepidermal patch designed to deliver nicotine, the addictive substance contained in cigarettes, directly through the skin and into the blood stream. The patch contains a drug reservoir sandwiched between a nonpermeable back layer and a permeable adhesive layer that attaches to the skin. The drug leeches slowly out of the reservoir, releasing small amounts of the drug at a constant rate for up to 24 hours. *(Illustration by Electronic Illustrators Group.)*

- cold sweat

- severe headache

- confusion

- severe weakness

Keep these drugs, including thrown-away patches and gum–out of the reach of children and pets. Even a small amount of nicotine can seriously harm a child or animal.

Nicotine in any form should not be used during **pregnancy**, as it may harm the fetus or cause **miscarriage**. Women who may become pregnant should use effective birth control while taking smoking cessation drugs. Women who become pregnant while taking this medicine should stop taking it immediately and check with their physicians.

Nicotine passes into breast milk and may cause problems for nursing babies. Women who are breast-feeding and want to use smoking cessation drugs may need to stop breastfeeding during treatment.

Anyone who has had unusual reactions to nicotine in the past should let his or her physician know before using a smoking cessation drug. The physician should also be told about any **allergies** to foods, dyes, preservatives, or other substances. People who have had a rash or irritation from adhesive bandages should check with a physician before using a nicotine patch.

The wheals on the arm of this patient was caused by an allergic reaction to nicotine patches used to help subdue the urge to smoke. *(Custom Medical Stock Photo. Reproduced by permission.)*

Smoking cessation patches, gum, and other products may make certain medical problems worse. Before using a smoking cessation drug, people with any of these medical problems should make sure their physicians are aware of their conditions:

- heart or blood vessel disease
- high blood pressure
- diabetes
- overactive thyroid
- skin rash or irritation
- stomach ulcer
- pheochromocytoma (pcc) (a tumor of the adrenal medulla)
- dental problems or mouth sores
- sore throat
- jaw pain or temporomandibular joint disorder (TMJ)

There are also precautions to take with bupropion and buspirone. Bupropion should not be taken by patients with a history of seizures, high blood pressure, anorexia, or **bulimia nervosa**. People taking buspirone should be careful about driving or operating heavy machinery until they can tell whether the drug makes them drowsy as a side effect. Although buspirone does not interact with alcohol as intensely as most

tranquilizers do, patients should still use alcohol cautiously if they are taking buspirone.

Side effects

Each type of smoking cessation product may cause minor side effects that usually go away as the body adjusts to the drug. These usually do not need medical attention unless they continue or they interfere with normal activities. For example, nicotine gum may cause belching, jaw aches, or sore mouth or throat. Nicotine patches may cause redness, **itching**, or burning where the patch is applied. The nasal spray may irritate the nose and sinuses, while the inhaler may cause throat irritation or coughing.

If nicotine gum injures the mouth, teeth, or dental work, check with a physician as soon as possible. Other side effects are possible. Anyone who has unusual symptoms while using smoking cessation drugs should get in touch with his or her physician.

The side effects of bupropion include **dry mouth** and difficulty sleeping. The possible side effects of buspirone include headaches and drowsiness.

Interactions

People taking certain drugs may need to change their doses when they stop smoking. Anyone who uses a smoking cessation drug should let the physician know all other medicines he or she is taking and should ask whether the doses need to be changed. Examples of drugs that may be affected when a person stops smoking are:

- insulin

- airway opening drugs (**bronchodilators**) such as aminophylline (Somophyllin), oxtriphylline (Choledyl) or theophylline (Somophyllin-T)

- opioid (narcotic) pain relievers such as propoxyphene (Darvon)

- the beta blocker propranolol (Inderal)

Other drugs may also interact with smoking cessation drugs. Be sure to check with a physician or pharmacist before combining smoking cessation drugs with any other prescription or nonprescription (over-the-counter) medicine.

Bupropion should not be used by patients who are also taking monoamine oxidase inhibitor (MAOI) medications. These include such drugs as furazolidone, isocarboxazid, and phenelzine. Bupropion may also interact with phenytoin, carbamazepine, and levodopa. Buspirone also interacts with MAOIs, as well as with trazadone and haloperidol.

Resources

BOOKS

American Cancer Society. *Quitting Smoking.* New York: American Cancer Society, 2000. < http://www.cancer.org/tobacco/quitting >.

Beers, Mark H., MD, and Robert Berkow, MD., editors. "Smoking Cessation." *The Merck Manual of Diagnosis and Therapy.* Whitehouse Station, NJ: Merck Research Laboratories, 2004.

United States Public Health Service. *You Can Quit Smoking.* Consumer Guide, June 2000. Government Publications Clearinghouse, P.O. Box 8547, Silver Spring, MD 20907. < http:www.surgeongeneral.gov/tobacco/consquits.htm >.

PERIODICALS

Okuyemi, K. S., et al. "Pharmacotherapy of Smoking Cessation." *Archives of Family Medicine* 9 (March 2000): 270-281.

ORGANIZATIONS

American Association for Respiratory Care. 11030 Ables Lane, Dallas, TX 75229. < http://www.aarc.org >.

American Cancer Society (ACS). 1599 Clifton Road, NE, Atlanta, GA 30329. (404) 320-3333 or (800) ACS-2345. Fax: (404) 329-7530. < http://www.cancer.org >.

American Lung Association. 1740 Broadway, 14th Floor, New York, NY 10019. (212) 315-8700 or (800) 586-4872 (LUNG USA).

Office on Smoking and Health. Centers for Disease Control and Prevention. Mailstop K-50, 4770 Buford Highway NE, Atlanta, GA 30341-3724. (800) 232-1311. < http://www.cdc.gov/tobacco/ >.

OTHER

de Guia, Nicole. *Rethinking Stop-Smoking Medications: Myths and Facts.* Position paper prepared for the Ontario Medical Association (OMA). OMA Health Policy Department, Ontario, Canada, June 1999.

Questions and Answers About Finding Smoking Cessation Services. Fact Sheet, National Cancer Institute. < http://www.nci.nih.gov >.

Smoking Cessation Guidelines. Agency for Health Care Policy and Research Publications Clearinghouse. PO Box 8547, Silver Spring, MD 20907.

Rebecca J. Frey, PhD

Smoking

Definition

Smoking is the inhalation of the smoke of burning tobacco encased in cigarettes, pipes, and cigars. Casual smoking is the act of smoking only occasionally, usually in a social situation or to relieve **stress**. A smoking habit is a physical **addiction** to tobacco products. Many health experts now regard habitual smoking as a psychological addiction, too, and one with serious health consequences.

Description

The U.S. Food and Drug Administration has asserted that cigarettes and smokeless tobacco should be considered nicotine delivery devices. Nicotine, the active ingredient in tobacco, is inhaled into the lungs, where most of it stays. The rest passes into the bloodstream, reaching the brain in about 10 seconds and dispersing throughout the body in about 20 seconds.

Depending on the circumstances and the amount consumed, nicotine can act as either a stimulant or tranquilizer. This can explain why some people report that smoking gives them energy and stimulates their mental activity, while others note that smoking relieves **anxiety** and relaxes them. The initial "kick" results in part from the drug's stimulation of the adrenal glands and resulting release of epinephrine into the blood. Epinephrine causes several physiological changes—it temporarily narrows the arteries, raises the blood pressure, raises the levels of fat in the blood, and increases the heart rate and flow of blood from the heart. Some researchers think epinephrine contributes to smokers' increased risk of high blood pressure.

Nicotine, by itself, increases the risk of heart disease. However, when a person smokes, he or she is ingesting a lot more than nicotine. Smoke from a cigarette, pipe, or cigar is made up of many additional toxic chemicals, including tar and carbon monoxide. Tar is a sticky substance that forms into deposits in the lungs, causing lung **cancer** and respiratory distress. Carbon monoxide limits the amount of oxygen that the red blood cells can convey throughout your body. Also, it may damage the inner walls of the arteries, which allows fat to build up in them.

Besides tar, nicotine, and carbon monoxide, tobacco smoke contains 4,000 different chemicals. More than 200 of these chemicals are known be toxic. Nonsmokers who are exposed to tobacco smoke also take in these toxic chemicals. They inhale the smoke exhaled by the smoker as well as the more toxic *sidestream smoke*—the smoke from the end of the burning cigarette, cigar, or pipe.

Here's why sidestream smoke is more toxic than exhaled smoke: When a person smokes, the smoke he or she inhales and then breathes out leaves harmful deposits inside the body. But because lungs partially cleanse the smoke, exhaled smoke contains fewer poisonous chemicals. That's why exposure to tobacco smoke is dangerous even for a nonsmoker.

Causes and symptoms

No one starts smoking to become addicted to nicotine. It isn't known how much nicotine may be consumed before the body becomes addicted. However, once smoking becomes a habit, the smoker faces a lifetime of health risks associated with one of the strongest addictions known to man.

About 70% of smokers in the United States would like to quit; in any given year, however, only about 3.6% of the country's 47 million smokers quit successfully.

Although specific genes have not yet been identified as of 2003, researchers think that genetic factors contribute substantially to developing a smoking habit. Several twin studies have led to estimates of 46–84% heritability for smoking. It is thought that some genetic variations affect the speed of nicotine metabolism in the body and the activity level of nicotinic receptors in the brain.

Symptoms That Occur After Quitting Smoking

Symptom	Cause	Duration	Relief
Craving for cigarette	nicotine craving	first week can linger for months	distract yourself with other activity
Irritability, impatience	nicotine craving	2 to 4 weeks	Exercise, relaxation techniques, avoid caffeine
Insomnia	nicotine craving temporarily reduces deep sleep	2 to 4 weeks	Avoid caffeine after 6 PM relaxation techniques; exercise
Fatigue	lack of nicotine stimulation	2 to 4 weeks	Nap
Lack of concentration	lack of nicotine stimulation	A few weeks	Reduce workload; avoid stress
Hunger	cigarettes craving confused hunger pangs	Up to several weeks	Drink water or low calorie drinks; eat low-calorie snacks
Coughing, dry throat, nasal drip	Body ridding itself of mucus in lungs and airways	Several weeks	Drink plenty of fluids; use cough drops
Constipation, gas	Intestinal movement decreases with lack of nicotine	1 to 2 weeks	Drink plenty of fluids; add fiber to diet; exercise

Smoking risks

Smoking is recognized as the leading preventable cause of **death**, causing or contributing to the deaths of approximately 430,700 Americans each year. Anyone with a smoking habit has an increased chance of lung, cervical, and other types of cancer; respiratory diseases such as **emphysema**, **asthma**, and chronic **bronchitis**; and cardiovascular disease, such as **heart attack**, high blood pressure, **stroke**, and **atherosclerosis** (narrowing and hardening of the arteries). The risk of stroke is especially high in women who take birth control pills.

Smoking can damage fertility, making it harder to conceive, and it can interfere with the growth of the fetus during **pregnancy**. It accounts for an estimated 14% of premature births and 10% of infant deaths. There is some evidence that smoking may cause **impotence** in some men.

Because smoking affects so many of the body's systems, smokers often have vitamin deficiencies and suffer oxidative damage caused by free radicals. Free radicals are molecules that steal electrons from other molecules, turning the other molecules into free radicals and destabilizing the molecules in the body's cells.

Smoking is recognized as one of several factors that might be related to a higher risk of hip **fractures** in older adults.

Studies reveal that the more a person smokes, the more likely he is to sustain illnesses such as cancer, chronic bronchitis, and emphysema. But even smokers who indulge in the habit only occasionally are more prone to these diseases.

Some brands of cigarettes are advertised as "low tar," but no cigarette is truly safe. If a smoker switches to a low-tar cigarette, he is likely to inhale longer and more deeply to get the chemicals his body craves. A smoker has to quit the habit entirely in order to improve his health and decrease the chance of disease.

Though some people believe chewing tobacco is safer, it also carries health risks. People who chew tobacco have an increased risk of heart disease and mouth and throat cancer. Pipe and cigar smokers have increased health risks as well, even though these smokers generally do not inhale as deeply as cigarette smokers do. These groups haven't been studied as extensively as cigarette smokers, but there is evidence that they may be at a slightly lower risk of cardiovascular problems but a higher risk of cancer and various types of circulatory conditions.

Recent research reveals that passive smokers, or those who unavoidably breathe in second-hand tobacco smoke, have an increased chance of many health problems such as lung cancer and asthma, and in children, **sudden infant death syndrome**.

Smokers' symptoms

Smokers are likely to exhibit a variety of symptoms that reveal the damage caused by smoking. A nagging morning **cough** may be one sign of a tobacco habit. Other symptoms include **shortness of breath, wheezing**, and frequent occurrences of respiratory illness, such as bronchitis. Smoking also increases **fatigue** and decreases the smoker's sense of smell and taste. Smokers are more likely to develop poor circulation, with cold hands and feet and premature wrinkles.

Sometimes the illnesses that result from smoking come on silently with little warning. For instance, **coronary artery disease** may exhibit few or no symptoms. At other times, there will be warning signs, such as bloody discharge from a woman's vagina, a sign of cancer of the cervix. Another warning sign is a hacking cough, worse than the usual smoker's cough, that brings up phlegm or blood—a sign of lung cancer.

Withdrawal symptoms

A smoker who tries to quit may expect one or more of these withdrawal symptoms: **nausea, constipation** or **diarrhea**, drowsiness, loss of concentration, **insomnia, headache**, nausea, and irritability.

Diagnosis

It's not easy to quit smoking. That's why it may be wise for a smoker to turn to his physician for help. For the greatest success in quitting and to help with the withdrawal symptoms, the smoker should talk over a treatment plan with his doctor or alternative practitioner. He should have a general **physical examination** to gauge his general health and uncover any deficiencies. He should also have a thorough evaluation for some of the serious diseases that smoking can cause.

Treatment

Research shows that most smokers who want to quit benefit from the support of other people. It helps to quit with a friend or to join a group such as those organized by the American Cancer Society. These groups provide support and teach behavior modification methods that can help the smoker quit. The smoker's physician can often refer him to such groups.

Other alternatives to help with the withdrawal symptoms of kicking the habit include nicotine replacement therapy in the form of gum, patches, nasal sprays, and oral inhalers. These are available by prescription or over the counter. A physician can provide advice on how to use them. They slowly release a small amount of nicotine into the bloodstream, satisfying the smoker's physical craving. Over time, the amount of gum the smoker chews is decreased and the amount of time between applying the patches is increased. This helps wean the smoker from nicotine slowly, eventually beating his addiction to the drug. But there's one important caution: If the smoker lights up while taking a nicotine replacement, a nicotine overdose may cause serious health problems.

The prescription drug Zyban (bupropion hydrochloride) has shown some success in helping smokers quit. This drug contains no nicotine, and was originally developed as an antidepressant. It isn't known exactly how bupropion works to suppress the desire for nicotine. A five-year study of bupropion reported in 2003 that the drug has a very good record for safety and effectiveness in treating tobacco dependence. Its most common side effect is insomnia, which can also result from nicotine withdrawal.

Researchers are investigating two new types of drugs as possible treatments for tobacco dependence as of 2003. The first is an alkaloid known as 18-methoxycoronaridine (18-MC), which selectively blocks the nicotinic receptors in brain tissue. Another approach involves developing drugs that inhibit the activity of cytochrome P450 2A6 (CYP2A6), which controls the metabolism of nicotine.

Expected results

Research on smoking shows that most smokers desire to quit. But smoking is so addictive that fewer than 20% of the people who try ever successfully kick the habit. Still, many people attempt to quit smoking over and over again, despite the difficulties—the cravings and withdrawal symptoms, such as irritability and restlessness.

For those who do quit, the benefits to health are well worth the effort. The good news is that once a smoker quits the health effects are immediate and dramatic. After the first day, oxygen and carbon monoxide levels in the blood return to normal. At two days, nerve endings begin to grow back and the senses of taste and smell revive. Within two weeks to three months, circulation and breathing improve. After one year of not smoking, the risk of heart disease is reduced by 50%. After 15 years of abstinence, the risks of health problems from smoking virtually vanish. A smoker who quits for good often feels a lot better too, with less fatigue and fewer respiratory illnesses.

Alternative treatment

There are a wide range of alternative treatments that can help a smoker quit the habit, including **hypnotherapy**, herbs, **acupuncture**, and **meditation**. For example, a controlled trial demonstrated that self-massage can help smokers crave less intensely, smoke fewer cigarettes, and in some cases completely give them up.

Hypnotherapy

Hypnotherapy helps the smoker achieve a trance-like state, during which the deepest levels of the mind are accessed. A session with a hypnotherapist may begin with a discussion of whether the smoker really wants to and truly has the motivation to stop smoking. The therapist will explain how hypnosis can reduce the stress-related symptoms that sometimes come with kicking the habit.

Often the therapist will discuss the dangers of smoking with the patient and begin to "reframe" the patient's thinking about smoking. Many smokers are convinced they can't quit, and the therapist can help persuade them that they can change this behavior. These suggestions are then repeated while the smoker is under hypnosis. The therapist may also suggest while the smoker is under hypnosis that his feelings of worry, anxiety, and irritability will decrease.

In a review of 17 studies of the effectiveness of hypnotherapy, the percentage of people treated by hypnosis who still were not smoking after six months ranged from 4–8%. In programs that included several hours of treatment, intense interpersonal interaction, individualized suggestions, and follow-up treatment, success rates were above 50%.

Aromatherapy

One study demonstrated that inhaling the vapor from black pepper extract can reduce symptoms associated with smoking withdrawal. Other essential oils can be used for relieving the anxiety a smoker often experiences while quitting.

Herbs

A variety of herbs can help smokers reduce their cravings for nicotine, calm their irritability, and even reverse the oxidative cellular damage done by smoking. Lobelia, sometimes called Indian tobacco, has historically been used as a substitute for tobacco. It contains a substance called lobeline, which decreases the craving for nicotine by bolstering the nervous system and calming the smoker. In high doses, lobelia can cause **vomiting**, but the average dose—about 10 drops per day—should pose no problems.

Herbs that can help relax a smoker during withdrawal include wild oats and kava kava.

To reduce the oral fixation supplied by a nicotine habit, a smoker can chew on licorice root—the plant, not the candy. Licorice is good for the liver, which is a major player in the body's **detoxification** process. Licorice also acts as a tonic for the adrenal system, which helps reduce stress. And there's an added benefit: If a smoker tries to light up after chewing on licorice root, the cigarette tastes like burned cardboard.

Other botanicals that can help repair free-radical damage to the lungs and cardiovascular system are those high in flavonoids, such as hawthorn, gingko biloba, and bilberry, as well as antioxidants such as vitamin A, vitamin C, zinc, and selenium.

Acupuncture

This ancient Chinese method of healing is used commonly to help beat addictions, including smoking. The acupuncturist will use hair-thin needles to stimulate the body's *qi*, or healthy energy. Acupuncture is a sophisticated treatment system based on revitalizing qi, which supposedly flows through the body in defined pathways called meridians. During an addiction like smoking, qi isn't flowing smoothly or gets stuck, the theory goes.

Points in the ear and feet are stimulated to help the smoker overcome his addiction. Often the acupuncturist will recommend keeping the needles in for five to seven days to calm the smoker and keep him balanced.

Vitamins

Smoking seriously depletes vitamin C in the body and leaves it more susceptible to infections. Vitamin C can prevent or reduce free-radical damage by acting as an antioxidant in the lungs. Smokers need additional C, in higher dosage than nonsmokers. Fish in the diet supplies **Omega-3 fatty acids**, which are associated with a reduced risk of chronic obstructive pulmonary disease (emphysema or chronic bronchitis) in smokers. Omega-3 fats also provide cardiovascular benefits as well as an anti-depressive effect. Vitamin therapy doesn't reduce craving but it can help beat some of the damage created by smoking. Vitamin B$_{12}$ and **folic acid** may help protect against smoking-induced cancer.

Prevention

How do you give up your cigarettes for good and never go back to them again?

Here are a few tips from the experts:

- Have a plan and set a definite quit date.
- Get rid of all the cigarettes and ashtrays at home or in your desk at work.
- Don't allow others to smoke in your house.
- Tell your friends and neighbors that you're quitting. Doing so helps make quitting a matter of pride.
- Chew sugarless gum or eat sugar-free hard candy to redirect the oral fixation that comes with smoking. This will prevent weight gain, too.
- Eat as much as you want, but only low-calorie foods and drinks. Drink plenty of water. This may help with the feelings of tension and restlessness that quitting can bring. After eight weeks, you'll lose your craving for tobacco, so it's safe then to return to your usual eating habits.
- Stay away from social situations that prompt you to smoke. Dine in the nonsmoking section of restaurants.
- Spend the money you save not smoking on an occasional treat for yourself.

KEY TERMS

Antioxidant—Any substance that reduces the damage caused by oxidation, such as the harm caused by free radicals.

Chronic bronchitis—A smoking-related respiratory illness in which the membranes that line the bronchi, or the lung's air passages, narrow over time. Symptoms include a morning cough that brings up phlegm, breathlessness, and wheezing.

Cytochrome—A substance that contains iron and acts as a hydrogen carrier for the eventual release of energy in aerobic respiration.

Emphysema—An incurable, smoking-related disease, in which the air sacs at the end of the lung's bronchi become weak and inefficient. People with emphysema often first notice shortness of breath, repeated wheezing and coughing that brings up phlegm.

Epinephrine—A nervous system hormone stimulated by the nicotine in tobacco. It increases heart rate and may raise smokers' blood pressure.

Flavonoid—A food chemical that helps to limit oxidative damage to the body's cells, and protects against heart disease and cancer.

Free radical—An unstable molecule that causes oxidative damage by stealing electrons from surrounding molecules, thereby disrupting activity in the body's cells.

Nicotine—The addictive ingredient of tobacco, it acts on the nervous system and is both stimulating and calming.

Nicotine replacement therapy—A method of weaning a smoker away from both nicotine and the oral fixation that accompanies a smoking habit by giving the smoker smaller and smaller doses of nicotine in the form of a patch or gum.

Sidestream smoke—The smoke that is emitted from the burning end of a cigarette or cigar, or that comes from the end of a pipe. Along with exhaled smoke, it is a constituent of second-hand smoke.

Resources

PERIODICALS

"AAAAI, EPA Mount Effort to Raise Awareness to Dangers of Secondhand Smoke." *Immunotherapy Weekly* November 30, 2001: 30.

Batra, V., A. A. Patkar, W. H. Berrettini, et al. "The Genetic Determinants of Smoking." *Chest* 123 (May 2003): 1338–1340.

Ferry, L., and J. A. Johnston. "Efficacy and Safety of Bupropion SR for Smoking Cessation: Data from Clinical Trials and Five Years of Postmarketing Experience." *International Journal of Clinical Practice* 57 (April 2003): 224–230.

Janson, Christer, Susan Chinn, Deborah Jarvis, et al. "Effect of Passive Smoking on Respiratory Symptoms, Bronchial Responsiveness, Lung Function, and Total Serum IgE in the European Community Respiratory Health Survey: A Cross-Sectional Study." *Lancet* 358 (December 22, 2001): 2103.

Lerman, C., and W. Berrettini. "Elucidating the Role of Genetic Factors in Smoking Behavior and Nicotine Dependence." *American Journal of Medical Genetics* 118-B (April 1, 2003): 48–54.

Maisonneuve, I. M., and S. D. Glick. "Anti-Addictive Actions of an Iboga Alkaloid Congener: A Novel Mechanism for a Novel Treatment." *Pharmacology, Biochemistry, and Behavior* 75 (June 2003): 607–618.

Richmomd, R., and N. Zwar. "Review of Bupropion for Smoking Cessation." *Drug and Alcohol Review* 22 (June 2003): 203–220.

Sellers, E. M., R. F. Tyndale, and L. C. Fernandes. "Decreasing Smoking Behaviour and Risk through CYP2A6 Inhibition." *Drug Discovery Today* 8 (June 1, 2003): 487–493.

"Study Shows Link Between Asthma and Childhood Exposure to Smoking." *Immunotherapy Weekly* October 10, 2001: np.

Yochum, L., L. H. Kushi, and A. R. Folsom. "Dietary Flavonoid Intake and Risk of Cardiovascular Disease in Postmenopausal Women." *American Journal of Epidemiology* 149, no. 10 (May 1999): 943–9.

ORGANIZATIONS

American Association of Oriental Medicine. 5530 Wisconsin Avenue, Suite 1210, Chevy Chase, MD 20815. (301) 941-1064 or (888) 500-7999. < http://www.aaom.org >.

American Cancer Society. Contact the local organization or call (800) 227-2345. < http://www.cancer.org >.

American Lung Association. 1740 Broadway, New York, NY 10019. (800) 586-4872 or (212) 315-8700. < http:// www.lungusa.org >.

Herb Research Foundation. 1007 Pearl St., Suite 200, Boulder CO 80302. (303) 449-2265. < http:// www.herbs.org >.

National Heart, Lung, and Blood Institute (NHLBI). Building 31, Room 5A52, 31 Center Drive, MSC 2486, Bethesda, MD 20892. (301) 592-8573. < http:// www.nhlbi.nih.gov >.

Smoking, Tobacco, and Health Information Line. Centers for Disease Control and Prevention. Mailstop K-50, 4770 Buford Highway NE, Atlanta, GA 30341-3724. (800) 232-1311. < http://www.cdc.gov/tobacco >.

OTHER

Virtual Office of the Surgeon General: Tobacco Cessation Guideline. < http://www.surgeongeneral.gov/ tobacco >.

Barbara Boughton

Snoring

Definition

Snoring is a sound generated during sleep by vibration of loose tissue in the upper airway.

Description

Snoring is one symptom of a group of disorders known as sleep disordered breathing. It occurs when the soft palate, uvula, tongue, tonsils, and/or muscles in the back of the throat rub against each other and generate a vibrating sound during sleep. Twenty percent of all adults are chronic snorers, and 45% of normal adults snore occasionally. As people grow older, their chance of snoring increases. Approximately half of all individuals over 60 snore regularly.

In some cases, snoring is a symptom of a more serious disorder called obstructed **sleep apnea** (OSA). OSA occurs when part of the airway is closed off (usually at the back of the throat) while a person is trying to inhale during sleep, and breathing stops for more than 10 seconds before resuming again. These breathless episodes can occur as many as several hundred times a night.

People with OSA almost always snore heavily, because the same narrowing of the airway that causes snoring can also cause OSA. Snoring may actually attribute to OSA as well, because the vibration of the throat tissues which occurs in snoring can cause the tissue to swell.

Snoring is associated with physical problems as well as social **stress**. People who do not suffer from OSA may be diagnosed with socially unacceptable snoring (SUS), which refers to snoring that is loud enough to prevent the sleeper's bed partner or roommate from sleeping. SUS is a factor in the breakup of some marriages and other long-term relationships.

Moreover, a study published in 2002 indicates that people who snore are at increased risk of developing type 2 diabetes. Snoring appears to be a risk factor that is independent of body weight or a family history of diabetes.

Causes and symptoms

There are several major causes of snoring, including:

- Excessively relaxed throat muscles. Alcohol, drugs, and sedatives can cause the throat muscles to become lax, and/or the tongue to pull back into the airway.

- Large uvula. The piece of tissue that hangs from the back of the throat is called the uvula. Individuals with a large or longer than average uvula can suffer from snoring when the uvula vibrates in the airway.

- Large tonsils and/or adenoids. The tonsils (tissue at the back of either side of the throat) can also vibrate if they are larger than normal, as can the adenoids.

- Excessive weight. Overweight people are more likely to snore. This is frequently caused by the extra throat and neck tissue they are carrying around.

- Nasal congestion. Colds and **allergies** can plug the nose, creating a vacuum in the throat that results in snoring as airflow increases.

- Cysts and tumors. Cysts and/or tumors of the throat can trigger snoring.

- Structural problems of the nose. A **deviated septum** or other nasal problems can also cause snoring.

Diagnosis

A patient interview, and possibly an interview with the patient's spouse or anyone else in the household who has witnessed the snoring, is usually enough for a diagnosis of snoring. A medical history that includes questions about alcohol or tranquilizer use; past ear, nose, and throat problems; and the pattern and degree of snoring will be completed, and a physical exam will be performed to determine the cause of the problem. This will typically include examination of the throat to look for narrowing, obstruction, or malformations. If the snoring is suspected to be a symptom of a more serious disorder such as obstructive sleep apnea, the patient will require further testing. This testing is called a **polysomnography** study, and is conducted during an overnight stay in a specialized sleep laboratory. The polysomnography study include measurements of heart rate, airflow at the mouth and nose, respiratory effort, sleep stage (light sleep, deep sleep, dream sleep, etc.), and oxygen level in the blood.

In some cases the patient may be referred to a dentist or orthodontist for evaluation of the jaw structure and dentition.

In addition, the patient may be examined by sleep endoscopy. In this procedure, the patient is given a medication (midazolam) to induce sleep. His or her throat and nasal passages are then examined with a flexible laryngoscope. In many cases, sleep endoscopy reveals obstructions that are not apparent during a standard **physical examination** of the throat. Many patients are found to have obstructions at more than one level in their breathing passages.

Treatment

Several surgical procedures are available for treating chronic snoring. These include:

- Uvulopalathopharyngoplasty (UPPP), a surgical procedure which involves removing excess throat tissues (e.g., tonsils, parts of the soft palate) to expand the airway.

- Laser-assisted uvulopalatoplasty (LAUP) uses a surgical laser to remove part of the uvula and palate.

- Palatal stiffening is a minimally-invasive surgical technique where a laser or a cauterizer is used to produce scar tissue in the soft palate in order to stop the vibrations that produce snoring.

- Radiofrequency ablation is another technique which uses scarring to shrink the uvula and/or soft palate. A needle electrode is used to shrink and scar the mouth and throat tissues.

Alternative treatment

There are a number of remedies for snoring, but few are proven clinically effective. Popular treatments include:

- Mechanical devices. Many splints, braces, and other devices are available which reposition the nose, jaw, and/or mouth in order to clear the airways. Other devices are designed to wake an individual when snoring occurs. Patients should consult a dentist or orthodontist about these devices, as most require custom fitting. In addition, persons with certain types of gum disease or dental problems should not be fitted with oral appliances to stop snoring.

- Nasal strips. Nasal strips that attach like an adhesive bandage to the bridge of the nose are available at most drugstores, and can help stop snoring in some individuals by opening the nasal passages.

- Continuous positive airway pressure (CPAP). Some chronic snorers find relief by sleeping with a nasal mask which provides air pressure to the throat.

- **Decongestants**. Snoring caused by nasal congestion may be successfully treated with decongestants. Some effective herbal remedies that clear the nasal passages include golden rod (*Solidago virgauria*) and golden seal (*Hydrastis canadensis*). Steam inhalation of essential oils of eucalyptus blue gum (*Eucalyptus globulus*) or peppermint (*Mentha x piperata*) can also relieve congestion.

- Weight loss. Snoring thought to be caused by excessive weight may be curtailed by a sensible weight loss and **exercise** program.

- Sleep position. Snoring usually worsens when an individual sleeps on his or her back, so sleeping on one's side may alleviate the problem. Those who have difficulty staying in a side sleeping position may find sleeping with pillows behind them helps them maintain the position longer. Other devices include a new vest designed to prevent the sleeper from lying on his or her back.

- Bed adjustments. For some people, raising the head of the bed solves their snoring problem. A slight incline can prevent the tongue from retracting into the back of the throat. Bricks, wooden blocks, or specially designed wedges can be used to elevate the head of the bed approximately 4–16 in (10–41 cm).

Alternative treatments that have been reported to be effective for patients whose snoring is caused by colds or allergies include **acupuncture**, homeopathy, and **aromatherapy** treatments. Aromatherapy treatments for snoring typically make use of marjoram oil, which is thought to be particularly effective in clearing the nasal passages.

Prevention

Adults with a history of snoring may be able to prevent snoring episodes with the following measures:

- avoid alcohol and sedatives before bedtime

- remove allergens from the bedroom

- use a decongestant before bed

- sleep on the side, not the back

Resources

BOOKS

Beers, Mark H., MD, and Robert Berkow, MD., editors. "Disorders of the Oral Region." Section 9, Chapter 105 In *The Merck Manual of Diagnosis and Therapy*.

Whitehouse Station, NJ: Merck Research Laboratories, 2004.

Beers, Mark H., MD, and Robert Berkow, MD., editors. "Sleep Disorders." Section 14, Chapter 173 In *The Merck Manual of Diagnosis and Therapy*. Whitehouse Station, NJ: Merck Research Laboratories, 2004.

Pelletier, Kenneth R., MD. *The Best Alternative Medicine*, Part I, Chapter 5, "Acupuncture," and Chapter 8, "Homeopathy." New York: Simon & Schuster, 2002.

PERIODICALS

Al-Delaimy, W. K., J. E. Manson, W. C. Willett, et al. "Snoring as a Risk Factor for Type II Diabetes Mellitus: A Prospective Study." *American Journal of Epidemiology* 155 (March 1, 2002): 394-395.

Ayappa, I., and D. M. Rapoport. "The Upper Airway in Sleep: Physiology of the Pharynx." *Sleep Medicine Reviews* 7 (February 2003): 3–7.

Blumen, M. B., S. Dahan, I. Wagner, et al. "Radiofrequency Versus LAUP for the Treatment of Snoring." *Otolaryngology and Head and Neck Surgery* 126 (January 2002): 67-73.

Ellis, S. G., N. W. Craik, R. F. Deans, and C. D. Hanning. "Dental Appliances for Snoring and Obstructive Sleep Apnoea: Construction Aspects for General Dental Practitioners." *Dental Update* 30 (January-February 2003): 16–22, 24–26.

Hassid, S., A. H. Afrapoli, C. Decaesteker, and G. Choufani. "UPPP for Snoring: Long-Term Results and Patient Satisfaction." *Acta Otorhinolaryngologica Belgica* 56 (2002): 157-162.

Hessel, N. S., and N. de Vries. "Diagnostic Work-Up of Socially Unacceptable Snoring. II. Sleep Endoscopy." *European Archives of Otorhinolaryngology* 259 (March 2002): 158-161.

Maurer, J. T., B. A. Stuck, G. Hein, et al. "Treatment of Obstructive Sleep Apnea with a New Vest Preventing the Supine Position." [in German] *Deutsche medizinische Wochenschrift* 128 (January 17, 2003): 71–75.

Nakano, H., T. Ikeda, M. Hayashi, et al. "Effects of Body Position on Snoring in Apneic and Nonapneic Snorers." *Sleep* 26 (March 15, 2003): 169–172.

Remacle, M., E. Jouzdani, G. Lawson, and J. Jamart. "Laser-Assisted Surgery Addressing Snoring Long-Term Outcome Comparing CO_2 Laser vs. CO_2 Laser Combined with Diode Laser." *Acta Otorhinolaryngologica Belgica* 56 (2002): 177-182.

Stevenson, J. E. "Diagnosis of Sleep Apnea." *Wisconsin Medical Journal* 102 (2003): 25–27, 46.

Trotter, M. I., A. R. D'Souza, and D. W. Morgan. "Medium-Term Outcome of Palatal Surgery for Snoring Using the Somnus Unit." *Journal of Laryngology and Otology* 116 (February 2002): 116-118.

ORGANIZATIONS

American Academy of Otolaryngology, Head and Neck Surgery, Inc. One Prince Street, Alexandria, VA 22314-3357. (703) 836-4444. < http://www.entnet.org >.

American Academy of Sleep Medicine (AASM). One Westbrook Corporate Center, Suite 920, Westchester, IL 60154. (708) 492-0930. < http://www.aasmnet.org >.

American Dental Association. 211 East Chicago Avenue, Chicago, IL 60611. (312) 440-2500. < http://www.ada.org >.

American Sleep Apnea Association. *Wake-Up Call: The Wellness Letter for Snoring and Apnea.* 1424 K Street NW, Suite 302, Washington, DC 20005. (202) 293-3650. < http://www.sleepapnea.org >.

National Sleep Foundation. 1522 K Street, NW, Suite 500, Washington, DC 20005. < http://www.sleepfoundation.org >.

OTHER

American Sleep Apnea Association (ASAA). *Considering Surgery for Snoring?* < http://www.sleepapnea.org/snoring.html >.

National Heart, Lung, and Blood Institute (NHLBI). *Facts About Sleep Apnea.* NIH Publication No. 95-3798.

[cited April 13, 2003]. < http://www.nhlbi.nih.gov/health/public/sleep/sleepapn.htm >.

Paula Anne Ford-Martin
Rebecca J. Frey, PhD

Sodium imbalance *see* **Hypernatremia; Hyponatremia**

Somatization disorder *see* **Somatoform disorders**

Somatoform disorders

Definition

The somatoform disorders are a group of mental disturbances placed in a common category on the basis of their external symptoms. These disorders are characterized by physical complaints that appear to be medical in origin but that cannot be explained in terms of a physical disease, the results of **substance abuse**, or by another mental disorder. In order to meet the criteria for a somatoform disorder, the physical symptoms must be serious enough to interfere with the patient's employment or relationships, and must be symptoms that are not under the patient's voluntary control.

It is helpful to understand that the present classification of these disorders reflects recent historical changes in the practice of medicine and psychiatry. When psychiatry first became a separate branch of medicine at the end of the nineteenth century, the term *hysteria* was commonly used to describe mental disorders characterized by altered states of consciousness (for example, sleepwalking or trance states) or physical symptoms (for example, a "paralyzed" arm or leg with no neurologic cause) that could not be fully explained by a medical disease. The term *dissociation* was used for the psychological mechanism that allows the mind to split off uncomfortable feelings, memories, or ideas so that they are lost to conscious recall. Sigmund Freud and other pioneering psychoanalysts thought that the hysterical patient's symptoms resulted from dissociated thoughts or memories reemerging through bodily functions or trance states. Prior to the categorization all mental disorders that were considered to be forms of **hysteria** were grouped together on the basis of this theory about their cause. Since 1980, however, the somatoform disorders and the so-called **dissociative disorders** have been placed in separate categories on the basis of their chief symptoms. In general, the somatoform disorders are characterized by disturbances in the patient's physical sensations or ability to move the limbs or walk, while the dissociative disorders are marked by disturbances in the patient's sense of identity or memory.

Description

As a group, the somatoform disorders are difficult to recognize and treat because patients often have long histories of medical or surgical treatment with several different doctors. In addition, the physical symptoms are not under the patient's conscious control, so that he or she is not intentionally trying to confuse the doctor or complicate the process of diagnosis. Somatoform disorders are, however, a significant problem for the health care system because patients with these disturbances overuse medical services and resources.

Somatization disorder (Briquet's syndrome)

Somatization disorder was formerly called Briquet's syndrome, after the French physician who first recognized it. The distinguishing characteristic of this disorder is a group or pattern of symptoms in several different organ systems of the patient's body that cannot be accounted for by medical illness. The criteria for this disorder require four symptoms of **pain**, two symptoms in the digestive tract, one symptom involving the sexual organs, and one symptom related to the nervous system. Somatization disorder usually begins before the age of 30. It is estimated that 0.2% of the United States population will develop this disorder in the course of their lives. Another researcher estimates that 1% of all women in the United States have symptoms of this disorder. The female-to-male ratio is estimated to range between 5:1 and 20:1.

Somatization disorder is considered to be a chronic disturbance that tends to persist throughout the patient's life. It is also likely to run in families. Some psychiatrists think that the high female-to-male ratio in this disorder reflects the cultural pressures on women in North American society and the social "permission" given to women to be physically weak or sickly.

Conversion disorder

Conversion disorder is a condition in which the patient's senses or ability to walk or move are impaired without a recognized medical or neurological disease or cause and in which psychological factors (such as **stress** or trauma) are judged to be temporarily related to onset or exacerbation. The disorder gets its name from the notion that the patient is converting a psychological conflict or problem into an inability to move specific parts of the body or to use the senses normally. An example of a conversion reaction would be a patient who loses his or her voice in a situation in which he or she is afraid to speak. The symptom simultaneously contains the **anxiety** and serves to get the patient out of the threatening situation. The resolution of the emotion that underlies the physical symptom is called the patient's *primary gain*, and the change in the patient's social, occupational, or family situation that results from the symptom is called a *secondary gain*. Doctors sometimes use these terms when they discuss the aftereffects of conversion disorder or of other somatoform disorders on the patient's emotional adjustment and lifestyle.

The specific physical symptoms of conversion disorder may include a loss of balance or **paralysis** of an arm or leg; the inability to swallow or speak; the loss of touch or pain sensation; going blind or deaf; seeing double; or having **hallucinations**, seizures, or convulsions.

Unlike somatization disorder, conversion disorder may begin at any age, and it does not appear to run in families. It is estimated that as many as 34% of the population experiences conversion symptoms over a lifetime, but that the disorder is more likely to occur among less educated or sophisticated people. Conversion disorder is not usually a chronic disturbance; 90% of patients recover within a month, and most do not have recurrences. The female-to-male ratio is between 2:1 and 5:1. Male patients are likely to develop conversion disorders in occupational settings or military service.

Pain disorder

Pain disorder is marked by the presence of severe pain as the focus of the patient's concern. This category of somatoform disorder covers a range of patients with a variety of ailments, including chronic headaches, back problems, arthritis, muscle aches and cramps, or pelvic pain. In some cases the patient's pain appears to be largely due to psychological factors, but in other cases the pain is derived from a medical condition as well as the patient's psychology.

Pain disorder is relatively common in the general population, partly because of the frequency of work-related injuries in the United States. This disorder appears to be more common in older adults, and the sex ratio is nearly equal, with a female-to-male ratio of 2:1.

Hypochondriasis

Hypochondriasis is a somatoform disorder marked by excessive fear of or preoccupation with having a serious illness that persists in spite of medical testing and reassurance. It was formerly called hypochondriacal neurosis.

Although hypochondriasis is usually considered a disorder of young adults, it is now increasingly recognized in children and adolescents. It may also develop in elderly people without previous histories of health-related fears. The disorder accounts for about 5% of psychiatric patients, and is equally common in men and women. Hypochondriasis may persist over a number of years but usually occurs as a series of episodes rather than continuous treatment-seeking. The flare-ups of the disorder are often correlated with stressful events in the patient's life.

Body dysmorphic disorder

Body dysmorphic disorder is a new category of somatoform disorders. It is defined as a preoccupation with an imagined or exaggerated defect in appearance. Most cases involve features on the patient's face or head, but other body parts–especially those associated with sexual attractiveness, such as the breasts or genitals–may also be the focus of concern.

Body dysmorphic disorder is regarded as a chronic condition that usually begins in the patient's late teens and fluctuates over the course of time. It was initially considered to be a relatively unusual disorder, but may be more common than was formerly thought. It appears to affect men and women with equal frequency. Patients with body dysmorphic disorder frequently have histories of seeking or obtaining **plastic surgery** or other procedures to repair or treat the supposed defect. Some may even meet the criteria for a delusional disorder of the somatic type.

Somatoform disorders in children and adolescents

The most common somatoform disorders in children and adolescents are conversion disorders, although body dysmorphic disorders are being reported more frequently. Conversion reactions in this age group usually reflect stress in the family or problems with school rather than long-term psychiatric disturbances. Some psychiatrists speculate that adolescents with conversion disorders frequently have overprotective or overinvolved parents with a subconscious need to see their child as sick; in many cases the son or daughter's symptoms become the center of family attention. The rise in body dysmorphic disorders in adolescents is thought to reflect the increased influence of media preoccupation with physical perfection.

Causes and symptoms

Because groups the somatoform disorders are categorized on the basis of symptom patterns, their causes as presently understood include several different factors.

Family stress

Family stress is believed to be one of the most common causes of somatoform disorders in children and adolescents. Conversion disorders in this age group may also be connected with physical or sexual **abuse** within the family of origin.

Parental modeling

Somatization disorder and hypochondriasis may result in part from the patient's unconscious reflection or imitation of parental behaviors. This "copycat" behavior is particularly likely if the patient's parent derived considerable secondary gain from his or her symptoms.

Cultural influences

Cultural influences appear to affect the gender ratios and body locations of somatoform disorders, as well as their frequency in a specific population. Some cultures (for example, Greek and Puerto Rican) report higher rates of somatization disorder among men than is the case for the United States. In addition, researchers found lower levels of somatization disorder among people with higher levels of education. People in Asia and Africa are more likely to report certain types of physical sensations (for example, burning hands or feet, or the feeling of ants crawling under the skin) than are Westerners.

Biological factors

Genetic or biological factors may also play a role. For example, people who suffer from somatization disorder may also differ in how they perceive and process pain.

Diagnosis

Accurate diagnosis of somatoform disorders is important to prevent unnecessary surgery, laboratory tests, or other treatments or procedures. Because somatoform disorders are associated with physical symptoms, patients are often diagnosed by primary care physicians as well as by psychiatrists. In many cases the diagnosis is made in a general medical clinic. Children and adolescents with somatoform disorders are most likely to be diagnosed by pediatricians. Diagnosis of somatoform disorders requires a thorough physical workup to exclude medical and neurological conditions, or to assess their severity in patients with pain disorder. A detailed examination is especially necessary when conversion disorder is a possible diagnosis, because some neurological conditions–including **multiple sclerosis** and myasthenia gravis–have on occasion been misdiagnosed as conversion disorder. Some patients who receive a diagnosis of somatoform disorder ultimately go on to develop neurologic disorders.

In addition to ruling out medical causes for the patient's symptoms, a doctor who is evaluating a patient for a somatization disorder will consider the possibility of other psychiatric diagnoses or of overlapping psychiatric disorders. Somatoform disorders often coexist with **personality disorders** because of the chicken-and-egg relationship between physical illness and certain types of character structure or personality traits. At one time, the influence of Freud's theory of hysteria led doctors to assume that the patient's hidden emotional needs "cause" the illness. But in many instances, the patient's personality may have changed over time due to the stresses of adjusting to a chronic disease. This gradual transformation is particularly likely in patients with pain disorder. Patients with somatization disorder often develop panic attacks or **agoraphobia** together with their physical symptoms. In addition to anxiety or personality disorders, the doctor will usually consider major depression as a possible diagnosis when evaluating a patient with symptoms of a somatoform disorder. Pain disorders may be associated with depression, and body dismorphic disorder may be associated with obsessive-compulsive disease.

Treatment

Relationship with primary care practitioner

Because patients with somatoform disorders often have lengthy medical histories, a long-term relationship with a trusted primary care practitioner (PCP) is a safeguard against unnecessary treatments as well as a comfort to the patient. Many PCPs prefer to schedule brief appointments on a regular basis with the patient and keep referrals to specialists to a minimum. This practice also allows them to monitor the patient for any new physical symptoms or diseases. However, some PCPs work with a psychiatric consultant.

Medications

Patients with somatoform disorders are sometimes given **antianxiety drugs** or **antidepressant drugs** if they have been diagnosed with a coexisting mood or anxiety disorder. In general, however, it is considered better practice to avoid prescribing medications for these patients since they are likely to become psychologically dependent on them. However, body dysmorphic disorder as been successfully treated with **selective serotonin reuptake inhibitors (SSRI)** antidepressants.

Psychotherapy

Patients with somatoform disorders are not considered good candidates for **psychoanalysis** and other forms of insight-oriented psychotherapy. They can benefit, however, from supportive approaches to treatment that are aimed at symptom reduction and stabilization of the patient's personality. Some patients with pain disorder benefit from **group therapy** or support groups, particularly if their social network has been limited by their pain symptoms. **Cognitive-behavioral therapy** is also used sometimes to treat pain disorder.

Family therapy is usually recommended for children or adolescents with somatoform disorders, particularly if the parents seem to be using the child as a focus to divert attention from other difficulties. Working with families of chronic pain patients also helps avoid reinforcing dependency within the family setting.

Hypnosis is a technique that is sometimes used as part of a general psychotherapeutic approach to conversion disorder because it may allow patients to recover memories or thoughts connected with the onset of the physical symptoms.

Alternative treatment

Patients with somatization disorder or pain disorder may be helped by a variety of alternative therapies including **acupuncture**, **hydrotherapy**, therapeutic massage, **meditation**, botanical medicine, and homeopathic treatment. Relief of symptoms, including pain, can occur on the physical level, as well as on the mental, emotional, and spiritual levels.

Prognosis

The prognosis for somatoform disorders depends, as a rule, on the patient's age and whether the disorder is chronic or episodic. In general, somatization

KEY TERMS

Briquet's syndrome—Another name for somatization disorder.

Conversion disorder—A somatoform disorder characterized by the transformation of a psychological feeling or impulse into a physical symptom. Conversion disorder was previously called hysterical neurosis, conversion type.

Dissociation—A psychological mechanism in which the mind splits off certain aspects of a traumatic event from conscious awareness. Dissociation can affect the patient's memory, sense of reality, and sense of identity.

Hysteria—The earliest term for a psychoneurotic disturbance marked by emotional outbursts and/or disturbances of movement and sense perception. Some forms of hysteria are now classified as somatoform disorders and others are grouped with the dissociative disorders.

Hysterical neurosis—An older term for conversion disorder or dissociative disorder.

Primary gain—The immediate relief from guilt, anxiety, or other unpleasant feelings that a patient derives from a symptom.

Repression—A unconscious psychological mechanism in which painful or unacceptable ideas, memories, or feelings are removed from conscious awareness or recall.

Secondary gain—The social, occupational, or interpersonal advantages that a patient derives from symptoms. A patient's being relieved of his or her share of household chores by other family members would be an example of secondary gain.

Somatoform disorder—A category of psychiatric disorder characterized by physical complaints that appear to be medical in origin but that cannot be explained in terms of a physical disease, the results of substance abuse, or by another mental disorder.

disorder and body dysmorphic disorder rarely resolve completely. Hypochondriasis and pain disorder may resolve if there are significant improvements in the patient's overall health and life circumstances, and people with both disorders may go through periods when symptoms become less severe (remissions) or become worse (exacerbations). Conversion disorder tends to be rapidly resolved, but may recur in about 25% of all cases.

Prevention

Generalizations regarding prevention of somatoform disorders are difficult because these syndromes affect different age groups, vary in their symptom patterns and persistence, and result from different problems of adjustment to the surrounding culture. In theory, allowing expression of emotional pain in children, rather than regarding it as "weak," might reduce the secondary gain of physical symptoms that draw the care or attention of parents.

Resources

BOOKS

Eisendrath, Stuart J. "Psychiatric Disorders." In *Current Medical Diagnosis and Treatment, 1998*, edited by Stephen McPhee, et al., 37th ed. Stamford: Appleton & Lange, 1997.

Rebecca J. Frey, PhD

Somatotrophic hormone test *see* **Growth hormone tests**

▮ Sore throat

Definition

Sore throat, also called pharyngitis, is a painful inflammation of the mucous membranes lining the pharynx. It is a symptom of many conditions, but most often is associated with colds or **influenza**. Sore throat may be caused by either viral or bacterial infections or environmental conditions. Most sore throats heal without complications, but they should not be ignored because some develop into serious illnesses.

Description

Almost everyone gets a sore throat at one time or another, although children in child care or grade school have them more often than adolescents and adults. Sore throats are most common during the winter months when upper respiratory infections (colds) are more frequent.

Sore throats can be either acute or chronic. Acute sore throats are the more common. They appear suddenly and last from three to about seven days. A chronic sore throat lasts much longer and is a symptom of an unresolved underlying condition or disease, such as a sinus infection.

Causes and symptoms

Sore throats have many different causes, and may or may not be accompanied by cold symptoms, **fever**, or swollen lymph glands. Proper treatment depends on understanding the cause of the sore throat.

Viral sore throat

Viruses cause 90–95% of all sore throats. Cold and flu viruses are the main culprits. These viruses cause an inflammation in the throat and occasionally the tonsils (**tonsillitis**). Cold symptoms almost always accompany a viral sore throat. These can include a runny nose, **cough**, congestion, hoarseness, **conjunctivitis**, and fever. The level of throat **pain** varies from uncomfortable to excruciating, when it is painful for the patient to eat, breathe, swallow, or speak.

Another group of viruses that cause sore throat are the adenoviruses. These may also cause infections of the lungs and ears. In addition to a sore throat, symptoms that accompany an adenovirus infection include cough, runny nose, white bumps on the tonsils and throat, mild **diarrhea**, **vomiting**, and a rash. The sore throat lasts about one week.

A third type of virus that can cause severe sore throat is the coxsackie virus. It can cause a disease called herpangina. Although anyone can get herpangina, it is most common in children up to age ten and is more prevalent in the summer or early autumn. Herpangina is sometimes called summer sore throat.

Three to six days after being exposed to the virus, an infected person develops a sudden sore throat that is accompanied by a substantial fever usually between 102–104°F (38.9–40°C). Tiny grayish-white blisters form on the throat and in the mouth. These fester and become small ulcers. Throat pain is often severe, interfering with swallowing. Children may become dehydrated if they are reluctant to eat or drink because of the pain. In addition, people with herpangina may vomit, have abdominal pain, and generally feel ill and miserable.

One other common cause of a viral sore throat is mononucleosis. Mononucleosis occurs when the Epstein-Barr virus infects one specific type of lymphocyte. The infection spreads to the lymphatic system, respiratory system, liver, spleen, and throat. Symptoms appear 30–50 days after exposure.

Mononucleosis, sometimes called the kissing disease, is extremely common. It is estimated that by the age of 35–40, 80–95% of Americans will have had mononucleosis. Often, symptoms are mild, especially in young children, and are diagnosed as a cold. Since symptoms are more severe in adolescents and adults, more cases are diagnosed as monomucleosis in this age group. One of the main symptoms of mononucleosis is a severe sore throat.

Although a runny nose and cough are much more likely to accompany a sore throat caused by a virus than one caused by a bacteria, there is no absolute way to tell what is causing the sore throat without a laboratory test. Viral sore throats are contagious and are passed directly from person to person by coughing and sneezing.

Bacterial sore throat

From 5–10% of sore throats are caused by bacteria. The most common bacterial sore throat results from an infection by group A *Streptococcus*. This type of infection is commonly called **strep throat**. Anyone can get strep throat, but it is most common in school age children.

Pharyngeal **gonorrhea**, a sexually transmitted bacterial disease, causes a severe sore throat. Gonorrhea in the throat is transmitted by having oral sex with an infected person.

Noninfectious sore throat

Not all sore throats are caused by infection. Postnasal drip can irritate the throat and make it sore. It can be caused by hay fever and other **allergies** that irritate the sinuses. Environmental and other conditions, such as heavy **smoking** or breathing second-hand smoke, heavy alcohol consumption, breathing polluted air or chemical fumes, or swallowing substances that burn or scratch the throat can also cause pharyngitis. Dry air, like that in airplanes or from forced hot air furnaces, can make the throat sore. People who breathe through their mouths at night because of nasal congestion often get sore throats that improve as the day progresses. Sore throat caused by environmental conditions is not contagious.

Diagnosis

It is easy for people to tell if they have a sore throat, but difficult to know what has caused it without laboratory tests. Most sore throats are minor and heal without any complications. A small number of bacterial sore throats do develop into serious diseases. Because of this, it is advisable to see a doctor if a sore throat lasts more than a few days or is accompanied by fever, **nausea**, or abdominal pain.

Diagnosis of a sore throat by a doctor begins with a **physical examination** of the throat and chest. The doctor will also look for signs of other illness, such as a

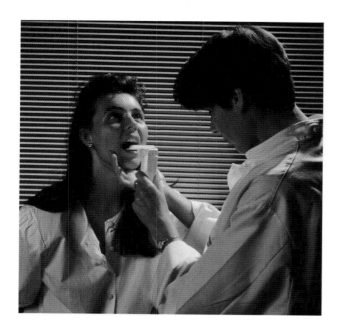

This young woman is having her sore throat examined by a medical practitioner using a fiber-optic tongue depressor. *(Custom Medical Stock Photo. Reproduced by permission.)*

sinus infection or **bronchitis**. Since both bacterial and viral sore throat are contagious and pass easily from person to person, the doctor will seek information about whether the patient has been around other people with flu, sore throat, colds, or strep throat. If it appears that the patient may have strep throat, the doctor will do laboratory tests.

If mononucleosis is suspected, the doctor may do a mono spot test to look for antibodies indicating the presence of the Epstein-Barr virus. The test in inexpensive, takes only a few minutes, and can be done in a physician's office. An inexpensive blood test can also determine the presence of antibodies to the mononucleosis virus.

Treatment

Effective treatment varies depending on the cause of the sore throat. As frustrating as it may be to the patient, viral sore throat is best left to run its course without drug treatment. **Antibiotics** have no effect on a viral sore throat. They do not shorten the length of the illness, nor do they lessen the symptoms.

Sore throat caused by a streptococci or another bacteria must be treated with antibiotics. Penicillin is the preferred medication. Oral penicillin must be taken for 10 days. Patients need to take the entire amount of antibiotic prescribed, even after symptoms of the sore throat improve. Stopping the antibiotic

early can lead to a return of the sore throat. Occasionally a single injection of long-acting penicillin G is given instead of 10 days of oral treatment. These medications generally cost under $15.

Because mononucleosis is caused by a virus, there is no specific drug treatment available. Rest, a healthy diet, plenty of fluids, limiting heavy **exercise** and competitive sports, and treatment of aches with **acetaminophen** (Datril, Tylenol, Panadol) or ibuprofen (Advil, Nuprin, Motrin, Medipren) will help the illness pass. Nearly 90% of mononucleosis infections are mild. The infected person does not normally get the disease again.

In the case of chronic sore throat, it is necessary to treat the underlying disease to heal the sore throat. If a sore throat caused by environmental factors, the aggravating stimulus should be eliminated from the sufferer's environment.

Home care for sore throat

Regardless of the cause of a sore throat, there are some home care steps that people can take to ease their discomfort. These include:

- taking acetaminophen or ibuprofen for pain; **aspirin** should not be given to children because of its association with increased risk for **Reye's Syndrome**, a serious disease

- gargling with warm double strength tea or warm salt water made by adding 1 tsp of salt to 8 oz (237 ml) of water

- drinking plenty of fluids, but avoiding acid juices like orange juice, which can irritate the throat (sucking on popsicles is a good way to get fluids into children)

- eating soft, nutritious foods like noodle soup and avoiding spicy foods

- refraining from smoking

- resting until the fever is gone, then resuming strenuous activities gradually

- a room humidifier may make sore throat sufferers more comfortable

- antiseptic lozenges and sprays may aggravate the sore throat rather than improve it

Alternative treatment

Alternative treatment focuses on easing the symptoms of sore throat using herbs and botanical medicines.

- Aromatherapists recommend inhaling the fragrances of essential oils of lavender (Lavandula officinalis), thyme (*Thymus vulgaris*), eucalyptus (*Eycalyptus globulus*), sage (*Salvia officinalis*), and sandalwood.

- Ayurvedic practitioners suggest gargling with a mixture of water, salt, and tumeric (*Curcuma longa*) powder or astringents such as alum, sumac, sage, and bayberry (*Myrica* spp.).

- Herbalists recommend taking osha root (*Ligusticum porteri*) internally for infection or drinking ginger (*Zingiber officinale*) or slippery elm (*Ulmus fulva*) tea for pain.

- Homeopaths may treat sore throats with superdilute solutions *Lachesis*, *Belladonna*, *Phytolacca*), yellow jasmine (*Gelsemium*), or mercury.

- Nutritional recommendations include zinc lozenges every two hours along with vitamin C with bioflavonoids, vitamin A, and beta-carotene supplements.

Prognosis

Sore throat caused by a viral infection generally clears up on its own within one week with no complications. The exception is mononucleosis. Ninety percent of cases of mononucleosis clear up without medical intervention or complications, so long as **dehydration** does not occur. In young children the symptoms may last only a week, but in adolescents the symptoms last longer. Adults over age 30 have the most severe and long lasting symptoms. Adults may take up to six months to recover. In all age groups **fatigue** and weakness may continue for up to six weeks after other symptoms disappear.

In rare cases of mononucleosis, breathing may be obstructed because of swollen tonsils, adenoids, and lymph glands. If this happens, the patient should immediately seek emergency medical care.

Patients with bacterial sore throat begin feeling better about 24 hours after starting antibiotics. Untreated strep throat has the potential to cause **scarlet fever**, kidney damage, or **rheumatic fever**. Scarlet fever causes a rash, and can cause high fever and convulsions. Rheumatic fever causes inflammation of the heart and damage to the heart valves. Taking antibiotics within the first week of a strep infection will prevent these complications. People with strep throat remain contagious until after they have been taking antibiotics for 24 hours.

Prevention

There is no way to prevent a sore throat; however, the risk of getting one or passing one on to another person can be minimized by:

KEY TERMS

Antigen—A foreign protein to which the body reacts by making antibodies

Conjunctivitis—An inflammation of the membrane surrounding the eye; also known as pinkeye.

Lymphocyte—A type of white blood cell. Lymphocytes play an important role in fighting disease.

Pharynx—The pharynx is the part of the throat that lies between the mouth and the larynx or voice box.

Toxin—A poison. In the case of scarlet fever, the toxin is secreted as a byproduct of the growth of the streptococcus bacteria and causes a rash.

- washing hands well and frequently

- avoiding close contact with someone who has a sore throat

- not sharing food and eating utensils with anyone

- not smoking

- staying out of polluted air

Resources

BOOKS

Berktow, Robert, editor. *The Merck Manual of Diagnosis and Therapy*. 16th ed. Rahway, NJ: Merck Research Laboratories, 1992.

Tish Davidson, A.M.

Sotalol *see* **Antiarrhythmic drugs**

Sound therapy *see* **Music therapy**

South American blastomycosis

Definition

South American **blastomycosis** is a potentially fatal, chronic fungus infection that occurs more often in men. The infection may affect different parts of the body, including the lungs or the skin, and may cause ulcers of the mouth, voicebox, and nose.

Description

South American blastomycosis occurs primarily in Brazil, although cases crop up in Mexico, Central America, or other parts of South America. It affects men between ages 20 and 50 about 10 times more often than women.

The disease is far more serious than its North American variant (North American blastomycosis), which is endemic to the eastern United States, southern Canada, and the midwest.

South American blastomycosis is known medically as paracoccidioidal granuloma, or paracoccidioidomycosis. The infection has a very long incubation period (at least five years).

Causes and symptoms

South American blastomycosis is caused by the yeast-like fungus *Paracoccidioides brasiliensis* that is acquired by breathing in the spores of the fungus, which is commonly found in old wood and soil. It may appear very similar to **tuberculosis**; in fact, both diseases may infect a patient at the same time.

Symptoms include ulcers in the mouth, larynx and nose, in addition to large, draining lymph nodes, **cough**, chest **pain**, swollen lymph glands, weight loss, and lesions on the skin, genitals, and intestines. There may also be lesions in the liver, spleen, intestines, and adrenal glands.

Diagnosis

A physician can diagnose the condition by microscopic examination of a smear prepared from a lesion or sputum (spit). Biopsy specimens may also reveal the infection. While blood tests are helpful, they can't determine the difference between past and active infection.

Treatment

The primary goal of treatment is to control the infection. The best treatment has been amphotericin B. Sulfonamide drugs have been used and can stop the progress of the infection, but they don't kill the fungus.

Scientists are studying new treatments for the fungal infection, including ketoconazole, fluconazole, and itraconazole, which appear to be equally effective as amphotericin B, according to research.

Prognosis

The disease is chronic and often fatal. Because blastomycosis may be recurrent, patients should continue follow-up care for several years.

Prevention

There is no way to prevent the disease.

Resources

ORGANIZATIONS

National Institute of Allergy and Infectious Disease. Building 31, Room 7A-50, 31 Center Drive MSC 2520, Bethesda, MD 20892-2520. (301) 496-5717. <http://www.niaid.nih.gov/default.htm>.

National Organization for Rare Disorders. P.O. Box 8923, New Fairfield, CT 06812-8923. (800) 999-6673. <http://www.rarediseases.org>.

Carol A. Turkington

Space medicine *see* **Aviation medicine**

Spanish flu *see* **Influenza**

Spastic colitis *see* **Irritable bowel syndrome**

Spastic colon *see* **Irritable bowel syndrome**

Speech disorders

Definition

According to the American Speech-Language-Hearing Association (ASHA), a language disorder is an impairment in comprehension use of the spoken, written, or other symbol system.

Description

Speech disorders affect the language and mechanics, the content of speech, or the function of language in communication. Because speech disorders affect a person's ability to communicate effectively, every aspect of the person's life can be affected, for example, the person's ability to make friends, and to communicate at school or at work.

Amyotrophic lateral sclerosis (ALS)

Amyotrophic lateral sclerosis (ALS), also known as Lou Gehrig's disease, is a neurological disease that attacks the nerve cells in the brain that control voluntary muscles. ALS causes motor neurons to die so that the brain and spinal cord are unable to send messages to the muscles telling them to move. Because the muscles are not functioning, they begin to atrophy. Muscles in the face and jaw can be affected, and thereby affecting a person's speech.

Aphasia

Aphasia results from damage to the language centers of the brain, which affects a person's ability to communicate through speaking, listening, and writing.

Persons with aphasia have trouble with expressive language, what is said, or receptive language, what is understood. Not only are speech and understanding speech affected, but also reading and writing is affected. The severity of aphasia varies from person to person, but in the most severe cases, a person may not be able to understand speech at all. Persons with mild aphasia may only become confused when speech becomes lengthy and complicated.

Developmental apraxia of speech

Developmental **apraxia** is a disorder that affects the nervous system and affects a person's ability to sequence and say sounds, syllables, and words. The brain does not send the correct messages to the mouth and jaw so that the person can say what he or she wants to say.

Children who are suffering from this disorder don't babble as an infant and first words are delayed. Older children may have more difficulty with longer phrases, and may appear to be searching for words to express a thought. Listeners will likely have a difficult time understanding the child.

Laryngeal cancer

Laryngeal cancer is characterized by a malignant growth in the larynx, or the voice box, which sometimes requires removal of the larynx or part of it.

Cancer anywhere in the throat affects speech, swallowing, and chewing. Depending on the size of the growth, a person may have trouble moving the mouth and lips. Therefore, speech sounds and eating will be affected and a person will have trouble communicating.

Orofacial myofunctional disorders

Orofacial myofunctional disorder (OMD) causes the tongue to move forward in an exaggerated manner while a person is speaking or swallowing. The tongue also may protrude when resting in the mouth.

Because heredity contributes to the size and shape of a person's mouth, there may be genetic reasons for the disorder. **Allergies** also affect the mouth and face muscles, which make it difficult to breathe because of nasal congestion. Because a person may sleep with the tongue protruding, lip muscles weaken. Enlarged tonsils also can block airways, creating the same breathing problems. Additionally, thumb-sucking, nail-biting, and teeth-clenching and grinding also can contribute to the disorder.

Stuttering

Stuttering is a disorder of speech fluency that frequently interrupts the flow of speech.

Because children typically stumble and confuse their words as speech develops, stuttering is not immediately evident. It is usually when children become older and continue to stumble that stuttering becomes evident.

Causes and symptoms

Amyotrophic lateral sclerosis (ALS)

Initial symptoms include weakness in any part of the body, and appendages begin to tire easily. Occasionally the disease affects only one appendage rather than both at the same time. Persons with ALS may have trouble maintaining balance and may stumble or have difficulty with tasks that require manual dexterity, such as buttoning a shirt or tying a shoe.

Eventually, the diaphragm and chest wall become so weak that a person cannot breathe on his or her own and needs the help of a ventilator. Because of the lack of muscle strength, a person with ALS will experience difficulty speaking loudly and clearly until the person is unable to speak at all using the vocal cords. The person will have difficulty pronouncing words and have difficulty completing lengthy sentences.

Along with the difficulty in speaking also comes difficulty in chewing and swallowing. Food can be broken down and pureed to make it easier to chew and swallow. However, a person eventually will have difficulty chewing and swallowing foods that are broken down or pureed. When ability to eat is affected, proper **nutrition** and body weight also are affected, and medical professionals may decide that it is best to put in a feeding tube.

Aphasia

Stroke is the most common cause of aphasia, although other injuries, such as a **brain tumor** or gunshot wound, also can cause aphasia.

Developmental apraxia of speech

Developmental apraxia is a disorder that affects the nervous system and affects a person's ability to sequence and say sounds, syllables, and words. The brain does not send the correct messages to the mouth and jaw so that the person can say what he or she wants to say.

Children who are suffering from this disorder don't babble as an infant and first words are delayed. Older children may have more difficulty with longer phrases, and may appear to be searching for words to express a thought. Listeners will likely have a difficult time understanding the child.

There is no known cause for developmental apraxia of speech. Symptoms include weakness of the jaw, tongue, and lips, and delayed speech development. Persons with the disorder also may have trouble identifying an object in the mouth using the sense of touch, which is known as oral-sensory perception.

Laryngeal cancer

Any kind of **smoking** of cigarettes, cigars, or tobacco and alcohol **abuse** contribute to oral cancer, including smokeless tobacco. Persons with laryngeal cancer or another type of oral cancer may have a red or white patch or lump in the mouth. Symptoms also include difficulty chewing, swallowing, or chewing.

Stuttering

There is no known cause for stuttering, although poor muscle coordination and the rate of language development are believed to contribute to it.

Stuttering is characterized by repetition of sounds, syllables, portions of a word, words, and complete phrases; stretching the sounds and syllables; hesitation between words; words spoken in spurts; tense muscles in the jaw and mouth; and a feeling of loss of control.

Diagnosis

Amyotrophic lateral sclerosis (ALS)

About 20,000 people in the United States have ALS at any given time with 5,000 new cases diagnosed every year. ALS is in the same family of disorders as **multiple sclerosis**, Parkinson's disease, and **muscular dystrophy**. Persons of all races and ethic groups are afflicted by the disease, although men are more likely to have it than women.

Aphasia

About 700,000 persons in the United States have strokes every year, and one million are estimated to have aphasia.

Developmental apraxia of speech

A child suspected to have apraxia should first have his or her hearing tested to determine if the child has any deafness. Muscle development in the face and jaw should be evaluated and speech exercises tested. Articulation of words should be tested as well as the person's expressive and receptive language skills.

Laryngeal cancer

It is likely that a dentist or physician will first detect signs of possible cancer. Oral cancer makes up about 2–5% of all cancers, and about 30,000 cases are diagnosed each year. Twice as many men than women are diagnosed with cancer typically between the ages of 50 and 70.

Orofacial myofunctional disorders

The diagnosis of orofacial myofunctional disorder affects speech sounds because of weak tongue tip muscles, although a person's speech may not be affected at all.

Stuttering

Stuttering is a problem that most likely will manifest itself during childhood rather than adulthood.

Treatment

Amyotrophic lateral sclerosis (ALS)

In addition to treatments such as a feeding tube, a person with ALS would likely enlist the help of a speech therapist to help him or her determine ways in which he or she can maintain vocal control. A person also may enlist the help of an occupational therapist, a medical professional trained to help persons who have trouble with activities of daily living such as dressing, bathing, and eating.

Aphasia

A speech-language pathologist can perform drills and exercises with a person that include practice in naming objects and following directions to try to improve skills. The person learns the best way to express himself of herself. **Group therapy** also is an option, which focuses on structured discussions.

Developmental apraxia of speech

Treatment should focus on the coordination of motor movements necessary during speech production, which includes controlling breathing. A speech-language pathologist teaches exercises to a person with apraxia that will strengthen the jaws, lips, and tongue to improve coordination during speech. The therapist uses tactile, auditory, and visual feedback to direct the brain to move the muscles used during speech.

Laryngeal cancer

Depending on when the cancer is first detected, and depending on the size of the cancer, the entire larynx may not need to be removed. Radiation, **chemotherapy**, or partial removal can be done in lieu of complete removal. In these cases, the voice may be preserved although the quality likely will be affected.

Orofacial myofunctional disorders

In cases where speech is affected, a speech pathologist should be consulted to help control breathing problems and work on speech articulation. The lip, palate, tongue, and facial muscles should be evaluated so that errors in speech can be detected. Therapy includes increasing awareness of the mouth and facial muscles, as well as the posture of the mouth and tongue. Muscle **exercise** can be done to increase strength and control.

Stuttering

A treatment plan by a speech therapist includes improving fluency and ease with which a person speaks. Strategies include reducing the rate of speech and using slower speech movements; articulating lightly; and starting air flow for speech before any other muscle movement.

Alternative treatment

Developmental apraxia of speech

Some persons with apraxia may decide to use alternative communication systems, such as a computer that transcribes and "speaks" what a person is directing it to say. These augmentative systems should only be used when a person is so severely impaired that effective speech or communication isn't possible.

Laryngeal cancer

In cases of a full **laryngectomy**, a hole is made in the neck and, rather than using the mouth and nose to talk and breath, the person must use the hole.

Once the larynx is removed, the person needs to develop a new speech system without a voice. A speech pathologist should follow one of three plans: esophageal speech, artificial larynx, or tracheoesophageal puncture (TEP).

- Esophageal speech. Without a larynx, a person is no longer able to exhale air from the lungs through the mouth to speak. Using esophageal speech, the person inhales and traps the air in the throat, causing the esophagus to vibrate and create sound.

- Artificial larynx. A mechanical instrument can be used that produces sound for some speech. These devices can be held against the neck or used by inserting a tube in the mouth.

- Tracheoesophageal puncture. This is a popular method in restoring speech production. During surgery, a hole is made between the trachea and esophagus and a valve is inserted into the hole. The person breathes air into the lungs and then covers the hole in the throat. During exhalation, the esophagus vibrates and creates speech.

Stuttering

A person suffering from stuttering may employ distraction strategies to help him or her stop stuttering. Typically, a person stuttering becomes frustrated and embarrassed; subsequently, encouraging the person to think of something or do something else may break the stuttering cycle.

Prognosis

Amyotrophic lateral sclerosis (ALS)

ALS patients often die of **respiratory failure** within three to five years of being diagnosed, although some persons have been known to survive as many as 10 years or longer.

KEY TERMS

Neurons—Nerve cells in the brain, brain stem, and spinal cord that connect the nervous system and the muscles.

Aphasia

Persons with aphasia can improve and eventually function in more typical public settings, and possibly return to school or work.

Developmental apraxia of speech

With proper treatment, apraxia can be brought under control and the person will be able to function normally as an adult.

Laryngeal cancer

Full removal of the larynx removes the risk of a cancer relapse, although other parts of the throat and mouth can be affected.

Orofacial myofunctional disorders

A person can learn to control this disorder with proper treatment and maintain normal speech and breathing patterns.

Stuttering

With proper speech therapy, stuttering can be controlled or eliminated.

Prevention

Laryngeal cancer

Persons should not engage in smoking or drug abuse to decrease the risk of oral cancer.

Orofacial myofunctional disorders

In cases where the cause is evident, such as allergies or enlarged tonsils, a person should first remedy that problem; perhaps have the tonsils removed and treat allergies with medication.

Resources

BOOKS

Paul, Rhea. *Language Disorders from Infancy through Adolescence*. 2nd ed. St. Louis: Mosby, Inc., 2001.

ORGANIZATIONS

American Speech-Language-Hearing Association. 1801 Rockville Pike, Rockville, MD 20852. (800) 638-8255. < http://www.asha.org >.

Meghan Gourley

Speech disturbance *see* **Aphasia**
Speech therapy *see* **Rehabilitation**
Sperm count *see* **Semen analysis**

Spina bifida

Definition

Spina bifida is a serious birth abnormality in which the spinal cord is malformed and lacks its usual protective skeletal and soft tissue coverings.

Description

Spina bifida may appear in the body midline anywhere from the neck to the buttocks. In its most severe form, termed spinal rachischisis, the entire spinal canal is open, exposing the spinal cord and nerves. More commonly, the abnormality appears as a localized mass on the back that is covered by skin or by the meninges, the three-layered membrane that envelopes the spina cord. Spina bifida is usually readily apparent at birth because of the malformation of the back and **paralysis** below the level of the abnormality.

Various forms of spina bifida are known as meningomyelocele, myelomeningocele, spina bifida aperta, open spina bifida, myelodysplasia, spinal dysraphism, spinal rachischisis, myelocele, and meningocele. The term meningocele is used when the spine malformation contains only the protective covering (meninges) of the spinal cord. The other terms indicate involvement of the spinal cord and nerves in the malformation. A related term, spina bifida occulta, indicates that one or more of the bony bodies in the spine are incompletely hardened, but that there is no abnormality of the spinal cord itself.

Spina bifida occurs worldwide, but there has been a steady downward trend in occurrence rates over the past 50–70 years, particularly in regions of high prevalence. The highest prevalence rates, about one in 200 pregnancies, have been reported from certain northern provinces in China. Intermediate prevalence rates, about one in 1,000 pregnancies, have been found in

Central and South America. The lowest prevalence rates, less than one in 2,000 pregnancies, have been found in the European countries. The highest regional prevalence in the United States of about one in 500 pregnancies has occurred in the Southeast.

Causes and symptoms

Spina bifida may occur as an isolated abnormality or in the company of other malformations. As an isolated abnormality, spina bifida is caused by the combination of genetic factors and environmental influences that bring about malformation of the spine and spinal column. The specific genes and environmental influences that contribute to the many-factored causes of spina bifida are not completely known. An insufficiency of **folic acid** is known to be one influential nutritional factor. Changes (mutations) in genes involving the metabolism of folic acid are believed to be significant genetic risk factors. The recurrence risk after the birth of an infant with isolated spina bifida is 3–5%. Recurrence may be for spina bifida or another type of spinal abnormality.

Spina bifida may arise because of chromosome abnormalities, single gene mutations, or specific environmental insults such as maternal **diabetes mellitus** or prenatal exposure to certain **anticonvulsant drugs**. The recurrence risk varies with each of these specific causes.

In most cases, spina bifida is obvious at birth because of malformation of the spine. The spine may be completely open, exposing the spinal cord and nerves. More commonly, the spine abnormality appears as a mass on the back covered by membrane (meninges) or skin. Spina bifida may occur anywhere from the base of the skull to the buttocks. About 75% of abnormalities occur in the lower back (lumbar) region. In rare instances, the spinal cord malformation may occur internally, sometimes with a connection to the gastrointestinal tract.

In spina bifida, many complications arise, dependent in part on the level and severity of the spine malformation. As a rule, the nerves below the level of the abnormality develop in a faulty manner and fail to function, resulting in paralysis and loss of sensation below the level of the spine malformation. Since most abnormalities occur in the lumbar region, the lower limbs are paralyzed and lack sensation. Furthermore, the bowel and bladder have inadequate nerve connections, causing an inability to control bowel and bladder function. Most infants also develop hydrocephaly, an accumulation of excess fluid in the four cavities of the brain. At least one of every seven cases develop

findings of Chiari II malformation, a condition in which the lower part of the brain is crowded and may be forced into the upper part of the spinal cavity.

There are a number of mild variant forms of spina bifida, including multiple vertebral abnormalities, skin dimples, tufts of hair, and localized areas of skin deficiency over the spine. Two variants, lipomeningocele and lipomyelomeningocele, typically occur in the lower back area (lumbar or sacral) of the spine. In these conditions, a tumor of fatty tissue becomes isolated among the nerves below the spinal cord, which may result in tethering of the spinal cord and complications similar to those with open spina bifida.

Diagnosis

Few disorders are to be confused with open spina bifida. The diagnosis is usually obvious based on the external findings at birth. Paralysis below the level of the abnormality and fluid on the brain (hydrocephaly) may contribute to the diagnosis. Other spine abnormalities such as congenital **scoliosis** and **kyphosis**, or soft tissue tumors overlying the spine, are not likely to have these accompanying findings. In cases in which there are no external findings, the diagnosis is more difficult and may not become evident until neurological abnormalities or hydrocephaly develop weeks, months, or years following birth.

Prenatal diagnosis may be made in most cases with ultrasound examination after 12–14 weeks of **pregnancy**. Many cases are also detected by the testing of the mother's blood for the level of alpha-fetoprotein at about 16 weeks of pregnancy. If the spine malformation is not skin covered, alpha-fetoprotein from the fetus' circulation may leak into the surrounding amniotic fluid, a small portion of which is absorbed into the mother's blood.

Treatment

Aggressive surgical and medical management have improved the survival and function of infants with spina bifida. Initial surgery may be carried out during the first days of life, providing protection against injury and infection. Subsequent surgery is often necessary to protect against excessive curvature of the spine, and in the presence of hydrocephaly, to place a mechanical shunt to decrease the pressure and amount of cerebrospinal fluid in the cavities of the brain. Because of weakness or paralysis below the level of the spine abnormality, most children will require physical therapy, bracing, and other orthopedic assistance to enable them to walk. A variety of

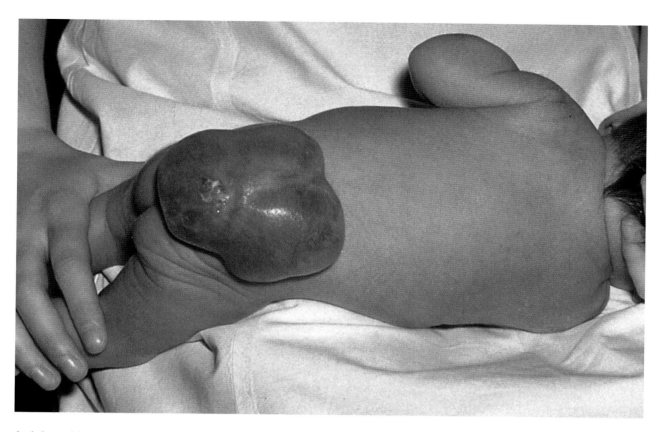

An infant with spina bifida. *(Photograph by Biophoto Associates, Photo Researchers, Inc. Reproduced by permission.)*

approaches including periodic bladder catheterization, surgical diversion of urine, and **antibiotics** are used to protect urinary function.

Although most individuals with spina bifida have normal intellectual function, learning disabilities or **mental retardation** occur in a minority. This may result, in part, from hydrocephaly and/or infections of the nervous system. Children so affected may benefit from early educational intervention, physical therapy, and occupational therapy. Counseling to improve self-image and lessen barriers to socialization becomes important in late childhood and adolescence.

Open fetal surgery has been performed for spina bifida during the last half of pregnancy. After direct closure of the spine malformation, the fetus is returned to the womb. By preventing chronic intrauterine exposure to mechanical and chemical trauma, **prenatal surgery** improves neurological function and leads to fewer complications after birth. Fetal surgery is considered experimental, and results have been mixed.

Prevention of isolated spina bifida and other spinal abnormalities has become possible during recent decades. The major prevention is through the

---

KEY TERMS

Chiari II anomaly—A structural abnormality of the lower portion of the brain (cerebellum and brain stem) associated with spina bifida. The lower structures of the brain are crowded and may be forced into the foramen magnum, the opening through which the brain and spinal cord are connected.

Fetus—The term used to describe a developing human infant from approximately the third month of pregnancy until delivery. The term embryo is used prior to the third month.

Hydrocephalus—The excess accumulation of cerebrospinal fluid around the brain, often causing enlargement of the head.

---

use of a B vitamin, folic acid, for several months prior to and following conception. The Centers for Disease Control and Prevention recommend the intake of 400 micrograms of synthetic folic acid every day for all women of childbearing years.

Prognosis

More than 80% of infants born with spina bifida survive with surgical and medical management. Although complications from paralysis, hydrocephaly, Chiari II malformation, and urinary tract deterioration threaten the well-being of the survivors, the outlook for normal intellectual function is good.

Resources

ORGANIZATIONS

March of Dimes Birth Defects Foundation. 1275 Mamaroneck Ave., White Plains, NY 10605. (888) 663-4637. < http://www.modimes.org >.

National Birth Defects Prevention Network. Atlanta, GA (770) 488-3550. < http://www.nbdpn.org >.

Shriners Hospitals for Children. International Shrine Headquarters, 2900 Rocky Point Dr., Tampa, FL 33607-1460. (813) 281-0300. < http://www.shrinershq.org >.

Spina Bifida Association of America. 4590 MacArthur Blvd. NW, Suite 250, Washington, DC 20007-4226. (800) 621-3141 or (202) 944-3285. Fax: (202) 944-3295.

Roger E. Stevenson

Spina bifida occulta *see* **Spina bifida**

Spinal cord injury

Definition

Spinal cord injury is damage to the spinal cord that causes loss of sensation and motor control.

Description

Approximately 10,000 new spinal cord injuries (SCIs) occur each year in the United States. About 250,000 people are currently affected. Spinal cord injuries can happen to anyone at any time of life. The typical patient, however, is a man between the ages of 19 and 26, injured in a motor vehicle accident (about 50% of all SCIs), a fall (20%), an act of violence (15%), or a sporting accident (14%). Alcohol or other drug **abuse** plays an important role in a large percentage of all spinal cord injuries. Six percent of people who receive injuries to the lower spine die within a year, and 40% of people who receive the more frequent higher injuries die within a year.

Short-term costs for hospitalization, equipment, and home modifications are approximately $140,000 for an SCI patient capable of independent living. Lifetime costs may exceed one million dollars. Costs may be three to four times higher for the SCI patient who needs long-term institutional care. Overall costs to the American economy in direct payments and lost productivity are more than $10 billion per year.

Causes and symptoms

Causes

The spinal cord is about as big around as the index finger. It descends from the brain down the back through hollow channels of the backbone. The spinal cord is made of nerve cells (neurons). The nerve cells carry sensory data from the areas outside the spinal cord (periphery) to the brain, and they carry motor commands from brain to periphery. Peripheral neurons are bundled together to make up the 31 pairs of peripheral nerve roots. The peripheral nerve roots enter and exit the spinal cord by passing through the spaces between the stacked vertebrae. Each pair of nerves is named for the vertebra from which it exits. These are known as:

- C1-8. These nerves enter from the eight cervical or neck vertebrae.
- T1-12. These nerves enter from the thoracic or chest vertebrae.
- L1-5. These nerves enter from the lumbar vertebrae of the lower back.
- S1-5. These nerves enter through the sacral or pelvic vertebrae.
- Coccygeal. These nerves enter through the coccyx or tailbone.

Peripheral nerves carry motor commands to the muscles and internal organs, and they carry sensations from these areas and from the body's surface. (Sensory data from the head, including sight, sound, smell, and taste, do not pass through the spinal cord and are not affected by most SCIs.) Damage to the spinal cord interrupts these signals. The interruption damages motor functions that allow the muscles to move, sensory functions such as feeling heat and cold, and autonomic functions such as urination, sexual function, sweating, and blood pressure.

Spinal cord injuries most often occur where the spine is most flexible, in the regions of C5-C7 of the neck, and T10-L2 at the base of the rib cage. Several physically distinct types of damage are recognized. Sudden and violent jolts to nearby tissues can jar the cord. This jarring causes a temporary spinal **concussion**. Concussion symptoms usually disappear completely within several hours. A spinal contusion or bruise is bleeding within the spinal column. The pressure from the excess fluid may kill spinal cord neurons. Spinal compression is caused by some object, such as a tumor, pressing on the cord. Lacerations or tears cause direct damage to cord neurons. Lacerations can be caused by bone fragments or missiles such as bullets. Spinal transection describes the complete severing of the cord. Most spinal cord injuries involve two or more of these types of damage.

Symptoms

PARALYSIS AND LOSS OF SENSATION. The extent to which movement and sensation are damaged depends on the level of the spinal cord injury. Nerves leaving the spinal cord at different levels control sensation and movement in different parts of the body. The distribution is roughly as follows:

• C1-C4: head and neck.

• C3-C5: diaphragm (chest and breathing).

• C5-T1: shoulders, arms and hands.

• T2-T12: chest and abdomen (excluding internal organs).

• L1-L4: abdomen (excluding internal organs), buttocks, genitals, and upper legs.

• L4-S1: legs.

• S2-S4: genitals and muscles of the perineum.

Damage below T1, which lies at the base of the rib cage, causes **paralysis** and loss of sensation in the legs and trunk below the injury. Injury at this level usually does no damage to the arms and hands. Paralysis of the legs is called paraplegia. Damage above T1 involves the arms as well as the legs. Paralysis of all four limbs is called quadriplegia or tetraplegia. Cervical or neck injuries not only cause quadriplegia but also may cause difficulty in breathing. Damage in the lower part of the neck may leave enough diaphragm control to allow unassisted breathing. Patients with damage at C3 or above, just below the base of the skull, require mechanical assistance to breathe.

Symptoms also depend on the extent of spinal cord injury. A completely severed cord causes paralysis and loss of sensation below the wound. If the cord is only partially severed, some function will remain below the injury. Damage limited to the front portion of the cord causes paralysis and loss of sensations of **pain** and temperature. Other sensation may be preserved. Damage to the center of the cord may spare the legs but paralyze the arms. Damage to the right or left half causes loss of position sense, paralysis on the side of the injury, and loss of pain and temperature sensation on the opposite side.

DEEP VENOUS THROMBOSIS. Blood does not flow normally to a paralyzed limb that is inactive for long periods. The blood pools in the deep veins and forms clots, a condition known as **deep vein thrombosis**. A clot or thrombus can break free and lodge in smaller arteries in the brain, causing a **stroke**, or in the lungs, causing **pulmonary embolism**.

PRESSURE ULCERS. Inability to move also leads to pressure ulcers or bed sores. Pressure ulcers form where skin remains in contact with a bed or chair for a long time. The most common sites of pressure ulcers are the buttocks, hips, and heels.

SPASTICITY AND CONTRACTURE. A paralyzed limb is incapable of active movement, but the muscle still has tone, a constant low level of contraction. Normal muscle tone requires communication between the muscle and the brain. Spinal cord injury prevents the brain from telling the muscle to relax. The result is prolonged muscle contraction or spasticity. Because the muscles that extend and those that bend a joint are not usually equal in strength, the involved joint is bent, often severely. This constant pressure causes deformity. As the muscle remains in the shortened position over several weeks or months, the tendons remodel and cause permanent muscle shortening or contracture. When muscles have permanently shortened, the inner surfaces of joints, such as armpits or palms, cannot be cleaned and the skin breaks down in that area.

HETEROTOPIC OSSIFICATION. Heterotopic ossification is an abnormal deposit of bone in muscles and tendons that may occur after injury. It is most common in the hips and knees. Initially heterotopic ossification causes localized swelling, warmth, redness, and stiffness of the muscle. It usually begins one to four months after the injury and is rare after one year.

AUTONOMIC DYSREFLEXIA. Body organs that regulate themselves, such as the heart, gastrointestinal tract, and glands, are controlled by groups of nerves called autonomic nerves. Autonomic nerves emerge from three different places: above the spinal column, in the lower back from vertebrae T1-L4, and from the lowest regions of the sacrum at the base of the spine. In general, these three groups of autonomic nerves operate in balance. Spinal cord injury can disrupt this balance, a condition called autonomic dysreflexia or autonomic hyperreflexia. Patients with injuries at T6 or above are at greatest risk.

In autonomic dysreflexia, irritation of the skin, bowel, or bladder causes a highly exaggerated

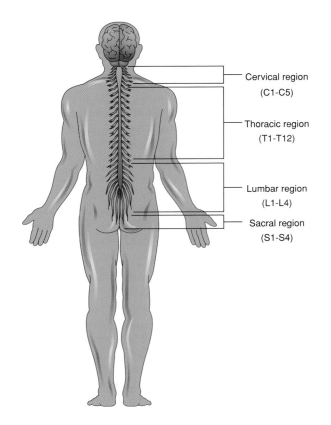

Cervical region
(C1-C5)

Thoracic region
(T1-T12)

Lumbar region
(L1-L4)

Sacral region
(S1-S4)

The extent of sensory and motor loss resulting from a spinal cord injury depends on the level of the injury because nerves at different levels control sensation and movement in different parts of the body. The distribution is as follows: C1-C4: head and neck; C3-C5: diaphragm; C5-T1: shoulders, arms, and hands; T2-T12: chest and abdomen (excluding internal organs); L1-L4: abdomen (excluding internal organs), buttocks, genitals, upper legs; L4-S3: legs; S2-S4: genitals, muscles of the perineum. (*Illustration by Electronic Illustrators Group.*)

response from autonomic nerves. This response is caused by the uncontrolled release of norepinephrine, a hormone similar to adrenaline. Uncontrolled release of norepinephrine causes a rapid rise in blood pressure and a slowing of the heart rate. These symptoms are accompanied by throbbing **headache**, **nausea**, **anxiety**, sweating, and goose bumps below the level of the injury. The elevated blood pressure can rapidly cause loss of consciousness, seizures, cerebral hemorrhage, and **death**. Autonomic dysreflexia is most often caused by an over-full bladder or bladder infection, impaction or hard impassable fecal mass in the bowel, or skin irritation from tight clothing, **sunburn**, or other irritant. Inability to sense these irritants before the autonomic reaction begins is a major cause of dysreflexia.

LOSS OF BLADDER AND BOWEL CONTROL. Bladder and bowel control require both motor nerves and the autonomic nervous system. Both of these systems may be damaged by SCI. When the autonomic nervous system triggers an urge to urinate or defecate, continence is maintained by contracting the anal or urethral sphincters. A sphincter is a ring of muscle that contracts to close off a passage or opening in the body. When the neural connections to these muscles are severed, conscious control is lost. In addition, loss of feeling may prevent sensations of fullness from reaching the brain. To compensate, the patient may help empty the bowel or bladder by using physical maneuvers that stimulate autonomic contractions before they would otherwise begin. However, the patient may not be able to relax the sphincters. If the sphincters cannot be relaxed, the patient will retain urine or feces.

Retention of urine may cause muscular changes in the bladder and urethral sphincter that make the problem worse. Urinary tract infection is common. Retention of feces can cause impaction. Symptoms of impaction include loss of appetite and nausea. Untreated impaction may cause perforation of the large intestine and rapid overwhelming infection.

SEXUAL DYSFUNCTION. Men who have sustained SCI may be unable to achieve an erection or ejaculate. Sperm formation may be abnormal too, reducing fertility. Fertility and the ability to achieve orgasm are less impaired for women. Women may still be able to become pregnant and deliver vaginally with proper medical care.

Diagnosis

The location and extent of spinal cord injury is determined with **computed tomography scans** (CT scans), **magnetic resonance imaging** (MRI) scans, and x rays. X rays may be enhanced with an injected contrast dye.

Treatment

A person who may have a spinal cord injury should not be moved. Treatment of SCI begins with **immobilization**. This strategy prevents partial injuries of the cord from severing it completely. Use of splints to completely immobilize suspected SCI at the scene of the injury has helped reduce the severity of spinal cord injuries in the last two decades. Intravenous methylprednisone, a steroidal anti-inflammatory drug, is given during the first 24 hours to reduce inflammation and tissue destruction.

Rehabilitation after spinal cord injury seeks to prevent complications, promote recovery, and make the most of remaining function. Rehabilitation is a complex and long-term process. It requires a team of professionals, including a neurologist, physiatrist or rehabilitation specialist, physical therapist, and occupational therapist. Other specialists who may be needed include a respiratory therapist, vocational rehabilitation counselor, social worker, speech-language pathologist, nutritionist, special education teacher, recreation therapist, and clinical psychologist. Support groups provide a critical source of information, advice, and support for SCI patients.

Paralysis and loss of sensation

Some limited mobility and sensation may be recovered, but the extent and speed of this recovery cannot be predicted. Experimental electrical stimulation has been shown to allow some control of muscle contraction in paraplegia. This experimental technique offers the possibility of unaided walking. Further development of current control systems will be needed before useful movement is possible outside the laboratory.

The physical therapist focuses on mobility, to maintain range of motion of affected limbs and reduce contracture and deformity. Physical therapy helps compensate for lost skills by using those muscles that are still functional. It also helps to increase any residual strength and control in affected muscles. A physical therapist suggests adaptive equipment such as braces, canes, or wheelchairs.

An occupational therapist works to restore ability to perform the activities of daily living, such as eating and grooming, with tools and new techniques. The occupational therapist also designs modifications of the home and workplace to match the individual impairment.

A pulmonologist or respiratory therapist promotes airway hygiene through instruction in assisted coughing techniques and postural drainage. The respiratory professional also prescribes and provides instruction in the use of ventilators, facial or nasal masks, and tracheostomy equipment where necessary.

Pressure ulcers

Pressure ulcers are prevented by turning in bed at least every two hours. The patient should be turned more frequently when redness begins to develop in sensitive areas. Special mattresses and chair cushions can distribute weight more evenly to reduce pressure.

Electrical stimulation is sometimes used to promote muscle movement to prevent pressure ulcers.

Spasticity and contracture

Range of motion (ROM) exercises help to prevent contracture. Chemicals can be used to prevent **contractures** from becoming fixed when ROM **exercise** is inadequate. Phenol or alcohol can be injected onto the nerve or botulinum toxin directly into the muscle. Botulinum toxin is associated with fewer complications, but it is more expensive than phenol and alcohol. Contractures can be released by cutting the shortened tendon or transferring it surgically to a different site on the bone where its pull will not cause as much deformity. Such tendon transfers may also be used to increase strength in partially functional extremities.

Heterotopic ossification

Etidronate disodium (Didronel), a drug that regulates the body's use of calcium, is used to prevent heterotopic ossification. Treatment begins three weeks after the injury and continues for 12 weeks. Surgical removal of ossified tissue is possible.

Autonomic dysreflexia

Autonomic dysreflexia is prevented by bowel and bladder care and attention to potential irritants. It is treated by prompt removal of the irritant. Drugs to lower blood pressure are used when necessary. People with SCI should educate friends and family members about the symptoms and treatment of dysreflexia, because immediate attention is necessary.

Loss of bladder and bowel control

Normal bowel function is promoted through adequate fluid intake and a diet rich in fiber. Evacuation is stimulated by deliberately increasing the abdominal pressure, either voluntarily or by using an abdominal binder.

Bladder care involves continual or intermittent catheterization. The full bladder may be detected by feeling its bulge against the abdominal wall. Urinary tract infection is a significant complication of catheterization and requires frequent monitoring.

Sexual dysfunction

Counseling can help in adjusting to changes in sexual function after spinal cord injury. Erection may be enhanced through the same means used to treat **erectile dysfunction** in the general population.

KEY TERMS

Autonomic nervous system—The part of the nervous system that controls involuntary functions such as sweating and blood pressure.

Botulinum toxin—Any of a group of potent bacterial toxins or poisons produced by different strains of the bacterium *Clostridium botulinum*.

Computed tomography (CT)—An imaging technique in which cross-sectional x rays of the body are compiled to create a three-dimensional image of the body's internal structures.

Magnetic resonance imaging (MRI)—An imaging technique that uses a large circular magnet and radio waves to generate signals from atoms in the body. These signals are used to construct images of internal structures.

Motor—Of or pertaining to motion, the body apparatus involved in movement, or the brain functions that direct purposeful activity.

Motor nerve—Motor or efferent nerve cells carry impulses from the brain to muscle or organ tissue.

Peripheral nervous system—The part of the nervous system that is outside the brain and spinal cord. Sensory, motor, and autonomic nerves are included.

Postural drainage—The use of positioning to drain secretions from the bronchial tubes and lungs into the trachea or windpipe.

Range of motion (ROM)—The range of motion of a joint from full extension to full flexion (bending) measured in degrees like a circle.

Sensory nerves—Sensory or afferent nerves carry impulses of sensation from the periphery or outward parts of the body to the brain. Sensations include feelings, impressions, and awareness of the state of the body.

Voluntary—An action or thought undertaken or controlled by a person's free will or choice.

Prognosis

The prognosis of SCI depends on the location and extent of injury. Injuries of the neck above C4 with significant involvement of the diaphragm hold the gravest prognosis. Respiratory infection is one of the leading causes of death in long-term SCI. Overall, 85% of SCI patients who survive the first 24 hours are alive 10 years after their injuries. Recovery of function is impossible to predict. Partial recovery is more likely after an incomplete wound than after the spinal cord has been completely severed.

Prevention

Risk of spinal cord injury can be reduced through prevention of the accidents that lead to it. Chances of injury from automobile accidents, the major cause of SCIs, can be significantly reduced by driving at safe speeds, avoiding alcohol while driving, and using seat belts.

Resources

ORGANIZATIONS

National Spinal Cord Injury Association. 8300 Colesville Road, Silver Spring, Maryland 20910. (301) 588-6959. < http://www.erols.com/nscia >.

Richard Robinson

Spinal cord tumors

Definition

A spinal cord tumor is a benign or cancerous growth in the spinal cord, between the membranes covering the spinal cord, or in the spinal canal. A tumor in this location can compress the spinal cord or its nerve roots; therefore, even a noncancerous growth can be disabling unless properly treated.

Description

The spinal cord contains bundles of nerves that carry messages between the brain and the body. Because the spinal cord is rigidly encased in bone, any tumor that grows on or near it can compress the nerves, and interfere in this communication. About 10,000 Americans develop spinal cord tumors each year, and about 40% of these are cancerous. Similar to brain tumors, spinal cord growths are rare.

Newly formed tumors that begin within the spinal cord are unusual, especially among children and the elderly. More typically, tumors originate elsewhere in the body and move through the bloodstream (metastasize) to the spinal cord.

Causes and symptoms

Scientists don't know what causes these tumors, although the noncancerous growths may be hereditary or present since birth.

When the tumor presses on the spinal cord, it causes symptoms including;

- back **pain**
- severe or burning pain in other parts of the body
- numbness or cold
- progressive loss of muscle strength or sensation in the legs
- loss of bladder or bowel control

A tumor in the top of the spinal column can cause pain radiating from the arms or neck; a tumor in the lower spine may cause leg or back pain. If there are several tumors in different areas of the spinal cord at the same time, it may cause symptoms in a variety of spots on the body.

Diagnosis

Suspected spinal cord compression, by tumor, is a medical emergency. Prompt intervention may prevent **paralysis**.

If a neurological exam and review of symptoms suggest a spinal cord tumor, the doctor may order some of these additional tests:

- MRI or CT scan
- myelography
- blood and spinal fluid studies
- x rays of the spine
- biopsy
- radionuclide bone scan

Treatment

If the tumor is malignant and has metastasized, treatment depends on the type of the primary **cancer**. Surgery is usually the first step in treating benign and malignant tumors outside the spinal cord. Tumors inside the spinal cord may not be able to be completely removed with surgery. If they can not be, radiation and **chemotherapy** treatments may be effective. Treatment also may include pain relievers and cortisone drugs to lessen swelling around the tumor, and ease pressure on the spinal cord.

KEY TERMS

Computed tomography scans (CT Scan)—The CT scan combines an X-ray with a computer to create a detailed picture of the spinal cord. It may help to determine the type of tumor, locate swelling or bleeding, and check results of treatment.

Magnetic resonance imaging (MRI) — MRI is an imaging technique that uses a magnetic field to scan the body's tissues and structures. It gives a better picture of tumors located near bone than does a CT scan, without the risk of radiation, and can provide a three-dimensional image of the tumor.

Myelogram—A myelogram is an x ray exam of the spinal cord, nerves and other tissues within the spinal cord that are highlighted by injected contrast dye.

Prognosis

Early diagnosis and treatment can produce a higher success rate. Long-term survival also depends on the tumor's type, location, and size. Surgery to remove the bone around the cord can ease pressure on the spinal nerves and nerve pathways, which will usually ease pain and other symptoms; however, it may make walking more difficult. Physical therapy and **rehabilitation** may help.

Prevention

Since spinal cord tumors usually are the result of a cancer that has first appeared elsewhere in the body, early detection of cancer in other organs may prevent spinal cord tumors. Lifestyle changes, as stopping **smoking**, to lower the risk of the development of other types of cancer, may also help.

Resources

ORGANIZATIONS

National Institute of Neurological Disorders and Stroke. P.O. Box 5801, Bethesda, MD 20824. (800) 352-9424. < http://www.ninds.nih.gov/index.htm >.

Carol A. Turkington

Spinal fluid analysis *see* **Cerebrospinal fluid (CSF) analysis**

Spinal fusion *see* **Disk removal**

Spinal instrumentation

Definition

Spinal instrumentation is a method of straightening and stabilizing the spine after spinal fusion, by surgically attaching hooks, rods, and wire to the spine in a way that redistributes the stresses on the bones and keeps them in proper alignment.

Purpose

Spinal instrumentation is used to treat instability and deformity of the spine. Instability occurs when the spine no longer maintains its normal shape during movement. Such instability results in nerve damage, spinal deformities, and disabling **pain**. Spinal deformities may be caused by:

- birth defects
- fractures
- marfan syndrome
- neurofibromatosis
- neuromuscular diseases
- severe injuries
- tumors

Curvature of the spine (**scoliosis**) is usually treated with spinal fusion and spinal instrumentation. Scoliosis is a disorder of unknown origin. It causes bending and twisting of the spine that eventually results in distortion of the chest and back. About 85% of cases occur in girls between the ages of 12 and 15, who are experiencing adolescent growth spurt.

Spinal instrumentation serves three purposes. It provides a stable, rigid column that encourages bones to fuse after spinal-fusion surgery. Second, it redirects the stresses over a wider area. Third, it restores the spine to its proper alignment.

Different types of spinal instrumentation are used to treat different spinal problems. Several common types of spinal instrumentation are explained below. Although the details of the insertion of rods, wires, and hooks varies, the purpose of all spinal instrumentation is the same—to correct and stabilize the backbone.

Harrington rod

The Harrington Rod is one of the oldest and most proven forms of spinal instrumentation. It is used to straighten and stabilize the spine when curvature is greater than 60 degrees. It is an appropriate treatment for scoliosis.

Advantages of the Harrington rod are its relative simplicity of installation, the low rate of complications, and a proven record of reducing curvature of the spine. The main disadvantage is that the patient must remain in a body cast for about six months, then wear a brace for another three to six months while the bone fusion solidifies.

Luque rod

Luque rods are custom contoured metal rods that are fixed to each segment (vertebra) in the affected part of the spine. The main advantage is that the patient may not need to wear a cast or brace after the procedure. The main disadvantage is that the risk of injury to the nerves and spinal cord is higher than with a some other forms of instrumentation. This is because wires must be threaded through each vertebra near the spinal column, increasing the risk of such damage. Luque rods are sometimes used to treat scoliosis.

Drummond instrumentation

Drummond instrumentation, also called Harri-Drummond instrumentation, uses a Harrington rod on the concave side of the spine and a Luque rod on the convex side. The advantage is that each vertebra segment is fixed, with the risk of nerve injury decreased over Luque rod instrumentation. The disadvantage is that, like Harrington rod instrumentation, the patient must wear a cast and a brace after surgery.

Cotrel-Dubousset instrumentation

Cotrel-Dubousset instrumentation uses hooks and rods in a cross-linked pattern to realign the spine and redistribute the biomechanical **stress**. The main advantage of Cotrel-Dubousset instrumentation is that, because of the extensive cross-linking, the patient may have to wear a cast or brace after surgery. The disadvantage is the complexity of the operation and the number of hooks and cross-links that may fail.

Zeilke instrumentation

Zeilke instrumentation is similar to Cotrel-Dubousset instrumentation, but is used to treat double curvature of the spine. It requires wearing a brace for many months after surgery.

Other forms of instrumentation

The Kaneda device is used to treat fractured thoracic or lumbar vertebrae when it is suspected that bone fragments are present in the spinal canal. Variations on the basic forms of spinal instrumentation, such as Wisconsin instrumentation, are being refined as technology improves. A physician chooses the proper type of instrumentation based on the type of disorder, the age and health of the patient, and on the physician's experience.

Precautions

Since the hooks and rods of spinal instrumentation are anchored in the bones of the back, spinal instrumentation should not be performed on people with serious **osteoporosis**. To overcome this limitation, techniques are being explored that help anchor instrumentation in fragile bones.

Description

Spinal instrumentation is performed by a neuro and/or orthopedic surgical team with special experience in spinal operations. The surgery is done in a hospital under **general anesthesia**. It is done at the same time as spinal fusion.

The surgeon strips the muscles away from the area to be fused. The surface of the bone is peeled away. A piece of bone is removed from the hip and placed along side the area to be fused. The stripping of the bone helps the bone graft to fuse.

After the fusion site is prepared, the rods, hooks, and wires are inserted. There is some variation in how this is done based on the spinal instrumentation chosen. In general, Harrington rods are the simplest instrumentation to install, and Cotrel-Dubousset instrumentation is the most complex and risky. Once the rods are in place, the incision is closed.

Preparation

Spinal fusion with spinal instrumentation is major surgery. The patient will undergo many tests to determine that nature and exact location of the back problem. These tests are likely to include x rays, **magnetic resonance imaging** (MRI), **computed tomography scans** (CT scans), and myleograms. In addition, the patient will undergo a battery of blood and urine tests, and possibly an electrocardiogram to provide the surgeon and anesthesiologist with information that will allow the operation to be performed safely. In Harrington rod instrumentation, the patient may be placed in **traction** or an upper body cast to stretch contracted muscles before surgery.

> ## KEY TERMS
>
> **Lumbar vertebrae**—The vertebrae of the lower back below the level of the ribs.
>
> **Marfan syndrome**—A rare hereditary defect that affects the connective tissue.
>
> **Neurofibromatosis**—A rare hereditary disease that involves the growth of lesions that may affect the spinal cord.
>
> **Osteoporosis**—A bone disorder, usually seen in the elderly, in which the boned become increasingly less dense and more brittle.
>
> **Spinal fusion**—An operation in which the bones of the lower spine are permanently joined together using a bone graft obtained usually from the hip.
>
> **Thoracic vertebrae**—The vertebrae in the chest region to which the ribs attach.

Aftercare

After surgery, the patient will be confined to bed. A catheter is inserted so that the patient can urinate without getting up. Vital signs are monitored, and the patient's position is changed frequently so that **bedsores** do not develop.

Recovery from spinal instrumentation can be a long, arduous process. Movement is severely limited for a period of time. In certain types of instrumentation, the patient is put in a cast to allow the realigned bones to stay in position until healing takes place. This can be as long as six to eight months. Many patients will need to wear a brace after the cast is removed.

During the recovery period, the patient is taught respiratory exercises to help maintain respiratory function during the time of limited mobility. Physical therapists assist the patient in learning self-care and in performing strengthening and range of motion exercises. Length of hospital stay depends on the age and health of the patient, as well as the specific problem that was corrected. The patient can expect to remain under a physician's care for many months.

Risks

Spinal instrumentation carries a significant risk of nerve damage and **paralysis**. The skill of the surgeon can affect the outcome of the operation, so patients should look for a hospital and surgical team that has a lot of experience doing spinal procedures.

After surgery there is a risk of infection or an inflammatory reaction due to the presence of the foreign material in the body. Serious infection of the membranes covering the spinal cord and brain can occur. In the long-term, the instrumentation may move or break, causing nerve damage and requiring a second surgery. Some bone grafts do not heal well, lengthening the time the patient must spend in a cast or brace, or necessitating additional surgery. Casting and wearing a brace may take an emotional toll, especially on young people. Patients who have had spinal instrumentation must avoid contact sports, and, for the rest of their lives, eliminate situations that will abnormally put stress on their spines.

Normal results

Many young people with scoliosis heal with significantly improved alignment of the spine. Results of spinal instrumentation done for other conditions vary widely.

Resources

ORGANIZATIONS

National Scoliosis Foundation. 5 Cabot Place, Stoughton, MA 020724. (800) 673-6922. < http:// www.scoliosis.org >.

OTHER

Orthogate. < http://owl.orthogate.org/ >.

Tish Davidson, A.M.

Spinal meningitis *see* **Meningitis**

Spinal stenosis

Definition

Spinal stenosis is any narrowing of the spinal canal that causes compression of the spinal nerve cord. Spinal stenosis causes **pain** and may cause loss of some body functions.

Description

Spinal stenosis is a progressive narrowing of the opening in the spinal canal. The spine is a long series of bones called vertebrae. Between each pair of vertebra is a fibrous intervertebral disk. Collectively, the vertebrae and disks are called the backbone. Each vertebra has a hole through it. These holes line up to form the spinal canal. A large bundle of nerves called the spinal cord runs through the spinal canal. This bundle of 31 nerves carries messages between the brain and the various parts of the body. At each vertebra, some smaller nerves branch out from these nerve roots to serve the muscles and tissue in the immediate area. When the spinal canal narrows, nerve roots in the spinal cord are squeezed. Pressure on the nerve roots causes chronic pain and loss of control over some functions because communication with the brain is interrupted. The lower back and legs are most affected by spinal stenosis. The nerve roots that supply the legs are near the bottom of the spinal cord. The pain gets worse after standing for a long time and after some forms of **exercise**. The posture required by these physical activities increases the **stress** on the nerve roots. Spinal stenosis usually affects people over 50 years of age. Women have the condition more frequently than men do.

Cervical spinal stenosis is a narrowing of the vertebrae of the neck (cervical vertebrae). The disease and its effects are similar to stenosis in the lower spine. A narrower opening in the cervical vertebrae can also put pressure on arteries entering the spinal column, cutting off the blood supply to the remainder of the spinal cord.

Causes and symptoms

Spinal stenosis causes pain in the buttocks, thigh, and calf and increasing weakness in the legs. The patient may also have difficulty controlling bladder and bowel functions. The pain of spinal stenosis seems more severe when the patient walks downhill. Spinal stenosis can be congenital, acquired, or a combination. Congenital spinal stenosis is a birth defect. Acquired spinal stenosis develops after birth. It is usually a consequence of tissue destruction (degeneration) caused by an infectious disease or a disease in which the immune system attacks the body's own cells (autoimmune disease). The two most common causes of spinal stenosis are birth defect and progressive degeneration of the tissue of the joints (**osteoarthritis**). Other causes include improper alignment of the vertebrae as in spondylolisthesis, destruction of bone tissue as in Paget's disease, or an overgrowth of bone tissue as in diffuse idiopathic skeletal hyperostosis. The spinal canal is usually more than 0.5 in (12 mm) in diameter. A smaller diameter indicates stenosis. The diameter of the cervical spine ranges is 0.6–1 in (15–12 mm). Any opening under 0.5 in (13 mm)in diameter is considered evidence of stenosis. Acquired spinal stenosis usually begins with degeneration of the intervertebral disks or the surfaces of the vertebrae or both. In trying to heal this degeneration, the body builds up the spinal column. In the process, the spinal canal can become narrower.

Diagnosis

The physician must determine that the symptoms are caused by spinal stenosis. Conditions that can cause similar symptoms include a slipped (herniated) intervertebral disk, spinal tumors, and disorders of the blood flow (circulatory disorders). Spinal stenosis causes back and leg pain. The leg pain is usually worse when the patient is standing or walking. Some forms of spinal stenosis are less painful when the patient is riding an exercise bike because the forward tilt of the body changes the pressure in the spinal column. Doppler scanning can trace the flow of blood to determine whether the pain is caused by circulatory problems. X-ray images, **computed tomography scans** (CT scans), and **magnetic resonance imaging** (MRI) scans can reveal any narrowing of the spinal canal. **Electromyography**, nerve conduction velocity, or **evoked potential studies** can locate problems in the muscles indicating areas of spinal cord compression.

Treatment

Mild cases of spinal stenosis may be treated with rest, **nonsteroidal anti-inflammatory drugs** (such as **aspirin**), and **muscle relaxants**. Spinal stenosis can be a progressive disease, however, and the source of pressure may have to be surgically removed (surgical decompression) if the patient is losing control over bladder and bowel functions. The surgical procedure removes bone and other tissues that have entered the spinal canal or put pressure on the spinal cord. Two vertebrae may be fused, to eliminate improper alignment, such as that caused by spondylolisthesis. For surgery, patients lie on their sides or in a modified kneeling position. This position reduces bleeding and places the spine in proper alignment. Alignment is especially important if vertebrae are to be fused. Surgical decompression can eliminate leg pain and restore control of the legs, bladder, and bowels, but usually does not eliminate lower back pain. Physical therapy and massage can help reduce the symptoms of spinal stenosis. An exercise program should be developed to increase flexibility and mobility. A brace or corset may be worn to improve posture. Activities that place stress on the lower back muscles should be avoided.

Prognosis

Surgical decompression does not stop the degenerative processes that cause spinal stenosis, and the condition can develop again. Nevertheless, most

---

KEY TERMS

Computed tomography (CT) Scans—An imaging technique in which cross-sectional x rays of the body are compiled to create a three-dimensional image of the body's internal structures.

Congenital—Present before birth. The term is used to describe disorders that developed in the fetal stage.

Doppler scanning—A procedure in which ultrasound images are used to watch a moving structure such as the flow of blood or the beating of the heart.

Electromyography—A test that uses electrodes to record the electrical activity of muscle. The information gathered is used to find disorders of the nerves that serve the muscles.

Evoked potential—A test of nerve response that uses electrodes placed on the scalp to measure brain reaction to a stimulus such as a touch.

Magnetic resonance imaging (MRI)—An imaging technique that uses a large circular magnet and radio waves to generate signals from atoms in the body. These signals are used to construct images of internal structures.

Nerve conduction velocity test—A test that measures the time it takes a nerve impulse to travel a specific distance over the nerve after electronic stimulation.

Stenosis—The narrowing or constriction of a channel or opening.

---

patients achieve good results with surgical decompression. The patient will probably continue to have lower back pain after the surgical procedure.

Resources

BOOKS

Berkow, Robert, editor. *Merck Manual of Medical Information.* Whitehouse Station, NJ: Merck Research Laboratories, 2004.

John T. Lohr, PhD

Spinal tap *see* **Cerebrospinal fluid (CSF) analysis**

Spirometry *see* **Pulmonary function test**

Spleen, enlarged *see* **Hypersplenism**

Spleen removal *see* **Splenectomy**

Splenectomy

Definition

Splenectomy is the surgical removal of the spleen, which is an organ that is part of the lymphatic system. The spleen is a dark-purple, bean-shaped organ located in the upper left side of the abdomen, just behind the bottom of the rib cage. In adults, the spleen is about 4.8 X 2.8 X 1.6 in (12 X 7 X 4 cm) in size, and weighs about 4–5 oz (113–14 zg). Its functions include a role in the immune system; filtering foreign substances from the blood; removing worn-out blood cells from the blood; regulating blood flow to the liver; and sometimes storing blood cells. The storage of blood cells is called sequestration. In healthy adults, about 30% of blood platelets are sequestered in the spleen.

Purpose

Splenectomies are performed for a variety of different reasons and with different degrees of urgency. Most splenectomies are done after the patient has been diagnosed with **hypersplenism**. Hypersplenism is not a specific disease but a group of symptoms, or syndrome, that can be produced by a number of different disorders. It is characterized by enlargement of the spleen (splenomegaly), defects in the blood cells, and an abnormally high turnover of blood cells. It is almost always associated with splenomegaly caused by specific disorders such as **cirrhosis** of the liver or certain cancers. The decision to perform a splenectomy depends on the severity and prognosis of the disease that is causing the hypersplenism.

Splenectomy always necessary

There are two diseases for which splenectomy is the only treatment—primary cancers of the spleen and a blood disorder called hereditary spherocytosis (HS). In HS, the absence of a specific protein in the red blood cell membrane leads to the formation of relatively fragile cells that are easily damaged when they pass through the spleen. The cell destruction does not occur elsewhere in the body and ends when the spleen is removed. HS can appear at any age, even in newborns, although doctors prefer to put off removing the spleen until the child is five or six years old.

Splenectomy usually necessary

There are some disorders in which splenectomy is usually recommended. They include:

- Immune (idiopathic) thrombocytopenic purpura (ITP). ITP is a disease involving platelet destruction.

Splenectomy has been regarded as the definitive treatment for this disease and is effective in about 70% of chronic ITP cases. More recently, however, the introduction of new drugs in the treatment of ITP has reopened the question as to whether splenectomy is always the best treatment option.

- Trauma. The spleen can be ruptured by blunt as well as penetrating injuries to the chest or abdomen. Car accidents are the most common cause of blunt traumatic injury to the spleen.

- Abscesses in the spleen. These are relatively uncommon but have a high mortality rate.

- Rupture of the splenic artery. Rupture sometimes occurs as a complication of pregnancy.

- Hereditary elliptocytosis. This is a relatively rare disorder. It is similar to HS in that it is characterized by red blood cells with defective membranes that are destroyed by the spleen.

Splenectomy sometimes necessary

In other disorders, the spleen may or may not be removed.

- Hodgkin's disease, a serious form of **cancer** that causes lymph nodes to enlarge. Splenectomy is often performed in order to find out how far the disease has progressed.

- Thrombotic thrombocytopenic purpura (TTP). TTP is a rare disorder marked by **fever**, kidney failure, and an abnormal decrease in the number of platelets. Splenectomy is one part of treatment for TTP.

- Autoimmune hemolytic disorders. These disorders may appear in patients of any age but are most common in patients over 50. The red blood cells are destroyed by antibodies produced by the patient's own body (autoantibodies).

- **Myelofibrosis**. Myelofibrosis is a disorder in which bone marrow is replaced by fibrous tissue. It produces severe and painful splenomegaly. Splenectomy does not cure myelofibrosis but may be performed to relieve **pain** caused by the swollen spleen.

- **Thalassemia**. Thalassemia is a hereditary form of anemia that is most common in people of Mediterranean origin. Splenectomy is sometimes performed if the patient's spleen has become painfully enlarged.

Precautions

Patients should be carefully assessed regarding the need for a splenectomy. Because of the spleen's role in protecting people against infection, it should not be removed unless necessary. The operation is relatively safe for young and middle-aged adults. Older adults, especially those with cardiac or pulmonary disease, are more vulnerable to post-surgical infections. Thromboembolism following splenectomy is another complication for this patient group, which has about 10% mortality following the surgery. Splenectomies are performed in children only when the benefits outweigh the risks.

The most important part of the assessment is the measurement of splenomegaly. The normal spleen cannot be felt when the doctor examines the patient's abdomen. A spleen that is large enough to be felt indicates splenomegaly. In some cases the doctor will hear a dull sound when he or she thumps (percusses) the patient's abdomen near the ribs on the left side. Imaging studies that can be used to demonstrate splenomegaly include ultrasound tests, technetium-99m sulfur colloid imaging, and CT scans. The rate of platelet or red blood cell destruction by the spleen can be measured by tagging blood cells with radioactive chromium or platelets with radioactive indium.

Description

Complete splenectomy

REMOVAL OF ENLARGED SPLEEN. Splenectomy is performed under **general anesthesia**. The most common technique is used to remove greatly enlarged spleens. After the surgeon makes a cut (incision) in the abdomen, the artery to the spleen is tied to prevent blood loss and reduce the spleen's size. It also helps prevent further sequestration of blood cells. The surgeon detaches the ligaments holding the spleen in place and removes it. In many cases, tissue samples will be sent to a laboratory for analysis.

REMOVAL OF RUPTURED SPLEEN. When the spleen has been ruptured by trauma, the surgeon approaches the organ from its underside and fastens the splenic artery.

In some cases, the doctor may prefer conservative (nonsurgical) management of a ruptured spleen, most often when the patient's blood pressure is stable and there are no signs of other abdominal injuries. In the case of multiple abdominal trauma, however, the spleen is usually removed.

Partial splenectomy

In some cases the surgeon removes only part of the spleen. This procedure is considered by some to be a useful compromise that reduces pain from an enlarged spleen while leaving the patient less vulnerable to infection. Long-term follow-up of the results of partial splenectomies has not yet been done.

Laparoscopic splenectomy

Laparoscopic splenectomy, or removal of the spleen through several small incisions, has been more frequently used in recent years. Laparoscopic surgery involves the use of surgical instruments, with the assistance of a tiny camera and video monitor. Laparoscopic procedures reduce the length of hospital stay, the level of post-operative pain, and the risk of infection. They also leave smaller **scars**. Laparoscopic splenectomy is not, however, the best option for many patients.

Laparoscopic splenectomy is gaining increased acceptance in the early 2000s as an alternative to open splenectomy for a wide variety of disorders, although splenomegaly still presents an obstacle to laparoscopic splenectomy; massive splenomegaly has been considered a contraindication. In patients with enlarged spleens, however, laparoscopic splenectomy is associated with less morbidity, decreased **transfusion** rates, and shorter hospital stays than when the open approach is used. Patients with enlarged spleens usually have more severe hematologic diseases related to greater morbidity; therefore, laparoscopic splenectomy has potential advantages.

The most frequent serious complication following laparoscopic splenectomy is damage to the pancreas. Application of a hydrogel sealant to the pancreas during surgery, however, appears to significantly reduce the risk of leakage from the pancreas.

Splenic embolization

Splenic embolization is an alternative to splenectomy that is used in some patients who are poor surgical risks. Embolization involves plugging or blocking the splenic artery to shrink the size of the spleen. The substances that are injected during this procedure include polyvinyl alcohol foam, polystyrene, and silicone. Embolization is a technique that needs further study and refinement.

Preparation

Preoperative preparation for nonemergency splenectomy includes:

- Correction of abnormalities of blood clotting and the number of red blood cells.

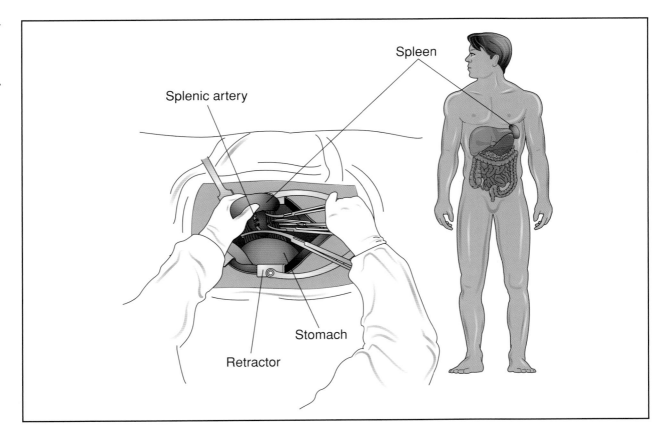

Spleen

Splenic artery

Stomach

Retractor

Splenectomy is the surgical removal of the spleen. This procedure is performed as a last result in most diseases involving the spleen. In some cases, however, splenectomy does not address the underlying causes of splenomegaly or other conditions affecting the spleen. *(Illustration by Electronic Illustrators Group.)*

- Treatment of any infections.
- Control of immune reactions. Patients are usually given protective vaccinations about a month before surgery. The most common vaccines used are Pneumovax or Pnu-Imune 23 (against pneumococcal infections) and Menomune-A/C/Y/W-135 (against meningococcal infections).

Aftercare

Immediately following surgery, patients should follow the physician's instructions and take all medications intended to prevent infection. Blood transfusions may be indicated for some patients to replace defective blood cells. The most important part of aftercare, however, is long-term caution regarding vulnerability to infection. Patients should see their doctor at once if they have a fever or any other sign of infection, and avoid travel to areas where exposure to **malaria** or similar diseases is likely. Children with splenectomies may be kept on antibiotic therapy until they are 16 years old. All patients can be given a booster dose of pneumococcal vaccine five to 10 years after splenectomy.

Risks

The chief risk following splenectomy is over-whelming bacterial infection, or postsplenectomy **sepsis**. This vulnerability results from the body's decreased ability to clear bacteria from the blood, and lowered levels of a protein in blood plasma that helps to fight viruses (immunoglobulin M). The risk of dying from infection after splenectomy is highest in children, especially in the first two years after surgery. The risk of postsplenectomy sepsis can be reduced by vaccinations before the operation. Some doctors also recommend a two-year course of penicillin following splenectomy or long-term treatment with ampicillin.

Other risks following splenectomy include inflammation of the pancreas and collapse of the lungs. In some cases, splenectomy does not address the underlying causes of splenomegaly or other conditions. Excessive bleeding after the operation is an additional

KEY TERMS

Embolization—An alternative to splenectomy that involves injecting silicone or similar substances into the splenic artery to shrink the size of the spleen.

Hereditary spherocytosis (HS)—A blood disorder in which the red blood cells are relatively fragile and are damaged or destroyed when they pass through the spleen. Splenectomy is the only treatment for HS.

Hypersplenism—A syndrome marked by enlargement of the spleen, defects in one or more types of blood cells, and a high turnover of blood cells.

Immune or idiopathic thrombocytopenic purpura (ITP)—A blood disease that results in destruction of platelets, which are blood cells involved in clotting.

Laparoscope—An instrument used to view the abdominal cavity through a small incision and perform surgery on a small area, such as the spleen.

Pneumovax—A vaccine that is given to splenectomy patients to protect them against bacterial infections. Other vaccines include Pnu-Imune and Menomune.

Sepsis—A generalized infection of the body, most often caused by bacteria.

Sequestration—A process in which the spleen withdraws some normal blood cells from circulation and holds them in case the body needs extra blood in an emergency. In hypersplenism, the spleen sequesters too many blood cells.

Splenomegaly—Abnormal enlargement of the spleen.

Thromboembolism—A clot in the blood that forms and blocks a blood vessel. It can lead to infarction, or death of the surrounding tissue due to lack of blood supply.

possible complication, particularly for ITP patients. Infection immediately following surgery may also occur.

Normal results

Results depend on the reason for the operation. In blood disorders, the splenectomy will remove the cause of the blood cell destruction. Normal results for patients with an enlarged spleen are relief of pain and of the complications of splenomegaly. It is not always possible, however, to predict which patients will respond well or to what degree.

Resources

BOOKS

Beers, Mark H., MD, and Robert Berkow, MD., editors. "Disorders of the Spleen." Section 11, Chapter 141 In *The Merck Manual of Diagnosis and Therapy.* Whitehouse Station, NJ: Merck Research Laboratories, 2004.

Wilkins, Bridget S., and Dennis H. Wright. *Illustrated Pathology of the Spleen.* Cambridge, UK:Cambridge University Press, 2000.

PERIODICALS

Balague, C., E. M. Targarona, G. Cerdan, et al. "Long-Term Outcome after Laparoscopic Splenectomy Related to Hematologic Diagnosis." *Surgical Endoscopy* 18 (August 2004): 1283–1287.)

Bemelman, W. A., et al. "Hand-assisted Laparoscopic Splenectomy." *Surgical Endoscopy* 14, no. 11 (November 2000): 997–8.

Bjerke, H. Scott, MD, and Janet S. Bjerke, MSN. "Splenic Rupture." *eMedicine* June 19, 2002. < http://www.e-medicine.com/med/topic2792.htm > .

Bolton-Maggs, P. H., R. F. Stevens, N. J. Dodd, et al. "Guidelines for the Diagnosis and Management of Hereditary Spherocytosis." *British Journal of Haematology* 126 (August 2004): 455–474.

Brigden, M.L. "Detection, Education and Management of the Asplenic or Hyposplenic Patient." *American Family Physician* 63, no. 3: 499–506, 508.

Kahn, M. J., and K. R. McCrae. "Splenectomy in Immune Thrombocytopenic Purpura: Recent Controversies and Long-term Outcomes." *Current Hematology Reports* 3 (September 2004): 317–323.

Lo, A., A. M. Matheson, and D. Adams. "Impact of Concomitant Trauma in the Management of Blunt Splenic Injuries." *New Zealand Medical Journal* 117 (September 10, 2004): U1052.

Rosen, M., R. M. Walsh, and J. R. Goldblum. "Application of a New Collagen-Based Sealant for the Treatment of Pancreatic Injury." *Surgical Laparoscopy, Endoscopy and Percutaneous Techniques* 14 (August 2004): 181–185.

ORGANIZATIONS

Leukaemia Research Fund. 43 Great Ormond Street, London, WC1N 3JJ. (020) 7405-0101. < http://dspace.dial.pipex.com/lrf-// > .

National Heart, Lung and Blood Institute. P.O. Box 30105, Bethesda, MD 20824-0105. (301) 251-1222. < http://www.nhlbi.nih.gov > .

OTHER

"Laparoscopic Splenectomy." *Foxhall Surgical Page.* < http://www.foxhall.com/lap_sple.htm > .

Non-emergency Surgery Hotline. (800) 638-6833.

Teresa Odle
Rebecca J. Frey, PhD

Splenic trauma

Definition

Splenic trauma is physical injury to the spleen, the lymphatic organ located in the upper left side of the abdomen just under the rib cage. The spleen weighs between 75 and 150 grams (between 0.16 and 0.33 pounds) in adults.

Description

The spleen is an organ that produces white blood cells, filters the blood (10–15% of the total blood supply every minute), stores red blood cells and platelets, and destroys those that are **aging**. It is located near the stomach on the left side of the abdomen. A direct blow to the abdomen may bruise, tear or shatter the spleen. Trauma to the spleen can cause varying degrees of damage, the major problem associated with internal bleeding. Mild splenic subcapsular hematomas are injuries in which bleeding is limited to small areas on and immediately around the spleen. Splenic contusions refer to bruising and bleeding on and around larger areas of the spleen. Lacerations (tears) are the most common splenic trauma injuries. Tears tend to occur on the areas between the three main blood vessels of the spleen. Because of the abundant blood supply, splenic trauma may cause serious internal bleeding. Most injuries to the spleen in children heal spontaneously. Severe trauma can cause the spleen or its blood vessels to rupture or fragment.

Splenic trauma is more common in children than in adults. In general, children are prone to abdominal injuries due to accidents and falls and because their abdominal organs are less protected by bone, muscle and fat. Abdominal injuries including splenic trauma are the most common cause of preventable deaths in children.

Causes and symptoms

The most common cause of injury to the spleen is blunt abdominal trauma. Blunt trauma is often caused by a direct blow to the belly, car and motorcycle accidents, falls, sports mishaps, and fights. The spleen is the most commonly injured organ in blunt abdominal trauma; splenic injury occurs in nearly 25% of injuries of this type. Penetrating injuries such as those from stabbing, gunshot **wounds**, and accidental impaling also account for cases of splenic trauma, although far less frequently than blunt trauma.

In adults, ruptured spleens may have been preceded by conditions causing rapid splenic enlargement, such as infections, particularly those caused by the Epstein-Barr virus (EBV); **cancer**; immune system disorders; diseases of the spleen; or circulatory problems. In a very few cases the spleen may be injured by a spell of violent coughing. This type of rupture is known as an atraumatic rupture.

A spleen that has become enlarged and fragile from disease is sometimes ruptured by a doctor or medical student in the course of palpating (feeling) the patient's abdomen, or damaged by a surgeon in the course of an operation on other abdominal organs.

Damage to the spleen may cause localized or general abdominal **pain**, tenderness, and swelling. Fractured ribs may be present. Splenic trauma may cause mild or severe internal bleeding, leading to **shock** and for which symptoms include rapid heartbeat, **shortness of breath**, thirst, pale or clammy skin, weak pulse, low blood pressure, **dizziness**, **fainting**, sweating. **Vomiting** blood, blood in the stools or urine, deterioration of vital signs, and loss of consciousness are other symptoms.

Diagnosis

The goal of diagnosis of all abdominal traumas is to detect and treat life-threatening injuries as quickly as possible. The physician will determine the extent of organ damage and whether surgery will be necessary while providing appropriate emergency care. Initial diagnosis consists of detailing all circumstances of the injury from the patient and bystanders as well as the close **physical examination** of the patient and measurement of vital signs. Blood tests, **urinalysis**, stool samples and x rays of the chest and abdomen are usually performed. Plain x rays may show abdominal air pockets that indicate internal ruptures, but are rarely helpful because they do not show splenic and intra-abdominal damage.

Several other diagnostic tests may be used for the noninvasive and accurate assessment of splenic damage: **computed tomography scans** (CT), of **magnetic resonance imaging** (MRI), radionuclide scanning, and ultrasonography. Ultrasonography—particularly focused abdominal sonographic technique (FAST)—has now become a standard bedside technique in many hospitals to check for bleeding in the abdomen. Imaging tests allow doctors to determine the necessity and type of surgery required. The CT scan has been shown to be the most available and accurate test for abdominal trauma. MRI tests are accurate but costly and less available in some hospitals, while radionuclide scanning requires more time and patient stability. Peritoneal lavage is another diagnostic technique in which the abdominal cavity is entered and flushed to check for bleeding. When patients exhibit shock, infection, or prolonged internal bleeding, exploratory **laparoscopy** is used for emergency diagnosis.

Treatment

Not long ago nearly all cases of splenic trauma were treated by laparoscopy, opening the abdomen, and by **splenectomy**, the surgical removal of the spleen. This approach resulted from the difficulty in assessing the severity of the injury, the potential dangers of shock and **death**, and the beliefs that the spleen healed poorly and that it was not an important organ. Nowadays, improved techniques of diagnosis and monitoring (particularly the introduction of CT scans), as well as understanding that removal of the spleen creates future risk of a lowered capacity to fight infection has modified treatment approaches. Research over the past two decades has shown that the spleen has high healing potential, and confirmed that children are more susceptible to infection after splenectomy (post splenectomy **sepsis**, PSS). PSS has a mortality rate of over 50% and standard procedure now avoids splenectomy as much as possible. Adult splenic trauma is treated by splenectomy more often than children's; for unknown reasons, the adult spleen more frequently spontaneously ruptures after injury. Adults are also less susceptible to PSS.

Nonoperative treatment

In nonoperative therapy, splenic trauma patients are monitored closely, often in intensive care units for several days. Fluid and blood levels are observed and maintained by intravenous fluid and possible blood transfusions. Follow-up scans may be used to observe the healing process.

Operative treatment

Splenic trauma patients require surgery when nonoperative treatment fails, when major or prolonged internal bleeding exists and for gunshot and many stab wounds. Whenever possible, surgeons try to preserve at least part of the spleen and try to repair its blood vessels.

Prognosis

The ample blood supply to the spleen can promote rapid healing. Studies have shown that intra-abdominal bleeding associated with splenic trauma stops without surgical intervention in up to two out of three cases in children. When trauma patients stabilize

---

KEY TERMS

Computed tomography (CT) scan—Computer-aided x-ray examination that allows cross-sectional views of organs and tissues.

Laparoscope—An optical or fiberoptic instrument that is inserted by incision in the abdominal wall and is used to view the interior of the peritoneal cavity.

Laparoscopy—Procedure using a laparoscope to view organs, obtain tissue samples and perform surgery.

Magnetic resonance imaging (MRI)—Imaging technique using magnets and radio waves to provide internal pictures of the body.

Radionuclide scanning—Diagnostic test in which a radioactive dye is injected into the bloodstream and photographed to display internal vessels, organs and tissues.

Ultrasonography—Imaging test using sound waves to view internal organs and tissues.

---

during nonoperative therapy, chances are high that surgery will be avoided and that spleen injuries will heal themselves. Splenic trauma patients undergoing diagnostic tests such as CT and MRI scans have improved chances of avoiding splenectomy and retaining whole or partial spleens.

Resources

BOOKS

Beers, Mark H., MD, and Robert Berkow, MD., editors. "Splenic Rupture." Section 11, Chapter 141 In *The Merck Manual of Diagnosis and Therapy*. Whitehouse Station, NJ: Merck Research Laboratories, 2004.

PERIODICALS

Bjerke, H. Scott, MD, and Janet S. Bjerke, MSN. "Splenic Rupture." *eMedicine* June 19, 2002. < http://www.e-medicine.com/med/topic2792.htm >.

Dixon, E., J. S. Graham, R. Sutherland, and P. C. Mitchell. "Splenic Injury Following Endoscopic Retrograde Cholangiopancreatography: A Case Report and Review of the Literature." *Journal of the Society of Laparoendoscopic Surgeons* 8 (July-September 2004): 275–277.

Kara, E., Y. Kaya, R. Zeybek, et al. "A Case of a Diaphragmatic Rupture Complicated with Lacerations of Stomach and Spleen Caused by a Violent Cough Presenting with Mediastinal Shift." *Annals of the Academy of Medicine, Singapore* 33 (September 2004): 649–650.

Laseter, T., and T. McReynolds. "Spontaneous Splenic Rupture." *Military Medicine* 169 (August 2004): 673–674.

ORGANIZATIONS

American Trauma Society. 8903 Presidential Pkwy Suite 512, Upper Marlboro, MD 20227. (800) 556-7890. <http://www.amtrauma.org>.

OTHER

American Association for the Surgery of Trauma home page. <http://www.aast.org>.

Douglas Dupler, MA
Rebecca J. Frey, PhD

Split personality *see* **Multiple personality disorder**

Spontaneous abortion *see* **Miscarriage**

Sporothrix schenckii infection *see* **Sporotrichosis**

Sporotrichosis

Definition

Sporotrichosis is a chronic infection caused by the microscopic fungus *Sporothrix schenckii*. The disease causes ulcers on the skin that are painless but do not heal, as well as nodules or knots in the lymph channels near the surface of the body. Infrequently, sporotrichosis affects the lungs, joints, or central nervous system and can cause serious illness.

Description

The fungus that causes sporotrichosis is found in spagnum moss, soil, and rotting vegetation. Anyone can get sporotrichosis, but it is most common among nursery workers, farm laborers, and gardeners handling spagnum moss, roses, or barberry bushes. Cases have also been reported in workers whose jobs took them under houses into crawl spaces contaminated with the fungus. Children who played on baled hay have also gotten the disease. Sporotrichosis is sometimes called spagnum moss disease or alcoholic rose gardener's disease.

Causes and symptoms

The fungus causing sporotrichosis enters the body through scratches or cuts in the skin.

Therefore, people who handle plants with sharp thorns or needles, like roses, barberry, or pines, are more likely to get sporotrichosis. Sporotrichosis is not passed directly from person to person, so it is not possible to catch sporotrichosis from another person who has it.

The first signs of sporotrichosis are painless pink, red, or purple bumps usually on the finger, hand, or arm where the fungus entered the body. These bumps may appear anywhere from one to 12 weeks after infection, but usually appear within three weeks. Unlike many other fungal infections sporotrichosis does not cause **fever** or any feelings of general ill health.

The reddish bumps eventually expand and fester, creating skin ulcers that do not heal. In addition, the infection often moves to nearby lymph nodes. Although most cases of sporotrichosis are limited to the skin and lymph channels, occasionally the joints, lungs, and central nervous system become infected. In rare cases, **death** may result.

People who have weakened immune systems, either from a disease such as acquired immune deficiency syndrome (**AIDS**) or leukemia, or as the result of medications they take (**corticosteroids**, **chemotherapy** drugs), are more likely to get sporotrichosis and are more at risk for the disease to spread to the internal organs. Alcoholics and people with **diabetes mellitus** or a pre-existing lung disease are also more likely to become infected. Although sporotrichosis is painless, it is important for people with symptoms to see a doctor and receive treatment.

Diagnosis

The preferred way to diagnose sporotrichosis is for a doctor to obtain a sample of fluid from a freshly opened sore and send it to a laboratory to be cultured. The procedure is fast and painless. It is possible to confirm the presence of advanced sporotrichosis through a blood test or a biopsy. Doctors may also take a blood sample to perform tests that rule out other fungal infections or diseases such as **tuberculosis** or bacterial **osteomyelitis**.

Dermatologists and doctors who work with AIDS patients are more likely to have experience in diagnosing sporotrichosis. In at least one state, New York, the laboratory test to confirm this disease is provided free through the state health department. In other cases, diagnosis should be covered by health insurance at the same level as other diagnostic laboratory tests.

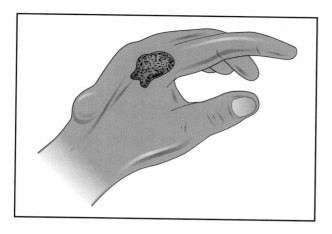

Sporotrichosis is a chronic infection caused by the microscopic fungus *Sporothrix schenckii*. It produces ulcers on the skin that are painless but do not heal, and nodules or knots in the lymph channels near the surface of the body. *(Illustration by Electronic Illustrators Group.)*

Treatment

When sporotrichosis is limited to the skin and lymph system, it is usually treated with a saturated solution of potassium iodine that the patient dilutes with water or juice and drinks several times a day. The iodine solution can only be prescribed by a physician. This treatment must be continued for many weeks. Skin ulcers should be treated like any open wound and covered with a clean bandage to prevent a secondary bacterial infection. The drug itraconazol (Sporanox), taken orally, is also available to treat sporotrichosis.

In serious cases of sporotrichosis, when the internal organs are infected, the preferred treatment is the drug amphotericin B. Amphotericin B is a strong anti-fungal drug with potentially severe toxic side effects. It is given intravenously, so hospitalization is required for treatment. The patient may also receive other drugs to minimize the side effects of the amphotericin B.

Alternative treatment

Alternative treatment for fungal infections focuses on maintaining general good health and eating a diet low in dairy products, sugars, including honey and fruit juice, and foods, such as beer, that contain yeast. This is complemented by a diet high in raw food. Supplements of and **vitamins** C, E, and A, B complex, and pantothenic acid may also be added to the diet, as may *Lactobacillus acidophilus*, bifidobacteria, and garlic capsules.

Fungicidal herbs such as myrrh (*Commiphora molmol*), tea tree oil (*Melaleuca* spp.), citrus seed extract, pau d'arco tea, and garlic (*Allium sativum*) may also be applied directly to the infected skin.

Prognosis

Most cases of sporotrichosis are confined to the skin and lymph system. With treatment, skin sores begin healing in one to two months, but complete recovery often takes six months or more. People who have AIDS are also more likely to have the fungus spread throughout the body, causing a life-threatening infection. In people whose bones and joints are infected or who have pulmonary lesions, surgery may be necessary.

Prevention

Since an opening in the skin is necessary for the sporotrichosis fungus to enter the body, the best way to prevent the disease is to avoid accidental scrapes and cuts on the hands and arms by wearing gloves and long sleeves while gardening. Washing hands and arms well after working with roses, barberry, spagnum moss, and other potential sources of the fungus may also provide some protection.

Resources

PERIODICALS

Dillon, Gary P., et. al. "Handyperson's Hazard: Crawl Space Sporotrichosis." *The Journal of the American Medical Association* 274 (December 6, 1995): 1673+.

Tish Davidson, A.M.

Sports injuries

Definition

Sports injuries result from acute trauma or repetitive **stress** associated with athletic activities. Sports injuries can affect bones or soft tissue (ligaments, muscles, tendons).

Professional dancers are increasingly recognized as performing athletes, and many of the treatments and preventive measures utilized in sports medicine are now applied to dance-related injuries.

It is also important to remember that many types of injuries that affect athletes may also occur in workers in certain occupations; for example, many people in the building trades develop **tennis elbow** or golfer's elbow. The principles of sports medicine can be applied in the treatment of most common musculoskeletal injuries.

Description

Adults are less likely to suffer sports injuries than children, whose vulnerability is heightened by immature reflexes, an inability to recognize and evaluate risks, and underdeveloped coordination.

In 2002, about 20.3 million Americans suffered a sports injury. Of those, 53% were minor enough to be self-treated or left untreated. However, about 10 million Americans annually receive medical attention for their sports-related injuries. That equates to almost 26 per 1,000 people. The highest rate is among children age five to 14 years old (59.3 per 1,000 people). As many as 20% of children who play sports get hurt, and about 25% of their injuries are classified as serious. Boys aged 12 to 17 are the highest risk group. More than 775,000 boys and girls under age 14 are treated in hospital emergency rooms for sports-related injuries.

Injury rates are highest for athletes who participate in contact sports, but the most serious injuries are associated with individual activities. Between one-half and two-thirds of childhood sports injuries occur during practice, or in the course of unorganized athletic activity.

Baseball and softball are the leading causes of sports-related facial trauma in the United States, with 68% of these injuries caused by contact with the ball rather than player-player collision or being hit by a swung bat.

Types of sports injuries

About 95% of sports injuries are minor soft tissue traumas.

The most common sports injury is a bruise (contusion). It is caused when blood collects at the site of an injury and discolors the skin.

Sprains account for one-third of all sports injuries. A sprain is a partial or complete tear of a ligament, a strong band of tissue that connects bones to one another and stabilizes joints.

A strain is a partial or complete tear of:

- muscle (tissue composed of cells that enable the body to move)
- tendon (strong connective tissue that links muscles to bones)

Inflammation of a tendon (**tendinitis**) and inflammation of one of the fluid-filled sacs that allow tendons to move easily over bones (**bursitis**) usually result from minor stresses that repeatedly aggravate the same part of the body. These conditions often occur at the same time.

SKELETAL INJURIES. **Fractures** account for 5–6% of all sports injuries. The bones of the arms and legs are most apt to be broken. Sports activities rarely involve fractures of the spine or skull. The bones of the legs and feet are most susceptible to stress fractures, which occur when muscle **strains** or contractions make bones bend. Stress fractures are especially common in ballet dancers, long-distance runners, and in people whose bones are thin.

Shin splints are characterized by soreness and slight swelling of the front, inside, and back of the lower leg, and by sharp **pain** that develops while exercising and gradually intensifies. Shin splints are caused by overuse or by stress fractures that result from the repeated foot pounding associated with activities such as aerobics, long-distance running, basketball, and volleyball.

A compartment syndrome is a potentially debilitating condition in which the muscles of the lower leg grow too large to be contained within membranes that enclose them. This condition is characterized by **numbness and tingling**. Untreated compartment syndrome can result in long-term loss of function.

BRAIN INJURIES. Brain injury is the primary cause of fatal sports-related injuries. **Concussion**, which is also called mild traumatic brain injury or MTBI, can result from even minor blows to the head. A concussion can cause loss of consciousness and may affect:

- balance
- comprehension
- coordination
- hearing

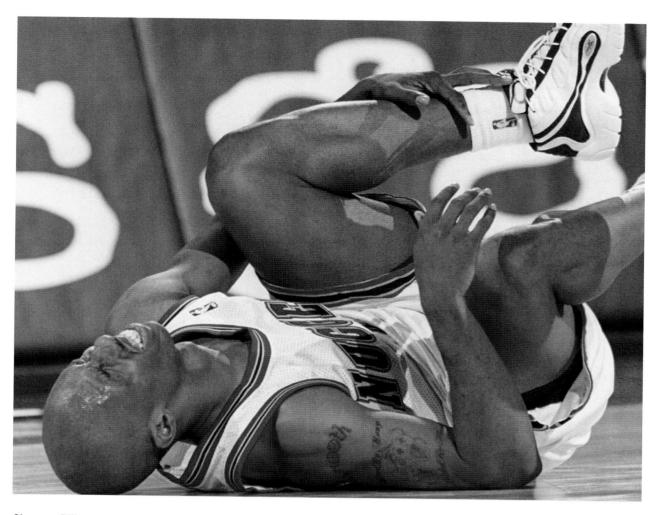

Chauncy Billups, a guard for the Denver Nuggets, grimaces after spraining his ankle during a game. *(AP/Wide World Photos. Reproduced by permission.)*

- memory
- vision
- swelling
- weakness

Causes and symptoms

Common causes of sports injuries include:

- athletic equipment that malfunctions or is used incorrectly
- falls
- forceful high-speed collisions between players
- wear and tear on areas of the body that are continually subjected to stress

Symptoms include:

- instability or obvious dislocation of a joint
- pain

Diagnosis

Symptoms that persist, intensify, or reduce the athlete's ability to play without pain should be evaluated by an orthopedic surgeon. Prompt diagnosis often can prevent minor injuries from becoming major problems, or causing long-term damage.

An orthopedic surgeon should examine anyone:

- who is prevented from playing by severe pain associated with acute injury
- whose ability to play has declined due to chronic or long-term consequences of an injury
- whose injury has caused visible deformities in an arm or leg.

The physician will perform a **physical examination**, ask how the injury occurred, and what symptoms the patient has experienced. X rays and other imaging studies of bones and soft tissues may be ordered.

Anyone who has suffered a blow to the head should be examined immediately, and at five-minute intervals until normal comprehension has returned. The initial examination measures the athlete's:

- awareness
- concentration
- short-term memory

Subsequent evaluations of concussion assess:

- dizziness
- headache
- nausea
- visual disturbances

Treatment

Treatment for minor soft tissue injuries generally consists of:

- compressing the injured area with an elastic bandage
- elevation
- ice
- rest.

Anti-inflammatories, taken by mouth or injected into the swelling, may be used to treat bursitis. Anti-inflammatory medications and exercises to correct muscle imbalances usually are used to treat tendinitis. If the athlete keeps stressing inflamed tendons, they may rupture, and casting or surgery is sometimes necessary to correct this condition.

Orthopedic surgery may be required to repair serious **sprains and strains**.

Controlling inflammation as well as restoring normal use and mobility are the goals of treatment for overuse injuries.

Athletes who have been injured are usually advised to limit their activities until their injuries are healed. The physician may suggest special exercises or behavior modifications for athletes who have had several injuries. Athletes who have been severely injured may be advised to stop playing altogether.

Prevention

Every child who plans to participate in organized athletic activity should have a pre-season sports physical. This special examination is performed by a pediatrician or family physician who:

- carefully evaluates the site of any previous injury
- may recommend special stretching and strengthening exercises to help growing athletes create and preserve proper muscle and joint interaction
- pays special attention to the cardiovascular and skeletal systems.

Telling the physician which sport the athlete plays will help that physician determine which parts of the body will be subjected to the most stress. The physician then will be able to suggest to the athlete steps to take to minimize the chance of getting hurt.

Other injury-reducing game plans include:

- being in shape
- knowing and obeying the rules that regulate the activity
- not playing when tired, ill, or in pain
- not using steroids, which can improve athletic performance but cause life-threatening problems
- taking good care of athletic equipment and using it properly
- wearing appropriate protective equipment

On a larger scale, sports injuries are becoming a public health concern in America. Prevention efforts include wearing protective devices (such as bicycle helmets and pads when skating or skateboarding), and educating both children and adults about safety. Other preventive efforts include changes in the rules of the game or sport to minimize injuries. For example, wearing goggles will be mandatory in women's lacrosse as of 2005 in order to reverse the rising rate of eye and other facial injuries in that sport. Research also continues on improving equipment. For example, thick rubber insoles can help prevent against repetitive injuries from running, but scientists recently observed that they can add to injuries in sports such as soccer, where athletes need to make quick changes of direction. On the other hand, recent improvements in the design and construction of football helmets have been credited with a significant decline in the frequency and severity of head injuries among football players.

Resources

BOOKS

Beers, Mark H., MD, and Robert Berkow, MD., editors. "Common Sports Injuries." Section 5, Chapter 62 In *The Merck Manual of Diagnosis and Therapy*. Whitehouse Station, NJ: Merck Research Laboratories, 2004.

PERIODICALS

Bak, M. J., and T. D. Doerr. "Craniomaxillofacial Fractures during Recreational Baseball and Softball." *Journal of Oral and Maxillofacial Surgery* 62 (October 2004): 1209–1212.

Bernhardt, David T., MD. "Concussion." *eMedicine* July 6, 2004. < http://www.emedicine.com/sports/topic27htm >.

Chaudry, Samena. "Insoles Help Prevent Sports Injuries.." *Student BMJ* May 2003: 137.

Conne, J.M., J.L. Annest, and J. Gilchrist. "Sports and Recreation Related Injury Episodes in the U.S. Population." *Injury Prevention* June 2003: 117.

Koutedakis, Y., and A. Jamurtas. "The Dancer as a Performing Athlete: Physiological Considerations." *Sports Medicine* 34, no. 10 (2004): 651–661.

Levy, M. L., B. M. Ozgur, C. Berry, et al. "Analysis and Evolution of Head Injury in Football." *Neurosurgery* 55 (September 2004): 649–655.

Matz, S. O., and G. Nibbelink. "Injuries in Intercollegiate Women's Lacrosse." *American Journal of Sports Medicine* 32 (April-May 2004): 608–611.

Rupp, Timothy J., MD, Marian Bednar, MD, and Stephen Karageanes, DO. "Facial Fractures." *eMedicine* August 29, 2004. < http://www.emedicine.com/sports/topic33.htm >.

ORGANIZATIONS

American Academy of Orthopedic Surgeons. 6300 North River Road, Rosemont, IL 60018-4262. (800) 346-2267. < http://www.aaos.org >.

American Academy of Otolaryngology—Head and Neck Surgery. One Prince Street, Alexandria, VA 22314-3357. (703) 836-4444. < http://www.entnet.org >.

American College of Sports Medicine (ACSM). 401 West Michigan Street, Indianapolis, IN 46202-3233. (317) 637-9200. Fax: (317) 634-7817. < http://www.acsm.org >.

Institute for Preventative Sports Medicine. P.O. Box 7032, Ann Arbor, MI 48107 (313) 434-3390. < http://www.ipsm.org >.

Maureen Haggerty
Teresa G. Odle
Rebecca J. Frey, PhD

Sports vision *see* **Vision training**

Spouse abuse *see* **Abuse**

Sprains and strains

Definition

Sprain refers to damage or tearing of ligaments or a joint capsule. Strain refers to damage or tearing of a muscle.

Description

When excessive force is applied to a joint, the ligaments that hold the bones together may be torn or damaged. This results in a sprain, and its seriousness depends on how badly the ligaments are torn. Any joint can be sprained, but the most frequently injured joints are the ankle, knee, and finger.

Strains are tears in the muscle. Sometimes called pulled muscles, they usually occur because of overexertion or improper lifting techniques. Sprains and strains are common. Anyone can have them.

Children under age eight are less likely to have sprains than are older people. Childrens' ligaments are tighter, and their bones are more apt to break before a ligament tears. People who are active in sports suffer more strains and sprains than less active people. Repeated sprains in the same joint make the joint less stable and more prone to future sprains.

Causes and symptoms

There are three grades of sprains. Grade I sprains are mild injuries where there is no tearing of the ligament, and no joint function is lost, although there may be tenderness and slight swelling.

Grade II sprains are caused by a partial tear in the ligament. These sprains are characterized by obvious swelling, extensive bruising, **pain**, difficulty bearing weight, and reduced function of the joint.

Grade III, or third degree, sprains are caused by complete tearing of the ligament where there is severe pain, loss of joint function, widespread swelling and bruising, and the inability to bear weight. These symptoms are similar to those of bone **fractures**.

Strains can range from mild muscle stiffness to great soreness. Strains result from overuse of muscles, improper use of the muscles, or as the result of injury in another part of the body when the body compensates for pain by altering the way it moves.

Diagnosis

Grade I sprains and mild strains are usually self-diagnosed. Grade II and III sprains are often seen by a physician, who x rays the area to differentiate between a sprain and a fracture.

Treatment

Grade I sprains and mild strains can be treated at home. Basic first aid for sprains consists of RICE: Rest, Ice for 48 hours, Compression (wrapping in an elastic bandage), and Elevation of the sprain above the level of the heart. Over-the-counter pain medication such as **acetaminophen** (Tylenol) or ibuprofen (Motrin) can be taken for pain.

In addition to RICE, people with grade II and grade III sprains in the ankle or knee usually need to use crutches until the sprains have healed enough to bear weight. Sometimes, physical therapy or home exercises are needed to restore the strength and flexibility of the joint.

Grade III sprains are usually immobilized in a cast for several weeks to see if the sprain heals. Pain medication is prescribed. Surgery may be necessary to relieve pain and restore function. Athletic people under age 40 are the most likely candidates for surgery, especially with grade III knee sprains. For complete healing, physical therapy usually will follow surgery.

Alternative treatment

Alternative practitioners endorse RICE and conventional treatments. In addition, nutritional therapists recommend vitamin C and bioflavonoids to supplement a diet high in whole grains, fresh fruits, and vegetables. Anti-inflammatories, such as bromelain (a proteolytic enzyme from pineapples) and tumeric (*Curcuma longa*), may also be helpful. The homeopathic remedy arnica (*Arnica montana*) may be used initially for a few days, followed by ruta (*Ruta graveolens*) for joint-related injuries or *Rhus toxicodendron* for muscle-related injuries. If surgery is needed, alternative practitioners can recommend pre- and post-surgical therapies that will enhance healing.

Prognosis

Moderate sprains heal within two to four weeks, but it can take months to recover from severe ligament tears. Until recently, tearing the ligaments of the knee meant the end to an athlete's career. Improved surgical and rehabilitative techniques now offer the possibility of complete recovery. However, once a joint has been sprained, it will never be as strong as it was before.

Prevention

Sprains and strains can be prevented by warming-up before exercising, using proper lifting techniques, wearing properly fitting shoes, and taping or bracing the joint.

Resources

PERIODICALS

Wexler, Randall K. "The Injured Ankle." *American Family Physician* 57 (February 1, 1998): 474.

Tish Davidson, A.M.

Sputum culture

Definition

Sputum is material coughed up from the lungs and expectorated (spit out) through the mouth. A sputum culture is done to find and identify the microorganism causing an infection of the lower respiratory tract such as **pneumonia** (an infection of the lung). If a microorganism is found, more testing is done to determine which **antibiotics** will be effective in treating the infection.

Purpose

A person with a **fever** and a continuing **cough** that produces pus-like material and/or blood may have an infection of the lower respiratory tract. Infections of the lungs and bronchial tubes are caused by several types of microorganisms, including bacteria, fungi (molds and yeast), and viruses. **A chest x ray** provides visual evidence of an infection; a culture can grow the microorganism causing the infection. The microorganism is grown in the laboratory so it can be identified, and tested for its response to medications, such as antifungals and antibiotics.

Description

Based on the clinical condition of the patient, the physician determines what group of microorganism is likely to be causing the infection, and then orders one or more specific types of cultures: bacterial, viral, or fungal (for yeast and molds). For all culture types, the sputum must be collected into a sterile container. The sputum specimen must be collected carefully, so that bacteria that normally live in the mouth and saliva don't contaminate the sputum and complicate the process of identifying the cause of the infectious agent. Once in the laboratory, each culture type is handled differently.

Bacterial culture

A portion of the sputum is smeared on a microscope slide for a Gram stain. Another portion is spread over the surface of several different types of culture plates, and placed in an incubator at body temperature for one to two days.

A Gram stain is done by staining the slide with purple and red stains, then examining it under a microscope. Gram staining checks that the specimen does not contain saliva or material from the mouth. If many epithelial (skin) cells and few white blood cells are seen, the specimen is not pure sputum and is not adequate for culture. Depending on laboratory policy, the specimen may be rejected and a new specimen requested. If many white blood cells and bacteria of one type are seen, this is an early confirmation of infection. The color of stain picked up by the bacteria (purple or red), their shape (such as round or rectangular), and their size provide valuable clues as to their identity and helps the physician predict what antibiotics might work best before the entire test is completed. Bacteria that stain purple are called gram-positive; those that stain red are called gram-negative.

During incubation, bacteria present in the sputum sample multiply and will appear on the plates as visible colonies. The bacteria are identified by the appearance of their colonies, by the results of biochemical tests, and through a Gram stain of part of a colony.

A sensitivity test, also called antibiotic susceptibility test, is also done. The bacteria are tested against different antibiotics to determine which will treat the infection by killing the bacteria.

The initial result of the Gram stain is available the same day, or in less than an hour if requested by the physician. An early report, known as a preliminary report, is usually available after one day. This report will tell if any bacteria have been found yet, and if so, their Gram stain appearance–for example, a gram-negative rod, or a gram-positive cocci. The final report, usually available in one to three days, includes complete identification and an estimate of the quantity of the bacteria and a list of the antibiotics to which they are sensitive.

Fungal culture

To look for mold or yeast, a fungal culture is done. The sputum sample is spread on special culture plates that will encourage the growth of mold and yeast. Different biochemical tests and stains are used to identify molds and yeast. Cultures for fungi may take several weeks.

Viral culture

Viruses are a common cause of pneumonia. For a viral culture, sputum is mixed with commercially-prepared animal cells in a test tube. Characteristic changes to the cells caused by the growing virus help identify the virus. The time to complete a viral culture varies with the type of virus. It may take from several days to several weeks.

Special procedures

Tuberculosis is caused by a slow-growing bacteria called *Mycobacterium tuberculosis*. Because it does not easily grow using routine culture methods, special procedures are used to grow and identify this bacteria. When a sputum sample for tuberculosis first comes into the laboratory, a small portion of the sputum is smeared on a microscope slide and stained with a special stain, called an acid-fast stain. The stained sputum is examined under a microscope for tuberculosis organisms, which pick-up the stain, making them visible. This smear is a rapid screen for the organism, and allows the physician to receive a preliminary report within 24 hours.

To culture for tuberculosis, portions of the sputum are spread on and placed into special culture plates and tubes of broth that promote the growth of the organism. Growth in broth is faster than growth on culture plates. Instruments are available that can detect growth in broth, speeding the process even further. Growth and identification may take two to four weeks.

Other microorganisms that cause various types of lower respiratory tract infections also require special culture procedures to grow and identify. *Mycoplasma pneumonia* causes a mild to moderate form of pneumonia, commonly called walking pneumonia; *Bordetella pertussis* causes **whooping cough**; *Legionella pneumophila*, Legionnaire's disease; *Chlamydia pneumoniae*, an atypical pneumonia; and *Chlamydia psittaci*, **parrot fever**.

Pneumocystis carinii causes pneumonia in people with weakened immune systems, such as people with **AIDS**. This organism does not grow in culture. Special stains are done on sputum when pneumonia caused by this organism is suspected. The diagnosis is based on the results of these stains, the patient's symptoms, and medical history.

Sputum culture is also called sputum culture and sensitivity.

It is possible that sputum cultures will eventually be replaced in the diagnosis of tuberculosis by newer molecular techniques. These advanced methods speed the diagnostic process as well as improve its accuracy. As of late 2002, four molecular techniques are increasingly used in laboratories around the world to diagnose TB. They include polymerase chain reaction to detect mycobacterial DNA in patient specimens; nucleic acid probes to identify mycobacteria in culture; restriction fragment length polymorphism analysis to compare different strains of TB for epidemiological studies; and genetic-based susceptibility testing to identify drug-resistant strains of mycobacteria.

Preparation

The specimen for culture should be collected before antibiotics are begun. Antibiotics in the person's system may prevent microorganisms present in the sputum from growing in culture.

The best time to collect a sputum sample is early in the morning, before having anything to eat or drink. The patient should first rinse his or her mouth with water to decrease mouth bacteria and dilute saliva. Through a deep cough, the patient must cough up sputum from within the chest. Taking deep breaths and lowering the head helps bring up the sputum. Sputum must not be held in the mouth but immediately spat into a sterile container. For tuberculosis, the physician may want the patient to collect sputum samples on three consecutive mornings.

If coughing up sputum is difficult, a health care worker can have the patient breathe in sterile saline produced by a nebulizer. This nebulized saline coats the respiratory tract, loosening the sputum, and making it easier to cough up. Sputum may also be collected by a physician during a **bronchoscopy** procedure. Bronchoscopy, however, is not regarded as a cost-effective way of obtaining a useful sample.

If tuberculosis is suspected, collection of sputum should be carried out in an **isolation** room, with all attending healthcare workers wearing masks.

KEY TERMS

Acid-fast stain—A special stain done to microscopically identify the bacteria that cause tuberculosis.

Culture—A laboratory test done to grow and identify microorganisms causing infection.

Gram stain—Microscopic examination of a portion of a bacterial colony or sample from an infection site after it has been stained by special stains. Certain bacteria pick up and retain the purple stain; these bacteria are called gram-positive. Other bacteria loose the purple stain and retain the red stain; these bacteria are called gram-negative. The color of the bacteria, in addition to their size and shape, provide clues as to the identity of the bacteria.

Normal flora—The mixture of bacteria normally found at specific body sites.

Pneumonia—An infection of the lungs.

Sputum—Material coughed up from the lower respiratory tract and expectorated through the mouth.

Sensitivity test—A test that determines which antibiotics will kill the bacteria that has been isolated from a culture.

In addition to special precautions in collecting sputum when tuberculosis is suspected, workers in hospital laboratories must take extra care to inactivate unstained smear preparations that may contain *M. tuberculosis*. As of 2002, the most effective deactivation technique is the use of a solution of 5% phenol in ethanol.

Normal results

Sputum from a healthy person would have no growth on culture. A mixture of microorganisms, however, normally found in a person's mouth and saliva often contaminate the culture. If these microorganisms grow in the culture, they may be reported as normal flora contamination.

Abnormal results

The presence of bacteria and white blood cells on the Gram stain and the isolation of a microorganism from culture, other than normal flora contamination, is evidence of a lower respiratory tract infection.

Microorganisms commonly isolated from sputum include: *Streptococcus pneumoniae, Haemophilus* influenzae, *Staphylococcus aureus*, *Legionella pneumophila*, *Mycoplasma pneumonia*, *Klebsiella pneumoniae*, *Pseudomonas aeruginosa*, *Bordetella pertussis*, and ***Escherichia coli***.

Resources

BOOKS

Beers, Mark H., MD, and Robert Berkow, MD., editors. "Infectious Diseases Caused by Mycobacteria." In *The Merck Manual of Diagnosis and Therapy*. Whitehouse Station, NJ: Merck Research Laboratories, 2004.

Beers, Mark H., MD, and Robert Berkow, MD., editors. "Pneumonia." In *The Merck Manual of Diagnosis and Therapy*. Whitehouse Station, NJ: Merck Research Laboratories, 2004.

PERIODICALS

Chedore, P., C. Th'ng, D. H. Nolan, et al. "Method for Inactivating and Fixing Unstained Smear Preparations of *Mycobacterium tuberculosis* for Improved Laboratory Safety." *Journal of Clinical Microbiology* 40 (November 2002): 4077–4080.

McWilliams, T., A. U. Wells, A. C. Harrison, et al. "Induced Sputum and Bronchoscopy in the Diagnosis of Pulmonary Tuberculosis." *Thorax* 57 (December 2002): 1010–1014.

Su, W. J. "Recent Advances in the Molecular Diagnosis of Tuberculosis." *Journal of Microbiology, Immunology, and Infection* 35 (December 2002): 209–214.

Wattal, C. "Improving Bacteriological Diagnosis of Tuberculosis." *Indian Journal of Pediatrics* 69, Supplement 1 (November 2002): S11–S19.

ORGANIZATIONS

American Lung Association. 432 Park Avenue South, New York, NY 10016. (800) LUNG-USA. < www.lungusa.org >.

National Heart, Lung, and Blood Institute (NHLBI). P. O. Box 30105, Bethesda, MD 20824-0105. (301) 592-8573. < www.nhlbi.nih.gov >.

Nancy J. Nordenson
Rebecca J. Frey, PhD

Squam *see* **Skin cancer, non-melanoma**

Squint *see* **Strabismus**

SSPE *see* **Subacute sclerosing panencephalitis**

SSRIs *see* **Selective serotonin reuptake inhibitors**

SSSS *see* **Staphylococcal scalded skin syndrome**

Stanford-Binet intelligence scales

Definition

The Stanford-Binet intelligence scale is a standardized test that assesses intelligence and cognitive abilities in children and adults aged two to 23.

Purpose

The Stanford-Binet intelligence scale is used as a tool in school placement, in determining the presence of a learning disability or a developmental delay, and in tracking intellectual development. In addition, it is sometimes included in neuropsychological testing to assess the brain function of individuals with neurological impairments.

Precautions

Although the Stanford-Binet was developed for children as young as two, examiners should be cautious in using the test to screen very young children for developmental delays or disabilities. The test cannot be used to diagnose **mental retardation** in children aged three and under, and the scoring design may not detect developmental problems in preschool-age children.

Intelligence testing requires a clinically trained examiner. The Stanford-Binet intelligence scale should be administered and interpreted by a trained professional, preferably a psychologist.

Description

The Stanford-Binet intelligence scale is a direct descendent of the Binet-Simon scale, the first intelligence scale created in 1905 by psychologist Alfred Binet and Dr. Theophilus Simon. This revised edition, released in 1986, was designed with a larger, more diverse, representative sample to minimize the gender and racial inequities that had been criticized in earlier versions of the test.

The Stanford-Binet scale tests intelligence across four areas: verbal reasoning, quantitative reasoning, abstract/visual reasoning, and short-term memory. The areas are covered by 15 subtests, including vocabulary, comprehension, verbal absurdities, pattern analysis, matrices, paper folding and cutting, copying, quantitative, number series, equation building, memory for sentences, memory for digits, memory for objects, and bead memory.

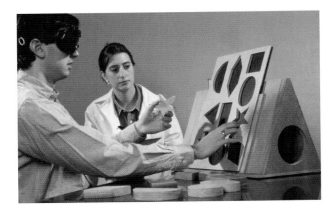

The Stanford-Binet intelligence scale. *(Photo Researchers Inc. Reproduced by permission.)*

All test subjects take an initial vocabulary test, which along with the subject's age, determines the number and level of subtests to be administered. Total testing time is 45–90 minutes, depending on the subject's age and the number of subtests given. Raw scores are based on the number of items answered, and are converted into a standard age score corresponding to age group, similar to an IQ measure.

The 1997 Medicare reimbursement rate for psychological and neuropsychological testing, including intelligence testing, is $58.35 an hour. Billing time typically includes test administration, scoring and interpretation, and reporting. Many insurance plans cover all or a portion of diagnostic psychological testing.

Normal results

The Stanford-Binet is a standardized test, meaning that norms were established during the design phase of the test by administering the test to a large, representative sample of the test population. The test has a mean, or average, standard score of 100 and a standard deviation of 16 (subtests have a mean of 50 and a standard deviation of 8). The standard deviation indicates how far above or below the norm the subject's score is. For example, an eight-year-old is assessed with the Stanford-Binet scale and achieves a standard age score of 116. The mean score of 100 is the average level at which all eight-year-olds in the representative sample performed. This child's score would be one standard deviation above that norm.

While standard age scores provide a reference point for evaluation, they represent an average of a variety of skill areas. A trained psychologist will evaluate and interpret an individual's performance on the

---

scale's subtests to discover strengths and weaknesses and offer recommendations based upon these findings.

Resources

ORGANIZATIONS

American Psychological Association (APA). 750 First St. NE, Washington, DC 20002-4242. (202) 336-5700. < ttp://www.apa.org >.

Paula Anne Ford-Martin

Stapedectomy

Definition

Stapedectomy is a surgical procedure in which the innermost bone (stapes) of the three bones (the stapes, the incus, and the malleus) of the middle ear is removed, and replaced with a small plastic tube of stainless-steel wire (a prosthesis) to improve the movement of sound to the inner ear.

Purpose

A stapedectomy is used to treat progressive **hearing loss** caused by **otosclerosis**, a condition in which spongy bone hardens around the base of the stapes. This condition fixes the stapes to the opening of the inner ear, so that the stapes no longer vibrates

---

properly; therefore, the transmission of sound to the inner ear is disrupted. Untreated otosclerosis eventually results in total deafness, usually in both ears.

Description

With the patient under local or **general anesthesia**, the surgeon opens the ear canal and folds the eardrum forward. Using an operating microscope, the surgeon is able to see the structures in detail, and evaluates the bones of hearing (ossicles) to confirm the diagnosis of otosclerosis.

Next, the surgeon separates the stapes from the incus; freed from the stapes, the incus and malleus bones can now move when pressed. A laser (or other tiny instrument) vaporizes the tendon and arch of the stapes bone, which is then removed from the middle ear.

The surgeon then opens the window that joins the middle ear to the inner ear and acts as the platform for the stapes bone. The surgeon directs the laser's beam at the window to make a tiny opening, and gently clips the prosthesis to the incus bone. A piece of tissue is taken from a small incision behind the ear lobe and used to help seal the hole in the window and around the prosthesis. The eardrum is then gently replaced and repaired, and held there by absorbable packing ointment or a gelatin sponge. The procedure usually takes about an hour and a half.

Good candidates for the surgery are those who have a fixed stapes from otosclerosis, and a conductive hearing loss at least 20 dB. Patients with a severe hearing loss might still benefit from a stapedectomy, if only to improve their hearing to the point where a hearing aid can be of help. The procedure can improve hearing in more than 90% of cases.

Preparation

Prior to admission to the hospital, the patient will be given a hearing test to measure the degree of deafness, and a full ear, nose, and throat exam.

Most surgeons prefer to use general anesthesia; in this case, an injection will be given to the patient before surgery.

Aftercare

The patient is usually discharged the morning after surgery. **Antibiotics** are given up to five days after surgery to prevent infection; packing and sutures are removed about a week after surgery.

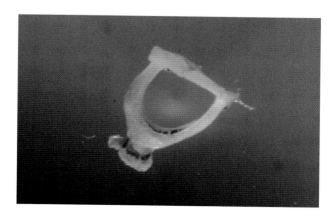

A human stapes bone (located in middle ear) extracted during a stapedectomy. *(Custom Medical Stock Photo. Reproduced by permission.)*

It is important that the patient not put pressure on the ear for a few days after surgery. Blowing one's nose, lifting heavy objects, swimming underwater, descending rapidly in high-rise elevators, or taking an airplane flight should be avoided.

Right after surgery, the ear is usually quite sensitive, so the patient should avoid loud noises until the ear retrains itself to hear sounds properly.

It is extremely important that the patient avoid getting the ear wet until it has completely healed. Water in the ear could cause an infection; most seriously, water could enter the middle ear and cause an infection within the inner ear, which could then lead to a complete hearing loss. When taking a shower, and washing the hair, the patient should plug the ear with a cotton ball or lamb's wool ball, soaked in Vaseline. The surgeon should give specific instructions about when and how this can be done.

Usually, the patient may return to work and normal activities about a week after leaving the hospital, although if the patient's job involves heavy lifting, three weeks of home rest is recommend. Three days after surgery, the patient may fly in pressurized aircraft.

Risks

The most serious risk is an increased hearing loss, which occurs in about one percent of patients. Because of this risk, a stapedectomy is usually performed on only one ear at a time.

Less common complications include:

- temporary change in taste (due to nerve damage) or lack of taste

KEY TERMS

Cochlea—The hearing part of the inner ear. This snail-shaped structure contains fluid and thousands of microscopic hair cells tuned to various frequencies, in addition to the organ of Corti (the receptor for hearing).

Conductive hearing loss—A type of medically treatable hearing loss in which the inner ear is usually normal, but there are specific problems in the middle or outer ears that prevent sound from getting to the inner ear in a normal way.

Incus—The middle of the three bones of the middle ear. It is also known as the "anvil."

Malleus—One of the three bones of the middle ear. It is also known as the "hammer."

Ossicles—The three small bones of the middle ear: the malleus (hammer), the incus (anvil) and the stapes (stirrup). These bones help carry sound from the eardrum to the inner ear.

Vertigo—A feeling of dizziness together with a sensation of movement and a feeling of rotating in space.

- perforated eardrum
- vertigo that may persist and require surgery
- damage to the chain of three small bones attached to the eardrum
- temporary facial nerve **paralysis**
- ringing in the ears

Severe **dizziness** or vertigo may be a signal that there has been an incomplete seal between the fluids of the middle and inner ear. If this is the case, the patient needs immediate bed rest, an exam by the ear surgeon, and (rarely) an operation to reopen the eardrum to check the prosthesis.

Normal results

Most patients are slightly dizzy for the first day or two after surgery, and may have a slight **headache**. Hearing improves once the swelling subsides, the slight bleeding behind the ear drum dries up, and the packing is absorbed or removed, usually within two weeks. Hearing continues to get better over the next three months.

About 90% of patients will have a completely successful surgery, with markedly improved hearing. In 8% of cases, hearing improves, but not quite as patients usually expect. About half the patients who had ringing in the ears (**tinnitus**) before surgery will have significant relief within six weeks after the procedure.

Resources

ORGANIZATIONS

American Academy of Otolaryngology-Head and Neck Surgery, Inc. One Prince St., Alexandria VA 22314-3357. (703) 836-4444. < http://www.entnet.org >.

Better Hearing Institute. 515 King Street, Suite 420, Alexandria, VA 22314. (703) 684-3391.

Carol A. Turkington

Staphylococcal infections

Definition

Staphylococcal (staph) infections are communicable conditions caused by certain bacteria and generally characterized by the formation of abscesses. They are the leading cause of primary infections originating in hospitals (nosocomial infections) in the United States.

Description

Classified since the early twentienth century as among the deadliest of all disease-causing organisms, staph exists on the skin or inside the nostrils of 20–30% of healthy people. It is sometimes found in breast tissue, the mouth, and the genital, urinary, and upper respiratory tracts.

Although staph bacteria are usually harmless, when injury or a break in the skin enables the organisms to invade the body and overcome the body's natural defenses, consequences can range from minor discomfort to **death**. Infection is most apt to occur in:

- newborns
- women who are breastfeeding
- individuals whose immune systems have been undermined by radiation treatments, **chemotherapy**, or medication
- intravenous drug users
- those with surgical incisions, skin disorders, and serious illness like **cancer**, diabetes, and lung disease

Types of infections

Staph infections produce pus-filled pockets (abscesses) located just beneath the surface of the skin or deep within the body. Risk of infection is greatest among the very young and the very old.

A localized staph infection is confined to a ring of dead and dying white blood cells and bacteria. The skin above it feels warm to the touch. Most of these abscesses eventually burst, and pus that leaks onto the skin can cause new infections.

A small fraction of localized staph infections enter the bloodstream and spread through the body. In children, these systemic (affecting the whole body) or disseminated infections frequently affect the ends of the long bones of the arms or legs, causing a bone infection called **osteomyelitis**. When adults develop invasive staph infections, bacteria are most apt to cause abscesses of the brain, heart, kidneys, liver, lungs, or spleen.

Staphylococcus aureus

Named for the golden color of the bacteria grown under laboratory conditions, S. aureus is a hardy organism that can survive in extreme temperatures or other inhospitable circumstances. About 70–90% of the population carry this strain of staph in the nostrils at some time. Although present on the skin of only 5–20% of healthy people, as many as 40% carry it elsewhere, such as in the throat, vagina, or rectum, for varying periods of time, from hours to years, without developing symptoms or becoming ill.

S. aureus flourishes in hospitals, where it infects healthcare personnel and patients who have had surgery; who have acute **dermatitis**, insulin-dependent diabetes, or dialysis-dependent **kidney disease**; or who receive frequent allergy-desensitization injections. Staph bacteria can also contaminate bedclothes, catheters, and other objects.

S. aureus causes a variety of infections. **Boils** and inflammation of the skin surrounding a hair shaft (**folliculitis**) are the most common. Toxic **shock** (TSS) and scalded skin syndrome (SSSS) are among the most serious.

TOXIC SHOCK. Toxic shock syndrome is a life-threatening infection characterized by severe **headache**, **sore throat**, **fever** as high as 105°F, and a sunburn-like rash that spreads from the face to the rest of the body. Symptoms appear suddenly; they also include **dehydration** and watery **diarrhea**.

Inadequate blood flow to peripheral parts of the body (shock) and loss of consciousness occur within the first 48 hours. Between the third and seventh day of illness, skin peels from the palms of the hands, soles of the feet, and other parts of the body. Kidney, liver, and muscle damage often occur.

SCALDED SKIN SYNDROME. Rare in adults and most common in newborns and other children under the age of five, scalded skin syndrome originates with a localized skin infection. A mild fever and/or an increase in the number of infection-fighting white blood cells may occur.

A bright red rash spreads from the face to other parts of the body and eventually forms scales. Large, soft blisters develop at the site of infection and elsewhere. When they burst, they expose inflamed skin that looks as if it had been burned.

MISCELLANEOUS INFECTIONS. S. aureus can also cause:

- arthritis
- bacteria in the bloodstream (**bacteremia**)
- pockets of infection and pus under the skin (**carbuncles**)
- tissue inflammation that spreads below the skin, causing **pain** and swelling (cellulitis)
- inflammation of the valves and walls of the heart (**endocarditis**)
- inflammation of tissue that enclosed and protects the spinal cord and brain (**meningitis**)
- inflammation of bone and bone marrow (osteomyelitis)
- pneumonia

Other strains of staph

S. EPIDERMIDIS. Capable of clinging to tubing (as in that used for intravenous feeding, etc.), prosthetic devices, and other non-living surfaces, S. epidermidis is the organism that most often contaminates devices that provide direct access to the bloodstream.

The primary cause of bacteremia in hospital patients, this strain of staph is most likely to infect cancer patients, whose immune systems have been compromised, and high-risk newborns receiving intravenous supplements.

S. epidermidis also accounts for two of every five cases of prosthetic valve endocarditis. Prosthetic valve endocarditis is endocarditis as a complication of the implantation of an artificial valve in the heart. Although contamination usually occurs during surgery, symptoms of infection may not become evident until a year after the operation. More than

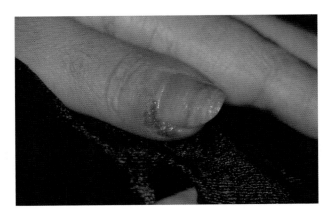

A close-up of a woman's finger and nail cuticle infected with *Staphyloccus aureus*. (Custom Medical Stock Photo. Reproduced by permission.)

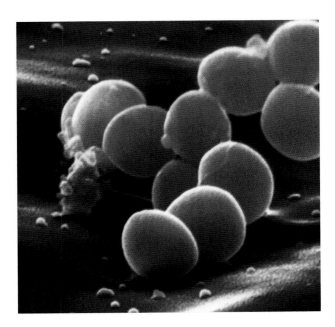

A micrographic image of *Staphylococcus aureus*. (Photograph by Oliver Meckes, Photo Researchers, Inc. Reproduced by permission.)

half of the patients who develop prosthetic valve endocarditis die.

STAPHYLOCOCCUS SAPROPHYTICUS. Existing within and around the tube-like structure that carries urine from the bladder (urethra) of about 5% of healthy males and females, *S. saprophyticus* is the second most common cause of unobstructed urinary tract infections (UTIs) in sexually active young women. This strain of staph is responsible for 10–20% of infections affecting healthy outpatients.

Causes and symptoms

Staph bacteria can spread through the air, but infection is almost always the result of direct contact with open sores or body fluids contaminated by these organisms.

Staph bacteria often enter the body through inflamed hair follicles or oil glands. Or they penetrate skin damaged by **burns**, cuts and scrapes, infection, insect bites, or **wounds**.

Multiplying beneath the skin, bacteria infect and destroy tissue in the area where they entered the body. Staph infection of the blood (staphylococcal bacteremia) develops when bacteria from a local infection infiltrate the lymph glands and bloodstream. These infections, which can usually be traced to contaminated catheters or intravenous devices, usually cause persistent high fever. They may cause shock. They also can cause death within a short time.

Warning signs

Common symptoms of staph infection include:

- pain or swelling around a cut, or an area of skin that has been scraped
- boils or other skin abscesses
- blistering, peeling, or scaling of the skin; this is most common in infants and young children
- enlarged lymph nodes in the neck, armpits, or groin

A family physician should be notified whenever:

- Lymph nodes in the neck, armpits, or groin become swollen or tender.
- An area of skin that has been cut or scraped becomes painful or swollen, feels hot, or produces pus. These symptoms may mean the infection has spread to the bloodstream.
- A boil or carbuncle appears on any part of the face or spine. Staph infections affecting these areas can spread to the brain or spinal cord.
- A boil becomes very sore. Usually a sign that infection has spread, this condition may be accompanied by fever, chills, and red streaks radiating from the site of the original infection.
- Boils that develop repeatedly. This type of recurrent infection could be a symptom of diabetes.

Diagnosis

Blood tests that show unusually high concentrations of white blood cells can suggest staph infection, but diagnosis is based on laboratory analysis of material removed from pus-filled sores, and on analysis of normally uninfected body fluids, such as, blood and urine. Also, x rays can enable doctors to locate internal abscesses and estimate the severity of infection. Needle biopsy (removing tissue with a needle, then examining it under a microscope) may be used to assess bone involvement.

Treatment

Superficial staph infections can generally be cured by keeping the area clean, using soaps that leave a germ-killing film on the skin, and applying warm, moist compresses to the affected area for 20–30 minutes three or four times a day.

Severe or recurrent infections may require a seven to 10 day course of treatment with penicillin or other oral **antibiotics**. The location of the infection and the identity of the causal bacteria determines which of several effective medications should be prescribed.

In case of a more serious infection, antibiotics may be administered intravenously for as long as six weeks. Intravenous antibiotics are also used to treat staph infections around the eyes or on other parts of the face.

Surgery may be required to drain or remove abscesses that form on internal organs, or on shunts or other devices implanted inside the body.

Alternative treatment

Alternative therapies for staph infection are meant to strengthen the immune system and prevent recurrences. Among the therapies believed to be helpful for the person with a staph infection are **yoga** (to stimulate the immune system and promote relaxation), **acupuncture** (to draw heat away from the infection), and herbal remedies. Herbs that may help the body overcome, or withstand, staph infection include:

• Garlic (*Allium sativum*). This herb is believed to have anitbacterial properties. Herbalists recommend consuming three garlic cloves or three garlic oil capsules a day, starting when symptoms of infection first appear.

• Cleavers (*Galium aparine*). This anti-inflammatory herb is believed to support the lymphatic system. It may be taken internally to help heal staph abscesses and reduce swelling of the lymph nodes. A cleavers compress can also be applied directly to a skin infection.

• Goldenseal (*Hydrastis canadensis*). Another herb believed to fight infection and reduce imflammation,

goldenseal may be taken internally when symptoms of infection first appear. Skin infections can be treated by making a paste of water and powdered goldenseal root and applying it directly to the affected area. The preparation should be covered with a clean bandage and left in place overnight.

• Echinacea (*Echinacea* spp.). Taken internally, this herb is believed to have antibiotic properties and is also thought to strengthen the immune system.

• Thyme (*Thymus vulgaris*), lavender (*Lavandula officinalis*), or bergamot (*Citrus bergamot*) oils. These oils are believed to have antibacterial properties and may help to prevent the scarring that may result from skin infections. A few drops of these oils are added to water and then a compress soaked in the water is applied to the affected area.

• Tea tree oil (*Melaleuca* spp.). Another infection-fighting herb, this oil can be applied directly to a boil or other skin infection.

Prognosis

Most healthy people who develop staph infections recover fully within a short time. Others develop repeated infections. Some become seriously ill, requiring long-term therapy or emergency care. A small percentage die.

Prevention

Healthcare providers and patients should always wash their hands thoroughly with warm water and soap after treating a staph infection or touching an open wound or the pus it produces. Pus that oozes onto the skin from the site of an infection should be removed immediately. This affected area should then be cleansed with antiseptic or with antibacterial soap.

To prevent infection from spreading from one part of the body to another, it is important to shower rather than bathe during the healing process. Because staph infection is easily transmitted from one member of a household to others, towels, washcloths, and bed linens used by someone with a staph infection should not be used by anyone else. They should be changed daily until symptoms disappear, and laundered separately in hot water with bleach.

Children should frequently be reminded not to share:

- brushes, combs, or hair accessories
- caps
- clothing
- sleeping bags
- sports equipment
- other personal items

A diet rich in green, yellow, and orange vegetables can bolster natural immunity. A doctor or nutritionist may recommend **vitamins** or mineral supplements to compensate for specific dietary deficiencies. Drinking eight to 10 glasses of water a day can help flush disease-causing organisms from the body.

Because some strains of staph bacteria are known to contaminate artificial limbs, prosthetic devices implanted within the body, and tubes used to administer medication or drain fluids from the body, catheters and other devices should be removed on a regular basis, if possible, and examined for microscopic signs of staph. Symptoms may not become evident until many months after contamination has occurred, so this practice should be followed even with patients who show no sign of infection.

Resources

BOOKS

Civetta, Joseph M., et al., editors. *Critical Care.* Philadelphia: Lippincott-Raven Publishers, 1997.

Maureen Haggerty

Staphylococcal scalded skin syndrome

Definition

Staphylococcal scalded skin syndrome (SSSS) is a disease, caused by a type of bacteria, in which large sheets of skin may peel away.

Description

SSSS primarily strikes children under the age of five, particularly infants. Clusters of SSSS cases (epidemics) can occur in newborn nurseries, when staff in those nurseries accidentally pass the causative bacteria between patients. It can also strike other age groups who have weakened immune systems. Such immunocompromised patients include those with **kidney disease**, people undergoing **cancerchemotherapy**, organ transplant patients, and individuals with acquired **immunodeficiency** syndrome (**AIDS**).

Causes and symptoms

SSSS is caused by a type of bacteria called *Staphylococcus aureus.* This bacteria produces a chemical called an epidermolytic toxin ("epiderm," deriving from the Greek words *epi,* meaning on, and *derma,* meaning skin, refers to the top layer of skin; "-lytic," deriving from the Greek word *lysis,* which literally denotes the act of undoing, means breaking or destroying; a toxin is a poison). While the bacteria itself is not spread throughout the body, it affects all of the skin by sending this toxin through the bloodstream.

SSSS begins with a small area of infection. In newborn babies, this may appear as a crusted area around the umbilicus, or in the diaper area. In children between the ages of one and six, a small, red, crusty bump appears near the nose or ear. The child may have no energy, and may have a **fever.** The skin becomes sensitive and uncomfortable even before the rash is fully visible. The rash starts out as bright red patches around the original area of crusting. Blisters may appear, and the skin may look wrinkled. When the blisters pop, they leave pitted areas. Even gently touching these red patches of skin may cause them to peel away in jagged sheets. The skin below is shiny, moist, and bright pink. Within a day or two, the top layer of skin all over the body is peeling off in large sheets.

The dangers of this illness include the chance that a different kind of bacteria will invade through the open areas in the skin and cause a serious systemic infection (**sepsis**). A lot of body fluid is lost as the skin peels away, and the layer underneath dries. **Dehydration** is a danger at this point.

Diagnosis

Although good patient care includes taking specimens of blister fluid and smears from the nose or throat, no bacteria are usually demonstrated. SSSS is usually diagnosed on the basis of the typical progression of symptoms in a child of this age, prone to this disorder. A sample of skin (**skin biopsy**) should be taken, prepared, and examined under a microscope. If the patient's disease is truly SSSS, the biopsy will show a characteristic appearance. There will be no accumulation of those cells usually present in the case of a bacterial infection. Instead, there will be evidence of disruption of only the top layer of skin (epidermis).

Treatment

Treatment involves careful attention to avoid the development of dehydration. A variety of lotions and creams are available to apply to areas where the epidermis has peeled away. This both soothes the sensitive areas, and protects against drying and further moisture loss.

Prognosis

Most patients heal from SSSS within about 10–14 days. Healing occurs without scarring in the majority of patients. **Death** may occur if severe dehydration or sepsis complicate the illness. About 3% of children die of these complications; about 50% of immunocompromised adults die of these complications.

Prevention

As always, good hygiene can prevent the passage of the causative bacteria between people. In the event of an outbreak in a newborn nursery, members of the staff should have nasal smears taken to identify an adult who may be unknowingly carrying the bacteria and passing it on to the babies.

Resources

BOOKS

Deresiewicz, Robert L., and Jeffrey Parsonnet. In *Harrison's Principles of Internal Medicine*, edited by Anthony S. Fauci, et al. New York: McGraw-Hill, 1997.

Rosalyn Carson-DeWitt, MD

Staphylococcal food poisoning *see* **Food poisoning**

Starvation

Definition

Starvation is the result of a severe or total lack of nutrients needed for the maintenance of life.

Description

Adequate **nutrition** has two components, necessary nutrients and energy in the form of calories. It is possible to ingest enough energy without a well-balanced selection of individual nutrients and produce diseases that are noticeably different from those resulting from an overall insufficiency of nutrients and energy. Although all foods are a source of energy for the human body, it is possible to consume a seemingly adequate amount of food without getting the required minimum of energy (calories). For example, marasmus is the result of a diet that is deficient mainly in energy. Children who get enough calories, but not enough protein have kwashiorkor. This is typical in cultures with a limited variety of foods that eat mostly a single staple carbohydrate like maize or rice. These conditions overlap and are associated with multiple vitamin and mineral deficits, most of which have specific names and set of problems associated with them.

- Marasmus produces a very skinny child with stunted growth.

- Children with kwashiorkor have body fat, an enlarged liver, and edema—swelling from excess water in the tissues. They also have growth retardation.

- Niacin deficiency produces **pellagra** characterized by **diarrhea**, skin **rashes**, brain dysfunction, tongue, mouth and vaginal irritation, and trouble swallowing.

- Thiamine (Vitamin B_1) deficiency causes **beriberi**, which can appear as **heart failure** and **edema**, a brain and nerve disease, or both.

- Riboflavin deficiency causes a sore mouth and throat, a skin rash, and anemia.

- Lack of vitamin C (ascorbic acid)—scurvy—causes hair damage, bleeding under the skin, in muscles and joints, gum disease, poor wound healing, and in severe cases convulsions, **fever**, loss of blood pressure, and **death**.

- Vitamin B_{12} is needed to keep the nervous system working properly. It and pyridoxine (vitamin B_6) are both necessary for blood formation.

- Vitamin A deficiency causes at first loss of night vision and eventually blindness from destruction of the cornea, a disease called keratomalacia.

- Vitamin K is necessary for blood clotting.
- Vitamin D regulates calcium balance. Without it, children get **rickets** and adults get osteomalacia.

Causes and symptoms

Starvation may result from a number of factors. They include:

- anorexia nervosa, which is an eating disorder characterized by extreme calorie restriction
- intentional fasting
- coma
- stroke
- inability to obtain food (famine; **child abuse**; aftermath of war or other disaster; being lost in wilderness or desert areas)
- severe gastrointestinal disease

Since the body will combat **malnutrition** by breaking down its own fat and eventually its own tissue, a whole host of symptoms can appear. The body's structure, as well as its functions, are affected. Starved adults may lose as much as 50% of their normal body weight.

Characteristic symptoms of starvation include:

- shrinkage of such vital organs as the heart, lungs, ovaries, or testes, and gradual loss of their functions
- chronic diarrhea
- anemia
- reduction in muscle mass and consequent weakness
- lowered body temperature combined with extreme sensitivity to cold
- decreased ability to digest food because of lack of digestive acid production
- irritability and difficulty with mental concentration
- immune deficiency
- swelling from fluid under the skin
- decreased sex drive

Complete starvation in adults leads to death within eight to 12 weeks. In the final stages of starvation, adult humans experience a variety of neurological and psychiatric symptoms, including **hallucinations** and convulsions, as well as severe muscle **pain** and disturbances in heart rhythm.

In children, chronic malnutrition is marked by growth retardation. Anemia is the first sign to appear in an adult. Swelling of the legs is next, due to a drop in the protein content of the blood. Loss of resistance to

infection follows next, along with poor wound healing. There is also progressive weakness and difficulty swallowing, which may lead to inhaling food. At the same time, the signs of specific nutrient deficiencies may appear.

Treatment

If the degree of malnutrition is severe, the intestines may not tolerate a fully balanced diet. They may, in fact, not be able to absorb adequate nutrition at all. Carefully prepared elemental **diets** or intravenous feeding must begin the treatment. A formula consisting of 42% dried skim milk, 32% edible oil, and 25% sucrose plus electrolyte, mineral, and vitamin supplements is recommended for the first phase of refeeding. The treatment back to health is long and first begins with liquids. Gradually, solid foods are introduced and a daily diet providing 5,000 calories or more is instituted.

Prognosis

People can recover from severe degrees of starvation to a normal stature and function. Children, however, may suffer from permanent **mental retardation** or growth defects if their deprivation was long and extreme.

Resources

BOOKS

Beers, Mark H., MD, and Robert Berkow, MD., editors. "Starvation." In *The Merck Manual of Diagnosis and Therapy*. Whitehouse Station, NJ: Merck Research Laboratories, 2004.

PERIODICALS

Btaiche, I. F., and N. Khalidi. "Metabolic Complications of Parenteral Nutrition in Adults, Part 1." *American Journal of Health-System Pharmacy* 61 (September 15, 2004): 1938–1949.

Nagao, M., Y. Maeno, H. Koyama, et al. "Estimation of Caloric Deficit in a Fatal Case of Starvation Resulting from Child Neglect." *Journal of Forensic Science* 49 (September 2004): 1073–1076.

J. Ricker Polsdorfer, MD
Rebecca J. Frey, PhD

Stasis dermatitis *see* **Dermatitis**

Static encephalopathy *see* **Cerebral palsy**

STDs *see* **Sexually transmitted diseases**

Steatosis *see* **Fatty liver**

Steele-Richardson-Olszewski syndrome *see* **Progressive supranuclear palsy**

Stein-Leventhal syndrome *see* **Polycystic ovary syndrome**

Steinert's disease *see* **Myotonic dystrophy**

Stem cell therapy *see* **Bone marrow transplantation**

Stem cell transplantation

Definition

Stem cells are basic human cells that reproduce (replicate) easily, providing a continuous source of new, sometimes different types of cells. A stem cell transplant is a procedure that replaces unhealthy stem cells with healthy ones.

Purpose

Physicians use stem cell transplants to treat many diseases that damage or destroy bone marrow, found in the soft fatty tissue inside the bones. Examples of these diseases are leukemia and **multiple myeloma**. Some patients lack bone marrow because of aggressive **cancer** treatments or diseases such as **aplastic anemia**, which causes abnormal blood cell production.

Recent advances in stem cell research have made it a treatment possibility for patients with certain types of lymphomas, genetic disorders, and **autoimmune disorders** as well. Researchers are hoping to eventually harvest stem cells to treat diseases such as Parkinson's disease, type 1 diabetes, Alzheimer's disease, **liver disease**, arthritis, and spinal cord injuries.

Precautions

The physician will weigh many factors when determining if a patient is a candidate for stem cell transplantation, including overall health and function of many vital organ systems. Stem cell transplantation is an aggressive treatment and may not be recommended for some patients, including those with heart, kidney, or lung disorders. If the patient has an aggressive cancer that has spread throughout the body, he or she may not be considered for a stem cell transplant. It once was thought that stem cell transplants were not safe in patients over age 60, but new research shows that elderly patients can safely receive stem cells from donors.

Many ethical and legal factors are impacting the research and development into stem cell transplantation. Much debate surrounds scientific advances. For example, human embryos, fetal tissues and umbilical cords are sources of stem cells that may be transplanted or used for disease research. Some people have ethical problems with the use of embryos in fertility clinics for stem cell research or transplantation. Some link stem cell transplantation for disease with cloning and want to stop funding for stem cell research over fear of human cloning. A study released in 2005 stated that 63% of Americans back embryonic stem cell research and 70% support federal legislation to promote more research. Meanwhile, scientists continue to develop new and exciting possibilities for transplanting stem cells into the human body that may one day lead to new treatments for previously incurable diseases. Many do so with private funding.

Description

Stem cell transplants sometimes are called bone marrow transplants. Nearly 100 years ago, physicians tried to give patients with leukemia and anemia bone marrow by mouth. These treatments were not successful, but led to experiments showing healthy bone marrow transfused into the blood stream could restore damaged bone marrow.

Today, two types of stem cell transplants are performed most often. When a patient's own stem cells are collected (harvested) before they are destroyed by high-dose **chemotherapy** or **radiation therapy** treatments, then returned to the same patient's body, it is called an autologous transplant. Using stem cells from another person, or a donor, is called allogenic transplant. In many cases, donor cells come from a relative, such as a brother or sister. However, the likelihood that a sibling will match the patient is only about 25%. Stem cells may need to come from a person not related to the recipient.

To find out if a patient could receive stem cells from a donor, physicians developed human leukocyte antigen (HLA) testing to match tissue types. The next challenge became finding donors. Throughout the 1980s and 1990s, private individuals, hospitals, foundations, and states worked to set up a nationwide registry of bone marrow donors. The National Marrow Donor Program (NMDP) now has the largest stem cell donor registry in the world. In July 2003, more than five million volunteer donors and more than 28,000 units of umbilical cord blood were listed on the NMDP registry. More than 16,000 bone marrow transplants have been performed since the NMDP was founded in 1986.

Stem cell transplants normally take place at specialized centers. Donor cells are taken from the donor in an operating room while the patient is unconscious and under **general anesthesia**. Bone marrow normally is harvested from the top of the hip bone. The marrow usually is filtered, treated, and either transplanted immediately or frozen for later use. Stem cells are transfused through an intravenous (IV) catheter that physicians insert in the patient's neck or chest. Physicians refer to this step as the "rescue process." The stem cells replace old cells. For example, the transplanted cells travel to the bone cavities and begin replacing old bone marrow.

Preparation

Standard preparation involves getting rid of the remaining disease and damaged cells. The exact process depends on the patient. In many cases, the patient will receive chemotherapy. Some also receive radiation therapy. Another goal of preparation is to depress the immune system. This makes it less likely that the patient's body will reject the new stem cells. New advances have been made that allow some of the patient's diseased cells to remain and mix with the new cells. Immediately before transplantation, the treating physician and staff will give the patient special instructions and precautions, depending on his or her disease and exact procedure.

Aftercare

Stem cells take up to three weeks to begin producing new cells or bone marrow, a process called

---

KEY TERMS

Catheter—A medical device shaped like a tube that physicians can insert into vessels, canals, or passageways to more easily inject or withdraw fluids.

Embryo—A developing human from the time of conception to the end of the eighth week after conception.

Engraftment—The process of transplanted stem cells reproducing new cells.

---

engraftment. Until engraftment is complete, patients may bleed easily and are at risk for infections. They may be required to stay in the hospital at least one week following surgery until blood cell counts reach a safe level. Once home, patients usually must be closely monitored, be careful not to risk infection, and may be anemic and sleep most of the time. They may receive **antibiotics** to prevent infection and will receive specific instructions for care from the transplant center staff. Most stem cell transplant patients cannot return to work or normal activities for up to six months following the transplant.

Risks

In addition to the risk of a life-threatening infection following a stem cell transplant, patients receiving stem cells from donors risk serious complications from graft-versus-host disease (GVHD). GVHD is caused when the donor's cells react against the patient's (recipient s) tissue. Sometimes, the patient's body simply rejects the new cells. Researchers continue to explore ways to lessen risks of complications following stem cell transplants. For example, recent studies recommend a **measles vaccination** after stem cell transplantation to prevent measles in recipients, who are at risk because of their low immunity.

Normal results

When **bone marrow transplantation** is successful, it prolongs the life of a person who might have otherwise died from the disease that caused damage to the bone marrow. People with more siblings have a higher chance of finding a compatible donor, though successful stem cell transplants also occur with donors who are not related to the recipients. Patients usually can return to normal activities within six months to one year after the transplant.

Resources

PERIODICALS

"Allogenic Stem Cell Transplantation Is Safe in Elderly Patients." *Immunotherapy Weekly* (Sept. 22, 2004):195.

"More Americans Backing Stem Cell Research, Says Study." *Pharma Marketletter* (Feb. 21, 2005).

"Patients Should Receive Measles Vaccine After Stem Cell Transplantation." *Life Science Weekly* (Nov. 23, 2004):883.

ORGANIZATIONS

International Myeloma Foundation. 12650 Riverside Drive, Suite 206. North Hollywood, CA 91607-3421. 800-452-CURE. http://www.myeloma.org.

National Marrow Donor Program. Suite 500, 3001 Broadway St. NE, Minneapolis, MN 55413-1753. 800-627-7692. http://www.marrow.org.

OTHER

Advances in Stem Cell Transplants: A Primer for Patients. Web page. National Marrow Donor Program, 2005. http://www.marrow.org/PATIENT/ advances_stem_cell_transplants_primer_patients.html.

Teresa G. Odle

Sterilization *see* **Tubal ligation; Vasectomy**

Stillbirth

Definition

A stillbirth is defined as the **death** of a fetus at any time after the twentieth week of **pregnancy**. Stillbirth is also referred to as intrauterine fetal death (IUFD).

Description

It is important to distinguish between a stillbirth and other words that describe the unintentional end of a pregnancy. A pregnancy that ends before the twentieth week is called a **miscarriage** rather than a stillbirth, even though the death of the fetus is a common cause of miscarriage. After the twentieth week, the unintended end of a pregnancy is called a stillbirth if the infant is dead at birth and premature delivery if it is born alive.

Factors that increase a mother's risk of stillbirth include: age over 35, **malnutrition**, inadequate prenatal care, **smoking**, and alcohol or drug **abuse**.

Causes and symptoms

Causes

A number of different disorders can cause stillbirth. They include:

- Pre-eclampsia and **eclampsia**. These are disorders of late pregnancy characterized by high blood pressure, fluid retention, and protein in the urine.
- Diabetes in the mother.
- Hemorrhage.
- Abnormalities in the fetus caused by infectious diseases, including **syphilis**, **toxoplasmosis**, German **measles (rubella)**, and **influenza**.
- Severe **birth defects**, including **spina bifida**. Birth defects are responsible for about 20% of stillbirths.
- Postmaturity. Postmaturity is a condition in which the pregnancy has lasted 41 weeks or longer.
- Unknown causes. These account for about one-third of stillbirths.

Symptoms

In most cases the only symptom of stillbirth is that the mother notices that the baby has stopped moving. In some cases, the first sign of fetal death is **premature labor**. Premature labor is marked by a rush of fluid from the vagina, caused by the tearing of the membrane around the baby; and by abdominal cramps or contractions.

Diagnosis

When the mother notices that fetal movement has stopped, the doctor can use several techniques to evaluate whether the baby has died. The doctor can listen for the fetal heartbeat with a stethoscope, use Doppler ultrasound to detect the heartbeat, or give the mother an electronic fetal nonstress test. In this test, the mother lies on her back with electronic monitors attached to her abdomen. The monitors record the baby's heart rate, movements, and contractions of the uterus.

Treatment

Medical

In most cases of intrauterine death, the mother will go into labor within two weeks of the baby's death. If the mother does not go into labor, the doctor will bring on (induce) labor in order to prevent the risk of hemorrhage. Labor is usually induced by giving the mother a drug (oxytocin) that cause the uterus to contract.

Follow-up therapy

Emotional support from family and friends, self-help groups, and counseling by a mental health professional can help bereaved parents cope with their loss.

Prognosis

With the exception of women with diabetes, women who have a stillbirth have as good a chance of carrying a future pregnancy to term as women who are pregnant for the first time.

Prevention

The risk of stillbirth can be lowered to some extent by good prenatal care and the mother's avoidance of exposure to infectious diseases, smoking, alcohol abuse, or drug consumption. Tests before delivery (**antepartum testing**), such as ultrasound, the alpha-fetoprotein blood test, and the electronic fetal nonstress test, can be used to evaluate the health of the fetus before there is a stillbirth.

Resources

BOOKS

Johnson, Robert V. *Mayo Clinic Complete Book of Pregnancy and Baby's First Year.* New York: William Morrow and Co., Inc.

ORGANIZATIONS

Compassionate Friends. P.O. Box 3696, Oak Brook, IL 60522. (877) 969-0010. < http:www/ compassionatefriends.org >.

GriefNet. P.O. Box 3272, Ann Arbor, MI 48106. < http:// rivendell.org >.

Hannah's Prayer. P.O. Box 5016, Auburn CA 95604. (775) 852-9202. < http://www.hannah.org >.

M.E.N.D. (Mommies Enduring Neonatal Death). P.O. Box 1007, Coppell, TX 75067. (972) 459-2396; (888) 695-6363. < http://www.mend.org/home_index.asp >.

Pregnancy and Infant Loss Support (SHARE). St. Joseph Health Center, 300 First Capitol Dr., St. Charles, MO 63301. (800) 821-6819. < http:// www.nationalshareoffice.com/index.html >.

Carol A. Turkington

Stings *see* **Bites and stings**

Stockholm syndrome

Definition

Stockholm syndrome refers to a group of psychological symptoms that occur in some persons in a captive or hostage situation. It has received considerable media publicity in recent years because it has been used to explain the behavior of such well-known kidnapping victims as Patty Hearst (1974) and Elizabeth Smart (2002). The term takes its name from a bank robbery in Stockholm, Sweden, in August 1973. The robber took four employees of the bank (three women and one man) into the vault with him and kept them hostage for 131 hours. After the employees were finally released, they appeared to have formed a paradoxical emotional bond with their captor; they told reporters that they saw the police as their enemy rather than the bank robber, and that they had positive feelings toward the criminal. The syndrome was first named by Nils Bejerot (1921–1988), a medical professor who specialized in **addiction** research and served as a psychiatric consultant to the Swedish police during the standoff at the bank. Stockholm syndrome is also known as Survival Identification Syndrome.

Description

Stockholm syndrome is considered a complex reaction to a frightening situation, and experts do not agree completely on all of its characteristic features or on the factors that make some people more susceptible than others to developing it. One reason for the disagreement is that it would be unethical to test theories about the syndrome by experimenting on human beings. The data for understanding the syndrome are derived from actual hostage situations since 1973 that differ considerably from one another in terms of location, number of people involved, and time frame. Another source of disagreement concerns the extent to which the syndrome can be used to explain other historical phenomena or more commonplace types of abusive relationships. Many researchers believe that Stockholm syndrome helps to explain certain behaviors of survivors of World War II concentration camps; members of religious cults; battered wives; incest survivors; and physically or emotionally abused children as well as persons taken hostage by criminals or terrorists.

Most experts, however, agree that Stockholm syndrome has three central characteristics:

- The hostages have negative feelings about the police or other authorities.

- The hostages have positive feelings toward their captor(s).

- The captors develop positive feelings toward the hostages.

Causes & symptoms

Stockholm syndrome does not affect all hostages (or persons in comparable situations); in fact, a Federal Bureau of Investigation (FBI) study of over 1200 hostage-taking incidents found that 92% of the hostages did *not* develop Stockholm syndrome. FBI researchers then interviewed flight attendants who had been taken hostage during airplane hijackings, and concluded that three factors are necessary for the syndrome to develop:

- The crisis situation lasts for several days or longer.

- The hostage takers remain in contact with the hostages; that is, the hostages are not placed in a separate room.

- The hostage takers show some kindness toward the hostages or at least refrain from harming them. Hostages abused by captors typically feel anger toward them and do not usually develop the syndrome.

In addition, people who often feel helpless in other stressful life situations or are willing to do anything in order to survive seem to be more susceptible to developing Stockholm syndrome if they are taken hostage.

People with Stockholm syndrome report the same symptoms as those diagnosed with posttraumatic

stress disorder (PTSD): **insomnia**, nightmares, general irritability, difficulty concentrating, being easily startled, feelings of unreality or confusion, inability to enjoy previously pleasurable experiences, increased distrust of others, and flashbacks.

Diagnosis

Stockholm syndrome is a descriptive term for a pattern of coping with a traumatic situation rather than a diagnostic category. Most psychiatrists would use the diagnostic criteria for **acute stress disorder** or posttraumatic stress disorder when evaluating a person with Stockholm syndrome.

Treatment

Treatment of Stockholm syndrome is the same as for PTSD, most commonly a combination of medications for short-term sleep disturbances and psychotherapy for the longer-term symptoms.

Prognosis

The prognosis for recovery from Stockholm syndrome is generally good, but the length of treatment needed depends on several variables. These include the nature of the hostage situation; the length of time the crisis lasted, and the individual patient's general coping style and previous experience(s) of trauma.

Prevention

Prevention of Stockholm syndrome at the level of the larger society includes further development of crisis intervention skills on the part of law enforcement as well as strategies to prevent kidnapping or hostage-taking incidents in the first place. Prevention at the individual level is difficult as of the early 2000s because researchers have not been able to identify all the factors that may place some persons at greater risk than others; in addition, they disagree on the specific psychological mechanisms involved in Stockholm syndrome. Some regard the syndrome as a form of regression (return to childish patterns of thought or action) while others explain it in terms of emotional **paralysis** ("frozen fright") or identification with the aggressor.

Resources

BOOKS

American Psychiatric Association.*Diagnostic and Statistical Manual of Mental Disorders*, 4th edition, text revision. Washington, DC: American Psychiatric Association, 2000.

Graham, Dee L. R., with Edna I. Rawlings and Roberta K. Rigsby. *Loving to Survive*, Chapter 1, "Love Thine Enemy: Hostages and Classic Stockholm Syndrome." New York and London: New York University Press, 1994.

Herman, Judith, MD. *Trauma and Recovery*, 2nd ed., revised. New York: Basic Books, 1997. Chapter 4, "Captivity," is particularly helpful in understanding Stockholm syndrome.

PERIODICALS

Bejerot, Nils. "The Six-Day War in Stockholm." *New Scientist* 61 (1974): 486–487.

Fuselier, G. Dwayne, PhD. "Placing the Stockholm Syndrome in Perspective." *FBI Law Enforcement Bulletin* (July 1999): 23–26.

Grady, Denise. "Experts Look to Stockholm Syndrome on Why Girl Stayed." *International Herald Tribune*, 17 March 2003. A newspaper article about the Elizabeth Smart kidnapping case.

ORGANIZATIONS

American Psychiatric Association. 1400 K Street, NW, Washington, DC 20005. < www.psych.org >.

Federal Bureau of Investigation (FBI). J. Edgar Hoover Building, 935 Pennsylvania Avenue, NW, Washington, DC 20535-0001. (202) 324-3000. < http://www.fbi.gov >.

OTHER

Carver, Joseph M., PhD. *Love and Stockholm Syndrome: The Mystery of Loving an Abuser*. < http://www.drjoe-carver.com/stockholm.html >.

Rebecca Frey, PhD

Stomach acid determination *see* **Gastric acid determination**

▌Stomach cancer

Definition

Stomach **cancer** (also known as gastric cancer) is a disease in which the cells forming the inner lining of the stomach become abnormal and start to divide uncontrollably, forming a mass called a tumor.

Description

The stomach is a J-shaped organ that lies in the left and central portion of the abdomen. The stomach produces many digestive juices and acids that mix with food and aid in the process of digestion. There are five regions of the stomach that doctors refer to when determining the origin of stomach cancer. These are:

- the cardia, area surrounding the cardiac sphincter which controls movement of food from the esophagus into the stomach,
- the fundus, upper expanded area adjacent to the cardiac region,
- the antrum, lower region of the stomach where it begins to narrow,
- the prepyloric, region just before or nearest the pylorus,
- and the pylorus, the terminal region where the stomach joins the small intestine

Cancer can develop in any of the five sections of the stomach. Symptoms and outcomes of the disease will vary depending on the location of the cancer.

Based on previous data from the National Cancer Institute and the United States Census, the American Cancer Society estimates that 21,700 Americans will be diagnosed with stomach cancer during 2001 and approximately 13,000 deaths will result from the disease. In most areas, men are affected by stomach cancer nearly twice as often as women. Most cases of stomach cancer are diagnosed between the ages of 50 and 70, but in families with a hereditary risk of stomach cancer, younger cases are more frequently seen.

Stomach cancer is one of the leading causes of cancer deaths in several areas of the world, most notably Japan and other Asian countries. In Japan it appears almost ten times as frequently as in the United States. The number of new stomach cancer cases is decreasing in some areas, however, especially in developed countries. In the United States, incidence rates have dropped from 30 individuals per 100,000 in the 1930s, to only 8 in 100,000 individuals developing stomach cancer by the 1980s. The use of refrigerated foods and increased consumption of fresh fruits and vegetables, instead of preserved foods with high salt content, may be a reason for the decline.

Causes and symptoms

While the exact cause for stomach cancer has not been identified, several potential factors have lead to increased numbers of individuals developing the disease and therefore, significant risk has been associated. Diet, work environment, exposure to the bacterium *Helicobacter pylori*, and a history of stomach disorders such as ulcers or polyps are some of these believed causes.

Studies have shown that eating foods with high quantities of salt and nitrites increases the risk of stomach cancer. The diet in a specific region can have a great impact on its residents. Making changes to the types of foods consumed has been shown to decrease likelihood of disease, even for individuals from countries with higher risk. For example, Japanese people who move to the United States or Europe and change the types of foods they eat have a far lower chance of developing the disease than do Japanese people who remain in Japan and do not change their dietary habits. Eating recommended amounts of fruit and vegetables may lower a person's chances of developing this cancer.

A high risk for developing stomach cancers has been linked to certain industries as well. The best proven association is between stomach cancer and persons who work in coal mining and those who work processing timber, nickel, and rubber. An unusually large number of these workers have been diagnosed with this form of cancer.

Several studies have identified a bacterium (*Helicobacter pylori*) that causes stomach ulcers (inflammation in the inner lining of the stomach). Chronic (long-term) infection of the stomach with these bacteria may lead to a particular type of cancer (lymphomas or mucosa-associated lymphoid tissue [MALT]) in the stomach.

Another risk factor is the development of polyps, benign growths in the lining of the stomach. Although polyps are not cancerous, some may have the potential to turn cancerous. People in blood group A are also at elevated risk for this cancer for unknown reasons. Other speculative causes of stomach cancer include previous stomach surgery for ulcers or other conditions, or a form of anemia known as **pernicious anemia**.

Stomach cancer is a slow-growing cancer. It may be years before the tumor grows very large and produces distinct symptoms. In the early stages of the disease, the patient may only have mild discomfort, **indigestion**, **heartburn**, a bloated feeling after eating, and mild **nausea**. In the advanced stages, a patient will have loss of appetite and resultant weight loss, stomach pains, **vomiting**, difficulty in swallowing, and blood in the stool. Stomach cancer often spreads (metastasizes) to adjoining organs such as the esophagus, adjacent lymph nodes, liver, or colon.

Diagnosis

Unfortunately, many patients diagnosed with stomach cancer experience **pain** for two or three years before informing a doctor of their symptoms. When a doctor suspects stomach cancer from the symptoms described by the patient, a complete medical history will be taken to check for any risk factors. A thorough **physical examination** will be conducted to assess all the symptoms. Laboratory tests may be ordered to check for blood in the stool (**fecal occult blood test**) and anemia (low red blood cell count), which often accompany gastric cancer.

In some countries, such as Japan, it is appropriate for patients to be given routine screening examinations for stomach cancer, as the risk of developing cancer in that society is very high. Such screening might be useful for all high-risk populations. Due to the low prevalence of stomach cancer in the United States, routine screening is usually not recommended unless a family history of the disease exists.

Whether as a screening test or because a doctor suspects a patient may have symptoms of stomach cancer, endoscopy or barium x rays are used in diagnosing stomach cancer. For a barium x ray of the upper gastrointestinal tract, the patient is given a chalky, white solution of barium sulfate to drink. This solution coats the esophagus, the stomach, and the small intestine. Air may be pumped into the stomach after the barium solution in order to get a clearer picture. Multiple x rays are then taken. The barium coating helps to identify any abnormalities in the lining of the stomach.

In another more frequently used test, known as upper gastrointestinal endoscopy, a thin, flexible, lighted tube (endoscope) is passed down the patient's throat and into the stomach. The doctor can view the lining of the esophagus and the stomach through the tube. Sometimes, a small ultrasound probe is attached at the end of the endoscope. This probe sends high frequency sound waves that bounce off the stomach wall. A computer creates an image of the stomach wall by translating the pattern of echoes generated by the reflected sound waves. This procedure is known as an endoscopic ultrasound or EUS.

Endoscopy has several advantages, in that the physician is able to see any abnormalities directly. In addition, if any suspicious-looking patches are seen, biopsy forceps can be passed painlessly through the tube to collect some tissue for microscopic examination. This is known as a biopsy. EUS is beneficial because it can provide valuable information on depth of tumor invasion.

After stomach cancer has been diagnosed and before treatment starts, another type of x-ray scan is taken. Computed tomography (CT) is an imaging procedure that produces a three-dimensional picture of organs or structures inside the body. CT scans are used to obtain additional information in regard to how large the tumor is and what parts of the stomach it borders; whether the cancer has spread to the lymph nodes; and whether it has spread to distant parts of the body (metastasized), such as the liver, lung, or bone. A CT scan of the chest, abdomen, and pelvis is taken. If the tumor has gone through the wall of the stomach and extends to the liver, pancreas, or spleen, the CT will often show this. Although a CT scan is an effective way of evaluating whether cancer has spread to some of the lymph nodes, it is less effective than EUS in evaluating whether the nodes closest to the stomach are free of cancer. However, CT scans, like barium x-rays, have the advantage of being less invasive than upper endoscopy.

Laparoscopy is another procedure used to stage some patients with stomach cancer. This involves a medical device similar to an endoscope. A laparoscopy is a minimally invasive surgery technique with one or a few small incisions, which can be performed on an outpatient basis, followed by rapid recovery. Patients who may receive **radiation therapy** or **chemotherapy** before surgery may undergo a laparoscopic procedure to determine the precise stage of cancer. The patient

with bone pain or with certain laboratory results should be given a bone scan.

Benign gastric neoplasms are tumors of the stomach that cause no major harm. One of the most common is called a submucosal leiomyoma. If a leiomyoma starts to bleed, surgery should be performed to remove it. However, many leiomyomas require no treatment. Diagnosis of stomach cancers should be conducted carefully so that if the tumor does not require treatment the patient is not subjected to a surgical operation.

Treatment

More than 95% of stomach cancers are caused by adenocarcinomas, malignant cancers that originate in glandular tissues. The remaining 5% of stomach cancers include lymphomas and other types of cancers. It is important that gastric lymphomas be accurately diagnosed because these cancers have a much better prognosis than stomach adenocarcinomas. Approximately half of the people with gastric lymphomas survive five years after diagnosis. Treatment for gastric lymphoma involves surgery combined with chemotherapy and radiation therapy.

Staging of stomach cancer is based on how deep the growth has penetrated the stomach lining; to what extent (if any) it has invaded surrounding lymph nodes; and to what extent (if any) it has spread to distant parts of the body (metastasized). The more confined the cancer, the better the chance for a cure.

One important factor in the staging of adenocarcinoma of the stomach is whether or not the tumor has invaded the surrounding tissue and, if it has, how deep it has penetrated. If invasion is limited, prognosis is favorable. Disease tissue that is more localized improves the outcome of surgical procedures performed to remove the diseased area of the stomach. This is called a resection of the stomach.

Several distinct ways of classifying stomach cancer according to cell type have been proposed. The Lauren classification is encountered most frequently. According to this classification system, gastric adenocarcinomas are either called intestinal or diffuse. Intestinal cancers are much like a type of intestinal cancer called intestinal carcinoma. Intestinal tumors are more frequently found in males and in older patients. The prognosis for these tumors is better than that for diffuse tumors. Diffuse tumors are more likely to infiltrate, that is, to move into another organ of the body.

cannot be removed with surgery, an attempt will be made to remove blockage and control symptoms such as pain or bleeding. Depending on the location of the cancer, a portion of the stomach may be removed, a procedure called a partial **gastrectomy**. In a surgical procedure known as total gastrectomy, the entire stomach may be removed. However, doctors prefer to leave at least part of the stomach if possible. Patients who have been given a partial gastrectomy achieve a better quality of life than those having a total gastrectomy and typically lead normal lives. Even when the entire stomach is removed, the patients quickly adjust to a different eating schedule. This involves eating small quantities of food more frequently. High-protein foods are generally recommended.

Partial or total gastrectomy is often accompanied by other surgical procedures. Lymph nodes are frequently removed and nearby organs, or parts of these organs, may be removed if cancer has spread to them. Such organs may include the pancreas, colon, or spleen.

Preliminary studies suggest that patients who have tumors that cannot be removed by surgery at the start of therapy may become candidates for surgery later. Combinations of chemotherapy and radiation therapy are sometimes able to reduce disease for which surgery is not initially appropriate. Preliminary studies are being performed to determine if some of these patients can become candidates for surgical procedures after such therapies are applied.

Chemotherapy

Whether or not patients undergoing surgery for stomach cancer should receive chemotherapy is a controversial issue. Chemotherapy involves administering anti-cancer drugs either intravenously (through a vein in the arm) or orally (in the form of pills). This can either be used as the primary mode of treatment or after surgery to destroy any cancerous cells that may have migrated to distant sites. Most cancers of the gastrointestinal tract do not respond well to chemotherapy, however, adenocarcinoma of the stomach and advanced stages of cancer are exceptions.

Chemotherapy medicines such as doxorubicin, mitomycin C, and 5-fluorouracil, used alone, provide benefit to at least one in five patients. Combinations of agents may provide even more benefit, although it is not certain that this includes longer survival. For example, some doctors use what is called the FAM regimen, which combines 5-fluorouacil, doxorubicin, and mitomycin. Some doctors prefer using 5-fluorouracil alone to FAM since side effects are more moderate. Another combination some doctors are using involve high doses

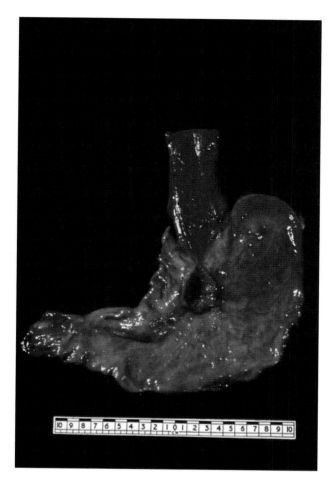

An excised section of a human stomach showing a cancerous tumor (center, triangular shape). *(Custom Medical Stock Photo. Reproduced by permission.)*

Because symptoms of stomach cancer are so mild, treatment often does not commence until the disease is well advanced. The three standard modes of treatment for stomach cancer include surgery, radiation therapy, and chemotherapy. While deciding on the patient's treatment plan, the doctor takes into account many factors. The location of the cancer and its stage are important considerations. In addition, the patient's age, general health status, and personal preferences are also taken into account.

Surgery

In the early stages of stomach cancer, surgery may be used to remove the cancer. Surgical removal of adenocarcinoma is the only treatment capable of eliminating the disease. Laparoscopy is often used before surgery to investigate whether or not the tumor can be removed surgically. If the cancer is widespread and of the medications methotrexate, 5- fluorouracil, and doxorubicin. Other combinations that have shown benefit include the ELF regimen, a combination of leucovorin, 5- fluorouracil, and etoposide. The EAP regimen, a combination of etoposide, doxorubicin, and cisplatin is also used.

Although chemotherapy using a single medicine is sometimes used, the best response rates are often achieved with combinations of medicines. Therefore, in addition to studies exploring the effectiveness of new medicines there are other studies attempting to evaluate how to best combine existing forms of chemotherapy to bring the greatest degree of help to patients.

Radiation therapy

Radiation therapy is often used after surgery to destroy the cancer cells that may not have been completely removed during surgery. To treat stomach cancer, external beam radiation therapy is generally used. In this procedure, high-energy rays from a machine that is outside of the body are concentrated on the area of the tumor. In the advanced stages of gastric cancer, radiation therapy is used to ease symptoms such as pain and bleeding. However, studies of radiation treatment for stomach cancer have shown that the way it has been used it has been ineffective for many patients.

Researchers are actively assessing the role of chemotherapy and radiation therapy used before a surgical procedure is conducted. They are searching for ways to use both chemotherapy and radiation therapy so that they increase the length of survival of patients more effectively than current methods are able to do.

Prognosis

Overall, approximately 20% of patients with stomach cancer live at least five years following diagnosis. Patients diagnosed with stomach cancer in its early stages have a far better prognosis than those for whom it is in the later stages. In the early stages, the tumor is small, lymph nodes are unaffected, and the cancer has not migrated to the lungs or the liver. Unfortunately, only about 20% of patients with stomach cancer are diagnosed before the cancer had spread to the lymph nodes or formed a distant metastasis.

It is important to remember that statistics on prognosis may be misleading. Newer therapies are being developed rapidly and five-year survival has not yet been measured with these. Also, the largest

KEY TERMS

Adenocarcinoma—Malignant cancers that originate in the tissues of glands or that form glandular structures.

Anemia—A condition in which iron levels in the blood are low.

Barium x ray (upper GI)—An x-ray test of the upper part of the gastrointestinal (GI) tract (including the esophagus, stomach, and a small portion of the small intestine) after the patient is given a white, chalky barium sulfate solution to drink. This substance coats the upper GI and the x rays reveal any abnormality in the lining of the stomach and the upper GI.

Biopsy—Removal of a tissue sample for examination under the microscope to check for cancer cells.

Chemotherapy—Treatment of cancer with synthetic drugs that destroy the tumor either by inhibiting the growth of the cancerous cells or by killing the cancer cells.

Endoscopic ultrasound (EUS)—A medical procedure in which sound waves are sent to the stomach wall by an ultrasound probe attached to the end of an endoscope. The pattern of echoes generated by the reflected sound waves are translated into an image of the stomach wall by a computer.

External radiation therapy—Radiation therapy that focuses high-energy rays from a machine on the area of the tumor.

Infiltrate—A tumor that moves into another organ of the body.

Polyp—An abnormal growth that develops on the inside of a hollow organ such as the colon, stomach, or nose.

Radiation therapy—Treatment using high-energy radiation from x-ray machines, cobalt, radium, or other sources.

Total gastrectomy—Surgical removal (excision) of the entire stomach.

Upper endoscopy—A medical procedure in which a thin, lighted, flexible tube (endoscope) is inserted down the patient's throat. Through this tube the doctor can view the lining of the esophagus, stomach, and the upper part of the small intestine.

group of people diagnosed with stomach cancer are between 60 and 70 years of age, suggesting that some of these patients die not from cancer but from other age-related diseases. As a result, some patients with stomach cancer may be expected to have longer survival than did patients just ten years ago.

Prevention

Avoiding many of the risk factors associated with stomach cancer may prevent its development. Excessive amounts of salted, smoked, and pickled foods should be avoided, as should foods high in nitrates. A diet that includes recommended amounts of fruits and vegetables is believed to lower the risk of several cancers, including stomach cancer. The American Cancer Society recommends eating at least five servings of fruits and vegetables daily and choosing six servings of food from other plant sources, such as grains, pasta, beans, cereals, and whole grain bread.

Abstaining from tobacco and excessive amounts of alcohol will reduce the risk for many cancers. In countries where stomach cancer is common, such as Japan, early detection is important for successful treatment.

Resources

BOOKS

Braunwald, Eugene, et al. *Harrison's Principles of Internal Medicine.* 15th ed. New York: McGraw-Hill, 2001.

Herfindal Eric T., and Dick R. Gourley. *Textbook of Therapeutics: Drug and Disease Management.* 7th ed. Philadelphia: Lippincott Williams & Wilkins, 2000.

Humes, H. David, editor. *Kelley's Textbook of Internal Medicine.* Philadelphia: Lippincott Williams & Wilkins, 2000.

Pazdur, Richard, et al. *Cancer Management: A Multidisciplinary Approach: Medical, Surgical, & Radiation Oncology.* 4th ed. Melville, NY: PRR, 2000.

Steen, Grant, and Joseph Mirro. *Childhood Cancer: A Handbook from St. Jude Children's Research Hospital.* Cambridge, MA: Perseus Publishing, 2000.

ORGANIZATIONS

National Coalition for Cancer Survivorship. 1010 Wayne Ave., 7th Floor, Silver Spring, MD 20910-5600. (301) 650-9127 or (877) NCCS-YES. <http://www.cansearch.org>.

Lata Cherath, PhD
Bob Kirsch

Stomach flu *see* **Gastroenteritis**

Stomach flushing

Definition

Stomach flushing is the repeated introduction of fluids into the stomach through a nasogastric tube, and their subsequent withdrawal by **nasogastric suction**.

Purpose

Stomach flushing is performed to aid in controlling gastrointestinal bleeding or to cleanse the stomach of poisons.

Controlling stomach bleeding

Bleeding from the esophagus due to ruptured veins or bleeding from the stomach due to ulcers is a medical emergency. In an attempt to stop the bleeding, the stomach is flushed with large quantities of body-temperature saline solution or ice water. This procedure is called stomach flushing or gastric lavage.

Stomach flushing to control bleeding is not uniformly accepted, and some experts believe it is of little benefit and exposes the patient to unnecessary risks. It is usually done in conjunction with the administration of drugs to constrict the blood vessels.

Stomach flushing to remove poisons

At one time, stomach flushing was common practice to remove certain poisons. Recent thinking by the American Academy of Clinical Toxicology is that stomach flushing should not be used routinely with poisoned patients. It is useful only if the patient has swallowed a life-threatening quantity of poison, and when the flushing can be done within 60 minutes of having swallowed the poison.

Precautions

In **poisoning** cases, stomach flushing should not be used if the poison is a strong corrosive acid (hydrochloric acid, sulfuric acid), alkali (lye, ammonia), or a volatile hydrocarbon such as gasoline. Stomach flushing should also not be done on patients who are having convulsions. Patients who are losing or have lost consciousness must have their airways intubated before a nasogastric tube is inserted.

Description

Stomach flushing is performed in a hospital emergency room or intensive care unit by an emergency room physician or gastroenterologist. A nasogastric tube is inserted, and small amounts of saline or ice water are introduced into the stomach and withdrawn. The procedure is repeated until the withdrawn fluid is clear.

Preparation

Little preparation is necessary for this procedure other than educating the patient as to what will happen. The patient should remove dental appliances before the nasogastric tube is inserted.

Aftercare

After stomach flushing, the patient's vital signs will be monitored. Checks will be made for fluid and electrolyte imbalances. If necessary, additional treatment to prevent gastrointestinal bleeding or poisoning will be done.

Risks

In poisoning cases, stomach flushing delays the administration of **activated charcoal**, which may be more beneficial to treating the patient than flushing the stomach. In addition, stomach flushing may stimulate bleeding from the esophagus or stomach. The patient may inhale some of the stomach contents, causing aspiration, **pneumonia**, or infection in the lungs. Fluid and electrolyte imbalances are more likely to occur in older, sicker patients. Mechanical damage to the throat is more likely in patients who are uncooperative.

Normal results

Stomach flushing is usually tolerated by patients and is a temporary treatment, performed in conjunction with other therapies.

Resources

PERIODICALS

"Gastric Lavage (The AACT/EAPCCT Position Statements on Gastrointestinal Decontamination)." *Journal of Toxicology: Clinical Toxicology* 35, no. 7 (December 1997): 771.

Tish Davidson, A.M.

Stomach removal *see* **Gastrectomy**

Stomach resection *see* **Gastrectomy**

Stomatitis

Definition

Inflammation of the mucous lining of any of the structures in the mouth, which may involve the cheeks, gums, tongue, lips, and roof or floor of the mouth. The word "stomatitis" literally means inflammation of the mouth. The inflammation can be caused by conditions in the mouth itself, such as poor **oral hygiene**, poorly fitted dentures, or from mouth **burns** from hot food or drinks, or by conditions that affect the entire body, such as medications, allergic reactions, or infections.

Description

Stomatitis is an inflammation of the lining of any of the soft-tissue structures of the mouth. Stomatitis is usually a painful condition, associated with redness, swelling, and occasional bleeding from the affected area. **Bad breath** (halitosis) may also accompany the condition. Stomatitis affects all age groups, from the infant to the elderly.

Causes and symptoms

A number of factors can cause stomatitis; it is a fairly common problem in the general adult population in North America. Poorly fitted oral appliances, cheek biting, or jagged teeth can persistently irritate the oral structures. Chronic mouth breathing due to plugged nasal airways can cause dryness of the mouth tissues, which in turn leads to irritation. Drinking beverages that are too hot can burn the mouth, leading to irritation and **pain**. Diseases, such as herpetic infections (the **common cold** sore), **gonorrhea**, **measles**, leukemia, **AIDS**, and lack of vitamin C can present with oral signs. Other systemic diseases associated with stomatitis include inflammatory bowel disease (IBD) and Behçet's syndrome, an inflammatory multisystem disorder of unknown cause.

Aphthous stomatitis, also known as recurrent aphthous ulcers (RAU) or **canker sores**, is a specific type of stomatitis that presents with shallow, painful ulcers that are usually located on the lips, cheeks, gums, or roof or floor of the mouth. These ulcers can range from pinpoint size to up to 1 in (2.5 cm) or more in diameter. Though the causes of canker sores are unknown, nutritional deficiencies, especially of vitamin B_{12}, folate, or iron is suspected. Generalized or contact stomatitis can result from excessive use of alcohol, spices, hot food, or tobacco products. Sensitivity to mouthwashes, toothpastes, and lipstick can irritate the lining of the mouth. Exposure to heavy metals, such as mercury, lead, or bismuth can cause stomatitis. Thrush, a fungal infection, is a type of stomatitis.

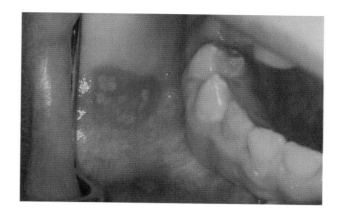

This patient is afflicted with stomatitis, a common inflammatory disease of the mouth. (Photograph by Edward H. Gill, Custom Medical Stock Photo. Reproduced by permission.)

Diagnosis

Diagnosis of stomatitis can be difficult. A patient's history may disclose a dietary deficiency, a systemic disease, or contact with materials causing an allergic reaction. A **physical examination** is done to evaluate the oral lesions and other skin problems. Blood tests may be done to determine if any infection is present. Scrapings of the lining of the mouth may be sent to the laboratory for microscopic evaluation, or cultures of the mouth may be done to determine if an infectious agent may be the cause of the problem.

Treatment

The treatment of stomatitis is based on the problem causing it. Local cleansing and good oral hygiene are fundamental. Sharp-edged foods such as peanuts, tacos, and potato chips should be avoided. A soft-bristled toothbrush should be used, and the teeth and gums should be brushed carefully; the patient should avoid banging the toothbrush into the gums. Local factors, such as ill-fitting dental appliances or sharp teeth, can be corrected by a dentist. An infectious cause can usually be treated with medication. Systemic problems, such as AIDS, leukemia, and anemia are treated by the appropriate medical specialist. Minor mouth burns from hot beverages or hot foods will usually resolve on their own in a week or so. Chronic problems with aphthous stomatitis are treated by first correcting any vitamin B_{12}, iron, or folate deficiencies. If those therapies are unsuccessful, medication can be prescribed which can be applied to each aphthous ulcer with a cotton-tipped applicator. This therapy is successful with a limited number of patients. More recently, low-power treatment with a carbon dioxide laser has been found to relieve the discomfort of recurrent aphthae. Major outbreaks of aphthous stomatitis can be treated with tetracycline **antibiotics** or **corticosteroids**. Valacyclovir has been shown to be effective in treating stomatitis caused by herpesviruses.

Patients may also be given topical anesthetics (usually a 2% lidocaine gel) to relieve pain and a protective paste (Orabase) or a coating agent like Kaopectate to protect eroded areas from further irritation from dentures, braces, or teeth.

Alternative treatment

Alternate treatment of stomatitis mainly involves prevention of the problem. Patients with such dental appliances as dentures should visit their dentist on a regular basis. Patients with systemic diseases or chronic medical problems need to ask their health care provider what types of oral problems they can expect from their particular disease. These patients must also contact their medical clinic at the first sign of problems. Common sense needs to be exercised when consuming hot foods or drinks. Use of tobacco products should be discouraged. Alcohol should be used in moderation. Mouthwashes and toothpastes known to the patient to cause problems should be avoided.

Botanical medicine can assist in resolving stomatitis. One herb, calendula (*Calendula officinalis*), in tincture form (an alcohol-based herbal extract) and diluted for a mouth rinse, can be quite effective in treating aphthous stomatitis and other manifestations of stomatitis.

Mirowski, Ginat W., DMD, MD, and Christy L. Nebesio. "Aphthous Stomatitis." *eMedicine* September 24, 2004. < http://www.emedicine.com/derm/topic486.htm >.

Sciubba, James J., DMD, PhD. "Denture Stomatitis." *eMedicine* June 11, 2002. < http://www.emedicine.com/derm/topic642.htm >.

Shulman, J. D., M. M. Beach, and F. Rivera-Hidalgo. "The Prevalence of Oral Mucosal Lesions in U.S. Adults: Data from the Third National Health and Nutrition Examination Survey, 1988–1994." *Journal of the American Dental Association* 135 (September 2004): 1279–1286.

Wohlschlaeger, A. "Prevention and Treatment of Mucositis: A Guide for Nurses." *Journal of Pediatric Oncology Nursing* 21 (September-October 2004): 281–287.

ORGANIZATIONS

American Dental Association. 211 E. Chicago Ave., Chicago, IL 60611. (312) 440-2500. < http://www.ada.org >.

American Medical Association. 515 N. State St., Chicago, IL 60612. (312) 464-5000. < http://www.ama-assn.org >.

Joseph Knight, PA
Rebecca J. Frey, PhD

Stone removal *see* **Gallstone removal**

Stool culture

Definition

Stool culture is a test to identify bacteria in patients with a suspected infection of the digestive tract. A sample of the patient's feces is placed in a special medium where bacteria is then grown. The bacteria that grow in the culture are identified using a microscope and biochemical tests.

Purpose

Stool culture is performed to identify bacteria or other organisms in persons with symptoms of gastrointestinal infection, most commonly **diarrhea**. Identification of the organism is necessary to determine the treatment of the patient's infection or to trace the cause of an outbreak or epidemic of certain types of diarrhea.

According to the Centers for Disease Control and Prevention (CDC), doctors are most likely to order a stool culture for patients with any of the following characteristics: **AIDS**, bloody stools, diarrhea lasting

---

More recently, a group of researchers in Brazil have reported that an extract made from the leaves of *Trichilia glabra*, a plant found in South America, is effective in killing several viruses that cause stomatitis.

Prognosis

The prognosis for the resolution of stomatitis is based on the cause of the problem. Many local factors can be modified, treated, or avoided. Infectious causes of stomatitis can usually be managed with medication, or, if the problem is being caused by a certain drug, by changing the offending agent.

Prevention

Stomatitis caused by local irritants can be prevented by good oral hygiene, regular dental checkups, and good dietary habits. Problems with stomatitis caused by systemic disease can be minimized by good oral hygiene and closely following the medical therapy prescribed by the patient's health care provider.

Resources

BOOKS

Beers, Mark H., MD, and Robert Berkow, MD., editors. "Disorders of the Oral Region." In *The Merck Manual of Diagnosis and Therapy*. Whitehouse Station, NJ: Merck Research Laboratories, 2004.

PERIODICALS

Cella, M., D. A. Riva, F. C. Coulombie, and S. E. Mersich. "Virucidal Activity Presence in *Trichilia glabra* Leaves." *Revista Argentina de microbiologia* 36 (July-September 2004): 136–138.

Miller, C. S., L. L. Cunningham, J. E. Lindroth, and S. A. Avdiushko. "The Efficacy of Valacyclovir in Preventing Recurrent Herpes Simplex Virus Infections Associated with Dental Procedures." *Journal of the American Dental Association* 135 (September 2004): 1311–1318.

longer than three days, high **fever**, history of recent travel abroad, or severe **dehydration**.

Precautions

Stool culture is performed only if an infection of the digestive tract is suspected. The test has no harmful effects.

Description

Stool culture may also be called fecal culture. To obtain a specimen for culture, the patient is asked to collect a stool sample into a special sterile container. In some cases, the container may contain a transport solution. Specimens may need to be collected on three consecutive days. It is important to return the specimen to the doctor's office or the laboratory in the time specified by the physician or nurse. Laboratories do not accept stool specimens contaminated with water, urine, or other materials.

The culture test involves placing a sample of the stool on a special substance, called a medium, that provides nutrients for certain organisms to grow and reproduce. The medium is usually a thick gel-like substance. The culture is done in a test tube–or on a flat round culture plate–which is incubated at the proper temperature for growth of the bacteria. After a colony of bacteria grows in the medium, the type of bacteria is identified by observing the colony's growth, its physical characteristics, and its microscopic features. The bacteria may be dyed with special stains that make it easier to identify features specific to particular bacteria.

The length of time needed to perform a stool culture depends on the laboratory where it is done and the culture methods used. Stool culture usually takes 72 hours or longer to complete. Some organisms may take several weeks to grow in a culture.

An antibiotic sensitivity test may be done after a specific bacterium is identified. This test shows which **antibiotics** will be most effective for treating the infection.

Although most intestinal infections are caused by bacteria, in some cases a fungal or viral culture may be necessary. The most common bacterial infections of the digestive tract are caused by *Shigella*, *Salmonella*, *Campylobacter*, and *Yersinia*. Patients taking certain antibiotics may be susceptible to infection with *Clostridium difficile*. In some cases, as with *Clostridium difficile*, the stool culture is used to detect the toxin (poison or harmful chemical) produced by the bacteria.

Patients with AIDS, or other immune system diseases, may also have gastrointestinal infections caused by such fungi as *Candida*, or viral organisms including cytomegalovirus.

Several intestinal parasites may cause gastrointestinal infection and diarrhea. Parasites are not cultured, but are identified microscopically in a test called "Stool Ova and Parasites."

Insurance coverage for stool culture may vary among different insurance plans. This common test usually is covered if ordered by a physician approved by the patient's insurance plan, and if it is done at an approved laboratory.

Alternative methods

Newer methods of testing stool samples for specific disease organisms include various forms of polymerase chain reaction (PCR) assays. One type that has been used to test for several different types of intestinal viruses at the same time is the RT-PCR, which stands for reverse transcriptase polymerase chain reaction. This assay measures changes in an organism's messenger RNA. RT-PCR assays have several advantages over standard stool cultures: they require only very small samples of material; they can be performed much more rapidly; and they can be used to test environmental water for virus contamination as well as human stool samples.

Preparation

The physician or other healthcare provider will ask the patient for a complete medical history and perform a **physical examination** to determine possible causes of the gastrointestinal problem. Information about the patient's diet, any medications taken, and recent travel may provide clues to the identity of possible infectious organisms.

Stool culture normally doesn't require any special preparation. Patients do not need to change their diet before collecting the specimen. Intake of some substances can contaminate the stool specimen and should not be taken the day before collection. These substances include castor oil, bismuth, and laxative preparations containing psyllium hydrophilic mucilloid.

Normal results

Bacteria that are normally found in the intestines include *Pseudomonas* and ***Escherichia coli***. These enteric bacteria (bacteria of the gastrointestinal system) are considered normal flora and usually do not cause infection in the digestive tract.

Abnormal results

Bacteria that do not normally inhabit the digestive tract, and that are known to cause gastrointestinal infection include *Shigella*, *Salmonella*, *Campylobacter*, and *Yersinia*. *Clostridium difficile* produces a toxin that can cause severe diarrhea. Other bacteria that produce toxins are *Staphylococcus aureus*, *Bacillus cereus*, and enterotoxigenic (producing disease in the digestive system) *Escherichia coli*. Although *Escherichia coli* is a normal bacteria found in the intestines, the enterotoxigenic type of this bacteria can be acquired from eating contaminated meat, juice, or fruits. It produces a toxin that causes severe inflammation and bleeding of the colon.

Resources

BOOKS

Beers, Mark H., MD, and Robert Berkow, MD., editors. "Disturbances in Newborns and Infants." In *The Merck Manual of Diagnosis and Therapy*. Whitehouse Station, NJ: Merck Research Laboratories, 2004.

PERIODICALS

Grimm, A. C., J. L. Cashdollar, F. P. Williams, and G. S. Fout. "Development of an Astrovirus RT-PCR Detection Assay for Use with Conventional, Real-Time, and Integrated Cell Culture/RT-PCR." *Canadian Journal of Microbiology* 50 (April 2004): 269–278.

Hennessy, T. W., R. Marcus, V. Deneen, et al. "Survey of Physician Diagnostic Practices for Patients with Acute Diarrhea: Clinical and Public Health Implications." *Clinical Infectious Diseases* 38, Supplement 3 (April 15, 2004): s203–S211.

Heryford, A. G., and S. A. Seys. "Outbreak of Occupational Campylobacteriosis Associated with a Pheasant Farm." *Journal of Agricultural Safety and Health* 10 (May 2004): 127–132.

Rohayem, J., S. Berger, T. Juretzek, et al. "A Simple and Rapid Single-Step Multiplex RT-PCR to Detect Norovirus, Astrovirus and Adenovirus in Clinical Stool Samples." *Journal of Virological Methods* 118 (June 1, 2004): 49–59.

Sloan, L. M., J. R. Uhl, E. A. Vetter, et al. "Comparison of the Roche LightCycler vanA/vanB Detection Assay and Culture for Detection of Vancomycin-Resistant Enterococci from Perianal Swabs." *Journal of Clinical Microbiology* 42 (June 2004): 2636–2643.

ORGANIZATIONS

Centers for Disease Control and Prevention. 1600 Clifton Rd., NE, Atlanta, GA 30333. (800) 311-3435, (404) 639-3311. < http://www.cdc.gov >.

Toni Rizzo
Rebecca J. Frey, PhD

Stool fat test

Definition

Stool fats, also known as fecal fats, or fecal lipids, are fats that are excreted in the feces. When secretions from the pancreas and liver are adequate, emulsified dietary fats are almost completely absorbed in the small intestine. When a malabsorption disorder or other cause disrupts this process, excretion of fat in the stool increases.

Purpose

This test evaluates digestion of fats by determining excessive excretion of lipids in patients exhibiting signs of malabsorption, such as weight loss, abdominal distention, and scaly skin.

Precautions

Drugs that may increase fecal fat levels include **enemas** and **laxatives**, especially mineral oil. Drugs that may decrease fecal fat include Metamucil and barium. Other substances that can affect test results include alcohol, potassium chloride, calcium carbonate, neomycin, kanamycin, and other broad-spectrum **antibiotics**.

Description

Excessive excretion of fecal fat is called steatorrhea, a condition that is suspected when the patient has large, "greasy," and foul-smelling stools. Both digestive and absorptive disorders can cause steatorrhea. Digestive disorders affect the production and release of the enzyme lipase from the pancreas, or bile from the liver, which are substances that aid digestion of fats; absorptive disorders disturb the absorptive and enzyme functions of the intestine. Any condition that causes malabsorption or maldigestion is also associated with increased fecal fat. As an example, children with **cystic fibrosis** have mucous plugs that block the pancreatic ducts. The absence or significant decrease of the pancreatic enzymes, amylase, lipase, trypsin, and chymotrypsin limits fat protein and carbohydrate digestion, resulting in steatorrhea due to fat malabsorption.

Both qualitative and quantitative tests are used to identify excessive fecal fat. The qualitative test involves staining a specimen of stool with a special dye, then examining it microscopically for evidence of malabsorption, such as undigested muscle fiber and various fats. The quantitative test involves drying and weighing a 72-hour stool specimen, then using an extraction technique to separate the fats, which are subsequently evaporated and weighed. This measurement of the total output of fecal fat per 24 hours in a three-day specimen is the most reliable test for steatorrhea.

Preparation

This test requires a 72-hour stool collection. The patient should abstain from alcohol during this time and maintain a high-fat diet (100 g/day) for three days before the test, and during the collection period. The patient should call the laboratory for instructions on how to collect the specimen.

Normal results

Reference values vary from laboratory to laboratory, but are generally found within the range of 5–7 g/24 hr.

It should be noted that children, especially infants, cannot ingest the 100 g/day of fat that is suggested for the test. Therefore, a fat retention coefficient is determined by measuring the difference between ingested fat and fecal fat, and expressing that difference as a percentage. The figure, called the fat retention coefficient, is 95% or greater in healthy children and adults. A low value is indicative of steatorrhea.

Abnormal results

Increased fecal fat levels are found in cystic fibrosis, malabsorption secondary to other conditions like Whipple's disease or **Crohn's disease**, maldigestion secondary to pancreatic or bile duct obstruction, and "short-gut" syndrome secondary to surgical resection, bypass, or congenital anomaly.

Resources

BOOKS

Pagana, Kathleen Deska. *Mosby's Manual of Diagnostic and Laboratory Tests*. St. Louis: Mosby, Inc., 1998.

Janis O. Flores

Stool O & P test

Definition

The stool O & P test is the stool ova and parasites test. In this test, a stool sample is examined for the presence of intestinal parasites and their eggs, which are called ova.

Purpose

The ova and parasites test is performed to look for and identify intestinal parasites and their eggs in persons with symptoms of gastrointestinal infection. Patients may have no symptoms, or experience **diarrhea**, blood in the stools, and other gastrointestinal distress. Identification of a particular parasite indicates the cause of the patient's disease and determines the medication needed to treat it.

Precautions

Stool O & P is performed if an infection of the digestive tract is suspected. The test has no harmful effects.

Description

Examination of the stool for ova and parasites is done to diagnose parasitic infection of the intestines.

The test may be done in the doctor's office or a laboratory. The patient collects a stool sample in one or more sterile containers containing special chemical fixatives. The feces should be collected directly into the container. It must not be contaminated with urine, water, or other materials. Three specimens are often needed–collected every other day, or every third day. However, as many as six specimens may be needed to diagnose the amoeba *Entamoeba histolytica*. The specimen does not need to be refrigerated. It should be delivered to the doctor's office or laboratory within 12 hours.

In the laboratory, the stool sample is observed for signs of parasites and their eggs. Some parasites are large enough to be seen without a microscope. For others, microscope slides are prepared with fresh unstained stool, and with stool dyed with special stains. These preparations are observed with a microscope for the presence of parasites or their eggs.

An unstained stool examination for ova and parasites normally only takes a few minutes. If specimen staining and other preparation is done, the test may take longer. When the specimen is sent to a laboratory, the results may take eight to 24 hours to be reported.

The most common intestinal parasites in North America that cause infections are:

- roundworms: *Ascaris lumbricoides*
- hookworms: *Necator americanus*
- pinworms: *Enterobius follicularis*
- tapeworms: *Diphyllobothrium latum*, *Taenia saginata*, and *Taenia solium*
- protozoa: *Entamoeba histolytica* (an amoeba), and *Giardia lamblia* (a flagellate)

Numerous other parasites are found in other parts of the world. These may be contracted by travelers to other countries. Patients with acquired immune deficiency syndrome (**AIDS**) or other immune system disorders are commonly infected with the parasites in the *Microsporidia* family, *Cryptosporidium*, and *Isospora belli*.

Insurance coverage for stool ova and parasites may vary among different insurance plans. This test usually is covered if ordered by a physician approved by the patient's insurance plan, and if it is done at an approved laboratory.

Preparation

The physician, or other healthcare provider, will ask the patient for a complete medical history, and perform a **physical examination** to determine possible

---

KEY TERMS

Amoeba—A type of protozoa (one-celled animal) that can move or change its shape by extending projections of its cytoplasm.

Bismuth—A substance used in medicines to treat diarrhea, nausea, and indigestion.

Cryptosporidium—A type of parasitic protozoa.

Feces—Material excreted by the intestines.

Flagellate—A microorganism that uses flagella (hair-like projections) to move.

Gastrointestinal—Referring to the digestive tract; the stomach and intestines.

Isospora belli—A type of parasitic protozoa.

Microsporida—A type of parasitic protozoa.

Ova—Eggs.

Parasite—An organism that lives on or inside another living organism (host), causing damage to the host.

Pathogenic—Disease-causing.

Protozoa—One-celled eukaryotic organisms belonging to the kingdom Protista.

Sterile—Free of microorganisms.

---

causes of the gastrointestinal symptoms. Information about the patient's diet, any medications taken, and recent travel may provide clues to the identity of possible infectious parasites.

Collecting a stool sample for ova and parasite detection normally doesn't require any special preparation. Patients do not need to change their diet before collecting the specimen. Patients should avoid taking any medications or treatments containing mineral oil, castor oil, or bismuth, magnesium or other antidiarrheal medicines, or **antibiotics** for seven to 10 days before collecting the specimen.

Normal results

Normally, parasites and eggs should not be found in stools. Some parasites are not pathogenic, which means they do not cause disease. If these are found, no treatment is necessary.

Abnormal results

The presence of any pathogenic parasite indicates an intestinal parasitic infection. Depending on the parasite identified, other tests may need to be performed to determine if the parasite has invaded other parts of the body. Some parasites travel from the intestines to other parts of the body and may already have caused damage to other tissues by the time a diagnosis is made. For example, the roundworm, *Ascaris* penetrates the intestinal wall and can cause inflammation in the abdomen. It can also migrate to the lungs and cause **pneumonia**. This kind of injury can occur weeks before the roundworm eggs show up in the stool.

Other types of damage caused by intestinal parasites include anemia due to hemorrhage caused by hookworms, and anemia caused by depletion of vitamin B_{12} through the action of tapeworms.

When a parasite is identified, the patient can be treated with the appropriate medications to eliminate the parasite.

Resources

BOOKS

Zaret, Barry L., et al., editors. *The Patient's Guide to Medical Tests.* Boston: Houghton Mifflin, 1997.

Toni Rizzo

Stool occult blood test *see* **Fecal occult blood test**

Stool ova and parasites test *see* **Stool O & P test**

Strabismus

Definition

Strabismus is a condition in which the eyes do not point in the same direction. It can also be referred to as a tropia or squint.

Description

Strabismus occurs in 2–5% of all children. About half are born with the condition, which causes one or both eyes to turn:

- inward (esotropia or "crossed eyes")
- outward (exotropia or "wall eyes")
- upward (hypertropia)
- downward (hypotropia)

Strabismus is equally common in boys and girls. It sometimes runs in families.

Types of strabismus

Esotropia is the most common type of strabismus in infants. Accommodative esotropia develops in children under age two who cross their eyes when focusing on objects nearby. This usually occurs in children who are moderately to highly farsighted (hyperopic).

Another common form of strabismus, exotropia, may only be noticeable when a child looks at far-away objects, daydreams, or is tired or sick.

Sometimes the eye turn is always in the same eye; however sometimes the turn alternates from one eye to the other'.

Most children with strabismus have comitant strabismus. No matter where they look, the degree of deviation does not change. In incomitant strabismus, the amount of misalignment depends upon which direction the eyes are pointed.

False strabismus (pseudostrabismus)

A child may appear to have a turned eye, however this appearance may actually be due to:

- extra skin that covers the inner corner of the eye
- a broad, flat nose
- eyes set unusually close together or far apart

This condition, false strabismus, usually disappears as the child's face grows. An eye doctor needs to determine whether the eyeturn is true or pseudostrabismus.

With normal vision, both eyes send the brain the same message. This binocular fixation (both eyes looking directly at the same object) is necessary to see three-dimensionally and to aid in depth perception. When an eye is misaligned, the brain receives two different images. Young children learn to ignore distorted messages from a misaligned eye, but adults with strabismus often develop double vision (diplopia).

A baby's eyes should be straight and parallel by three or four months of age. A child who develops strabismus after the age of eight or nine years is said to have adult-onset strabismus.

Causes and symptoms

Strabismus can be caused by a defect in muscles or the part of the brain that controls eye movement. It is especially common in children who have:

- brain tumors
- cerebral palsy
- Down syndrome
- hydrocephalus
- other disorders that affect the brain

Diseases that cause partial or total blindness can cause strabismus. So can extreme farsightedness, **cataracts**, eye injury, or having much better vision in one eye than the other.

In adults, strabismus is usually caused by:

- diabetes
- head trauma
- stroke
- brain tumor
- other diseases affecting nerves that control eye muscles

The most obvious symptom of strabismus is an eye that isn't always straight. The deviation can vary from day to day or during the day. People who have strabismus often squint in bright sunlight or tilt their heads to focus their eyes.

Diagnosis

Every baby's eyes should be examined by the age of six months. A baby whose eyes have not straightened by the age of four months should be examined to rule out serious disease.

A pediatrician, family doctor, ophthalmologist, or optometrist licensed to use diagnostic drugs uses drops that dilate the pupils and temporarily paralyze eye-focusing muscles to evaluate visual status and ocular health. Early diagnosis is important. Some eye turns may be a result of a tumor. Untreated strabismus can damage vision in the unused eye and possibly result in lazy eye (**amblyopia**).

Treatment

Preserving or restoring vision and improving appearance may involve one or more of the following:

- glasses to aid in focusing and straighten the eye(s)
- patching to force infants and young children to use and straighten the weaker eye
- eye drops or ointments as a substitute for patching or glasses, or to make glasses more effective
- surgery to tighten, relax, or reposition eye muscles

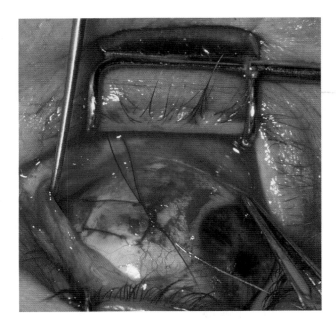

A close-up of ophthalmic surgery being performed to correct strabismus. *(Photograph by Michael English, M.D. Custom Medical Stock Photo. Reproduced by permission.)*

- medication injected into an overactive eye muscle to allow the opposite muscle to straighten the eye
- vision training (also called eye exercises)

Prognosis

Early consistent treatment usually improves vision and appearance. The most satisfactory results are achieved if the condition is corrected before the age of seven years old.

Resources

ORGANIZATIONS

American Academy of Ophthalmology. 655 Beach Street, P.O. Box 7424, San Francisco, CA 94120-7424. < http://www.eyenet.org >.

American Academy of Pediatric Ophthalmology and Strabismus (AAPOS). < http://med-aapos.bu.edu >.

American Optometric Association. 243 North Lindbergh Blvd., St. Louis, MO 63141. (314) 991-4100. < http://www.aoanet.org >.

Maureen Haggerty

Strawberry marks *see* **Birthmarks**

Strengthening exercises *see* **Exercise**

Strep culture *see* **Throat culture**

Strep test *see* **Streptococcal antibody tests**

Strep throat

Definition

Streptococcal **sore throat**, or strep throat as it is more commonly called, is an infection of the mucous membranes lining the pharynx. Sometimes the tonsils are also infected (**tonsillitis**). The disease is caused by group A *Streptococcus* bacteria. Untreated strep throat may develop into **rheumatic fever** or other serious conditions.

Description

Strep throat accounts for between 5–10% of all sore throats. Although anyone can get strep throat, it is most common in school-age children. People who smoke, who are fatigued, run down, or who live in damp, crowded conditions are also more likely to become infected. Children under age two and adults who are not around children are less likely to get the disease.

Strep throat occurs most frequently from November to April. The disease passes directly from person to person by coughing, sneezing, and close contact. Very occasionally the disease is passed through food, when a food handler infected with strep throat accidentally contaminates food by coughing or sneezing. Statistically, if someone in the household is infected, one out of every four other household members may get strep throat within two to seven days.

Causes and symptoms

A person with strep throat suddenly develops a painful sore throat one to five days after being exposed to the streptococcus bacteria. The **pain** is indistinguishable from sore throats caused by other diseases.

The infected person usually feels tired and has a **fever**, sometimes accompanied by chills, **headache**, muscle aches, swollen lymph glands, and **nausea**. Young children may complain of abdominal pain. The tonsils look swollen and are bright red, with white or yellow patches of pus on them. Sometimes the roof of the mouth is red or has small red spots. Often a person with strep throat has **bad breath**.

Despite these common symptoms, strep throat can be deceptive. It is possible to have the disease and not show any of these symptoms. Many young children complain only of a headache and stomachache, without the characteristic sore throat.

Occasionally, within a few days of developing the sore throat, an individual may develop a fine, rough, sunburn-like rash over the face and upper body, and have a fever of 101–104°F (38.3–40°C). The tongue becomes bright red, with a flecked, strawberry-like appearance. When a rash develops, this form of strep throat is called **scarlet fever**. The rash is a reaction to toxins released by the streptococcus bacteria. Scarlet fever is no more dangerous than strep throat, and is treated the same way. The rash disappears in about five days. One to three weeks later, patches of skin may peel off, as might occur with a **sunburn**, especially on the fingers and toes.

Untreated strep throat can cause rheumatic fever. This is a serious illness, although it occurs rarely. The most recent outbreak appeared in the United States in the mid-1980s. Rheumatic fever occurs most often in children between the ages of five and 15, and may have a genetic component, since it seems to run in families. Although the strep throat that causes rheumatic fever is contagious, rheumatic fever itself is not.

Rheumatic fever begins one to six weeks after an untreated streptococcal infection. The joints, especially the wrists, elbows, knees, and ankles become red, sore, and swollen. The infected person develops a high fever, and possibly a rapid heartbeat when lying down, paleness, **shortness of breath**, and fluid retention. A red rash over the trunk may come and go for weeks or months. An acute attack of rheumatic fever lasts about three months.

Rheumatic fever can cause permanent damage to the heart and heart valves. It can be prevented by promptly treating **streptococcal infections** with **antibiotics**. It does not occur if all the streptococcus bacteria are killed within the first 10–12 days after infection.

In the 1990s, outbreaks of a virulent strain of group A *Streptococcus* were reported to cause a toxic-shock-like illness and a severe invasive infection called necrotizing fasciitis, which destroys skin and muscle tissue. Although these diseases are caused by group A *Streptococci*, they rarely begin with strep throat. Usually the streptococcus bacteria enters the body through a skin wound. These complications are rare. However, since the **death** rate in necrotizing fasciitis is 30–50%, it is wise to seek prompt treatment for any streptococcal infection.

Diagnosis

Diagnosis of a strep throat by a doctor begins with a **physical examination** of the throat and chest. The doctor will also look for signs of other illness, such as a sinus infection or **bronchitis**, and seek information about whether the patient has been around other people with strep throat. If it appears that the patient may have strep throat, the doctor will do laboratory tests.

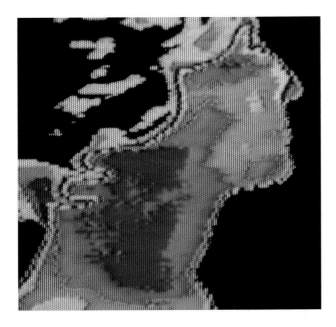

A thermographic image showing a streptococcal sore throat, or strep throat. *(Photograph by Howard Sochurek, The Stock Market. Reproduced by permission.)*

There are two types of tests to determine if a person has strep throat. A rapid strep test can only determine the presence of streptococcal bacteria, but will not tell if the sore throat is caused by another kind of bacteria. The results are available in about 20 minutes. The advantage of this test is the speed with which a diagnosis can be made.

The rapid strep test has a false negative rate of about 20%. In other words, in about 20% of cases where no strep is detected by the rapid strep test, the patient actually does have strep throat. Because of this, when a rapid strep test is negative, the doctor often does a **throat culture**.

For a rapid strep test or a throat culture, a nurse will use a sterile swab to reach down into the throat and obtain a sample of material from the sore area. The procedure takes only a few seconds, but may cause gagging.

For a throat culture a sample of swabbed material is cultured, or grown, in the laboratory on a medium that allows technicians to determine what kind of bacteria are present. Results take 24–48 hours. The test is very accurate and will show the presence of other kinds of bacteria besides *Streptococci*. It is important not to take any leftover antibiotics before visiting the doctor and having a throat culture. Even small amounts of antibiotics can suppress the bacteria and mask its presence in the throat culture.

In the event that rheumatic fever is suspected, the doctor does a blood test. This test, called an antistreptolysin-O test, will tell the doctor whether the person has recently been infected with strep bacteria. This helps the doctor distinguish between rheumatic fever and **rheumatoid arthritis**.

Treatment

Strep throat is treated with antibiotics. Penicillin is the preferred medication. Oral penicillin must be taken for 10-days. Patients need to take the entire amount of antibiotic prescribed and not discontinue taking the medication when they feel better. Stopping the antibiotic early can lead to a return of the strep infection. Occasionally, a single injection of long-acting penicillin (Bicillin) is given instead of 10 days of oral treatment.

About 10% of the time, penicillin is not effective against the strep bacteria. When this happens a doctor may prescribe other antibiotics such as amoxicillin (Amoxil, Pentamox, Sumox, Trimox), clindamycin (Cleocin), or a cephalosporin (Keflex, Durocef, Ceclor). Erythromycin (Eryzole, Pediazole, Ilosone), another inexpensive antibiotic, is given to people who are allergic to penicillin. Scarlet fever is treated with the same antibiotics as strep throat.

Without treatment, the symptoms of strep throat begin subsiding in four or five days. However, because of the possibility of getting rheumatic fever, it is important to treat strep throat promptly with antibiotics. If rheumatic fever does occur, it is also treated with antibiotics. Anti-inflammatory drugs, such as steroids, are used to treat joint swelling. **Diuretics** are used to reduce water retention. Once the rheumatic fever becomes inactive, children may continue on low doses of antibiotics to prevent a reoccurrence. Necrotizing fasciitis is treated with intravenous antibiotics.

Home care for strep throat

There are home care steps that people can take to ease the discomfort of their strep symptoms.

- Take **acetaminophen** or ibuprofen for pain. **Aspirin** should not be given to children because of its association with an increase in **Reye's Syndrome**, a serious disease.

- Gargle with warm double strength tea or warm salt water, made by adding one teaspoon of salt to eight ounces of water, to relieve sore throat pain.

- Drink plenty of fluids, but avoid acidic juices like orange juice because they irritate the throat.

- Eat soft, nutritious foods like noodle soup. Avoid spicy foods.

- Avoid smoke and smoking.

- Rest until the fever is gone, then resume strenuous activities gradually.

- Use a room humidifier, as it may make sore throat sufferers more comfortable.

- Be aware that antiseptic lozenges and sprays may aggravate the sore throat rather than improve it.

Alternative treatment

Alternative treatment focuses on easing the symptoms of strep throat through herbs and botanical medicines. Some practitioners suggest using these treatments in addition to antibiotics, since they primarily address the comfort of the patient and not the underlying infection. Many practitioners recommend *Lactobacillus acidophilus* to offset the suppressive effects of antibiotics on the beneficial bacteria of the intestines.

Some suggested treatments include:

- Inhaling fragrances of the essential oils of lavender (*Lavandula officinalis*), thyme (*Thymus vulgaris*), eucalyptus (*Eucalyptus globulus*), sage (*Salvia officinalis*), and sandalwood (Aromatherapy).

- Gargling with a mixture of water, salt, and tumeric (*Curcuma longa*) powder or astringents, such as alum, sumac, sage, and bayberry (Ayurvedic medicine).

- Taking osha root (*Ligusticum porteri*) internally for infection or drinking tea made of sage, **echinacea** (*Echinacea* spp.) and cleavers (*Gallium aparine*) Osha root has an unpleasant taste many children will not accept (Botanical medicine).

Prognosis

Patients with strep throat begin feeling better about 24 hours after starting antibiotics. Symptoms rarely last longer than five days.

People remain contagious until after they have been taking antibiotics for 24 hours. Children should not return to school or childcare until they are no longer contagious. Food handlers should not work for the first 24 hours after antibiotic treatment, because strep infections are occasionally passed through contaminated food. People who are not treated with antibiotics can continue to spread strep bacteria for several months.

About 10% of strep throat cases do not respond to penicillin. People who have even a mild sore throat after a 10 day treatment with antibiotic should return to their doctor. An explanation for this may be that the person is just a carrier of strep, and that something else is causing the sore throat.

Taking antibiotics within the first week of a strep infection will prevent rheumatic fever and other complications. If rheumatic fever does occur, the outcomes vary considerably. Some cases may be cured. In others there may be permanent damage to the heart and heart valves. In rare cases, rheumatic fever can be fatal.

Necrotizing fasciitis has a death rate of 30–50%. Patients who survive often suffer a great deal of tissue and muscle loss. Fortunately, this complication of a streptococcus infection is very rare.

Prevention

There is no way to prevent getting a strep throat. However, the risk of getting one or passing one on to another person can be minimized by:

- sashing hands well and frequently, especially after nose blowing or sneezing and before food handling

- disposing of used tissues properly

- avoiding close contact with someone who has a strep throat

- not sharing food and eating utensils with anyone

- not smoking

Resources

OTHER

"Group A Streptococcal Infections." *National Institute of Allergy and Infectious Diseases Page.* February 22, 1998. < http://www.niaid.nih.govfactsheets/ strep.htm. >.

Tish Davidson, A.M.

Streptobacillary rat-bite fever *see* **Rat-bite fever**

Streptococcal antibody tests

Definition

Streptococcal infections are caused by a micro-organism called *Streptococcus*. Three streptococcal antibody tests are available: the antistreptolysin O titer (ASO), the antideoxyribonuclease-B titer (anti-Dnase-B, or ADB), and the streptozyme test.

Purpose

The antistreptolysin O titer, or ASO, is ordered primarily to determine whether a previous group A *Streptococcus* infection has caused a poststreptococcal disease, such as **scarlet fever**, **rheumatic fever**, or a **kidney disease** called **glomerulonephritis**.

The anti-DNase-B (ADB) test is performed to determine a previous infection of a specific type of *Streptococcus*, group A beta-hemolytic *Streptococcus*. Identification of infections of this type are particularly important in suspected cases of acute rheumatic **fever** (ARF) or acute glomerulonephritis.

Streptozyme is a screening test used to detect antibodies to several streptococcal antigens. An antigen is a substance that can trigger an immune response, resulting in production of an antibody as part of the body's defense against infection and disease.

Precautions

For the ASO test, increased levels of fats, called beta lipoproteins, in the blood can neutralize streptolysin O and cause a false-positive ASO titer. **Antibiotics**, which reduce the number of streptococci and thereby suppress ASO production, may decrease ASO levels. Steroids, which suppress the immune system, consequently may also suppress ASO production. Also Group A streptococcal infections of the skin may not produce an ASO response. Antibiotics also may decrease anti-DNase-B (ADB) levels.

Description

Streptococcal infections are caused by bacteria known as *Streptococcus*. There are several disease-causing strains of streptococci (groups A, B, C, D, and G), which are identified by their behavior, chemistry, and appearance. Each group causes specific types of infections and symptoms. These antibody tests are useful for group A streptococci. Group A streptococci are the most virulent species for humans and are the cause of **strep throat**, **tonsillitis**, wound and skin infections, blood infections (septicemia), scarlet fever, **pneumonia**, rheumatic fever, **Sydenham's chorea** (formerly called St. Vitus' dance), and glomerulonephritis.

Although symptoms may suggest a streptococcal infection, the diagnosis must be confirmed by tests. The best procedure, and one that is used for an acute infection, is to take a sample from the infected area for culture, a means of growing bacteria artificially in the laboratory. However, cultures are useless about two to three weeks after initial infection, so the ASO, anti-DNase-B, and streptozyme tests are used to determine if a streptococcal infection is present.

Antistreptolysin O titer (ASO)

The ASO titer is used to demonstrate the body's reaction to an infection caused by group A beta-hemolytic streptococci. Group A streptococci produce the enzyme streptolysin O, which can destroy (lyse) red blood cells. Because streptolysin O is antigenic (contains a protein foreign to the body), the body reacts by producing antistreptolysin O (ASO), which is a neutralizing antibody. ASO appears in the blood serum one week to one month after the onset of a strep infection. A high titer (high levels of ASO) is not specific for any type of poststreptococcal disease, but it does indicate if a streptococcal infection is or has been present.

Serial (several given in a row) ASO testing is often performed to determine the difference between an acute or convalescent blood sample. The diagnosis of a previous strep infection is confirmed when serial titers of ASO rise over a period of weeks, then fall slowly. ASO titers peak during the third week after the onset of acute symptoms of a streptococcal disease; at six months after onset, approximately 30% of patients exhibit abnormal titers.

Antideoxyribonuclease-B titer (anti-DNase B, or ADB)

Anti-DNase-B, or ADB, also detects antigens produced by group A strep, and is elevated in most patients with rheumatic fever and poststreptococcal glomerulonephritis. This test is often done concurrently with the ASO titer, and subsequent testing is usually performed to detect differences in the acute and convalescent blood samples. When ASO and ADB are performed concurrently, 95% of previous strep infections are detected. If both are repeatedly negative, the likelihood is that the patient's symptoms are not caused by a poststreptococcal disease.

When evaluating patients with acute rheumatic fever, the American Heart Association recommends the ASO titer rather than ADB. Even though the ADB is more sensitive than ASO, its results are too variable. It also should be noted that, while ASO is the recommended test, when ASO and ADB are done together, the combination is better than either ASO or ADB alone.

Streptozyme

The streptozyme test is often used as a screening test for antibodies to the streptococcal antigens NADase, DNase, streptokinase, streptolysin O, and hyaluronidase. This test is most useful in evaluating suspected poststreptococcal disease following *Streptococcus pyogenes* infection, such as rheumatic fever.

Streptozyme has certain advantages over ASO and ADB. It can detect several antibodies in a single assay, it is technically quick and easy, and it is unaffected by factors that can produce false-positives in the ASO test. The disadvantages are that, while it detects different antibodies, it does not determine which one has been detected, and it is not as sensitive in children as in adults. In fact, borderline antibody elevations, which could be significant in children, may not be detected at all. As with the ASO and ADB, a serially rising titer is more significant than a single determination.

Preparation

These tests are performed on blood specimens drawn from the patient's vein. The patient does not need to fast before these tests.

Risks

The risks associated with these tests are minimal, but may include slight bleeding from the blood-drawing site, **fainting** or feeling lightheaded after the blood is drawn, or blood accumulating under the puncture site (hematoma).

Normal results

Antistreptolysin O titer:

- adult: 160 Todd units/ml
- child: six months to two years: 50 Todd units/ml; two to four years: 160 Todd units/ml; five to 12 years: 170–330 Todd units/ml
- newborn: similar to the mother's value

Antideoxyribonuclease-B titer:

- adult: 85 units
- child (preschool): 60 units
- child (school age): 170 units

KEY TERMS

Antibody—A protein manufactured by a type of white blood cells called lymphocytes, in response to the presence of an antigen, or foreign protein, in the body. Because bacteria, viruses, and other organisms commonly contain many antigens, antibodies are formed against these foreign proteins to neutralize or destroy the invaders.

Antigen—A substance that can trigger a defensive response in the body, resulting in production of an antibody as part of the body's defense against infection and disease. Many antigens are foreign proteins not found naturally in the body, and include bacteria, viruses, toxins, and tissues from another person used in organ transplantation.

Glomerulonephritis—An inflammation of the glomeruli, the filtering units of the kidney. Damage to these structures hampers removal of waste products, salt, and water from the bloodstream, which may cause serious complications. This disorder can be mild and cause no symptoms, or so severe enough to cause kidney failure.

Rheumatic fever—A disease that causes inflammation in various body tissues. Rare in most developed countries, but reported to be on the increase again in parts of the United States. Joint inflammation occurs, but more serious is the frequency with which the disease permanently damages the heart. The nervous system may also be affected, causing Sydenham's chorea.

Sydenham's chorea—A childhood disorder of the central nervous system. Once called St. Vitus' dance, the condition is characterized by involuntary, jerky movements that usually follow an attack of rheumatic fever. Rare in the United States today, but a common disorder in developing countries. Usually resolves in two to three months with no long-term adverse effects.

Streptozyme: less than 100 streptozyme units.

Abnormal results

Antistreptolysin O titer: Increased levels are seen after the second week of an untreated infection in acute streptococcal infection, and are also increased with acute rheumatic fever, acute glomerulonephritis (66% of patients will not have high ASO titers), and scarlet fever.

Antideoxyribonuclease-B titer: Increased titers are seen in cases of acute rheumatic fever and post-streptococcal glomerulonephritis.

Streptozyme: As this is a screening test for antibodies to streptococcal antigens, increased levels require more definitive tests to confirm diagnosis.

Resources

BOOKS

Pagana, Kathleen Deska. *Mosby's Manual of Diagnostic and Laboratory Tests*. St. Louis: Mosby, Inc., 1998.

Janis O. Flores

Streptococcal gangrene *see* **Gangrene**

Streptococcal infections

Definition

Streptococcal (strep) infections are communicable diseases that develop when bacteria normally found on the skin or in the intestines, mouth, nose, reproductive tract, or urinary tract invade other parts of the body and contaminate blood or tissue.

Some strep infections don't produce symptoms. Some are fatal.

Description

Most people have some form of strep bacteria in their body at some time. A person who hosts bacteria without showing signs of infection is considered a carrier.

Types of infection

Primary strep infections invade healthy tissue, and most often affect the throat. Secondary strep infections invade tissue already weakened by injury or illness. They frequently affect the bones, ears, eyes, joints, or intestines.

Both primary and secondary strep infections can travel from affected tissues to lymph glands, enter the bloodstream, and spread throughout the body.

Numerous strains of strep bacteria have been identified. Types A, B, C, D, and G are most likely to make people sick.

Group A

Group A strep (GAS) is the form of strep bacteria most apt to be associated with serious illness.

Between 10,000 and 15,000 GAS infections occur in the United States every year. Most are mild inflammations of the throat or skin, where the bacteria are normally found; however, GAS infections can be deadly.

Two of the most severe invasive GAS infections are necrotizing fasciitis or flesh-eating bacteria (destruction of muscle tissue and fat) and **toxic shock syndrome** (a rapidly progressive disorder that causes **shock** and damages internal organs).

GROUP B. Group B strep (GBS) most often affects pregnant women, infants, the elderly, and chronically ill adults.

Since first emerging in the 1970s, GBS has been the primary cause of life-threatening illness and **death** in newborns. GBS exists in the reproductive tract of 20-25% of all pregnant women. Although no more than 2% of these women develop invasive infection, 40-73% transmit bacteria to their babies during delivery.

About 12,000 of the 3.5 million babies born in the United States each year develop GBS disease in infancy. About 75% of them develop early-onset infection. Sometimes evident within a few hours of birth and always apparent within the first week of life, this condition causes inflammation of the membranes covering the brain and spinal cord (**meningitis**), **pneumonia**, blood infection (**sepsis**) and other problems.

Late-onset GBS develops between the ages of seven days and three months. It often causes meningitis. About half of all cases of this rare condition can be traced to mothers who are GBS carriers. The cause of the others is unknown.

GBS has also been linked to a history of **breast cancer**.

GROUP C. Group C strep (GCS) is a common source of infection in animals. It rarely causes human illness.

GROUP D. Group D strep (GDS) is a common cause of wound infections in hospital patients. GDS is also associated with:

- abnormal growth of tissue in the gastrointestinal tract
- urinary tract infection (UTI)
- womb infections in women who have just given birth

GROUP G. Normally present on the skin, in the mouth and throat, and in the intestines and genital tract, Group G strep (GGS) is most likely to lead to infection in alcoholics and in people who have **cancer**, **diabetes mellitus**, **rheumatoid arthritis**, and other conditions that suppress immune-system activity.

GGS can cause a variety of infections, including:

• bacteria in the bloodstream (bacteremia)

• inflammation of the connective tissue structure surrounding a joint (bursitis)

• endocarditis (a condition that affects the lining of the heart chambers and the heart valves)

• meningitis

• inflammation of bone and bone marrow (osteomyelitis)

• inflammation of the lining of the abdomen (peritonitis)

Causes and symptoms

Streptococcal infection occurs when bacteria contaminate cuts or open sores or otherwise penetrate the body's natural defenses.

GAS

GAS is transmitted by direct contact with saliva, nasal discharge, or open **wounds** of someone who has the infection. Chronic illness, **kidney disease** treated by dialysis, and steroid use increase vulnerability to infection.

About one of five people with GAS infection develops a sore, inflamed throat, and pus on the tonsils. The majority of those infected by GAS either have no symptoms or develop enlarged lymph nodes, **fever**, **headache**, **nausea**, **vomiting**, weakness, and a rapid heartbeat.

Flesh-eating bacteria is characterized by fever, extreme **pain**, and swelling and redness at a site where skin is broken.

Symptoms of toxic shock include abdominal pain, confusion, **dizziness**, and widespread red skin rash.

GBS

A pregnant woman who has GBS infection can develop infections of the bladder, blood, and urinary tract, and deliver a baby who is infected or stillborn. The risk of transmitting GBS infection during birth is highest in a woman whose labor begins before the 37th week of **pregnancy** or lasts more than 18 hours or who:

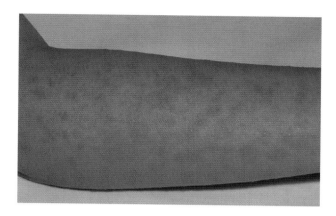

The scarlet fever rash on this person's arm was caused by a streptococcal infection. *(Custom Medical Stock Photo. Reproduced by permission.)*

• becomes a GBS carrier during the final stages of pregnancy

• has a GBS urinary-tract infection

• has already given birth to a baby infected with GBS

• develops a fever during labor

More than 13% of babies who develop GBS infection during birth or within the first few months of life develop neurologic disorders. An equal number of them die.

Among men, and in women who are not pregnant, the most common consequences of GBS infection are pneumonia and infections of blood, skin, and soft tissue.

Miscellaneous symptoms

Other symptoms associated with strep infection include:

• anemia

• elevated white blood cell counts

• inflammation of the epiglottis (epiglottitis)

• heart murmur

• high blood pressure

• infection of the heart muscle

• kidney inflammation (**nephritis**)

• swelling of the face and ankles

Diagnosis

Strep bacteria can be obtained by swabbing the back of the throat or the rectum with a piece of sterile cotton. Microscopic examination of the smear can identify which type of bacteria has been collected.

Treatment

Penicillin and other **antibiotics** are used to treat strep infections.

It takes less than 24 hours for antibiotics to eliminate an infected person's ability to transmit GAS.

Guidelines developed by the American Academy of Obstetrics and Gynecology (AAOG), the American Academy of Pediatrics (AAP), and the Centers for Disease Control and Prevention (CDC) recommend administering intravenous antibiotics to a woman at high risk of passing GBS infection on to her child, and offering the medication to any pregnant woman who wants it.

Initiating antibiotic therapy at least four hours before birth allows medication to become concentrated enough to protect the baby during passage through the birth canal.

Babies infected with GBS during or shortly after birth may die. Those who survive often require lengthy hospital stays and develop vision or **hearing loss** and other permanent disabilities.

Alternative treatment

Conventional medicine is very successful in treating strep infections. However, several alternative therapies, including homeopathy and botanical medicine, may help relieve symptoms or support the person with a strep infection. For example, several herbs, including garlic (*Allium sativum*), **echinacea** (*Echinacea* spp.), and goldenseal (*Hydrastis canadensis*), are believed to strengthen the immune system, thus helping the body fight a current infection, as well as helping prevent future infections.

Prognosis

GAS is responsible for more than 2,000 deaths a year. About 20% of people infected with flesh-eating bacteria die. So do three of every five who develop toxic shock syndrome.

Early-onset GBS kills 15% of the infants it affects. Late-onset disease claims the lives of 10% of babies who develop it.

GBS infections are fatal in about 20% of the men and non-pregnant women who develop them.

About 10–15% of non-GAS strep infections are fatal. Antibiotic therapy, begun when symptoms first appear, may increase a patient's chance of survival.

Prevention

Washing the hands frequently, especially before eating and after using the bathroom, and keeping wounds clean can help prevent strep infection. Exposure to infected people should be avoided, and a family physician should be notified by anyone who develops an extremely **sore throat** or pain, redness, swelling, or drainage at the site of a wound or break in the skin.

Until vaccines to prevent strep infection become available, 12 monthly doses of oral or injected antibiotics may prevent some types of recurrent infection.

Resources

OTHER

"Infectious Diseases." *The Merck Page.* June 17, 1998. < http://www.merck.com >.

Maureen Haggerty

Streptococcal sore throat *see* **Strep throat**

Streptococcal toxic shock syndrome *see* **Toxic shock syndrome**

Streptomycin *see* **Aminoglycosides**

Streptozyme test *see* **Streptococcal antibody tests**

Stress

Definition

Stress is defined as an organism's total response to environmental demands or pressures. When stress was first studied in the 1950s, the term was used to denote both the causes and the experienced effects of these pressures. More recently, however, the word stressor has been used for the stimulus that provokes a stress response. One recurrent disagreement among researchers concerns the definition of stress in humans. Is it primarily an external response that can be measured by changes in glandular secretions, skin reactions, and other physical functions, or is it an internal interpretation of, or reaction to, a stressor; or is it both?

Description

Stress in humans results from interactions between persons and their environment that are perceived as straining or exceeding their adaptive

Top Ten Stressful Life Events
Death of spouse
Divorce
Marital separation
Jail term or death of close family member
Personal injury or illness
Marriage
Loss of job due to termination
Marital reconciliation or retirement
Pregnancy
Change in financial state

capacities and threatening their well-being. The element of perception indicates that human stress responses reflect differences in personality, as well as differences in physical strength or general health.

Risk factors for stress-related illnesses are a mix of personal, interpersonal, and social variables. These factors include lack or loss of control over one's physical environment, and lack or loss of social support networks. People who are dependent on others (e.g., children or the elderly) or who are socially disadvantaged (because of race, gender, educational level, or similar factors) are at greater risk of developing stress-related illnesses. Other risk factors include feelings of helplessness, hopelessness, extreme fear or anger, and cynicism or distrust of others.

Causes and symptoms

Causes

The causes of stress can include any event or occurrence that a person considers a threat to his or her coping strategies or resources. Researchers generally agree that a certain degree of stress is a normal part of a living organism's response to the inevitable changes in its physical or social environment, and that positive, as well as negative, events can generate stress as well as negative occurrences. Stress-related disease, however, results from excessive and prolonged demands on an organism's coping resources. It is now believed that 80–90% of all disease is stress-related.

Recent research indicates that some vulnerability to stress is genetic. Scientists at the University of Wisconsin and King's College London discovered that people who inherited a short, or stress-sensitive, version of the serotonin transporter gene were almost three times as likely to experience depression following

a stressful event as people with the long version of the gene. Further research is likely to identify other genes that affect susceptibility to stress.

One cause of stress that has affected large sectors of the general population around the world since 2001 is terrorism. The events of September 11, 2001, the sniper shootings in Virginia and Maryland and the Bali nightclub bombing in 2002, the **suicide** bombings in the Middle East in 2003, have all been shown to cause short-term symptoms of stress in people who read about them or watch television news reports as well as those who witnessed the actual events. Stress related to terrorist attacks also appears to affect people in countries far from the location of the attack as well as those in the immediate vicinity. It is too soon to tell how stress related to episodes of terrorism will affect human health over long periods of time, but researchers are already beginning to investigate this question. In 2004 the Centers for Disease Control and Prevention (CDC) released a report on the aftereffects of the World Trade Center attacks on rescue and recovery workers and volunteers. The researchers found that over half the 11,700 people who were interviewed met threshold criteria for a mental health evaluation. A longer-term evaluation of these workers is underway.

A new condition that has been identified since 9/11 is childhood traumatic grief, or CTG. CTG refers to an intense stress reaction that may develop in children following the loss of a parent, sibling, or other loved one during a traumatic event. As defined by the National Child Traumatic Stress Network (NCTSN), "Children with childhood traumatic grief experience the cause of [the loved one's] **death** as horrifying or terrifying, whether the death was sudden and unexpected (for example, due to homicide, suicide, motor vehicle accident,drug overdose, natural disaster, war, terrorism, and so on) or due to natural causes (**cancer, heart attack**, and so forth). Even if the manner of death does not appear to others to be sudden, shocking, or frightening, children who perceive the death in this way may develop childhood traumatic grief. In this condition, even happy thoughts and memories of the deceased person remind children of the traumatic way in which the deceased died." More information on the identification and treatment of childhood traumatic grief can be obtained from the NCTSN web site, < http://www.nctsnet.org/nccts/nav.do?pid = hom_main > .

Symptoms

The symptoms of stress can be either physical or psychological. Stress-related physical illnesses, such as **irritable bowel syndrome**, heart attacks, arthritis, and chronic headaches, result from long-term overstimulation of a part of the nervous system that regulates the heart rate, blood pressure, and digestive system. Stress-related emotional illness results from inadequate or inappropriate responses to major changes in one's life situation, such as marriage, completing one's education, becoming a parent, losing a job, or retirement. Psychiatrists sometimes use the term adjustment disorder to describe this type of illness. In the workplace, stress-related illness often takes the form of burnout—a loss of interest in or ability to perform one's job due to long-term high stress levels. For example, palliative care nurses are at high risk of burnout due to their inability to prevent their patients from dying or even to relieve their physical suffering in some circumstances.

Diagnosis

When the doctor suspects that a patient's illness is connected to stress, he or she will take a careful history that includes stressors in the patient's life (family or employment problems, other illnesses, etc.). Many physicians will evaluate the patient's personality as well, in order to assess his or her coping resources and emotional response patterns. There are a number of personality inventories and **psychological tests** that doctors can use to help diagnose the amount of stress that the patient experiences and the coping strategies that he or she uses to deal with them. A variation on this theme is to identify what the patient perceives as threatening as well as stressful. Stress-related illness can be diagnosed by primary care doctors, as well as by those who specialize in psychiatry. The doctor will need to distinguish between **adjustment disorders** and **anxiety** or **mood disorders**, and between psychiatric disorders and physical illnesses (e.g., thyroid activity) that have psychological side effects.

Treatment

Recent advances in the understanding of the many complex connections between the human mind and body have produced a variety of mainstream approaches to stress-related illness. Present treatment regimens may include one or more of the following:

- Medications. These may include drugs to control blood pressure or other physical symptoms of stress, as well as drugs that affect the patient's mood (tranquilizers or antidepressants).

- Stress management programs. These may be either individual or group treatments, and usually involve analysis of the stressors in the patient's life. They often focus on job or workplace-related stress.

- Behavioral approaches. These strategies include relaxation techniques, breathing exercises, and physical **exercise** programs including walking.

- Massage. Therapeutic massage relieves stress by relaxing the large groups of muscles in the back, neck, arms, and legs.

- Cognitive therapy. These approaches teach patients to reframe or mentally reinterpret the stressors in their lives in order to modify the body's physical reactions.

- Meditation and associated spiritual or religious practices. Recent studies have found positive correlations between these practices and stress hardiness.

Alternative treatment

Treatment of stress is one area in which the boundaries between traditional and alternative therapies have changed in recent years, in part because some forms of physical exercise (**yoga**, **tai chi**, aikido) that were once associated with the counterculture have become widely accepted as useful parts of mainstream **stress reduction** programs. Other alternative therapies for stress that are occasionally recommended by mainstream medicine include **aromatherapy**, dance therapy, **biofeedback**, nutrition-based treatments (including dietary guidelines and **nutritional supplements**), **acupuncture**, homeopathy, and herbal medicine.

Prognosis

The prognosis for recovery from a stress-related illness is related to a wide variety of factors in a person's life, many of which are genetically determined (race, sex, illnesses that run in families) or beyond the individual's control (economic trends, cultural stereotypes and prejudices). It is possible, however, for humans to learn new responses to stress and, thus, change their experiences of it. A person's ability to remain healthy in stressful situations is sometimes referred to as stress hardiness. Stress-hardy people have a cluster of personality traits that strengthen their ability to cope. These traits include believing in the importance of what they are doing; believing that they have some power to influence their situation; and viewing life's changes as positive opportunities rather than as threats.

Prevention

Complete prevention of stress is neither possible nor desirable, because stress is an important stimulus

KEY TERMS

Adjustment disorder—A psychiatric disorder marked by inappropriate or inadequate responses to a change in life circumstances. Depression following retirement from work is an example of adjustment disorder.

Biofeedback—A technique in which patients learn to modify certain body functions, such as temperature or pulse rate, with the help of a monitoring machine.

Burnout—An emotional condition, marked by tiredness, loss of interest, or frustration, that interferes with job performance,. Burnout is usually regarded as the result of prolonged stress.

Stress hardiness—A personality characteristic that enables persons to stay healthy in stressful circumstances. It includes belief in one's ability to influence the situation; being committed to or fully engaged in one's activities; and having a positive view of change.

Stress management—A category of popularized programs and techniques intended to help people deal more effectively with stress.

Stressor—A stimulus, or event, that provokes a stress response in an organism. Stressors can be categorized as acute or chronic, and as external or internal to the organism.

of human growth and creativity, as well as an inevitable part of life. In addition, specific strategies for stress prevention vary widely from person to person, depending on the nature and number of the stressors in an individual's life, and the amount of control he or she has over these factors. In general, however, a combination of attitudinal and behavioral changes works well for most patients. The best form of prevention appears to be parental modeling of healthy attitudes and behaviors within the family.

Resources

BOOKS

Beers, Mark H., MD, and Robert Berkow, MD., editors. "Psychiatry in Medicine. " In *The Merck Manual of Diagnosis and Therapy*. Whitehouse Station, NJ: Merck Research Laboratories, 2004.

Pelletier, Kenneth R., MD. *The Best Alternative Medicine*, Part I, "Spirituality and Healing." New York: Simon & Schuster, 2002.

PERIODICALS

Blumenthal, J. A., M. Babyak, J. Wei, et al. "Usefulness of Psychosocial Treatment of Mental Stress-Induced Myocardial Ischemia in Men." *American Journal of Cardiology* 89 (January 15, 2002): 164-168.

Cardenas, J., K. Williams, J. P. Wilson, et al. "PSTD, Major Depressive Symptoms, and Substance Abuse Following September 11, 2001, in a Midwestern University Population" *International Journal of Emergency Mental Health* 5 (Winter 2003): 15–28.

Centers for Disease Control and Prevention. "Mental Health Status of World Trade Center Rescue and Recovery Workers and Volunteers—New York City, July 2002–August 2004." *Morbidity and Mortality Weekly Report* 53 (September 10, 2004): 812–815.

Gallo, L. C., and K. A. Matthews. "Understanding the Association Between Socioeconomic Status and Physical Health: Do Negative Emotions Play a Role?" *Psychological Bulletin* 129 (January 2003): 10–51.

Goodman, R. F., A. V. Morgan, S. Juriga, and E. J. Brown. "Letting the Story Unfold: A Case Study of Client-Centered Therapy for Childhood Traumatic Grief." *Harvard Review of Psychiatry* 12 (July-August 2004): 199–212.

Hawkley, L. C., and J. T. Cacioppo. "Loneliness and Pathways to Disease." *Brain, Behavior, and Immunity* 17, Supplement 1 (February 2003): S98–S105.

Latkin, C. A., and A. D. Curry. "Stressful Neighborhoods and Depression: A Prospective Study of the Impact of Neighborhood Disorder." *Journal of Health and Social Behavior* 44 (March 2003): 34–44.

Ottenstein, R. J. "Coping with Threats of Terrorism: A Protocol for Group Intervention." *International Journal of Emergency Mental Health* 5 (Winter 2003): 39–42.

Ritchie, L. J. "Threat: A Concept Analysis for a New Era." *Nursing Forum* 39 (July-September 2004): 13–22.

Surwit, R. S., M. A. van Tilburg, N. Zucker, et al. "Stress Management Improves Long-Term Glycemic Control in Type 2 Diabetes." *Diabetes Care* 25 (January 2002): 30-34.

West, P., and H. Sweeting. "Fifteen, Female and Stressed: Changing Patterns of Psychological Distress Over Time." *Journal of Child Psychology and Psychiatry* 44 (March 2003): 399–411.

White, K., L. Wilkes, K. Cooper, and M. Barbato. "The Impact of Unrelieved Patient Suffering on Palliative Care Nurses." *International Journal of Palliative Nursing* 10 (September 2004): 438–444.

ORGANIZATIONS

The American Institute of Stress. 124 Park Avenue, Yonkers, NY 10703 (914) 963-1200. Fax: (914) 965-6267. < http://www.stress.org >.

Centers for Disease Control and Prevention. 1600 Clifton Rd., NE, Atlanta, GA 30333. (800) 311-3435, (404) 639-3311. < http://www.cdc.gov >.

National Child Traumatic Stress Initiative. Center for Mental Health Services, Substance Abuse and Mental

Health Services Administration, Department of Health and Human Services, 5600 Fishers Lane, Parklawn Building, Room 17C-26, Rockville, MD 20857. (301) 443-2940. < http://www.nctsnet.org/nccts/ nav.do?pid = hom_main >.

National Institute of Mental Health (NIMH). 6001 Executive Boulevard, Room 8184, MSC 9663, Bethesda, MD 20892-9663. (301) 443-4513. < http:// www.nimh.nih.gov >.

OTHER

National Center for Post-Traumatic Stress Disorder, Department of Veterans Affairs. *Fact Sheet: Survivors of Human-Caused and Natural Disasters.* < http:// www.ncptsd.org/facts/disasters/ fs_survivors_disaster.html >.

National Institute of Mental Health (NIMH) news release, July 17, 2003. "Gene More Than Doubles Risk of Depression Following Life Stresses." < http:// www.nimh.nih.gov/events/prgenestress.cfm >.

Rebecca J. Frey, PhD

Stress reduction

Definition

Stress is the body's normal response to anything that disturbs its natural physical, emotional, or mental balance. Stress reduction refers to various strategies that counteract this response and produce a sense of relaxation and tranquility.

Purpose

Although stress is a natural phenomenon of living, stress that is not controlled and that continues for a long period of time can seriously compromise health. For this reason, stress must be understood, managed and appropriately reduced. Several very different strategies and therapies are available that help with relaxation and stress management.

Precautions

Stress reduction can only present a problem if an individual attributes an actual, serious condition or disease to being simply a stress-related response and avoids consulting a physician.

People who have undergone a severe trauma (criminal assault, combat, natural or transportation disaster, etc.) may experience symptoms of **post-traumatic stress disorder** (PTSD) or **acute stress disorder** (ASD). These disorders are defined by their temporal connection to a traumatic event in the patient's life, and are characterized by a cluster of **anxiety** and dissociative symptoms. They interfere with the patient's normal level of functioning, and require some form of supportive therapy. People who experience a sense of detachment or unreality, emotional numbing, a general feeling of being dazed, **amnesia** for part of the traumatic event, or similar symptoms should consult a medical doctor in addition to using other approaches to stress reduction.

Description

Everyone encounters stress every day. Although most people think of it as something negative that happens to them, in fact stress itself is really neither good nor bad but is neutral or nonspecific. Stress may be internal (from within ourselves) or external (such as noise from the environment) and does not always result from something unpleasant. A certain amount of stress in our lives is actually essential to being sufficiently stimulated to meet the challenges of everyday life, but when stress is constant and acute, it can have dangerous consequences. Since stress is both natural and unavoidable, it is necessary to understand it and to learn how to deal with it, particularly how to reduce it.

The specific and immediate cause of stress is called the stressor. A stressor can be something dramatic or terrible, such as a violent experience or the **death** of a loved one, or it can be a positive and rewarding event, like marriage or a promotion. The stressor can be internal, such as feelings of guilt or anger felt in a relationship, or it can be external, such as a natural disaster or the ordinary rigors and frustrations of commuting. It can also have a physical source, like simple **exercise** or hard work, or it can be strictly mental, like worry. Our bodies react the same way physiologically no matter what the source and reasons for stress might be.

From a physical standpoint, the body reacts to stress in a standard and predictable manner. When stress occurs, the brain immediately receives nerve impulses. These impulses initiate an automatic sequence carried out by the body's sympathetic nervous system: it begins with stimulation of the brain's hypothalamus, which sends nerve impulses to both the adrenal and the pituitary glands. Also called the "fight or flight" response, this automatic physiological process is known to have evolved in humans and animals to enable them to cope with sudden life-threatening emergencies. When faced with a major stressor, the body's biochemistry instantly hurtles into a ready mode that marshals all the possible resources necessary to either escape or do battle. Thus, the adrenal glands located on top of the kidneys provide an instant surge of adrenaline, the body's rocket fuel, quickening the heart rate and blood flow and providing every cell with extra oxygen. They also release cortisol or hydrocortisone, causing an increase in both amino acids (the building blocks of proteins) and blood sugar. These will be needed if tissue repair must take place. Finally, the pituitary gland at the base of the brain releases a variety of hormones, endorphins among them, that act as natural painkillers and permit the body to do things it ordinarily cannot do. Thus, at just about the same time a stressor is recognized by the body, the heart and breathing rate spikes, the pupils dilate to let in more light, perspiration increases and digestion slows, and the body is aroused, energized, and temporarily feels no **pain**. This sequence of events allows individuals to do whatever is required to save themselves, whether it is to flee from a predator or engage in combat and fend off an attack.

While these automatic physiological responses served early man well and were essential to survival of the species, today's men and women rarely must literally fight for their lives or dodge and elude a predator. Yet their bodies' automatic response to stress has remained unchanged in a radically changed, modern world. Whether caveman or corporate executive, when the fight-or-flight response kicks in, a three-stage process begins. Stage one is the alarm stage in which the body releases hormones and prepares for extreme physical action. Resistance is stage two in which the body attempts to resist yet adapt to the stress and to repair any damage done. The final stage, exhaustion, occurs if the stress remains constant. It is especially dangerous since stage one's physical response may begin all over again. The persistence of stress and stage three's exhaustion is the point at which disease can occur. The body may then experience severe debilitating conditions like migraine, heart irregularities, and mental illness. The body's functions may even shut down altogether.

Although different individuals may have different levels of tolerance to stress, chronic stress will eventually wear down even the strongest of people. Prolonged stress can cause biochemical imbalances that weaken the immune system and invite serious illness. Overall, stress that persists is known to interfere with digestion and, more seriously, alter brain chemistry, create hormonal imbalances, increase heart rate, raise blood pressure, and negatively affect both metabolic and immune function. It is also important to recognize that although stress itself is not a disease, it can worsen any number of already serious physical conditions. Many physicians feel that chronic stress can so overtax an individual's physical resources and ways of coping that **cancer**, **stroke**, and heart disease can occur. While long-term stress can seriously affect one's quality of life and lead to major, sometimes fatal, diseases, prolonged stress also results in the everyday miseries of **headache** and allergy, digestive disorders and **fatigue**, irritable bladder and **impotence**, **insomnia**, anxiety, depression, and simple aches and pains. Researchers exploring the connection between stress and susceptibility to colds exposed stressed individuals (who had experienced a death in the family, become divorced, or had recently moved) to cold viruses and then tested for antibodies a month later. Results indicated that severely stressed individuals were four times more likely to become infected.

It follows that if stress can cause or contribute to illness, then reducing stress should have the opposite effect and perhaps even encourage healing. Probably the most important step toward reducing the stress in everyone's life is to understand the nature of stress and to learn how to condition ourselves to be able to gain some control over it. Being able to recognize that we are stressed is probably the first step toward understanding. Of the many signs and symptoms that alert us, some are obvious and require only common sense to recognize. Short-term noticeable effects of stress include sweaty palms and other types of perspiration, dilated pupils, and difficulty in swallowing ("a lump in the throat"). Tightness in the chest is another stress signal as are stomach problems and some skin conditions. Stress that is the result of prolonged anxiety (a sense of apprehension) often results in feelings of panic or actual trembling, fatigue, insomnia, and **shortness of breath**, heart **palpitations** and **dizziness**, and sometimes simple irritability. Although none of these symptoms is pleasant, they are relatively minor compared to the silent but much more serious internal effects that can lead to immune-related disorders and even cancer and heart disease.

Fortunately, stress and the negative effects it creates can be reduced by a wide variety of therapeutic approaches. When successfully applied, many of these therapies or strategies can both reduce stress and reverse its damage. Before selecting a particular therapy, it is important to be able distinguish bad or unhealthy stress from the type that is not bad. Researchers have found that the most important variable among types of stress is an individual's sense of control in a given situation. The least harmful stress scenario is one in which an individual has a sufficient degree of control or some idea of predictability. Put simply, predictable pain is less stressful because individuals know when to relax (gaining relief from pain as well as protecting themselves from its damaging effects). But when individuals have no warning of pain, they are in a state of constant stress. An example from daily life might be the difference between the stress experienced by top executives who are in control of their fate and their middle-level managers who are not. The former can pick and choose when to enter or engage a stressful situation or problem, but the latter have no control nor any ability to predict when such a situation will arise and are constantly on alert or in a state of anxiety.

For those with little control over situations that make them anxious, there are basically two ways to deal with their stress. One is to remove or at least reduce the stressor, and the other is to increase their resistance to it. Although there are many strategies to achieve each of these, all of them can be reduced to some variation of a single simple concept—relaxation. While there is no one single technique or therapy for everyone to use to manage and reduce stress, there is certainly some combination of lifestyle change, diet, exercise, and relaxation that will allow all types of individuals to better manage the stress in their lives. Although relaxation is at the core of most stress reduction methods, it is not something that everyone can fully achieve without assistance and guidance. Interestingly, our modern life experiences often do not provide us with the coping skills needed to deal with stressful stimuli, and increasingly, people find that simple relaxing is something that they must learn how to do.

Fortunately, there are a number of relaxation therapies that enable the willing individual to achieve deep, beneficial relaxation. In fact, there are almost too many from which to choose. A 1997 book on stress remedies cowritten by the editors of *Prevention* magazine and published by Rodale Press is organized alphabetically and lists fifty-nine separate stress-reducing techniques and subjects, from Acceptance to **Yoga**. These and many other methods of reducing stress can be grouped into the following general categories: mind-body therapies, body work and movement therapies, and herbal-based **diets** and natural regimens. Many of the specific techniques in these categories can be part of a self-help or self-care approach, although some require the help of an experienced practitioner.

Therapies that focus on the mind/body connection are based on the fact that thinking and emotions can have physical effects on the body. These techniques encourage the individual to take control and learning how to cope with stressors rather than trying to eliminate them. Such therapies range from individual counseling and **meditation** or involvement with a support group to the mystery of **guided imagery** and the technology of **biofeedback**. They all have the common goal of evoking the physiological relaxation response, in which a person can achieve such beneficial internal results as lowering blood pressure and decreasing gastric acid secretion.

Body work and movement therapies include techniques ranging from dance therapy and the gentleness of massage to **reflexology** and the rigors of **rolfing**. Body work is based partly on the therapeutic power of human touch and can also include manipulation, realignment, and posture correction. Movement therapies are a particular form of physical exercise, although they attempt to do much more than simply get a person into shape. Most usually emphasize the mind/body connection and strive to put people in better touch with both their bodies and their feelings. Body work and movement therapies can be as vigorous as deep tissue manipulation or as simple and minimal as the Alexander technique's light posture corrections.

Herbal remedies for stress are usually part of a larger system of natural, **holistic medicine**. Whether Chinese traditional medicine, its counterpart from India, or the homeopathy of the West, all these systems of natural medicine have a holistic focus and emphasize the need for inner balance. All demonstrate how the individual's physical, emotional, mental, and spiritual states are connected and use natural substances as part of the treatment for reducing stress. Such therapies range from the occasional purging (cleansing) of **Ayurvedic medicine** to the sleep-inducing properties of chamomile tea. They also can include the use of cayenne to relieve pain, fragrant essential oils from flowers to evoke a pleasing response and relieve tension, or aloe vera to soothe burned skin.

A list of some of the more common therapies and techniques available for reducing stress includes:

- Acupuncture. Insertion of needles at certain spots under the skin for the purpose of attaining balance by either releasing blocked energy or draining off excess energy.

- Alexander technique. Improving the alignment of head, neck, and back claims to achieve efficient posture and movement.

- Aromatherapy. Massage with essential oils from flowers claims to affect mood and produce a sense of well-being.

- Art therapy. Creating something allows free expression and results in feelings of achievement and mood change.

- Autogenic training therapy. A form of deep meditation or self-hypnosis.

- Autosuggestion therapy. A form of verbal therapy involving repetition of a positive idea.

- Ayurvedic medicine. A complete system of daily living based on awareness of one's particular constitution.

- Behavioral therapy. A variety of psychotherapies that are based on changing ourselves by retraining.

- Bach flower therapy. Herbal remedies that are prepared from flowers acting energetically to soothe the mind and body.

- Bioenergetics. A practice that encourages sudden release of tensions by crying or kicking.

- Biofeedback. Monitoring rates of body functions and using data to influence and gain control over autonomic functions.

- Breathing for relaxation. Stylized breathing technique to control and lower body functions.

- Counseling. Work with a therapist trained in talking-based therapy.

- Dance **movement therapy**. Freedom of expression through movement.

- Feldenkrais method. Slow, light movements alter habits and reeducate neuromuscular system.

- Flotation therapy. Floating in a soundproof tank with no external stimulation.

- Guided imagery. Creating a mental picture of what is desired. Also called Creative imagery or Visualization.

- Herbal medicine. Uses substances derived from plants as treatment instead of synthetic drugs.

- Homeopathy. Uses minute doses of plant, animal, and mineral substances to stimulate the body's natural healing.

- Hydrotherapy. Use of water internally and externally for healing purposes.

- Hypnotherapy. Hypnosis in order to identify and release patterns that keep an individual from a personal balance point.

- Kinesiology. Uses muscle testing to correct imbalances in the body's "energy system." Also called Touch for Health.

- Massage. Use of touch and manipulation to soothe. Can also employ vigorous deep tissue manipulation.

- Meditation. Deep, relaxed, receptive, and focused concentration on a single object, sound, or word.

- Music therapy. Playing or listening to music to create an emotional reaction.

- Naturopathy. A complete health care system that uses a variety of natural healing therapies.

- Psychotherapy. A talking-based therapy with a mental health professional to get at the root of a conflict, modify behavior and disruptive negative thought patterns.

- Reflexology. Manipulation of zones of the feet that relate to the major organs, glands, and areas of the body.

- Rolfing. Vigorous manipulation of the body's connective tissue to restore "balance."

- Shiatsu. Traditional Japanese finger pressure massage therapy.

- Sound therapy. Uses sound waves to slow the body's autonomic system.

- Tai chi chuan. System of slow, continuous exercises based on rhythm and equilibrium.

- Yoga. System of exercises that combines certain positions with deep breathing and meditation.

These and many other techniques, systems, and therapies are available to the person searching for some way to reduce and manage the stress of everyday life. Some methods are very simple and can be easily learned, while others are high-tech and often involve a practitioner. A search for common elements among most of these stress-reducing systems reveals several obvious strategies that nearly everyone can employ on their own. However, it is important to know and recognize the signals of stress. Further, it is easier to resist the negative effects of stress by eating properly and getting sufficient sleep and exercise.

Nearly all stress-reducing systems are geared to evoking some degree of beneficial mind/body relaxation, and most include some version of the following:

- mental time out

- deep breathing

- meditation and singular focus

- gentle, repetitive exercise

The best stress reduction system is the one that works for the individual. Whether stress can be relieved by laughter, mellow music, repetition of a single word, self-massage, vigorous activity, or simply by doing everyday chores in a mindful state of heightened awareness, it is important that stress be recognized and managed every day. Studies have shown that regular relaxation eventually makes the body less responsive to its stress hormones and acts as a sort of natural tranquilizer. People can build their own immune defense against the stress response.

Many companies have introduced workplace stress management programs to improve their employees' health. These programs typically include instruction on emotional refocusing or restructuring, and have been shown to be beneficial in reducing the participants' blood pressure, heart rate, and other signs of emotional upset. In addition, stress management programs designed for persons in specific high-stress occupations (medicine, law enforcement, emergency response, etc.) have proved to be effective in reducing burnout and helping members of these professions cope with the specific stresses of their respective jobs.

An additional general strategy for handling stress in family life or the workplace is the cultivation of a group of character traits that has been termed "psychological hardiness." These traits include believing in the importance of what one is doing; believing that one has some power to influence the immediate situation; and viewing life's changes as positive opportunities rather than as threats. These qualities are sometimes referred to as the "3 Cs," which stand for commitment, control and challenge. Approaches to stress reduction that enhance these qualities are especially beneficial to people.

Newer trends in stress reduction

One trend in stress reduction in the early 2000s is the development of stress management programs or stress reduction strategies tailored to specific categories of people, often defined by their occupation or by a chronic health condition. For example, journalists who cover traumatic events are increasingly recognized as susceptible to developing posttraumatic stress disorder. With regard to specific diseases, stress management programs have been pioneered as of 2004 for patients with **asthma** or lupus erythematosus.

Another new trend in stress reduction is the development of programs designed for communities as well as individuals. After the events of September 11, 2001, many mental health professionals recognized that acts of terrorism or mass violence affect large groups of people, and that psychiatric interventions need to address stress as a group experience as well as an individual one.

Risks

All relaxation-based therapies to reduce stress are virtually free of serious risk.

Normal results

Learning how to manage stress has the short-term benefits of giving people some sense of control in their lives, providing them with positive coping strategies, and making them more relaxed and healthier. The long-term benefits can be a stronger immune system, proper hormonal balance, and reduced susceptibility to such serious, life-threatening diseases as heart disease and cancer.

Resources

BOOKS

American Psychiatric Association. *Diagnostic and Statistical Manual of Mental Disorders.* 4th ed., revised. Washington, DC: American Psychiatric Association, 2000.

Beers, Mark H., MD, and Robert Berkow, MD., editors. "Anxiety Disorders." In *The Merck Manual of Diagnosis and Therapy.* Whitehouse Station, NJ: Merck Research Laboratories, 2004.

Beers, Mark H., MD, and Robert Berkow, MD., editors. "Psychiatry in Medicine. " In *The Merck Manual of Diagnosis and Therapy.* Whitehouse Station, NJ: Merck Research Laboratories, 2004.

Pelletier, Kenneth R., MD. *The Best Alternative Medicine,* Part I. "Spirituality and Healing." New York: Simon & Schuster, 2002.

PERIODICALS

Collins, P. A., and A. C. Gibbs. "Stress in Police Officers: A Study of the Origins, Prevalence and Severity of Stress-Related Symptoms Within a County Police Force." *Occupational Medicine (London)* 53 (June 2003): 256–264.

Czech, T. "Journalists and Trauma: A Brief Overview." *International Journal of Emergency Mental Health* 6 (Summer 2004): 159–162.

Greco, C. M., T. E. Rudy, and S. Manzi. "Effects of a Stress-Reduction Program on Psychological Function, Pain, and Physical Function of Systemic Lupus Erythematosus Patients: A Randomized Controlled Trial." *Arthritis and Rheumatism* 51 (August 15, 2004): 625–634.

Lambert, V. A., C. E. Lambert, and H. Yamase. "Psychological Hardiness, Workplace Stress and Related Stress Reduction Strategies." *Nursing and Health Sciences* 5 (June 2003): 181–184.

KEY TERMS

Adrenal gland—A pair of glands that rest on the top of each kidney that produce steroids, such as sex hormones and those concerned with metabolic functions.

Amino acid—Organic acids that are the main components of proteins and are synthesized by living cells.

Antibody—A type of protein produced in the blood in response to a foreign substance that destroys the intruding substance; it is responsible for immunity.

Burnout—An emotional condition marked by tiredness, loss of interest, or frustration that interferes with job performance. Burnout is usually regarded as the result of prolonged stress.

Chronic—Long-term or frequently recurring.

Debilitating—Weakening, or reducing the strength of.

Dilate—To enlarge, open wide, or distend.

Endorphins—A group of proteins with powerful pain-killing properties that originate naturally in the brain.

Holistic—That which pertains to the entire person, involving the body, mind, and spirit.

Hydrocortisone—A steroid hormone produced by the adrenal glands that provides resistance to stress.

Hypothalamus—A part of the brain that controls some of the body's automatic regulatory functions.

Immune function—The state in which the body recognizes foreign materials and is able to neutralize them before they can do any harm.

Impotence—The inability of the male to engage in sexual intercourse because of insufficient erection.

Insomnia—Inability to sleep under normal conditions.

Metabolic function—Those processes necessary for the maintenance of a living organism.

Neuromuscular—Relating to nerve and muscle or their interaction.

Physiological—Dealing with the functions and processes of the body.

Pituitary gland—A gland at the base of the brain responsible for growth, maturation, and reproduction.

Sympathetic nervous system—That part of the autonomic nervous system that affects contraction of muscles and blood vessels. Stimulation of this system by a stressor triggers the production of hormones that prepare the body for fight or flight

Therapeutic—Curative or healing.

Macy, R. D., L. Behar, R. Paulson, et al. "Community-Based, Acute Posttraumatic Stress Management: A Description and Evaluation of a Psychosocial-Intervention Continuum." *Harvard Review of Psychiatry* 12 (July-August 2004): 217–228.

McCraty, R., M. Atkinson, and D. Tomasino. "Impact of a Workplace Stress Reduction Program on Blood Pressure and Emotional Health in Hypertensive Employees." *Journal of Alternative and Complementary Medicine* 9 (June 2003): 355–369.

Ritchie, E. C., M. Friedman, P. Watson, et al. "Mass Violence and Early Mental Health Intervention: A Proposed Application of Best-Practice Guidelines to Chemical, Biological, and Radiological Attacks." *Military Medicine* 169 (August 2004): 575–579.

Sotile, W. M., and M. O. Sotile. "Beyond Physician Burnout: Keys to Effective Emotional Management." *Journal of Medical Practice Management* 18 (May-June 2003): 314–318.

Wright, R. J. "Alternative Modalities for Asthma That Reduce Stress and Modify Mood States: Evidence for Underlying Psychobiologic Mechanisms." *Annals of Allergy, Asthma and Immunology* 93, no. 2, Supplement 1 (August 2004): S18–S23.

ORGANIZATIONS

American Institute of Stress. 124 Park Avenue. Yonkers, NY 10703. (914) 963-1200. < http://www.stress.org >.

American Psychiatric Association (APA). 1400 K Street, NW, Washington, DC 20005. (888) 357-7924. < http://www.psych.org >.

Center for Mindfulness. University of Massachusetts Medical Center, 55 Lake Avenue North, Worcester, MA 01655. (508) 856-2656. < http://www.umassmed.edu/cfm >.

National Institute of Mental Health (NIMH) Office of Communications. 6001 Executive Boulevard, Room 8184, MSC 9663, Bethesda, MD 20892-9663. (866) 615-NIMH or (301) 443-4513. < http://www.nimh.nih.gov >.

OTHER

National Institute of Mental Health (NIMH). *Anxiety Disorders.* NIH Publication No. 02-3879. Bethesda, MD: NIMH, 2002.

Leonard C. Bruno, PhD
Rebecca J. Frey, PhD

Stress test

Definition

Used to evaluate heart function, a **stress** test requires that a patient exercises on a treadmill or **exercise** bicycle while his or her heart rate, breathing, blood pressure, electrocardiogram (ECG), and feeling of well being are monitored.

Purpose

When the body is active, it requires more oxygen than when it is at rest, and, therefore, the heart has to pump more blood. Because of the increased stress on the heart, exercise can reveal coronary problems that are not apparent when the body is at rest. This is why the stress test, though not perfect, remains the best initial, noninvasive, practical coronary test.

The stress test helps doctors determine how well the heart handles the increased demands imposed by physical activity. It is particularly useful for evaluating possible **coronary artery disease**, detecting inadequate supply of oxygen-rich blood to the tissues of the heart muscle (**ischemia**), and determining safe levels of exercise in people with existing heart disease.

Precautions

The exercise stress test carries a very slight risk (1 in 100,000) of causing a **heart attack**. For this reason, the exercise stress test should be attended by a health care professional with a defibrillator and other emergency equipment on standby.

The patient must be aware of the symptoms of a heart attack and stop the test if he or she develops any of the following symptoms:

- an unsteady gait
- confusion
- skin is grayish or cold and clammy
- **dizziness** or **fainting**
- a drop in blood pressure
- chest **pain** (**angina**)
- irregular heart beat (cardiac arrhythmias)

Description

The technician affixes electrodes to specific areas of the patient's chest, using special adhesive patches with a special gel that conducts electrical impulses. Typically, electrodes are placed under each collarbone and each bottom rib, and six electrodes are placed across the chest in a rough outline of the heart. Then the technician attaches wires from the electrodes to an ECG, which records the electrical activity picked up by the electrodes.

The technician runs resting ECG tests while the patient is lying down, then standing up, and then breathing heavily for half a minute. These tests can later be compared with the ECG tests performed while the patient is exercising. The patient's blood pressure is taken and the blood pressure cuff is left in place, so that blood pressure can be measured periodically throughout the test.

The patient begins riding a stationary bicycle or walking on a treadmill. Gradually the intensity of the exercise is increased. For example, if the patient is walking on a treadmill, the speed of the treadmill increases and the treadmill is tilted upward to simulate an incline. If the patient is on an exercise bicycle, the resistance or "drag" is gradually increased. The patient continues exercising at increasing intensity until he or she reaches his or her target heart rate (generally set at a minimum of 85% of the maximal predicted heart rate based on the patient's age) or experiences severe **fatigue**, dizziness, or chest pain. During this time, the patient's heart rate, ECG pattern, and blood pressure are continually monitored.

In some cases, other tests, such as **echocardiography** or thallium scanning, are also used in conjunction with the exercise stress test. For instance, recent studies suggest that women have a high rate of false negatives (results showing no problem when one exists) and false positives (results showing a problem when one does not exist) with the stress test. They may benefit from another test, such as exercise echocardiography. People who are unable to exercise may be injected with drugs that mimic the effects of exercise on the heart and given a thallium scan, which can detect the same abnormalities that an exercise test can.

Preparation

Patients are usually instructed not to eat or smoke for several hours before the test. They should also tell the doctor about any medications they are taking. They should wear comfortable sneakers and exercise clothing.

Aftercare

After the test, the patient should rest until blood pressure and heart rate return to normal. If all goes

KEY TERMS

Angina—Chest pain from a poor blood supply to the heart muscle due to narrowing of the coronary arteries.

Cardiac arrhythmia—An irregular heart rate or rhythm.

Coronary arteries—Two arteries that branch off from the aorta and supply blood to the heart.

Defibrillator—A device that delivers an electric shock to the heart muscle through the chest wall in order to restore a normal heart rate.

False negative—Test results showing no problem when one exists.

False positive—Test results showing a problem when one does not exist.

Hypertrophy—The overgrowth of muscle.

Ischemia—Dimished supply of oxygen-rich blood to an organ or area of the body.

well, and there are no signs of distress, the patient may return to his or her normal daily activities.

Risks

There is a very slight risk of a heart attack from the exercise, as well as cardiac arrhythmia (irregular heart beats), angina, or cardiac arrest (about one in 100,000).

Normal results

A normal result of an exercise stress test shows normal electrocardiogram tracings and heart rate, blood pressure within the normal range, and no angina, unusual dizziness, or **shortness of breath**.

Abnormal results

A number of abnormalities may show up on an exercise stress test. An abnormal electrocardiogram (ECG) may indicate deprivation of oxygen-rich blood to the heart muscle (ST wave segment depression, for example), heart rhythm disturbances, or structural abnormalities of the heart, such as overgrowth of muscle (hypertrophy). If the blood pressure rises too high or the patient experiences distressing symptoms during the test, the heart may be unable to handle the increased workload. Stress test abnormalities usually require further evaluation and therapy.

Resources

ORGANIZATIONS

American Heart Association. 7320 Greenville Ave. Dallas, TX 75231. (214) 373-6300. < http://www.americanheart.org > .

National Heart, Lung and Blood Institute. P.O. Box 30105, Bethesda, MD 20824-0105. (301) 251-1222. < http://www.nhlbi.nih.gov > .

Robert Scott Dinsmoor

Stridor

Definition

Stridor is a term used to describe noisy breathing in general, and to refer specifically to a high-pitched crowing sound associated with **croup**, respiratory infection, and airway obstruction.

Description

Stridor occurs when erratic air currents attempt to force their way through breathing passages narrowed by:

- illness
- infection
- the presence of **foreign objects**
- throat abnormalities

Stridor can usually be heard from a distance but is sometimes audible only during deep breathing. Someone who has stridor may crow and wheeze when:

- inhaling
- exhaling
- inhaling and exhaling

Most common in young children, whose naturally small airways are easily obstructed, stridor can be a symptom of a life-threatening respiratory emergency.

Causes and symptoms

During childhood, stridor is usually caused by infection of the cartilage flap (epiglottis) that covers the opening of the windpipe to prevent **choking** during swallowing. It can also be caused by a toy or other tiny object the child has tried to swallow.

Laryngomalacia is a common cause of a rapid, low-pitched form of stridor that may be heard when a baby inhales. This harmless condition does not require medical attention. It usually disappears by the time the child is 18 months old.

The most common causes of stridor in adults are:

- abscess or swelling of the upper airway
- paralysis or malfunction of the vocal cords
- tumor.

Other common causes of stridor include:

- enlargement of the thyroid gland (**goiter**)
- swelling of the voice box (largyngeal **edema**)
- narrowing of the windpipe (tracheal stenosis)

When stridor is caused by a condition that slowly narrows the airway, crowing and **wheezing** may not develop until the obstruction has become severe.

Diagnosis

When stridor is present in a newborn, pediatricians and neonatologists look for evidence of:

- heart defects inherent at birth (congenital)
- neurological disorders
- General toxicity.

If examinations do not reveal the reasons for the baby's noisy breathing, the air passages are assumed to be the cause of the problem.

Listening to an older child or adult breathe usually enables pediatricians, family physicians, and pulmonary specialists to estimate where an airway obstruction is located. The extent of the obstruction can be calculated by assessing the patient's:

- complexion
- chest movements
- breathing rate
- level of consciousness

X rays and direct examination of the voice box (larynx) and breathing passages indicate the exact location of the obstruction or inflammation. Flow-volume loops and pulse oximetry are diagnostic tools used to measure how much air flows through the breathing passages, and how much oxygen those passages contain.

Pulmonary function tests may also be performed.

Treatment

The cause of this condition determines the way it is treated.

Life-threatening emergencies may require:

- the insertion of a breathing tube through the mouth and nose (tracheal intubation)
- the insertion of a breathing tube directly into the windpipe (tracheostomy)

Resources

BOOKS

Berkow, Robert, editor. *The Merck Manual of Medical Information: Home Edition.* Whitehouse Station, NJ: Merck & Co., Inc., 1997.

Maureen Haggerty

Stroke

Definition

A stroke is the sudden death of brain cells in a localized area due to inadequate blood flow.

Description

A stroke occurs when blood flow is interrupted to part of the brain. Without blood to supply oxygen and nutrients and to remove waste products, brain cells quickly begin to die. Depending on the region of the brain affected, a stroke may cause **paralysis**, speech impairment, loss of memory and reasoning ability, **coma**, or death. A stroke also is sometimes called a brain attack or a cerebrovascular accident (CVA).

Some important stroke statistics include:

- more than one-half million people in the United States experience a new or recurrent stroke each year
- stroke is the third leading cause of death in the United States and the leading cause of disability
- stroke kills about 160,000 Americans each year, or almost one out of three stroke victims
- three million Americans are currently permanently disabled from stroke
- in the United States, stroke costs about $30 billion per year in direct costs and loss of productivity
- two-thirds of strokes occur in people over age 65 but they can occur at any age
- strokes affect men more often than women, although women are more likely to die from a stroke

- strokes affect blacks more often than whites, and are more likely to be fatal among blacks

Stroke is a medical emergency requiring immediate treatment. Prompt treatment improves the chances of survival and increases the degree of recovery that may be expected. A person who may have suffered a stroke should be seen in a hospital emergency room without delay. Treatment to break up a blood clot, the major cause of stroke, must begin within three hours of the stroke to be effective. Improved medical treatment of all types of stroke has resulted in a dramatic decline in death rates in recent decades. In 1950, nine in ten died from stroke, compared to slightly less than one in three in the twenty-first century. However, about two-thirds of stroke survivors will have disabilities ranging from moderate to severe.

Causes and symptoms

Causes

There are four main types of stroke. Cerebral thrombosis and cerebral **embolism** are caused by **blood clots** that block an artery supplying the brain, either in the brain itself or in the neck. These account for 70–80% of all strokes. **Subarachnoid hemorrhage** and intracerebral hemorrhage occur when a blood vessel bursts around or in the brain.

Cerebral thrombosis occurs when a blood clot, or thrombus, forms within the brain itself, blocking the flow of blood through the affected vessel. Clots most often form due to "hardening" (**atherosclerosis**) of brain arteries. Cerebral thrombosis occurs most often at night or early in the morning. Cerebral thrombosis is often preceded by a **transient ischemic attack**, or TIA, sometimes called a "mini-stroke." In a TIA, blood flow is temporarily interrupted, causing short-lived stroke-like symptoms. Recognizing the occurrence of a TIA, and seeking immediate treatment, is an important step in stroke prevention.

Cerebral embolism occurs when a blood clot from elsewhere in the circulatory system breaks free. If it becomes lodged in an artery supplying the brain, either in the brain or in the neck, it can cause a stroke. The most common cause of cerebral embolism is atrial fibrillation, a disorder of the heart beat. In atrial fibrillation, the upper chambers (atria) of the heart beat weakly and rapidly, instead of slowly and steadily. Blood within the atria is not completely emptied. This stagnant blood may form clots within the atria, which can then break off and enter the circulation. Atrial fibrillation is a factor in about 15% of all strokes. The risk of a stroke from atrial fibrillation can be dramatically reduced with daily use of anticoagulant medication.

Hemorrhage, or bleeding, occurs when a blood vessel breaks, either from trauma or excess internal pressure. The vessels most likely to break are those with preexisting defects such as an aneurysm. An aneurysm is a "pouching out" of a blood vessel caused by a weak arterial wall. Brain aneurysms are surprisingly common. According to **autopsy** studies, about 6% of all Americans have them. Aneurysms rarely cause symptoms until they burst. Aneurysms are most likely to burst when blood pressure is highest, and controlling blood pressure is an important preventive strategy.

Intracerebral hemorrhage affects vessels within the brain itself, while subarachnoid hemorrhage affects arteries at the brain's surface, just below the protective arachnoid membrane. Intracerebral hemorrhages represent about 10% of all strokes, while subarachnoid hemorrhages account for about 7%.

In addition to depriving affected tissues of blood supply, the accumulation of fluid within the inflexible skull creates excess pressure on brain tissue, which can quickly become fatal. Nonetheless, recovery may be more complete for a person who survives hemorrhage than for one who survives a clot, because the blood deprivation effects usually are not as severe.

Death of brain cells triggers a chain reaction in which toxic chemicals created by cell death affect other nearby cells. This is one reason why prompt treatment can have such a dramatic effect on final recovery.

Risk factors

Risk factors for stroke involve age, sex, heredity, predisposing diseases or other medical conditions, use of certain medications, and lifestyle choices:

- Age and sex. The risk of stroke increases with age, doubling for each decade after age 55. Men are more likely to have a stroke than women.

- Heredity. Blacks, Asians, and Hispanics have higher rates of stroke than do whites, related partly to higher blood pressure. People with a family history of stroke are at greater risk.

- Diseases. Stroke risk is increased for people with diabetes, heart disease (especially atrial fibrillation), high blood pressure, prior stroke, or TIA. Risk of stroke increases tenfold for someone with one or more TIAs.

- Other medical conditions. Stroke risk increases with **obesity**, high blood cholesterol level, or high red blood cell count.

- **Hormone replacement therapy**. In mid-2003, a large clinical trial called the Women's Health Initiative was halted when researchers discovered several potentially dangerous effects of combined hormone replacement therapy on postmenopausal women. In addition to increasing the risk of some cancers and **dementia**, combined estrogen and progesterone therapy increased risk of ischemic stroke by 31% among study participants.

- Lifestyle choices. Stroke risk increases with cigarette **smoking** (especially if combined with the use of **oral contraceptives**), low level of physical activity, alcohol consumption above two drinks per day, or use of **cocaine** or intravenous drugs.

Symptoms

Symptoms of an embolic stroke usually come on quite suddenly and are at their most intense right from the start, while symptoms of a thrombotic stroke come on more gradually. Symptoms may include:

- blurring or decreased vision in one or both eyes
- severe **headache**, often described as "the worst headache of my life"
- weakness, **numbness**, or paralysis of the face, arm, or leg, usually confined to one side of the body
- dizziness, loss of balance or coordination, especially when combined with other symptoms

Diagnosis

The diagnosis of stroke is begun with a careful medical history, especially concerning the onset and distribution of symptoms, presence of risk factors, and the exclusion of other possible causes. A brief neurological exam is performed to identify the degree and location of any deficits, such as weakness, incoordination, or visual losses.

Once stroke is suspected, a computed tomography scan (CT scan) or **magnetic resonance imaging** (MRI) scan is performed to distinguish a stroke caused by blood clot from one caused by hemorrhage, a critical distinction that guides therapy. Blood and urine tests are done routinely to look for possible abnormalities.

Other investigations that may be performed to guide treatment include an electrocardiogram, **angiography**, ultrasound, and electroencephalogram.

Treatment

Emergency treatment

Emergency treatment of stroke from a blood clot is aimed at dissolving the clot. This "thrombolytic therapy" currently is performed most often with tissue plasminogen activator, or t-PA. t-PA must be administered within three hours of the stroke event. Therefore, patients who awaken with stroke symptoms are ineligible for t-PA therapy, as the time of onset cannot be accurately determined. t-PA therapy has been shown to improve recovery and decrease long-term disability in selected patients. t-PA therapy carries a 6.4% risk of inducing a cerebral hemorrhage, and is not appropriate for patients with bleeding disorders, very high blood pressure, known aneurysms, any evidence of intracranial hemorrhage, or incidence of stroke, head trauma, or intracranial surgery within the past three months. Patients with clot-related (thrombotic or embolic) stroke who are ineligible for t-PA treatment may be treated with heparin or other blood thinners, or with **aspirin** or other anti-clotting agents in some cases.

Emergency treatment of hemorrhagic stroke is aimed at controlling intracranial pressure. Intravenous urea or mannitol plus hyperventilation is the most common treatment. **Corticosteroids** also may be used. Patients with reversible bleeding disorders, such as those due to anticoagulant treatment, should have these bleeding disorders reversed, if possible.

Surgery for hemorrhage due to aneurysm may be performed if the aneurysm is close enough to the cranial surface to allow access. Ruptured vessels are closed off to prevent rebleeding. For aneurysms that are difficult to reach surgically, endovascular treatment may be used. In this procedure, a catheter is guided from a larger artery up into the brain to reach the aneurysm. Small coils of wire are discharged into the aneurysm, which plug it up and block off blood flow from the main artery.

Rehabilitation

Rehabilitation refers to a comprehensive program designed to regain function as much as possible and compensate for permanent losses. Approximately 10% of stroke survivors are without any significant disability and able to function independently. Another 10% are so severely affected that they must remain institutionalized for severe disability. The remaining 80% can return home with appropriate therapy, training, support, and care services.

Rehabilitation is coordinated by a team of medical professionals and may include the services of a neurologist, a physician who specializes in rehabilitation medicine (physiatrist), a physical therapist, an occupational therapist, a speech-language pathologist, a nutritionist, a mental health professional, and a social worker. Rehabilitation services may be provided in an acute care hospital, rehabilitation hospital, long-term care facility, outpatient clinic, or at home.

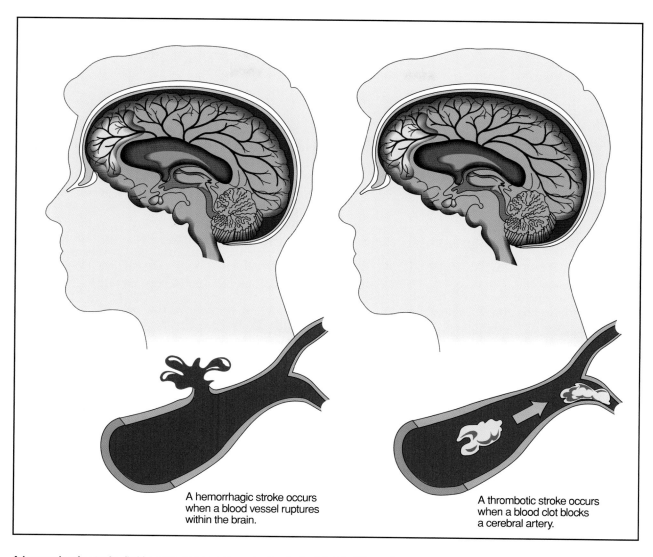

A hemorrhagic stroke occurs when a blood vessel ruptures within the brain.

A thrombotic stroke occurs when a blood clot blocks a cerebral artery.

A hemorrhagic stroke (left) compared to a thrombotic stroke (right). *(Illustration by Hans &Cassady, Inc.)*

The rehabilitation program is based on the patient's individual deficits and strengths. Strokes on the left side of the brain primarily affect the right half of the body, and vice versa. In addition, in left brain dominant people, who constitute a significant majority of the population, left brain strokes usually lead to speech and language deficits, while right brain strokes may affect spatial perception. Patients with right brain strokes also may deny their illness, neglect the affected side of their body, and behave impulsively.

Rehabilitation may be complicated by cognitive losses, including diminished ability to understand and follow directions. Poor results are more likely in patients with significant or prolonged cognitive changes, sensory losses, language deficits, or incontinence.

PREVENTING COMPLICATIONS. Rehabilitation begins with prevention of stroke recurrence and other medical complications. The risk of stroke recurrence may be reduced with many of the same measures used to prevent stroke, including quitting smoking and controlling blood pressure.

One of the most common medical complications following stroke is deep venous thrombosis, in which a clot forms within a limb immobilized by paralysis. Clots that break free often become lodged in an artery feeding the lungs. This type of **pulmonary embolism** is a common cause of death in the weeks following a stroke. Resuming activity within a day or two after the stroke is an important preventive measure, along with use of elastic stockings on the lower limbs. Drugs that prevent clotting may be given, including intravenous heparin and oral warfarin.

Weakness and loss of coordination of the swallowing muscles may impair swallowing (dysphagia), and allow food to enter the lower airway. This may lead to aspiration **pneumonia**, another common cause of death shortly after a stroke. Dysphagia may be treated with retraining exercises and temporary use of pureed foods.

Depression occurs in 30–60% of stroke patients. Antidepressants and psychotherapy may be used in combination.

Other medical complications include urinary tract infections, pressure ulcers, falls, and seizures.

TYPES OF REHABILITATIVE THERAPY. Brain tissue that dies in a stroke cannot regenerate. In some cases, the functions of that tissue may be performed by other brain regions after a training period. In other cases, compensatory actions may be developed to replace lost abilities.

Physical therapy is used to maintain and restore range of motion and strength in affected limbs, and to maximize mobility in walking, wheelchair use, and transferring (from wheelchair to toilet or from standing to sitting, for instance). The physical therapist advises on mobility aids such as wheelchairs, braces, and canes. In the recovery period, a stroke patient may develop muscle spasticity and **contractures**, or abnormal contractions. Contractures may be treated with a combination of stretching and splinting.

Occupational therapy improves self-care skills such as feeding, bathing, and dressing, and helps develop effective compensatory strategies and devices for activities of daily living. A speech-language pathologist focuses on communication and swallowing skills. When dysphagia is a problem, a nutritionist can advise alternative meals that provide adequate **nutrition**.

Mental health professionals may be involved in the treatment of depression or loss of thinking (cognitive) skills. A social worker may help coordinate services and ease the transition out of the hospital back into the home. Both social workers and mental health professionals may help counsel the patient and family during the difficult rehabilitation period. Caring for a person affected with stroke requires learning a new set of skills and adapting to new demands and limitations. Home caregivers may develop **stress**, **anxiety**, and depression. Caring for the caregiver is an important part of the overall stroke treatment program.

Support groups can provide an important source of information, advice, and comfort for stroke patients and for caregivers. Joining a support group can be one of the most important steps in the rehabilitation process.

Prognosis

Stroke is fatal for about 27% of white males, 52% of black males, 23% of white females, and 40% of black females. Stroke survivors may be left with significant deficits. Emergency treatment and comprehensive rehabilitation can significantly improve both survival and recovery. A 2003 study found that treating people who have had a stroke with certain antidepressant medications, even if they were not depressed, could increase their chances of living longer. People who received the treatment were less likely to die from cardiovascular events than those who did not receive **antidepressant drugs**.

Prevention

Damage from stroke may be significantly reduced through emergency treatment. Knowing the symptoms of stroke is as important as knowing those of a **heart attack**. Patients with stroke symptoms should seek emergency treatment without delay, which may mean dialing 911 rather than their family physician.

The risk of stroke can be reduced through lifestyle changes:

• quitting smoking

• controlling blood pressure

• getting regular exercise

• keeping body weight down

• avoiding excessive alcohol consumption

• getting regular checkups and following the doctor's advice regarding diet and medicines, particularly hormone replacement therapy.

Treatment of atrial fibrillation may significantly reduce the risk of stroke. Preventive anticoagulant therapy may benefit those with untreated atrial fibrillation. Warfarin (Coumadin) has proven to be more effective than aspirin for those with higher risk. A new drug called ximelagatran (Exanta) with fewer side effects has been introduced in Europe. The drug's manufacturer was applying for FDA approval to market the drug for use in preventing stroke and other thromboembolic complications in early 2004.

In 2003, physicians at the Framingham Heart Study derived new risk scores to help physicians determine which patients with new onset of atrial fibrillation are at higher risk for stroke alone or for stroke or

KEY TERMS

Aneurysm—A pouchlike bulging of a blood vessel. Aneurysms can rupture, leading to stroke.

Atrial fibrillation—A disorder of the heart beat associated with a higher risk of stroke. In this disorder, the upper chambers (atria) of the heart do not completely empty when the heart beats, which can allow blood clots to form.

Cerebral embolism—A blockage of blood flow through a vessel in the brain by a blood clot that formed elsewhere in the body and traveled to the brain.

Cerebral thrombosis—A blockage of blood flow through a vessel in the brain by a blood clot that formed in the brain itself.

Intracerebral hemorrhage—A cause of some strokes in which vessels within the brain begin bleeding.

Subarachnoid hemorrhage—A cause of some strokes in which arteries on the surface of the brain begin bleeding.

Tissue plasminogen activator (tPA)—A substance that is sometimes given to patients within three hours of a stroke to dissolve blood clots within the brain.

death. Screening for aneurysms may be an effective preventive measure in those with a family history of aneurysms or autosomal **polycystic kidney disease**, which tends to be associated with aneurysms.

Resources

PERIODICALS

"HRT Increases Risk of Dementia and Stroke." *Contemporary OB/GYN* July 2003: 16–21.

"New Classification Scheme Helpful to Predict Risk of Stroke or Death." *Heart Disease Weekly* September 14, 2003: 3.

"New Drug Application Submitted to FDA for Exanta." *Heart Disease Weekly* January 25, 2004: 79.

"New Stroke Prevention Drug." *Chemist & Druggist* September 13, 2003: 24.

"Post-stroke Antidepressant Treatment Appears to Reduce Death Rate." *Heart Disease Weekly* October 26, 2003: 56.

ORGANIZATIONS

American Heart Association. 7320 Greenville Ave. Dallas, TX 75231. (214) 373-6300. <http://www.americanheart.org>.

National Stroke Association. 9707 E. Easter Lane, Englewood, Co. 80112. (800) 787-6537. <http://www.stroke.org>.

Richard Robinson
Teresa G. Odle

Strongyloidiasis *see* **Threadworm infection**

Structural integration *see* **Rolfing**

Stupor *see* **Coma**

Stuttering

Definition

Stuttering is a speech problem characterized by repetitions, pauses, or drawn out syllables, words, and phrases. Stutterers are different than people experiencing normal fluency problems because a stutterer's disfluency is more severe and consistent than that of people who do not stutter.

Description

Normal language development in a child can include a period of disfluency. Children might repeat syllables or words once or twice. Sometimes, children experiencing normal disfluencies hesitate during speech or use fillers, including "um," with frequency. These developmental problems usually happen between one and five years of age. Often, parents are concerned about the disfluency they hear in their children. In fact, about 25% of all children experience speech disfluencies during development concern their parents because of their severity.

A child with mild stuttering, however, will repeat sounds more than twice. Parents and teachers often notice the child's facial muscles become tense and he or she might struggle to speak. The child's voice pitch might rise with repetitions, and some children experience occasional periods when airflow or voice stops for seconds at a time. Children with more severe stuttering stutter through more than 10% of their speech. This child exhibits considerable tension and tries to avoid stuttering by using different words. In these children, complete blocks of speech are more common than repetitions or prolongations, during which children lengthen syllables or words.

Stuttering usually begins in childhood when the child is developing language skills, and it rarely develops in adulthood with only 1% of the population affected by the disorder. Stuttering does not affect intelligence. Teens often experience more noticeable problems with stuttering as they enter the dating scene and increase their social interactions. Stuttering can severely affect one's life. Often, adults who are concerned about stuttering choose their careers based on the disability.

The degree of stuttering is often inconsistent. Stutterers can be fluent in some situations. Many find that they stop stuttering when singing or doing other activities involving speech. Some have good and bad days when it comes to stuttering. On good days, a stutterer might be able to talk fluently using words that usually cause him to repeat, pause or prolongate sounds, syllables, parts of words, entire words, or phrases.

Causes and symptoms

There is no known cause of stuttering. Some believe that it has a physical cause and that it might be related to a breakdown in the neurological system. Stuttering starts early in life and often is inherited. Brain scan research has revealed that there might be abnormalities in the brains of stutterers, while they are stuttering. Myths about why stuttering occurs abound. Some cultures believe that stuttering is caused by emotional problems, tickling an infant too much or because a mother ate improperly during breastfeeding. None have been proven to be true. It is believed that some drugs might induce stuttering-like conditions. These include antidepressants, **antihistamines**, tranquilizers and **selective serotonin reuptake inhibitors**.

Diagnosis

Speech and language therapists diagnose stuttering by asking stutterers to read out loud, pronounce specific words, and talk. Some also order hearing tests. The tests will determine whether or not a person needs speech therapy.

Treatment

Researchers don't understand what causes stuttering. However, progress has been made into what contributes to the development of the disability and, therefore, in some cases it can be prevented in childhood with the help of therapy early on. Therapy can help people of all ages suffering from the speech disability. While not an overnight cure, therapy can offer positive results and more fluent speech patterns. The goals of therapy are to reduce stuttering frequency,

KEY TERMS

Antipsychotics—A class of drugs used to treat psychotic or neurotic behavior.

Disfluency—An interruption in speech flow.

Neuroleptics—Antipsychotic drugs that affect psychomotor activity.

decrease the tension and struggle of stuttering, become educated about stuttering, and learn to use effective communications skills, such as making eye contact, to further enhance speech. The therapy focuses on helping stutterers to discover easier and different ways of producing sounds and expressing thoughts. The success of therapy depends largely on the stutterer's willingness to work at getting better.

The duration of stuttering therapy needed varies among stutterers. Sometimes, it helps stutterers if they have therapy intermittently throughout their lives.

Parents, teachers and others can do things to help ease stuttering. These include: talking slowly, but normally, clearly, and in a relaxed manner to a stutterer: answering questions after a pause to encourage a relaxed transaction; trying not to make stuttering worse by getting annoyed by a person's stuttering; giving stutterers reassurance about their stuttering; and encourage the stutterer to talk about his or her stuttering.

Electronic fluency aids help some stutterers when used as an adjunct to therapy. Medications, such as antipsychotics and neuroleptics, have been used to treat stuttering with limited success.

Alternative treatment

Some use relaxation techniques to help their stuttering.

Prognosis

More than three million Americans stutter and four times more males are affected than females. Winston Churchill, Marilyn Monroe, Carly Simon, James Earl Jones and King George VI are among the many people who stuttered but went on to live successful professional lives. Decades of research have yielded no answers to the causes of stuttering; still much has been learned about what contributes to stuttering's development and how to prevent it in children. People who stutter can get better through therapy.

Prevention

New and exciting developments are occurring in researchers' understanding of the genetics of stuttering. Researchers are finding the locations of genes that predispose people to stuttering. While genetic factors will not explain all stuttering, genetics will help to uncover the disability's causes. Speech therapy, especially that performed at a young age, can stop the progression of stuttering.

Resources

ORGANIZATIONS

National Stuttering Foundation of America. 1-(800) 992-9392. < http://www.stutteringhelp.org >.

OTHER

The Stuttering Home Page. Minnesota State University, Mankato. < http://www.mandato.msus.edu/deprt/comdis/kuster/stutter.html >.

"Stuttering." The Nemours Foundation, KidsHealth.org. < http://kidshealth.org >.

"What is Stuttering?" Robert W. Quesal, PhD, Professor and Program Director. Communications Sciences and Disorders. Western Illinois University. < http://www.wiu.edu >.

Lisette Hilton

Stye *see* **Eyelid disorders**

Subacute sclerosing panencephalitis

Definition

Subacute sclerosing panencephalitis is a rare, progressive brain disorder caused by an abnormal immune response to the **measles** virus.

Description

This fatal condition is a complication of measles, and affects children and young adults before the age of 20. It usually occurs in boys more often than in girls, but is extremely rare, appearing in only one out of a million cases of measles.

Causes and symptoms

Experts believe this condition is a form of measles **encephalitis** (swelling of the brain), caused by an improper response by the immune system to the measles virus.

KEY TERMS

Measles encephalitis—A serious complication of measles occurring in about one out of every 1,000 cases, causing headache, drowsiness, and vomiting seven to ten days after the rash appears. Seizures and coma can follow, which may lead to retardation and death.

The condition begins with behavioral changes, memory loss, irritability, and problems with school work. As the neurological damage increases, the child experiences seizures, involuntary movements, and further neurological deterioration. Eventually, the child starts suffering from progressive **dementia**. The optic nerve begins to shrink and weaken (atrophy) and subsequently the child becomes blind.

Diagnosis

Blood tests and spinal fluid reveal high levels of antibodies to measles virus, and there is a characteristically abnormal electroencephalogram (EEG), or brain wave test. Typically, there is a history of measles infection two to ten years before symptoms begin.

Treatment

There is no standard treatment, and a number of **antiviral drugs** have been tested with little success. Treatment of symptoms, including the use of **anticonvulsant drugs**, can be helpful.

Prognosis

While there may be periodic remissions during the course of this disease, it is usually fatal (often from **pneumonia**) within one to three years after onset.

Resources

ORGANIZATIONS

National Institute of Allergy and Infectious Disease. Building 31, Room 7A-50, 31 Center Drive MSC 2520, Bethesda, MD 20892-2520. (301) 496-5717. < http://www.niaid.nih.gov/default.htm >.

National Organization for Rare Disorders. P.O. Box 8923, New Fairfield, CT 06812-8923. (800) 999-6673. < http://www.rarediseases.org >.

Carol A. Turkington

Subacute spongiform encephalopathy *see* **Creutzfeldt-Jakob disease**

Subacute thyroiditis *see* **Thyroiditis**

Subarachnoid hemorrhage

Definition

A subarachnoid hemorrhage is an abnormal and very dangerous condition in which blood collects beneath the arachnoid mater, a membrane that covers the brain. This area, called the subarachnoid space, normally contains cerebrospinal fluid. The accumulation of blood in the subarachnoid space can lead to **stroke**, seizures, and other complications. Additionally, subarachnoid hemorrhages may cause permanent brain damage and a number of harmful biochemical events in the brain. A subarachnoid hemorrhage and the related problems are frequently fatal.

Description

Subarachnoid hemorrhages are classified into two general categories: traumatic and spontaneous. Traumatic refers to brain injury that might be sustained in an accident or a fall. Spontaneous subarachnoid hemorrhages occur with little or no warning and are frequently caused by ruptured aneurysms or blood vessel abnormalities in the brain.

Traumatic brain injury is a critical problem in the United States. According to annual figures compiled by the Brain Injury Association, approximately 373,000 people are hospitalized, more than 56,000 people die, and 99,000 survive with permanent disabilities due to traumatic brain injuries. The leading causes of injury are bicycle, motorcycle, and automobile accidents, with a significant minority due to accidental falls, and sports and recreation mishaps.

Exact statistics are not available on traumatic subarachnoid hemorrhages, but several large clinical studies have found an incidence of 23–39% in relation to severe **head injury**. Furthermore, subarachnoid hemorrhages have been described in the medical literature as the most common brain injury found during **autopsy** investigations of head trauma.

Spontaneous subarachnoid hemorrhages are often due to an aneurysm (a bulge or sac-like projection from a blood vessel) which bursts. **Arteriovenous malformations** (AVMs), which are abnormal interfaces between arteries and veins, may also rupture and release blood into the subarachnoid space. Both aneurysms and AVMs are associated with weak spots in the walls of blood vessels and account for approximately 60% of all spontaneous subarachnoid hemorrhages. The rest may be attributed to other causes, such as **cancer** or infection, or are of unknown origin.

In industrialized countries, it is estimated that there are 6.5–26.4 cases of spontaneous subarachnoid hemorrhage per 100,000 people annually. Certain factors raise the risk of suffering a hemorrhage. Aneurysms are acquired over a person's lifetime and are rarely a factor in subarachnoid hemorrhage before age 20. Conversely, AVMs are present at birth. In some cases, there may be a genetic predisposition for aneurysms or AVMs. Other factors that have been implicated, but not definitively linked to spontaneous subarachnoid hemorrhages, include **atherosclerosis**, cigarette use, extreme alcohol consumption, and the use of illegal drugs, such as **cocaine**. The exact role of high blood pressure is somewhat unclear, but since it does seem linked to the formation of aneurysms, it may be considered an indirect risk factor.

The immediate danger due to subarachnoid hemorrhage, whether traumatic or spontaneous, is **ischemia**. Ischemia refers to tissue damage caused by restricted or blocked blood flow. The areas of the brain that do not receive adequate blood and oxygen can suffer irreparable injury, leading to permanent brain damage or **death**. An individual who survives the initial hemorrhage is susceptible to a number of complications in the following hours, days, and weeks.

The most common complications are intracranial **hypertension**, vasospasm, and **hydrocephalus**. Intracranial hypertension, or high pressure within the brain, can lead to further bleeding from damaged blood vessels; a complication associated with a 70% fatality rate. Vasospasm, or blood vessel constriction, is a principal cause of secondary ischemia. The blood vessels in the brain constrict in reaction to chemicals released by blood breaking down within the subarachnoid space. As the blood vessels become narrower, blood flow in the brain becomes increasingly restricted. Approximately one third of spontaneous subarachnoid hemorrhages and 30-60% of traumatic bleeds are followed by vasospasm. Hydrocephalus, an accumulation of fluid in the chambers of the brain (ventricles) due to restricted circulation of cerebrospinal fluid, follows approximately 15% of subarachnoid hemorrhages. Because cerebrospinal fluid cannot drain properly, pressure accumulates on the brain, possibly prompting further ischemic complications.

Causes and symptoms

Whether through trauma or disease, subarachnoid hemorrhages are caused by blood being released by a damaged blood vessel and accumulating in the subarachnoid space. Symptoms associated with traumatic subarachnoid hemorrhage may or may not resemble those associated with spontaneous hemorrhage, as trauma can involve multiple injuries with overlapping symptoms.

Typically, a spontaneous subarachnoid hemorrhage is indicated by a sudden, severe **headache**. **Nausea**, **vomiting**, and **dizziness** frequently accompany the **pain**. Loss of consciousness occurs in about half the cases of spontaneous hemorrhage. A **coma**, usually brief, may occur. A stiff neck, **fever**, and aversion to light may appear following the hemorrhage. Neurologic symptoms may include partial **paralysis**, loss of vision, seizures, and speech difficulties.

Spontaneous subarachnoid hemorrhages may be preceded by warning signs prior to the initial bleed. Sentinel, or warning, headaches may be present in the days or weeks before an aneurysm or AVM ruptures. These headaches can be accompanied by dizziness, nausea, and vomiting, and possibly neurologic symptoms. Approximately 50% of AVMs are discovered before they bleed significantly; however, most aneurysms are not diagnosed before they rupture.

Diagnosis

To make a diagnosis, a health-care provider takes a detailed history of the symptoms and does a **physical examination**. The symptoms may mimic other disorders and diagnosis can be complicated, especially if the individual is unconscious. The sudden, severe headache can fuel suspicion of a subarachnoid hemorrhage or similar event, and a computed tomography scan (CT scan) or **magnetic resonance imaging** (MRI) scan is considered essential to a quick diagnosis. The MRI is less sensitive than the CT in detecting acute subarachnoid bleeding, but more sensitive in diagnosing AVM or aneurysm.

A CT scan reveals blood that has escaped into the subarachnoid space. For the best results, the scan should be done within 12 hours of the hemorrhage. If this is not possible, lumbar puncture and examination of the cerebrospinal fluid is advised. Lumbar puncture is also done in cases in which the CT scan doesn't reveal a hemorrhage, but there is a high suspicion that one has occurred. In subarachnoid hemorrhage, cerebrospinal fluid shows red blood cells and/or xanthochromia, a yellowish tinge caused by blood

breakdown products. Xanthochromia first appears six to 12 hours after subarachnoid hemorrhage, making it advisable to delay lumbar puncture until at least 12 hours after the onset of symptoms for a more definite diagnosis.

Once a hemorrhage, AVM, or aneurysm has been diagnosed, further tests are done to pinpoint the damage. The CT scan may be useful in giving the general location, but cerebral **angiography** maps out the exact details. This procedure involves injecting a special dye into the blood stream. This dye makes blood vessels visible in x rays of the area.

Treatment

The initial course of treatment focuses on stabilizing the hemorrhage victim. Depending on the individual's condition, this may involve intubation and mechanical ventilation, supplemental oxygen, intravenous fluids, and close monitoring of vital signs. If the person suffers seizures, an anticonvulsant, such as phenytoin (Dilantin), is administered. Nimodipine, a calcium channel blocker, may be given to prevent vasospasm and its complications. Sedatives and medications for pain, nausea, and vomiting are administered as needed.

Once the individual is stabilized, cerebral angiography is done to locate the damaged blood vessel. This information and the individual's condition are considered before attempting surgical treatment. Surgery is necessary to remove the damaged area of the blood vessel and prevent a second hemorrhage. The specific neurosurgical procedures depend on the location and type of blood vessel damage. Typically, clip ligation is the preferred means of treating an aneurysm, and surgical excision, radiosurgery, or endovascular embolization are used to manage an AVM.

Prognosis

Individuals who are conscious and demonstrate few neurologic symptoms when they reach medical help have the best prognosis. However, the overall prospects for subarachnoid hemorrhage patients are generally not good. Of the individuals who suffer an aneurysmal hemorrhage, approximately 15% do not live long enough to get medical treatment. Another 20-40% will not survive the complications caused by the hemorrhage, and approximately 12% of the survivors will experience permanent neurologic disability. Neurologic disabilities may include partial paralysis, weakened or numbed areas of the body, cognitive or speech difficulties, and vision problems. Individuals

KEY TERMS

Aneurysm—A weak point in a blood vessel where the pressure of the blood causes the vessel wall to bulge outwards. An aneurysm may also appear as a sac-like projection from the blood vessel wall.

Arachnoid mater—One of three membranes that encase the brain and spinal cord. The arachnoid mater is the middle membrane.

Arteriovenous malformation—An abnormal tangle of arteries and veins in which the arteries feed directly into the veins without a normal intervening capillary bed.

Atherosclerosis—An abnormal condition in which lipids, or fats, form deposits on the inside walls of blood vessels.

Cerebral angiography—A medical test in which an x-ray visible dye is injected into blood vessels to allow them to be imaged on an x ray.

Cerebrospinal fluid—The clear, normally colorless fluid found within the subarachnoid space.

Computerized tomography (CT) scan—Cross-sectional x rays of the body compiled to create a three-dimensional image of the body's internal structures.

Hemorrhage—The escape of blood from blood vessels.

Hydrocephalus—Englargement of the chambers in the brain (ventricles) caused by an accumulation of cerebrospinal fluid.

Intracranial hypertension—Abnormally high pressure within the brain.

Ischemia—A condition in which blood flow is cut off or restricted from a particular area. The tissue becomes starved of oxygen and nutrients, resulting in tissue death.

Ischemic—Referring to ischemia.

Lumbar puncture—A diagnostic procedure in which a needle is inserted into the lower spine to withdraw a small amount of cerebrospinal fluid. This fluid is examined to assess trauma to the brain.

Subarachnoid—Referring to the space underneath the arachnoid mater.

Vasospasm—The constriction or narrowing of blood vessels. In cases of hemorrhage, the constriction is prompted by chemical signals from the escaped blood as it breaks down.

whose subarachnoid hemorrhages occur as a result of AVMs have a slightly better prognosis, although the risk of death is approximately 10–15% for each hemorrhage.

Subarachnoid hemorrhage associated with traumatic brain injury has a poor prognosis. In clinical studies, 46–78% of head injury cases involving subarachnoid hemorrhage resulted in severe disability, vegetative survival, or death. Furthermore, it is possible that traumatic subarachnoid hemorrhages are accompanied by additional injuries, which would further diminish survival and recovery rates.

Prevention

Traumatic brain injury is the leading cause of subarachnoid hemorrhages, so it follows that efforts to prevent head injury would prevent these hemorrhages. Since accidents cannot always be prevented, measures to minimize potential damage are always advisable. Use of activity-appropriate protective gear, such as bicycle helmets, motorcycle helmets, and sports head gear, is strongly encouraged and promoted by medical associations, consumer organizations, advocacy groups, and health-care professionals. These same groups also advise using seat belts in automobiles.

Spontaneous subarachnoid hemorrhages are more difficult to prevent. Since there may be a genetic component to aneurysms and AVMs, close relatives to individuals with these conditions may consider being screened to assess their own status. Quitting **smoking** and keeping blood pressure within normal limits may also reduce the risk of suffering a spontaneous subarachnoid hemorrhage.

Resources

ORGANIZATIONS

Brain Injury Association of America. 105 North Alfred St., Alexandria, VA 22314. (800) 444-6443. < http://www.biausa.org >.

National Stroke Association. 9707 E. Easter Lane, Englewood, Co. 80112. (800) 787-6537. < http://www.stroke.org >.

Julia Barrett

Subdural empyema *see* **Central nervous system infections**

Subdural hematoma

Definition

A subdural hematoma is a collection of blood in the space between the outer layer (dura) and middle layers of the covering of the brain (the meninges). It is most often caused by torn, bleeding veins on the inside of the dura as a result of a blow to the head.

Description

Subdural hematomas most often affect people who are prone to falling. Only a slight hit on the head or even a fall to the ground without hitting the head may be enough to tear veins in the brain, often without fracturing the skull. There may be no external evidence of the bruising on the brain's surface.

Small subdural hematomas may not be very serious, and the blood can be slowly absorbed over several weeks. Larger hematomas, however, can gradually enlarge over several weeks, even though the bleeding has stopped. This enlargement can compress the brain itself, possibly leading to **death** if the blood is not drained.

The time between the injury and the appearance of symptoms can vary from less than 48 hours to several weeks, or more. Symptoms appearing in less than 48 hours are due to an acute subdural hematoma. This type of bleeding is often fatal, and results from tearing of the venous sinus. If more than two weeks have passed before symptoms appear, the condition is called a chronic subdural hematoma, resulting from tearing of the smaller vein. The young and the old are most likely to experience a chronic condition. This chronic form is less risky, as pressure of the veins against the skull lessens the bleeding. Prompt medical care can reduce the probability of permanent brain damage.

Causes and symptoms

A subdural hematoma is caused by an injury to the head that tears blood vessels. In childhood, hematomas are a common complication of falls. A subdural hematoma also may be an indication of **child abuse**, as evidenced by **shaken baby syndrome**.

Symptoms tend to fluctuate, and include:

- **headache**
- episodes of confusion and drowsiness

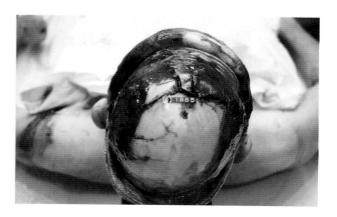

Subdural hematoma present on autopsied body. *(Custom Medical Stock Photo. Reproduced by permission.)*

- one-sided weakness or **paralysis**
- lethargy
- enlarged or asymmetric pupils
- convulsions or loss of consciousness after **head injury**
- coma

A doctor should be contacted immediately if symptoms appear. Because these symptoms mimic the signs of a **stroke**, the patient should tell the doctor about any head injury within the previous few months.

In an infant, symptoms may include increased pressure within the skull, growing head size, bulging fontanelle (one of two soft spots on a infant's skull), **vomiting**, irritability, lethargy, and seizures. In cases of child **abuse**, there may be **fractures** of the skull or other bones.

Diagnosis

A chronic subdural hematoma can be difficult to diagnose, but a slow loss of consciousness after a head injury is assumed to be a hematoma unless proven otherwise. The hematoma can be confirmed with **magnetic resonance imaging** (MRI), which is the preferred type of scan; a hematoma can be hard to detect on a computed tomography scan (CT scan), depending on how long after the hemorrhage the CT is done.

Treatment

Small hematomas that do not cause symptoms may not need to be treated. Otherwise, the hematoma should be surgically removed. Liquid blood can be drained from burr holes drilled into the skull. The surgeon may have to open a section of skull to remove a large hematoma or to tie off the bleeding vein.

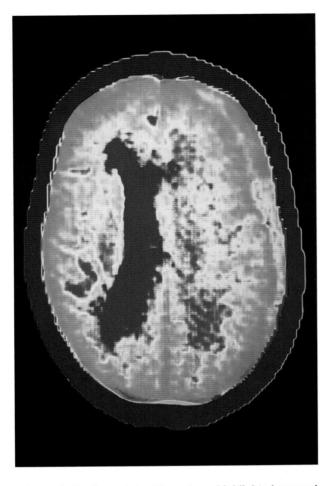

CT scan indicating subdural hematoma highlighted as a red mass on the center left of the brain. *(Photo Researchers. Reproduced by permission.)*

Corticosteroids and **diuretics** can control brain swelling. After surgery, **anticonvulsant drugs** (such as phenytoin) may help control or prevent seizures, which can begin as late as two years after the head injury.

Prognosis

If treatment is provided soon enough, recovery is usually complete. Headache, **amnesia**, attention problems, **anxiety**, and giddiness may continue for some time after surgery. Most symptoms in adults usually disappear within six months, with further improvement over several years. Children tend to recover much faster.

Prevention

Because a subdural hematoma usually follows a head injury, preventing head injury can prevent a hematoma.

Resources

ORGANIZATIONS

American Academy of Neurology. 1080 Montreal Ave., St. Paul, MN 55116. (612) 695-1940. < http://www.aan.com >.

Brain Injury Association of America. 105 North Alfred St., Alexandria, VA 22314. (800) 444-6443. < http://www.biausa.org >.

Head Injury Hotline. P.O. Box 84151, Seattle WA 98124. (206) 621- 8558. < http://www.headinjury.com >.

Head Trauma Support Project, Inc. 2500 Marconi Ave., Ste. 203, Sacramento, CA 95821. (916) 482-5770.

Carol A. Turkington

Subdural hemorrhage *see* **Subdural hematoma**

Subluxations *see* **Dislocations and subluxations**

Substance abuse and dependence

Definition

Substance **abuse** and dependence refer to any continued pathological use of a medication, non-medically indicated drug (called drugs of abuse), or toxin. They normally are distinguished as follows.

Substance abuse is any pattern of substance use that results in repeated adverse social consequences related to drug-taking—for example, interpersonal conflicts, failure to meet work, family, or school obligations, or legal problems. Substance dependence, commonly known as **addiction**, is characterized by physiological and behavioral symptoms related to substance use. These symptoms include the need for increasing amounts of the substance to maintain desired effects, withdrawal if drug-taking ceases, and a great deal of time spent in activities related to substance use.

Substance abuse is more likely to be diagnosed among those who have just begun taking drugs and is often an early symptom of substance dependence. However, substance dependence can appear without substance abuse, and substance abuse can persist for extended periods of time without a transition to substance dependence.

Description

Substance abuse and dependence are disorders that affect all population groups although specific patterns of abuse and dependence vary with age, gender, culture, and socioeconomic status. According to data from the National Longitudinal Alcohol Epidemiologic Survey, 13.3% of a survey group of Americans exhibited symptoms of alcohol dependence during their lifetime, and 4.4% exhibited symptoms of alcohol dependence during the past 12 months. According to the 1997 National Household Survey on Drug Abuse, 6.4% of those surveyed had used an illicit drug in the past month.

Although substance dependence can begin at any age, to people aged 18 to 24 have relatively high substance use rates, and dependence often arises sometime during the ages of 20 to 49. Gender proportions vary according to the class of drugs, but substance use disorders are in general more frequently seen in men. A 2004 report revealed that in a 2002 national survey, more than 2.6 million youths age 12 to 17 had used inhalants more than once.

In addition to being an individual health disorder, substance abuse and dependence may be viewed as a public health problem with far-ranging health, economic, and adverse social implications. Substance-related disorders are associated with teen **pregnancy** and the transmission of **sexually transmitted diseases** (STDs), as well as failure in school, unemployment, domestic violence, homelessness, and crimes such as

rape and sexual assault, aggravated assault, robbery, burglary, and larceny. According to the National Institute on Alcohol Abuse and **Alcoholism** (NIAAA), the estimated cost of alcohol-related disorders alone (including health care expenditures, lost productivity, and premature **death**) was $166.5 billion in 1995.

The term substance, when discussed in the context of substance abuse and dependence, refers to medications, drugs of abuse, and toxins. These substances have an intoxicating effect, desired by the user, which can have either stimulating (speeding up) or depressive/sedating (slowing down) effects on the body. Substance dependence and/or abuse can involve any of the following 10 classes of substances:

- alcohol

- amphetamines (including "crystal meth," some medications used in the treatment of attention deficit disorder [ADD], and amphetamine-like substances found in appetite suppressants)

- cannibis (including **marijuana** and hashish)

- **cocaine** (including "crack")

- hallucinogens (including **LSD**, mescaline, and MDMA ["ecstasy"])

- inhalants (including compounds found in gasoline, glue, and paint thinners)

- nicotine (substance dependence only)

- opioids (including morphine, heroin, codeine, **methadone**, oxycodone [Oxycontin (TM)])

- phencyclidine (including PCP, angel dust, ketamine)

- sedative, hypnotic, and anxiolytic (anti-anxiety) substances (including **benzodiazepines** such as valium, **barbiturates**, prescription sleeping medications, and most prescription anti-anxiety medications)

Caffeine has been identified as a substance in this context, but as yet there is insufficient evidence to establish whether caffeine-related symptoms fall under substance abuse and dependence.

Substances of abuse may thus be illicit drugs, readily available substances such as alcohol or glue, over-the-counter drugs, or prescription medications. In many cases, a prescription medication that becomes a substance of abuse may have been a legal, medically indicated prescription for the user, but the pattern of use diverges from the use prescribed by the physician.

Frequency Of Substance Abuse By Gender And Age	
Men	
Ages 18 to 29	17 to 24 percent
Ages 30 to 44	11 to 14 percent
Ages 45 to 64	6 to 8 percent
Over age 65	1 to 3 percent
Women	
Ages 18 to 29	4 to 10 percent
Ages 30 to 44	2 to 4 percent
Ages 45 to 64	1 to 2 percent
Over age 65	less than 1 percent

Causes and symptoms

Causes

The causes of substance dependence are not well established, but three factors are believed to contribute to substance-related disorders: genetic factors, psychopathology, and social learning. In genetic epidemiological studies of alcoholism, the probability of identical twins both exhibiting alcohol dependence was significantly greater than with fraternal twins, thus suggesting a genetic component in alcoholism. It is unclear, however, whether the genetic factor is related to alcoholism directly, or whether it is linked to other psychiatric disorders that are known to be associated with substance abuse. For example, there is evidence that alcoholic males from families with **depressive disorders** tend to have more severe courses of substance dependence than alcoholic men from families without such family histories.

These and other findings suggest substance use may be way to relieve the symptoms of a psychological disorder. In this model, unless the underlying pathology is treated, attempts to permanently stop substance dependence are ineffective. Psychopathologies that are associated with substance dependence include antisocial personality disorder, **bipolar disorder**, depression, **anxiety** disorder, and **schizophrenia**.

A third factor related to substance dependence is social environment. In this model, drug-taking is essentially a socially learned behavior. Local social norms determine the likelihood that a person is exposed to the substance and whether continued use is reinforced. For example, individuals may, by observing family or peer role models, learn that substance use is a normal way to relieve daily stresses. External

penalties, such as legal or social sanctions, may reduce the likelihood of substance use.

At the level of neurobiology, it is believed that substances of abuse operate through similar pathways in the brain. The chemical changes induced by the stimulation of these pathways by initial use of the substance lead to the desire to continue substance use, and eventual substance dependence.

Symptoms

The DSM-IV-TR identifies seven criteria (symptoms), at least three of which must be met during a given 12-month period, for the diagnosis of substance dependence:

- Tolerance, as defined either by the need for increasing amounts of the substance to obtain the desired effect or by experiencing less effect with extended use of the same amount of the substance.

- Withdrawal, as exhibited either by experiencing unpleasant mental, physiological, and emotional changes when drug-taking ceases or by using the substance as a way to relieve or prevent withdrawal symptoms.

- Longer duration of taking substance or use in greater quantities than was originally intended.

- Persistent desire or repeated unsuccessful efforts to stop or lessen substance use.

- A relatively large amount of time spent in securing and using the substance, or in recovering from the effects of the substance.

- Important work and social activities reduced because of substance use.

- Continued substance use despite negative physical and psychological effects of use.

Although not explicitly listed in the DSM-IV-TR criteria, "craving," or the overwhelming desire to use the substance regardless of countervailing forces, is a universally-reported symptom of substance dependence.

Symptoms of substance abuse, as specified by DSM-IV-TR, include one or more of the following occurring during a given 12-month period:

- Substance use resulting in a recurrent failure to fulfill work, school, or home obligations (work absences, substance-related school suspensions, neglect of children).

- Substance use in physically hazardous situations such as driving or operating machinery.

- Substance use resulting in legal problems such as drug-related arrests.
- Continued substance use despite negative social and relationship consequences of use.

In addition to the general symptoms, there are other physical signs and symptoms of substance abuse that are related to specific drug classes:

- Signs and symptoms of alcohol intoxication include such physical signs as slurred speech, lack of coordination, unsteady gait, memory impairment, and stupor, as well as behavior changes shortly after alcohol ingestion, including inappropriate aggressive behavior, mood volatility, and impaired functioning.
- Amphetamine users may exhibit rapid heartbeat, elevated or depressed blood pressure, dilated (enlarged) pupils, weight loss, as well as excessively high energy, inability to sleep, confusion, and occasional paranoid psychotic behavior.
- Cannibis users may exhibit red eyes with dilated pupils, increased appetite, **dry mouth**, and rapid pulse; they may also be sluggish and slow to react.
- Cocaine users may exhibit rapid heart rate, elevated or depressed blood pressure, dilated pupils, weight loss, in addition to wide variations in their energy level, severe mood disturbances, **psychosis**, and **paranoia**.
- Users of hallucinogens may exhibit anxiety or depression, paranoia, and unusual behavior in response to **hallucinations** (imagined sights, voices, sounds, or smells that appear real). Signs include dilated pupils, rapid heart rate, **tremors**, lack of coordination, and sweating. Flashbacks, or the re-experiencing of a hallucination long after stopping substance use, are also a symptom of hallucinogen use.
- Users of inhalants experience **dizziness**, spastic eye movements, lack of coordination, slurred speech, and slowed reflexes. Associated behaviors may include belligerence, tendency toward violence, apathy, and impaired judgment.
- Opioid drug users exhibit slurred speech, drowsiness, impaired memory, and constricted (small) pupils. They may appear slowed in their physical movements.
- Phencyclidine users exhibit spastic eye movements, rapid heartbeat, decreased sensitivity to **pain**, and lack of muscular coordination. They may show belligerence, predisposition to violence, impulsiveness, and agitation.

- Users of sedative, hypnotic, or anxiolytic drugs show slurred speech, unsteady gait, inattentiveness, and impaired memory. They may display inappropriate behavior, mood volatility, and impaired functioning.

Other signs are related to the form in which the substance is used. For example, heroin, certain other opioid drugs, and certain forms of cocaine may be injected. A person using an injectable substance may have "track marks" (outwardly visible signs of the site of an injection, with possible redness and swelling of the vein in which the substance was injected). Furthermore, poor judgment brought on by substance use can result in the injections being made under dangerously unhygienic conditions. These unsanitary conditions and the use of shared needles are risk factors for major infections of the heart, as well as infection with HIV (the virus that causes **AIDS**), certain forms of hepatitis (a liver infection), and **tuberculosis**.

Cocaine is often taken as a powdery substance which is "snorted" through the nose. This can result in frequent nosebleeds, sores in the nose, and even erosion (an eating away) of the nasal septum (the structure that separates the two nostrils).

Overdosing on a substance is a frequent complication of substance abuse. **Drug overdose** can be purposeful (with **suicide** as a goal), or due to carelessness, the unpredictable strength of substances purchased from street dealers, mixing of more than one type of substance, or as a result of the increasing doses that a person must take to experience intoxicating effects. Substance overdose can be a life-threatening emergency, with the specific symptoms depending on the type of substance used. Substances with depressive effects may dangerously slow the breathing and heart rate, drop the body temperature, and result in a general unresponsiveness. Substances with stimulatory effects may dangerously increase the heart rate and blood pressure, produce abnormal heart rhythms, increase body temperature, induce seizures, and cause erratic behavior.

Diagnosis

Tools used in the diagnosis of substance dependence include screening questionnaires and patient histories, **physical examination**, and laboratory tests. A simple and popular screening tool is the CAGE questionnaire. CAGE refers to the first letters of each word that forms the basis of each of the four questions of the screening exam:

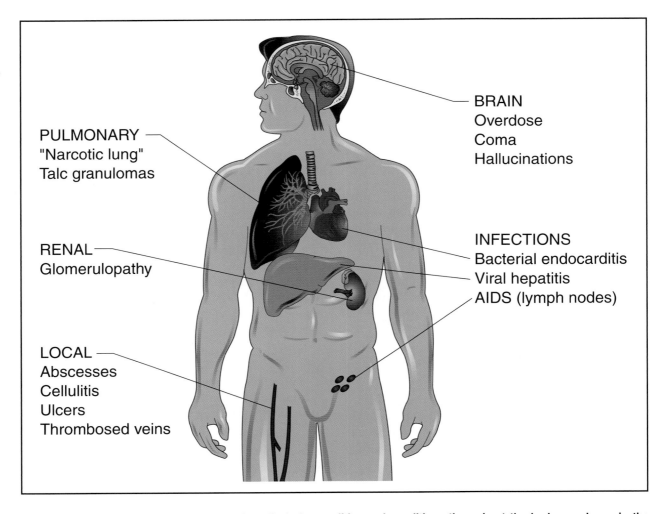

PULMONARY
"Narcotic lung"
Talc granulomas

RENAL
Glomerulopathy

LOCAL
Abscesses
Cellulitis
Ulcers
Thrombosed veins

BRAIN
Overdose
Coma
Hallucinations

INFECTIONS
Bacterial endocarditis
Viral hepatitis
AIDS (lymph nodes)

Substance abuse often causes a variety of medical abnormalities and conditions throughout the body, as shown in the illustration above. *(Illustration by Electronic Illustrators Group.)*

- Have you ever tried to Cut down on your substance use?
- Have you ever been Annoyed by people trying to talk to you about your substance use?
- Do you ever feel Guilty about your substance use?
- Do you ever need an Eye opener (use of the substance first thing in the morning) in order to start your day?

A "yes" answer to two or more of these questions is an indication that the individual should be referred for more thorough work-up for substance dependency or abuse.

In addition to CAGE, other screening questionnaires are available. Some are designed for particular population groups such as pregnant women, and others are designed to more thoroughly assess the severity of substance dependence. These questionnaires, known by their acronyms, include AUDIT, HSS, HSQ, PRIME-MD, ACE, TWEAK, s-MAST, and SADD. There is some variability among questionnaires in terms of how accurately and comprehensively they can identify individuals as substance dependent.

Patient history, as taken through the direct interview, is important for identifying physical symptoms and psychiatric factors related to substance use. Family history of alcohol or other substance dependency is also useful for diagnosis.

A physical examination may reveal signs of substance abuse. These signs are specific to the substances used, as well as needle marks, tracks, or nasal erosion.

With the individual's permission, substance use can be detected through laboratory testing of his or her blood, urine, or hair. Laboratory testing, however, may be limited by the sensitivity and specificity of the testing method, and by the time elapsed since the person last used the drug.

One of the most difficult aspects of diagnosis involves overcoming the patient's denial. Denial is a psychological state during which a person is unable to acknowledge the (usually negative) circumstances of a situation. In this case, denial leads a person to underestimate the degree of substance use and of the problems associated with substance use.

Treatment

According to the American Psychiatric Association, there are three goals for the treatment of people with substance use disorders: (1) the patient abstains from or reduces the use and effects of the substance; (2) the patient reduces the frequency and severity of relapses; and (3) the patient develops the psychological and emotional skills necessary to restore and maintain personal, occupational, and social functioning.

In general, before treatment can begin, many treatment centers require that the patient undergo **detoxification**. Detoxification is the process of weaning the patient from his or her regular substance use. Detoxification can be accomplished "cold turkey," by complete and immediate cessation of all substance use, or by slowly decreasing (tapering) the dose which a person is taking, to minimize the side effects of withdrawal. Some substances must be tapered because "cold turkey" methods of detoxification are potentially life threatening. In some cases, medications may be used to combat the unpleasant and threatening physical and psychological symptoms of withdrawal. For example, methadone is used to help patients adjust to the tapering of heroin use.

Treatment itself consists of three parts: (1) assessment; (2) formulation of a treatment plan; (3) psychiatric management. The first step in treatment is a comprehensive medical and psychiatric evaluation of the patient. This evaluation includes:

- a history of the patient's past and current substance use, and its cognitive, psychological, physiological, and behavioral effects
- a medical and psychiatric history and examination
- a history of psychiatric treatments and outcomes
- a family and social history
- screening of blood, breath, or urine for substances
- other laboratory tests to determine the presence of other conditions commonly found with substance use disorders

After the assessment is made, a treatment plan is formulated. Treatment plans vary according to the needs of the specific patient and can change for the same patient as he or she undergoes different phases of the disorder. Plans typically involve the following elements: (1) a strategy for the psychiatric management of the patient; (2) a strategy for reducing effects or use of substances, or for abstinence; (3) efforts to ensure compliance with the treatment program and to prevent relapse; (4) treatments for other conditions associated with substance use. Initial therapy and treatment setting (hospital, residential treatment, partial hospitalization, outpatient) decisions are made as part of the treatment plan, but because substance use disorders are considered a chronic condition requiring long-term care, these plans can and do change through the course of treatment.

The third step, psychiatric management of the patient, is the implementation of the treatment plan. Psychiatric management of the patient includes establishing a trusting relationship between clinician and patient; monitoring the patient's progress; managing the patient's relapses and withdrawal; diagnosing and treating associated psychiatric disorders; and helping the patient adhere to the treatment plan through therapy and the development of skills and social interactions that reinforce a drug-free lifestyle.

As part of the treatment process, patients typically undergo psychosocial therapy and, in some cases, pharmacologic treatment. Psychosocial therapeutic modalities include **cognitive-behavioral therapy**, behavioral therapy, individual psychodynamic or interpersonal therapy, **group therapy**, **family therapy**, and self-help groups. Pharmacologic treatment may include medications that ease withdrawal symptoms, reduce craving, interact negatively with substances of abuse to discourage drug-taking, or treat associated psychiatric disorders.

Alternative treatment

The efficacy of alternative treatments for substance use disorders remains for the most part ambiguous. One treatment that has been recently shown to have variable success is the use of **acupuncture** in treating substance dependence. In 2000, a randomized controlled trial of the effect of acupuncture on cocaine addiction reported that acupuncture significantly reduced the cocaine use of study participants. A 1999 meta-analysis (summary analysis of studies), however, reported that acupuncture had no statistically significant effect on **smoking** cessation.

There has been movement toward examining some touted treatments in more rigorous clinical trials. In particular, there has been some interest in *Pueraria lobata*, or kudzu, an herb that has reputedly been used in Chinese medicine to treat alcoholism. Preclinical trials of an herbal formula with kudzu have shown that increased consumption of the herbal formula is associated with decreased consumption of alcohol. Toxicity studies show few ill effects of the formula, and human trials are currently being undertaken to more fully evaluate the efficacy of this treatment.

The effectiveness of electroacupuncture (the practice of acupuncture accompanied by the application of low levels of electrical current at acupuncture points) in alleviating opiate withdrawal symptoms is also being examined. Preclinical trials suggest that electroacupuncture treatment given prior to the administration of naxolone seems to alleviate the withdrawal effects of naxolone.

Prognosis

Recovery from substance use is notoriously difficult, even with exceptional treatment resources. Although relapse rates are difficult to accurately obtain, the NIAAA cites evidence that 90% of alcohol dependent users experience at least one relapse within the 4 years after treatment. Relapse rates for heroin and nicotine users are believed to be similar. Certain pharmacological treatments, however, have been shown to reduce relapse rates.

Relapses are most likely to occur within the first 12 months of having discontinued substance use. Triggers for relapses can include any number of life stresses (problems on the job or in the marriage, loss of a relationship, death of a loved one, financial stresses), in addition to seemingly mundane exposure to a place or an acquaintance associated with previous substance use.

The development of adaptive life skills and ongoing drug-free social support are believed to be two important factors in avoiding relapse. The effect of the support group Alcoholics Anonymous has been intensively studied, and a 1996 meta-analysis noted that long-term sobriety appears to be positively related to Alcoholics Anonymous attendance and involvement. Support for family members in addition to support for the individual in recovery is also important. Because substance dependence has a serious impact on family functioning, and because family members may inadvertently maintain behaviors that initially led to the substance dependence, ongoing therapy and support for family members should not be neglected.

KEY TERMS

Addiction—The state of being both physically and psychologically dependent on a substance.

Dependence—A state in which a person requires a steady concentration of a particular substance to avoid experiencing withdrawal symptoms.

Detoxification—A process whereby an addict is withdrawn from a substance.

Intoxication—The desired mental, physical, or emotional state produced by a substance.

Street drug—A substance purchased from a drug dealer; may be a legal substance, sold illicitly (without a prescription, and not for medical use), or it may be a substance that is illegal to possess.

Tolerance—A phenomenon whereby a drug user becomes physically accustomed to a particular dose of a substance, and requires increasing dosages in order to obtain the same effects.

Withdrawal—Those side effects experienced by a person who has become physically dependent on a substance, upon decreasing the substance's dosage or discontinuing its use.

Prevention

Prevention is best aimed at teenagers and young adults aged 18–24 who are at very high risk for substance experimentation. Prevention programs should include an education component that outlines the risks and consequences of substance use and a training component that gives advice on how to resist peer pressure to use drugs.

Furthermore, prevention programs should work to identify and target children who are at relatively higher risk for substance abuse. This group includes victims of physical or sexual abuse, children of parents who have a history of substance abuse, and children with poor school performance and/or attention deficit disorder. These children may require more intensive intervention.

Resources

BOOKS

American Psychiatric Association. *Diagnostic and Statistical Manual of Mental Disorders.* 4th ed., revised. Washington, DC: American Psychiatric Association, 2000.

PERIODICALS

"Inhalant Abuse Becomes Focus of SAMHSA Guidelines, Prevention Effors." *Alcoholism &Drug Abuse Weekly* March 22, 2004: 1–4.

Schneider, Robert K., James L. Levenson, and Sidney H. Schnoll. "Update in Addiction Medicine." *Annals of Internal Medicine* 134 (March 6, 2001): 387-395.

Genevieve Pham-Kanter
Teresa G. Odle

Substance dependence *see* **Substance abuse and dependence**

Sucralfate *see* **Antiulcer drugs**

Sucrose intolerance *see* **Carbohydrate intolerance**

Sudden cardiac death

Definition

Sudden cardiac **death** (SCD) is an unexpected death due to heart problems, which occurs within one hour from the start of any cardiac-related symptoms. SCD is sometimes called cardiac arrest.

Description

When the heart suddenly stops beating effectively and breathing ceases, a person is said to have experienced sudden cardiac death.

SCD is not the same as actual death. In actual death, the brain also dies. The important difference is that sudden cardiac death is potentially reversible. If it is reversed quickly enough, the brain will not die.

Sudden cardiac death is also not the same as a **heart attack**. A heart attack (myocardial infarction) is the result of a blockage in an artery which feeds the heart, so the heart becomes starved for oxygen. The part that has been starved is damaged beyond repair, but the heart can still beat effectively.

Causes and symptoms

Sudden cardiac death is usually caused by **ventricular fibrillation** (the lower chamber of the heart quivers instead of pumping in an organized rhythm). Ventricular fibrillation almost never returns to normal by itself, so the condition requires immediate intervention. **Ventricular tachycardia** can also lead to sudden

---

cardiac death. The risk for SCD is higher for anyone with heart disease.

When the heart stops beating effectively and the brain is being deprived of oxygenated blood, a medical emergency exists.

Diagnosis

Diagnosis of sudden cardiac death is made when there is a sudden loss of consciousness, breathing stops, and there is no effective heart beat.

Treatment

When sudden cardiac death occurs, the first priority is to establish the flow of oxygenated blood to the brain. The next priority is to restore normal rhythm to the heart. Forcing air into the mouth will get oxygen into the lungs. Compressing the chest simulates a pumping heart and will get some blood flow to the lungs, brain, and coronary arteries. This method is called **cardiopulmonary resuscitation (CPR)**. When trained help arrives, they will attempt to establish a normal heart beat by using a device called a defibrillator.

When If sudden cardiac death occurs outside the hospital setting, **cardiopulmonary resuscitation (CPR)** must begin within four to six minutes and advanced **life support** measures must begin within eight minutes, to avoid brain death. CPR requires no special medical skills and training is available for the ordinary person nationwide.

Prognosis

Sudden cardiac death is reversible in most people if treatment is begun quickly. However, of the people who are resuscitated, 40% will have another SCD within two years if they do not receive appropriate treatment for the underlying cause of the episode.

Prevention

When In order to prevent sudden cardiac death, underlying heart conditions must be addressed. Medications and implantable cardioverter-defibrillators may be used.

Resources

ORGANIZATIONS

American Heart Association. 7320 Greenville Ave. Dallas, TX 75231. (214) 373-6300. < http://www.americanheart.org >.

Dorothy Elinor Stonely

Sudden infant death syndrome

Definition

Sudden infant **death** syndrome (SIDS) is the unexplained death without warning of an apparently healthy infant, usually during sleep.

Description

Also known as crib death, SIDS has baffled physicians and parents for years. In the 1990s, advances have been made in preventing the occurrence of SIDS, which killed more than 4,800 babies in 1992 and 3,279 infants in 1995. Education programs aimed at encouraging parents and caregivers to place babies on their backs and sides when putting them to bed have helped contribute to a lower mortality rate from SIDS.

In the United States, SIDS strikes one or two infants in every thousand, making it the leading cause of death in newborns. It accounts for about 10% of deaths occurring during the first year of life. SIDS most commonly affects babies between the ages of two months and six months; it almost never strikes infants younger than two weeks of age or older than eight months. Most SIDS deaths occur between midnight and 8 A.M.

Causes and symptoms

Risk factors for SIDS

The exact causes of SIDS are still unknown, although studies have shown that many of the infants had recently been under a doctor's care for a cold or other illness of the upper respiratory tract. Most SIDS deaths occur during the winter and early spring, which are the peak times for respiratory infections. The most common risk factors for SIDS include:

Ten Leading Causes Of Infant Death (U.S.)

Congenital anomalies
Pre-term/Low birthweight
Sudden Infant Death Syndrome (SIDS)
Respiratory Distress Syndrome
Problems related to complications of pregnancy
Complications of placenta, cord, and membrane Accidents
Perinatal infections
Pneumonia/Influenza
Intrauterine hypoxia and birth asphyxia

- sleeping on the stomach (in the prone position)
- mother who smokes during **pregnancy**; smokers are as much as three times more likely than nonsmokers to have a SIDS baby
- the presence of passive smoke in the household
- male sex; the male/female ratio in SIDS deaths is 3:2;
- belonging to an economically deprived or minority family
- mother under 20 years of age at pregnancy
- mother who abuses drugs
- mother with little or no prenatal care
- prematurity or low weight at birth
- family history of SIDS

Most of these risk factors are associated with significantly higher rates of SIDS; however, none of them are exact enough to be useful in predicting which specific children may die from SIDS.

Theories about SIDS

MEDICAL DISORDERS. Currently, it is not known whether the immediate cause of death from SIDS is a heart problem or a sudden interruption of breathing. The most consistent **autopsy** findings are pinpoint hemorrhages inside the baby's chest and mild inflammation or congestion of the nose, throat, and airway. Some doctors have thought that the children stop breathing because their upper airway gets blocked. Others have suggested that the children have an abnormally high blood level of the chemicals that transmit nerve impulses to the brain, or that there is too much fetal hemoglobin in the blood. A third theory concerns the possibility that SIDS infants have an underlying abnormality in the central nervous system. This suggestion is based on the assumption that normal infants sense when their air supply is inadequate and wake up. Babies with an abnormal nervous

KEY TERMS

Congenital—Existing or present at the time of birth.

Crib death—Another name for SIDS.

Prone—Lying on the stomach with the face downward.

Supine—Lying on the back with the face upward.

system, however, do not have the same alarm mechanism in their brains. Other theories about the cause of death in SIDS include immune system disorders that cause changes in the baby's heart rate and breathing patterns during sleep, or a metabolic disorder that causes a buildup of fatty acids in the baby's system.

PHYSICAL SURROUNDINGS. A recent theory proposes that SIDS is connected to the child's rebreathing of stale air trapped in soft bedding. In addition to the infant's sleeping in the prone position, pillows, sheepskins, and other soft items may contribute to trapping air around the baby's mouth and nose, which causes the baby to breathe in too much carbon dioxide and not enough oxygen. Wrapping a baby too warmly has also been proposed as a factor.

Diagnosis

The diagnosis of SIDS is primarily a diagnosis of exclusion. This means that it is given only after other possible causes of the baby's death have been ruled out. Known risk factors aid in the diagnosis. Unlike the pattern in other diseases, however, the diagnosis of SIDS can only be given post-mortem. It is recommended that all infants who die in their sleep receive an autopsy to determine the cause. Autopsies indicate a definite explanation in about 20% of cases of sudden infant death. In addition, an autopsy can often put to rest any doubts the parents may have. Investigation of the location of the death is also useful in determining the child's sleeping position, bedding, room temperature, and similar factors.

Treatment

There is no treatment for SIDS, only identification of risk factors and preventive measures. The baby's parents may benefit from referral to counseling and support groups for parents of SIDS victims.

Prevention

SIDS appears to be at least partly preventable, which has been shown by a substantial decrease in the case rate. The following are recommended as preventive measures:

- Sleep position. The United States Department of Health and Human Services initiated a "Back-to-Sleep" campaign in 1994 to educate the public about sleep position. Prior to that time, an estimated 70% of infants slept on their stomachs, since parents had been taught that a "back down" position contributed to **choking** during sleep. There are some conditions for which doctors will recommend the prone position, but for normal infants, side or back (supine) positions are better. When placing an infant on his or her side, the parent should pull the child's lower arm forward so that he or she is less likely to roll over onto the stomach. When babies are awake and being observed, they should be placed on their stomachs frequently to aid in the development of the muscles and skills involved in lifting the head. Once a baby can roll over to his or her stomach, he or she has developed to the point where the risk of SIDS is minimal.

- Good prenatal care. Proper prenatal care can help prevent the abnormalities that put children at higher risk for SIDS. Mothers who do not receive prenatal care are also more likely to have premature and low birth-weight babies. Expectant mothers should also be warned about the risks of **smoking**, alcohol intake, and drug use during pregnancy.

- Proper bedding. Studies have shown that soft bedding, such as beanbags, waterbeds and soft mattresses, contributes to SIDS. Babies should sleep on firm mattresses with no soft or fluffy materials underneath or around them– including quilts, pillows, thick comforters or lambskin. Soft stuffed toys should not be placed in the crib while babies sleep.

- Room temperature. Although babies should be kept warm, they do not need to be any warmer than is comfortable for the caregiver. An overheated baby is more likely to sleep deeply, perhaps making it more difficult to wake when short of breath. Room temperature and wrapping should keep the baby warm and comfortable but not overheated.

- Diet. Some studies indicate that breastfed babies are at lower risk for SIDS. It is thought that the mother's milk may provide additional immunity to the infections that can trigger sudden death in infants.

- Bedsharing with parents. Opinions differ on whether or not bedsharing of infant and mother increases or decreases the risk of SIDS. Bedsharing may encourage breastfeeding or alter sleep patterns, which could lower the risk of SIDS. On the other hand, some studies suggest that bedsharing increases the risk of SIDS. In any case, mothers who choose to bring their babies to bed should observe the following cautions: Soft sleep surfaces, as well as quilts, blankets, comforters or pillows should not be placed under the baby. Parents who sleep with their infants should not smoke around the baby, or use alcohol or other drugs which might make them difficult to arouse. Parents should also be aware that adult beds are not built with the same safety features as infant cribs.

- Secondhand smoke. It is as important to keep the baby's environment smoke-free during infancy as it was when the mother was pregnant with the baby.

- Electronic monitoring. Electronic monitors are available for use in the home. These devices sound an alarm for the parents if the child stops breathing. There is no evidence, however, that these monitors prevent SIDS. In 1986, experts consulted by the National Institutes of Health (NIH) recommended monitors only for infants at risk. These infants include those who have had one or more episodes of breath stopping; premature infants with breathing difficulties; and babies with two or more older siblings that died of SIDS. Parents who use monitors should know how to use them properly and what to for the baby if the alarm goes off.

- Immunizations. There is no evidence that immunizations increase the risk of SIDS. In fact, babies who receive immunizations on schedule are less likely to die of SIDS.

Resources

ORGANIZATIONS

Association of SIDS and Infant Mortality Programs. MN SID Center, Children's Hospitals and Clinics, 2525 Chicago Ave. So., Minneapolis, MN 55404. (612) 813-6285. < http://www.asip1.org >.

National Institute of Child Health and Human Development. Bldg 31, Room 2A32, MSC 2425, 31 Center Drive, Bethesda, MD 20892-2425. (800) 505-2742. < http://www.nichd.nih.gov/sids/sids.htm >.

National SIDS Resource Center. 2070 Chain Bridge Road, Suite 450, Vienna, VA 22181. (703) 821-8955. < http://www.circsol.com/SIDS/ >.

Sudden Infant Death Syndrome Alliance. 1314 Bedford Avenue, Suite 210, Baltimore, MD 21208. (800) 221-7437. < http://www.sidsalliance.org >.

Teresa Odle

Sugar diabetes *see* **Diabetes mellitus**

Sugar intolerance *see* **Carbohydrate intolerance**

Suicide

Definition

Suicide is defined as the intentional taking of one's own life. Prior to the late nineteenth century, suicide was legally defined as a criminal act in most Western countries. In the social climate of the early 2000s, however, suicidal behavior is most commonly regarded and responded to as a psychiatric emergency.

Description

Suicide is considered a major public health problem around the world as well as a personal tragedy. According to the National Institute of Mental Health (NIMH), suicide was the eleventh leading cause of **death** in the United States in 2000, and the third leading cause of death for people between the ages of 15 and 24. About 10.6 out of every 100,000 persons in the United States and Canada die by their own hands. There are five suicide victims for every three homicide deaths in North America as of the early 2000s. There are over 30,000 suicides per year in the United States, or about 86 per day; and each day about 1900 people attempt suicide.

The demographics of suicide vary considerably within Canada and the United States, due in part to differences among age groups and racial groups, and between men and women. Adult males are three to five times more likely to commit suicide than females, but females are more likely to attempt suicide. Most suicides occur in persons below the age of 40; however, elderly Caucasians are the sector of the population with the highest suicide rate. Americans over the age of 65 accounted for 18 percent of deaths by suicide in the United States in 2000. Geographical location is an additional factor; according to the Centers for Disease Control and Prevention (CDC), suicide rates in the United States are slightly higher than the national average in the western states, and somewhat lower than average in the East and the Midwest.

Race is also a factor in the demographics of suicide. Between 1979 and 1992, Native Americans had a suicide rate 1.5 times the national average, with young males between 15 and 24 accounting for 64% of Native American deaths by suicide. Asian American women have the highest suicide rate among all women over the age of 65. And between 1980 and 1996 the suicide rate more than doubled for black males between the ages of 15 and 19.

Causes & symptoms

Causes

Suicide is a complex act that represents the end result of a combination of factors in any individual. These factors include biological vulnerabilities, life history, occupation, present social circumstances, and the availability of means for committing suicide. While these factors do not "cause" suicide in the strict sense, some people are at greater risk of self-harm than others. Risk factors for suicide include:

- Male sex.

- Age over 75.

- A family history of suicide.

- A history of previous suicide attempts.

- A history of **abuse** in childhood.

- A local cluster of recent suicides or a local landmark associated with suicides. Examples of the latter include the Golden Gate Bridge in San Francisco; Sydney Harbor Bridge in Australia; St. Peter's Basilica in Rome; the Eiffel Tower in Paris; Prince Edward Viaduct in Toronto; and Mount Mihara, a volcano in Japan.

- Recent stressful events: separation or divorce, job loss, bankruptcy, upsetting medical diagnosis, death of spouse.

- Medical illness. Persons in treatment for such serious or incurable diseases as **AIDS**, Parkinson's disease, and certain types of **cancer** are at increased risk of suicide.

- Employment as a police officer, firefighter, physician, dentist, or member of another high-stress occupation.

- Presence of firearms in the house. Death by firearms is the most common method for women as well as men as of the early 2000s. In 2001, 55% of reported suicides in the United States were committed with guns.

- Alcohol or **substance abuse**. Mood-altering substances are a factor in suicide because they weaken a person's impulse control.

- Presence of a psychiatric illness. Over 90% of Americans who commit suicide have a significant mental illness. Major depression accounts for 60% (especially in the elderly), followed by **schizophrenia**, **alcoholism**, substance abuse, borderline personality disorder, Huntington's disease, and epilepsy. The lifetime mortality due to suicide in psychiatric patients is 15% for major depression; 20% for **bipolar disorder**; 18% for alcoholism; 10% for schizophrenia; and 5–10% for borderline and certain other personality disorders.

Neurobiological factors may also influence a person's risk of suicide. Post-mortem studies of the brains of suicide victims indicate that the part of the brain associated with aggression and other impulsive behaviors (the frontal cortex) has a significantly lower level of serotonin, a neurotransmitter associated with **mood disorders**. Low serotonin levels are correlated with major depression. In addition, suicide victims have higher than normal levels of cortisol, a hormone produced in stressful situations, in the tissues of their central nervous system. Other research has indicated that abuse in childhood may have permanent effects on the level of serotonin in the brain, possibly "resetting" the level abnormally low. In addition, twin studies have suggested that there may be a genetic susceptibility to both suicidal ideation and suicide attempts which cannot be explained by inheritance of common psychiatric disorders.

Some psychiatrists propose psychodynamic explanations of suicide. According to one such theory, suicide is "murder in the 180th degree" that is, the suicidal person really wants to kill someone else but turns the anger against the self instead. Another version of this idea is that the suicidal person has incorporated the image of an abusive parent or other relative in their own psyche and then tries to eliminate the abuser by killing the self.

Diagnosis

When a person consults a doctor because they are thinking of committing suicide, or they are taken to a doctor's office or emergency room after a suicide attempt, the doctor will evaluate the patient's potential for acting on their thoughts or making another attempt. The physician's assessment will be based on several different sources of information:

- The patient's history, including a history of previous attempts or a family history of suicide.

- A clinical interview in which the physician will ask whether the patient is presently thinking of suicide; whether they have made actual plans to do so; whether they have thought about the means; and what they think their suicide will accomplish. These questions help in evaluating the seriousness of the patient's intentions.

- A suicide note, if any.

- Information from friends, relatives, or first responders who may have accompanied the patient.

- Short self-administered psychiatric tests that screen people for depression and suicidal ideation. The most commonly used screeners are the Beck Depression Inventory (BDI), the Depression Screening Questionnaire, and the Hamilton Depression Rating Scale.

- The doctor's own instinctive reaction to the patient's mood, appearance, vocal tone, and similar factors.

Treatment of attempted suicide

Suicide attempts range from well-planned attempts involving a highly lethal method (guns, certain types of poison, jumping from high places, throwing oneself in front of trains or subway cars) that fail by good fortune to impulsive or poorly planned attempts using a less lethal method (medication overdoses, cutting the wrists). Suicide attempts at the less lethal end of the spectrum are sometimes referred to as suicide gestures or pseudocide. These terms should not be taken to indicate that suicide gestures are only forms of attention-seeking; they should rather be understood as evidence of serious emotional and mental distress.

A suicide attempt of any kind is treated as a psychiatric emergency by the police and other rescue personnel. Treatment in a hospital emergency room includes a complete psychiatric evaluation; a **mental status examination**; blood or urine tests if alcohol or drug abuse is suspected; and a detailed assessment of the patient's personal circumstances (occupation, living situation, family or friends nearby, etc.). The patient will be kept under observation while decisions are made about the need for hospitalization.

A person who has attempted suicide can be legally hospitalized against his or her will if he or she seems to be a danger to the self or others. The doctor will base decisions about hospitalization on the severity of the patient's depression; the availability of friends, relatives, or other social support; and the presence of other suicide risk factors, including a history of previous suicide attempts, substance abuse, and **psychosis** (loss of contact with reality, often marked by **delusions** and **hallucinations**). If the attempt is judged to be a nonlethal suicide gesture, the patient may be released after the psychiatric assessment is completed. According to CDC figures, 132,353 Americans were hospitalized in 2002 following suicide attempts while 116,639 were released following emergency room treatment.

Related issues

Survivors of suicide

One group of people that is often overlooked in discussions of suicide is the friends and family left behind by the suicide. It is estimated that each person who kills him- or herself leaves six survivors to deal with the aftermath; thus there are at least 4.5 million survivors of suicide in the United States. In addition to the grief that ordinarily accompanies death, survivors of suicide often struggle with feelings of guilt and shame as well. They often benefit from group or individual psychotherapy in order to work through such issues as wondering whether they could have prevented the suicide or whether they are likely to commit suicide themselves. The American Foundation for Suicide Prevention (AFSP) has a number of online resources available for survivors of suicide.

Assisted suicide

One question that has been raised in developed countries as the average life expectancy increases is the legalization of assisted suicide for persons suffering from a painful terminal illness. Physician-assisted suicide has become a topic of concern since it was legalized in the Netherlands in 2001 and in the state of Oregon in 1997. It is important to distinguish between physician-assisted suicide and euthanasia, or "mercy killing.". Assisted suicide, which is often called "self-deliverance" in Britain, refers to a person's bringing about his or her own death with the help of another person. Because the other person is often a physician, the act is often called "doctor-assisted suicide." Euthanasia strictly speaking means that the physician or other person is the one who performs the last act that causes death. For example, if a physician injects a patient with a lethal overdose of a pain-killing medication, he or she is performing euthanasia. If the physician leaves the patient with a loaded syringe and the patient injects himself or herself with it, the act is an assisted suicide. As of early 2005 assisted suicide is illegal everywhere in the United States except for Oregon, and euthanasia is illegal in all fifty states.

Media treatment of suicide

The Centers for Disease Control and Prevention (CDC) sponsored a national workshop in April 1994 that addressed the connection between sensationalized media treatments of suicide and the rising rate of suicide among American youth. The CDC and the American Association of Suicidology subsequently adopted a set of guidelines for media coverage of suicide intended to reduce the risk of suicide by contagion.

The CDC guidelines point out that the following types of reporting may increase the risk of "copycat" suicides:

- Presenting oversimplified explanations of suicide, when in fact many factors usually contribute to a person's decision to take their own life.

- Excessive or repetitive local news coverage.

- Sensationalizing the suicide by inclusion of morbid details or dramatic photographs.

- Giving "how-to" descriptions of the method of suicide.

- Describing suicide as an effective coping strategy or as a way to achieve certain goals.

- Glorifying the act of suicide or the person who commits suicide.

Alternative treatment

Some alternative treatments may help to prevent suicide by preventing or relieving depression. **Meditation** practice or religious faith and worship have been shown to lower a person's risk of suicide. In addition, any activity that brings people together in groups and encourages them to form friendships helps to lower the risk of suicide, as people with strong social networks are less likely to give up on life.

Prognosis

The prognosis for a person who has attempted suicide is generally favorable, although further research needs to be done. A 1978 follow-up study of 515 people who had attempted suicide between 1937 and 1971 reported that 94% were either still alive or had died of natural causes. This finding has been taken to indicate that suicidal behavior is more likely to be a passing response to an acute crisis than a reflection of a permanent state of mind.

Prevention

One reason that suicide is such a tragedy is that most self-inflicted deaths are potentially preventable. Many suicidal people change their minds if they can be helped through their immediate crisis; Dr. Richard Seiden, a specialist in treating survivors of suicide attempts, puts the high-risk period at 90 days after the crisis. Some potential suicides change their minds during the actual attempt; for example, a number of people who survived jumping off the Golden Gate Bridge told interviewers afterward that they regretted their action even as they were falling and that they were grateful they survived.

Brain research is another important aspect of suicide prevention. Since major depression is the single most common psychiatric diagnosis in suicidal people, earlier and more effective recognition of depression is a necessary preventive measure. Known biological markers for an increased risk of suicide can now be correlated with personality profiles linked to suicidal behavior under **stress** to help identify individuals at risk. In addition, brain imaging studies using **positron emission tomography** (**PET**) are presently in use to detect abnormal patterns of serotonin uptake in specific regions of the brain. Genetic studies are also yielding new information about inherited predispositions to suicide.

Another major preventive measure is education of clinicians, media people, and the general public. In 2002 the CDC, the National Institutes of Health (NIH), and several other government agencies joined together to form the National Strategy for Suicide Prevention, or NSSP. Education of the general public includes a growing number of medical and government websites posting information about suicide, publications available for downloading, lists of books for further reading, tips for identifying symptoms of depressed and suicidal thinking, and advice about helping friends or loved ones who may be at risk. Many of these websites also have direct connections to suicide hotlines.

The National Institute of Mental Health (NIMH) recommends the following action steps for anyone dealing with a suicidal person:

- Make sure that someone is with them at all times; do not leave them alone even for a short period of time.

- Persuade them to call their family doctor or the nearest hospital emergency room.

- Call 911 yourself.

- Keep the person away from firearms, drugs, or other potential means of suicide.

Resources

BOOKS

Alvarez, A. *The Savage God: A Study of Suicide*. New York: Random House, Inc., 1972. A now-classic study of suicide written for general readers. The author includes a historical overview of suicide along with accounts of his own suicide attempt and the suicide of his friend, the poet Sylvia Plath.

American Psychiatric Association. *Diagnostic and Statistical Manual of Mental Disorders*, 4th edition, text revision.

KEY TERMS

Assisted suicide—A form of self-inflicted death in which a person voluntarily brings about his or her own death with the help of another, usually a physician, relative, or friend.

Cortisol—A hormone released by the cortex (outer portion) of the adrenal gland when a person is under stress. Cortisol levels are now considered a biological marker of suicide risk.

Euthanasia—The act of putting a person or animal to death painlessly or allowing them to die by withholding medical services, usually because of a painful and incurable disease. Mercy killing is another term for euthanasia.

Frontal cortex—The part of the human brain associated with aggressiveness and impulse control. Abnormalities in the frontal cortex are associated with an increased risk of suicide.

Psychodynamic—A type of explanation of human behavior that regards it as the outcome of interactions between conscious and unconscious factors.

Serotonin—A chemical that occurs in the blood and nervous tissue and functions to transmit signals across the gaps between neurons in the central nervous system. Abnormally low levels of serotonin are associated with depression and an increased risk of suicide.

Suicide gesture—Attempted suicide characterized by a low-lethality method, low level of intent or planning, and little physical damage. Pseudocide is another term for a suicide gesture.

Washington, DC: American Psychiatric Association, 2000.

"Depression." In *The Merck Manual of Geriatrics*, edited by Mark H. Beers, MD, and Robert Berkow, MD. Whitehouse Station, NJ: Merck Research Laboratories, 2004.

"Psychiatric Emergencies." In *The Merck Manual of Diagnosis and Therapy*, edited by Mark H. Beers, MD, and Robert Berkow, MD. Whitehouse Station, NJ: Merck Research Laboratories, 2004.

"Suicidal Behavior." In *The Merck Manual of Diagnosis and Therapy*, edited by Mark H. Beers, MD, and Robert Berkow, MD. Whitehouse Station, NJ: Merck Research Laboratories, 2004.

"Suicide in Children and Adolescents." In *The Merck Manual of Diagnosis and Therapy*, edited by Mark H. Beers, MD, and Robert Berkow, MD.

Whitehouse Station, NJ: Merck Research Laboratories, 2004.

PERIODICALS

Friend, Tad "Letter from California: Jumpers." *New Yorker*, 10 November 2003. < http://newyorker.com/printable/?fact/031013fa_fact > . A journalist's account of the Golden Gate Bridge in San Francisco, the world's leading location for suicide.

Fu, Q., A. C. Heath, K. K. Bucholz, et al. "A Twin Study of Genetic and Environmental Influences on Suicidality in Men." *Psychology in Medicine* 32 (January 2002): 11-24.

Plunkett, A., B. O'Toole, H. Swanston, et al. "Suicide Risk Following Child Sexual Abuse." *Ambulatory Pediatrics* 1 (September-October 2001): 262-266.

Soreff, Stephen, MD. "Suicide." *eMedicine*, 3 September 2004. < http://www.emedicine.com/med/topic3004.htm > .

ORGANIZATIONS

American Academy of Child and Adolescent Psychiatry. 3615 Wisconsin Avenue, NW, Washington, DC 20016-3007. (202) 966-7300. Fax: (202) 966-2891. < http://www.aacap.org. > .

American Association of Suicidology. Suite 408, 4201 Connecticut Avenue, NW, Washington, DC 20008. (202) 237-2280. Fax: (202) 237-2282. < http://www.suicidology.org. > .

American Foundation for Suicide Prevention (AFSP). 120 Wall Street, 22nd Floor, New York, NY 10005. (888) 333-2377 or (212)

Centers for Disease Control and Prevention (CDC), National Center for Injury Prevention and Control (NCIPC). Mailstop K60, 4770 Buford Highway, Atlanta, GA 30341-3724. (770) 488-4362. Fax: (770) 488-4349. < http://www.cdc.gov/ncipc.htm > .

National Institute of Mental Health (NIMH). 6001 Executive Boulevard, Room 8184, MSC 9663, Bethesda, MD 20892-9663. (301) 443-4513 or (886) 615-NIMH. < www.nimh.nih.gov. > .

OTHER

American Academy of Child and Adolescent Psychiatry (AACAP). *Teen Suicide*. AACAP Facts for Families #10. Washington, DC: AACAP, 2004.

Centers for Disease Control and Prevention, National Center for Injury Prevention and Control. "Suicide Contagion and the Reporting of Suicide: Recommendations from a National Workshop." *Morbidity and Mortality Weekly Report* 43 (22 April 1994): 9–18. < http://www.cdc.gov/mmwr/preview/mmwrhtml/00031539.htm. > .

Centers for Disease Control and Prevention, National Center for Injury Prevention and Control. *Suicide: Fact Sheet*. < http://www.cdc.gov/ncipc/factsheets/suifacts.htm. > .

National Institute of Mental Health (NIMH). *In Harm's Way: Suicide in America*. NIH Publication No. 03-

4594. Bethesda, MD: NIMH, 2003. <http:// www.nimh.nih.gov/publicat/NIMHharmsway.pdf>.

National Suicide Hotline: (800) 273-TALK (1-800-273-8255).

Rebecca Frey, PhD

Sulfacetamide *see* **Antibiotics, ophthalmic**

Sulfamethoxazole and trimethoprim *see* **Sulfonamides**

Sulfinpyrazone *see* **Gout drugs**

Sulfisoxazole *see* **Sulfonamides**

Sulfonamides

Definition

Sulfonamides are medicines that prevent the growth of bacteria in the body.

Purpose

Sulfonamides are used to treat many kinds of infections caused by bacteria and certain other microorganisms. Physicians may prescribe these drugs to treat urinary tract infections, ear infections, frequent or long-lasting **bronchitis**, bacterial **meningitis**, certain eye infections, *Pneumocystis carinii* **pneumonia**, **traveler's diarrhea**, and a number of other kinds of infections. These drugs will *not* work for colds, flu, and other infections caused by viruses.

Description

Sulfonamides, also called sulfa medicines, are available only with a physician's prescription. They are sold in tablet and liquid forms. Some commonly used sulfonamides are sulfisoxazole (Gantrisin) and the combination drug sulfamethoxazole and trimethoprim (Bactrim, Cotrim).

Recommended dosage

The recommended dosage depends on the type of sulfonamide, the strength of the medicine, and the medical problem for which it is being taken. Check with the physician who prescribed the drug or the pharmacist who filled the prescription for the correct dosage.

Always take sulfonamides exactly as directed. To make sure the infection clears up completely, take the medicine for as long as it has been prescribed. Do not stop taking the drug just because symptoms begin to improve. Symptoms may return if the drug is stopped too soon.

Sulfonamides work best when they are at constant levels in the blood. To help keep levels constant, take the medicine in doses spaced evenly through the day and night. Do not miss any doses. For best results, take the medicine with a full glass of water and drink several more glasses of water every day. This will help prevent some of the medicine's side effects.

Precautions

Symptoms should begin to improve within a few days of beginning to take this medicine. If they do not, or if they get worse, check with the physician who prescribed the medicine.

Although such side effects are rare, some people have had severe and life-threatening reactions to sulfonamides. These include sudden, severe liver damage, serious blood problems, breakdown of the outer layer of the skin, and a condition called Stevens-Johnson syndrome, in which people get blisters around the mouth, eyes, or anus. Call a physician immediately if any of these signs of a dangerous reaction occur:

- skin rash or reddish or purplish spots on the skin
- other skin problems, such as blistering or peeling
- fever
- sore throat
- cough
- shortness of breath
- joint **pain**
- pale skin
- yellow skin or eyes

This medicine may cause **dizziness**. Anyone who takes sulfonamides should not drive, use machines or do anything else that might be dangerous until they have found out how the drugs affect them.

Sulfonamides may cause blood problems that can interfere with healing and lead to additional infections. Avoid injuries while taking this medicine. Be especially careful not to injure the mouth when brushing or flossing the teeth or using a toothpick. Do not have dental work done until the blood is back to normal.

This medicine may increase sensitivity to sunlight. Even brief exposure to sun can cause a severe **sunburn** or a rash. While being treated with this medicine, avoid being in direct sunlight, especially between 10 A.M. and 3 P.M.; wear a hat and tightly woven clothing that covers the arms and legs; use a sunscreen with a skin protection factor (SPF) of at least 15; protect the lips with a sun block lipstick; and do not use tanning beds, tanning booths, or sunlamps.

Babies under 2 months should not be given sulfonamides unless their physician has ordered the medicine.

Older people may be especially sensitive to the effects of sulfonamides, increasing the chance of unwanted side effects, such as severe skin problems and blood problems. Patients who are taking water pills (**diuretics**) at the same time as sulfonamides may also be more likely to have these problems.

Special conditions

People with certain medical conditions or who are taking certain other medicines can have problems if they take sulfonamides. Before taking these drugs, be sure to let the physician know about any of these conditions:

ALLERGIES. Anyone who has had unusual reactions to sulfonamides, water pills (diuretics), diabetes medicines, or **glaucoma** medicine in the past should let his or her physician know before taking sulfonamides. The physician should also be told about any **allergies** to foods, dyes, preservatives, or other substances.

PREGNANCY. In studies of laboratory animals, some sulfonamides cause **birth defects**. The drugs' effects on human fetuses have not been studied. However, pregnant women are advised not to use this medicine around the time of labor and delivery, because it can cause side effects in the baby. Women who are pregnant or who may become pregnant should check with their physicians about the safety of using sulfonamides during **pregnancy**.

BREASTFEEDING. Sulfonamides pass into breast milk and may cause liver problems, anemia, and other problems in nursing babies whose mothers take the medicine. Because of those problems, women should not breastfeed when they are under treatment with this drug. Women who are breastfeeding and who need to take this medicine should check with their physicians to find out how long they need to stop breastfeeding.

OTHER MEDICAL CONDITIONS. Before using sulfonamides, people with any of these medical problems should make sure their physicians are aware of their conditions:

- anemia or other blood problems
- kidney disease
- liver disease
- asthma or severe allergies
- alcohol **abuse**
- poor **nutrition**
- abnormal intestinal absorption
- porphyria
- folic acid deficiency
- deficiency of the enzyme glucose-6-phosphate dehydrogenase (G6PD)

USE OF CERTAIN MEDICINES. Taking sulfonamides with certain other drugs may affect the way the drugs work or may increase the chance of side effects.

Side effects

The most common side effects are mild **diarrhea**, **nausea**, **vomiting**, dizziness, **headache**, loss of appetite, and tiredness. These problems usually go away as the body adjusts to the drug and do not require medical treatment.

More serious side effects are not common, but may occur. If any of the following side effects occur, check with a physician immediately:

- itching or skin rash
- reddish or purplish spots on the skin
- other skin problems, such as redness, blistering, peeling
- severe, watery or bloody diarrhea
- muscle or joint aches
- fever
- sore throat
- cough
- shortness of breath
- unusual tiredness or weakness
- unusual bleeding or bruising
- pale skin
- yellow eyes or skin
- swallowing problems

Other rare side effects may occur. Anyone who has unusual symptoms while taking sulfonamides should get in touch with his or her physician.

KEY TERMS

Anemia—A lack of hemoglobin–the compound in blood that carries oxygen from the lungs throughout the body and brings waste carbon dioxide from the cells to the lungs, where it is released.

Bronchitis—Inflammation of the air passages of the lungs.

Fetus—A developing baby inside the womb.

Inflammation—Pain, redness, swelling, and heat that usually develop in response to injury or illness.

Meningitis—Inflammation of tissues that surround the brain and spinal cord.

***Pneumocystis carinii* pneumonia**—A lung infection that affects people with weakened immune systems, such as people with AIDS or people taking medicines that weaken the immune system.

Porphyria—A disorder in which porphyrins build up in the blood and urine.

Porphyrin—A type of pigment found in living things.

Urinary tract—The passage through which urine flows from the kidneys out of the body.

Interactions

Sulfonamides may interact with a large number of other medicines. When this happens, the effects of one or both of the drugs may change or the risk of side effects may be greater. Anyone who takes sulfonamides should let the physician know all other medicines he or she is taking. Among the drugs that may interact with sulfonamides are:

- acetaminophen (Tylenol)
- medicine for overactive thyroid
- male hormones (androgens)
- female hormones (estrogens)
- other medicines used to treat infections
- birth control pills
- medicines for diabetes such as glyburide (Micronase)
- anticoagulants such as warfarin (Coumadin)
- disulfiram (Antabuse), used to treat alcohol abuse
- amantadine (Symmetrel), used to treat flu and also Parkinson's disease
- water pills (diuretics) such as hydrochlorothiazide (HCTZ, HydroDIURIL)

- the anticancer drug methotrexate (Rheumatrex)
- antiseizure medicines such as valproice acid (Depakote, Depakene)

The list above does not include every drug that may interact with sulfonamides. Be sure to check with a physician or pharmacist before combining sulfonamides with any other prescription or nonprescription (over-the-counter) medicine.

Nancy Ross-Flanigan

Sumatriptan *see* **Antimigraine drugs**

Sunburn

Definition

Inflammation of the skin caused by overexposure to the sun.

Description

Sunburn is caused by exposure to the ultraviolet (UV) rays of the sun. There are two types of ultraviolet rays, UVA and UVB. UVA rays penetrate the skin more deeply and can cause melanoma in susceptible people. UVB rays, which don't penetrate as deeply, cause sunburn and wrinkling. Most UVB rays are absorbed by **sunscreens**, but only about half the UVA rays are absorbed.

Skin **cancer** from sun overexposure is a serious health problem in the United States, affecting almost a million Americans each year. One out of 87 will develop **malignant melanoma**, the most serious type of skin cancer, and 7,300 of them will die each year.

Fair-skinned people are most susceptible to sunburn, because their skin produces only small amounts of the protective pigment called melanin. People trying to get a tan too quickly in strong sunlight are also more vulnerable to sunburn. While they have a lower risk, even the darkest-skinned people can get skin cancer.

Repeated sun overexposure and burning can prematurely age the skin, causing yellowish, wrinkled skin. Overexposure can increase the risk of skin cancer, especially a serious burn in childhood.

Causes and symptoms

The ultraviolet rays in sunlight destroy cells in the outer layer of the skin, damaging tiny blood vessels

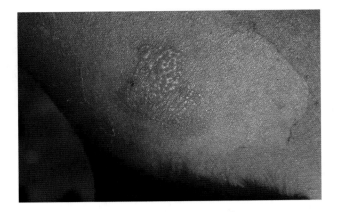

This person has a second-degree sunburn on the back of the neck. *(Custom Medical Stock Photo. Reproduced by permission.)*

underneath. When the skin is burned, the blood vessels dilate and leak fluid. Cells stop making protein. Their DNA is damaged by the ultraviolet rays. Repeated DNA damage can lead to cancer.

When the sun **burns** the skin, it triggers immune defenses which identify the burned skin as foreign. At the same time, the sun transforms a substance on the skin which interferes with this immune response. While this substance keeps the immune system from attacking a person's own skin, it also means that any malignant cells in the skin will be able to grow freely.

Sunburn causes skin to turn red and blister. Several days later, the dead skin cells peel off. In severe cases, the burn may occur with sunstroke (**vomiting, fever** and collapse).

Diagnosis

Visual inspection and a history of exposure to the sun.

Treatment

Aspirin can ease **pain** and inflammation. Tender skin should be protected against the sun until it has healed. In addition, apply:

- calamine lotion
- sunburn cream or spray
- cool tap water compress
- colloidal oatmeal (Aveeno) baths
- dusting powder to reduce chafing

People who are severely sunburned should see a doctor, who may prescribe corticosteroid cream to speed healing.

Alternative treatment

Over-the-counter preparations containing aloe (*Aloe barbadensis*) are an effective treatment for sunburn, easing pain and inflammation while also relieving dryness of the skin. A variety of topical herbal remedies applied as lotions, poltices, or compresses may also help relieve the effects of sunburn. Calendula (*Calendula officinalis*) is one of the most frequently recommended to reduce inflammation.

Prognosis

Moderately burned skin should heal within a week. While the skin will heal after a sunburn, the risk of skin cancer increases with exposure and subsequent burns. Even one bad burn in childhood carries an increased risk of skin cancer.

Prevention

Everyone from age six months on should use a water-resistant sunscreen with a sun protective factor (SPF) of at least 15. Apply at least an ounce 15–30 minutes before going outside. It should be reapplied every two hours (more often after swimming). Babies should be kept completely out of the sun for the first six months of life, because their skin is thinner than older children. Sunscreens have not been approved for infants.

In addition, people should:

- limit sun exposure to 15 minutes the first day, even if the weather is hazy, slowly increasing exposure daily
- reapply sunscreen every two hours (more often if sweating or swimming)
- reapply waterproof sunscreen after swimming more than 80 minutes, after toweling off, or after perspiring heavily
- avoid the sun between 10 A.M. and 3 P.M.

- use waterproof sunscreen on legs and feet, since the sun can burn even through water

- wear an opaque shirt in water, because reflected rays are intensified

If using a sunscreen under SPF 15, simply applying more of the same SPF won't prolong allowed time in the sun. Instead, patients should use a higher SPF in order to lengthen exposure safely. A billed cap protects 70% of the face; a wide-brimmed hat is better. People at very high risk for skin cancer can wear clothing that blocks almost all UV rays, but most people can simply wear white cotton summer-weight clothing with a tight weave.

Resources

PERIODICALS

Tyler, Varro. "Aloe: Nature's Skin Soother." *Prevention Magazine* April 1, 1998: 94-96.

Carol A. Turkington

Sunscreens

Definition

Sunscreens are products applied to the skin to protect against the harmful effects of the sun's ultraviolet (UV) rays.

Purpose

Everyone needs a little sunshine. About 15 minutes of exposure a day helps the body make Vitamin D, which is important for healthy bones and teeth. But longer exposure may cause many problems, from wrinkles to skin **cancer**. One particularly deadly form of skin cancer, **malignant melanoma**, has been on the rise in recent decades, as tanning has become more popular. Over the same period, scientists have warned that the thin layer of ozone that protects life on Earth from the sun's ultraviolet (UV) radiation is being depleted. This allows more UV radiation to get through, adding to the risk of overexposure.

Sunscreens help protect against the sun's damaging effects. But just how much protection they provide is a matter of debate. The sun gives off two kinds of ultraviolet radiation, called UV-A and UV-B. For many years, experts thought that only UV-B was harmful. However, recent research suggests that UV-A may be just as dangerous as UV-B, although its

effects may take longer to show up. In particular, UV-A may have a role in causing melanoma. Most sunscreen products contain ingredients that provide adequate protection only against UV-B rays. Even those labeled as broad-spectrum sunscreens may offer only partial protection against UV-A radiation. Those containing the ingredient avobenzone give the most protection against UV-A rays.

Some medical experts are concerned that sunscreens give people a false sense of security, allowing them to stay in the sun longer than they should. Although sunscreens protect the skin from burning, they may not protect against other kinds of damage. A number of studies suggest that people who use sunscreens may actually increase their risk of melanoma because they spend too much time in the sun. This does not mean that people should stop using sunscreens. It means that they should not rely on sunscreens *alone* for protection. According to the American Academy of Dermatology, sunscreens should be one part of sun protection, along with wide-brimmed hats and tightly-woven clothing that covers the arms and legs.

Sunscreens are also recommended for patients with **rosacea** or other skin disorders that are aggravated by exposure to sunlight.

Description

Many brands of sunscreens are available, containing a variety of ingredients. The active ingredients work by absorbing, reflecting, or scattering some or all of the sun's rays. Most sunscreen products contain combinations of ingredients.

The U.S. Food and Drug Administration (FDA) has required sunscreen products to carry a sun protection factor (SPF) rating on their labels since 1999. This number tells the consumer how well the sunscreen protects against burning. The higher the number, the longer a person can stay in the sun without burning.

Sunscreens are usually grouped into two major categories, namely chemical absorbers and physical blockers. Chemical absorbers absorb high-intensity UV rays while physical blockers reflect or scatter them. Chemical absorber compounds include avobenzone, padimate O, octyl methoxycinnamate, octisalate, and octocrylene. Physical blocker compounds include titanium dioxide and zinc oxide. The chief drawback of the physical blockers is their tendency to leave a white film on the skin, causing many people to use less of the product than they should for full sun protection.

A plant-derived compound that shows promise as a sunscreen is nobiletin, a flavonoid extracted from *Citrus depressa* or flat orange, a small citrus fruit native to Taiwan and Okinawa. Topical application of nobiletin has been shown to be effective in preventing the swelling and reddening of the skin associated with overexposure to sunlight.

Sunscreen products are sold as lotions, creams, gels, oils, sprays, sticks, and lip balms, and can be bought without a physician's prescription.

Recommended dosage

One should be sure to read the instructions that come with the product. Some need to be applied as long as one or two hours before sun exposure. Others should be applied 15–30 minutes before exposure, and reapplied frequently during exposure.

People should apply sunscreen liberally to all exposed parts of the skin, including the hands, feet, nose, ears, neck, scalp (if the hair is thin or very short), and eyelids. They should take care not to get sunscreen in the eyes, as it can cause irritation. People should also use a lip balm containing sunscreen to protect the lips, and reapply sunscreen liberally every 1–2 hours—more frequently when perspiring heavily or after swimming.

Precautions

Sunscreen alone will not provide full protection from the sun. When possible, one should wear a hat, long pants, long-sleeved shirts or blouses, and sunglasses. Try to stay out of the sun between 10 A.M. and 2 P.M. (11 A.M. to 3 P.M. Daylight Saving Time), when the sun's rays are strongest. The sun can damage the skin even on cloudy days, so get in the habit of using a sunscreen every day. Be especially careful at high elevations or in areas with surfaces that reflect the sun's rays, such as sand, water, concrete, or snow.

Sunlamps, tanning beds, and tanning booths were once thought to be safer than the sun, because they give off mainly UV-A rays. However, UV-A rays are now known to cause serious skin damage and may increase the risk of melanoma. Heatlh experts advise people not to use these tanning devices.

People with fair skin, blond, red or light-brown hair, and blue or light-colored eyes are at greatest risk for developing skin cancer. So are people with many large skin **moles**. These people should avoid exposure to the sun as much as possible. However, even dark-skinned people, including African Americans and Hispanic Americans may suffer skin damage from the sun and should be careful about exposure.

Other groups of people who should minimize sun exposure are those who have had organ transplants or recent **plastic surgery**. Patients who have received organ transplants have a greatly increased risk of developing skin cancer, and the facial skin of people who have had face lifts or similar plastic surgery procedures sunburns more easily than intact skin.

Sunscreens should not be used on infants under 6 months of age because of the risk of side effects. Instead, children this young should be kept out of the sun. Children over 6 months should be protected with clothing and sunscreens of at least SPF 15, preferably lotions. Sunscreens containing alcohol should not be used on children because they may irritate the skin.

Older people who stay out of the sun and use sunscreens may not produce enough vitamin D in their bodies. They may need to increase the vitamin D in their **diets** by including foods such as fortified milk and salmon. A health care professional can help decide if this precaution is necessary.

Anyone who has had unusual reactions to any sunscreen ingredients in the past should check with a physician or pharmacist before using a sunscreen. The physician or pharmacist should also be told about any **allergies** to foods, dyes, preservatives, or other substances, especially the following:

- artificial sweeteners
- such anesthetics as benzocaine, procaine, or tetracaine
- diabetes medicine taken by mouth
- hair dyes
- sulfa medicines
- water pills
- cinnamon flavoring

People with skin conditions or diseases should check with their physicians before using a sunscreen. This is especially true of people with conditions that get worse with exposure to light.

Side effects

The most common side effects are drying or tightening of the skin. This problem does not need medical attention unless it does not improve.

KEY TERMS

Hair follicle—A tiny pit in the skin from which hair grows.

Melanoma—A rapidly spreading and deadly form of cancer that usually occurs on the skin.

Ozone—A gas found in the atmosphere. A layer of ozone about 15 mi (24 km) above Earth's surface helps protect living things from the damaging effects of the sun's ultraviolet rays.

Pus—Thick, whitish or yellowish fluid that forms in infected tissue.

Rosacea—A chronic skin disease characterized by persistent redness of the skin and periodic outbreaks of pustules, usually affecting the middle third of the face.

Ultraviolet rays—Invisible light rays with a wavelength shorter than that of visible light but longer than that of x rays.

Other side effects are rare, but possible. If any of the following symptoms occur, check with a physician as soon as possible:

- acne
- burning, **itching**, or stinging of the skin
- redness or swelling of the skin
- rash, with or without blisters that ooze and become crusted
- pain in hairy parts of body
- pus in hair follicles

Interactions

Anyone who is using a prescription or nonprescription (over-the-counter) drug that is applied to the skin should check with a physician before using a sunscreen.

Resources

BOOKS

Beers, Mark H., MD, and Robert Berkow, MD., editors. "Pigmentation Disorders." In *The Merck Manual of Diagnosis and Therapy*. Whitehouse Station, NJ: Merck Research Laboratories, 2004.

Beers, Mark H., MD, and Robert Berkow, MD., editors. "Reactions to Sunlight." In *The Merck Manual of Diagnosis and Therapy*. Whitehouse Station, NJ: Merck Research Laboratories, 2004.

PERIODICALS

Levy, Stanley B., MD. "Sunscreens and Photoprotection." *eMedicine* November 25, 2002. < http://www.emedicine.com/derm/topic510.htm >.

Mahe, E., E. Morelon, J. Fermanian, et al. "Renal-Transplant Recipients and Sun Protection." *Transplantation* 78 (September 15, 2004): 741–744.

Murphy, G. "Ultraviolet Light and Rosacea." *Cutis* 74, Supplement 3 (September 2004): 13–16, 32–34.

Tanaka, S., T. Sato, N. Akimoto, et al. "Prevention of UVB-Induced Photoinflammation and Photoaging by a Polymethoxy Flavonoid, Nobiletin, in Human Keratinocytes in Vivo and in Vitro." *Biochemical Pharmacology* 68 (August 1, 2004): 433–439.

ORGANIZATIONS

American Academy of Dermatology (AAD). P. O. Box 4014, Schaumburg, IL 60168-4014. (847) 330-0230. < http://www.aad.org >.

American Society of Plastic Surgeons (ASPS). 444 East Algonquin Road, Arlington Heights, IL 60005. (847) 228-9900. < htpp://www.plasticsurgery.org >.

National Institutes of Health. National Cancer Institute. 9000 Rockville Pike, Bethesda, MD 20982. Cancer Information Service: (800) 4-CANCER. < http://cancernet.nci.nih.gov >.

United States Food and Drug Administration (FDA). 5600 Fishers Lane, Rockville, MD 20857-0001. (888) INFO-FDA. < http://www.fda.gov >.

Nancy Ross-Flanigan
Rebecca J. Frey, PhD

Sunstroke *see* **Heat disorders**

Superficial phlebitis *see* **Thrombophlebitis**

Superior vena cava syndrome

Definition

The superior vena cava is the major vein in the chest that carries blood from the upper part of the body in to the heart. A restriction of the blood flow (occlusion) through this vein can cause superior vena cava syndrome (SVCS).

Description

Superior vena cava syndrome is a partial occlusion of the superior vena cava. This leads to a lower than normal blood flow through this major vein.

SVCS is also called superior mediastinal syndrome and/or superior vena cava obstruction.

Causes and symptoms

More than 95% of all cases of SVCS are associated with cancers involving the upper chest. The cancers most commonly associated with SVCS are advanced lung cancers, which account for nearly 80% of all cases of SVCS, and lymphoma. Cancers that have spread (metastasized) to the chest, such as metastatic **breast cancer** to the chest and metastatic **testicular cancer** to the chest have also been shown to cause SVCS.

Other causes of SVCS include: the formation of a blood clot in the superior vena cava, enlargement of the thyroid gland, **tuberculosis**, and **sarcoidosis**.

The symptoms of SVCS include:

- change in voice
- confusion
- cough
- enlargement of the veins in the upper body, particularly those in the arms
- headache
- light-headedness
- shortness of breath
- swelling of the arms
- swelling of the face
- trouble swallowing

Diagnosis

SVCS should be considered in any **cancer** patient with swelling of the face and arms. This diagnosis can be confirmed by x ray, computerized tomography (CT) scan, or medical resonance imaging (MRI) of the chest that reveals a partial occlusion of the superior vena cava.

Treatment

Treatment of SVCS depends on the underlying cancer that is causing it. This treatment may include radiation, **chemotherapy**, or a combination of both. In some cases, surgical procedures may be performed to open (dilate) the vessel. These procedures are generally performed by a trained radiologist or vascular surgeon.

Alternative treatment

Since treatment of SVCS is aimed at treating the underlying disorder that is causing SVCS, alternative treatments must also focus on treating these underlying causes. Alternative treatments for cancer include **acupuncture**, **aromatherapy**, herbal remedies, **hydrotherapy**, hypnosis, and massage, among many others.

Prognosis

The prognosis depends on the underlying cause of SVCS. In cases of SVCS caused by lung cancers, the prognosis is generally rather poor since SVCS does not generally occur until the later stages of these diseases.

Prevention

SVCS may be prevented by early medical intervention to halt and/or reverse the cancer which, in a later stage, would have lead to SVCS.

Resources

PERIODICALS

Haapoja, I.S., and C. Blendowski. "Superior Vena Cava Syndrome." *Seminars in Oncology Nursing* 15 (August 1999): 183-9.

Hemann, Rhonda. "Superior Vena Cava Syndrome." *Clinical Excellence for Nurse Practitioners* 5 (March 2001): 85-7.

ORGANIZATIONS

Alliance for Lung Cancer Advocacy, Support and Education. P.O. Box 849 Vancouver, WA 98666. (800) 298-2436. < http://www.alcase.org/ > .

OTHER

Beeson, Michael S. *eMedicine - Superior Vena Cava Syndrome*. May 12, 2001. < http://www.emedicine.com/emerg/topic561.htm >.

Paul A. Johnson, Ed.M.

Supportive cancer therapy *see* **Cancer therapy, supportive**

Surfactant

Definition

Surfactant is a complex naturally occurring substance made of six lipids (fats) and four proteins that is produced in the lungs. It can also be manufactured synthetically.

Purpose

Surfactant reduces the surface tension of fluid in the lungs and helps make the small air sacs in the lungs (alveoli) more stable. This keeps them from collapsing when an individual exhales. In preparation for breathing air, fetuses begin making surfactant while still in the womb. Babies that are born very prematurely often lack adequate surfactant and must receive surfactant replacement therapy immediately after birth in order to breathe.

Precautions

Babies are considered premature if they are born before 37 weeks gestation. Fetuses begin to produce surfactant between weeks 24 and 28. By about 35 weeks, most babies have enough naturally produced surfactant to keep the alveoli from collapsing. Babies born before 35 weeks, especially those born very prematurely (before 30 weeks), are likely to need surfactant replacement therapy. Over half the babies born before 28 weeks gestation need this treatment, while about one-third born between 32 and 36 weeks need supplemental surfactant. Some very premature infants may also need to be placed on a mechanical ventilator.

Description

The lungs consist of spongy tissue filled with air spaces called alveoli. In the alveoli, oxygen is taken up by the blood and carbon dioxide, a waste product of cellular metabolism, is released and exhaled. For efficient oxygen-carbon dioxide exchange to occur, the surface area of the alveoli must be as large as possible. Under normal conditions, when a person exhales, the alveoli would collapse into each other and form larger air sacs with less surface area. Surfactant prevents this collapse by reducing the surface tension of the fluids that line the lungs and helping to equalize the pressures between large and small air spaces.

Surface tension is a measure of the attraction molecules of a fluid have for each other. The attractive force pulls fluids into a shape with the smallest surface area. This is why a drop of water on a flat surface is rounded rather than flat. If the surface tension is lowered, the attraction among molecules of the fluid is decreased and the surface area of the fluid increases. For example, if a drop of detergent is added to a drop of water, the detergent reduces the surface tension and the drop of water flattens out.

In the lungs, surfactant reduces the surface tension and helps to maximize the surface area available for gas exchange. Without adequate surfactant, a baby works much harder to breathe, becomes exhausted, and does not get enough oxygen. Babies that do not have enough surfactant to breathe normally at birth are said to have infant **respiratory distress syndrome (RDS)** or hyaline membrane disease (HMD).

Babies with RDS are given replacement surfactant as soon as possible within the first six hours after birth. Manufactured surfactant is a white powder that is mixed with sterile water. It is given through a breathing tube (endotracheal tube) that is inserted in the baby's lungs. Multiple doses are usually required.

Surfactant replacement therapy continues until the baby's lungs have matured enough to make surfactant on their own. Some very premature babies are also put on mechanical respirators to help them breathe. Surfactant replacement therapy has reduced deaths due to respiratory distress by 50% since the early 1990s. This therapy is expensive, but it is normally covered by insurance.

Preparation

The administration of surfactant is often a neonatal emergency. The only way to prevent the need for surfactant replacement therapy is to prevent a premature birth. Mothers who are at known high risk to deliver prematurely are given drugs called **corticosteroids** toward the end of the **pregnancy** that stimulate the lungs of the fetus to mature and begin producing surfactant sooner. This helps reduce the need for

KEY TERMS

Alveolus (plural alveoli)—The terminal air sacs of the lungs where gas exchange occurs.

Hyaline membrane—A thin layer of cells that line the lung.

Surface tension—The attraction of molecules in a fluid for each other.

surfactant replacement therapy. Although babies of all races may be born prematurely, **prematurity** is more common if the mother is diabetic, is carrying multiple fetuses, or has delivered a previous premature baby. The decision to use surfactant replacement therapy is based on the condition of the baby, its blood oxygen level, and degree of respiratory distress.

Aftercare

Babies receiving surfactant therapy are normally cared for by a neonatologist, a pediatrician that specializes in newborn care. Premature newborns often have other health problems in addition to RDS. Aftercare varies depending on their other health risks.

Risks

Delivery of surfactant requires inserting a breathing tube into the baby's lungs. Complications of this therapy include air leaking into the area between the chest wall and the lungs and air leaking into the sac around the heart. Some infants also develop chronic lung disease.

Normal results

Normally surfactant replacement therapy keeps the infant alive until the lungs start producing their own surfactant.

Abnormal results

Surfactant replacement therapy is very effective if begun within six hours after birth. When it fails, **death** may result.

Resources

OTHER

Doctors Lounge, The. "Chronically Ventilated Premature Infants Need Continued Surfactant," 15 November 2004 [cited 16 February 2005]. < http://www.thedoctorslounge.net/pedlounge/articles/surfactant >.

Hyaline Membrane Disease/Respiratory Distress Syndrome. Lucile Packard Children's Hospital at Stanford. 2001-2005 [cited 16 February 2005]. < http://www.lpch.org/DiseaseHealthInfo/HealthLibrary/hrnewborn/hmd.html >.

Pramanik, Arun. *Respiratory Distress Syndrome,* 2 July 2002 [cited 16 February 2005]. < http://www.emedicine.com/ped/topic1993.htm >.

Surfactant. Johns Hopkins School of Medicine. 1995 [cited 16 February 2005]. < http://oac.med.jhmi.edu/res_phys/Encyclopedia/Surfactant/Surfactant.HTMLgt;

Tish Davidson, A.M.

Surgical debridement *see* **Debridement**

Swallowing disorders

Definition

Swallowing disorders include a number of diseases and conditions that cause difficulty in passing food or liquid from the mouth to the stomach.

Description

Although normally swallowing is automatic, it is a complex process involving several phases and 29 muscles. Saliva helps soften food as it is chewed. The tongue helps move food to the back of the mouth, triggering a swallowing reflex that passes food through the pharynx. The epiglottis helps keep food from mistakenly going down the windpipe and into the esophagus, the canal that carries food to the stomach. Swallowing disorders can occur at any phase in the swallowing process. The medical term for difficult swallowing is dysphagia.

Each year, about 10 million people in the United States require medical evaluation for swallowing problems. Some experts say that about 10% of Americans develop symptoms of swallowing disorders in adulthood. Elderly people are the most likely to have problems with swallowing.

Causes and symptoms

Swallowing disorders often result from other conditions and diseases. For example, Parkinson's disease, **cerebral palsy**, **stroke**, **head injury**, and other central nervous system conditions can damage the muscles and nerves involved in swallowing. Some people are born with abnormalities in the swallowing structures, such as infants with **cleft palate**.

Some cancers can lead to swallowing disorders. **Esophageal cancer** can cause narrowing and eventual blockage of the esophagus. Surgery and **radiation therapy** for **head and neck cancer** can restrict or weaken tongue motion, paralyze vocal cords, or cause muscle damage that affects swallowing. An inflamed esophagus, often resulting from gastroesophageal reflux disease (GERD), can cause painful or difficult swallowing. Infections of the esophagus also can inflame it and cause it to narrow. Swallowing difficulty may result from **aging**, though researchers are not certain why.

The most common symptoms people report are **choking** and the feeling that food feels stuck in the throat. Other symptoms include needing to swallow many times to clear food from the mouth and throat, a gurgly, wet sound to the voice after swallowing, having to clear the throat after eating, coughing, **pain** while swallowing, bringing food back up (regurgitation), food or acid backing up into the throat, unexpected weight loss, and not being able to swallow at all. Children also may gag during meals and may have excessive drooling or leaking of food or liquid from their mouths during meals. They may have difficulty breathing when eating or drinking, spit up frequently and lag behind in weight gain. They also may have recurring **pneumonia** or respiratory infections.

Diagnosis

A physician should perform a full head and neck examination based on the patient's symptoms. Speech-language pathologists may aid in the diagnosis. Physicians also might order a swallowing test to study how the patient swallows. The patient will be asked to drink a liquid with a contrast agent called barium that will show up on x rays of the throat and upper chest. The exam might be imaged with a technique called video fluoroscopy, which will take motion camera images in addition to still images. For this exam, the patient may be asked to swallow liquid, paste, and solids. A speech pathologist may work with the radiologist to perform this exam.

If the physician thinks the problem originates in the lower esophagus or has concerns about an abnormality in the esophagus, an endoscopy may be ordered. This test involves passing a thin, flexible instrument called an endoscope down the throat. The lighted endoscope helps the physician view the esophagus. Other tests may be used, including ultrasound.

KEY TERMS

Cleft palate—An opening or hole in the roof of the mouth that occurs at birth when the roof fails to fully develop in the infant.

Epiglottis—A thin layer of cartilage behind the tongue that helps block food from entering the windpipe.

Pharynx—The muscular cavity that leads from the mouth and nasal passages to the larynx and esophagus.

Treatment

Treatment will depend on the cause of the swallowing problem. Special exercises may help strengthen the muscles used for chewing and swallowing. Problems originating in the mouth may be treated with artificial saliva, improved hydration or better dental care. Esophageal problems will be treated depending on the cause. Patients with GERD will receive medications and instructions on how to better manage the disease. Esophageal **cancer** is a life-threatening disease that will involve coordinating care with an oncologist. Many patients will receive help with their disorders from speech pathologists. Special liquid **diets** may be ordered for patients who continue to have trouble chewing or swallowing. In severe cases, the patient may need a feeding tube that bypasses the part of the swallowing system that does not work.

Alternative treatment

Some herbs that may help improve swallowing include oil of peppermint and licorice. Valerian may be used as a tea. Homeopathic physicians may suggest some remedies aimed at improving bloating, **indigestion**, or **cough**. Alternative care should be sought from licensed practitioners and coordinated with physician care.

Prognosis

In many cases, these disorders can be corrected. If not treated, swallowing disorders can lead to serious complications, including **dehydration** and **malnutrition**. There also is a risk of food entering the airway (aspiration) as a person attempts to swallow, which can lead to aspiration pneumonia as the food particles enter the lungs.

Prevention

Many causes of swallowing disorders cannot be prevented. Slowly and fully chewing food helps. People with GERD should manage it to lower the risk of developing swallowing difficulties.

Resources

PERIODICALS

"Disorders of Swallowing." *Harvard Men's Health Watch* (Sept. 2003).

"The Evaluation and Management of Swallowing Disorders in the Elderly." *Geriatric Times* (Nov. 1, 2003): 17.

ORGANIZATIONS

American Academy of Otolaryngology-Head and Neck Surgery. One Prince St., Alexandria, VA 22314-3357. 703-836-4444. http://www.entnet.org.

American Speech-Language Association (ASHA). 10801 Rockville Pike, Rockville, MD 20852. 800-638-8255. http://www.asha.org.

National Institute of Dental and Craniofacial Research (NIDCR). 45 Center Dr., Rm 4AS19 MSC 6400, Bethesda, MD 20892-6400. 301-496-4261. http://www.nidr.nih.gov.

OTHER

Dysphagia. Web page. National Institute on Deafness and Other Communication Disorders, 2005. http://www.nidcd.nih.gov/health/voice/dysph.asp.

NINDS Swallowing Disorders Information Page. Web page. National Institute of Neurological Disorders and Stroke, 2005. http://www.ninds.nih.gov/disorders/swallowing_disorders/swallowing_disorders.htm.

Teresa G. Odle

Swan-Ganz catheterization *see* **Pulmonary artery catheterization**

Sweating, excessive *see* **Hyperhidrosis**

Swimmer's ear *see* **Otitis externa**

Swimming pool conjunctivitis *see* **Inclusion conjunctivitis**

Swollen glands *see* **Lymphadenitis**

Sydenham's chorea

Definition

Sydenham's chorea is an acute but self-limited movement disorder that occurs most commonly in children between the ages of 5 and 15, and occasionally in pregnant women. It is closely associated with **rheumatic fever** following a throat infection. The disorder is named for Thomas Sydenham (1624–1689), an English doctor who first described it in 1686. Other names for Sydenham's chorea include simple chorea, chorea minor, acute chorea, rheumatic chorea, juvenile chorea, and St. Vitus' dance. The English word "chorea" itself comes from the Greek word *choreia*, which means "dance." The disorder takes its name from the rapid involuntary jerking or twitching movements of the patient's face, limbs, and upper body.

Description

Sydenham's chorea is a disorder that occurs in children and is associated with rheumatic **fever**. Rheumatic fever is an acute infectious disease caused by certain types of streptococci bacteria. It usually starts with **strep throat** or **tonsillitis**. These types of streptococci are able to cause disease throughout the body. The most serious damage caused by rheumatic fever is to the valves in the heart. At one time, rheumatic fever was the most common cause of damaged heart valves, and it still is in most developing countries around the world. Rheumatic fever and rheumatic heart disease are still present in the industrialized countries, but the incidence has dropped substantially.

Both acute rheumatic fever and Sydenham's chorea are relatively uncommon disorders in the United States as of 2004. According to the Centers for Disease Control and Prevention (CDC), only 1%–3% of people with streptococcal throat infections develop acute rheumatic fever (ARF); thus the incidence of ARF in the United States is thought to be about 0.5 per 100,000 patients between 5 and 17 years of age.

With regard to age, the incidence of Sydenham's chorea is higher in childhood and adolescence than in adult life. It occurs more frequently in females than in males; the gender ratio is thought to be about 2 F: 1 M. Since the peak incidence of rheumatic fever in North America occurs in late winter and spring, Sydenham's chorea is more likely to occur in the summer and early fall. There is no evidence as of 2004 that the disorder selectively affects specific racial or ethnic groups.

Rheumatic fever may appear in several different forms. Sydenham's chorea is one of five major criteria for the diagnosis of rheumatic fever. There are also four minor criteria and two types of laboratory tests associated with the disease. The "Jones criteria" define the diagnosis. They require laboratory evidence of a streptococcal infection plus two or more of the criteria. The laboratory evidence may be identification of streptococci from a **sore throat** or antibodies to streptococcus in the blood. The most common criteria are arthritis and heart disease, occurring in half to three-quarters of the patients. Sydenham's chorea, characteristic nodules under the skin, and a specific type of skin rash occur only 10% of the time.

About 20% of patients diagnosed with Sydenham's chorea experience a recurrence of the disorder, usually within two years of the first episode. Most women who develop Sydenham's during **pregnancy** have a history of acute rheumatic fever in childhood or of using birth control pills containing estrogen.

Causes and symptoms

Sydenham's is caused by certain types of streptococci called Group A beta-hemolytic streptococci or GAS bacteria. In general, streptococci are spherical-shaped anaerobic bacteria that occur in pairs or chains. GAS bacteria belong to a subcategory known as pyogenic streptococci, which means that the infections they cause produce pus. These particular germs seem to be able to create an immune response that attacks the body's own tissues along with the germs. Those tissues are joints, heart valves, skin, and brain.

The initial throat infection that leads to Sydenham's chorea is typically followed by a symptom-free period of 1–5 weeks. The patient then develops an acute case of rheumatic fever (ARF), an inflammatory disease that affects multiple organ systems and tissues of the body. In most patients, ARF is characterized by fever, arthritis in one or more joints, and carditis, or inflammation of the heart. In about 20% of patients, however, Sydenham's chorea is the only indication of ARF. Sydenham's is considered a delayed complication of rheumatic fever; it may begin as late as 12 months after the initial sore throat, and it may start only after the patient's temperature and other physical signs have returned to normal. The average time interval between the pharyngitis and the first symptoms of Sydenham's, however, is eight or nine weeks.

It is difficult to describe a "typical" case of Sydenham's chorea because the symptoms vary in speed of onset as well as severity. Most patients have an acute onset of the disorder, but in others, the onset is insidious, which means that the symptoms develop slowly and gradually. In some cases, the child's physical symptoms are present for four to five weeks before they become severe enough for the parents to consult a doctor. In other cases, emotional or psychiatric symptoms precede the clumsiness and involuntary muscular movements that characterize the disorder. The psychiatric symptoms that may develop in patients with Sydenham's chorea are one reason why it is sometimes categorized as a PANDAS disorder. PANDAS stands for Pediatric Autoimmune Neuropsychiatric Disorders Associated with **Streptococcal Infections**.

Behavioral or emotional disturbances that have been observed with Sydenham's include:

- frequent mood changes
- episodes of uncontrollable crying
- behavioral regression; that is, acting like much younger children
- mental confusion
- general irritability
- difficulty concentrating
- impulsive behavior

Some researchers think that children who have had Sydenham's are at increased risk of developing **obsessive-compulsive disorder** (OCD). OCD is characterized by obsessions, which are unwanted recurrent thoughts, images, or impulses, and by compulsions, which are repetitive rituals, mental acts, or behaviors. Obsessions in children often take the form of fears of intruders or harm coming to a family member. Compulsions may include such acts as counting silently, washing the hands over and over, insisting on keeping items in a specific order, checking repeatedly to make sure a door is locked, and similar behaviors.

Diagnosis

Because rheumatic fever is such a damaging disease, a complete evaluation should be done whenever it is suspected. This includes cultures for streptococci, blood tests, and usually an electrocardiogram (heartbeat mapping to detect abnormalities).

The diagnosis of Sydenham's is also based on the doctor's observation of the patient's involuntary movements. Unlike tics, the movements associated with chorea are not repetitive; and unlike the behavior of hyperactive children, the movements are not intentional. The recent onset of the movements rules out a diagnosis of **cerebral palsy**. If the doctor suspects Sydenham's, he or she may ask the patient to stick out the tongue and keep it in that position, or to squeeze the doctor's hand. Many patients with Sydenham's cannot hold their mouth open and keep the tongue out for more than a second or two. Another characteristic of Sydenham's is an inability to grip with a steady pressure; when the patient squeezes the doctor's hand, the strength of the grip will increase and decrease in an erratic fashion. This characteristic is sometimes called the "milking sign."

Treatment

Suspected streptococcal infections must be treated. All the other manifestations of rheumatic fever, including Sydenham's chorea and excluding heart valve damage, remit with the acute disease and do not require treatment. Sydenham's chorea generally lasts for several months.

Most patients with Sydenham's chorea recover after a period of bed rest and temporary limitation of normal activities. In most cases the symptoms disappear gradually rather than stopping abruptly.

Most doctors recommend ongoing treatment with penicillin to prevent a recurrence of rheumatic fever or Sydenham's chorea, although there is some disagreement as to whether this treatment should continue for 5 years after an acute attack or for the rest of the patient's life. The penicillin may be given orally or by injection. Patients who cannot take penicillin may be given erythromycin or sulfadiazine.

Prognosis

Syndenham's chorea usually clears up without complications when the rheumatic fever is treated. The heart valve damage associated with rheumatic fever may lead to heart trouble and require a surgical valve repair or replacement.

In most cases of Sydenham's, the patient recovers completely, although a recurrence is possible. In a very few cases—about 1.5% of patients diagnosed with Sydenham's— there may be increasing muscle stiffness and loss of muscle tone resulting in disability. This condition is occasionally referred to as paralytic chorea

Prevention

All cases of strep throat in children should be treated with a full 10 days of **antibiotics** (penicillin or erythromycin). Treatment may best be delayed a day or two to allow the body to build up its own antibodies. In addition, for those who have had an episode of rheumatic fever or have damaged heart valves from any other cause, prophylactic antibiotics should be continued to prevent recurrence.

KEY TERMS

Arthralgia—Joint pain.

Chorea—A term that is used to refer to rapid, jerky, involuntary movements of the limbs or face that characterize several different disorders of the nervous system, including chorea of pregnancy and Huntington's chorea as well as Sydenham's chorea.

Electrocardiogram—Mapping the electrical activity of the heart.

Insidious—Developing in a stealthy or gradual manner. Sydenham's chorea may have an insidious onset.

PANDAS disorders—A group of childhood disorders associated with such streptococcal infections as scarlet fever and "strep throat." The acronym stands for Pediatric Autoimmune Neuropsychiatric Disorders Associated with Streptococcal Infections. Sydenham's chorea is considered a PANDAS disorder.

Pharyngitis—Inflammation of the throat, accompanied by dryness and pain. Pharyngitis caused by a streptococcal infection is the usual trigger of Sydenham's chorea.

Rheumatic fever—Chiefly childhood disease marked by fever, inflammation, joint pain, and Syndenham's chorea. It is often recurrent and can lead to heart valve damage.

St. Vitus' dance—Another name for Sydenham's chorea. St. Vitus was a fourth-century martyr who became the patron saint of dancers and actors during the Middle Ages. He was also invoked for protection against nervous disorders, epilepsy, and the disease that bears his name.

Streptococcus (plural, streptococci)—A genus of spherical-shaped anaerobic bacteria occurring in pairs or chains. Sydenham's chorea is considered a complication of a streptococcal throat infection.

Tonsillitis—Inflammation of the tonsils, which are in the back of the throat.

It is possible to eradicate dangerous GAS bacteria from a community by culturing everyone's throat and treating everyone who tests positive. This is worth doing wherever a case of rheumatic fever appears, but it is expensive and requires many resources.

Resources

BOOKS

Beers, Mark H., MD, and Robert Berkow, MD., editors. "Sydenham's Chorea (Chorea Minor; Rheumatic Fever; St. Vitus' Dance)." In *The Merck Manual of Diagnosis and Therapy.* Whitehouse Station, NJ: Merck Research Laboratories, 2004.

PERIODICALS

Bhidayasiri, R., and D. D. Truong. "Chorea and Related Disorders." *Postgraduate Medical Journal* 80 (September 2004): 527–534.

Bonthius, D. J., and B. Karacay. "Sydenham's Chorea: Not Gone and Not Forgotten." *Seminars in Pediatric Neurology* 10 (March 2003): 11–19.

Dale, R. C., I. Heyman, R. A. Surtees, et al. "Dyskinesias and Associated Psychiatric Disorders following Streptococcal Infections." *Archives of Disease in Childhood* 89 (July 2004): 604–610.

Herrera, Maria Alejandra, MD, and Nestor Galvez-Jiminez, MD. "Chorea in Adults." *eMedicine* February 1, 2002. < http://www.emedicine.com/neuro/topic62.htm >.

Kim, S. W., J. E. Grant, S. I. Kim, et al. "A Possible Association of Recurrent Streptococcal Infections and Acute Onset of Obsessive-Compulsive Disorder." *Journal of Neuropsychiatry and Clinical Neurosciences* 16 (Summer 2004): 252–260.

Korn-Lubetzki, I., A. Brand, and I. Steiner. "Recurrence of Sydenham Chorea: Implications for Pathogenesis." *Archives of Neurology* 61 (August 2004): 1261–1264.

Snider, L. A., and S. E. Swedo. "Post-Streptococcal Autoimmune Disorders of the Central Nervous System." *Current Opinion in Neurology* 16 (June 2003): 359–365.

ORGANIZATIONS

American Academy of Child and Adolescent Psychiatry (AACAP). 3615 Wisconsin Avenue, NW, Washington, DC 20016-3007. (202) 966-7300. Fax: (202) 966-2891. < http://www.aacap.org >.

American Academy of Family Physicians (AAFP). 11400 Tomahawk Creek Parkway, Leawood, KS 66211-2672. (800) 274-2237 or (913) 906-6000. *lt;http://www.aafp.org >.

National Institute of Neurological Disorders and Stroke (NINDS). NIH Neurological Institute, P. O. Box 5801, Bethesda, MD 20824. (800) 352-9424 or (301) 496-5751. < http://www.ninds.nih.gov >.

OTHER

American Academy of Child and Adolescent Psychiatry (AACAP). AACAP Facts for Families, No. 60. *Obsessive-Compulsive Disorder in Children and Adolescents.* < http://www.aacap.org/publications/factsfam/ocd.htm >.

National Institute of Neurological Disorders and Stroke (NINDS). *NINDS Sydenham Chorea Information Page.* < http://www.ninds.nih.gov/health_and_medical/disorders/sydenham.htm >.

J. Ricker Polsdorfer, MD
Rebecca J. Frey, PhD

Sympathectomy

Definition

Sympathectomy is a surgical procedure that destroys nerves in the sympathetic nervous system. The procedure is done to increase blood flow and decrease long-term **pain** in certain diseases that cause narrowed blood vessels. It can also be used to decrease excessive sweating. This surgical procedure cuts or destroys the sympathetic ganglia, collections of nerve cell bodies in clusters along the thoracic or lumbar spinal cord.

Purpose

The autonomic nervous system that controls unwilled (involuntary) body functions, such as breathing, sweating, and blood pressure, are divided into the sympathetic and the parasympathetic nervous systems. The sympathetic nervous system speeds the heart rate, narrows (constricts) blood vessels, and raises blood pressure. Blood pressure is controlled by means of nerve cells that run through sheaths around the arteries. The sympathetic nervous system can be described as the "fight or flight" system because it allows us to respond to danger by fighting off an attacker or by running away. When danger threatens, the sympathetic nervous system increases heart and respiratory rate, increases blood flow to muscles, and decreases blood flow to other areas, such as skin, digestive tract, and limb veins. The net effect is an increase in blood pressure.

Sympathectomy is performed to relieve intermittent constricting of blood vessels (**ischemia**) when the fingers, toes, ears, or nose are exposed to cold (Raynaud's phenomenon). In Raynaud's phenomenon, the affected extremities turn white, then blue, and red as the blood supply is cut off. The color changes are accompanied by **numbness**, **tingling**, burning, and pain. Normal color and feeling are restored when heat is applied. The condition sometimes occurs without direct cause but it is more often caused by an underlying medical condition, such as **rheumatoid arthritis**. Sympathectomy is usually less effective when Raynaud's is caused by an underlying medical condition. Narrowed blood vessels in the legs that cause painful cramping (claudication) are also treated with sympathectomy.

Sympathectomy may be helpful in treating **reflex sympathetic dystrophy** (RSD), a condition that sometimes develops after injury. In RSD, the affected limb is painful (causalgia) and swollen. The color, temperature, and texture of the skin change. These symptoms are related to prolonged and excessive activity of the sympathetic nervous system.

Because sweating is controlled by the sympathetic nervous system, sympathectomy is also effective in treating excessive sweating (**hyperhidrosis**) of the palms, armpits, or face.

Precautions

To determine whether sympathectomy is needed, a reversible block of the affected nerve cell (**ganglion**) should be done. A reversible ganglion block interrupts nerve impulses by means of steroid and anesthetic injected into it. If the block has a positive effect on pain and blood flow in the affected area, the sympathectomy will probably be helpful. The surgical procedure should be performed only if conservative treatment has not worked. Conservative treatment includes avoiding exposure to **stress** and cold, physical therapy, and medications.

Sympathectomy is most likely to be effective in relieving the pain of reflex sympathetic dystrophy if it is done soon after the injury occurs. However, increased benefit from early surgery should be balanced against time needed to promote spontaneous recovery and response to conservative treatment.

Description

Sympathectomy was traditionally done as an inpatient surgical procedure under **general anesthesia**. An incision was made on the mid-back, exposing the ganglia to be cut. Recent techniques are less invasive and may be done under **local anesthesia** and as outpatient surgery. If only one arm or leg is affected, it may be treated with a percutaneous radiofrequency technique. In this technique, the surgeon locates the ganglia by a combination of x ray and electrical stimulation. The ganglia are destroyed by applying radio waves through electrodes on the skin.

Sympathectomy for hyperhidrosis can be done by making a small incision under the armpit and introducing air into the chest cavity. The surgeon inserts a fiber optic tube (endoscope) that projects an image of the operation on a video screen. The ganglia can then be cut with fine scissors attached to the endoscope. Laser beams can also be used to destroy the ganglia.

Preparation

As with any surgery, patients should discuss expected results and possible risks with their surgeons. They should tell their surgeons all medications they are taking and all their medical problems, and they should be in good general health. To improve general health, the patient may be asked to lose weight, give up **smoking** or alcohol, and get the proper sleep, diet, and **exercise**. Immediately before the surgery, patients will not be permitted to eat or drink, and the surgical site will be cleaned and scrubbed.

Aftercare

The surgeon will inform the patient about specific aftercare needed for the technique used. **Doppler ultrasonography**, a test using sound waves to measure blood flow, can help to determine whether sympathectomy has had a positive result.

Risks

Side effects of sympathectomy may include decreased blood pressure while standing, which may cause **fainting** spells. After sympathectomy in men, semen is sometimes ejaculated into the bladder, which may impair fertility. After a sympathectomy done by inserting an endoscope in the chest cavity, patients may experience chest pain with deep breathing. This problem usually disappears within two weeks. They may also experience **pneumothorax** (air in the chest cavity).

In 30% of cases, surgery for hyperhidrosis may cause increased sweating on the chest. In 2% of cases, this surgery causes increased sweating in other areas, including increased facial sweating while eating. Other complications occur less frequently. These complications include Horner's syndrome, a condition of the nervous system that causes the pupil of the eye to close, the eyelid to droop, and sweating to decrease on one side of the face. Other rare complications are nasal blockage and pain of the nerves supplying the skin between the ribs.

Normal results

Some studies report that sympathectomy relieves causalgia in as many as 75% of cases. The studies also show that it relieves hyperhidrosis in more than 90%

KEY TERMS

Causalgia—A severe burning sensation sometimes accompanied by redness and inflammation of the skin. Causalgia is caused by injury to a nerve outside the spinal cord.

Claudication—Cramping or pain in a leg caused by poor blood circulation. This condition is frequently caused by hardening of the arteries (atherosclerosis). Intermittent claudication occurs only at certain times, usually after exercise, and is relieved by rest.

Fiberoptics—In medicine, fiberoptics uses glass or plastic fibers to transmit light through a specially designed tube. The tube is inserted into organs or body cavities where it transmits a magnified image of the internal body structures.

Hyperhidrosis—Excessive sweating. Hyperhidrosis can be caused by heat, overactive thyroid glands, strong emotion, menopause, or infection.

Parasympathetic nervous system—The division of the autonomic (involuntary or unwilled) nervous system that slows heart rate, increases digestive and gland activity, and relaxes the sphincter muscles that close off body organs.

Percutaneous—Performed through the skin, from the Latin *per*, meaning through and *cutis*, meaning skin.

Pneumothorax—A collection of air or gas in the chest cavity that causes a lung to collapse. Pneumothorax may be caused by an open chest wound that admits air.

of cases. The less invasive procedures cause very little scarring. Most patients stay in the hospital for less than one day and return to work within the week.

Resources

OTHER

The American Institute for Hyperhidrosis Page. < http://www.handsweat.com >.

Laurie Barclay, MD

Syncope *see* **Fainting**

Syndactyly *see* **Polydactyly and syndactyly**

Synergistic gangrene *see* **Flesh-eating disease**

Synovial fluid analysis *see* **Joint fluid analysis**

Synovial membrane biopsy *see* **Joint biopsy**

Syphilis

Definition

Syphilis is an infectious systemic disease that may be either congenital or acquired through sexual contact or contaminated needles.

Description

Syphilis has both acute and chronic forms that produce a wide variety of symptoms affecting most of the body's organ systems. The range of symptoms makes it easy to confuse syphilis with less serious diseases and ignore its early signs. Acquired syphilis has four stages (primary, secondary, latent, and tertiary) and can be spread by sexual contact during the first three of these four stages.

Syphilis, which is also called lues (from a Latin word meaning **plague**), has been a major public health problem since the sixteenth century. The disease was treated with mercury or other ineffective remedies until World War I, when effective treatments based on arsenic or bismuth were introduced. These were succeeded by **antibiotics** after World War II. At that time, the number of cases in the general population decreased, partly because of aggressive public health measures. This temporary decrease, combined with the greater amount of attention given to **AIDS** in recent years, leads some people to think that syphilis is no longer a serious problem. In actual fact, the number of cases of syphilis in the United States has risen since 1980. This increase affects both sexes, all races, all parts of the nation, and all age groups, including adults over 60. The number of women of childbearing age with syphilis is the highest that has been recorded since the 1940s. About 25,000 cases of infectious syphilis in adults are reported annually in the United States. It is estimated, however, that 400,000 people in the United States need treatment for syphilis every year, and that the annual worldwide total is 50 million persons.

In 1999, the Centers for Disease Control and Prevention (CDC) joined several other federal agencies in announcing the "National Plan to Eliminate Syphilis in the United States." Eliminating the disease was defined as the absence of transmission of the disease; that is, no transmission after 90 days following the report of an imported index case. The national goals for eliminating syphilis include bringing the annual number of reported cases in the United States below 1000, and increasing the number of syphilis-free counties to 90% by 2005. In November 2002, the CDC released figures for 2000–2001, which indicate that the number of reported cases of primary and secondary syphilis rose slightly. This rise, however, occurred only among men who have sex with other men. The CDC also stated that the number of new cases of syphilis has actually declined among women as well as among non-Hispanic blacks.

The increased incidence of syphilis since the 1970s is associated with drug **abuse** as well as changes in sexual behavior. The connections between drug abuse and syphilis include needle sharing and exchanging sex for drugs. In addition, people using drugs are more likely to engage in risky sexual practices. As of 2002, the risk of contracting syphilis is particularly high among those who abuse crack **cocaine**.

With respect to changing patterns of conduct, a sharp increase in the number of people having sex with multiple partners makes it more difficult for public health doctors to trace the contacts of infected persons. Women are not necessarily protected by having sex only with other women; in the past few years, several cases have been reported of female-to-female transmission of syphilis through oral-genital contact. In addition, the incidence of syphilis among men who have sex with other men continues to rise. Several studies in Latin America as well as in the United States reported in late 2002 that unprotected sexual intercourse is on the increase among gay and bisexual men.

Changing patterns of sexual behavior have led to a striking increase in the number of cases of syphilis in eastern Europe since the collapse of the Soviet Union; Slovenia reported an 18-fold increase in reported cases of syphilis just between 1993 and 1994. Over half of the new cases were linked to a source of infection in another European country.

In general, high-risk groups for syphilis in the United States and Canada include:

- sexually active teenagers
- people infected with another sexually transmitted disease (STD), including AIDS
- sexually abused children
- women of childbearing age
- prostitutes of either sex and their customers
- prisoners
- persons who abuse drugs or alcohol

The chances of contracting syphilis from an infected person in the early stages of the disease during unprotected sex are between 30–50%.

Causes and symptoms

Syphilis is caused by a spirochete, *Treponema pallidum*. A spirochete is a thin spiral- or coil-shaped bacterium that enters the body through the mucous membranes or breaks in the skin. In 90% of cases, the spirochete is transmitted by sexual contact. Transmission by blood **transfusion** is possible but rare; not only because blood products are screened for the disease, but also because the spirochetes die within 24 hours in stored blood. Other methods of transmission are highly unlikely because *T. pallidum* is easily killed by heat and drying.

Primary syphilis

Primary syphilis is the stage of the organism's entry into the body. The first signs of infection are not always noticed. After an incubation period ranging between 10 and 90 days, the patient develops a chancre, which is a small blister-like sore about 0.5 in (13 mm) in size. Most chancres are on the genitals, but may also develop in or on the mouth or on the breasts. Rectal chancres are common in male homosexuals. Chancres in women are sometimes overlooked if they develop in the vagina or on the cervix. The chancres are not painful and disappear in three to six weeks even without treatment. They resemble the ulcers of **lymphogranuloma venereum**, herpes simplex virus, or skin tumors.

About 70% of patients with primary syphilis also develop swollen lymph nodes near the chancre. The nodes may have a firm or rubbery feel when the doctor touches them but are not usually painful.

Secondary syphilis

Syphilis enters its secondary stage between six to eight weeks and six months after the infection begins. Chancres may still be present but are usually healing. Secondary syphilis is a systemic infection marked by the eruption of skin **rashes** and ulcers in the mucous membranes. The skin rash may mimic a number of other skin disorders such as drug reactions, **rubella**, **ringworm**, mononucleosis, and **pityriasis rosea**. Characteristics that point to syphilis include:

- a coppery color
- absence of **pain** or **itching**
- occurrence on the palms of hands and soles of feet

The skin eruption may resolve in a few weeks or last as long as a year. The patient may also develop condylomata lata, which are weepy pinkish or grey areas of flattened skin in the moist areas of the body.

The skin rashes, mouth and genital ulcers, and condylomata lata are all highly infectious.

About 50% of patients with secondary syphilis develop swollen lymph nodes in the armpits, groin, and neck areas; about 10% develop inflammations of the eyes, kidney, liver, spleen, bones, joints, or the meninges (membranes covering the brain and spinal cord). They may also have a flulike general illness with a low **fever**, chills, loss of appetite, headaches, runny nose, **sore throat**, and aching joints.

Latent syphilis

Latent syphilis is a phase of the disease characterized by relative absence of external symptoms. The term latent does not mean that the disease is not progressing or that the patient cannot infect others. For example, pregnant women can transmit syphilis to their unborn children during the latency period.

The latent phase is sometimes divided into early latency (less than two years after infection) and late latency. During early latency, patients are at risk for spontaneous relapses marked by recurrence of the ulcers and skin rashes of secondary syphilis. In late latency, these recurrences are much less likely. Late latency may either resolve spontaneously or continue for the rest of the patient's life.

Tertiary syphilis

Untreated syphilis progresses to a third or tertiary stage in about 35–40% of patients. Patients with tertiary syphilis cannot infect others with the disease. It is thought that the symptoms of this stage are a delayed hypersensitivity reaction to the spirochetes. Some patients develop so-called benign late syphilis, which begins between three and 10 years after infection and is characterized by the development of gummas. Gummas are rubbery tumor-like growths that are most likely to involve the skin or long bones but may also develop in the eyes, mucous membranes, throat, liver, or stomach lining. Gummas are increasingly uncommon since the introduction of antibiotics for treating syphilis. Benign late syphilis is usually rapid in onset and responds well to treatment.

CARDIOVASCULAR SYPHILIS. Cardiovascular syphilis occurs in 10–15% of patients who have progressed to tertiary syphilis. It develops between 10 and 25 years after infection and often occurs together with neurosyphilis. Cardiovascular syphilis usually begins as an inflammation of the arteries leading from the heart and causes heart attacks, scarring of the aortic valves, congestive **heart failure**, or the formation of an **aortic aneurysm**.

NEUROSYPHILIS. About 8% of patients with untreated syphilis will develop symptoms in the central nervous system that include both physical and psychiatric symptoms. Neurosyphilis can appear at any time, from 5-35 years after the onset of primary syphilis. It affects men more frequently than women and Caucasians more frequently than African Americans.

Neurosyphilis is classified into four types:

- Asymptomatic. In this form of neurosyphilis, the patient's spinal fluid gives abnormal test results but there are no symptoms affecting the central nervous system.

- Meningovascular. This type of neurosyphilis is marked by changes in the blood vessels of the brain or inflammation of the meninges (the tissue layers covering the brain and spinal cord). The patient develops headaches, irritability, and visual problems. If the spinal cord is involved, the patient may experience weakness of the shoulder and upper arm muscles.

- Tabes dorsalis. Tabes dorsalis is a progressive degeneration of the spinal cord and nerve roots. Patients lose their sense of perception of one's body position and orientation in space (proprioception), resulting in difficulties walking and loss of muscle reflexes. They may also have shooting pains in the legs and periodic episodes of pain in the abdomen, throat, bladder, or rectum. Tabes dorsalis is sometimes called locomotor ataxia.

- General paresis. General paresis refers to the effects of neurosyphilis on the cortex of the brain. The patient has a slow but progressive loss of memory, ability to concentrate, and interest in self-care. Personality changes may include irresponsible behavior, depression, **delusions** of grandeur, or complete **psychosis**. General paresis is sometimes called **dementia** paralytica, and is most common in patients over 40.

Special populations

CONGENITAL SYPHILIS. Congenital syphilis has increased at a rate of 400–500% over the past decade, on the basis of criteria introduced by the Centers for Disease Control (CDC) in 1990. In 1994, over 2,200 cases of congenital syphilis were reported in the United States. The prognosis for early congenital syphilis is poor: about 54% of infected fetuses die before or shortly after birth. Those who survive may look normal at birth but show signs of infection between three and eight weeks later.

Infants with early congenital syphilis have systemic symptoms that resemble those of adults with secondary syphilis. There is a 40-60% chance that the child's central nervous system will be infected. These infants may have symptoms ranging from **jaundice**, enlargement of the spleen and liver, and anemia to skin rashes, condylomata lata, inflammation of the lungs, "snuffles" (a persistent runny nose), and swollen lymph nodes.

CHILDREN. Children who develop symptoms after the age of two years are said to have late congenital syphilis. The characteristic symptoms include facial deformities (saddle nose), Hutchinson's teeth (abnormal upper incisors), saber shins, dislocated joints, deafness, **mental retardation, paralysis,** and seizure disorders.

PREGNANT WOMEN. Syphilis can be transmitted from the mother to the fetus through the placenta at any time during **pregnancy**, or through the child's contact with syphilitic ulcers during the birth process. The chances of infection are related to the stage of the mother's disease. Almost all infants of mothers with untreated primary or secondary syphilis will be infected, whereas the infection rate drops to 40% if the mother is in the early latent stage and 6–14% if she has late latent syphilis.

Pregnancy does not affect the progression of syphilis in the mother; however, pregnant women should not be treated with **tetracyclines**.

HIV PATIENTS. Syphilis has been closely associated with HIV infection since the late 1980s. Syphilis sometimes mimics the symptoms of AIDS. Conversely, AIDS appears to increase the severity of syphilis in patients suffering from both diseases, and to speed up the development or appearance of neurosyphilis. Patients with HIV are also more likely to develop lues maligna, a skin disease that sometimes occurs in secondary syphilis. Lues maligna is characterized by areas of ulcerated and dying tissue. In addition, HIV patients have a higher rate of treatment failure with penicillin than patients without HIV.

Diagnosis

Patient history and physical diagnosis

The diagnosis of syphilis is often delayed because of the variety of early symptoms, the varying length of the incubation period, and the possibility of not noticing the initial chancre. Patients do not always connect their symptoms with recent sexual contact. They may go to a dermatologist when they develop the skin rash of secondary syphilis rather than to their primary care

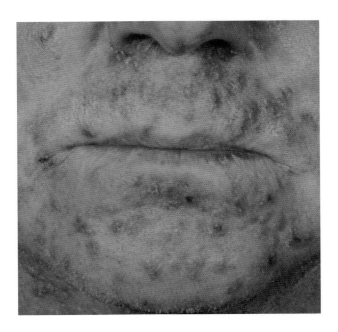

This patient has secondary syphilis, evidenced by the appearance of lesions on the skin. (*Custom Medical Stock Photo. Reproduced by permission.*)

doctor. Women may be diagnosed in the course of a gynecological checkup. Because of the long-term risks of untreated syphilis, certain groups of people are now routinely screened for the disease:

- pregnant women
- sexual contacts or partners of patients diagnosed with syphilis
- children born to mothers with syphilis
- patients with HIV infection
- persons applying for marriage licenses

When the doctor takes the patient's history, he or she will ask about recent sexual contacts in order to determine whether the patient falls into a high-risk group. Other symptoms, such as skin rashes or swollen lymph nodes, will be noted with respect to the dates of the patient's sexual contacts. Definite diagnosis, however, depends on the results of laboratory blood tests.

Blood tests

There are several types of blood tests for syphilis presently used in the United States. Some are used in follow-up monitoring of patients as well as diagnosis.

NONTREPONEMAL ANTIGEN TESTS. Nontreponemal antigen tests are used as screeners. They measure the presence of reagin, which is an antibody formed in reaction to syphilis. In the venereal disease research laboratory (VDRL) test, a sample of the patient's blood is mixed with cardiolipin and cholesterol. If the mixture forms clumps or masses of matter, the test is considered reactive or positive. The serum sample can be diluted several times to determine the concentration of reagin in the patient's blood.

The rapid plasma reagin (RPR) test works on the same principle as the VDRL. It is available as a kit. The patient's serum is mixed with cardiolipin on a plastic-coated card that can be examined with the naked eye.

Nontreponemal antigen tests require a doctor's interpretation and sometimes further testing. They can yield both false-negative and false-positive results. False-positive results can be caused by other infectious diseases, including mononucleosis, **malaria**, **leprosy**, **rheumatoid arthritis**, and lupus. HIV patients have a particularly high rate (4%, compared to 0.8% of HIV-negative patients) of false-positive results on reagin tests. False-negatives can occur when patients are tested too soon after exposure to syphilis; it takes about 14-21 days after infection for the blood to become reactive.

TREPONEMAL ANTIBODY TESTS. Treponemal antibody tests are used to rule out false-positive results on reagin tests. They measure the presence of antibodies that are specific for *T. pallidum*. The most commonly used tests are the microhemagglutination-*T. pallidum* (MHA-TP) and the fluorescent treponemal antibody absorption (FTA-ABS) tests. In the FTA-ABS, the patient's blood serum is mixed with a preparation that prevents interference from antibodies to other treponemal infections. The test serum is added to a slide containing *T. pallidum*. In a positive reaction, syphilitic antibodies in the blood coat the spirochetes on the slide. The slide is then stained with fluorescein, which causes the coated spirochetes to fluoresce when the slide is viewed under ultraviolet (UV) light. In the MHA-TP test, red blood cells from sheep are coated with *T. pallidum* antigen. The cells will clump if the patient's blood contains antibodies for syphilis.

Treponemal antibody tests are more expensive and more difficult to perform than nontreponemal tests. They are therefore used to confirm the diagnosis of syphilis rather than to screen large groups of people. These tests are, however, very specific and very sensitive; false-positive results are relatively unusual.

INVESTIGATIONAL BLOOD TESTS. Currently, ELISA, Western blot, and PCR testing are being studied as

additional diagnostic tests, particularly for congenital syphilis and neurosyphilis.

Other laboratory tests

MICROSCOPE STUDIES. The diagnosis of syphilis can also be confirmed by identifying spirochetes in samples of tissue or lymphatic fluid. Fresh samples can be made into slides and studied under darkfield illumination. A newer method involves preparing slides from dried fluid smears and staining them with fluorescein for viewing under UV light. This method is replacing darkfield examination because the slides can be mailed to professional laboratories.

SPINAL FLUID TESTS. Testing of cerebrospinal fluid (CSF) is an important part of patient monitoring as well as a diagnostic test. The VDRL and FTA-ABS tests can be performed on CSF as well as on blood. An abnormally high white cell count and elevated protein levels in the CSF, together with positive VDRL results, suggest a possible diagnosis of neurosyphilis. CSF testing is not used for routine screening. It is used most frequently for infants with congenital syphilis, HIV-positive patients, and patients of any age who are not responding to penicillin treatment.

Treatment

Medications

Syphilis is treated with antibiotics given either intramuscularly (benzathine penicillin G or ceftriaxone) or orally (doxycycline, minocycline, tetracycline, or azithromycin). Neurosyphilis is treated with a combination of aqueous crystalline penicillin G, benzathine penicillin G, or doxycycline. It is important to keep the levels of penicillin in the patient's tissues at sufficiently high levels over a period of days or weeks because the spirochetes have a relatively long reproduction time. Penicillin is more effective in treating the early stages of syphilis than the later stages.

In the fall of 2000, the CDC convened a group of medical advisors to discuss backup medications for treating syphilis. Although none of the newer drugs will displace penicillin as the primary drug, the doctors recommended azithromycin and ceftriaxone as medications that should have a larger role in the treatment of syphilis than they presently do.

Doctors do not usually prescribe separate medications for the skin rashes or ulcers of secondary syphilis. The patient is advised to keep them clean and dry, and to avoid exposing others to fluid or discharges from condylomata lata.

Pregnant women should be treated as early in pregnancy as possible. Infected fetuses can be cured if the mother is treated during the second and third trimesters of pregnancy. Infants with proven or suspected congenital syphilis are treated with either aqueous crystalline penicillin G or aqueous procaine penicillin G. Children who acquire syphilis after birth are treated with benzathine penicillin G.

Jarisch-Herxheimer reaction

The Jarisch-Herxheimer reaction, first described in 1895, is a reaction to penicillin treatment that may occur during the late primary, secondary, or early latent stages. The patient develops chills, fever, **headache**, and muscle pains within two to six hours after the penicillin is injected. The chancre or rash gets temporarily worse. The Jarisch-Herxheimer reaction, which lasts about a day, is thought to be an allergic reaction to toxins released when the penicillin kills massive numbers of spirochetes.

Alternative treatment

Antibiotics are essential for the treatment of syphilis. Recovery from the disease can be assisted by dietary changes, sleep, **exercise**, and **stress reduction**.

Homeopathy

Homeopathic practitioners are forbidden by law in the United States to claim that homeopathic treatment can cure syphilis. Given the high rate of syphilis in HIV-positive patients, however, some alternative practitioners who are treating AIDS patients with homeopathic remedies maintain that they are beneficial for syphilis as well. The remedies suggested most frequently are *Medorrhinum*, *Syphilinum*, *Mercurius vivus*, and *Aurum*. The historical link between homeopathy and syphilis is Hahnemann's theory of miasms. He thought that the syphilitic miasm was the second oldest cause of constitutional weakness in humans.

Prognosis

The prognosis is good for the early stages of syphilis if the patient is treated promptly and given sufficiently large doses of antibiotics. Treatment failures can occur and patients can be reinfected. There are no definite criteria for cure for patients with primary and secondary syphilis, although patients who are symptom-free and have had negative blood tests for two years after treatment are usually considered cured. Patients should be followed up with blood tests at one, three, six, and 12 months after treatment, or until the results are negative. CSF should be examined after one year. Patients with recurrences during the latency period should be tested for reinfection.

The prognosis for patients with untreated syphilis is spontaneous remission for about 30%; lifelong latency for another 30%; and potentially fatal tertiary forms of the disease in 40%.

Prevention

Immunity

Patients with syphilis do not acquire lasting immunity against the disease. Currently, no effective vaccine for syphilis has been developed. Prevention depends on a combination of personal and public health measures.

Lifestyle choices

The only reliable methods for preventing transmission of syphilis are sexual abstinence or monogamous relationships between uninfected partners. Condoms offer some protection but protect only the covered parts of the body.

Public health measures

CONTACT TRACING. The law requires reporting of syphilis cases to public health agencies. Sexual contacts of patients diagnosed with syphilis are traced and tested for the disease. This includes all contacts for the past three months in cases of primary syphilis and for the past year in cases of secondary disease. Neither the patients nor their contacts should have sex with anyone until they have been tested and treated.

Because of the rising incidence of syphilis abroad, a growing number of public health physicians are recommending routine screening of immigrants, refugees, and international adoptees for syphilis as of late 2002.

All patients who test positive for syphilis should be tested for HIV infection at the time of diagnosis.

PRENATAL TESTING OF PREGNANT WOMEN. Pregnant women should be tested for syphilis at the time of their first visit for prenatal care, and again shortly before delivery. Proper treatment of secondary syphilis in the mother reduces the risk of congenital syphilis in the infant from 90% to less than 2%.

As of late 2005, many obstetricians and gynecologists are recommending routine screening of non-pregnant as well as pregnant women for syphilis. At present, only about half of obstetricians and

KEY TERMS

Chancre—The initial skin ulcer of primary syphilis, consisting of an open sore with a firm or hard base.

Condylomata lata—Highly infectious patches of weepy pink or gray skin that appear in the moist areas of the body during secondary syphilis.

Darkfield—A technique of microscope examination in which light is directed at an oblique angle through the slide so that organisms look bright against a dark background.

General paresis—A form of neurosyphilis in which the patient's personality, as well as his or her control of movement, is affected. The patient may develop convulsions or partial paralysis.

Gumma—A symptom that is sometimes seen in tertiary syphilis, characterized by a rubbery swelling or tumor that heals slowly and leaves a scar.

Index case—The first case of a contagious disease in a group or population that serves to call attention to the presence of the disease.

Jarisch-Herxheimer reaction—A temporary reaction to penicillin treatment for syphilis that includes fever, chills, and worsening of the skin rash or chancre.

Lues maligna—A skin disorder of secondary syphilis in which areas of ulcerated and dying tissue are formed. It occurs most frequently in HIV-positive patients.

Spirochete—A type of bacterium with a long, slender, coiled shape. Syphilis is caused by a spirochete.

Tabes dorsalis—A progressive deterioration of the spinal cord and spinal nerves associated with tertiary syphilis.

gynecologists in the United States screen nonpregnant women for chlamydia and **gonorrhea**, while fewer than a third screen them for syphilis.

EDUCATION AND INFORMATION. Patients diagnosed with syphilis should be given information about the disease and counseling regarding sexual behavior and the importance of completing antibiotic treatment. It is also important to inform the general public about the transmission and early symptoms of syphilis, and provide adequate health facilities for testing and treatment.

Resources

BOOKS

Beers, Mark H., MD, and Robert Berkow, MD., editors. "Syphilis." In *The Merck Manual of Diagnosis and Therapy*. Whitehouse Station, NJ: Merck Research Laboratories, 2004.

PERIODICALS

Augenbraun, M. H. "Treatment of Syphilis 2001: Nonpregnant Adults." *Clinical Infectious Diseases* 35, Supplement 2 (October 15, 2002): S187–S190.

Campos-Outcalt, D., and S. Hurwitz. " Female-to-Female Transmission of Syphilis: A Case Report." *Sexually Transmitted Diseases* 29 (February 2002): 119–120.

Centers for Disease Control. "Primary and Secondary Syphilis—United States, 2000-2001." *Morbidity and Mortality Weekly Report* 51 (November 1, 2002): 971–973.

Dennis, L. K., and D. V. Dawson. "Meta-Analysis of Measures of Sexual Activity and Prostate Cancer." *Epidemiology* 13 (January 2002): 72–79.

Gibbs, R. S. "The Origins of Stillbirth: Infectious Diseases." *Seminars in Perinatology* 26 (February 2002): 75–78.

Grgic-Vitek, M., I Klavs, M. Potocnik, and M. Rogl-Butina. "Syphilis Epidemic in Slovenia Influenced by Syphilis Epidemic in the Russian Federation and Other Newly Independent States." *International Journal of STD and AIDS* 13, Supplement 2 (December 2002): 2–4.

Hagedorn, H. J., A. Kraminer-Hagedorn, K. de Bosschere, et al. "Evaluation of INNO-LIA Syphilis Assay as a Confirmatory Test for Syphilis." *Journal of Clinical Microbiology* 40 (March 2002): 973–978.

Hogben, M., J. S. Lawrence, D. Kasprzyk, et al. "Sexually Transmitted Disease Screening by United States Obstetricians and Gynecologists." *Obstetrics and Gynecology* 100 (October 2002): 801–807.

Kolivras, A., J. de Maubeuge, M. Song, et al. "A Case of Early Congenital Syphilis." *Dermatology* 204 (2002): 338–340.

Pao, D., B. T. Goh, and J. S. Bingham. "Management Issues in Syphilis." *Drugs* 62 (2002): 1447–1461.

Ross, M. W., L. Y. Hwang, C. Zack, et al. "Sexual Risk Behaviours and STIs in Drug Abuse Treatment Populations Whose Drug of Choice is Crack Cocaine." *International Journal of STD and AIDS* 13 (November 2002): 769–774.

Stauffer, W. M., D. Kamat, and P. F. Walker. "Screening of International Immigrants, Refugees, and Adoptees." *Primary Care* 29 (December 2002): 879–905.

Sutmoller, F., T. L. Penna, C. T. de Souza, et al. "Human Immunodeficiency Virus Incidence and Risk Behavior in the 'Projeto Rio': Results of the First 5 Years of the Rio de Janeiro Open Cohort of Homosexual and Bisexual Men, 1994–98." *International Journal of Infectious Diseases* 6 (December 2002): 259–265.

Whittington, W. L., T. Collis, C. Dithmer-Schreck, et al. "Sexually Transmitted Diseases and Human Immunodeficiency Virus-Discordant Partnerships

Among Men Who Have Sex With Men." *Clinical Infectious Diseases* 35 (October 15, 2002): 1010–1017.

ORGANIZATIONS

Centers for Disease Control and Prevention. 1600 Clifton Rd., NE, Atlanta, GA 30333. (800) 311-3435, (404) 639-3311. < http://www.cdc.gov >.

Rebecca J. Frey, PhD

Systemic antifungal drugs *see* **Antifungal drugs, systemic**

Systemic lupus erythematosus

Definition

Systemic lupus erythematosus (also called lupus or SLE) is a disease where a person's immune system attacks and injures the body's own organs and tissues. Almost every system of the body can be affected by SLE.

Description

The body's immune system is a network of cells and tissues responsible for clearing the body of invading foreign organisms, like bacteria, viruses, and fungi. Antibodies are special immune cells that recognize these foreign invaders, and begin a chain of events to destroy them. In an autoimmune disorder like SLE, a person's antibodies begin to recognize the body's own tissues as foreign. Cells and chemicals of the immune system damage the tissues of the body. The reaction that occurs in tissue is called inflammation. Inflammation includes swelling, redness, increased blood flow, and tissue destruction.

In SLE, some of the common antibodies that normally fight diseases are thought to be out of control. These include antinuclear antibodies and anti-DNA antibodies. Antinuclear antibodies are directed against the cell's central structure that contains genetic material (the nucleus). Anti-DNA antibodies are directed against the cell's genetic material. DNA is the chemical substance that makes up the chromosomes and genes.

SLE can occur in both males and females of all ages, but 90% of patients are women. The majority of these women are in their childbearing years. African Americans are more likely than Caucasians to develop SLE.

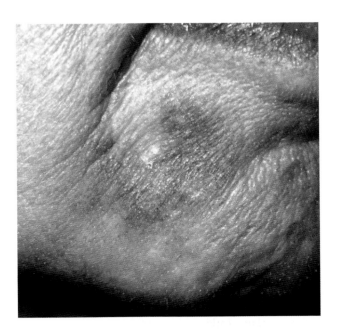

A close-up view of a woman's face with a lesion caused by systemic lupus erythematosus (SLE). One characteristic of this autoimmune disease is a butterfly rash present across the cheeks and nose. *(Photograph by Dr. P. Marazzi, Custom Medical Stock Photo. Reproduced by permission.)*

Occasionally, medications can cause a syndrome of symptoms very similar to SLE. This is called drug-induced lupus. Medications that may cause this syndrome include hydralazine (used for high blood pressure) and procainamide (used for abnormal heartbeats). Drug-induced lupus almost always disappears after the patient stops taking the medications that caused it.

Causes and symptoms

The cause of SLE is unknown. Because the vast majority of patients are women, some research is being done to determine what (if any) link the disease has to female hormones. SLE may have a genetic basis, although more than one gene is believed to be involved in the development of the disease. Because patients with the disease may suddenly have worse symptoms (called a flare) after exposure to things like sunlight, alfalfa sprouts, and certain medications, researchers suspect that some environmental factors may also be at work.

The severity of a patient's SLE varies over time. Patients may have periods with mild or no symptoms, followed by a flare. During a flare, symptoms increase in severity and new organ systems may become affected.

Many SLE patients have fevers, **fatigue**, muscle **pain**, weakness, decreased appetite, and weight loss. The spleen and lymph nodes are often swollen and enlarged. The development of other symptoms in SLE varies, depending on the organs affected.

- Joints. Joint pain and problems, including arthritis, are very common. About 90% of all SLE patients have these types of problems.

- Skin. A number of skin **rashes** may occur, including a red butterfly-shaped rash that spreads across the face. The "wings" of the butterfly appear across the cheekbones, and the "body" appears across the bridge of the nose. A discoid, or coin-shaped, rash causes red, scaly bumps on the cheeks, nose, scalp, ears, chest, back, and the tops of the arms and legs. The roof of the mouth may develop sore, irritated pits (ulcers). Hair loss is common. SLE patients tend to be very easily sunburned (photosensitive).

- When Lungs. Inflammation of the tissues that cover the lungs and line the chest cavity causes pleuritis, with fluid accumulating in the lungs. The patient frequently experiences coughing and shortness of breath.

- Heart and circulatory system. Inflammation of the tissue surrounding the heart causes **pericarditis**; inflammation of the heart itself causes **myocarditis**. These heart problems may result in abnormal beats (**arrhythmias**), difficulty pumping the blood strongly enough (**heart failure**), or even sudden **death**. **Blood clots** often form in the blood vessels and may lead to complications.

- Nervous system. Headaches, seizures, changes in personality, and confused thinking (**psychosis**) may occur.

- Kidneys. The kidneys may suffer significant destruction, with serious life-threatening effects. They may become unable to adequately filter the blood, leading to kidney failure.

- Gastrointestinal system. Patients may experience **nausea**, **vomiting**, **diarrhea**, and abdominal pain. The lining of the abdomen may become inflamed (peritonitis).

- Eyes. The eyes may become red, sore, and dry. Inflammation of one of the nerves responsible for vision may cause vision problems, and blindness can result from inflammation of the blood vessels (**vasculitis**) that serve the retina.

Diagnosis

Diagnosis of SLE can be somewhat difficult. There are no definitive tests for diagnosing SLE.

Many of the symptoms and laboratory test results of SLE patients are similar to those of patients with different diseases, including **rheumatoid arthritis**, **multiple sclerosis**, and various nervous system and blood disorders.

Laboratory tests that are helpful in diagnosing SLE include several tests for a variety of antibodies commonly elevated in SLE patients (including antinuclear antibodies, anti-DNA antibodies, etc.). SLE patients tend to have low numbers of red blood cells (anemia) and low numbers of certain types of white blood cells. The **erythrocyte sedimentation rate** (ESR), a measure of inflammation in the body, tends to be quite elevated. Samples of tissue (biopsies) from affected skin and kidneys show characteristics of the disease.

A test called the lupus erythematosus cell preparation (or LE prep) test is also performed. This test involves obtaining a sample of the patient's blood. Cells from the blood are damaged in the laboratory in order to harvest their nuclei. These damaged cells are then put together with the patient's blood serum, the liquid part of blood separated from the blood cells. Antinuclear antibodies within the patient's serum will clump together with the damaged nuclear material. A material called Wright's stain will cause these clumps to turn blue. These stained clumps are then reacted with some of the patient's white blood cells, which will essentially eat the clumps. LE cells are the white blood cells that contain the blue clumps. This test will be positive in about 70-80% of all patients with SLE.

The American Rheumatism Association developed a list of symptoms used to diagnose SLE. Research supports the idea that people who have at least four of the eleven criteria (not necessarily simultaneously) are extremely likely to have SLE. The criteria are:

- butterfly rash

- discoid rash

- photosensitivity

- mouth ulcers

- arthritis

- inflammation of the lining of the lungs or the lining around the heart

- kidney damage, as noted by the presence of protein or other abnormal substances called casts in the urine

- seizures or psychosis

- the presence of certain types of anemia and low counts of particular white blood cells

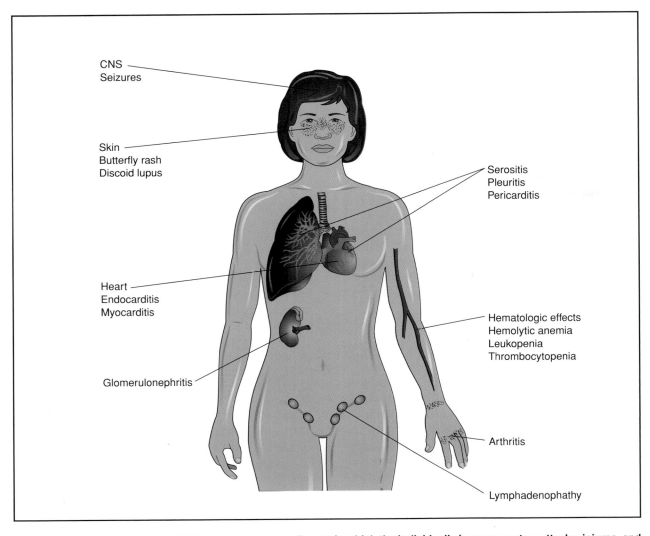

CNS
Seizures

Skin
Butterfly rash
Discoid lupus

Serositis
Pleuritis
Pericarditis

Heart
Endocarditis
Myocarditis

Hematologic effects
Hemolytic anemia
Leukopenia
Thrombocytopenia

Glomerulonephritis

Arthritis

Lymphadenophathy

Systemic lupus erythematosus (SLE) is an autoimmune disease in which the individual's immune system attacks, injures, and destroys the body's own organs and tissues. Nearly every system of the body can be affected by SLE, as depicted in the illustration above. *(Illustration by Electronic Illustrators Group.)*

- the presence of certain immune cells, anti-DNA antibodies, or a falsely positive test for **syphilis**

- the presence of antinuclear antibodies

Treatment

Treatment depends on the organ systems affected by SLE and the severity of the disease. Some patients have a mild form of SLE. Their mild symptoms of inflammation can be treated with **nonsteroidal anti-inflammatory drugs** like ibuprofen (Motrin, Advil) and **aspirin**. Severe skin rashes and joint problems may respond to a group of medications usually used to treat **malaria**. More severely ill patients with potentially life-threatening complications (including

kidney disease, pericarditis, or nervous system complications) will require treatment with more potent drugs, including steroid medications. Because steroids have serious side effects, they are reserved for more severe cases of SLE. Drugs that decrease the activity of the immune system (called **immunosuppressant drugs**) may also be used for severely ill SLE patients. These include azathioprine and cyclophosphamide.

Other treatments for SLE try to help specific symptoms. Clotting disorders will require blood thinners. Psychotic disorders will require specific medications. Kidney failure may require the blood to be cleaned outside the body through a machine (dialysis) or even a **kidney transplantation**.

KEY TERMS

Autoimmune disorder—A disorder in which the body's antibodies mistake the body's own tissues for foreign invaders. The immune system then attacks and causes damage to these tissues.

Chromosomes—Spaghetti-like structures located within the nucleus (or central portion) of each cell. Chromosomes contain genes, structures that direct the growth and functioning of all the cells and systems in the body. Chromosomes are responsible for passing on hereditary traits from parents to child.

Immune system—The system of specialized organs, lymph nodes, and blood cells throughout the body that work together to prevent foreign organisms (bacteria, viruses, fungi, etc.) from invading the body.

Psychosis—Extremely disordered thinking with a poor sense of reality; may include hallucinations (seeing, hearing, or smelling things that are not really there).

Alternative treatment

A number of alternative treatments have been suggested to help reduce the symptoms of SLE. These include **acupuncture** and massage for relieving the pain of sore joints and muscles. **Stress** management is key for people with SLE and such techniques as **meditation**, hynotherapy, and **yoga** may be helpful in promoting relaxation. Dietary suggestions include eating a whole foods diet with reduced amounts of red meat and dairy products in order to decrease pain and inflammation. **Food allergies** are believed either to contribute to SLE or to arise as a consequence of the digestive difficulties. Wheat, dairy products, and soy are the major offenders. An elimination/challenge diet can help identify the offending foods so that they can be avoided. Another dietary measure that may be beneficial is eating more fish that contain **omega-3 fatty acids**, like mackerel, sardines, and salmon. Because alfalfa sprouts have been associated with the onset of flares in SLE, they should be avoided. Supplements that have been suggested to improve the health of SLE patients include **vitamins** B, C, and E, as well as selenium, zinc, magnesium, and a complete trace mineral supplement. Vitamin A is believed to help improve discoid skin rashes. Botanical medicine can help the entire body through immune modulation and **detoxification**, as well as assisting individual organs and systems. Homeopathy and flower essences can work deeply on the emotional level to help people with this difficult disease.

Prognosis

The prognosis for patients with SLE varies, depending on the organ systems most affected and the severity of inflammation. Some patients have long periods of time with mild or no symptoms. About 90-95% of patients are still living after 2 years with the disease. About 82-90% of patients are still living after 5 years with the disease. After 10 years, 71-80% of patients are still alive, and 63-75% are still alive after 20 years. The most likely causes of death during the first 10 years include infections and kidney failure. During years 11-20 of the disease, the most likely cause of death involves the development of abnormal blood clots.

Because SLE frequently affects women of child-bearing age, **pregnancy** is an important issue. For pregnant SLE patients, about 30% of the pregnancies end in **miscarriage**. About 25% of all babies born to mothers with SLE are premature. Most babies born to mothers with SLE are normal. However, a rare condition called neonatal lupus causes a baby of a mother with SLE to develop a skin rash, liver or blood problems, and a serious heart condition.

Prevention

There are no known ways to avoid developing SLE. However, it is possible for a patient who has been diagnosed with SLE to prevent flares of the disease. Recommendations for improving general health to avoid flares include decreasing sun exposure, getting sufficient sleep, eating a healthy diet, decreasing stress, and exercising regularly. It is important for a patient to try to identify the early signs of a flare (like **fever**, increased fatigue, rash, **headache**). Some people believe that noticing and responding to these warning signs will allow a patient with SLE to prevent a flare, or at least to decrease its severity.

Resources

ORGANIZATIONS

American College of Rheumatology. 1800 Century Place, Suite 250, Atlanta, GA 30345. (404) 633-3777. <http://www.rheumatology.org>.

Lupus Foundation of America. 1300 Piccard Dr., Suite 200, Rockville, MD 20850. (800) 558-0121. <http://www.lupus.org>.

Rosalyn Carson-DeWitt, MD